AF575011

Handbook of BIOSENSORS and ELECTRONIC NOSES

Medicine, Food, and the Environment

Handbook of BIOSENSORS and ELECTRONIC NOSES
Medicine, Food, and the Environment

Edited by
Erika Kress-Rogers, D.Phil.
AEG
Frankfurt, Germany

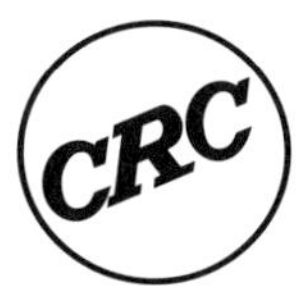

CRC Press
Boca Raton New York London Tokyo

The graphs on the front cover and back cover are based on: Aroma mapping, Figure 3 of Chapter 27 by Julian W. Gardner and Evor L. Hines; In-situ process biosensor, Figure 2 of Chapter 19 by Ursula Bilitewski and Ingrid Rohm; Artificial pancreas, Figure 2 of Chapter 18 by Danila Moscone and Marco Mascini; Olfactory receptor, Figure 1 of Chapter 22 by Heinz Breer.

Acquiring Editor:	Paul Petralia
Editorial Assistant:	Cindy Carelli
Assistant Managing Editor:	Gerry Jaffe
Marketing Manager:	Susie Carlisle
Direct Marketing Manager:	Becky McEldowney
Cover design:	Denise Craig
PrePress:	Carlos Esser
Manufacturing:	Sheri Schwartz

Library of Congress Cataloging-in-Publication Data

Handbook of biosensors and electronic noses : medicine, food, and the environment / edited by Erika Kress-Rogers
p. cm.
Includes bibliographical references and index.
ISBN 0-8493-8905-4 (alk. paper)
1. Biosensors—Handbooks, manuals, etc. 2. Molecular probes--Handbooks, manuals, etc. 3. Affinity labeling—Handbooks, manuals, etc. I. Kress-Rogers, Erika.
[DNLM: 1. Biosensors. 2. DNA Probes. 3. Microcomputers. QT 36 H236 1996]
R857.B54H36 1996
616′.28—dc20
DNLM/DLC
for Library of Congress 96-25899
CIP

This book contains information obtained from authentic and highly regarded sources. Reprinted material is quoted with permission, and sources are indicated. A wide variety of references are listed. Reasonable efforts have been made to publish reliable data and information, but the author and the publisher cannot assume responsibility for the validity of all materials or for the consequences of their use.

Neither this book nor any part may be reproduced or transmitted in any form or by any means, electronic or mechanical, including photocopying, microfilming, and recording, or by any information storage or retrieval system, without prior permission in writing from the publisher.

All rights reserved. Authorization to photocopy items for internal or personal use, or the personal or internal use of specific clients, may be granted by CRC Press, Inc., provided that $.50 per page photocopied is paid directly to Copyright Clearance Center, 27 Congress Street, Salem, MA 01970 USA. The fee code for users of the Transactional Reporting Service is ISBN 0-8493-8905-4/97/$0.00+$.50. The fee is subject to change without notice. For organizations that have been granted a photocopy license by the CCC, a separate system of payment has been arranged.

The consent of CRC Press does not extend to copying for general distribution, for promotion, for creating new works, or for resale. Specific permission must be obtained in writing from CRC Press for such copying.

Direct all inquiries to CRC Press, Inc., 2000 Corporate Blvd., N.W., Boca Raton, Florida 33431.

© 1997 by CRC Press, Inc.

No claim to original U.S. Government works

International Standard Book Number 0-8493-8905-4
Library of Congress Card Number 96-25899
Printed in the United States of America 1 2 3 4 5 6 7 8 9 0
Printed on acid-free paper

Preface

Biosensors provide high sensitivity and selectivity combined with a significant reduction in sample preparation, assay time, and in the use of expensive reagents. Commercial biosensors have demonstrated that these benefits can be realized in practical applications and that biosensors can be the basis of rapid, reliable, compact, and user-friendly instruments. Some of these are already being used by the patients themselves to improve the management of their chronic health disorders; others are providing tools for point-of-care testing and for the monitoring of patients during intensive care and surgery. Biosensors are also finding applications in quality assurance and process control in the biotechnology, food, drink, and cosmetics sectors; they are becoming available for applications in environmental protection.

Advanced commercial instruments based on biosensors, however, represent only a small fraction of the multitude of biochemical schemes and design principles; they cover only a small portion of the many analytes that can be measured with biosensors. Commercial instruments for a wider range of operating conditions remain to be developed — many more applications are waiting to be covered by fully optimized biosensor instruments.

For rapid progress in realizing the practical potential of biosensors, interested users need to identify the best approach towards solutions for their particular measurement problems. They need to be able to assess the feasibility and timescale for a biosensor development meeting analytical and other performance specifications, and moreover being economically viable. For the most effective dialogue between sensor users and developers, an overview on the principles, characteristics, and practical possibilities and limitations of competing and complementary sensors is needed and an awareness of the methods for the optimization of sensor performance is required.

In addition to a description of the components and configurations of biosensor devices, the authors have therefore addressed practical aspects such as cross-sensitivity (to changes in variables such as temperature, pH value, oxygen pressure, or the concentration of interfering chemical compounds) and stability (receptor and base device stability and their impact on the operational lifetime and calibration stability in real samples). Approaches leading to an extension of the analytical range, a reduction in cross-sensitivities and in deterioration by biofouling, and an improvement in biocompatibility are among the topics covered in the book.

Full biosensor optimization is frequently impractical within the technical and economic constraints of a development project. As an alternative, the scope for practical applications in surgery or in the processing industries is increased by systems connected to the medium to be analyzed and providing facilities for automatic intermittent sampling, conditioning, flow injection, or autocalibration. Increasingly important, are also, the applications of advanced software techniques for performance enhancement, signal interpretation (particularly for multisensor systems), control decisions on the basis of the measured data, and the smooth implementation of control actions.

In terms of analytes, base devices, and software techniques, there is an increasing overlap between biosensors and gas (or volatile) sensors with nonbiological sensing layers. This is particularly prominent in the approaches towards the electronic nose, where researchers are not only copying biochemical pathways but also are using nature's approach to signal interpretation as a blueprint for man-made sensing systems. By considering biosensors and electronic noses together, experience gained with shared base device designs and software techniques can be used synergistically to obtain the best effect.

The handbook begins with an introduction to the building blocks for biosensors and electronic noses. This is followed by a more detailed presentation of sensing layers and base devices for metabolism, affinity and recombinant biosensors including those using enzymes, whole bacterial cells, antibodies, and DNA probes as sensing agents immobilized onto microelectronic, optical, and acoustic base devices. Functional membranes for performance tailoring and protection are then treated.

Biosensor designs utilizing these building blocks for applications in medicine, food processing, and environmental protection are detailed in the following part of the handbook. Techniques for on-line and *in vivo* monitoring and control are discussed, including fuzzy logic control as an advanced software technique for the efficient implementation of control decisions.

The development of electronic noses is the subject of the concluding part of the handbook, beginning with an introduction to nature's approach to odor sensing as represented by the mammalian sense of smell. Devices used as elements in the sensor arrays employed in the construction of electronic noses are presented in detail, including those based on specially tailored metal oxide semiconductor gas sensors, conducting polymers, specifically sorbent polymers, and lipid membranes. Pattern analysis techniques including neural networks are a vital part of the electronic nose approach and are treated in a dedicated chapter.

Such techniques are also relevant for signal evaluation in heterogeneous multisensor systems, for example in assessing a set of data containing information on pressure, dissolved gases, and glucose concentration. Similarly, the fuzzy logic methods treated earlier in the handbook apply not only to control systems, but can also be used to enhance sensor performance by providing real-time compensation for complex cross-sensitivity relationships.

Sensor development for demanding operating environments is costly; the maximum benefit from this investment is gained by choosing the combination of sensors, sample handling, and signal processing that will provide the best performance under the prevalent conditions of the specific application.

Erika Kress-Rogers

Editor

Erika Kress-Rogers has carried out and coordinated a wide range of R&D projects in the area of instrumentation and sensors for process control and quality assurance for the food industry while at the LFRA (Leatherhead Food Research Association), an international food research association (based in Surrey, U.K.) that provides R&D, consultancy, and technical services to food companies, government bodies, and agencies. At the LFRA (from 1983 to 1992), her work has included a detailed technology transfer study on the principles and characteristics of novel sensors developed, or under development, for other sectors, with the brief of identifying and evaluating their potential applications in the food industry. Based on the results of her study, a collaborative R&D project on the development of novel sensors for the food industry was initiated.

This project was carried out by interdisciplinary teams at the LFRA in collaboration with industrial and university laboratories specializing in the chosen sensor technologies. The work, coordinated by Dr. Kress-Rogers, involved feasibility studies (supported by experimental trials and extensive surveys to assess the needs of the food industry) and prototype developments. Among the technologies investigated in the project were gas sensors (primarily CHEMFET), pH and ion sensors (ISFET and fiber-optic probes), acidity sensors (ISFET-based coulometric titrator devices), and enzyme-based biosensors (primarily amperometric mediated enzyme electrodes) as well as SPR immunosensor devices and SAW vapor sensors based on specific sorption.

For food industry applications where hostile conditions prevail (high temperatures and pressures, steam, inhomogeneous samples with fat and starch particles), alternative techniques were investigated. These included the *in situ* measurement of viscosity as an indicator of polymerization processes using a mechanically resonant probe, the monitoring of solute concentration with ultrasonic techniques, and the applications of dielectric measurements for the on-line monitoring of composite food properties. On the basis of this experience, companies and institutions were given the required input for their strategic planning in quality assurance.

After her ten-year period at the LFRA, she worked as a consultant with ATI Sensor Applications Ltd. before moving to Germany to take on a position as a Technical Editor with AEG (System Protection and Control) of Daimler-Benz Industrie. For seven years, she has served as Member of the International Editorial Board for the journal *Food Control*. Dr. Kress-Rogers is the editor of "Instrumentation and Sensors for the Food Industry", the first handbook to provide a detailed account of a wide range of on-line and at-line measurement technologies for the determination of physical, chemical, and microbial properties in the food industry, and to present an introduction to the principles together with a treatment of the practical potential and limitations. Her background is in experimental solid-state physics (Diplom der Physik, Universität Karlsruhe). Her doctorate (D.Phil.) was gained with a study in the field of semiconductor physics at the Clarendon Laboratory, University of Oxford, U.K., where she stayed as a Rhodes Scholar.

Contributors

Michael H. Abraham studied chemistry at the Northern Polytechnic London (B.Sc.) and then carried out research at University College London (Ph.D.). He was first lecturer at Battersea College of Technology, then lecturer and subsequently reader at the University of Surrey, and is now research fellow at University College London. He was awarded the D.Sc. degree in 1974 from London University. His research work has included mechanisms of reactions, solvent effects, the hydrophobic effect, and theoretical and experimental studies of electrolytes and of nonelectrolytes. Dr. Abraham has set out the first comprehensive scales of solute hydrogen-bond acidity and of solute hydrogen-bond basicity using 1:1 hydrogen-bond equilibrium constants, and more recently has developed scales of overall, or effective, hydrogen-bond acidity and hydrogen-bond basicity, and has used these and other descriptors in LSERs and QSARs in order to study a wide variety of physicochemical, biochemical, and toxicological processes. He has published a book, several reviews, and over 200 research papers, and was awarded the 1992 Ebert Prize of the American Pharmaceutical Association.

Eric Albone is Director of Clifton Scientific Trust, holds an honorary research appointment in the School of Chemistry at the University of Bristol, and teaches at Clifton College, Bristol. His current interests span research and education. He holds a doctorate in chemistry from the University of Oxford and has researched in the U.S. For a number of years, Dr. Albone directed research at the University of Bristol into mammalian chemical signaling, which led in 1984 to the publication of *Mammalian Semiochemistry,* the first volume to attempt a unified treatment of the subject from a chemical perspective.

Peter G. Berrie is a Technical Author at process instrumentation manufacturers Endress+Hauser, Maulburg, Germany. A graduate in metallurgy at Imperial College, London (degree, 1969; Ph.D., 1973), he spent five years in research — two years at the Institution for Transuranic Elements in Karlsruhe, Germany investigating the equation of state of mixed oxide fuels at very high temperatures; three years at Loughborough University, England working on laser cutting and drilling technology — before turning to technical communication. Dr. Berrie's responsibilities at Endress+Hauser, where he has worked for some six years, include writing on digital communication as well as on instrumentation employing fuzzy logic. "I work for the marketing department and was asked to observe the impact of fuzzy logic on process instrumentation. Fuzzy logic is a fascinating subject with a widening range of applications and I hope my contribution will encourage people to look more closely at its possibilities in biosensor optimization."

Ursula Bilitewski is head of the biosensor projects at the Gesellschaft für Biotechnologische Forschung mbH (GBF) in Braunschweig, Germany. She is interested in the development and application of biosensor systems based on enzymes, antibodies, whole cells, or receptors. The main fields of application are environmental analysis, food analysis, and process monitoring. Dr. Bilitewski's background is in chemistry (University of Münster, Germany).

Heinz Breer is Professor of Zoophysiology at the University of Stuttgart-Hohenheim, Germany. Projects there have included "Molecular Mechanisms of Olfactory Signal Transduction" and "Receptors and Ion Channels in Sensory and Neuronal Cells". Earlier, Professor

Breer worked at the University of Osnabrück, Germany. His background is in biology, studied at the University of Münster, Germany.

Karl Cammann received his Ph.D. at the University of Munich in 1975. Since 1979, he has been professor of Analytical Chemistry at the Universities of Ulm and Munich (Germany) and guest professor at the University of Delaware, (U.S.). In 1987 he received the Océ-van-der-Grinten Environmental Prize for Technology Transfer from the Ministry of Science and Education, Germany. He is now a Full Professor at the University of Münster and Head of the Institut für Chemo- und Biosensorik (ICB). He is mainly engaged in the development of chemical sensors and biosensors and in the development of spectroscopic and chromatographic methods.

Sang-Mok Chang is at the Department of Chemical Engineering, College of Engineering, Dong-A University, Pusan, Korea. He has also carried out research projects at the Research Centre for Advanced Science and Technology, University of Tokyo, Japan.

Arnaldo D'Amico is full Professor of Electronic Devices at the University of Rome "Tor Vergata", Italy. His main current activities concern the research and development of physical and chemical sensors, low-voltage electronics, noise measurements, and advanced devices. Earlier, he worked at the Institute of Solid State Electronics of the National Council of Research (CNR), leading the semiconductor group. He is Chairman of the steering committee of the International Meeting on Chemical Sensors, member of the steering committee of Eurosensors, and member of the editorial boards of the journals *Sensors* and *Actuators A&B*. Professor D'Amico is author of more than 150 papers in international journals.

Bengt Danielsson is an Associate Professor at the department of Pure and Applied Biochemistry at Lund University where he is leading a research group specializing in biosensor development and applications in bioanalysis. This work has been focused on thermometric and semiconductor gas sensors; however, current studies also include optical and optothermal techniques. Dr. Danielsson is seeking practically useful solutions for the application of biosensor systems in process control, including sterilizable sample handling devices, and in biomedical applications, for example, miniaturization for home monitoring.

Corrado Di Natale has been Research Assistant at the Department of Electronic Engineering at the University of Rome "Tor Vergata", Italy since 1990. He gained his Ph.D. in Physics at the University of Rome "La Sapienza" in 1987. Dr. Di Natale's main research activity concerns the utilization of sensor arrays for electronic nose applications and related topics such as sensor calibration techniques and the development of mathematical tools for the data analysis of sensor array signals.

Julian W. Gardner graduated from Birmingham University in 1979 with a first class honours degree and then studied the properties of thin films at the Cavendish Laboratory, Cambridge, U.K. for his Ph.D. From 1983 to 1987 he worked first at AEA Technology Ltd. and later at Molins Advanced Technology Unit on instrumentation. At Molins, Dr. Gardner developed a novel optoelectronic sensor that has been packaged in the U.K. and U.S. for implementation on high-speed packaging machinery. Since joining Warwick as a lecturer in 1987 his research interests have been sensor materials, the design of integrated gas sensor arrays, and associated signal processing techniques. In 1989, Dr. Gardner received the Esso Centenary Education Award sponsored by the Royal Society and Fellowship of Engineering to pursue his research interests. In 1992, he became a Senior Lecturer at Warwick and in 1994 was awarded an Alexander von Humboldt Fellowship in Germany. He is currently a Reader in Microengineering and the Director of the Sensors Research Laboratory in the Centre for Nanotechnology and Microengineering at Warwick University. He is the author of over 90 scientific papers and 3 books, including 1 on microsensors.

Norman J. Geddes received a B.Sc. in Physics from the University of Exeter (1985) and a Ph.D. (1988) for a study of the electrical properties of thin organic films. After visiting-scientist positions with GTE (Boston) and IBM (San Jose), he held a research scientist position with the C.S.I.R.O. (Australia) investigating piezoelectric and surface-plasmon-based transducers for the study of immuno-reactions for biosensing applications. Dr. Geddes currently holds a senior scientific officer position with the DRA, Malvern (U.K.) looking into applications for self-assembling organic systems for novel electronic and optoelectronic devices.

Jay W. Grate joined the Environmental Molecular Sciences Laboratory at the Pacific Northwest National Laboratory in 1992, where he leads a group in chemical sensor research. Prior to taking this position, he worked as a research chemist at the Naval Research Laboratory from 1984 to 1992, and spent a year's sabbatical at the Scripp's Research Institute. He received his Ph.D. in chemistry from the University of California, San Diego, in 1983. His interests include topics in organic and organometallic chemistry and surface science, with current research emphasizing the development of chemical sensors and microanalytical systems. Dr. Grate's research in sensors has focused primarily on acoustic wave devices such as SAW vapor sensors, where his studies have addressed issues including vapor/polymer interactions, sorption equilibria, polymer design and transduction mechanisms, models for sensor response, detection of polymer transition behavior, adhesion at the polymer/sensor interface, and the development of prototype sensor array systems with pattern recognition. Dr. Grate serves as a Member of the Executive Committee of the Sensors Group in the Electrochemical Society.

Alain Grisel is President and Executive Director of the Company MICROSENS located in Neuchâtel, Switzerland. MICROSENS specializes in the development and manufacturing of integrated chemical sensors. The products developed and currently manufactured by MICROSENS include pH-ISFET, specific Ion-Selective FET devices, amperometric sensors such as a dissolved oxygen sensor and a chlorine sensor for drinking water control, semiconductor, catalytic, and thermal conductivity gas sensors, as well as integrated electrodes for biosensor applications. Dr. Grisel has been leading projects in the field of biosensor development including research on "Insulating Thin Molecular Films and Biological Membranes on Solid State Surfaces" in the framework of a Swiss National Program between 1989 and 1992 on the physics and chemistry of surfaces, and the development of biosensors in a Swiss priority program on Bioelectronics since 1993. Among many sensor application studies, MICROSENS is also involved in the European Program MAST concerning the application of integrated chemical sensors for oceanographic and environmental analysis. Earlier, Dr. Grisel had worked at the Swiss Center for Electronics and Microtechnology, CSEM, in Neuchâtel, leading a department carrying out research and development in the field of integrated chemical sensors. His background is in physics, and he obtained a Ph.D. (1981) in solid state physics at the Federal Institute of Technology of Lausanne, Switzerland.

Evor L. Hines obtained his B.Sc. and Ph.D. in 1979 and 1983, respectively. He joined the Department of Engineering at the University of Warwick, Coventry, U.K. in 1984 and became a Senior Lecturer in Electronics in 1992. His main interest over the last 8 years has been Intelligent Systems Engineering and its application. Dr. Hines has been leading work in application areas such as computer vision, finance, water quality control, and electronic systems, among others, using neural networks, generic algorithms, and fuzzy logic. He has published over 70 papers.

Isao Karube is Professor of Bioelectronics and Biotechnology at the Research Centre for Advanced Science and Technology, University of Tokyo, Japan. He is Regional Editor of the international journals *Biocatalysis* and *Applied Biochemistry and Biotechnology* as well as an Editor or Editorial Board Member for 14 international journals in the biosensors and biotechnology field. His major research interests are the development of biosensors and bioreactor technologies, protein and chromosomal engineering, marine biotechnology, and environmental bioengineering. He holds the Divisional Award of the Chemical Society of Japan for 1966 and the Ichimura Prize in Technology for 1989. He was also awarded the Technologie Doctorem Honoris Causa from Lund University, Sweden in 1994, and the Chevalier dans Vordre des Palmes Academiques in 1994. Professor Karube is Director of the Biosensor Society and holds positions in many national and international scientific societies and committees. His background is in food science (B.Sc. from the Tokyo University of Fisheries) and in chemical engineering (M.Sc. and Dr.Eng. from the Tokyo Institute of Technology).

Claus-Dieter Kohl is Professor of Physics at Justus-Liebig University in Gießen, Germany. Projects there have included investigations of reaction mechanisms on sensor and catalyst surfaces and the development of signal evaluation algorithms. Sensor systems for alcohol in breath, air control, and the detection of smoldering fires have been developed. Previously, until 1991, he worked at the Physical Institute of the RWTH, Aachen, leading a team carrying out R&D in electrical properties of semiconductor interfaces and epitaxial growth processes. His background is in solid-state physics.

Rob P. H. Kooyman is Lecturer of Biophysics at Twente University, Enschede, The Netherlands. His main interests are optical characterization methods of biological interfaces, and waveguide methods for optical immunosensing. Prior to his present position, Dr. Kooyman has worked at the University of Utrecht and Agricultural University, Wageningen, where his research involved the structure of lipid layers and the molecular structure of photosynthetic pigment systems, respectively. Formal training in physics was at Leiden University, The Netherlands.

Silke Kröger studied Biology at the University of Bochum, Germany, finishing with a Diploma thesis in the field of microbial soil decontamination. She joined the department of Pure and Applied Biochemistry in Lund, Sweden as an Erasmus Scholar and investigated possibilities of incorporating calorimetric biosensors into environmental monitoring. This work was conducted in collaboration with the IFE GmbH (Institut für Angewandte Forschung und Entwicklung) in Recklinghausen, Germany. She then moved to Cranfield University, England were she is studying at the Biotechnology Centre for a Ph.D., developing an electrochemical immunosensor for herbicide detection in water and soil.

Chris R. Lawrence obtained his B.Sc. in Physics at the University of Exeter (1988) before joining The Thin Film & Interface Group within the physics department to obtain a Ph.D. (1992) for studies of the optical and electrical properties of Langmuir-Blodgett films. He is now a Research fellow within the same group, researching the design of composite materials exhibiting specific optical properties, as well as the detection and characterization of proteins and dielectric layers via the utilization of surface plasmon resonance techniques. The two chapters with Dr. Geddes in this book were researched and written during a four-month placement in Australia, where Dr. Lawrence was working for the Commonwealth Scientific and Industrial Research organization (C.S.I.R.O.) on a project involving the development of a novel grating-based biosensor.

Laura M. Lechuga is a Research Associate in the National Center for Microelectronics at the Spanish Council for Research. She is involved in projects on the development of sensors and biosensors based on III-V Semiconductors Technology. Earlier, she worked at the Biointerfaces Group of the MESA Research Institute (University of Twente, The Netherlands) in the field of Evanescent Field Immunosensors. Her background is in Chemistry (University of Cadiz, Spain) and III-V Semiconductor Devices (University Complutense of Madrid, Spain).

Marco Mascini is a Full Professor of Analytical Chemistry at the University of Florence (Italy). He has been one of the pioneers of biosensor research in Europe. His interests are the continuous development of electrochemical biosensors and applications of these devices in medicine, the environment, and in food chemistry. Recently, optical and piezoelectrical biosensors in the field of immunological biosensors have been realized and optimized as part of Professor Mascini's work.

R. Andrew McGill received his Ph.D. degree in Chemistry from the University of Surrey, England for physicochemical studies of solubility and sorption processes. From 1988 to 1990 at the University of Alabama, he conducted postdoctoral work including development of solvatochromic dye probe techniques to characterize polymer solubility properties, and silane studies for polymer immobilization techniques and their application in fiber-optic chemical/biochemical sensors. Since 1991 he has been working at the Naval Research Laboratory with Geo-Centers Inc. initially in Washington, D.C. His current interests cover several areas spanning basic to applied research related to chemical microsensors, including the development and applications of solubility theories to polymeric materials, and the design and application of prototype SAW chemical sensor systems.

Danila Moscone is a researcher at the University of Rome "Tor Vergata" (Italy). Dr. Moscone is carrying out biosensors research in the Analytical Chemistry group. Her special interests are related to medical applications with emphasis on microelectrodes for subcutaneous use. Her background is in electroanalytical chemistry.

David J. Newman (M.Sc., Ph.D., MCB, MRCPath) is a Senior Lecturer in Clinical Biochemistry at St. Bartholomew's and the Royal London School of Medicine and Dentistry, London, U.K. His research interests include optical immunoassay technologies (including optical sensors), kinetic rate analysis of Class 1 HLA molecular complexes, and the renal handling of proteins. Dr. Newman has previously worked at Addenbrooks Hospital, Cambridge; Northwick Park Hospital, Harrow, Middlesex; and St. Bartholomew's Hospital, London.

Yemi Olabiran (B.Sc., M.Sc., Ph.D.) is a postdoctoral scientist at St. Bartholomew's and the Royal London School of Medicine and Dentistry. She has a number of years of experience in the production of monoclonal antibodies using standard hybridoma techniques, and more recently she has initiated a project on the manipulation of antibody specificity using recombinant DNA technology. Dr. Olabiran's clinical research interests include markers of myocardial damage and tumor progression. Her background is in biochemistry (University of Sussex, U.K.).

Marjan Orban is currently pursuing a Ph.D. in Analytical Chemistry in Prof. Dr. K. Cammann's group at the University of Münster (Institut für Chemo- und Biosensorik). He works in the field of immunosensor development for pesticide detection in water by time-resolved fluorescence. His background is in Biophysical Chemistry (University of Münster, Germany).

Krishna C. Persaud is a senior lecturer at the Department of Instrumentation and Analytical Science, UMIST, Manchester, U.K. His background is in biochemistry and he specialized in the physiology and biochemistry of olfaction before entering into the field of artificial odor sensing. He gained his Ph.D. at the University of Warwick and subsequently worked in Italy and the U.S. in olfactory research before joining UMIST in 1988. Dr. Persaud currently runs a multidisciplinary research group dedicated to odor sensing.

Dorothea Pfeiffer is Managing Director of Research and Development of the company BST Bio Sensor Technology (Berlin, Germany) dealing with the development and production of biosensors for more than ten different substances with applications to medical diagnosis as well as food and environmental monitoring. In her earlier position as Senior Research Biophysicist of the Berlin Biosensor Group (Academy of Sciences) since 1975, her responsibilities have included the design and development of different generations of enzyme sensor-based autoanalyzers and portable analytical systems for the determination of glucose, lactate, amino acids, and disaccharides in the respective diluted and undiluted biological media (whole blood, serum, urine, food, fermentation solution). Her background is in biophysics (Humboldt University of Berlin, Germany).

Christopher P. Price (M.A., Ph.D., FRCPath, MCB, FRSC) is Professor of Clinical Biochemistry at St. Bartholomew's and the Royal London School of Medicine and Dentistry and Director of Clinical Biochemistry at the Royal Hospitals Trust. His research interests include optical immunoassay technologies (including biosensors), enzymology, and bone disease, and he has published extensively in these areas. He has previously worked at Addenbrooks Hospital, Cambridge; and University Hospital in Southampton and in Birmingham. Professor Price has a background in clinical biochemistry and in the research into novel analytical systems.

Subrayal M. Reddy obtained his B.Sc. (Hons.) in Chemistry from the University of Manchester and later went on to pursue his Ph.D. studies there in the field of membrane-based amperometric biosensors at the Department of Medicine. He is currently undertaking research at the School of Electronic Engineering and Computer Systems (Bangor, North Wales) where he is involved in the design and optimization of gel-based piezoelectric biosensors.

Reinhard Renneberg is Reader in Biosensorics at the University of Münster, Germany and Head of the Department of Immunosensors at the Institut für Chemo- und Biosensorik (ICB). He has worked in the field of biosensor development since 1975 and was involved in the construction of enzyme sensors for glucose, microbial sensors for biochemical oxygen demand (BOD), and immunosensors, for example, for early heart infarction markers and for pesticides. His background is in biochemistry (Universities of Moscow and Berlin). He is coeditor of *Biosensors & Bioelectronics* (Elsevier). At present, he has a position of Reader in Bioanalytical Chemistry at the new Hong Kong University of Science and Technology and is developing biomolecular sensors for environmental monitoring and health care.

Klaus Riedel is project manager of biosensor development for environmental control at the company Dr. Bruno Lange GmbH Berlin (Willstätterstr. 11, D-40549 Düsseldorf). His responsibilities have included the development of microbial sensors for the determination of biochemical oxygen demand (BOD) in waste water. Earlier, he worked at the department of Professor Scheller in Berlin Buch in the field of microbial sensors. His background is in biochemistry (Martin Luther University of Halle-Wittenberg).

Ingrid Rohm is a Ph.D. student in the biosensor group of the Gesellschaft für Biotechnologische Forschung mbH (GBF) in Braunschweig, Germany. Her main interest is the development of screen-printed enzyme electrodes to be used as detectors in automated flow injection analysis systems for application in animal cell cultivations. Earlier, she also worked on the development of immunoassays. Her background is in biology (University of Braunschweig, Germany).

Satoshi Sasaki is a Research Associate at the Research Centre for Advanced Science and Technology, University of Tokyo, Japan. He is currently working on several projects with Professor Isao Karube.

Frieder F. Scheller is Professor of Analytical Biochemistry at Potsdam University, Germany. Projects there have included coupled enzyme reactions, protein electrochemistry, and immunosensing. Earlier, he worked at the Max Delbrück Center of Molecular Medicine in Berlin, Germany, leading a team carrying out research and development in the field of biosensorics. His background is in physical chemistry (Humboldt University of Berlin).

Rolf D. Schmid received his B.Sc. degree in chemistry from the University of Munich and his M.Sc. degree in chemistry in 1967 from the University of Freiburg. He holds his Dr.rer.nat. since 1970 from the University of Freiburg. After postdoctoral training at the University of Freiburg, the Centre Nationale de la Recherche Scientifique in Gif-sur-Yvette, France, and the University of Texas in Austin, U.S., he worked as a research scientist at Henkel KGA in Düsseldorf from 1972 to 1987. From 1987 until 1993 he was Full Professor at the University of Braunschweig and head of the Division of Enzyme Technology at the Gesellschaft für Biotechnologische Forschung (GBF), the German National Research Centre for Biotechnology. Since 1993, he has been a Full Professor of Biotechnology at the University of Stuttgart. His current research interests include the design of proteins such as lipases, oxidases, and antibodies for applications in biocatalysis and biochemical analysis.

David J. Squirrell gained his first degree in the Biological Sciences department at Warwick University, England. He obtained a Ph.D. in 1979 in Warwick's Chemistry and Molecular Sciences department, having studied transduction mechanisms in olfaction. Moving to the Royal Arsenal in London, he worked on gas and vapor analysis and materials microbiology. Since transferring to the Chemical and Biological Defence Establishment at Porton Down in 1988, his research has been on rapid methods for microbial detection with particular interests in optical biosensors and bioluminescence.

Richard W. Titball graduated from the University of Plymouth with a degree in the Biological Sciences. His Ph.D. was also completed at Plymouth. In 1983, he moved to the Chemical and Biological Defence Establishment, Porton Down. He is now Head of the Microbiology group. His interests, in addition to the use of gene probes to detect microorganisms, concern mechanisms of pathogenicity and structure–function relationship in bacterial toxins.

Paul J. Travers is currently the manager of the sensor manufacturing group of Aromascan plc (Crewe, U.K.) responsible for the manufacture and development of the conducting polymer sensor arrays used in their gas- and odor-sensing equipment. Previously, he worked as a research associate at the University of Manchester Institute of Science and Technology (UMIST, Manchester, U.K.) and Coventry Polytechnic (Coventry, U.K.) carrying out research and development in the fields of heterocyclic chemistry, conducting polymers, and gas and odor detection. His background is in chemistry (University of Cambridge, U.K.).

Anthony P. F. Turner is Professor of Biosensor Technology and Head of Cranfield Biotechnology Centre at Cranfield University. He is the founder and Managing Director of Cranfield Diagnostics Ltd., a company manufacturing thick-film biosensors. He is Project Leader for an EU Concerted Action on Microsensors for Biomedical Applications, Editor-In-Chief of the international journal *Biosensors and Bioelectronics*, Editor of the annual series *Advances in Biosensors*, and has more than 200 publications and 20 U.K. patent applications. Professor Turner has received a variety of prizes and awards including being named 1994 winner of the National Physical Laboratory Award for Measurement Science. He has managed many industrial programs including the development of the world's most successful biosensor to date, the MediSense glucose monitor.

Gerald Urban is Assistant Professor at the Technische Universität Vienna and head of the Ludwig Boltzmann Institut for biomedical microengineering in Austria. Projects there have included development on integrated sensor systems for measurement of temperature, flow, perfusion, blood gas and electrolyte measurements, and biosensors for the detection of glucose, lactate, glutamate, and glutamine. Earlier, he worked at the Institute for Neurosurgery at the General Hospital, Vienna developing neurosurgical microprobes for EEG recordings on patients. He is leading a team of 20 co-workers carrying out research and development in sensors, thin-film and microsystem technology, electronic data acquisition, simulation, and chemistry. The group has considerable experience in clinical experiments and in cooperation with industry. His background is in Technical Physics (TU-Vienna), electrical engineering, and thin-film technology.

Pankaj M. Vadgama is Professor of Clinical Biochemistry at the University of Manchester, U.K. Projects there have included work on clinical *in vivo* enzyme electrodes, immunosensors, and sensors for sugar and acid measurement in citrus fruit. Professor Vadgama has had a longstanding interest in biosensors and has developed a range of membranes for improving biosensor performance. His background is in medical biochemistry, and he is an Honorary Chemical Pathologist at Hope Hospital, Salford.

Enrico Verona is Research Director at the Institute of Acoustics "O.M. Corbino" of the National Council of Research (CNR). He was awarded the Ph.D. degree in Electronic Engineering at the University of Rome "La Sapienza" in 1973. In 1975, he joined the "O.M. Corbino" Institute and has been leading the Acousto-Optics and Surface Acoustic Wave Group since 1983. In 1983 and 1984, he was visiting professor at the Department of Electronics of the University of Rome "La Sapienza" and in 1989/1990 at the Faculty of Engineering of the University of Perugia. His research interests include physical acoustic and acousto-optic devices, surface acoustic waves, nonlinear acoustics, and surface-acoustic-wave-based sensors.

Stephen F. White is a Research Officer at the Biotechnology Centre, Cranfield University. His main research interests include the design and fabrication of amperometric biosensors, with particular emphasis on methods of mass production. His background is in electromechanical engineering and biotechnology industries.

Christine Wittmann received her B.Sc. degree in chemistry from the Technical University of Darmstadt in 1984 and her M.Sc. degree in food chemistry in 1988 from the University of Frankfurt. She holds her Dr.rer.nat. degree since 1991 from the Technical University of Munich. After postdoctoral training at the Gesellschaft für Biotechnologische Forschung (GBF) at the Department of Enzyme Technology from 1991 to 1993, Dr. Wittmann worked as a research scientist at the University of Stuttgart, Institute for Technical Biochemistry, in the field of "Biochemical methods and biosensors for environmental analysis". Her current research interests include environmental and food analysis, antibody production, biosensors, immunochemical methods, flow injection systems, and protein designs of recombinant antibodies. She is now Professor of Food Technology at Fachhochschule Neubrandenburg.

Monika Wortberg is a Chemistry graduate from University of Münster, Germany. She conducted her Ph.D. research in Analytical Chemistry in Prof. Dr. K. Cammann's group, where she developed a flow-injection immunosensor for herbicides. Subsequently, she spent two years as a postdoctoral fellow in the Department of Entomology at the University of California, Davis (Prof. B. D. Hammock) on the development of multianalyte immunoassay methods for herbicides. Currently, she works at the BASF Agricultural Research Facility in Limburgerhof, Germany, in the field of chromatography.

Kenji Yokoyama is Associate Professor at the School of Materials Science, Japan Advanced Insititute of Science and Technology, Ishikawa, Japan. He is currently working on a cooperative research project with the group of Prof. Isao Karube, where he used to have a position as a Lecturer.

Table of Contents

PART III METABOLISM AND BIOAFFINITY SENSORS FOR MEDICINE, FOOD, AND THE ENVIRONMENT

PART IV ON-LINE AND *IN VIVO* MONITORING AND CONTROL

Part I

Introduction to the Handbook

1 Biosensors and Electronic Noses for Practical Applications

Erika Kress-Rogers

CONTENTS

1.1 INTRODUCTION

1.1.1 BIOSENSORS AND BIO-SENSES

Since Updike and Hicks[1] first created a biosensor for glucose monitoring in 1967 by mounting an enzyme membrane onto an oxygen probe, a rich and diverse range of biosensors of high

0-8493-8905-4/97/$0.00+$.50
© 1997 by CRC Press, Inc.

selectivity and sensitivity has been devised. Biosensors development has become a multidisciplinary field relying not only on biochemistry and biotechnology to provide a wide range of sensing agents, immobilization techniques, and membrane technologies, but also incorporating microelectronic, optical, and acoustic base devices and advanced signal processing techniques. Both in terms of the base devices and signal interpretation methods employed and of the analytes detected, an increasing overlap with the area of gas sensors has arisen, particularly in approaches towards the development of electronic noses. Not only biochemical pathways, but also the approaches of living systems to signal pattern analysis are being copied by researchers in this field.

Biosensors for volatile compounds compete with gas sensors based on chemically sensitive semiconductor materials or devices and with sensors carrying specifically sorbent films. There is a double benefit in considering such gas sensors together with biosensors. Firstly, the best choice for a given application can be made if the characteristics of alternative and complementary devices are known. Secondly, the experience gained with optical and acoustic base transducers used with specifically sorbent films can also be applied to the development of immunosensors and DNA probes. There is thus cross-fertilization between these two areas, and instrumentation for running the devices can advantageously be put to dual use. Similarly, some of the semiconductor gas sensors (CHEMFET) share design principles and manufacturing technologies with microelectronic ion sensors (ISFET) that form the base devices of some biosensor designs. Thirdly, common approaches to signal interpretation can be utilized.

Biosensors use catalysis and affinity interactions, generally using agents derived from biological systems (although efforts are being made to produce enzymes tailored to requirements). Electronic noses use a sensing approach copied from biological systems. Sophisticated signal interpretation is particularly important for the electronic noses but also has a role to play in enhancing the performance of biosensors. In both cases, software systems modelled on the function of biological systems have come to the aid of the sensors. Senses in living systems have provided the blueprint for sensors applied in living and other systems.

Where a wide range of biologically relevant compounds need to be screened simultaneously, the biochemical pathways and neural responses of animals have traditionally been harnessed to provide the ultimate biosensor and have been complemented rather than replaced by man-made sensors.

In water supply monitoring, fish fitted with probes to monitor physiological parameters can be used to raise the alarm on one or more of a wide range of potential toxic contaminants encountered in the water supply. As an alternative, not only sensors for specific target compounds but also biosensor systems based on a selection of microbe species, each immobilized onto an electrode that monitors the microbial metabolism, are being developed.

The caged canary has traditionally been used by miners to warn them of methane buildup. Today, gas sensors (Chapter 23) are a more convenient alternative for the detection of combustible gases. The caged canary, however, is still taken along when the presence of toxic gases of unknown composition is suspected, as in some terrorist incidents. Drug sniffer dogs and truffle pigs are not out of work yet although biosensors and electronic noses are being developed as more portable and lower-maintenance alternatives for many applications.

When the aroma of a new food for humans, a new pet food, or a new feed for farm animals is to be tested, only a panel of the mammals in question will do. Specially talented and trained human noses are needed for the assessment of new perfumes in personal care products such as eau de Cologne or soap. Once a product has been developed, however, this effort will only be needed for regular quality checks. In-between, deviations from the standard process pattern can be detected with electronic noses that don't tire, get bored, or catch cold.

An overview on the principles and characteristics of base devices for biosensors and electronic noses and their relevance to practical applications is given in the following section of this chapter (more details in Chapters 6 to 9). Signal interpretation techniques are the subject of the third section in this chapter (and later in the book the subject of Chapters 20 and 27). Sensing agents and functional membranes for biosensors are presented in Chapters 2 to 5. Chapters 10 to 19 discuss biosensor designs for applications in the health care, agriculture, food processing, biotechnology, and environmental protection sectors. Sensing layers for electronic noses are presented in Chapters 23 to 26 after an introduction to the mammalian sense of smell in Chapters 21 and 22. The framework for the commercial development of the sensors presented in this book is analyzed in the final section of this chapter.

1.2 BUILDING BLOCKS FOR BIOSENSORS AND ELECTRONIC NOSES

1.2.1 OVERVIEW

Biosensors have been variously defined as "a self-contained analytical device that responds selectively and reversibly to the concentration or activity of chemical species in biological samples", as "an analytical device that incorporates a biologically active material in intimate contact with an appropriate transduction element for the purpose of detecting — reversibly and selectively — the concentration or activity of chemical species in any type of sample". (Both definitions were proposed by Arnold and Meyerhoff in 1988.[2] Widened or narrowed variants of these definitions have also been used to suit particular fields of work.) For practical applications in medicine, environmental protection, and process monitoring, the second of these biosensor definitions (stipulating the incorporation of a biologically active material) has the advantage of encompassing a group of sensors that share potential performance characteristics governed by the biological sensor component.

Using this definition, biosensors can be further divided into metabolism biosensors, affinity biosensors, and recombinant biosensors depending on the sensing agent employed (Figure 1.1). For the first group, sensing agents include isolated enzymes, combinations of enzymes and cofactors, and whole biological cells such as bacteria or algae. Biosensors based on isolated enzymes provide high selectivity for specific saccharides, alcohols, amino acids, organic acids such as lactate, and many more compounds (see Chapter 2 in this book.) Whole cell biosensors are used particularly in the field of environmental monitoring to screen for analyte groups such as herbicides, fungicides, or pesticides, or to determine summary variables such as BOD (biological oxygen demand, see Chapter 14). Biosensors for BOD are commercially available and provide a measurement within 2 min compared with 5 days for the conventional method.[3,4] Plant and animal tissue containing the desired enzymes and cofactors have also been used.

For the second group of biosensors, monoclonal or polyclonal antibodies can be employed as sensing agents. The resulting "immunosensors" have the potential of providing a more rapid and simple-to-use alternative to immunoassays. For more on bioaffinity agents used for sensors, see Chapter 3 (a list of such agents is given in Table 3.1 of that chapter) and Chapter 17. Bioaffinity agents for environmental sensor applications are discussed in Chapter 15. In the third group, the sensing agents are DNA probes. A presentation of sensors based on DNA probes is given in Chapter 4. Rapid detection techniques based on DNA probes for foodborne pathogens have been described by Bsat et al.[5]

Affinity and recombinant biosensors share optical and acoustic base devices with sorption sensors for gases and volatiles and with lipid film odor sensors (Figure 1.2). These base devices measure the changes in the dielectric or elastic properties or in the mass loading of the sensing surface as binding, recombination, or sorption takes place. Sensors based on selective sorption (Chapter 25), lipid film sensors (Chapter 26), and chemically sensitive semiconductors (Chapters 23 and 24) are all used in the construction of electronic noses.

With the semiconductor gas sensors, changes in conductivity or surface charge density are usually measured using resistive or FET (field effect transistor) configurations. The resistor

Functional membrane

* prevents fouling
* improves biocompatibility
* reduces access by interfering chemicals (by size or charge discrimination)
* controls analyte diffusion rate (and thus analytical range in certain devices)

Sensing agent

Metabolism biosensors:
- isolated enzymes
- combinations of enzymes and cofactors
- whole biological cells such as bacteria or algae
- plant or animal tissue

Affinity biosensors:
- immunological bioaffinity agents such as monoclonal or polyclonal antibodies
- non-immunological bioaffinity agents such as lectins
- receptors such as photocentres isloated from bacteria

Recombinant biosensors:
- gene probes

Base Device

For metabolism biosensors:

◊ Carbon electrode modified with mediator compound
◊ Clark-type gas probe
◊ Planar micro-Clark gas probe
◊ ISE (ion-selective electrode)
◊ ISFET (ion-selective field effect transistor)
◊ Calorimetric devices or instruments
◊ FOP (fibre-optic probe) gas- or ion-selective probes
◊ FOP or compact optical instruments plus luminescent or fluorimetric labels

For affinity and recombinant biosensors:

◊ Optical devices such as SPR (surface plasmon resonance) devices or TIR (total internal reflection) devices
◊ Acoustic devices such as SAW (surface acoustic wave) devices
◊ FOP or compact optical instruments plus luminescent or fluorimetric labels

FIA (Flow injection analysis) arrangements can be used with metabolism or affinity agents.

FIGURE 1.1 Building blocks for biosensors. Base transducers and biologically active materials used in the construction of biosensors. A functional membrane can be added for the tailoring of analytical characteristics, device protection, and biocompatibility. (Note: Instruments such as bioluminometers do not match those biosensor definitions that stipulate an intimate contact between the sensing agent and transducer. However, they can be designed to be compact and user-friendly and utilize the same groups of sensing agents. From a practical point of view, therefore, it makes sense to treat them together with biosensors.)

gas sensors share the simplicity of their structure with one of the metabolism biosensor designs, namely, the mediated amperometric biosensors where electron transfer is measured without the need for a secondary chemical sensor.

Ideally, the sensor is combined with a reference element. This would carry an inactivated layer that was otherwise identical to the sensing layer. With a suitable referencing technique, one can then compensate for interfering variables such as variations in temperature or

Pattern recognition

* neural network
* conventional pattern analysis methods

Array of sensors

A. Arrays of sensors with broad selectivity

The sensing elements of the array are chosen, tailored and operated to exhibit distinct but overlapping broad selectivity profiles for the range of gases and/or volatiles of interest.

Set of sorption sensors:

- selectively sorbent polymer films
- odorant-selective lipid films

deposited onto an array of base devices:

◊ Optical devices such as SPR (surface plasmon resonance) devices
◊ Acoustic devices such as SAW (surface acoustic wave) devices

Set of chemically sensitive semiconductors:

- metal oxide (MeOx) semiconductors
- conducting polymers

◊ typically configured as simple resistor devices.
◊ Incorporation into microelectronic devices such as the FET is possible.

A heater film is incorporated for each MeOx gas sensing element.

B. Arrays of sensors with narrow selectivity

Gas sensors with narrow specificity profiles are used to form sensing arrays with pattern recognition for the analysis of certain gas mixtures.

- LB (Langmuir-Blodgett) or MBE (molecular beam epitaxy) films of MePb organic semiconductors; (where Pb stands for metal phthalocyanine and Me stands for Pb, Cu, Zn, Ni or Co, also for non-metal H_2)
- inorganic catalysts such as Pd, Pt, Ni and alloys

◊ These films are particularly suitable for CHEMFET (chemically selective field effect transistor) configurations.

Heater films are incorporated for the inorganic catalyst gas sensors.

FIGURE 1.2 Building blocks for electronic noses. In applications such as aroma assessment, a complex mixture of volatiles composed of many different chemical compounds needs to be analyzed. Electronic noses, consisting of arrays of sensors with broad, overlapping selectivity spectra combined with pattern analysis software are being developed for the identification and comparison of such volatile mixtures. (Note: The mechanism of interaction between analyte and sensing agent is still subject to research in some cases, for example, for odorant-sensitive lipids or conductive polymers.)

humidity by using, for example, a simple differential measurement, an algorithm, or a look-up table.

To eliminate drift problems, autocalibration can be implemented with actuators such as micropumps and -valves for calibration media. Both in autocalibration and in referencing for cross-sensitivity compensation, advanced software techniques can be applied advantageously (see Section 1.3.3 below).

In many practical applications, the highest performance can be achieved with flow injection analysis (FIA) systems. These are presented for process monitoring, clinical monitoring, and for pesticides detection in environmental protection in Chapters 19, 18, and

15, respectively. Flow injection immunoanalysis (FIIA) systems for herbicides, explosives, and drugs are presented in Chapter 17.

Reports on FIA biosensor systems intended for quality assurance in food processing and biotechnology hold a prominent position in the current literature. Examples include an FIA system with good long-term stability for the determination of glucose in beverages,[6] an FIA system for maltose and glucose determination in starch hydrolysate fermentation,[7] and an FIA biosensor system for essential fatty acids in fats and oils.[8] On-line monitoring applications include an FIA biosensor system determining glucose, fructose, and sucrose for cellulose hydrolysis control[9] and an FIA biosensor system for the monitoring of penicillin production.[10]

1.2.2 Base Devices for Metabolism Biosensors

In the first biosensor devices[1] the agent was glucose oxidase carried on a membrane held onto a Clark-type gas probe using an elastic ring. The concentration of glucose in the sample was indicated as a decrease in local oxygen pressure. Since then, a wide range of amperometric biosensors have been constructed on the basis of gas probes for oxygen, peroxide, or ammonia. Potentiometric biosensors have been based mainly on pH probes, but also on other ion-selective electrodes (ISE) and on microelectronic ion-sensitive devices (ISFET, Figure 1.3c) as base devices. Enzyme immobilization techniques for greater stability and compactness have been developed.

1.2.2.1 Amperometric and Potentiometric Biosensors

A simple, compact design for amperometric biosensors has been achieved by combining the enzyme with an electron mediator compound and monitoring electron transfer to a carbon electrode rather than using a gas probe for a secondary analyte. This mediated amperometric biosensor[11,12] has the further advantage of obviating the need for adequate oxygen pressures and of operating at low applied voltages compared with the Clark-type probes, thereby reducing the number of interfering electroactive compounds (Chapter 10). The mediated amperometric biosensor is the basis of the ExacTech glucose analyzer sold widely in the form of a disposable one-shot strip biosensor with a pen-type or card-type instrument.

The amperometric biosensors based on gas probes (often peroxide probes) remain a very active field of R & D. They lend themselves to performance tailoring with functional membranes[13] that reduce fouling, suppress interference from electroactive compounds, adjust the analytical range, and other functions (Chapter 5). They are dominant in the field of *in vivo* applications (Chapter 18) and continue to be important in other medical applications (Chapter 11). Miniaturization has been achieved by using Clark-type probes configured as planar devices manufactured in silicon technology (Chapter 6).

Whereas potentiometric devices based on conventional ISE are criticized as having a "noisy DC signal", this does not apply to the ENFET where the output signal is also related to the potential drop between an ion-sensitive membrane and the sample. One of the advantages of FET devices is the intrinsic preamplification, favoring good signal-to-noise ratios. The ISFET was first developed by Bergveld in 1970.[14] Together with a special reference ISFET device (the REFET), it forms a self-contained micro-unit without the need for conventional reference electrodes.

The robustness of FET sensors has been demonstrated with the direct insertion of ISFET/REFET probes into meat for the measurement of pH[15,16] and with other commercial uses.[17,18] (See also Chapter 6.)

The enzyme-sensitized field effect transistor (ENFET) is created by immobilizing an enzyme onto an ISFET device. The ENFET can be combined with an ISFET of the same type for reference. Examples include ENFET for lactose[19] and for protein characterization.[20]

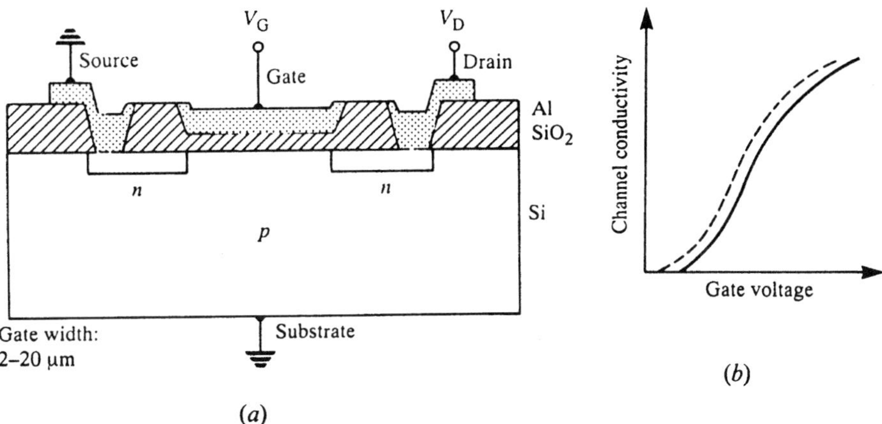

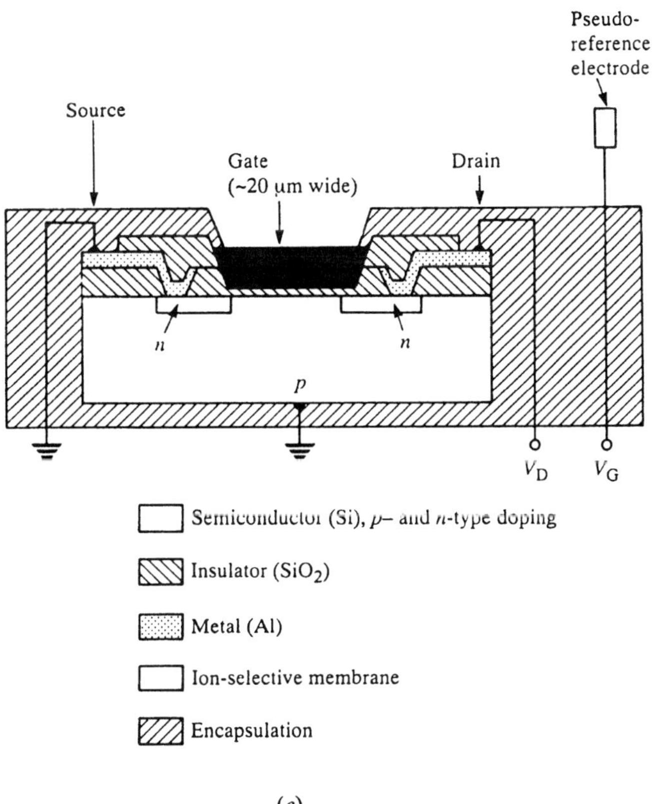

FIGURE 1.3 (a) Schematic diagram of the FET (field effect transistor) and the CHEMFET (chemically sensitive FET). The CHEMFET is derived from the transistor device by replacing the usual gate metal with a catalytic metal or metal alloy which is then left open rather than protected with passivating layers. (b) Shift of the CHEMFET characteristics when analyte gases interact with the gate metal film. (c) Schematic diagram of the ISFET (ion-selective FET). Here the gate metal film has been removed and the gate contact has been replaced by a pseudoreference electrode. An ion-selective membrane is deposited onto the gate insulator. The source and drain contacts are encapsulated to allow immersion into the sample. (From Kress-Rogers, E., *Instrumentation and Sensors for the Food Industry,* Butterworth-Heinemann, Boston, 1993, chap. 17. With permission.)

An interesting possibility is the further development of ENFET based on a pH-static ISFET where the pH is kept constant via a feedback circuit. The voltage needed to keep the pH at a constant value at any one time is an indicator for the analyte concentration. In combination with a separate pH sensor, there is the possibility of developing a measurement technique for which the sample pH is no longer an interfering variable.

The ISFET is also the basis of the coulometric microtitrator array which continuously maps out the titration curve for a liquid flowing through the cell, thus continuously quantifying titratable acidity in-line and helping to analyze acid mixtures. (For viscous samples, a dipstick configuration with pulsed mode operation was developed to monitor acidity.) The microtitrator arrangement was originally developed to provide a test signal for an *in situ* or *in vivo* ISFET pH sensor so as to provide autocalibration.[21] Low-cost production of all FET devices, however, depends on high production volumes.

Further designs for microelectronic metabolism biosensors have been devised including those employing CHEMFET gas sensors (Figure 1.3a) as base devices and those based on variants of the ISFET. The principles and characteristics of CHEMFET and ISFET are described in Reference 22, with special reference to food applications. For the manufacture and state of development of microelectronic devices see Chapters 6 and 12.

1.2.2.2 Calorimetric Biosensors

The enthalpy changes in enzymatic reactions used in conventional calorimetry and biosensors based on a calorimetric principle were pioneered by Mosbach and Danielsson in 1974.[23] Calorimetric biosensors are advantageous, particularly where several enzymes would otherwise be needed to produce a reaction product detectable with an electrochemical sensor. For example, in the assay of sucrose, invertase only is required with a calorimetric device, whereas both glucose oxidase and invertase would be needed with the electrochemical biosensors.

Calorimetric biosensors also have the advantage that a diverse range of analytes can be covered with a single instrument type and without the need for labels, where several optical and electrochemical instruments in conjunction with specially matched luminescent labels, electron mediators, or secondary chemical sensors would otherwise be required.

Conventional calorimeter designs are bulky due to the thermostatting provisions. In recent years, many designs for microcalorimetric biosensors have been devised where the enzyme is in close contact with the thermal sensor, a reference device carrying deactivated enzyme is included, and a reduction in the heat capacity of the sensor and sample volume is achieved through miniaturization. Calorimetric devices can be divided into three groups. The classic enzyme thermistor first designed by Mosbach and Danielsson[23] is in the second group, together with miniaturized enzyme thermistor designs developed in recent years. In the first group are the integrated Si thermopile biosensors[24] based on novel thermal sensors.[25] (Note: While the Si thermopile biosensors are indeed fabricated on silicon [Si] chips using planar Si technology, this is not the case for the bead thermistor devices sometimes referred to as "thermal biochip" or "bio-thermochip". Occasionally, confusion results from a minor misprint that turns silicone [used as a plastic support material in some sensing devices] into the semiconductor element silicon [Si] which forms the basis of microelectronic devices.)

The groups for calorimetric biosensor devices are summarized below. Calorimetric biosensors for specific analytes are discussed in Chapter 13.

1. *Heat conduction calorimeter*. The temperature differential between the reaction vessel and an isothermal heat sink is measured by a thermopile. (A thermopile consists of closely packed thermocouples in series. Alternate junctions are exposed

for receiving radiant heat, the EMF values for the junction pair of each thermocouple add up to provide the higher signal of the thermopile.)

- Calvet type: the reaction vessel is a thin metal cylinder surrounded by a wire-wound thermopile. The thermopile reference temperature is provided by contact with the surrounding heat sink. It is usually set up as a twin calorimeter differential system to compensate for temperature variations not related to the enzyme catalyzed reaction.
- Thermopile film: the thermopile is formed by metal films evaporated onto an insulating film, rolled up into a cylinder, and mounted onto a catheter. The enzyme is dip-coated onto the thermopile.[26]
- Integrated Si (silicon) thermopile: a thin-film thermopile comprising well over 100 thermocouples (providing a high signal output) is formed on a Si chip by planar silicon technology. The enzyme is coated onto the thermopile structure. Si technology lends itself to applications where miniaturization and reproducibility between devices are required. Si membrane structures can be used to reduce the heat capacity of the base device and thus increase sensitivity. The device can be used in a flow-through cell without bulky thermostatting provisions.

2. *Isoperibol calorimeter.* The reaction vessel is protected from variations in the environmental temperature by an isothermal jacket.
   - Two configurations were devised for the pioneering enzyme thermistor design. In the single-flow mode, one thermistor each is mounted on the sample inlet and outlet tubes attached to the enzyme column vessel. In the split-flow mode, one thermistor each is mounted on the enzyme and reference column flows. Finding a well-matched pair of thermistors can be a problem with conventional thermistor devices.
   - A number of miniaturized enzyme thermistor configurations have been developed in recent years, for example, consisting of microbead thermistors and flow injection systems (FIA). One has sample channels micromachined into Si chips and connected to miniature gold inlet and outlet tubes with attached bead thermistors.[27] Another consists of a microcolumn and bead thermistors mounted within a tubular jacket.[28] To increase enzyme loading and reaction heat capture, one device has the enzyme immobilized onto a cylindrical silicone tube frame mounted over a bead thermistor. This is used with a reference thermistor having a deactivated enzyme frame.[29]
3. *Isothermal calorimeter.* The temperature of the reaction vessel is kept constant by heat compensation in an adiabatic shield. The power required to stabilize the temperature by Joule heating or Peltier cooling provides the output signal.

1.2.2.3 Optical and Acoustic Biosensors

Further designs for metabolism biosensors have been devised including many designs based on fiber-optic probe (FOP) gas or ion sensors (sometimes called optrodes or optodes) or on fiber-optic probes in combination with fluorescent labeling techniques. One of the configurations for a fiber-optic pH sensor is shown in Figure 1.4. To form an FOP biosensor, an enzyme can be co-immobilized together with the pH-sensitive dye. The choice of the dye immobilization technique is crucial to ensure calibration stability. When the enzyme-catalyzed reaction which is to be monitored produces a wide range of pH values, several pH-sensitive dyes (covering one or two decades each) will need to be employed.

In clinical applications, FOP chemical sensors are already used for monitoring pH, dissolved oxygen, and carbon dioxide in blood during surgery. Biosensors based on such FOP gas and ion sensors could share the same optical instrument. FOP are also suited to the

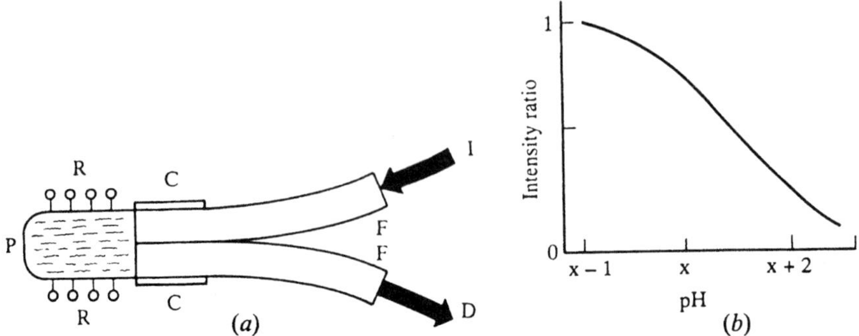

FIGURE 1.4 (a) Schematic diagram of a fiber-optic chemical sensor. F: optical fibers, C: cladding, I: input radiation, D: detected radiation, R: reagent immobilized onto polymer, P: polymer grown on fiber tip. (b) For the choice of a pH-sensitive dye as the reagent R, the typical response over two pH decades is shown for a single-fiber FOP (fiber-optic probe). The analytical range can be extended by combining several FOP sensors into a fiber-bundle. Biologically active agents can be immobilized onto FOP, either in combination with chemically sensitive agents such as pH-sensitive dyes or in combination with fluorescent or luminescent reagents. (From Kress-Rogers, E., *Instrumentation and Sensors for the Food Industry,* Butterworth-Heinemann, Boston, 1993. With permission.)

development of sensors for process monitoring as they can be designed to be robust, they are tolerant to high microwave intensities or electrical mains noise, and can be safely operated in environments where electrical connections are undesirable (spark hazard) or unreliable (steam ingress).

In principle, many colorimetric and fluorescent assays can be converted into FOP designs, provided that the reagent acts reversibly and can be immobilized reliably without loss of activity. Fiber-optic biosensor designs have been presented in some detail in the book by Wolfbeis[30] or in briefer form by Arnold[31] or by Blum et al.[32] An example for dual fructose/glucose analysis is given by Lee et al.[33]

Optical instruments used for bioluminescence assays can be developed into compact user-friendly instruments dedicated to a particular type of analysis and supplied with reagents in predosed kit form. Although such instruments do not conform to biosensor definitions stipulating an intimate contact between the enzyme and the transducer (here the light-sensitive element), they can be a useful alternative where a wide dynamic range is required.

Acoustic devices have also been employed as the basis of metabolism biosensors, for example, for pesticide detection using cholinesterase with a piezocrystal microbalance.[34,35] Generally, however, acoustic devices are more prominent in the area of immunosensors and sorption sensors and are discussed in more detail later in this chapter. These acoustic devices rely on detecting a change in the mass-loading of an oscillating piezoelectric crystal or on changes in the acoustic or electrical surface properties of surface acoustic wave devices.

They are sometimes confused with acoustic techniques involving the transmission of ultrasonic waves through the bulk of a sample where the speed of propagation of ultrasonic waves within the bulk of the sample (rather than just in the vicinity of the sensing layer) is measured. Such bulk ultrasonic measurements are very effective for biomass monitoring of cultures in fermentation or for sugar concentration measurements in process control. These ultrasonic techniques,[36,37] however, are quite different from the highly sensitive and selective acoustic biosensor devices considered in this handbook. A detailed presentation of acoustic devices for biosensors is given in Chapter 9 and a brief overview is found in the section below.

1.2.3 Base Devices for Bioaffinity, Recombinant, and Sorption Sensors

When antigens bind to an antibody layer, the dielectric properties such as the refractive index and the mechanical properties such as the thickness, mass, density, and elasticity of the surface layer change. If the antibody layer is immobilized onto a device which detects such surface properties sensitively and without being significantly affected by the properties of the bulk of the sample, then an immunosensor is created that provides a number of advantages compared to conventional immunoassays.

It is often possible to eliminate washing steps for the separation of bound from free antibodies, incubation times can be reduced, and in some circumstances it is even possible to monitor binding directly without waiting for the completion of the binding process and to gain additional information about the antigen from the binding kinetics. For example, a grating coupler has been applied to the real-time measurement of binding kinetics between herbicides and antibodies.[38]

These sensing techniques can be applied not only to antigens by using antibodies raised by immunological reactions, but other affinity binding agents such as lectins can also be employed as can DNA probes. The same base devices have earlier been used for the highly sensitive detection of certain gases and volatiles with the help of specifically sorbent layers, and further research is expanding the range of volatiles that can be monitored with these methods. They also play a significant role in the development of electronic noses.

Strictly speaking, the class of devices considered in this section are "affinity, recombinant, and sorption sensors", but for a less unwieldy term it is perhaps allowable to refer to them using a term for a part of this class, namely, the immunosensors. These cover only a part of the affinity sensors, but many of the considerations relevant for immunosensors also apply to the nonimmunological affinity biosensors, the gene probes, and the sorption sensors.

1.2.3.1 Optical Immunosensors

Considerable progress has already been achieved in the development of optical immunosensors. The surface plasmon resonance (SPR) device detects minute changes in the refractive index of the sensing surface and its immediate vicinity. This highly sensitive detection is based on a collective excitement of electrons (the surface plasmons) in a metal film on a substrate (such as glass), leading to total absorption of light at a particular angle of incidence which is dependent on the refractive indices on either side of the metal film. Thus, the refractive index of the sensitizing layer and a thin layer immediately adjacent to it can be measured as a shift in the angle of total absorption of light.

Laboratory prototypes of SPR devices may consist of a prism on a glass slide carrying the thin metal layer (Figure 1.5). For more compact devices, a diffraction grating structure can be formed to define the incident angle instead of using a prism. For SPR chemical sensors or immunosensors, the metal layer carries a sensitizing layer and this can be in contact with either a gas or a liquid sample. Rate-of-change mode (or kinetic mode) operation is possible with SPR devices so that the binding process can be monitored as it is progressing rather than waiting for the end of the incubation.

SPR prism devices were configured as sorption sensors for the clinically used gas halothane and for the determination of anti-IgG and anti-HSA in the early 1980s. Subsequent work has included diffraction grating devices, the development of techniques for enhancing the sensitivity of SPR devices, and applications development for particular assays. A detailed description of the principles and structures of SPR devices is given in Chapter 7 and the applications to biosensing are presented in Chapter 16. A system for specific DNA detection with SPR has been described.[39]

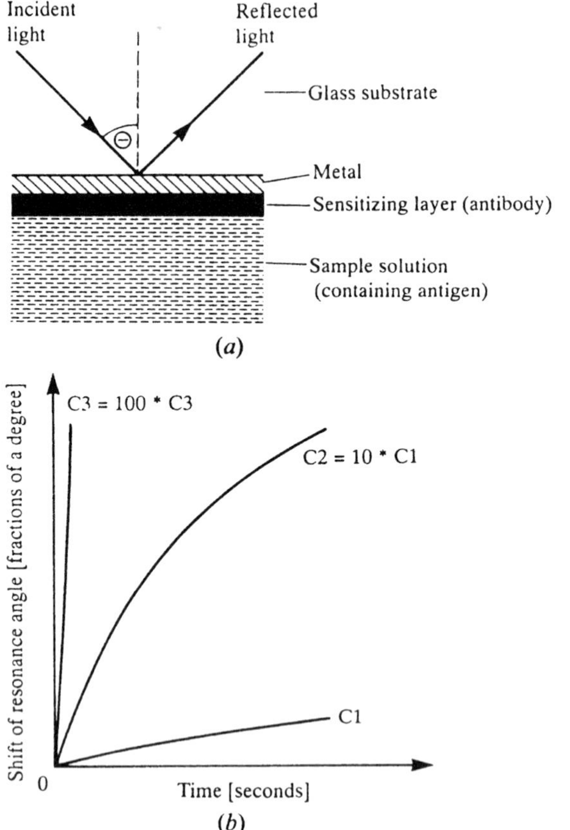

FIGURE 1.5 (a) Schematic diagram of the SPR (surface plasmon resonance) device for the measurement of minute changes in the refractive index. The device can be configured as a highly sensitive gas sensor or as an immunosensor by the immobilization of sensitizing layers on the device. (b) In the immunosensor configuration, it is possible to monitor the antibody-antigen binding process directly without a prior incubation period. The highest sensitivities are achieved after a brief incubation period; additional information on the nature of the analyte can be gained, however, by observing the time-resolved binding characteristics. (From Kress-Rogers, E., *Instrumentation and Sensors for the Food Industry,* Butterworth-Heinemann, Boston, 1993, chap. 17. With permission.)

Another successful immunosensor approach is based on total internal reflection (TIR). The TIR immunosensing device consists of a light guide (such as a thin slab of glass) carrying a sensitizing layer. When light from an optically denser medium (such as a light guide made of glass or heavy plastic) is incident on an optically rare medium (such as air or water), then light with an incidence angle above the critical angle will be totally reflected. Under reflection conditions, an evanescent wave penetrating only a fraction of a wavelength into the optically rarer medium will exist. In the field of this evanescent wave will be the sensing layer of a TIR immunosensor and the sample layer in its immediate vicinity. Hence, the technique is also known as an evanescent wave immunoassay (EWIA or EVIA).

One of the applications has been for the highly toxic *Clostridium botulinum* protein neurotoxin.[40] Food poisoning incidents of this source are very rare, but extremely serious when they occur. Usually, they are prevented by either ensuring a combination of adequately low water activity and pH value by the addition of preserving agents (i.e., curing and pickling), by providing adequate oxygen pressures (in modified atmosphere-packaging), or else by sterilization in a container that is microbe impermeable (i.e., canning and bottling).

When the refractive index or absorptivity in the sensing layer changes, total reflection conditions no longer apply, light will be lost by transmission into the sample or by absorption in the layer, and the light transmission through the wave guide will be reduced (Figure 1.6). The attenuated total reflection (ATR) technique provides a highly sensitive method for monitoring minute changes in the refractive index or absorptivity of the sensing surface.

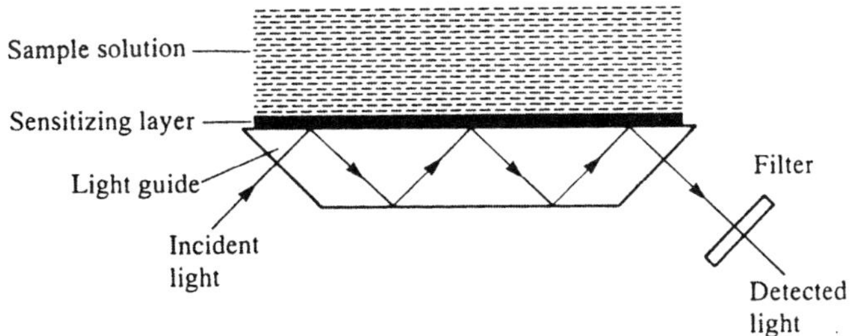

FIGURE 1.6 The TIR (total internal reflection) device makes use of the effect on the evanescent wave of analyte binding to an immobilized sensing layer. (From Kress-Rogers, E., *Instrumentation and Sensors for the Food Industry,* Butterworth-Heinemann, Boston, 1993, chap. 17. With permission.)

A variant of this method is total internal reflection fluorescence (TIRF) for enhanced fluorescence measurements. A fluorescent evanescent wave from fluorescent complexes in the sensing layer is coupled back into the light guide and a high fluorescence intensity can be measured at the angle of total internal reflection. On this basis, disposable immunosensor devices with automatic definition of sample volume by capillary tubes have been constructed. Separation of free labels in the sample solution is unnecessary and, by a suitable choice of capillary tube geometry, sensitive measurements with short incubation times can be achieved. Rather than measuring light intensity, one can also measure the phase with the help of interferometric techniques,[41] and this has been applied in the construction of further immunosensor designs.

Optical waveguide immunosensor principles and structures are presented in Chapter 8; immunosensors for pesticide determination are discussed in Chapter 15.

Fiber-optic probe (FOP) biosensors employing enzymes co-immobilized with pH-sensitive dyes, for example, were introduced in the previous section. Immunosensors can also be designed on the basis of FOP, including FOP bioluminescence sensors using immobilized firefly luciferase or FOP fluorescence sensors based on the fluorescence of NADH, for example. Fluorimetric immunosensors are presented in Chapter 17.

Many optical sensor designs can be realized in compact and robust FOP form including the SPR and TIR immunosensors introduced above (for example, an FOP-EVIA sensor for pollutants and food contaminants[42]). For continuous immunosensing, FOP with a continuous antibody supply to the sensing surface have been constructed using a controlled-release polymer.

1.2.3.2 Acoustic Immunosensors

One of the most widely used acoustic base devices for gas sensors and biosensors is the piezocrystal balance (also known as quartz microbalance or piezoelectric oscillator). Mechanical oscillations of the tiny piezocrystal slab (typically of quartz or lithium niobate) are excited by an AC voltage. The resonance frequency of the oscillating piezocrystal changes with its mass loading which in turn changes as binding or sorption at the sensing surface occurs. Frequency can be measured with a high degree of precision and lends itself as input to digital systems without the need for analogue-to-digital signal conversion. The device is thus a convenient and highly sensitive mass monitor down to picogram levels and has been the basis of many highly sensitive chemical sensors and biosensors. Detection limits have been discussed by Grate et al.[43]

The piezocrystal balance device has little in common with the far-less-sensitive methods for biomass monitoring based on measuring the velocity of propagation of ultrasound through bulk liquid. Piezoelectric crystals are also used in the latter method (as ultrasound transmitters/receiver transducers) but the measurement principle is quite different from the highly sensitive quartz microbalance technique. Both techniques are frequently simply referred to as acoustic sensors and it is advisable for potential users to identify the device actually involved.

The piezocrystal will also oscillate when immersed in a liquid. The signal will, however, depend on the mechanical and electrical properties of the liquid in this case, and the use of a reference crystal with an inactivated sensing layer is recommended. An example of a piezocrystal balance immunosensor is that used for the detection of herbicides[44] (see also Chapter 9).

A further highly sensitive acoustic device is the surface acoustic wave (SAW) device, and this is increasingly used, particularly in the field of odor sensing. The SAW device consists of a piezoelectric crystal, such as quartz or lithium niobate, carrying thin-film interdigital electrodes. A synchronous mechanical surface wave is excited by radio frequency excitation of the electrode pair and propagates on the surface of the piezoelectric substrate to a second electrode pair (for SAW delay lines) or back to the same electrode pair after reflection (for SAW resonator devices).

SAW devices are commonly used as VHF components in television circuits, but have been configured as sensors for many applications. Two SAW device configurations for chemical sensing are shown in Figure 1.7. Of these, the membrane configuration has the advantage of separating the electrical contacts from the sensing surface which is in contact with the sample. The propagation of the surface acoustic wave on the SAW device is highly sensitive to small changes in mechanical and electrical surface properties and this is the basis of highly sensitive sorption and affinity sensors.

SAW sensor arrays carrying a range of lipid membranes or specifically sorbent films are being used to construct electronic noses and this is an increasingly active area of research (see Chapters 25 and 26). Lipid membranes have also been employed in taste sensing, but here they were carried on electrodes for a measurement of the electrical potential in response to astringent acids such as tannic acid.[45]

A full presentation of the principles and configurations of acoustic devices is given in Chapter 9.

1.3 SENSING SYSTEMS

1.3.1 Choices in Biochemical Sensing

From the user's point of view, it is not decisive whether a sensor matches a chosen biosensor definition. Relevant is the functionality and performance of the sensor in fulfilling a monitoring, screening, or measurement task under the practical conditions prevailing for the application that the user has in mind. A biosensor based on the interaction of an enzyme interacting with the analyte inherently provides a high potential sensitivity and selectivity and, by a suitable choice of base transducer monitoring this enzyme-catalyzed interaction, a compact, simple, and inexpensive design as well as rapid direct measurement can be achieved. The sensitivity and selectivity of the biosensor, however, will be influenced by properties of the sample and environment of a specific application.

Variations in the background composition or viscosity of the sample, inhomogeneity within the sample, temperature or pH variations, ingredients or transient high temperatures that inactivate the enzyme, or particles fouling the sensor can all have a bearing on the

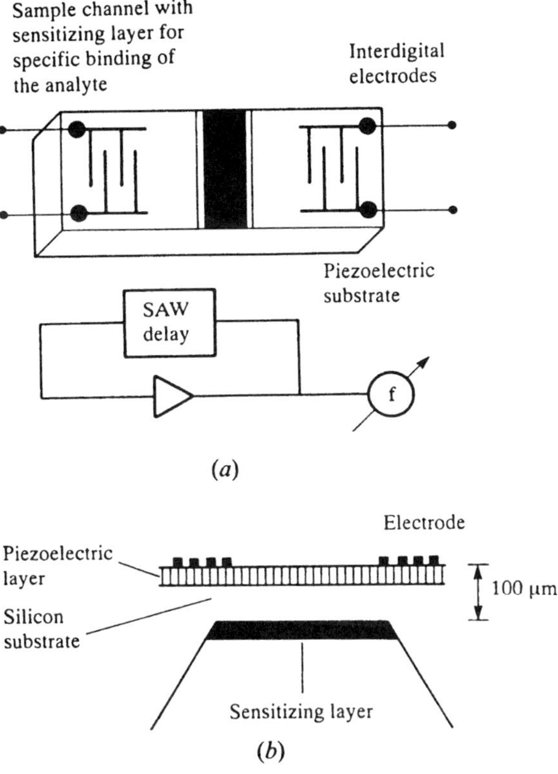

FIGURE 1.7 The SAW (surface acoustic wave) device. (a) Schematic diagram of a chemical sensor based on a SAW delay line device. The basic circuit for monitoring the sensor response is also shown. (b) Schematic design of a SAW membrane device. (From Kress-Rogers, E., *Instrumentation and Sensors for the Food Industry,* Butterworth-Heinemann, Boston, 1993, chap 17. With permission.)

performance of the sensor in a practical application. In some situations it is also difficult to replace enzyme membranes at the end of their operational lifetime, or mechanical stress may preclude the long-term use of sensors in direct contact with the sample. Only after taking into account all these operating conditions and considering the feasibility and cost of overcoming the associated problems, can the performance characteristics and cost-effectiveness in a specific application be estimated and compared with those of alternative techniques, keeping in mind the user's priorities.

In trace analysis, for example in pesticide determination in environmental monitoring, the achievement of a very high sensitivity is the overriding concern. The development of biosensors here competes with that of field instruments based on chromatography methods.

In process monitoring, real-time measurement and a high screening rate are important for a tight control of product specifications by a rapid feedback system. In general, special facilities are needed for the on-line application of biosensors in process monitoring. For example, when the sugar concentration of a hot syrup is to be measured on-line, the application of biosensors for glucose and sucrose would necessitate a bleed line to intermittently take small amounts of the flow volume and automatically dilute them before passing them over the biosensor. The cost of installing such a robotic bleed line conditioning and analysis system would be justified only if saccharide specificity was required, as would be the case, for example, in the control of sugar inversion processes (i.e., the conversion of sucrose into glucose). In other applications, a near-infrared (NIR) or ultrasound analysis system should be considered as an alternative for on-line sugar concentration monitoring.

In general, NIR, NMR (relaxation time measurement), ultrasound, and microwave composition measurement systems for on-line process control don't match biosensors in terms of selectivity or sensitivity. On the other hand, they are robust and capable of screening 100% of a process flow without pretreatment or dilution and can often be applied noncontacting through a suitable window. Thereby, errors due to nonrepresentative sampling or inaccurate dilution or due to sensor fouling are all eliminated and the sterility of the process is assured. Sensor configurations in process lines and batch process vessels are shown in Figures 1.8a to d. For the principles, advantages, and limitations see, for example, Reference 46 for NIR, References 36 and 37 for ultrasound methods, and Reference 47 for microwave techniques applied to on-line composition monitoring.

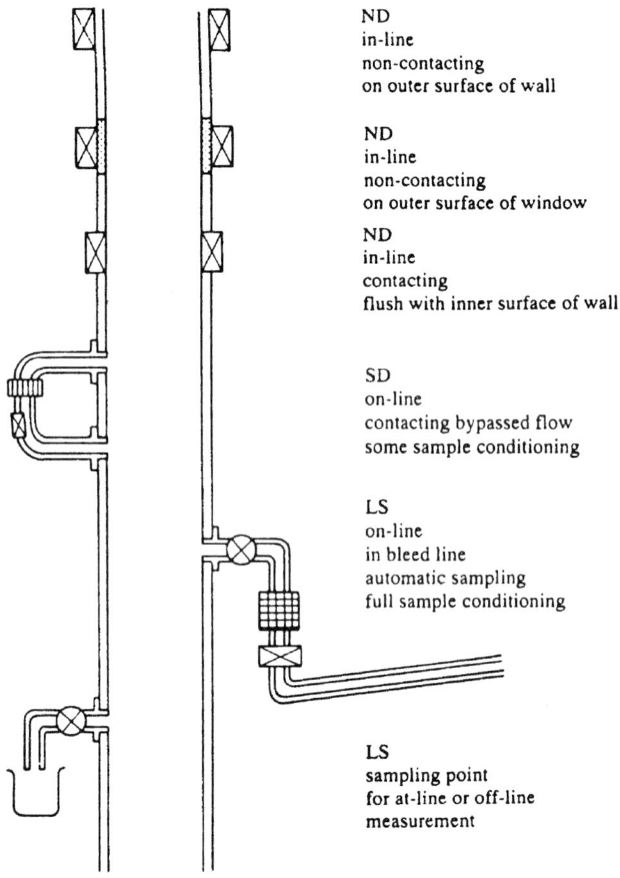

FIGURE 1.8 Sensor configurations in the food industry and in biotechnology. (a) Sensors on continuous processing lines, (b) sensors in batch processes, (c) handheld sensors. For a nondestructive measurement (ND) that is also noncontacting, it is usually necessary to employ an instrument based on the interaction of radiation (such as near-infrared, microwave, or ultrasound). However, a nondestructive noncontacting measurement is also possible with biosensors or electronic noses in the headspace, which can be separated from the sample by a membrane. Nondestructive measurements (ND) in liquid or volatile samples can often be carried out directly (or after light treatment in a bypass) with biosensors, and a measurement with only slight damage (SD) to semisolid samples is also possible with biosensors. Loss of sample (LS), as is the case in sampling from a process line can be minimized with biosensors that require only small sample volumes. For configurations in medical applications, see chapters 11, 12, and 18. ([a-c] From Kress-Rogers, E., *Instrumentation and Sensors for the Food Industry*, Butterworth-Heinemann, Boston, 1993, chap 1. With permission.) (d) Comparison of measurement modes in process control and quality assurance for continuous production processes.

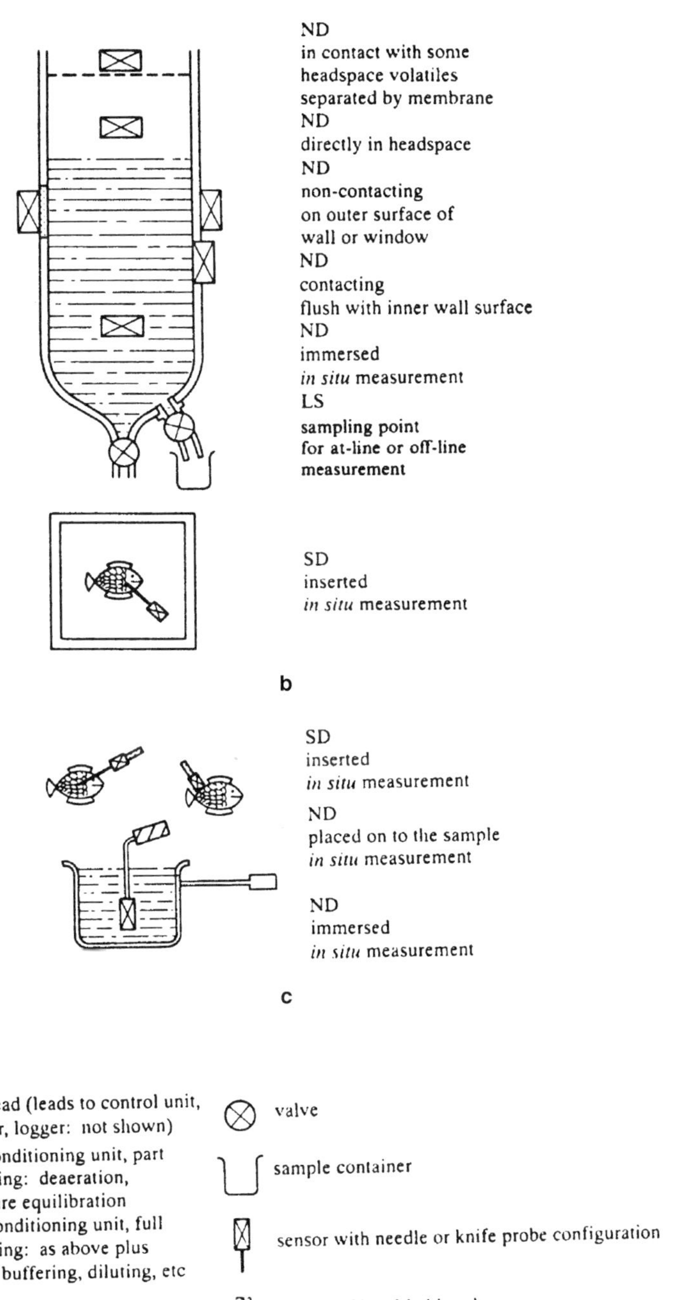

Key

sensing head (leads to control unit, transmitter, logger: not shown)

valve

sample conditioning unit, part conditioning: deaeration, temperature equilibration

sample container

sample conditioning unit, full conditioning: as above plus crushing, buffering, diluting, etc

sensor with needle or knife probe configuration

wall

handle of hand-held probe

window

---- membrane permeable for certain headspace volatiles

ND non-destructive measurement, sample unchanged

SD slight damage to sample (insertion mark of needle, deaeration of bypassed portion)

LS sample lost (to waste via bleed line after conditioning and measuring , or taken away for at-line or off-line measurement)

FIGURE 1.8b and c (continued) and Key to Figures 1.8a to 1.8c.

On-line Measurements for Process Control	At-line Measurements for Process Control	Off-line Measurements for Quality Control and Calibration
Characteristics	Characteristics	Characteristics
Data on a process stream segment available in 'real-time' (or with only a short delay after the segment has passed the measuring point). Measurements updated continuously or with a high repetition rate.	Samples are taken from the line and carried to a measurement point close to the line.	Samples are taken from the line and carried to a QC laboratory outside the production area.
Measurement Modes	Measurement Mode	Measurement Modes
• In-line (measurement point in the main process line), • In a bypass (to facilitate maintenance and improve measurement conditions) • In a bleed line (with the measurement point within the bleed line, often after some automated sample conditioning and/or with arrangements such as flow injection analysis/FIA)	• At-line measurements are taken after sampling with suitably robust and user-friendly instruments located in the production area.	• Off-line measurements are carried out in the QC laboratory on-site. • Off-site analysis is carried out in central laboratories with more specialized staff and more complex and expensive instrumentation.
Results	Results	Results
➲ Adjustment of process variables using rapid feedback or feed-forward control ➲ Product characteristics kept within a specified range to avoid reject product batches ➲ A high proportion of the product flow can be screened. Variations with time are identified.	➲ Process adjustments with longer response time but for a wider range of variables and measurement situations.	➲ Detailed QC data for quality control management ➲ Data with approved assay methods for compliance with labelling regulations, legal and customer specifications ➲ Data for the calibration of on-line and at-line instruments

Related terms in medical sensor applications: In-vivo (instead of on-line), point-of-care (instead of at-line).

d

FIGURE 1.8d (continued).

Noncontacting and nondestructive properties are important attributes not only in process control but also in clinical monitoring, and techniques such as ultrasound or NMR tomography are well known in this field (see Chapter 12). Depending on the measurement set-up, these techniques can be used to gain information not only on composition but also on characteristics such as texture. Ultrasound velocity is very sensitive to phase (gas, liquid, or solid) and to second phase inclusions (gas inclusions in a liquid, crystallites in a liquid phase), and NMR relaxation times indicate the mobility of water or fat molecules thus providing structural information. These techniques can provide information on the texture of body tissues or indicate the liquid/solid ratio of a semicrystallized fat in margarine processing. Using ultrasound or NMR imaging techniques, tissues can be mapped out nonintrusively.

In some applications, optical properties of the sample, including color and turbidity, are useful indicators of chemical processes. Translucency (measured as a scattering profile with an optical fiber bundle) is thought to be a highly sensitive indicator of yoghurt fermentation in the early stages. Many chemical processes are accompanied by a change in viscosity and this can be monitored with robust mechanical resonance probes.

Where the cost-effective application of a biosensor in a process line is feasible without unduly reducing its performance through a hostile environment, advantages accrue in terms of selectivity and sensitivity which in turn allow for satisfactory accuracy. A glucose sensor integrated into a self-calibrating system has been successfully mounted in the inner wall of a molasses processing line (where lower concentrations and temperatures prevail than in the hot syrup considered above). Strategies for process monitoring with biosensors are discussed in Chapter 19.

One possible solution for samples where cross sensitivity, poisoning, fouling, or abrasion pose problems can be the use of a biosensor in the headspace equilibrated with the sample. Although this is possible only for analytes that produce adequate vapor pressures and brings with it the problem of having to ensure a stable relationship between the concentration of the analyte in the solution and that in the headspace, it can solve many of the problems associated with hostile sample conditions. Alternatively, a functional and protective membrane at the interface between the sensing surface and sample may allow direct measurement by reducing adhesion of sample proteins on the sensing surface and reducing access by interfering chemical species to the enzyme layer (see Chapter 5).

Where headspace application is being considered or when the sample itself is volatile, gas sensors can be suitable for certain analytes and applications as an alternative to biosensors. For the monitoring of alcohol concentration in brewing, for example, gas sensors based on metal oxide (MeOx) semiconductors can be tailored and operated to optimize their response to alcohol (see Chapter 23 on semiconductor gas sensors). Their selectivity will generally be broader than that of biosensors and thus the effect of cross-sensitivity needs to be examined for the specific application. For liquid samples, a gas sensor for alcohol vapor can be positioned either in the equilibrated sample headspace or enclosed in a porous membrane for immersion in the sample. Compared to direct application in the liquid sample, less compounds will generally be present in the headspace to interfere with the sensor response or to damage the sensing surface and a MeOx sensor can more readily be kept at the optimum (usually elevated) temperature for selectivity tailoring. This strategy can, for example, be considered for the monitoring of alcohol development in controlling the process of beer brewing. In measuring the alcohol content of the finished product for the legal requirements including the labeling regulations, on the other hand, continuous monitoring is not needed, whereas higher selectivity and accuracy are required. Fortunately, the conditions for an accurate measurement are also more favorable in the stable clear conditions of many end products so that the development of a biosensor instrument for alcohol should be considered for applications that require a more portable alternative to distillation methods.

Progress has been achieved in tailoring the characteristics of MeOx gas sensors in recent years. On the other hand, there have also been advances in the on-line applications of FIA biosensor systems for alcohol, for example in the dealcoholization of beer,[48] and gas-phase biosensors for ethanol vapor have been developed.[49]

Gases and volatiles are produced in many processes including both desirable and unwanted microbial activity, oxidation processes, and other chemical reactions. Thus, fermentation processes can be controlled with the help of volatile monitoring, both microbial and rancid spoilage conditions may be assessed with the help of volatile measurements, and roasting or other heat-treatment processes can be followed by volatile measurement. The relationship between the condition to be assessed and the volatiles developed may be a quite complex one and require a major research effort just to identify the best indicator compound (or set of compounds). The sensing approach can then be investigated, deciding, for example, to develop a biosensor for particular aldehydes as a rancidity indicator or a gas sensor responding to hydrogen or ammonia as an indicator for certain microbial spoilage processes.

The development of gas sensors began in the early years of microelectronics development when the chemical sensitivity of semiconductor materials and devices was noted as an inconvenience to be overcome with passivating surface films. Later, this potential drawback was turned into a virtue by developing a range of chemical sensors for gases, volatiles, and ions. Gas and volatile sensors are now successfully applied in mining and industrial safety applications (detection of combustible or toxic gases, early fire detection) and in combustion control (air-fuel ratio). Further needs for volatile sensors were identified in security and defense (drugs, explosives, and nerve gases).

A wide range of sensors for gases and volatiles have been developed based on further optimization of chemically sensitive semiconductor devices and materials, including Langmuir-Blodgett films integrated into field effect transistors.[50] Research in the field of optical and acoustic sorption sensors has widened the spectrum and this has also provided new base devices for biosensors (Table 1.1).

TABLE 1.1
Sensors for Gases and Volatiles

Sensing agent	Device examples	Analyte examples
	High Specificity	
Enzyme	Amperometric enzyme electrode, ENFET, enzyme thermopile	Alcohols, aldehydes, amines
Inorganic catalyst	CHEMFET	Hydrogen, ammonia, methane, ethylene
Metal phthalocyanine	Thin film resistor	NO_2, Cl_2, O_2
Generally of Broader Specificity, Can Be Tailored By Film Composition and Impurities, Production Techniques and Operation Mode		
Metal oxide semiconductor	Heated resistor	Methane, oxygen, alcohols, aldehydes (broad specificity)
Conducting polymers (organic semiconductors)	Resistor	Alcohols, amines, ethyl acetate, pyridine (broad specificity)
Specifically sorbent polymer film	Optical devices (SPR, TIR) Acoustic devices (SAW, piezocrystal microbalance)	Solvent vapors, anesthetic gases (broad specificity)

Note: For more extensive listings see, e.g., Tables 17.1 and 17.5 of Reference 22.

1.3.2 Electronic Noses

A wide spectrum of volatiles needs to be analyzed in applications such as the monitoring of aroma or the detection of toxic contaminants such as solvent vapors. The development of an individual set of a number of quite different biosensors or chemical sensors specially designed for each of these applications would be prohibitively expensive. To overcome this problem, sensor researchers have copied nature's approach. Mammals use their sense of smell to detect both friend and foe, to decide on the suitability of mates for successful procreation, and to find and select food. Using their sense of smell, mammals can assess whether another mammal of their species is healthy, whether it is genetically closely related, and whether it is ready for breeding; they can judge which foods they can safely eat. The mammalian nose can identify and quantify a wide range of volatiles with high sensitivity and recognize substances by the combination and relative proportions of compounds. This is thought to be achieved by combining a set of sensing elements of broad, overlapping selectivity profiles producing a signal pattern that can be interpreted to identify the compound or set of compounds present (see Chapters 21 and 22).

The mammalian approach to the sense of smell is mimicked in the work aiming towards the development of electronic noses (see Chapter 24). In its simplest form, an "odor meter" as it is sometimes known, consists of an array of several MeOx gas sensors which are actually of identical design but kept at differing temperatures so that their selectivity profiles differ. As a refinement, an array of specially tailored MeOx devices can be used (see Chapter 23). In both cases, MeOx sensors can be used in a simple resistor configuration for a straightforward measurement set-up.

Alternatively, specifically sorbent films can be the sensing agents, particularly for the detection of contaminant volatiles (Chapter 25). Specifically sorbent films are usually applied to an acoustic (Chapter 9) or optical base sensor (Chapters 7 and 8) detecting changes in surface mass loading, or in the dielectric or elastic surface properties of the device on sorption of the analytes.

Acoustic devices have also been used as the basis for sensor arrays employing lipid films as sensing agents for odors (Chapter 26). This research has been inspired by lipid layers thought to play an important role in the detection of odorants in olfactory cells.

The signals from these gas (or volatile) sensors are then analyzed with a method for pattern recognition. Both conventional mathematical methods and neural networks have been used for this purpose (Chapter 27). The neural network is a computer software package mimicking the function of biological neurons. It is trained by presenting it with a large number of example patterns together with the associated interpretation. During training the response is adjusted by feedback until it corresponds to the "correct" response in a high proportion of the example patterns. Once trained, the neural network provides a rapid interpretation of complex patterns.

Even today, aroma is still monitored largely by human noses just as in the herb distillation plant of the middle ages (Figure 1.9). With electronic noses, this situation could change. It needs to be kept in mind, however, that the human nose has some idiosyncratic sensitivity priorities that may differ from those of an electronic nose.

Applications of the electronic nose are seen in the food, drinks, cosmetics, and fragrance sectors as monitoring aroma and fragrance as well as in detecting roasting or cooking end-points, freshness vs. spoilage status or taints. Authentication of products as containing specified ingredients or coming from a certain country of origin will be another application area.

There is interest in smoke detectors that are not triggered by volatiles or airborne particulates from regular cooking. Further uses are in the security sector by recognition of individual genetically determined body odor while ignoring soap or cosmetics smells. Environmental protection will offer many potential applications, from excessive wood-conserving chemicals in houses to gaseous effluent discharged from a faulty plant. Even in the diagnosis of medical conditions, there are potential applications for electronic noses: from the diagnosis of diabetic coma to the early detection and specification of wound infection.

Electronic noses do not tire nor do they become sensitized to particular smells; they are not affected by colds, allergies, or spicy food. They do not necessarily require comfortable or safe working conditions.

Careful selection of the training samples is essential. The chemical background of training samples needs to be matched to that of samples (often from a wide range of origins and storage histories) to be analyzed with a neural network system. Any short-cuts in training the network for the application in hand will entail the risk of errors. The requirement to take the chemical background and physical structure of a sample into account is not unique to

DISTILLATIO
In igne ſuccus omnium, arte, corporum
Vigens fit vnda, limpida et potiſsima.

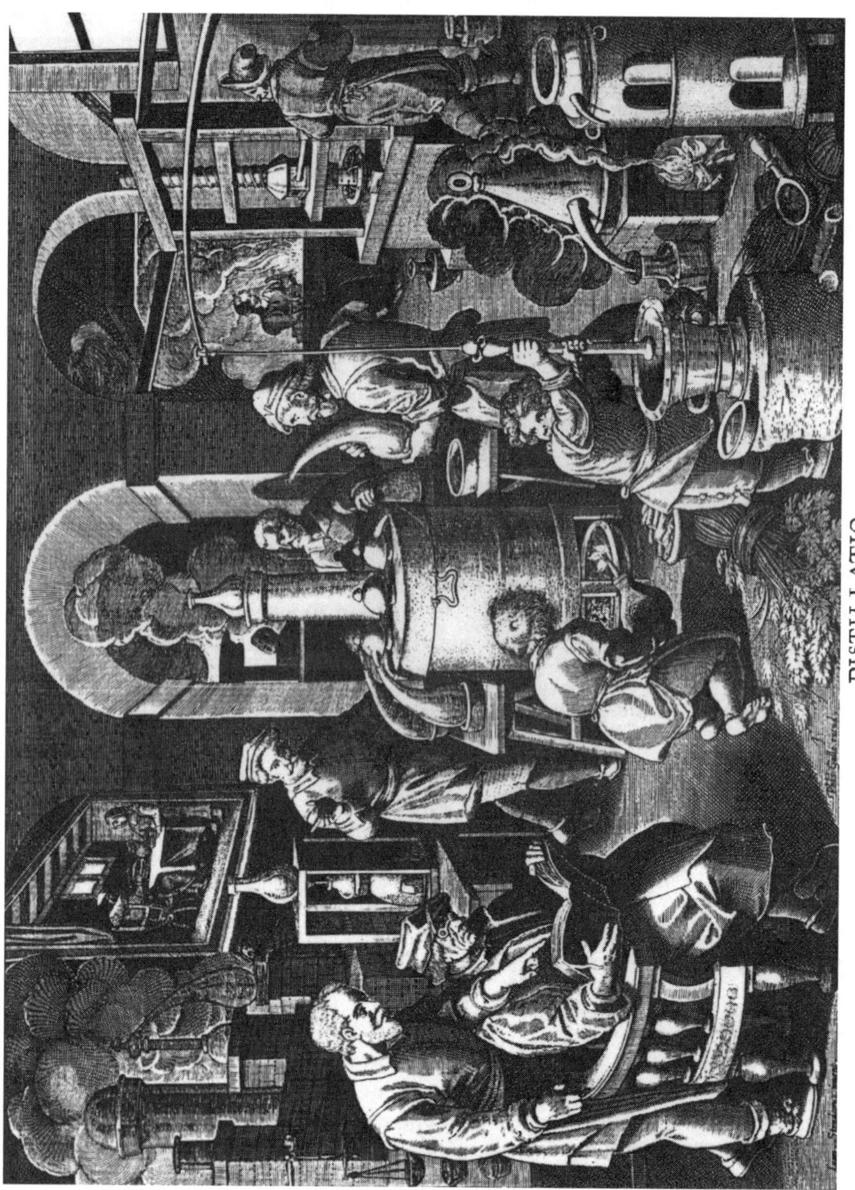

FIGURE 1.9 Process control in an earlier period. The production manager uses his own senses, feeling the temperature, listening to the bubbling, inspecting the color and turbidity, and smelling the aroma. (From the 1968 calendar of Scholven-Chemie AG, Gelsenkirchen, Germany.)

this type of analysis, however. Even with long-established assays such as moisture determination by titration or oven drying, the method of sample preparation and choice of the assay method need to be adapted to the sample type.

An anecdotal illustration of the importance of careful training in the application of neural networks is found in the interpretation of photographic images. Consider the experience of military personnel training a neural network for the automatic interpretation of aerial-view photographs to spot the presence of tanks or rocket launchers. As it turned out, the neural network had inadvertently been trained as a meteorological rather than a military aid in one experiment, since the photographs showing military maneuvers had been taken in cloudy autumn weather, whereas the control photographs had been taken in clear weather conditions. (Artificial intelligence can be outwitted by natural ignorance of its design principles.)

In addition to the selection of training samples, the careful choice of the applications suitable for a particular system of sensors and signal interpretation is also crucial. Larger arrays of 50 or more volatile sensors, each designed to provide a carefully tailored selectivity spectrum, have been constructed for the identification of aroma profiles by their sensor signal "fingerprint" patterns (Chapter 24). Alternatively, smaller arrays of devices of higher selectivity can be more successful in applications where a more limited number of compounds are encountered. Where one of the relevant compounds is well defined and can be measured with a specific sensor such as a particular biosensor, then the inclusion of this sensor into the measurement system will greatly increase the probability of correct identification of a substance or condition.

1.3.3 Software

There is thus no question of replacing specific sensors with software, but rather of software widening the scope for sensor applications. This concerns not only the analysis of complex combinations of chemical compounds; software systems can also help in optimizing the performance of an individual sensor or in providing control decisions based on the response of one sensor or of a set of sensors.

The response pattern of a sensor on exposure to the analyte, and subsequently the pattern of return to the baseline signal on withdrawal of the analyte, can be complex and be further complicated by a poor signal-to-noise ratio in nonequilibrium situations. Optimized signal pattern interpretation will increase the accuracy of the measurement in these situations. Also, the response pattern of the sensor or of a set of sensors can be indicative for the condition of the sensor; for example, it can indicate whether one or more sensing elements have reached the end of their operational life and need to be replaced, or whether a recalibration is due. This is particularly important with biosensors subject to loss of enzyme activity with time or more suddenly due to hostile operating conditions.

Sensors are ultimately used to provide a measurement as the basis of a decision on quality assessment or diagnosis, on process control actions, or on drug administration. Frequently, several variables need to be taken into account to arrive at such decisions. In a clinical application, for example, it may be necessary to monitor blood pressure, blood gases, blood glucose, etc. In food processing, variables such as pressure, temperature, pH value, acidity, salt content, proximate values (water, fat, protein, carbohydrate, and ash concentrations), and the concentration of a preservative compound may all need to be kept within narrow target bands. In environmental protection, synergetic effects in a mixture of pollutant gases may need to be taken into account; for water quality, the BOD value as well as the presence of pesticides and nitrite may need to be considered.

1.3.3.1 Fuzzy Logic for Clear Thinkers

There may be complex relationships between these variables and the conditions to be assessed or controlled. If a conventional mathematical model is used to handle the problem, a considerable development effort may be needed to adequately describe the system. Even then, there are many applications where several of the parameters used in the model are not known exactly and "empirical values" have to be used. In such cases, it can be preferable to use a "fuzzy logic" system instead, particularly when there are restrictions on the available computing capacity and time, as would be the case with real-time and field applications.

This is not to say that fuzzy logic techniques should be regarded as a replacement for mathematical models. On the contrary, the latter will continue to be used and find further applications in process optimization through the simulation of complex systems involving, for example, chemical reactions in multiphase flow systems with irregular geometries.

Fuzzy logic is based on the mathematical system "fuzzy set theory" that can handle variables with values that are not precisely defined but for which a band of values is assigned: in other words "fuzzy" rather than "crisp" variables. Fuzzy logic ties in well with the approach of a human operator faced with the control of a complex system. The car driver has neither the opportunity nor the necessity to measure the current distance to the curb accurately, to map out the geometry of the road boundaries, nor to define the position and speed of other road users accurately and to feed all this information into a mathematical model to calculate the direction and speed to be set for his or her own car. Instead, the driver will continuously adjust the vehicle controls based on continuous assessments and adjustments such as: "if I am slowly approaching the curb, I need to steer gently away from it." Using fuzzy logic control, it has been possible to implement this kind of approach for the control of robotic vehicles and thereby achieve good results much more quickly than with mathematical modeling. Fuzzy logic control with its ability to handle values such as "nearly full" or "warm" was initially used primarily in the control of industrial engineering plants.

1.3.3.2 Fuzzy-Assisted Sensors and Fuzzy-Assisted Experts

More recently, it has also been employed in enhancing sensor performance, for example, in optimizing ultrasonic level gauges by fuzzy logic interpretation of ultrasonic echo patterns.[51] Also, fuzzy logic has been used to enhance the precision of humidity gauges by rapid compensation of the sensor response for cross sensitivity to temperature variations measured with an ancillary sensor. Despite the complex relationship describing the cross sensitivity of the sensor to temperature, a highly accurate real-time reading was realized. Fuzzy-assisted sensors can be accommodated in hand-held instruments. To achieve the same response time and resolution specifications with a conventional program would require a powerful computer, resulting in a more expensive and less compact instrument.

A color sensor with embedded fuzzy logic has also become available. This is programmed by presenting acceptably colored products to the sensor and setting a tolerance level for acceptable deviation. Manufacturers of smart fuzzy-assisted sensors include, e.g., Endress & Hauser GmbH, Fisher Scientific, and Eaton Corp. Fuzzy logic may well play a significant role in future biosensor applications in diagnosing the condition of the sensing element(s), in compensating for cross sensitivity, in interpreting the signal, and in arriving at control decisions, be it for a food processing operation, for continuous automatic drug administration, or for triggering an alarm signal in environmental protection. An introduction to fuzzy logic is given in Chapter 20.

Fuzzy logic controllers for the control of temperatures, pressures, flow rates, and gas injection rates are already used industrially and have the advantage of exhibiting less under- and overshooting than conventional controllers. (For one of the many examples, see Reference 52.) This characteristic could also be of value in automatic sensor equilibration, for example.

Fuzzy logic has also been combined with expert systems and compared to their binary logic counterparts these fuzzy-assisted expert systems require less microprocessor hardware and less time for data exchange. Applications include fermentation management or the assessment of taste panel results, for example. Suppliers include Omron Electronics Inc., Yokogawa Corp., and Bailey Controls Co.

1.3.3.3 Sensors and Neural Networks + Fuzzy Logic and Actuators

Fuzzy logic differs from neural network analysis as used in the electronic nose (see Section 1.3.2 above). Fuzzy logic is based on the evaluation of inputs with a known preprogrammed, if "fuzzy" relationship between input variables and output signals. Neural network analysis is a pattern recognition technique that relies on the examination of large numbers of representative samples of known characteristics (the learning set) to find ("learn") a set of relationships connecting the input and output signals.

Fuzzy logic can, however, be combined with neural networks into "adaptive neuro-fuzzy inference systems" (ANFIS; Mathworks Inc.). Here the fuzzy system is further enhanced by taking into account training results from earlier runs using neural networks. Further, fuzzy clustering can assist with rapid pattern recognition.[53]

Combinations of neural networks and fuzzy logic are already seen in everyday household appliances such as baking ovens, washing machines, and vacuum cleaners. For example, for a smart washing machine (AEG Hausgeräte GmbH), measured values from four sensors are fed to a neural network in the form of an integrated circuit chip, which then derived the amount of water needed for the wash. The output from the neural net is fed to a fuzzy logic controller for the water flow control.[54]

Future applications for sensors combined with neural networks, fuzzy logic, and actuators are foreseen in home automation including heating, climatization, and a wider range of household appliances. This large market would result in a wider acceptance and reduced production costs of both sensors and associated supporting and enhancing software. Applications in intensive care systems and a wider range of industrial applications are expected.

1.3.3.4 Sensors and Actuators

A sensor is a device used to detect, locate, or quantify energy or matter, giving a signal for the detection of a physical or chemical property to which the device responds.

An actuator is a device which effects changes in physical or chemical properties in response to a signal. Actuators can, for example, be designed to operate a mechanical switch or valve in response to an electrical signal.

Sensors and actuators transduce between the signal domains Electrical, Optical, Thermal, Magnetic, Mechanical, and Chemical. For example, the glucose biosensor transduces from the chemical to the electrical domain, whereas the coulometric titrator is an actuator transducing in the opposite direction. A more familiar sensor/actuator pair are the photodiode and the LED indicator, transducing from the optical to the electrical domain and vice versa.

Actuators as well as sensors have benefitted from miniaturization, which is essential in medical applications such as portable drug administration systems. Miniaturized actuators are also used as part of sensors, for example in autocalibration.

Sensors and actuators together form the group of transducers. A term for sensors combined with displays, interfaces, etc. is transmitters, and this is encountered particularly with temperature and pressure sensors in the commercial literature.

1.3.3.5 Neural Networks

Prior to their application in electronic noses (see Section 3.2 above and Chapter 27), neural networks have been applied to image recognition and to forecasting on the basis of data collected earlier, with some favorite applications, for example, in playing the stock market or the timing of commodity purchasing.

Neural networks are particularly useful through their ability to "learn" from examples and subsequently to recognize and classify previously unknown patterns. Neural networks are effective mathematical instruments for the simultaneous modeling of a large number of parameters that are connected by nonlinear interactions. Neural networks are on the market in the form of both neurocomputers and software for standard computers (for example, by Siemens-Nixdorf).

In combination with sensors, neural networks are not only used to interpret multisensor signals to find derived variables, as in the case of the electronic nose (Chapter 27), or in the case of multi-inhibition biosensor arrays for pollutants.[55] They are also used to make predictions on the basis of sensor outputs, as in forecasting the breakdown of machine parts in time for preventive maintenance. It is not difficult to see how this function can be applied in medicine, for example, in intensive care.

Advanced software systems such as neural networks and fuzzy logic controllers play an increasing role both as part of an individual sensor and as part of systems for monitoring and control (Figure 1.10).

1.4 DEVELOPMENT PATTERNS

1.4.1 Stages in the Development of an Instrument

Three decades after development of the first biosensor, a growing number of commercial instruments based on biosensors have become available to doctors and to the patients themselves, providing a considerable improvement in the management of diabetes, for example. The application of biosensors in the monitoring and control of food-processing operations and in environmental protection has also been demonstrated. A market value of $10 billion has been estimated for commercial biosensors worldwide.[56] Yet, both researchers and potential users are sometimes disappointed when surveying the range of fully commercialized instruments, which compared with the flood of publications in the biosensors field, seems a mere trickle.

Years of research and development, however, lie between the laboratory prototype and production of a commercial instrument that will be successful through reliability, user-friendliness, compactness, and cost-effectiveness. At the beginning of a development programme, the performance and cost of the final instrument can rarely be predicted with absolute certainty. This means that it is difficult to definitively predict for which applications the instrument will be competitive and predictions for the achievable market volume will need to be adjusted in the course of the development programme. For a high probability of commercial success, therefore, an investor may need to support a portfolio of projects through months of R & D programmes before development can be focused onto the most promising approach.

Such hurdles have also played a role in other emerging and rapidly expanding technologies and generally result in a pyramidal pattern with a rich diversity of approaches being explored at the fundamental research level; from these a proportion is chosen to form the middle section of the pyramid where a wide range of approaches is followed up in more detail with potential applications in mind, and eventually in the top section of the pyramid there is a small but important range of mature commercial devices, often with considerable impact on wealth, health, and/or lifestyle.

The path through these development stages of a new technology is smoothed by the effective use of resources, and this depends on an informed interdisciplinary dialogue between the potential users and the developers, with an awareness of each other's needs, framework conditions, and limitations.

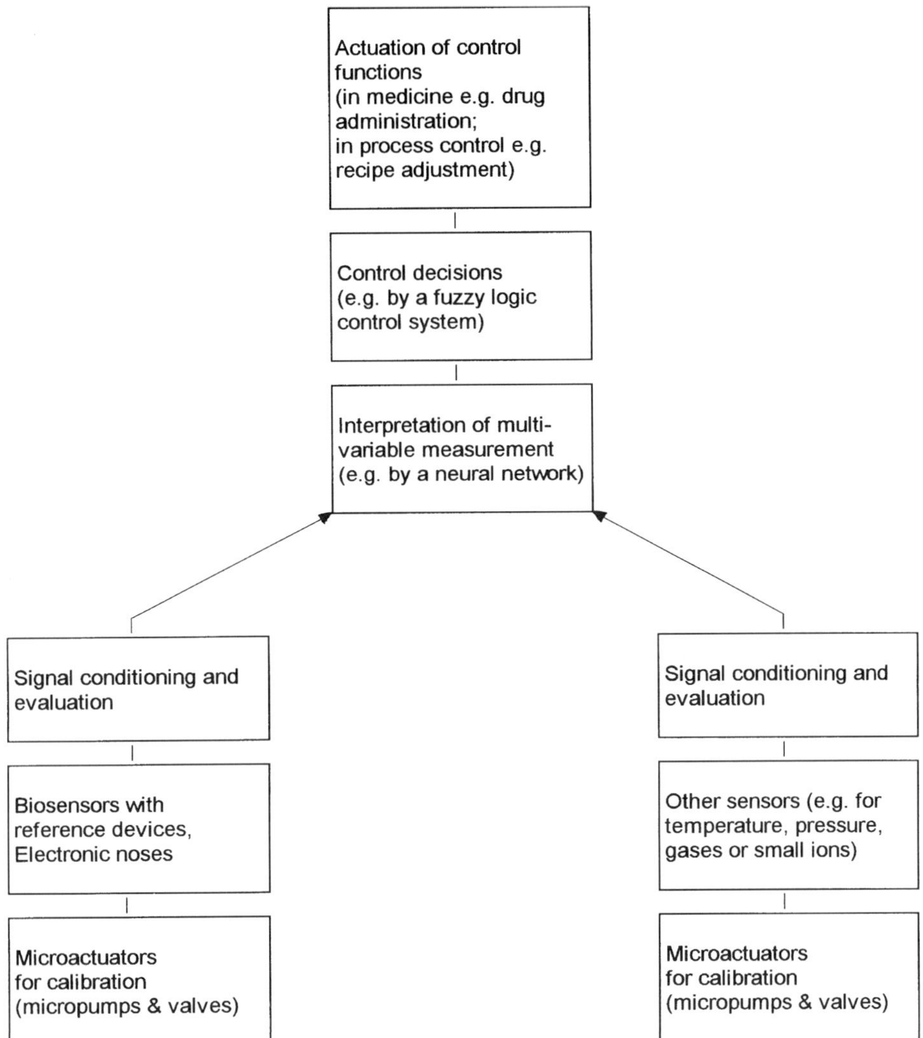

FIGURE 1.10 Building blocks for monitoring and control, combining sensors, actuators, and software. (Note: For electronic noses, signal evaluation in the form of pattern analysis, for example by a neural network, would already be included.)

A possible scheme for the development stages leading to a commercial instrument is shown in Figure 1.11. The initial concept is formed on the basis of a broad overview on sensing needs in a particular sector and on sensing technologies available and emerging. Wide-ranging studies and discussions with instrument users and instrument developers are important at this formative stage. In the later phases, experts in the sensing and application sector technologies involved will be drawn into the project. In the final stages, the input from business managers and financial and marketing advisers will increase.

1.4.2 Market Surveys

Frequently, there will be a demand from financial backers for market surveys and cost-benefit analyses even in the earlier phases of development and/or research. At this stage, estimates for the performance and cost of the instrument to be developed, or even the length and complexity of the development project, can only be regarded as a working premise to be adjusted later. This uncertainty will result in uncertainty about the instrument's applications

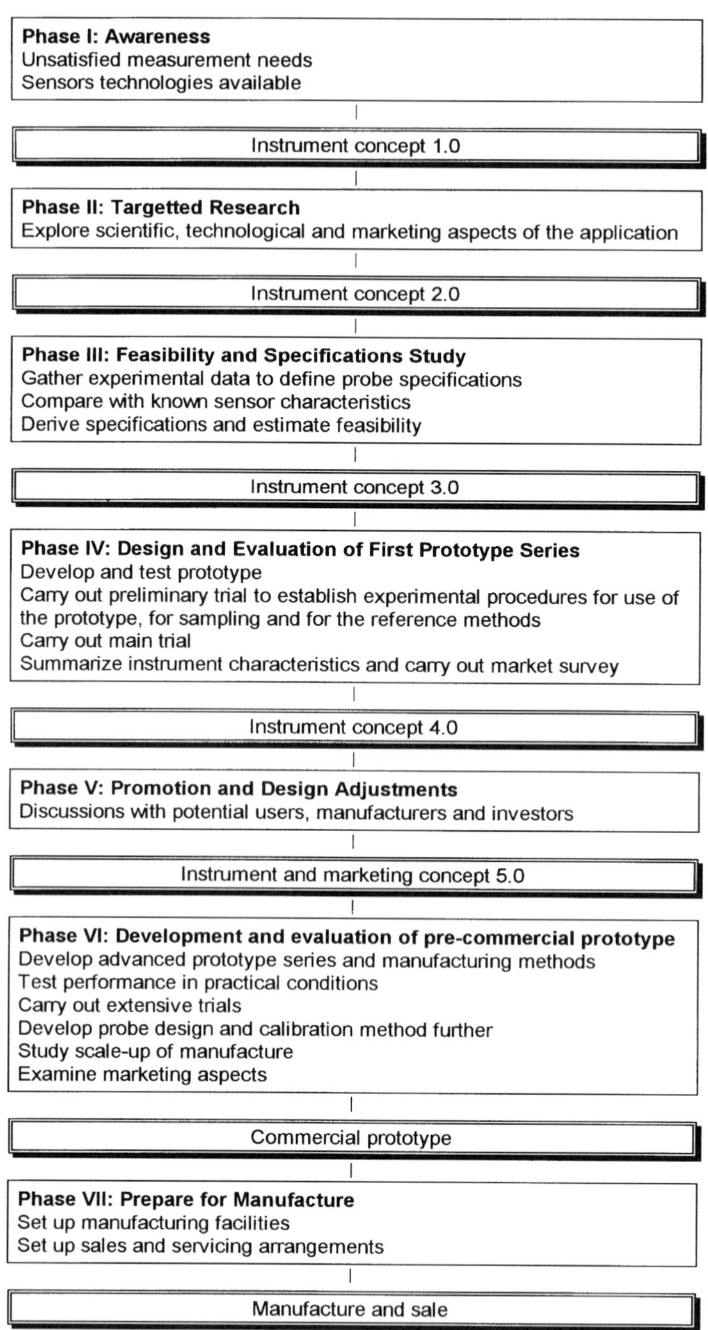

FIGURE 1.11 Possible stages in the development of a commercial instrument. The development of the laboratory prototype is only the first stage of a long process involving many disciplines of science and technology as well as business development analysis.

and about the group of potential users. There will thus be a certain latitude in the approach to a market survey. The chosen approach will, however, have a considerable impact on the result.

As an example, let's say you have developed a multisaccharide biosensor array. You have filed the patents, and now you are looking into the commercial potential. (Or, alternatively, you would like to see the development of a saccharide sensor to satisfy your measurement needs.) Fructose together with sucrose and glucose occur in produce and these sugars are an important factor both for the taste of a food product as well as in the browning and flavor development of fried or roasted produce by way of the Maillard reaction. You hear that monitoring and storage conditioning in order to control these sugars has an impact on processing efficiency and product quality, so you are planning to begin with a survey in the food industry. But to whom will you submit a questionnaire or interview? And what questions will you ask? What background information will you supply? The outcome of the survey will depend crucially on these choices.

At first glance, the obvious choice for the interviewee group might seem to be the managers of chemical quality control (QC) laboratories in the food industry. To avoid any suggestions of bias, you could just ask them open-ended questions such as which chemical sensors they would find useful, what concentrations would be of interest, what sample types would be relevant, and the cost and time of the current methods.

The advantage of this approach would be the absence of any undue influence in the interview that might result from more specific questions or background information. The disadvantage, on the other hand, would be that a full and thought-out response to such open-ended questions would take more time than most QC managers have available. Consequently, many would not respond at all, some would send in fairly random lists jotted down during the coffee break, a few would find the time to answer the question fully, but you would not necessarily end up with an industry-representative sample of chemical QC managers contributing to the result. Another problem is that every interviewee would be left to define "chemical sensor" according to his/her own best knowledge, and you would have to make a guess at the implied definitions later when interpreting the survey results.

In examining your results, keeping in mind all the reservations already outlined, you might find that saccharides do not figure highly on the list of analytes for which chemical sensors are wanted by the chemical QC managers. From the follow-up questions, you might gather that your interviewee is quite happy with the current laboratory instrumentation for sugars including, for example, the Dionex Ion Chromatograph or the enzyme-electrode-based Yellowsprings Analyzer.

You might well have received a different survey response if you had posed the same question to production managers or to managers responsible for total quality management (TQM). Instruments for the on-line or at-line (Figure 8a) determination of sugars are available, but are far less specific, far less sensitive, and are restricted in their application. It is, of course, possible to take samples periodically and carry them to the QC laboratory; however, firstly there will be a delay in obtaining the result. If the assay value turns out to be unfavorable, correction of the processing conditions may come too late for the tons of product that may have already passed through the line between the time of sampling and getting the result. Secondly, the samples taken will form only a tiny fraction of the product that has passed the line, and it may not be possible to ensure that the samples are representative of the product segment concerned.

If, for example, the measured component in the product flow varies by +/-5% with time, then a laboratory method with accuracy to 0.5% on samples taken every half hour may well be less accurate in assessing the component concentration in the product than a continuous on-line method with accuracy to 3%. If the product flow is sampled every half hour and the result of the laboratory assay becomes available half an hour after sampling, then the concentration may already have drifted away from the target value for one hour before corrective action is taken. If the component concentration in the product flow can drift by 10% within an hour, then an on-line method with 3% error is much more effective in controlling the relevant concentration in the product flow than a laboratory method of whatever precision (Table 1.2).

For the production manager then, an instrument that can sample the product flow continuously, or at least frequently, and give a rapid feedback of the results, is desirable even if

TABLE 1.2
On-Line Measurement

Disadvantages
Variable, non-optimum environment:
Reduced accuracy
Calibration and maintenance effort
May need to measure related variable
Advantages
Continuous and direct:
Shows time-dependent variation
Avoids sampling during nonrepresentative time interval — results representative for product flow
Rapid feedback — rapid correction — reduced product losses
Feed-forward possible with upstream measurement of precursor variables
Reduced labor cost

Note: Although this table is compiled for industrial process control, equivalent tables can be drawn up for in *vivo* monitoring during surgery or for the environmental monitoring of rivers, for example.

the accuracy under production line conditions is not as good as that of the corresponding laboratory instrument in a controlled environment. The situation is less critical for batch production, but here also, rapid results are valuable and can save a batch from having to be reworked or discarded.

Similar considerations on the assessment of instrument accuracy would apply in clinical applications where continuous monitoring during surgery with 1% accuracy of a metabolite in the patient's bloodstream may be more helpful than a laboratory assay with 0.1% accuracy. Not only does the laboratory result become available with a delay and the analytical value may no longer apply when it is received, but the *in vivo* value may actually change periodically and sampling at a particular time may be quite unrepresentative of the average value.

In environmental protection, too, a continuous monitoring system, even if less precise than the laboratory assay, can be invaluable in raising the alarm when a river is subject to pollution from a defective filter in an inflow pipe, for example.

1.4.3 Measurement Situations and Motivations

Biosensors are of interest not only for continuous monitoring but also for spot-check field applications in agriculture or environmental protection. For health applications, they are relevant not only to *in vivo* monitoring, but also to point-of-care measurements as, for example, with the ExacTech glucose analyzer (see Chapters 10 and 11).

Some food products depend largely on the properties of one principal ingredient for their quality. This is the case, for example, for tomato paste or ketchup, where the color, sweetness, and nonsoluble solids content of the fruit are crucial. Similarly, for fried potato or yam (sweet potato) products, the saccharide content and distribution within the tuber are important for browning and flavor development. For such food products, total quality management includes harvest, storage supervision and conditioning, control of the main ingredient, and can go right back to breeding programmes to obtain the best variety of the fruit or vegetable. There is much scope for measurements in the field and in storage areas for breeding efficiency or optimum quality assurance here. Portable, simple-to-use instrumentation is needed for these applications.

One step further towards processing is the quality control on purchase or delivery of ingredients. The negotation of commodity prices and the decision on the usability of an ingredient for a particular product line will depend on this assessment. Again, portability and simplicity are relevant here.

The motivation for continuous monitoring or frequent measurements is high whenever the measured component changes as a function of several parameters and cannot be predicted quantitatively. This occurs particularly during processing, for example: sucrose conversion to glucose, conversion of saccharides into alcohols or lactate, cooking processes involving protein denaturation, and aroma development. However, the composition of food ingredients and products can change at all stages of production.

Ripening, conditioning, intended fermentation, or spoilage of ingredients due to chemical interaction, bacterial, or fungal activity or due to physical migration can take place before the ingredients are processed. Similar changes can take place in the products after leaving the processing line. Control of these changes takes place at several levels. Ripening and conditioning changes are influenced by external factors such as temperature and ambient gas composition as well as by variety. These factors can be adjusted in response to a sensor measurement indicating the condition of interest.

In the important area of food safety, biosensors, gas sensors, and electronic noses can be applied either in monitoring factors influencing spoilage or in monitoring factors indicating spoilage. For example, solutes such as the traditional preserving agents sugar and salt will be a factor in determining the "water activity" (availability of water to microbial activity or chemical reactions). Together with the pH value and preserving additives such as nitrite, the water activity[57] is important for the stability of foods, cosmetics, and other perishable materials. Certain solutes in certain foods can also be indicators of the freshness or spoilage status. Similarly, ambient gas composition has an influence on spoilage and headspace gases or volatiles can indicate conditions such as microbial spoilage or oxidative rancidity. Improvements in stability towards spoilage and ultrarapid freshness testing are thus possible. Both these sensor functions make an important contribution to quality assurance concepts such as HACCP (Table 1.3).

The definition of food freshness and the perceived sensing needs are country dependent. Thus in countries where fish is eaten cooked, trimethylamine concentration can be used as an indicator, whereas compounds such as hypoxanthine and inosine would be looked at in assessing fish sold for raw consumption. Spoilage indicators also depend on source and storage conditions.

Temperature and humidity determine not only the quantitative growth of microbes in food, but also the nature and the type of metabolic activity of the microbial flora. Large fish trawled in tropical waters, for example, will retain a warm body temperature for a time before chilling becomes effective in the center portion of the fish, and this will affect the rates of microbial histamine production (in dark-fleshed fish) and of proteolytic changes. A rapid method using amine oxidase with an oxygen probe is described in Reference 58.

For the elimination of the most serious health risks it is necessary to detect specific pathogens in food. Immunoassay kits are in use for the specific detection of *Salmonella*, for example, and the construction of immunosensors is under investigation. Immunoassays and immunosensors are also of interest in the detection of bacterial and fungal toxins. Although molds can be identified and counted with conventional methods, this can be a considerable strain on the eyes of the evaluator, providing grounds for the development of immunoassay techniques to replace, for example, the tedious Howard mold count in tomato products.

Microbial contamination needs to be detected not just in the food itself but also on surfaces that come into contact with foods. The effectiveness of cleaning cycles, particularly in aseptic processing lines, needs to be monitored. Although in many food products the growth of pathogenic microbes is prevented by a low water activity and a low pH, there is still the need to avoid any contamination as the very young and the very old among the consumers are susceptible to even a very small number of pathogenic bacteria.

TABLE 1.3
Quality Assurance and Quality Control in the Food Industry

Chemical and Microbial Properties

Measurements for product quality
- Aroma, taste
- Nutritional value
- Functional properties
- Compliance with specifications

Screening for product safety
- Chemical contamination
  - Residues, toxins, taints
- Microbial contamination
  - Total load, pathogens, indicators of activity

Assessing product stability towards
- Chemical reactions and microbial growth:
  - Water activity, solute concentration, pH value, and preservative concentration
  - Local and volume-averaged values
  - Protective atmosphere composition
- Migration
  - Water activity gradient, solute concentration gradient

Process Management

Objectives
- Safety and continuity
- Compliance with product specifications
- Efficient use of resources
- Environmental protection

Established measurements
- Pressure, temperature, and pH value
- Volume and mass flow rates, fill level, density and weight
- Viscosity

Additional measurements wanted
- Chemical composition (gross and fine)
- Complex rheology and flow patterns
- Microsizing
- Volatiles (cooking, baking, roasting, drying)

HACCP — Hazard Analysis Critical Control Points

On-line measurement
- Pressure, temperature, local temperature-time integral $\int T(x,y,z)\,dt$
- Relative humidity (RH)
- pH value
- Solute concentration (related to the ERH or water activity)
- Cleaning solutions monitoring, strength and coverage

Off-line measurement
- Equilibrium relative humidity (ERH) (water activity)
- pH value
- Preservative concentration
- Microbial contamination of ingredients
- Microbial contamination of surfaces

Total quality management goes back to the farm and controls the rearing conditions that determine the presence of *Salmonella* in poultry, for example, and the cautious use of substances that could persist as agricultural residues, for example, antibiotics or hormones in meat, or pesticides in produce. The detection of residues is also a requirement in the quality control of ingredients on delivery.

Much of the discussion in this section is based on experience gained in the food industry. However, many of the considerations here have their equivalents in applications of biosensors and electronic noses in other areas, particularly in the medical, environmental, and biotechnology sector (Parts III and IV of this book). For an ultimately successful sensor development, the significance of a target analyte for the condition to be assessed or the process to be controlled needs to be examined. A comparison with potential alternatives should be made considering not only other methods for the determination of the same analyte, but also methods for the measurement of other variables indicative of the condition to be assessed or of the process to be controlled. Operating conditions specific to the intended application need to be taken into account and sensor optimization for this environment by means of, e.g., membrane technology, FIA, or software techniques would be investigated. On this basis, the viability of an envisaged sensor development can be examined (Table 1.4).

TABLE 1.4
Viability of Sensor Development

- Market volume of application sector
- Increase in market volume of application sector
- Price margins in the application sector

- Health and safety relevance of measurement
- Implications of measurement for legal or customer specifications
- Relevance to concepts such as total quality management (TQM) and good manufacturing practice (GMP)
- Relevance to national and international standards
- Support of quality assurance schemes

- Variability of samples within the application sector
- Harshness of the measurement environment
- Optimization of sensor performance through:
    - Choice and tailoring of the sensing layer
    - Membrane technology
    - Flow injection analysis
    - Multisensor systems
    - Software for calibration, interference compensation, and signal interpretation

1.4.4 Concluding Remarks

Where a biosensor offers advantages over existing laboratory instrumentation for the same analyte in terms of specificity, sensitivity, or rapidity, simplicity and savings in the cost of reagents and skilled labor (when applied in real samples), the framework for the commercial development of an instrument is comparatively straightforward. Where the biosensors measure an alternative variable that is thought to be equivalent, superior, or unique as an indicator for the condition of interest, there may be a need for additional research to prove that this equivalence holds for all samples of interest. There will also be obstacles in terms of overcoming traditional approaches and in adapting legislation.

Where the development of a particular biosensor for laboratory use would not be justified in itself, but the on-line, *in situ*, in-field, or point-of-care application would offer advantages compared with the sole application of laboratory instrumentation, the examination of development viability becomes more complex. It is no longer a comparison of novel sensor performance to conventional instrumentation in like conditions, but of benefits resulting from the direct and rapid application. One will also have to look at alternative on-line or field methods that have been or could be developed to compete with the biosensor in question (see Section 1.3.1 above).

Some caution is needed when comparing biosensor measurements with laboratory reference measurements. If the laboratory assay is based on homogenized samples, it is liable to differ systematically from a biosensor measurement which samples the concentration of a solute in a liquid, ignoring the presence of nonsoluble solids. Also a laboratory assay based on taking small samples infrequently may well not be representative for the time and volume average.

A biosensor should not necessarily be chosen as a replacement for a laboratory assay for the same analyte. The assay may have been chosen as the best alternative to an unavailable assay for a complex condition to be assessed. It pays, therefore, to look at the condition to be determined and then decide on the best variable to be measured. It may turn out that a set of laboratory assays can be replaced with a single summary variable such as BOD (biological oxygen demand) for waste waters that can be measured with a biosensor.

Conversely, the best replacement for a laboratory assay measuring the sum of reducing sugars in the prediction of Maillard browning may be a biosensor array measuring a set of individual saccharides, thus providing both a value for reducing sugars and also additional information. On the other hand, it may be found that just one of the saccharides needs to be measured for the intended application because its concentration correlates adequately with the Maillard browning potential for the produce in question.

Biosensors offer the potential of depth-profiling of concentration distributions in a semi-solid sample with a single measurement step by using multisensor arrays with several biosensors for the same analyte spread over a few millimeters. Such a depth profile can provide information on solute migration processes which in turn give information on properties such as diffusivity or on the activity of microbes or chemical processes at the sample surface. Depth-profiling probes can be configured as hand-held knife-type probes (Figure 1.12). Not only are they more convenient and rapid than slicing a sample and subsequently analyzing each slice, they can also be highly superior in accuracy to a laboratory assay performed on a thin sliver containing a minute amount of analyte.

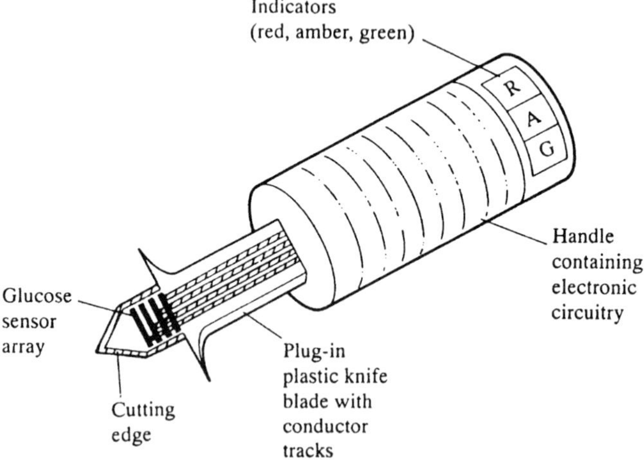

FIGURE 1.12 A possible configuration for a hand-held amperometric mediated enzyme biosensor array for analyte depth profiling, as developed in the collaboration between Leatherhead Food RA and Cranfield Biotechnology Centre (see Reference 60). The possibility of depth profiling with a single *in situ* measurement obviates the high labor costs associated with the preparation and assay of fine sample slivers for the assembly of a depth profile needed with laboratory assay methods. (From Kress-Rogers, E., *Instrumentation and Sensors for the Food Industry,* Butterworth-Heinemann, Boston, 1993, chap 16. With permission.)

REFERENCES

Note: For more references on individual biosensor designs, please see the reference lists of the following handbook chapters.

1. Updike, S. J. and Hicks, G. P., The enzyme electrode, *Nature,* 214, 986, 1967.
2. Arnold, M. A. and Meyerhoff, M. E., Recent advances in the development and analytical applications of biosensing probes, *CRC Crit. Rev. Anal. Chem.*, 20, 149, 1988.
3. Anon., BOD determination in minutes, *Lab News,* 95 (March), 26, 1995.
4. Anon., Lange's biosensor, *Brew. Guard.*, 95 (Jan.), 33, 1995.
5. Bsat, N., Wiedemann, M., Czajka, J., Barany, F., Piani, M., and Batt, C. A., Food safety applications of nucleic acid-based assays, *Food Technol.*, 48 (June) 142, 1994.
6. Mizutani F. and Yabuki, S., FIA for glucose using an amperometric enzyme electrode based on a lipid-modified glucose oxidase as the detector, *Biosens. Bioelectron.,* 9, 411, 1994.
7. Qu, H.-B., Zhang, X.-E., and Zhang, S.-Z., Simultaneous determination of maltose and glucose using a dual-electrode flow injection system, *Food Chem.,* 52, 187, 1995.
8. Schoemaker, M., Grundig, B., and Spener, F., Amperometric enzyme sensor for essential fatty acids, in *Biosensors 94*, Turner, A. P. F., Karube, I., Heineman, W. R., and Scheller, F., Eds., Elsevier, Oxford, 1994.
9. Park, J.-K., Shin, M.-C., Lee, S.-G., and Kim, H.-S., FIA of glucose, fructose and sucrose using a biosensor constructed with permeabilized Zymomonas mobilis and invertase, *Biotechnol. Prog.*, 11, 58, 1995.
10. Meier, H. and Tran-Minh, C., Biosensor for on-line monitoring of penicillin during its production by fermentation, in *Automatic Control of Food and Biological Processes. Proc. ACoFoP 3 Symposium Paris, Oct. 94*, Bimbinet, J. J., Dumoulin, E., and Trystram, G., Eds., Elsevier, Amsterdam, 1994, p. 83.
11. Turner, A. P. F., Applications of direct electron transfer bioelectrochemistry in sensors and fuel cells, *Biotech 83*, Online Publications, Northwood, U.K., 1983.
12. Cass, A. E .G., David, G., Francis, G. D., Hill, H. A. O., Aston, W. J., Higgins, I. J., Plotkin, E. V., Scott, L. D. L., and Turner, A. P. F., Ferrocene-mediated enzyme electrode for amperometric determination of glucose, *Anal. Chem.,* 56, 671, 1984.
13. MacDonnell, M. B. and Vadgama, P., Membrane: separation principles and sensing, *Sel. Electrodes Rev.,* 11, 17, 1989.
14. Bergveld, P., Development and application of an ion-sensitive solid-state device for neurophysical measurements, *Trans. Biomed. Eng.*, BME-14, 70-71, 1970
15. Roseiro, L. C., Santos, C., Almeida, J., and Melo, R. S., Measurements of pH-60 in pork using ISFET/REFET and glass electrode methods, *Meat Sci.*, 38, 347, 1994
16. Kress-Rogers, E., Chemosensors, biosensors and immunosensors, in *Instrumentation and Sensors for the Food Industry*, Kress-Rogers, E., Ed., Butterworth-Heinemann, Boston, 1993, chap. 17.
17. Anon., IFT '94 - Food Expo in print. Sentron 3001 pH system, *Food Technol.*, (August), 195, 1994.
18. Anon., Non-glass pH technology, *Food Trade Rev.*, 64, 705, 1994.
19. Sevilla, F., Kullick, T., and Scheper, T., A bio-FET sensor for lactose based on co-immobilized beta-galactosidase/glucose dehydrogenase, *Biosens. Bioelectron.*, 9, 275, 1994.
20. Bergveld, P., The intimate relationship between ISFETs and proteins, both theoretically and in practice, in *Biosensors 94*, Turner, A. P. F., Karube, I., Heineman, W. R., and Scheller, F., Eds., Elsevier, Oxford, 1994.
21. Van der Schoot, B. H. and Bergveld, P., Coulometric sensors, the applications of a sensor-actuator system for long-term stability in chemical sensing, *Sensors Actuators,* 13, 251, 1988.
22. Kress-Rogers, E., Chemosensors, biosensors and immunosensors, in *Instrumentation and Sensors for the Food Industry*, Kress-Rogers, E., Ed., Butterworth-Heinemann, Boston, 1993, chap. 17.
23. Mosbach, K. and Danielsson, B., An enzyme thermistor. *Biochim. Biophys. Acta,* 364, 140, 1974.

24. Muehlbauer, M. J., Guilbeau, E. J., and Towe, B. C., Applications and stability of a thermoelectric enzyme sensor, *Sensors Actuators,* B2, 223, 1990.
25. Nieveld, G. K., Thermopiles fabricated using silicon planar technology. *Sensors Actuators,* 3, 179, 1983.
26. Muehlbauer, M. J., Guilbeau, E. J., Towe, B. C., and Brandon, T. A., Thermoelectric enzyme sensor for measuring blood glucose, *Biosens. Bioelectron.* 5, 1, 1990.
27. Bin, Xie, Danielsson, B., Norberg, P., Winquist, F., and Lundström, I., Development of a thermal microbiosensor fabricated on a silicon chip, *Sensors Actuators,* B6, 127, 1992.
28. Bin, Xie, Hedberg, U., Mecklenburg, M., and Danielsson, B., Fast determination of whole blood glucose with a calorimetric microbiosensor, *Sensors Actuators,* B15-16, 141, 1993.
29. Shimohigoshi, M., Yokoyama, K., and Karube I., Development of a biothermochip and its application for the detection of glucose in urine, *Anal. Chim. Acta,* 303, 295, 1995.
30. Wolfbeis, O. S., *Fiber Optic Chemical Sensors and Biosensors,* Vols. I and II, CRC Press, Boca Raton, FL, 1991.
31. Arnold, M. A., Fibre-optic biosensors, *J. Biotechnol.,* 15, 219, 1990.
32. Blum, L. J., Gautier, S. M., and Coulet, P. R., Fiber-optic biosensors based on luminometric detection, in *Food Biosensor Analysis,* Wagner, G. and Guilbault, G. G., Eds., Marcel Dekker, New York, 1994, p. 101.
33. Lee, S.-J., Saleemuddin, M., Scheper, T., Loos, H., and Sahm, H., A fluorometric fiber-optic biosensor for dual analysis of glucose and fructose., *J. Biotechnol.,* 36, 39, 1994.
34. Sritongkham, P., Taravanit, N., Suwannakum, T., Tanticharoen, M., and Kirtikara, K., Piezoelectric crystal biosensor for the determination of organophosphorus pesticide, in *Biosensors 94,* Turner, A. P. F., Karube, I., Heineman, W. R., and Scheller, F., Eds., Elsevier, Oxford, 1994.
35. Osinkin, Y. A., Baranov, V. V., and Plate, N. A., Bifunctional polymeric reagents based on cholinesterases as piezoelectric crystal coating for detection of organophosphorous compounds, in *Biosensors 94,* Turner, A. P. F., Karube, I., Heineman, W. R., and Scheller, F., Eds., Elsevier, Oxford, 1994.
36. Denbow, N., Ultrasonic instrumentation in the food industry, in *Instrumentation and Sensors for the Food Industry,* Kress-Rogers, E., Ed., Butterworth-Heinemann, Boston, 1993, chap. 9.
37. Kress-Rogers, E., Ultrasound propagation in foods and ambient gases, principles and applications, in *Instrumentation and Sensors for the Food Industry,* Kress-Rogers, E., Ed., Butterworth-Heinemann, Oxford, Boston, 1993, chap. 8.
38. Bier, F. F. and Schmid, R. D., Real-time analysis of competitive binding using grating coupler immunosensors for pesticide detection. *Biosens. Bioelectron.,* 9, 125, 1994.
39. De Vries, E. F. A., Schasfoort, R. B. M., Van der Plas, J., and Greve, J., Development of latex-technology for specific DNA detection with surface plasmon resonance, in *Biosensors 94,* Turner, A. P. F., Karube, I., Heineman, W. R., and Scheller, F., Eds., Elsevier, Oxford, 1994.
40. Kumar, P., Colston, J. T., and Chambers, J. P., Detection of botulinum toxin using an evanescent wave immunosensor, *Biosens. Bioelectron.,* 9, 57, 1994.
41. Heideman, R. G., Kooyman, R. P. H., and Greve, J., Development of an optical waveguide interferometric immunosensor, *Sensors Actuators,* B4, 297, 1991.
42. Brown, C. W., Lin, J., and Chen, C.-S., Novel fiber optic evanescent wave sensor for pollutants and food contaminants, in *Biosensors 94,* Turner, A. P. F., Karube, I., Heineman, W. R., and Scheller, F., Eds., Elsevier, Oxford, 1994.
43. Grate, J. W., Martin, S. J., and White, R. M., Acoustic wave microsensors, *Anal. Chem.,* 65, 940A, 1993.
44. Yokoyama, K., Ikebukuro, K., Yano, K., Karube, I., and Arikawa, Y., Quartz crystal immunosensors for multisample detection of herbicides, in *Biosensors 94,* Turner, A. P. F., Karube, I., Heineman, W. R., and Scheller, F., Eds., Elsevier, Oxford, 1994.
45. Iiyama, S., Toko, K., Matsuno, T., and Yamafuji, K., Responses of lipid membranes of taste sensor to astringent and pungent substances, *Chem. Senses,* 19, 87, 1994.
46. Benson, I. B., Compositional analysis using near infrared absorption spectroscopy, in *Instrumentation and Sensors for the Food Industry,* Kress-Rogers, E., Ed., Butterworth-Heinemann, Boston, 1993, chap. 5.
47. Kent, M., Microwave measurements of product variables, in *Instrumentation and Sensors for the Food Industry,* Kress-Rogers, E., Ed., Butterworth-Heinemann, Boston, 1993, chap. 7.

48. Künnecke, W., Mohns, J., Rohm, I., and Bilitewski, U., Development of screen-printed biosensors for process monitoring, in *Biosensors 94*, Turner, A. P. F., Karube, I., Heineman, W. R., and Scheller, F., Eds., Elsevier, Oxford, 1994.
49. Yee, H.-J. and Park, J.-K., Gas-phase biosensors for the determination of ethanol vapor, in *Biosensors 94*, Turner, A. P. F., Karube, I., Heineman, W. R., and Scheller, F., Eds., Elsevier, Oxford, 1994.
50. Yamauchi, S., *Chemical Sensor Technology*, Vol. 4, Elsevier Science,, Amsterdam, 1992.
51. Berrie, P. G., Fuzzy-logic in ultrasonic fill measurement, *Alimenta,* 33, 21, 1994.
52. Mahjoub, M., Mosrati, R., Lamotte, M., Fonteix, C., and Marc I., Fuzzy control of baker's yeast fed-batch bioprocess: a robustness study, *Food Res. Int.*, 27, 145, 1994.
53. Anon., VDI-Nachrichten, 24 March 95, page 19.
54. Anon., VDI Nachrichten, 14 April 95, page 14.
55. Cowell, D. C., Dowman, A. A., Ashcroft, T., and Caffoor, I., The detection and identification of metal and organic pollutants in potable water using enzyme based sensors, in *Biosensors 94*, Turner, A. P. F., Karube, I., Heineman, W. R., and Scheller, F., Eds., Elsevier, Oxford, 1994.
56. Anon., VDI-Nachrichten, 20 Jan. 95.
57. Rödel, W., Water activity and its measurement in food, in *Instrumentation and Sensors for the Food Industry*, Kress-Rogers, E., Ed., Butterworth-Heinemann, Boston, 1993, chap. 12.
58. Ohashi, M., Nomura, F., Suzuk, M., Otsuka, M., Adachi, O., and Arakawa, N., Oxygen-sensor-based simple assay of histamine in fish using purified amine oxidase, *J. Food Sci.*, 59, 519-522, 1994.
59. Kress-Rogers, E., Instrumentation for food quality assurance, in *Instrumentation and Sensors for the Food Industry*, Kress-Rogers, E., Ed., Butterworth-Heinemann, 1993, Boston, chap. 1.
60. Kress-Rogers, E., The marker concept: frying oil monitor and meat freshness sensor, in *Instrumentation and Sensors for the Food Industry*, Kress-Rogers, E., Ed., Butterworth-Heinemann, Boston, 1993, chap. 16.

Part II

Receptors, Membranes, and Devices for Biosensors

2 Enzymes, Cofactors, and Mediators

Stephen F. White and Anthony P. F. Turner

CONTENTS

2.1 INTRODUCTION

One glance at the complex and intricate interactions that often go to make up even the simplest of metabolic pathways (frequently displayed on wall charts and adorning the walls of biochemistry departments) will graphically demonstrate the influence of enzymes on cellular processes. Enzymes are the cell's catalysts that permit a vast number and range of reactions to be carried out rapidly under mild conditions of constant temperature, pH, and pressure. One major characteristic of enzyme operation concerns the specific and selective nature of the reactions enhanced by their presence. At one extreme, many enzymes can only react with one of a pair of optical isomers, i.e., lactate dehydrogenase will catalyse (–) lactic acid to pyruvic acid, but is unreactive towards (+) lactic acid. In contrast, less-specific enzymes will react with a group of similar compounds, i.e., alcohol dehydrogenase can catalyze the oxidation of ethanol, methanol, 1-propanol, and 1-butanol.

All enzymes are composed of protein. Furthermore, many enzymes require a nonprotein component to combine with an otherwise inactive protein to produce a catalytically active complex. These nonprotein components are termed cofactors (more about cofactors in Section 2.3).

It is the individual or group specificity of enzymes that has been exploited and adapted for use in a range of analytical applications, including biosensors. One of the best examples of how enzymes can be used in an analytical role is illustrated by the widely used colourimetric "dipsticks". Generally, these are produced by impregnating filter paper with an appropriate

0-8493-8905-4/97/$0.00+$.50
© 1997 by CRC Press, Inc.

enzyme (determined by the analyte of interest) and a chromogen. Addition of a sample containing the substrate of interest will induce a colour change in the test strip. Comparing the colour with a standard chart will indicate the approximate concentration of analyte in the sample solution. A range of analytes, particularly in the clinical field, can be monitored using this method,[1] e.g., glucose and urea. A further development based on this was to substitute an artificial electron acceptor, such as hexacyanoferrate, for the chromogen to give an electrochemical method of detection.

Finally, in the field of biosensor research and development, another particular relationship between an enzyme and nonprotein component has been investigated and developed, namely, the interaction with mediators. These compounds facilitate the passage of electric charge between the enzyme and electrode (for enzymes belonging to a class known as oxidoreductases), hence providing a means of monitoring a desired analyte. This has formed the basis for the launch of a number of commercially available sensors, e.g., glucose sensors from Medisense and Kyoto Dauchi.

This chapter will give a brief overview of enzymes, cofactors, and mediators in relation to their role as components of biosensors. For a more extensive coverage the reader is referred to other general biochemistry publications (e.g., *Biochemistry*[2]) for details of enzymes and cofactors and texts such as *Biosensors: Fundamentals and Applications*[3] for further information on mediators.

2.2 ENZYMES

2.2.1 Basic Structure

Although the range and variety of reactions carried out by enzymes is enormous, the basic structure is chemically simple. A sequence of L-amino acids is linked together to form a polypeptide chain. There are 20 different types of amino acids, all of which are based on the same general structure:

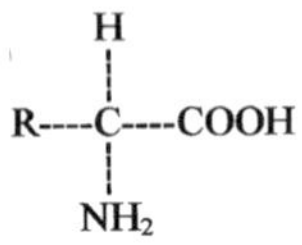

```
      H
      |
R----C----COOH
      |
     NH2
```

FIGURE 2.1 Basic amino acid structure.

Figure 2.1 represents the basic amino acid structure. The letter R denotes the particular side chain that determines the nature of the amino acid. All of the amino acids can be grouped into four categories according to their particular type of R group (see Table 2.1). Briefly, in the first two categories polar (hydrophilic) or nonpolar (hydrophobic) neutral R groups, respectively, are present. These two categories are distinguished by their ability to dissolve in water; the former being more readily soluble. The polar groups can form hydrogen bonds with water; cysteine and tyrosine being the most polar. The other two categories contain either positively charged (basic) groups or negatively charged (acidic) groups. Furthermore, because all the amino acids contain a carbon atom attached to four different groups they are chiral. That is to say (with the exception of glycine) each amino acid has a nonsuperimposable mirror image.

Polypeptide chains are formed via a condensation reaction between the amino acids. A peptide bond links the carboxyl and amino sites of two molecules, until eventually a long polypeptide chain is formed. The potential variation between proteins is enormous, both in the overall length of the chain and choice of amino acid. For example, a polypeptide of only 100 amino acids can be constructed using 1 of 20^{100} possible combinations.

TABLE 2.1
The 20 Naturally Occurring L-Amino Acids[2]

Enzyme name	Type of R group
Aspartic acid	Acidic hydrophilic
Glutamic acid	Acidic hydrophilic
Asparagine	Neutral
Glutamine	Neutral
Methionine	Neutral
Threonine	Neutral
Serine	Neutral
Tyrosine	Weak acid
Cysteine	Neutral
Histidine	Basic
Lysine	Basic
Arginine	Basic
Tryptophan	Basic
Glycine	Nonpolar hydrophobic
Alanine	Nonpolar hydrophobic
Valine	Nonpolar hydrophobic
Leucine	Nonpolar hydrophobic
Isoleucine	Nonpolar hydrophobic
Proline	Nonpolar hydrophobic
Phenylalanine	Nonpolar hydrophobic

The sequence of amino acids that constitute the polymer chain (termed the primary sequence), will also determine the three-dimensional shape of the enzyme. Interactions between the various amino acids result in a complex folding pattern. Generally these interactions involve ionic effects, hydrogen bonding, and hydrophobic bonds between nonpolar R groups. This can result in regions of the polypeptide chain where folding occurs in a regular manner (termed secondary structure). Furthermore, these regular forms are stabilized by weak interactions between the non-side chain components of the amino acids. Typical of this type of structure are the protein α-helix and B-pleated sheet.

The complete three-dimensional shape of the protein is termed the tertiary structure, usually determined by interactions among the R side chains of the constituent polypeptide chains. Finally, the highest order of structure (termed the quaternary structure) is observed when separate macromolecules come together in a specific order to form the final enzyme shape.

The protein conformation is a major determinant of biological activity; a definite three-dimensional shape is essential for the protein to work effectively.

2.2.2 Range and General Classification

The range of reactions catalysed by enzymes can be grouped under six major classifications (see Table 2.2).

Historically, many enzymes were named by adding the suffix "ase" to the substrate of interest. For example, the enzyme urease catalyses the hydrolysis of urea to CO_2 and ammonia. In order to catagorise the naming of enzymes, the Enzyme Commission system for classifying and assigning index numbers to all enzymes was introduced.[4] According to the system, each enzyme is given a recommendation name, a systematic name (describing the reaction it catalyses), and an identification number.

TABLE 2.2
Enzyme Commission Classnames[4]

1. Oxidoreductases (oxidation-reduction reactions).
2. Transferases (transfer of functional groups).
3. Hydrolases (hydrolysis reactions).
4. Lyases (addition to double bonds).
5. Isomerases (isomerization reactions).
6. Ligases (formation of bonds with ATP cleavage).

2.2.3 General Mechanism of Enzyme Reactions

In many cases the enzyme that catalyses a particular reaction is larger than the substrate(s) involved. Therefore, only a fraction of the total enzyme structure can be in contact with the substrate. The portion of the enzyme responsible for catalytic activity is termed the active site. If contact with the substrate is in the area of the active site, catalysis can occur. It is the precise shape of the enzyme's active site, determined by the complex three-dimensional shape of the protein, that initiates catalytic action. Small alterations (i.e., changes in the side chain of an amino acid) in the active site can lead to a complete loss of catalytic ability.

The activity of an enzyme can be described in terms of international units (IU). This is defined as "the amount of enzyme necessary to produce one micromole of product (or the loss of one micromolecule of substrate) per minute under specified conditions of substrate concentration, pH and temperature." The enzyme can be further characterised by its turnover number defined by the net number of substrate molecules reacted per catalyst site per unit time.

Like all catalysts, enzymes operate by lowering the energy of activation, thus increasing the number of substrate molecules capable of entering the transition state, in which the probability of a passage from substrate to product is very high. Generally, for any chemical reaction the concentration of the transition state species is proportional to the rate of reaction. All catalysts, including enzymes, increase the rate but do not change the reaction equilibrium.

2.2.4 Kinetics

Any investigation into the structure and function of an enzyme would certainly include a detailed look at the kinetic parameters that affect its activity. The methods adopted to carry out this investigation are exemplified by the work of Michaelis and Menten. The basis of their approach was that the rate or velocity of catalysis (v) by enzymes varies with the concentration of substrate. Increasing the concentration of substrate for a given reaction will lead to a linear increase in rate, up to a characteristic value. Beyond this point the rate increase declines until eventually it reaches a constant value, irrespective of higher concentration values. A simple model was proposed to define these observations. It was postulated that the enzyme (E) and substrate (S) combined to form a complex ES. The complex dissociates into product (P) and free enzyme.

$$\mathrm{S} + \mathrm{E} \underset{\mathrm{K}_{-1}}{\overset{\mathrm{K}_1}{\rightleftarrows}} \mathrm{ES} \tag{2.1}$$

Equation 2.1 represents the formation of a basic enzyme-substrate complex; where K_1 and K_{-1} are the rate of enzyme-substrate complex formation and dissociation, respectively.

$$ES \xrightarrow{K_2} P + E \tag{2.2}$$

Equation 2.2 represents dissociation of the enzyme-substrate complex to product, where K_2 is the rate of this reaction.

At high concentrations of substrate, all of the enzyme at any given time will be present as ES and hence no more S can be accommodated until some of the ES complex breaks down, hence the rate of reaction will be relatively slow. At this point the maximum velocity (V_{max}) is approached.

Michaelis and Menten derived an equation to describe the dependence of the velocity of reaction to the concentration of substrate:

$$v = \frac{V_{max} \cdot [S]}{K_m + [S]} \tag{2.3}$$

The value of K_m (the Michaelis constant) is defined operationally as that concentration of substrate at which the velocity of the reaction is half the maximum. Generally, using the equation to describe a particular reaction will result in a graph with a hyperbolic profile (Figure 2.2).

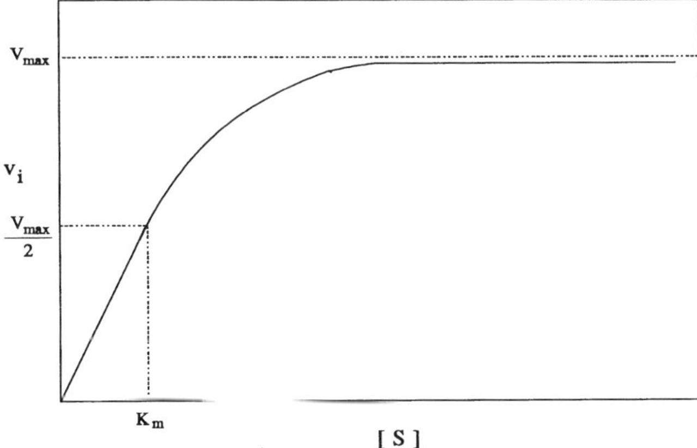

FIGURE 2.2 Plot showing Michaelis-Menton relationship between substrate concentration and initial velocity.

Determining the K_m value for an enzyme can be achieved by carrying out a relatively simple set of experiments, by measuring the initial velocity of the reaction at different substrate concentrations using a fixed amount of enzyme. At low concentrations the initial velocity will be proportional to the substrate value (first order). As the substrate concentration reaches V_{max} the rate will become less and less relative to the increase in substrate concentration, approaching zero order.

The rate of reaction is proportional to the total amount of enzyme present. Furthermore, the Michaelis constant is an indication of the relative affinity of the enzyme for the substrate. A low value for the constant is indicative of a high affinity. For an enzyme that has specificity for a range of similar compounds, the K_m value will differ with the substrate. An example of this is illustrated by alcohol oxidase, where a range of alcohols can be oxidised by the same enzyme.

Substrate	Relative activity (%)
Methanol	100
Ethanol	55.2
Propan-1-ol	20.7
Butan-1-ol	12.1

In addition, the K_m value for an enzyme will be influenced by a range of external influences.

In order to characterise the operating parameters of any enzyme it is necessary to determine the values of V_{max} and K_m by measuring the rate of reaction over a range of concentrations. These values would be difficult to determine, given the hyperbolic nature of the response. By modifying the general form of the Michaelis-Menten equation, a linear graph can be generated. One approach is to use a double reciprocal plot (Lineweaver-Burk plot). Taking the reciprocal of each side of the equation and rearranging the terms gives the following:

$$\frac{1}{v} = \frac{K_m}{V_{max}} \frac{1}{[S]} + \frac{1}{V_{max}} \tag{2.4}$$

Equation 4 is the Lineweaver-Burk equation. Plotting 1/v against 1/[S] gives a straight line with slope K_m/V_{max} and a y-intercept of $1/V_{max}$. Furthermore, by extrapolating the graph and crossing the x axis, a value of $-1/K_m$ can be determined. The main drawbacks to this method are that the rates obtained at low concentration will be affected by greater experimental error and the results from high concentrations will be confined to a small area near the y axis.

An alternative approach is based on dividing both sides of the rearranged Michaelis-Menten equation by [S]. This transforms the equation to give the following:

$$v = -K_m \frac{v}{[S]} v + V_{max} \tag{2.5}$$

Equation 2.5 is the Eadie-Hoftsee equation. Plotting v against v/[S] will generate a straight line graph whereby the y-intercept will give the value for V_{max}, the slope $-K_m$, and the x-intercept V_{max}/K_m. Using the Eadie-Hoftsee plot, the values of K_m and V_{max} can be obtained directly. In contrast to the double reciprocal plot, the data points will be spread out evenly, including the values for the high substrate concentrations.

2.2.5 External Influences on Activity

Enzymes, like most proteins, are subject to the effects from a number of external influences. Generally, they can only retain their activity within a limited range of parameters. One of the most important of these is pH. The protein structure on which enzymes are based contains a large number of ionizable groups from the amino acid side chains. Ionisation is dependent on the pKa value; thus at any particular pH some groups will be ionised and others neutral. Each enzyme will display a particular response to a range of pH values, many depicting a bell-shaped curve with an optimum value.

Temperature is another external influence that can affect the enzyme-catalysed reaction. As a rule of thumb, the reaction velocity doubles for every 10°C rise in temperature. However, in contrast with other types of chemical reactions, enzyme temperature reaction profiles follow a different shape. Increasing the temperature will lead to an increasing rate of reaction, up to an optimum degree range. Beyond this optimum, the enzyme rapidly loses activity due to thermal conformational (denaturation) changes.

Temperature optima are normally below 40°C. Once the temperature rises above 55 to 60°C most enzymes become inactivated. There are a number of thermophilic bacteria, however, containing thermostable enzymes that have increased activity at temperatures between 60 and 90°C or above. Experiments carried out to quantify the optimum temperature of an enzyme are based on determining the activity over a range of temperatures. The V_{max} value is obtained using the same amount of enzyme and saturating concentrations of substrate. Variations in these enzyme-catalysed reactions can be described by the Arrhenius expression which can be presented in the two forms

$$\begin{aligned} k &= A\exp\left(-E_a/RT\right) \\ \ln k &= \ln A - E_a/RT \end{aligned} \tag{2.6}$$

where ln k = $\log_e k$. The logarithm of the rate constant (k) is proportional to the activation energy (E_a) and inversely proportional to the absolute temperature (T); R is the gas constant and A can be regarded as constant. If $\log_{10}k$ is plotted against 1/T a straight line graph is generated for temperatures below denaturation and the activation energy can be determined from this plot.

Other major external factors that may influence the catalytic activity of enzymes include: chemical agents (e.g., hydrogen peroxide, a product of oxidase enzymes, can have a detrimental effect), fluid forces (e.g., hydrostatic tension), and irradiation (e.g., ionising radiation).

2.2.6 Inhibition

Enzymes are subject to different degrees of inhibition. Broadly these can be divided into two classes: irreversible and reversible inhibition. Irreversible inhibition results in "poisoning" of the enzyme by the formation of covalent bonds between catalyst and inhibitor. This can lead to complete incapacitation of the enzyme if the inhibitor cannot be removed. One graphical example of this effect is given by the action of nerve gases on the group of enzymes collectively termed cholinesterases. These enzymes play a vital role in the nervous system, therefore any inactivation will have disastrous consequences.

Reversible inhibition can be further subdivided into three major types: competitive, noncompetitive, and mixed. Each type has its own characteristic feature. As the name suggests, reversible inhibition can be reversed by removal of the inhibitor. With competitive inhibition the inhibitor competes with the substrate in binding to the active site of the enzyme. This results in a reduction in the number of enzyme-substrate complexes, leading to an apparent increase in the value for K_m. The V_{max} value remains unchanged. A number of competitive inhibitors are structually similar to the respective enzyme substrate. An example of this is given by the action of the antibiotic sulphanilamide. This compound can act as a competitive inhibitor with the bacterial growth substance *p*-aminobenzoic acid (the enzyme dihydrofolate synthetase converts the compound to folic acid), preventing binding of the substrate to the enzyme and disrupting bacterial production of folic acid (an essential cofactor used by enzymes catalysing the transfer of methyl groups). Because humans can obtain folic acid directly from their diet, the drug sulphanilamide can be safely used.

For noncompetitive inhibition, the inhibitor does not compete with the enzyme substrate. On the contrary, both compounds can bind simultaneously to the enzyme to give a ternary (enzyme-inhibitor-substrate) complex. The complex can then follow one of two routes; either the ternary structure will not decompose to give product, or it will break down into product but at a finite rate different from that of the conventional enzyme-substrate complex. In both instances there is no change in the K_m value, but there is a decrease in V_{max}. Furthermore, a noncompetitive inhibitor will bind to the enzyme in a manner that is independent of the concentration of substrate present.

Mixed inhibition occurs when either substrate can bind with an enzyme-inhibitor complex, or the inhibitor binds with an enzyme-substrate complex. Both reaction pathways lead to a nonproductive enzyme-substrate-inhibitor complex. This form of inhibition affects both the K_m and V_{max} values; the enzyme-inhibitor complex has a lower affinity for substrate compared to the free enzyme.

Many of the enzymes involved in metabolic pathways are under what is termed allosteric (other shape) control. This is a form of reversible inhibition where the inhibitor does not bind at the active site of the enzyme, but on other sites (allosteric sites). In this instance the other compound does not have to resemble the structure of the substrate, because binding occurs at a separate site from the active site. The result of allosteric control will be to either increase or reduce the catalytic activity of the enzyme. Usually, these enzymes do not follow Michaelis-Menten kinetics. Initial velocity vs. substrate concentration plots are sigmoidal rather than the usual hyperbolic shape.

2.2.7 Immobilised Enzymes

Because of their unique properties, particularly their specificity and the ability to operate under "mild" conditions, enzymes have been considered for use in a number of analytical devices, e.g., biosensors. To enhance these favourable characteristics, immobilisation of the desired enzyme has been adopted in a number of instances. By immobilising the enzyme in a fixed position, it can be used repeatedly. This has obvious benefits both in terms of expenditure and ease of operation, i.e., the cost of materials and labor, when compared to operating in a batch mode.

Enzyme immobilisation can lead to an increase in the stability of the enzyme,[5] although this cannot be taken as a general rule. It is assumed that an increased rigidity in the enzyme structure may enhance stability by reducing the opportunities for denaturation. Secondly, immobilising several enzymes in fixed positions near each other, principally those taking part in a catalytic sequence, can increase the efficiency of a multistep reaction pathway.

There are a number of methods applicable to enzyme immobilisation including:

1. Physical entrapment, e.g., enzymes may be immobilised within either an insoluble gel matrix or a microcapsule.
2. Chemical entrapment, e.g., enzymes can be immobilised to a support matrix via covalent bonds or by a multifunctional reagent.
3. Adsorption on a number of support materials, e.g., the enzyme can be adsorbed directly onto the surface by using a hydrophilic medium to dissolve the protein.

The method of choice will largely be determined by a number of factors, with simple adsorption giving the easiest route to immobilisation. Unfortunately this is probably the least stable method (the complex is mainly held together via van der Waals' forces), whereby the enzyme can be easily washed off the face of the support material, particularly when operating in an aqueous medium. Successful immobilisation should lead to a high enzyme loading with maximum retention of the enzyme activity. One consequence of immobilisation may be the effect on enzyme activity caused by the interaction between the support material and the catalyst. Changes in the microenvironment near the enzyme may lead to conformational changes. This would certainly be the case if positively or negatively charged groups were present on the support material, leading to a shift in the pH optimum of the enzyme.

Using low molecular weight bifunctional reagents, copolymerisation of enzymes can be accomplished through cross-linking. One of the most popular reagents in the field of biosensors has been glutaraldehyde. This compound couples the lysine residues present on the enzyme. Usually, a lysine-rich protein such as albumin is included in the immobilisation step. This increases the number of cross-linking sites available and provides mechanical strength to the resulting enzyme film.

Physical entrapment of the enzyme within a gel matrix (e.g., polyacrylamide, alginate, or polyvinyl alcohol) has been widely used. There are two methods applicable to this form of immobilisation; either the enzyme is immobilised directly onto the surface of the electrode, or it is fixed in a preformed matrix which is subsequently secured on the electrode face.

Immobilisation of an enzyme will inevitably lead to a change in the characteristics, particularly kinetics, of the catalyst. One immediate effect of immobilisation will concern how substrate reaches the enzyme support complex, compared to catalysis in the free state. The flow of substrate to the enzyme will be affected by mass transport, because the substrate must diffuse towards the enzyme for the reaction to occur. Furthermore, analytical instruments such as biosensors often include an outer protective membrane over the enzyme layer, leading to an even greater resistance to the diffusion of substrate to the catalyst. Not surprisingly, the overall effect will result in the enzyme operating below its maximum efficiency. One direct consequence will be that the K_m value increases, to give a K_m^{app} constant. Varying the thickness of the outer membrane will alter the K_m^{app} value. This has proved to be of enormous help in the development of biosensors where the enzyme is usually immobilised in close proximity to the sensing surface. Most applications of biosensors involve measuring a concentration range confined to the linear dynamic profile of the enzymatic response. In other words, the K_m constant of the enzyme will determine the useful limits of detection. Controlling the K_m value via the use of membranes can lead to sensors operating over a far greater analytical range.

2.3 COFACTORS

As briefly mentioned earlier, a cofactor is a nonprotein compound that combines with an inactive enzyme to produce a catalytically active complex. Cofactors can range from metal ions, e.g., Zn^{2+} (found in alcohol dehydrogenase), Mn^{2+} (found in arginase), and Fe^{2+} (found in catalase) to large, complex organic molecules such as nicotinamide adenine dinucleotide (NAD) and flavin adenine dinucleotide (FAD). Some enzymes require the presence of both types of cofactors. Enzymes that require the presence of a metal ion are termed metalloenzymes. The function of the metal ion can be either to provide the catalytic centre of the enzyme or it may form a bridging group to link enzyme and substrate together via a coordination complex. A further role may be as a stabilising factor, maintaining the conformation of the enzyme in a catalytically active form. In contrast to enzymes, cofactors tend to be more thermostable.

The class of enzymes termed oxidoreductases are an important group of compounds, frequently utilised in chemical analysis, particularly in biosensors. Usually, they are found to contain a tightly bound redox-active (catalytic) cofactor (see Table 2.2) such as flavin mononucleotide and FAD; such enzymes are termed flavoproteins. These enzymes function by oxidising the substrate (the prosthetic, nonproteinaceous, group becoming reduced as a result of this reaction) to product, resulting in the inactive reduced form of the enzyme. Reactivation of the enzyme is achieved by a reoxidation agent (usually oxygen). If oxygen is the oxidising agent, either H_2O_2 (a two-electron transfer) or H_2O (a four-electron transfer) is produced.

The use of oxidase enzymes has been exploited to great effect in the field of biosensors. A number of biosensors have been constructed based on either detecting the depletion of oxygen or on the production of hydrogen peroxide. An example of this is given by the oxidation of glucose by glucose oxidase:

$$\text{glucose} + O_2 \xrightarrow{\text{glucose oxidase}} \text{gluconic acid} + H_2O_2$$
$$H_2O_2 \longrightarrow 2H^+ + O_2 + 2e^- \qquad (2.7)$$

Equation 2.7 represents the reaction scheme for the oxidation of enzymatically generated hydrogen peroxide.

Other enzymes are activated by the presence of a soluble cofactor. Of these, the $NAD^+/NADH$ and $NAD(P)^+/NADPH$ cofactor-dependent dehydrogenases are by far the most abundant. These coenzymes are very important in cellular processes, where their primary function is to act as carriers of reducing equivalents (via the transfer of H atoms). One hydrogen atom is transferred as a hydride ion to the nicotinamide site of NAD, and the other atom enters solution as a proton. The general reaction scheme of dehydrogenase is as follows (this reaction is generally reversible):

$$\text{substrate} + NAD^+ \xrightarrow{\text{dehydrogenase}} \text{product} + NADH + H^+ \qquad (2.8)$$

Equation 2.8 represents the general reaction for dehydrogenase enzymes. Again, a large number of biosensors have been developed by using the product of this reaction as a basis for detecting the concentration of a desired analyte. A number of biosensor configurations have been constructed based on the electrochemical oxidation of either NADH or NADPH. Unfortunately these sensors are prone to a number of inherent problems. At concentrations above 0.5 mM, rapid poisoning of the electrode surface (e.g., platinum, gold, and glassy carbon) can occur, leading to an inaccurate monitoring step. The effects of poisoning can be reduced by pretreating the surface of the electrode either by mechanical polishing or by electrochemical methods, i.e., cycling in phosphate buffer over wide reducing and oxidising potentials. Furthermore, a high potential is required to carry out the reaction and the current response is subject to significant drift over a prolonged time.

To enhance the operation of biosensors based on either oxidase or dehydrogenase enzymes, a group of compounds termed mediators has been investigated.

2.4 MEDIATORS

Throughout this chapter a number of references have been made to the use of enzymes as the basis for a range of analytical devices termed biosensors. It must be stated that isolated purified enzymes are not the only form of biological material that lends itself to this particular application. Indeed, a whole range of species have been utilised including whole cells, tissues, and antibodies. To recap, the attraction of using enzymes for biosensors lies in the specific nature of their catalytic operation, their relatively small size, and the relative ease with which these compounds can be successfully immobilised. Furthermore, a number of different transducers can be used to convert the biochemical reaction, generated by the enzymatic reaction, into a quantifiable signal. Foremost amongst the various methods of transduction are those based on electrochemical methods of detection; in particular, amperometry.

Immobilising the enzyme onto an electrode and following the generation of a current leads to a method of determining the concentration of a desired analyte. Unfortunately, it is very difficult to achieve direct electron transfer from the reduced oxidase enzyme to the electrode. One of the major hindrances to accomplishing this concerns the unfavourable distance the electron would have to travel. A number of approaches have been used to circumvent the limitations imposed by direct electron transfer.

The initial work on enzyme electrodes was carried out by Clark and Lyons,[6] followed by Updike and Hicks,[7] using the enzyme glucose oxidase. By monitoring the depletion of oxygen (electrochemically) it proved possible to correlate this consumption with the concentration of glucose present in the sample. A second and highly successful (electrochemical) approach to monitoring the action of oxidase enzymes, is to oxidise the hydrogen peroxide generated and hence relate current to analyte concentration. Glucose oxidase (see Equation 2.7) has been the most widely used enzyme for both methods in the field of biosensors.[8]

Despite the widespread use of both approaches, a number of problems are encountered when put to practical use. Primarily, changes in the concentration of dissolved oxygen, affecting the local partial oxygen tension, can lead to erroneous signals. In other words, the depletion of oxygen detected by the system may not be the result of enzymatic reactions. Another source of error may be generated by the high potentials required to reduce oxygen or oxidise hydrogen peroxide. Other compounds present may also be electrochemically active at the same potential. Hence not only will there be a current from, e.g., the oxidation of hydrogen peroxide, but also from these other "contaminants".

To overcome these drawbacks, another approach was investigated: the use of mediating compounds. These compounds are able to replace oxygen as an electron acceptor (removing the problems caused by fluctuations in oxygen partial pressure) and to operate at a potential that greatly reduces the effects of other electrochemically active species. After oxidising the enzyme, the reduced mediator can diffuse to the electrode surface where it is subsequently reoxidised via a rapid charge transfer; consequently this current can be related to the concentration of analyte. The oxidised mediator is then ready to reenter the catalytic cycle.

In order to operate successfully, a mediator must be able to function under a number of constraints including:[9]

Reversible heterogeneous kinetics.
Rapid reaction with the reduced enzyme.
Stability in both the oxidised and reduced forms.
Nonreactivity towards oxygen.
A low potential for regeneration of the oxidised mediator.
For *in vivo* applications the compound must be nontoxic.

A wide range of compounds has been shown to be applicable for use as mediators. Broadly, these compounds can be divided into three major classes: organic, inorganic, and organometallic. The organic compounds that have been used include dyes such as phenazine methosulfate and 2,6-diclorophenolindophenol.[10] Overall, these compounds tend to exhibit poor stability and display a pH-dependent redox potential. An example of the use of an inorganic mediator was described by Taniguchi et al.[11] By coupling either the enzyme lactate oxidase or sarcosine oxidase, both of which are flavoproteins, to octacyanotungstate or octacyanomolybdate, effective electrochemical oxidation could be achieved.

Examples of the organometallic group include hexacyanoferrate III, ruthinium hexamine, and ferrocene and its derivatives. A range of ferrocenes[12] has been investigated and used in the fabrication of various biosensors. Ferrocene is a transition metal arene (aromatic compound) complex, consisting of an iron atom sandwiched between two cyclopentadiayl rings. One of the most notable sensors incorporating ferrocene was the glucose sensor described by Cass et al.[13] The sensor was constructed using the enzyme glucose oxidase immobilised onto the surface of a graphite foil electrode. Immobilisation was achieved by covalent binding of the enzyme using the carbodiimide reaction. One important feature of the ferrocene group is that demonstrated by the ability to carry out chemical substitution on either of the ring systems, leading to changes in the electrochemical characteristics of the compound. Of the range of derivatives investigated, 1,1-dimethylferrocene proved to be the most suitable for this application. Prior to the enzyme immobilisation, 1,1-dimethylferrocene was deposited onto the electrode face by adsorption. Finally, the enzyme layer was covered with an outer polycarbonate membrane.

The operation of this sensor provides a good example of some of the major points discussed in this chapter. Firstly, the enzyme K_m value increased as a result of both the immobilisation step and the outer membrane. The ultimate goal was to develop a glucose sensor that could measure the analyte in human blood. Glucose oxidase in a free state would not produce a sufficiently dynamic linear range to cover the full physiological scale.[8] Following construction, the sensor could operate over the 1 to 30 mM range required. The use of the mediator allowed the sensor to operate at the relatively low potential of +160 mV (vs. an Ag/AgCl reference electrode), reducing the effects of electrochemically active interferents. In addition, the sensors were found to be insensitive to changes in pH over a range of 6 to 9. Generally, if the electrochemical activity of the mediator does not involve protons it can reduce the pH sensitivity of the sensor. The use of carbon as a base material for the electrode also facilitated the inexpensive fabrication procedure later adopted. The experimental setup for sensor characterisation is shown in Figure 2.3.

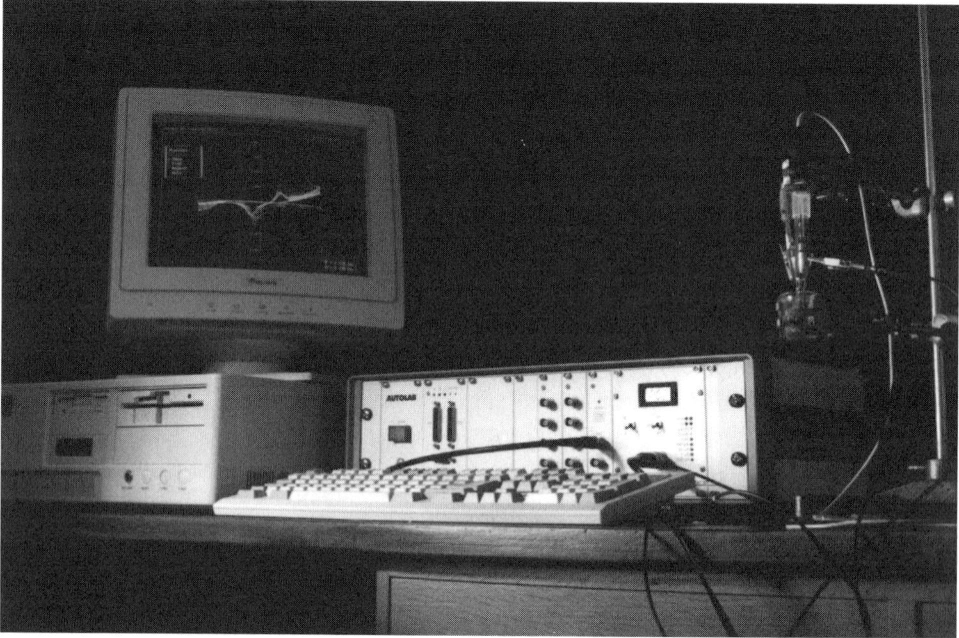

FIGURE 2.3 Modern analytical instruments are used to characterise the response from mediated biosensors.

Based on this mediator-enzyme configuration, a commercially successful glucose sensor for detecting the glucose in blood was launched.[14] The ExacTech one-shot disposable glucose sensor (the most commercially successful mediated product to date; Figure 2.4) is produced by using screen-printing technology to deposit both the mediator and enzyme onto a PVC substrate (see also Chapter 10).

Following the initial work with ferrocene derivatives, new approaches were investigated with the aim of increasing the stability of the mediator. One method has been to use carbon paste or carbon-epoxy resin substrate that can be mixed with the mediator and formed into a sensing surface.[15] Further work has looked at using covalent attachment to anchor the mediator and prevent leaching. An example of this was the approach of Dicks et al.[16] using ferrocene-modified n-type silicon electrodes for the anaerobic redox catalysis of glucose oxidase.

Another practical demonstration of a mediator in action was described by Hendry et al.[17] using the compound tetrathiafulvalene (TTF). The compound was shown to be an effective

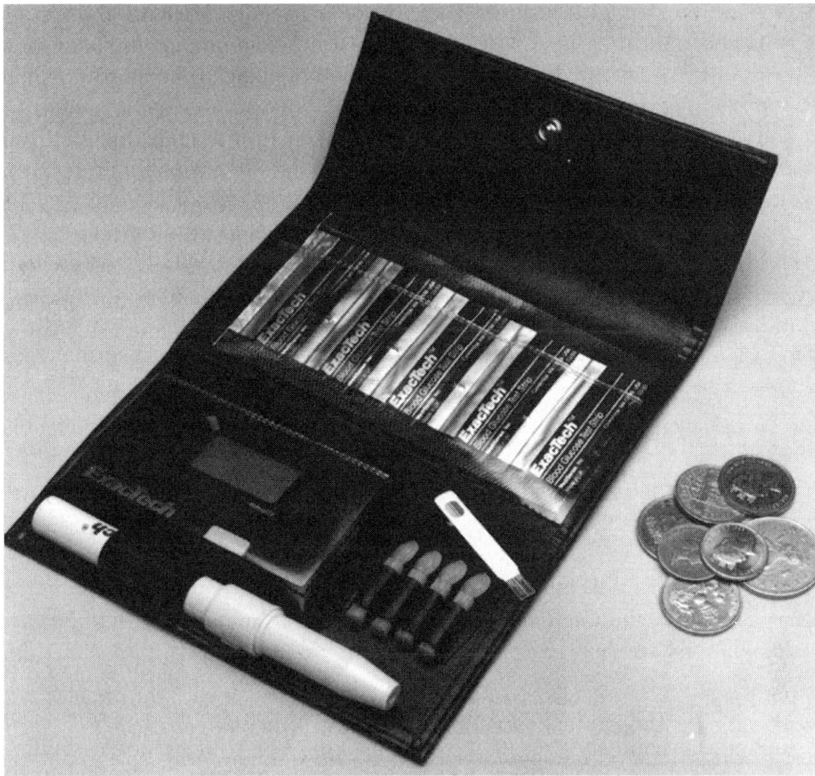

FIGURE 2.4 The ExacTech Glucose Sensor — the most successful commercial biosensor to date.

mediator for the enzymatic determination of glucose and lactate.[18,19] Palleschi and Turner[18] used the enzyme lactate oxidase (the substrate being lactate) immobilised onto carbon foil electrodes. At a relatively low potential of +200 mV, a range of lactate concentrations from 0.1 to 9 mM was detected. Tetracyanoquinodimethane (TCNQ) has also proved to be a useful mediator.[20,21] TCNQ was employed by Kulys and Schmid[20] to mediate the catalytic reaction between tyrosinase and phenol, with the aim of detecting this compound in water samples. In this instance the electrode was operated under cathodic conditions, through the reduction of TCNQ.

The examples mentioned here are only a very brief glimpse of the large amount of work that has been carried out investigating the use of mediators with oxidase enzymes. For a more in-depth study of this subject a number of review articles and publications are available.[3,12,22]

Work has also been carried out on mediating the oxidation of NADP(H). Again, a wide range of compounds has been investigated, including organic salts[22] and ferrocene derivatives. However, the efficiency of this approach is compromised by a poor selectivity for the electrocatalysis of NADH, coupled with an increasing response to other interfering (electro chemically) compounds. Another group of compounds that has been investigated extensively is the phenoxazines and their derivatives.[22] One example of their use is shown by the proposed reaction with the mediator Meldola Blue (7-dimethylamino-1,2-benzophenoxzium salt).[23]

$$\mathrm{NADH} + \mathrm{MB}^+ \rightarrow \mathrm{NADH.MB}^+$$

$$\mathrm{NADH.MB}^+ \rightarrow \mathrm{NAD}^+ + \mathrm{MBH}$$

$$\mathrm{MBH} \rightarrow \mathrm{MB}^+ + 2e^- + \mathrm{H}^+$$

The reaction involves the formation of a coenzyme-mediator complex. Overall, the second reaction is irreversible due to the fast oxidation of MBH.

Electrochemical immunoassays have also been developed to detect selected antigens.[24] Using enzyme-labelled (i.e., alkaline phosphatase, which dephosphorylates $NADP^+$ to NAD^+) antibodies plus a combination of other enzymes to drive a catalytic cycle, and the mediator ferricyanide to act as an oxidant, the authors demonstrated a sensitive method for detecting the amount of analyte present in a sample.

To overcome the drawbacks found with the direct mediation of NADH oxidation, one approach has been to use an NADH-specific enzyme: NADH oxidase. One form of the enzyme (from *Thermus aquaticus*) was used with a range of ferrocene derivatives.[25] The enzyme was used in solution, forming the basis of an enzyme amplification system for an electrochemical immunoassay, to reoxidise enzymatically generated NADH.

2.5 CONCLUSIONS

In summary, mediated amperometric enzyme electrodes have proved to be the most commercially successful approach to constructing biosensors to date. Limitations in terms of complexity, leaching of the mediator, and potential toxicity, however, bring into question whether mediators will continue to dominate the field. Advances in direct electrochemistry of proteins and improvements in the low potential catalytic oxidation of enzyme products suggest that for certain applications, such as *in vivo* and process monitoring, these approaches may displace the mediated sensor. In the disposable sensor market, however, considerable financial reward is still to be gained from the electrochemical strip and capillary-fill devices that have recently been launched onto the market.

REFERENCES

1. Coughlan, M. P., Marek, P. J. K., Border, P. M., and Turner, A. P. F., Analytical applications of immobilised proteins and cells, *J. Microb. Methods,* 8, 1, 1988.
2. Lehninger, A. L., *Biochemistry,* Worth Publishers, New York, 1981.
3. Turner, A. P. F., Karube, I., and Wilson, G. S., *Biosensors: Fundamentals and Applications,* Oxford University Press, New York, 1987.
4. Anon., *Enzyme Nomenclature,* the 1972 recommendations of the Commission on Enzyme Nomenclature, including units and kinetic symbols, Elsevier, New York, 1973.
5. Klibnov, A. M., Enzyme stabilisation by immobilisation, *Anal. Biochem.,* 93, 1, 1979.
6. Clark, L. C. and Lyons, C., Electrode systems for continuous monitoring in cardiovascular surgery, *Annu. N.Y. Acad. Sci.,* 102, 29, 1962.
7. Updike, S. J. and Hicks, G. P., The enzyme electrode, *Nature,* 214, 986, 1967.
8. Wilson, R. and Turner, A. P. F., Glucose oxidase: an ideal enzyme, *Biosens. Bioelectron.,* 7, 165, 1992.
9. Cardosi, M. F. and Turner, A. P. F., The realization of electron transfer from biological molecules to electrodes, in *Biosensors: Fundamentals and Applications,* Turner, A. P. F., Karube, I. and Wilson, G. S., Eds., Oxford University Press, New York, 1987, 257.
10. Aleksandrovski, Y. A., Bezhikina, L. V., and Rodinov, Y. V., Comparative study of reactions catalysed by glucose oxidase in the presence of different electron acceptors, *Biochemistry (USSR),* 46, 593, 1981.
11. Taniguchi, I., Miyamoto, S., Tomimura, S., and Hawkridge, F. M., Mediated electron transfer of lactate oxidase and sarcosine oxidase with octacyanotungstate (IV) and octacyanomolybdate, *J. Electroanal. Chem.,* 240, 333, 1988.
12. Turner, A. P. F., *Advances in Biosensors,* Suppl. 1, 2, 3, JAI Press, London, 1991, 1992, 1993, and 1994.

13. Cass, A. E. G., Davis, G., Francis, G. D., Hill, H. A. O., Aston, W. G., Higgins, I. J., Plotkin, E. V., Scott, L. D. L., and Turner, A. P. F., Ferrocene mediated enzyme electrode for amperometric determination of glucose, *Anal. Chem.*, 56, 667, 1984.
14. Cardosi, M. F. and Turner, A. P. F., Recent advances in enzyme based electrochemical glucose sensors. In the *Diabetes Annual 5,* Alberti, K. G. M. M. and Krall, L. P., Eds., Elsevier Science, Oxford, 1990, 254-272.
15. Wang, J., Modified electrodes for electrochemical sensors, *Electroanalysis*, 3, 255, 1991.
16. Dicks, J. M., Cardosi, M. F., Turner, A. P. F., and Karube, I., The application of ferrocene-modified *n*-type silicon in glucose biosensors, *Electroanalysis,* 5, 1, 1993.
17. Turner, A. P. F., Hendry, S. P., and Cardosi, M. F., Tetrathiafulvalene: a new mediator for amperometric biosensors, in *World Biotech. Report on Biosensors, Instrumentation and Processing, 1*, Online Publications, Pinner, U. K., 1987, 127.
18. Palleschi, G. and Turner, A. P. F., Amperometric tetrathiafulvalene-mediated lactate electrode using lactate oxidase adsorbed on carbon foil, *Anal. Chim. Acta*, 234, 459, 1990.
19. Gunasingham, H. and Tan, C.-H., Carbon paste-tetrathiafulvalene amperometric enzyme electrode for the determination of glucose in flowing streams, *Analyst*, 115, 35, 1990.
20. Kulys, J. and Schmid, R. D., A sensitive enzyme electrode for phenol monitoring, *Anal. Lett.*, 23, 589, 1990.
21. Hendry, S. P. and Turner, A. P. F., A glucose sensor utilising tetracyanoquinodimethane as a mediator, *Horm. Metab. Res. Suppl. Ser.,* 20, 37, 1988.
22. Wring, S. A. and Hart, J. P., Chemically modified carbon based electrodes and their application as electrochemical sensors for the analysis of biologically important compounds, *Analyst*, 117, 1215, 1992.
23. Gorton, L., Csoregi, E., Dominguez, E., Emneus, J., Jonsson-Pettersson, G., Marko-Varga, G., and Persson, L., Selective detection in flow analysis based on the combination of immobilised enzymes and chemically modified electrodes, *Anal. Chim. Acta*, 250, 203, 1991.
24. Cardosi, M. F., Birch, S. W., Stanley, C. J., Johannsson, A., and Turner, A. P. F., An electrochemical immunoassay for prostatic acid phosphatase incorporating enzyme amplification, *Am. Biotechnol. Lab.*, 7, 50, 1989.
25. McNeil, C. J., Spoors, J. A., Cocco, D., Cooper, J. M., and Bannister, J. V., Thermostable reduced nicotinamide adenine dinucleotide oxidase: application to amperometric enzyme assay, *Anal. Chem.*, 61, 25, 1989.

3 Bioaffinity Agents for Sensing Systems

David J. Newman, Yemi Olabiran, and Christopher P. Price

CONTENTS

0-8493-8905-4/97/$0.00+$.50
© 1997 by CRC Press, Inc.

3.1 INTRODUCTION

Molecular recognition is the first and arguably the most important step in the generation of a response by a biosensor device. The specificity and affinity of this step will determine the overall performance of an analytical system regardless of the detection technology employed. In this chapter the term bioaffinity agent will be used to describe the molecule providing the recognition component of a biosensor and includes a wide variety of molecules as shown in Table 3.1. The focus will be on the first two categories, and we will discuss structural and production aspects as well as strategies for selecting the appropriate bioaffinity agent for use in a sensor device.

TABLE 3.1
Bioaffinity Agents Used in Sensor Devices

Immunological
Intact primary antibodies
Polyclonal
Monoclonal
Fab_2 fragments
Fab fragments
sFv molecules
Second antibody systems
Nonimmunological
Biotin:streptavidin
Protein A and Protein G
Peptides
Oligonucleotides
Lectins
Receptors
Binding proteins
Antibody mimics
Enzymes

We have particular experience in the use of two commercially available optical sensor technologies, the BIAcore™ from Biosensor, Uppsala, Sweden and the IASys™ from Fisons Applied Sensor Technology, Cambridge, U.K. and we will give practical examples of how these systems have revolutionised the characterisation of bioaffinity agents and biomolecular interaction analysis in general over the last 4 years. Lessons learnt from these optical surface effect systems should be applicable to most other surface effect technologies when they are applied to biological matrices.

3.2 TYPES OF BIOAFFINITY AGENTS

A number of agents have been employed for studying bioaffinity interactions, of which antibody:antigen binding is perhaps the most well-studied example. The basis for the exploitation of these types of interactions in the development of biosensors is the ability of affinity interactions to separate an individual or a selected range of components from complex mixtures of biomolecules on the basis of chemical structure and/or biological function.

3.2.1 ANTIBODIES

Antibodies are proteins, called immunoglobulins, produced by the humoral immune system in response to a seemingly limitless array of antigenic structures and have widespread applications in clinical diagnostics and biotechnology. The basic structure is shown in Figure 3.1; a monomeric immunoglobulin molecule is constituted from two identical heavy (H) and light (L) polypeptide chains that are linked together by disulphide bonds.[1-3] Each chain is organised into domains that are approximately 110 amino acids in length. The amino terminal domains of each heavy and light chain comprise the variable (V) region within which there are three areas of greatest sequence variability: the hypervariable or complementarity determining regions (CDRs).[4]

Antibodies are produced by specialised cells of the immune system, the B-lymphocytes. Rearrangement of the immunoglobulin genes[5-7] combined with somatic mutation[8,9] within these cells following an antigenic challenge gives rise to the production of different antibody classes and specificities. Antibodies are available for *in vitro* use in a number of different forms as mentioned in Table 3.1. The conventional response of an immunised animal, usually a rabbit, sheep, goat, mouse, or rat, is to produce what is known as a polyclonal antiserum which contains many different antibody specificities recognising various epitopes on the antigen concerned. This is because this antiserum is the product of many different B-lymphocyte cells which develop and multiply giving rise to different clones of activated antibody-producing cells; the antiserum is heterogeneous in class of immunoglobulin, specificity, titre, and affinity.[10-12] Polyclonal antisera are therefore heterogeneous reagents, as a given antigen will consist of many epitopes to which an antibody can be generated. Even antibodies which bind to the same epitope may vary in their affinities and will thus compete for binding to the same epitope. The consequence of this heterogeneity is that each serum will be unique in its specific antibody composition and hence its performance in any particular immunoassay.

Affinity purification of polyclonal antisera using immobilised antigen on solid-phases is one way in which the performance of this type of antibody can be improved as this will remove nonspecific/low affinity antibodies. However the affinity purified product is still not monospecific and remains heterogeneous in nature; exposure of the immunoglobulin to a low pH during affinity purification can also cause structural alterations, making the molecule more sensitive to proteolytic degradation.

3.2.1.1 Production of Polyclonal Antibodies

Most proteins and polypeptides above about 10,000 Da molecular weight are naturally immunogenic in that they can stimulate an immune response upon injection into an animal. Molecules smaller than this may be antigenic but not immunogenic; these molecules, often called haptens, can stimulate a specific immune response but only when conjugated to a larger molecule prior to injection, e.g., bovine-serum albumin, ovalbumin, or keyhole limpet haemocyanin. Examples of haptens include many drugs, steroids, and vitamins, and by conjugation to a carrier protein and using a suitable conjugation chemistry, high affinity antibodies can be raised against these molecules. The molecular weight cut off quoted above is only a guide, as molecules smaller than this have been found to be immunogenic. It can be worth investigating the immunogenic potential of a novel antigen in this lower molecular

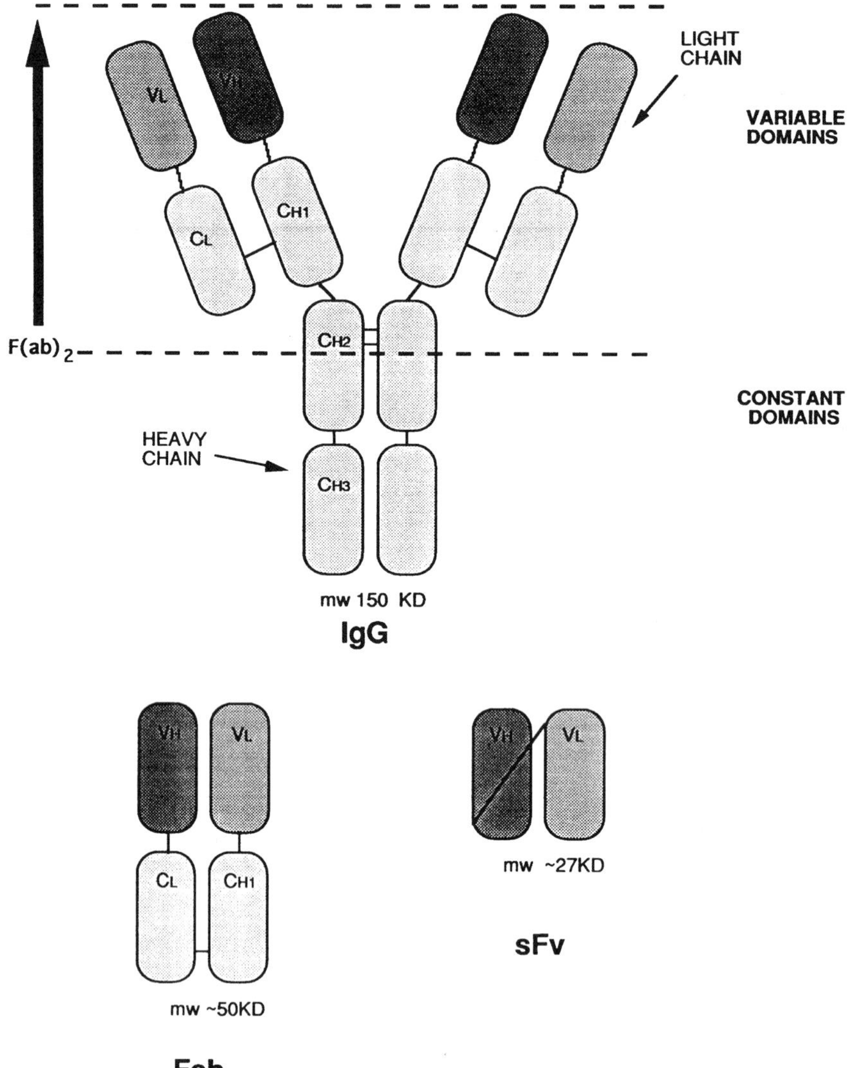

FIGURE 3.1 Structure of the immunoglobulin molecule.

weight range as conjugation to a carrier protein adds complexity to the process and results in the formation of antibodies to the hapten-carrier protein conjugation site and to the carrier protein itself — all of which may then have to be removed depending upon the use that is to be made of the antiserum.

A variety of animal species have been used to generate antibodies for experimental purposes and there is some suggestion that different species give different degrees of responsiveness to a given immunogen. There has been shown to be a genetic loci closely associated with a part of the major histocompatibility complex (MHC) which controls the immune response.[13] However, there are many additional sources of variation including the age of the animal and one of the major considerations in selecting a species is the cost of keeping it vs. the amount of serum required; for most in-house experimental work rabbits or guinea pigs are used, but larger animals such as sheep or goats are often used for commercial-scale production.

Animals can be immunised by a variety of routes and using a variety of immunogens; the use of subcutaneous or intramuscular injections of oily adjuvant emulsions is quite long-standing but there is increasing evidence suggesting that they are of limited benefit in comparison with the painful ulceration that is often to be found on the animal's skin. The commonest immunisation schedule probably involves the use of multiple site (30 to 50 sites) intradermal injection.[14]

Dosage and timing of immunisation is dependent upon individual opinion, there being little systematic investigation of the matter; however, some generally accepted guidelines can be made. Lower doses of immunogen are thought to favour the production of high affinity antibodies; a primary dose for a rabbit or a guinea pig would be of the order of 100 μg with second and subsequent booster injections of between 10 and 50% of this, the boosting injection being given after 4 to 6 weeks and the first harvesting of antiserum 10 to 14 days after the boost.[15] Trial bleeds can be used to assess the type and amount of the immune response and to predict the need for future booster injections if the titre (amount of antibody) is not high enough or is falling off.

Antiserum is usually harvested after the booster injections, as the primary response to the initial injection is usually predominantly a low affinity IgM response, whereas the secondary immune response results in the higher affinity IgG production. In order to obtain a suitable polyclonal antiserum, several animals, usually five or six, are immunised. In the case of a weakly immunogenic molecule, this number may have to be increased. Using this kind of protocol, a suitable polyclonal antiserum can usually be generated to most molecules within 3 to 6 months and if larger quantities or more consistent production is required then blending of antisera from different animals can be carried out using some defined desired characteristics such as titre and specificity.

3.2.1.2 Production of Monoclonal Antibodies

An alternative approach for the production of more specific and homogeneous antibodies is the use of hybridoma technology developed by Køhler and Milstein in 1975.[16,17] Using this approach, single antibody-producing B-lymphocytes can be immortalised by fusion with a B-cell tumour line to form a hybridoma cell line which by suitable selection can derive from a single clone of B-lymphocytes, hence the term "monoclonal". This hybrid cell line has the advantage that it secretes antibody which is homogeneous in specificity, affinity, and isotype. The applications of this type of antibody are widespread both in *in vitro* and *in vivo* diagnostics. Unlike polyclonal reagents, monoclonal antibodies can theoretically be produced in unlimited amounts in continuous supply and this is of considerable benefit in efforts to standardise reagents between laboratories. The only possible disadvantages of monoclonal antibodies are a consequence of their monospecificity and low epitope frequency; they are often only poor immunoaggregators and the individual epitope recognised may be more or less stable than the molecule that it is part of, leading to the immunological information no longer reflecting the biological activity of the molecule.

Monoclonal antibodies have now been produced from the spleen cells or peripheral lymphocytes of several animal species including human antibodies, but the most commonly used species are the mouse and the rat. The first stage in production is as described for polyclonal antibody production (Section 3.2.1.1). Where the processes diverge is that after the first booster injection the animals are screened for a polyclonal antibody response by taking a blood sample from their tail veins and selecting the animal which has shown the maximal response. The selected animal is then sacrificed and its spleen removed, under aseptic conditions. The spleen cells are washed out of the spleen by sieving and then mixed with a compatible strain of myeloma cells, e.g., NS1, NS0, or X63-Ag8.653 in the presence of a fusing agent, commonly polyethylene glycol,[18] although viruses and electroporation have also been used.

The process of fusion occurs relatively rarely, approximately with 1 in every 10,000 spleen cells, and only a few of these will secrete antibody with the desired characteristics.

The typical mouse spleen produces about 1×10^8 cells so an average fusion will result in potentially 500 to 1000 hybrids. Thus it is by no means certain that every fusion experiment will produce the desired antibody and, depending upon the immunogenic nature of the molecule used, from one to several hundred fusions can be required.

There are a variety of different protocols for each stage in monoclonal antibody production, but in general the fused cells, or hybridomas, are grown on a feeder layer of peritoneal macrophages supplemented with foetal calf serum, although the use of serum-free media with special growth supplements is now quite common. The selection of the successfully fused hybridomas depends on the use of hypoxanthine guanine phosphoribosyl transferase (HGPRT)-deficient myeloma cells. The unfused spleen cells die off in culture after a few days; the cells are grown in a medium containing aminopterin, which inhibits the main biosynthetic pathway for nucleic acid synthesis. Thus cells can only grow if they can use the HGPRT-dependent pathway and therefore only the hybridomas will be able to grow as they will receive HGPRT from the spleen cell component.

The successfully growing hybrids then need to be screened for antibody production in a rapid solid-phase assay that can identify the desired antibody-producing cells before they have multiplied too far. This is one area where immunosensors have played a role, especially the fully automated BIAcore™; microtitre plates can be placed in the instrument and the supernatants run over the antigen-coated sensor chip. The relative responses are used to identify the antibody-producing wells; furthermore, kinetic rate constant ranking is also possible, enabling the high affinity antibody-producing wells to be readily identified. However, at this initial stage of screening the wells in the microtitre plate may contain several different clones of hybridomas and in order to ensure monoclonality the positive wells in the first screen must be "cloned", usually by a process of limiting dilution which ensures that on average less than one cell is placed in each well of a microtitre plate. The cells grown under these conditions should be screened again and the positive wells taken through a second round of limiting dilutions; the resultant cells should be monoclonal.

The next stage in monoclonal antibody production is to identify the epitopes recognised by the panel of antibodies that will have been generated; this enables appropriate pairs of antibodies to be selected for the use in sandwich immunoassays. This will be discussed in more detail in Section 3.4.2 as this is another area where commercialised optical sensor systems have had an important impact.

The final stage is deciding upon the means of production of the monoclonal antibody, either *in vitro* or *in vivo*. The latter technique using ascitic fluid production in mice generated by initiating the growth of a solid tumour in the peritoneum is being used less and less. *In vitro* antibody generation using tissue culture techniques has received much attention in recent years and there are now a number of hollow fibre culture systems, e.g., Technomouse by Integra Biosciences, which enable the continuous production of monoclonal antibodies on the scale of grams per month. Smaller-scale production in roller bottles or other tissue culture vessels can produce several milligrams of antibody a month.

3.2.1.3 Intact vs. Antibody Fragments

Immunoassays using intact immunoglobulins can be prone to interferences that are unrelated to the specificity of the antigen binding site, for instance binding of rheumatoid factors and complement proteins to the F_c portion.[19] Removal of the F_c portion, leaving an $F(ab)_2$ or Fab fragment (Figure 3.1), can prevent this type of interference. These antibody fragments are generated by proteolytic cleavage (using papain) of the intact antibody and chromatographic purification of the cleaved products.[20,21] This process requires careful optimisation to ensure a high yield of pure antibody fragment and adds significantly to the cost of the final antibody reagent; thus clear evidence of an interference with a particular antibody is needed before such a procedure should be considered. Not all assays that use intact immunoglobulins are prone to these interferences and there is some evidence that this may be due to the reaction conditions selected; furthermore, there is the possibility of using sulphydryl reagents such as dithiothreitol to eliminate the interference at a more reasonable cost.[22]

3.2.1.4 Genetic Engineering and Production of Single-Chain Antibodies

Antibody fragments can also be generated by means of recombinant DNA technology; this allows the production of novel antibody molecules even without the use of laboratory animals[23,24] (also see Chapter 4). Antibodies to self antigens have been generated, as well as human antibodies with a wide range of specificities. The genes encoding for the variable chains of immunoglobulins can be amplified by use of the polymerase chain reaction (PCR) and sequence-specific oligonucleotide primers.[25] The starting material for isolation of antibody genes is the mRNA transcript from antibody-producing cells which can be used as a template for the preparation of cDNA for amplification in the PCR reaction. Generally, any tissue containing antibody-producing cells can be used as a source of RNA including β-lymphocytes from immunised mouse spleens or cultured hybridoma cells. For amplification of antibody genes by PCR the main approach has been to use oligonucleotides hybridizing to sequences in the signal peptide encoding part of the immunoglobulin molecule, together with oligonucleotides annealing with sequences encoding the constant region. Amplified variable heavy (V_H) and light (V_L) sequences can be purified by agarose gel electrophoresis which can also be used to confirm the size (300 bps) of these fragments. Following purification, cloning into a suitable vector for sequencing is necessary. Having sequenced these amplified V_H and V_L sequences they can be recombined, again using the PCR reaction, by linkage with a short (approximately 15-amino-acid) spacer which allows the structure to assume a conformation capable of antigen binding.[26,27] This structure is a single-chain antibody fragment or sFv (see Figure 3.2). Production of large quantities of this single-chain antibody is achieved by cloning of the gene construct into a plasmid for expression in a suitable strain of *E. coli*. Following lysis of the cells, sFv protein can be purified from the cell extract by affinity chromatography against antigen or it is also possible to incorporate a peptide tag into the gene construct which can be used for purification using an anti-peptide antibody. Another variant of this approach is the incorporation of a hexahistidine tag into the sFv construct which allows purification of the protein by metal chelate affinity chromatography using zinc or nickel columns. Once purified sFv is available it is very important to check that the sFv retains the binding specificity of the original antibody. It is not uncommon during the manipulation of DNA that unintended mutations could arise. Certainly, Taq polymerase used in the PCR reaction is error prone and hence it is necessary to avoid too many rounds of amplification to reduce the error risk. The beauty of this technology is that the affinity and specificity of the sFv can be altered by site-directed mutagenesis, potentially generating higher affinity and more specific immunoreagents.

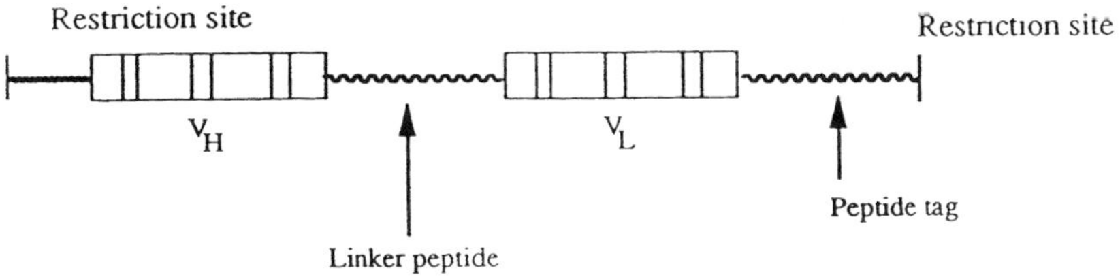

FIGURE 3.2 sFv gene construct.

Biosensors such as the BIAcore™ certainly have a major role to play in the determination of structure/function relationships of both intact and fragmented antibodies. Manipulation of antibodies at the DNA level for improvement of characteristics such as specificity and affinity does require a means of assessment of the effect of what might be subtle changes in structure on the antibody's function. If this is combined with the potential of generating very large antibody libraries using phage display technology[28] then it is evident that biosensors will increasingly be of use for rapid determination of changes in kinetic parameters of antibody-to-antigen binding studies. There are limitations to the improvements that can be made and although the use of sFv's in tumour imaging and therapy is now well established, the impact that this technology will have on *in vitro* immunodiagnostics is not yet clear.

3.2.2 Antibody Mimics

Over the last few years there have been a series of papers from Sweden exploring the potential of nonimmunological bioaffinity agents prepared by molecular imprinting.[29] In this process functional monomers are polymerised in the presence of a "print" molecule, and following the removal of the molecule from the now rigid polymer there remain sites in the polymer which will specifically bind the original "print" molecule. These polymeric bioaffinity agents have been used to develop assays for drugs such as theophylline, but it is suggested that they might be applicable to proteins and nucleic acids. The assays that have so far been developed have been cumbersome in the extreme, but if polymerisation could be carried out on the surface of a sensor chip or the final polymer could be coated onto the surface, it is possible that these antibody mimics might find a more widespread use. The appropriate regeneration conditions would still need to be optimised, but there is the potential for an extremely robust sensor surface if there are no nonspecific binding difficulties.

3.2.3 Lectins

Lectins are a class of carbohydrate-binding proteins of nonimmune origin which agglutinate cells or precipitate polysaccharides and exhibit antibody-like sugar binding specificity.[30] They are multivalent and structurally very diverse, being found in animals, plants, and bacteria, with widely varying molecular weights, metal ion requirements, and three-dimensional structure. The most well known and best studied lectin is that of the jack bean (*Canavalia ensiformis*) better known as Concanavalin A or more usually con A; this lectin is a member of the mannose/glucose-binding family and was first isolated by Sumner and Howell in 1936.[31] Examples of other lectins and their specificities are given in Table 3.2. Con A is composed of four identical carbohydrate-free subunits (mol wt 26,500 Da); there is a pH-dependent association of the subunits and at pH values less than 5.6 a dimer is the predominant form. Each subunit contains one Ca^{2+} and one Mn^{2+} and both are required for carbohydrate binding; the ions are removed by acid washing, e.g., 0.1 M HCl. Several hundred lectins with different specificities can now be found in commercial catalogues and a number of specialised articles and reviews describe their utility.[32,33]

The multisubunit nature and metal ion requirement are common features of lectins, and due to their heterogeneity in structure each has to be considered separately if they are to be used as a bioaffinity agent in a sensor system. The running buffer and regeneration buffer will have to be individually optimised and may need, at least in the case of the former, to contain excess metal ions. Lectins have been much employed in the study of blood group antigens and other cellular interactions, but have as yet received little use as bioaffinity agents in sensors; with the correct design of the flow cell or cuvette, cellular interactions including cell lysis could be monitored using lectins.

3.2.4 Receptors[34,35]

In drug discovery work it can be very important to screen large numbers of candidate molecules for their binding to a particular receptor. In the investigation of novel hormones,

TABLE 3.2
Examples of the Binding Specificity of Lectins

Lectin	Specificity group	Nominal specificity
Canavalia ensiformis (Concanavalin A)	Glucose/mannose	Man > Glc > GlcNAc
Vicia faba	Glucose/mannose	Man > Glc = GlcNAc
Lens culinaris	Glucose/mannose	Man > Glc > GlcNAc
Triticum vulgare	*N*-acetylglucosamine	$GlcNAc(1,4GlcNAc)_{1\text{-}2}$ > GlcNAc
Riccinus communis	*N*-acetylgalactosamine/galactose	Gal > Gal >> GalNAc
Ulex europeus I	L-Fucose	L-Fuc
Limax flavus	Sialic Acid	Neu5Ac > Neu5Gc

receptor identification and characterisation can be of vital importance. These investigations can pose a number of difficulties, as in many cases the receptor molecule can be poorly characterised and unavailable in pure form or there is a requirement for other membrane proteins for receptor stabilisation and function. Receptors are proteins which can consist of one or more subunits, and whilst varying significantly in molecular weight, they are generally 100,000 Da or larger. However, it can be important to investigate the receptor *in situ*, either in an intact cell or as part of a membrane preparation, and this can cause stability problems. An alternative approach would be to couple a ligand of known function and affinity to the sensor and to monitor the competitive behaviour of other candidate molecules using a liquid-phase receptor preparation, but this will still be time-consuming and expensive in the case of screening for new drugs.

Indirect coupling of the receptor to the sensor surface is possible using an antibody that recognises an epitope distinct from the active site, although care must be taken to investigate whether antibody binding causes any conformational changes in the receptor that could alter the function of the active site. Finally, and with the same proviso that direct coupling doesn't cause large conformational changes, partially purified receptors can be coupled to sensor surfaces as long as the binding of the drug or hormone, which are likely to be small molecules, can be detected.

3.2.5 Binding Proteins[36]

The main value of binding proteins as bioaffinity agents lies in their use in indirect coupling techniques, enabling a standardised surface to be produced for use in a number of different applications. Secondly, the use of a binding protein that is specific for a particular part of a bioaffinity agent, such as the F_c region of an immunoglobulin in the case of the bacterial proteins, Proteins A and G, can result in a more favourable orientation of the bioaffinity molecule than direct coupling would allow. Thirdly, binding protein:ligand interactions, e.g., cortisol binding to cortisol binding globulin, are biomolecular interactions that require investigation for their physiological significance and their uniqueness is more a matter of semantics than functionality.

3.2.5.1 Proteins A and G

Bacterial proteins with nonimmune binding specificities for the F_c portion of immunoglobulins have been found on the surface of a variety of Streptococci and Staphylococci. Proteins A and G are examples of this type of bioaffinity agent.[37] Protein A is a component of the cell wall of *Staphylococcus aureus*. It has a molecular weight of 42,000 Da and six independent binding sites for the F_c region of immunoglobulins from most mammalian species (see

Table 3.3). Some binding to the Fab region also occurs, resulting in binding of IgA, M, and E; specificity of binding is enhanced by careful selection of the reaction conditions used for binding, particularly the pH.

Protein A is the prototype IgG-binding protein and has been used extensively for many immunochemical procedures, although the major use has been purification of IgG.[38] Protein A reagents are extremely versatile, one Protein A reagent can be used as a secondary reagent for primary antibodies of different species, and may be radiolabeled, and fluorochrome or enzyme conjugated.

TABLE 3.3
Binding Specificities of Proteins A and G

Polyclonal immunoglobulin	Protein A	Protein G
Human albumin	++	+++
Human alpha$_2$-macroglobulin	+++	+++
Human	+++	+++
Mouse	+++	+++
IgG$_1$	+	++
IgG$_{2a}$	+++	+++
IgG$_{2b}$	+++	+++
IgG$_3$	+++	+++
IgG$_4$	+	+++
Rabbit	+++	+++
Goat	+	+
Rat	+	+/–
Sheep	+	+++
Cow	+	+++
Guinea Pig	+++	+
Pig	+++	+
Horse	+	+++
Dog	+++	+
Chicken	–	–
Human IgM	+	–
Human IgD	–	–
Human IgA	+	–

Note: Key: +++ very strong binding, ++ strong binding, + weak binding, +/– negligible binding.

Protein G,[39] a cell surface protein of group G streptococci is of the type III F_c receptor binding proteins and binds to immunoglobulins by a similar manner to that of Protein A; however, its binding profile differs from that of Protein A, depending on the species origin of the immunoglobulin (see Table 3.3).

3.2.5.2 Avidin:Biotin

The avidin:biotin system has been widely used in biology and is particularly attractive as a sandwich system used in conjunction with antibodies.[40] Avidin is a tetrameric protein with identical subunits, each of molecular weight 15,000 Da, found in egg white, with extremely high affinity (10^{-15} M^{-1}) for the water-soluble vitamin B6, biotin.[41] Biotin is relatively polar and can be coupled to antibodies under very mild conditions with little disruption to their structure. Avidin, coupled to fluorochromes, enzymes, and other molecules, may then be used as a stable high-affinity detection system.

Both avidin and biotin are readily available commercially at little cost. The disadvantage of the system is the extremely basic nature of avidin (pI = 10.5) and thus it may bind nonspecifically by electrostatic forces. Another potential problem with this system is the fact that most cell culture media contain biotin and thus it is important to wash cells thoroughly in medium lacking biotin before addition of avidin.

Streptavidin, a binding protein isolated from *Streptomyces,* is an alternative to avidin. It has four identical chains, but amino acid analysis shows that streptavidin has only half the number of basic amino acids and therefore it would be expected to have a much less basic isoelectric point and correspondingly less nonspecific binding.[41] The streptavidin:biotin system can also be used as an enhancement technique as four biotin molecules can in theory be bound by each streptavidin molecule.

3.2.6 Nucleic Acids

DNA:DNA, DNA:RNA, and DNA:protein interactions can be treated in the same way as any other biomolecular interaction in that the forces involved in the interaction are identical and the same questions of affinity and specificity are also pertinent. Oligonucleotides and longer lengths of DNA can be coupled to sensor surfaces particularly by means of the biotin:streptavidin interaction, as nucleotides can be easily biotinylated and streptavidin conjugated to the sensor surface. This approach has been used to study the interaction of the *E. coli lac* repressor with immobilised *lac* operator DNA sequences enabling the binding kinetics to be determined.[42] Hybridisation reactions have also been monitored looking at the effects of single base mismatches and different length probes upon hybridisation kinetics; both association and dissociation can be monitored if the appropriate conditions are selected.[43]

3.2.7 Enzymes

The selection and conjugation of enzymes have been discussed in Chapter 2 in this volume, but it is perhaps pertinent in this section to mention them again for the sake of completeness even if they may not usually be considered as bioaffinity molecules in this particular context of binding interactions. Enzyme reactions can be monitored in several ways, but the two that will be mentioned here are the use and measurement of proteases and the effect of enzyme modifiers of binding interactions. Measurement of serum proteases can be carried out by means of their effect on immobilised substrates.[44] The effect of phosphatases and phosphorylating enzymes upon multicomponent binding interactions can also be elegantly investigated using immunosensors — the enzyme reaction being carried out on the sensor surface and the change in response monitored.[45]

3.3 IMMUNOASSAYS AND OTHER BINDING ASSAYS

Binding assays, and immunoassays in particular, are now widely used in the biotechnology and diagnostic industries due to their high sensitivity and specificity, the former now being limited by the detection technology employed and the latter by the care with which the bioaffinity agent is chosen. Immunoassays are used to measure the concentration of molecules across the whole range of biological interest from whole cells and large proteins to individual amino acids, and from the millimole/litre range down to attomole/litre. There is a complex panoply of manual to fully automated immunoassay systems already crowding the diagnostics market and it is against these that any new sensing technology will need to be judged.[46] The various assay formats that can be used on a sensor surface are shown in Figure 3.3, and are the same as can be used in the investigation of all binding interactions.

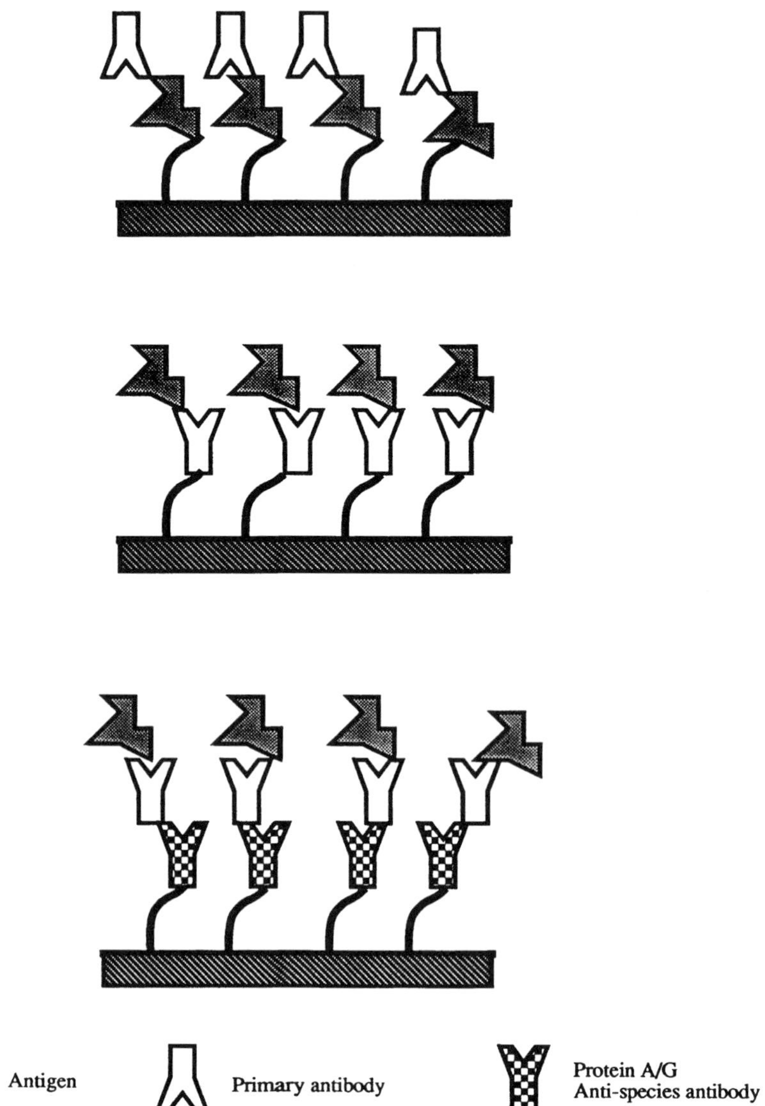

FIGURE 3.3 Assay formats on a sensor surface.

Immunosensors will need to offer something different, and it is unlikely that they will offer improvements either in terms of sensitivity or specificity and if it is to be in terms of convenience, then this will have now to be measured against the use of fully automated systems.[47] One potential area is in multianalyte testing using technologies such as that of Professor Roger Ekins of the Middlesex Hospital in London. The Multispot system utilises microfabrication technology to eliminate the need for accurate sample volume measurement and enables the simultaneous measurement of potentially hundreds of different molecules.[48]

A further advantage of sensor technologies is the potential for real-time monitoring of a binding event. The advantages of this have been exploited by the BIAcore™ and IASys™ optical sensor systems where real-time monitoring has revolutionised kinetic rate analysis of bimolecular interactions.[49,50] The possibilities of characterising the affinity and specificity of interactions both qualitatively and quantitatively are now being widely explored. Real-time analysis also enables continuous monitoring of fermentation systems, whereas metabolites have been monitored for a number of years, bioaffinity agents enable the production of more complicated molecules to be followed *in situ*.

There needs to be careful characterisation of the affinity, specificity, and stability of bioaffinity agents for use in quantitative analytical sensing systems and the best way to do this is rapidly becoming the focus of particular sensing technologies.

3.4 CHARACTERISATION OF BINDING SPECIFICITY AND AFFINITY

All of the above-mentioned bioaffinity agents have been used in different sensor systems, but the widest experience has been with the commercially available optical systems. Complicated receptor ligand interactions involving multiple components and even DNA:DNA interactions have been monitored, their kinetic rate constants determined, or the complex formed quantified. The possibilities of real-time kinetic rate analysis and automated epitope mapping have resulted in the use of the BIAcore™ and IASys™ to characterise and select antibody combinations for use in other immunological systems. The fundamental characteristics of any ligand:affinity agent interaction are specificity and affinity. The minimum affinity that will be required for a particular analytical task will depend upon the design of the analytical system and upon the concentration of the ligand to be measured; in the latter case the equilibrium rate constant K_A will need to be at least the same order of magnitude as the molarity of the ligand of interest.

For a measurement to be termed specific it is necessary to define the molecular or biological characteristic that a system should exclusively recognise. In the biosensors field this can be a particular molecular weight, a particular molecular charge, a particular molecular shape or epitope, or a particular chemical or biological activity. In some cases a less "specific" bioaffinity agent may be required, for instance if it is necessary to monitor the metabolites, e.g., of a drug as well as the parent molecule if they retain biological activity. The ability to recognise the selected molecular characteristic will be in part determined by the bioaffinity agent and partly by the detection technology employed. The specificity of the bioaffinity agent can be characterised and one with the desired behaviour selected; whilst affinity and specificity are intimately linked they need to be separately investigated. The best way to do this at present is to use the BIAcore™ and IASys™ sensor systems.

3.4.1 Kinetic Rate Analysis

Classical methods of kinetic rate analysis have been based around the original work of Scatchard[51] using equilibrium conditions which require days to achieve, during which any amount of degradation of the reactant molecules can occur and in any case only the equilibrium and dissociation rate constants could be measured directly. Furthermore, one of the reaction partners was required to be labelled, thus introducing an alteration from the natural state. The two commercialised optical sensor systems described above, and in particular the BIAcore™, have revolutionised our understanding of the kinetic interactions of biomolecular interactions in that they enable automated, real-time (i.e., continuous) monitoring of interactions, do not require the labelling of a ligand and can, in a matter of minutes to hours, provide direct quantification of both association and dissociation rate constants.[49] Many groups have now published kinetic rate constants for a variety of biomolecular interactions using one of these systems, and particularly due to the automation of the BIAcore™, vast amounts of kinetic data can now be generated.[49]

Kinetic rate analysis in these sensor systems uses genuine rate equations with sophisticated computer curve fitting and due to the continuous monitoring capabilities vast numbers of data points can be collected to improve the precision and accuracy of measurement. There are a number of authoritative reviews on the use of kinetic rate constant analysis so only a brief introduction will be given here.[52,53] The general rate equation used is shown below:

$$A_{bulk} \underset{k_m}{\overset{k_m}{\rightleftarrows}} A_{surface} + B \underset{k_{diss}}{\overset{k_{ass}}{\rightleftarrows}} AB$$

The observed rate of complex formation is as follows if $k_{ass}B << k_m$, i.e., mass transport is not rate limiting:

$$\frac{d[AB]}{dt} = k_{ass}[A][B] - k_{diss}[AB]$$

If $[B] = [B]_0 - [AB]$ then substituting

$$\frac{d[AB]}{dt} = k_{ass}[A]([B]_0 - [AB]) - k_{diss}[AB]$$

and if the complex formation is replaced by signal response R and $[B]_0 = R_{max}$, then this becomes:

$$\frac{dR}{dt} = k_{ass}[A](R_{max} - R) - k_{diss}R$$

on rearranging this becomes

$$\frac{dR}{dt} = k_{ass}[A]R_{max} - (k_{ass}[A] + k_{diss})R$$

which is in the form $y = mX + C$ if dR/dt is plotted against R and there are no mass transport problems. The degree of linearity of this plot can thus be used as part of the assessment of how large the contribution of mass transport is to the observed reaction rate (this is the first-derivative plot, see Figure 3.4). Because R_{max} is very rarely determined then k_{ass} and k_{diss} cannot be determined directly from this plot, so up to five different concentrations of A are used to determine slopes of the dR/dt vs. R plot and the slopes are then replotted against their respective [A]. The slope of this plot (the second-derivative plot, see Figure 3.4) gives the k_{ass} and the y intercept approximates to the k_{diss}. The plot should be linear and in both cases some assessment of fit of the plots to the data should be provided in the software. As most biomolecular interactions are neither univalent nor homogeneous there is usually some degree of nonlinearity in the first-derivative plot; this has been accommodated by use of nonlinear curve-fitting routines that enable an assessment of the number of components involved in the binding interaction, a further refinement not often used in equilibrium rate constant analysis.

Association rate constant measurement involves coupling the ligand to the sensor surface at a relatively low concentration in comparison with concentration measurement conditions. This is to reduce the impact of mass transport from the bulk phase to the boundary layer in contact with the sensor; if the boundary layer of the ligand is depleted too rapidly then the reaction kinetics monitored can reflect the transport from the bulk phase rather than the biomolecular interaction. Using efficient mixing, either flow or stirring, and relatively low

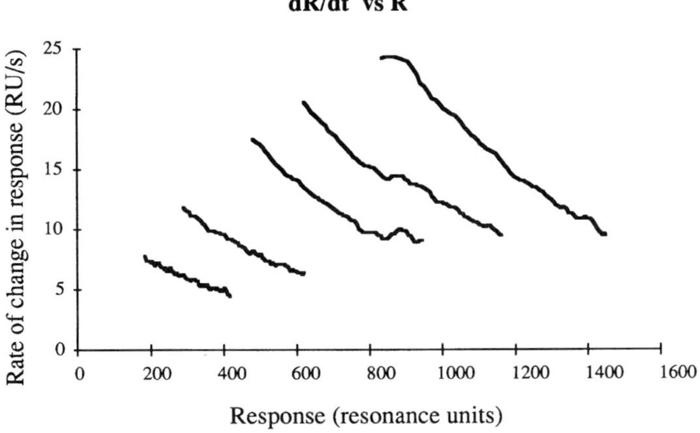

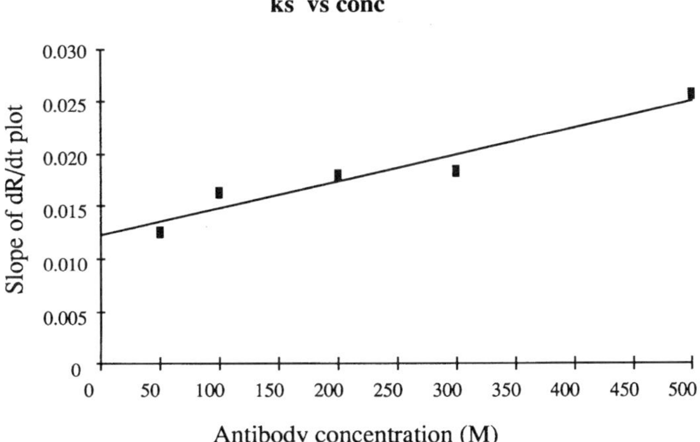

FIGURE 3.4 Kinetic rate analysis sensogram. First-derivative and second-derivative plots for phenytoin conjugated to the BIAcore™ sensor chip interacting with different concentrations of a Fab_2 fragment of a monoclonal antibody to phenytoin. The experiment was carried out in 10 mM HEPES buffer, pH 7.4, containing 150 mM NaCl.

ligand concentrations on the sensor, these problems can be reduced, but it should be recognised that it is extremely difficult to eliminate them completely.[54]

The value of k_{diss} obtained from the intercept of the second-derivative plot is not fully reliable due to the error in fitting the line. It is best to determine k_{diss} directly in a separate calculation although it can be a later part of the same experiment. The problem in measuring k_{diss} is to prevent reassociation of the binding partner. This is best prevented by the injection of an excess of the immobilised ligand in free form and then monitoring the dissociation reaction. Under these conditions

$$\frac{dR}{dt} = -k_{diss}R$$

On integration this becomes

$$R_t = R_0 \cdot e^{-k_{diss}(t-t_0)} \quad \text{or} \quad \ln\frac{R_0}{R_t} = k_{diss}(t - t_0)$$

where R_0 is a signal generated at an early stage in the dissociation reaction and R_t a signal generated "t" seconds later. Using nonlinear regression analysis k_{diss} can be calculated from the first version of the above equations. Alternatively plotting $\ln(R_0/R_t)$ vs. $(t - t_0)$ gives a straight line the slope of which equals k_{diss} (see Figure 3.5). The measurement of k_{diss} should be independent of the concentration of "A" used and thus only needs to be calculated from one experiment; if there are significant differences between values calculated from different "A" concentrations it is likely that some rebinding is occurring.

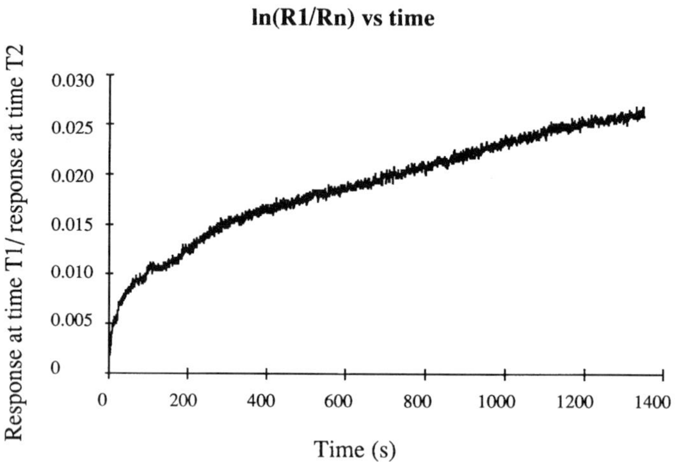

FIGURE 3.5 Dissociation rate constant analysis for the same model system as described in Figure 3.4.

There is a continuing discussion over the difference in values for k_{ass} and k_{diss} measured using surface effect devices such as BIAcore™ and IASys™ as compared to other more classical techniques, as each approach has its own artifacts and limitations. A pragmatic resolution to the controversy may be to accept that absolute rate constants cannot be measured; the values obtained using one system may not be equal to those from another, but there should be a proportionality between the different systems. This argument can be extended further to state that the value for an individual rate constant is only valid under the experimental conditions used to measure it, as has long been recognised to be the case with enzyme kinetics.[55] Experimental work in our own laboratory has shown significant influences of reaction buffer ionic strength, detergent concentration, and viscosity upon the values obtained for k_{ass}, k_{diss} and even K_{eq} using the BIAcore™ and IASys™ systems (see Figures 3.6 and 3.7). This is in addition to the well-known influences of reaction temperature on kinetic rate constants.[56]

The automated capabilities of these instruments with computerised data analysis has enabled a large expansion in the use of kinetic rate constant measurement that at times has appeared to be perhaps a little uncritical with regards to the limitations and difficulties of the experiments. Considerable care is required in the selection of experimental conditions, time points for data analysis, and in the assessment of the goodness of fit in the derivative plots, even when nonlinear routines are used. If these factors are taken care of then very reproducible results (CV of less than 10%) can be achieved, as shown in Figure 3.8 for a model anti-hapten:hapten interaction.

If quantitative assessment of rate constants is not required then qualitative assessments can be made even more rapidly as, for instance, in the selection of monoclonal antibodies, where affinity ranking can be very useful. However, it can also be extended to the analysis of receptor mutants, to drug arrays, and peptide and oligonucleotide variants. Such is the flexibility of these systems; it remains to be seen what the impact of other sensor systems

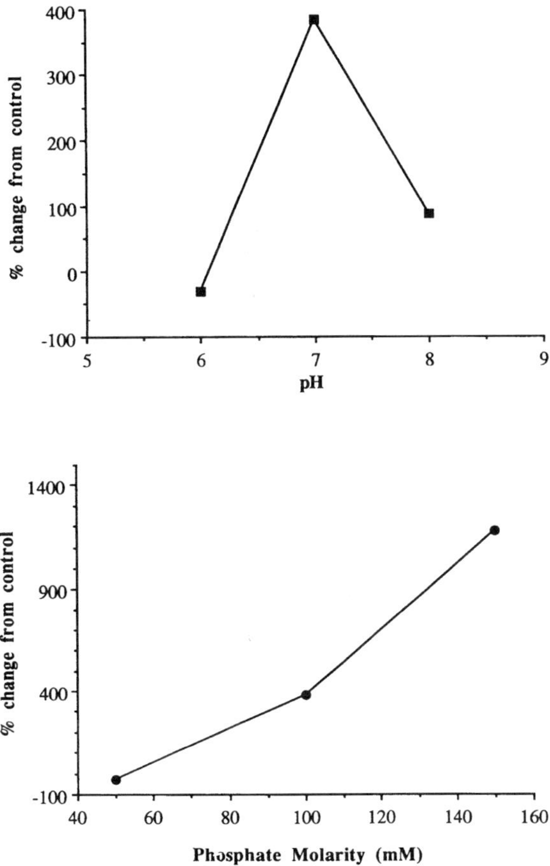

FIGURE 3.6 Influence of reaction conditions on equilibrium constant measurement (BIAcore™), the effects of reaction pH and phosphate buffer molarity on a model anti-phenytoin:phenytoin system. The control buffer is 10 mM HEPES buffer, pH 7.4, containing 150 mM NaCl, reference $K_A = 9.58 \times 10^8 M^{-1}$.

may be, as not all will be able to monitor reactions in real time, but the introduction of the optical systems described above has genuinely caused a revolution in kinetic rate constants analysis.

3.4.2 Epitope Mapping

Epitope mapping is the assessment of a panel of antibodies so as to determine which structural region of the antigen each individual antibody recognises; this enables complementary pairs of antibodies to be recognised so that they can be selected for use in sandwich immunoassays of enhanced specificity. This has classically been carried out using solid-phase ELISA techniques, but here too the introduction of automated optical immunosensor systems has revolutionised the mapping of large arrays of monoclonal antibodies and the effects of systematic peptide and oligonucleotide sequence alterations.

Essentially, either the antigen of interest is conjugated to the sensor or an antispecies antibody or Protein A/G surface is prepared (in this case the antibodies under investigation are captured and the antigen binding is monitored in a second reaction). Then, different antibodies are allowed to react with the surface with and without the other antibodies in the panel. With a sequential analysis of the type illustrated in Figure 3.9 the pattern of interactions can be elucidated and the antibodies grouped into different epitopic groups.

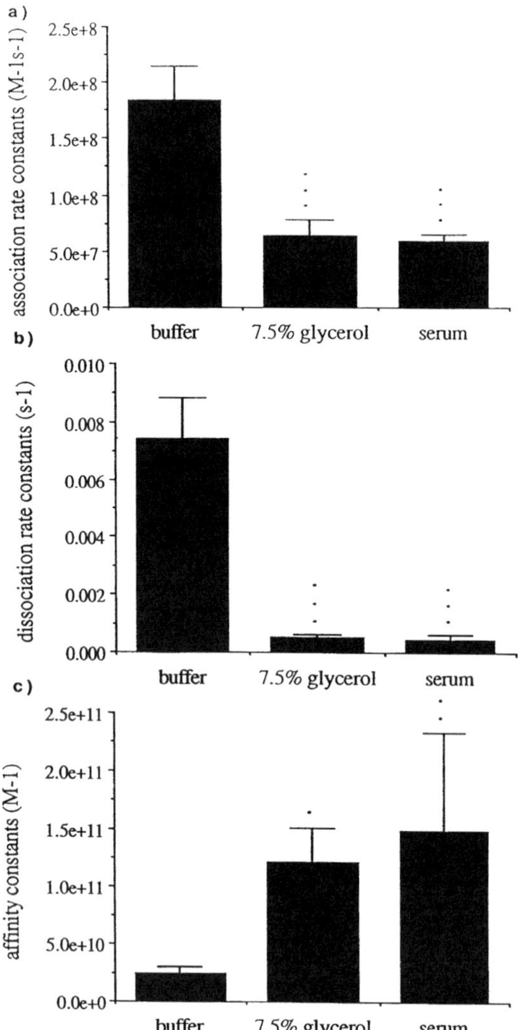

FIGURE 3.7 Influence of reaction conditions on equilibrium constant measurement (IASys™). The influence of sample matrix viscosity on the K_A for anti-$\beta_2$microgloblin:$\beta_2$microgloblin interaction.

Combining automated epitopic mapping and kinetic rate constant ranking enables rapid and more complete analysis of hybridomas at an earlier stage than in the usual screening cycle. Peptide and oligonucleotide series in which sequential mutations are introduced can be readily investigated for differences in binding affinity and specificity, by binding one sequence to the sensor surface and looking at competition for binding with the bioaffinity agent.

3.4.3 Selection of a Bioaffinity Molecule

The primary characteristic of a bioaffinity molecule is that it should be specific for the desired molecular characteristic or biological function. The characterisation of the specificity and affinity of the bioaffinity agent has been described in the previous section. It should be borne in mind that absolute specificity is not always required. It can be beneficial to have an antibody that recognises a group of metabolites as well as the parent compound. Having obtained the desired specificity and affinity there are several other characteristics that can help in the

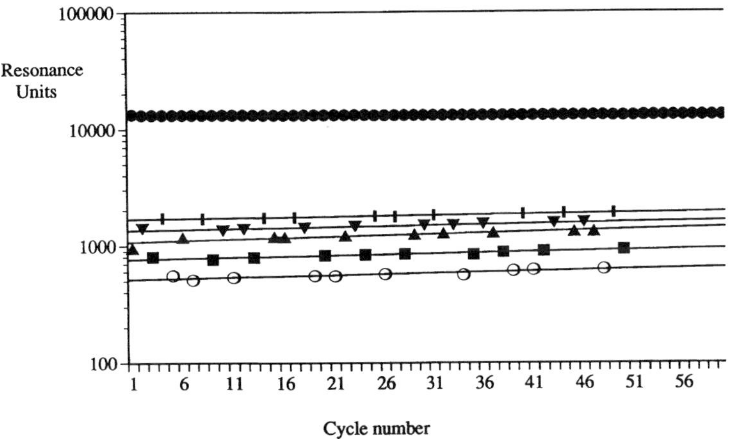

FIGURE 3.8 Stability of hapten:antihapten sensor surface for rate constant measurement. This represents 41 cycles of regeneration over a period of 1 month across 4 different sensor chip surfaces. The baseline is given in absolute resonance units (the highest plot) and the remainder are the resonance signals for different concentrations of monoclonal antibody. The model anti-phenytoin:phenytoin system in a buffer of 10 mM HEPES buffer, pH 7.4, containing 150 mM NaCl, mean $K_A = 9.58 \times 10^8$ M^{-1} with a CV of 37%. However, using only one sensor chip the CV is significantly better at 8.6%. Regeneration of the surface used 50 mM NaOH in 20% acetonitrile; the phenytoin was conjugated to the sensor surface.

selection of the most appropriate agent for use in a particular sensor system, that is, stability, tolerance to pH, purity, cost of production, and coupling chemistry (see Table 3.4).

When an impure bioaffinity molecule is all that is available, e.g., for measuring an antibody concentration and affinity in a human serum sample, then it can be more appropriate to couple the ligand of interest to the sensor surface. The same can apply when hapten interactions are being investigated as the binding signal from such a small molecule can be hard to detect, depending upon the sensor detection system. The coupling of the ligand will be much more idiosyncratic than binding the bioaffinity agent and can increase the possibility of nonspecific binding reactions. This, however, may also be the only choice if the bioaffinity agent itself is very unstable or prone to conformational changes upon coupling to the sensor surface.

3.4.3.1 Stability

Immunoglobulin molecules are generally very robust and when conjugated to solid phases retain their immunological activity for several years;[57,58] oligonucleotides and peptides can also be more stable conjugated to a solid phase than in free solution. The long-term stability of lectins on a solid phase is also likely to be good although there are little actual data. The least stable of the bioaffinity agents discussed are likely to be the receptor molecules, and their actual stability will be an individual characteristic.

The coupling of proteins to a solid phase per se has been shown to enhance the stability of a wide range of proteins; the difficulties lie not with the storage of the coupled proteins but in their ability to retain their activity in multi-use systems when regeneration cycles are required. The primary determinant of the stability of the bioaffinity agent under regeneration conditions will be the care with which these conditions have been optimised. Information on the likely stability of different bioaffinity molecules to regeneration can often be obtained from publications concerning their use in affinity chromatography systems. Thus stability is inherently interlinked with tolerance to pH as modulation of pH is one of the most important dissociation factors. The coupling of enzymes and immunoglobulins to solid phases has been

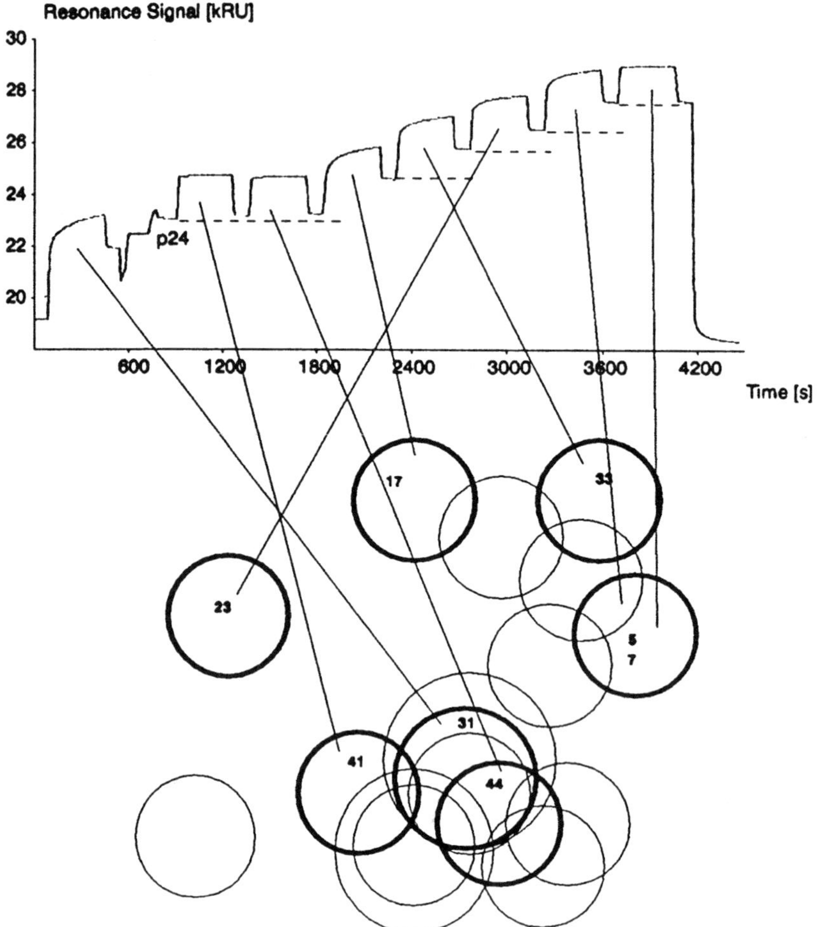

FIGURE 3.9 Epitope mapping using an optical biosensor. An automated epitope analysis of 30 monoclonal antibodies to recombinant HIV core protein p24 was carried out by pair-wise binding tests dividing the 30 antibodies into 17 groups representing 17 epitopes on the antigen. Anti-mouse IgG:Fc was immobilised on the chip and the surface regenerated with 100 mM HCl. Circles represent epitopic regions of the protein.

TABLE 3.4
Strategy for Selection of Bioaffinity Agent

Decide whether system is to be qualitative or quantitative.
Quantitative systems can be more demanding of the affinity of the bioaffinity agent.
Decide whether system is to be single or multiple use.
Stability of bioaffinity agent is vital if multiple use is required.
What is the molar concentration of ligand?
Equilibrium constant should be of the same order of magnitude.
What is the molecular characteristic that is important?

shown to enhance their tolerance to pH to include short exposure to pHs between 1 and 13.[59] The pH range used can be reduced by inclusion of chaotropic agents such as acetonitrile[60] and the use of high ionic strength and detergents.[61] These same factors will need optimisation if the ligand molecule is conjugated to the sensor surface.

3.4.3.2 Purity

It is best to couple a purified bioaffinity agent to the surface of the sensor in order to ensure good control over coupling density and to minimise nonspecific interactions; if one is not available but a pure source of the ligand is, then it is better that this is conjugated to the surface. In the case of polyclonal antibodies it is better that either an immunoglobulin fraction or an affinity purified preparation is used. For monoclonal antibodies, antibody fragments, and sFv's, chromatographically pure preparations should be made; for lectins and proteins A and G the commercial sources should already be pure, but there are always possibilities of batch to batch variations. A further alternative is to use purified second-antibody systems to capture primary antibody from a tissue culture supernatant. Oligonucleotides synthesised automatically can be obtained 90% pure. The purity requirement is perhaps more relevant to the specificity of the interaction to be monitored as the contaminants are likely to be of similar structure to the target sequence. The greatest difficulty can come with the purification of membrane-bound receptors; it is probably more appropriate with receptors to use purified ligands on the sensor surface and this may also be true for novel binding proteins.

3.4.3.3 Cost of Production

The cost of a bioaffinity agent will be a combination of the cost of production and ease of reuse; thus an expensive agent can be more cost-effective if it can withstand a large number of regeneration cycles. Commercial sources of monoclonal antibodies, lectins, proteins A/G, and oligonucleotides can all be expensive, costing hundreds of dollars per milligram. These costs can apparently be reduced by in-house production, but usually only if the true labour costs are defrayed. The relative cost of antibodies is fragments > intact monoclonals = affinity purified intact polyclonals > immunoglobulin fractions > antiserum. One of the advantages of antibody production using recombinant DNA technology is the cost benefit compared with other methods of production.

3.4.3.4 Coupling Techniques[62-64]

The technique used to couple a bioaffinity agent can have a profound effect on its utility. Most workers would agree that a covalent coupling technique is required for immobilisation to the sensor surface and a wide range is available, some of which are listed in Table 3.5. These can be complemented by techniques that enable spacers of various length to be introduced; the general aim of these techniques is to ensure a stable conjugation with an appropriate orientation of the molecules to enable fully functional interactions. These all require the molecule to be conjugated to have a suitable active residue for conjugation — most commonly a free amino group, but carboxyl, aldehyde, and sulphydryl groups can also be used. The different conjugation techniques use a range of pHs and reagents and these can have a profound effect upon the activity and stability of the conjugated bioaffinity agent. If an appropriate orientation or activity cannot be obtained using direct coupling techniques then an indirect one such as second antibody, Proteins A/G, or biotin:streptavidin should be used. Further possibilities of protecting or stabilising unstable macromolecules include adding the antigen/ligand to the antibody/receptor to form a more stable complex which can then be conjugated to the sensor surface.

TABLE 3.5
Coupling Techniques for Use With Sensor Devices

Sensor active group	Ligand active group	Conjugation chemistry
$-COOH$	$-NH_2$	Carbodiimide, e.g., EDC/NHS
$-NH_2$	$-NH_2$	Glutaraldehyde
	$-SH$	Sulphydryl
$-OH$	$-NH_2$	Cyanogen bromide, tosyl chloride
$-CONH_2$	$-NH_2$	Hydrazide
$-CONHNH_2$	$-CHO$	Hydrazine

3.5 OPTIMISATION OF BINDING ASSAYS

All immunoassays and other binding assays require careful optimisation of the reaction conditions under which the molecular interactions are allowed to occur. The same general approaches can be taken whether the reactions occur in the liquid phase or on a solid phase as the intermolecular forces are common to all interactions and it is only the balance between them that will be different. The overall aim is to promote a rapid and specific interaction with minimal nonspecific binding and, if multiple use is envisaged, suitable baseline stability and functional activity following regeneration (see Table 3.6).

TABLE 3.6
Factors Influencing Performance of Binding Assays

Concentration and conformation of the bioaffinity molecule on the sensor surface
- Conjugation chemistry
- Use of spacer sequences

Reaction buffer: pH, ionic strength, and nature of anion
Reaction temperature
Nonspecific binding
Sample viscosity, pH, ionic strength, etc.
Mixing of sample and buffer and delivery to bioaffinity molecule
Interfering substances: rheumatoid factor, metabolites of parent compound
Regeneration of bioaffinity surface

3.5.1 Concentration of Bioaffinity Agent

The amount of bioaffinity agent or ligand coupled to the sensor surface requires some optimisation, as the optimal amount will depend upon the use to which the sensor is to be put. For concentration measurement using a noncompetitive binding assay a high concentration of bioaffinity agent is required to ensure the rapid attainment of the binding equilibrium that will give maximal response. For competitive binding assays and kinetic rate constant measurement a much lower concentration of ligand or bioaffinity agent is required. The actual amounts conjugated will depend upon the individual sensor design.

3.5.2 Reaction Buffer

The choice of the reaction buffer and its constituents is of paramount importance; different bioaffinity agents will have different pH and ionic strength optima. These have to be balanced against the nonspecific interactions that can be caused by the biological matrix that is to be used, and which can be minimal at reaction conditions a long way away from the optimum for the binding activity of the bioaffinity agent. This can result in a need to include other constituents in the buffer: chaotropes such as acetonitrile or potassium chloride, detergents such as SDS or Tween 20, and accelerators of binding interactions such as polyethylene glycol and various dextran polymers. The balance between these parameters will need to be empirically optimised for each bioaffinity agent and matrix combination.

Additional buffer constituents such as dithiothreitol may need to be added if specific interferences from the matrix are encountered. In other instances, when matrix interferences cannot be eliminated by appropriate buffer optimisation, then as a last resort a sample pretreatment such as protein precipitation may be necessary (see Section 3.5.4).

3.5.3 Nonspecific Binding

Surface effect technologies are particularly prone to the phenomenon of nonspecific binding and this includes all solid phase immunoassay technologies. Nonspecific binding leads to the generation of a signal response independent of the bioaffinity agent:ligand interaction; this can be hydrophobic and/or electrostatic in nature and is predominantly determined by the substrate to which the bioaffinity agent is conjugated at the sensor surface. The dextran polymers that have been used in the BIAcore™ and IASys™ systems have proved very successful in reducing the nonspecific binding (that can be a significant problem in biological matrices such as serum) to an insignificant level when used in combination with the selection of appropriate running buffers. Other surfaces e.g., gold films, may be significantly more prone to nonspecific binding; another example of this is the protein fouling that occurs with ion-selective electrode membranes.

3.5.4 Matrix Effect and Sample Preparation

Currently there are relatively few sensor technologies that have achieved reliable performance in biological matrices. This has been less due to the bioaffinity agents employed than the sensing technologies; the biological matrix, in particular the blood serum matrix, has caused significant difficulties in the field of biosensors. However, there are some common features of the biological matrix that need to be contemplated and need careful optimisation of the analytical system. These are listed in Table 3.6.

Highly proteinaceous fluids give rise to significant viscosity effects that will reduce rates of reaction even with careful attention to adequate mixing, either by stirring or flow.[65] For accurate quantification and kinetic rate constant measurement a constant dilution of a serum sample should be used and the calibrator, if an external one is used, should be prepared in the same matrix as the sample. This assumes that a sample is analysed directly; if this is not the case and a preparative procedure is required, then whilst the convenience of a sensor will be diminished so will the matrix effects.

3.5.5 Single Use as Compared to Regeneration

Single use sensor devices will engender different problems than multiple use devices, but they have one significant advantage in that no regeneration of the sensor surface is required. The antibody:antigen complex is highly stable and requires moderately stringent conditions to disrupt it. The binding forces involved are well described elsewhere[66,67] and their disruption using chaotropic agents, ionic strength, low pH, detergents, etc. are as one would expect from the common reagents used during affinity chromatography experiments (see Table 3.7). The selection of the appropriate regeneration conditions is intimately associated with the selection of an appropriate bioaffinity agent that can withstand them. For instance it may be more appropriate to use a second-antibody system, where an excess of second antibody can be coupled to the sensor surface rather than a fixed amount of primary antibody, resulting in a greater number of reuse cycles. The use of a common second antibody or Proteins A/G system can also reduce fabrication costs and enable a common regeneration system to be used with a number of different primary antibody systems.

TABLE 3.7
Regeneration Conditions

Low pH
High ionic strength
Ionic detergents
Chaotropic buffers, e.g., containing acetonitrile
Excess free ligand, e.g., glucose in the case of a lectin

3.5.6 Examples of Bioaffinity Ligands in use on Optical Sensor Devices

3.5.6.1 β2m: Measurement of Antibody Binding

Purified β2microglobulin (11,800 Da, pI 5.4) is coupled to the carboxylated dextran on the surface of the IASys™ sensor chip using a two-step carbodiimide chemistry in sodium formate buffer pH 4.5, followed by blocking of the remaining active groups using ethanolamine. Serum β2microglobulin can be measured using a competitive inhibition assay format with regeneration of the surface between binding cycles using 10 mM HCl. Figure 3.10 gives a representative standard curve; approximately 50 repeat cycles can be used.[65]

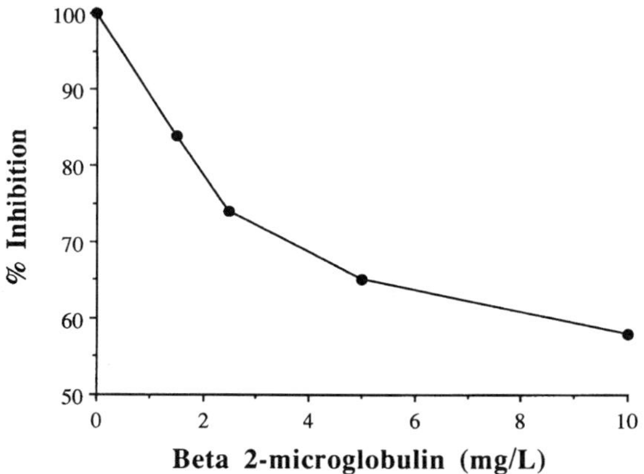

FIGURE 3.10 Serum β2m assay on the FAST IASys™. Human β2m was immobilised on the surface of a cuvette using EDC/NHS chemistry. Polyclonal anti-β2m is mixed with a serum sample containing free β2m which competes with the β2m bound to the surface. The assay takes 3 min and the surface is regenerated with 10 mM HCl.

3.5.6.2 Lectin Interactions with Immobilised Glycoproteins[68]

Four glycoproteins:thyroglobulin, fetuin, IgG and GP120 were conjugated to a BIAcore™ sensor chip using an amine coupling protocol (Figure 3.11). Seven lectins were evaluated for the relative specificity and affinity of binding to each of the four glycoproteins; control experiments used a blank sensor surface exposed to the coupling procedure and a nonglycosylated recombinant protein. All kinetic interactions were performed in 10 mM HEPES buffer with surface regeneration using 10 mM HCl.

3.5.6.3 DNA:DNA Interactions[69]

Oligonucleotides of varying lengths (19 to 50 mer) were synthesised by phosphoramidite chemistry with a 5′ biotin tail. Streptavidin was conjugated to the surface of an IASys™ cuvette using EDC/NHS chemistry in acetate buffer at pH 5. The hybridisation reaction between different complementary oligonucleotides was monitored by capturing a biotinylated partner to the sensor surface and then passing over this a complementary but nonbiotinylated oligonucleotide, as shown in Figure 3.12. Hybridisation was carried out at 25°C at pH 6.8 in a sodium citrate/phosphate buffer containing 0.1% Tween 20, sodium chloride, and Denhardt's solution; control experiments with noncomplementary oligonucleotides showed no hybridisation. Both association and dissociation kinetics could be monitored; regeneration of the streptavidin surface could be achieved by 10 mM HCl.

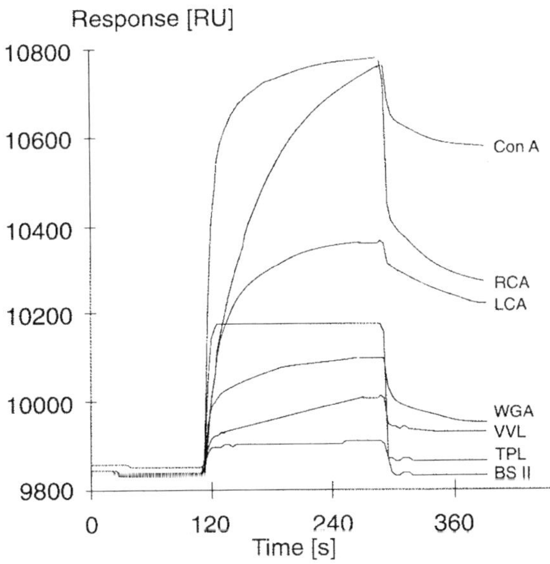

FIGURE 3.11 Lectin interactions with immobilised glycoproteins. Human thyroglobulin was immobilised on the surface of a BIAcore™ flow cell using an amine coupling procedure. Seven different lectins were passed over the thyroglobulin surface at 50 μg/ml in 10 mM HEPES buffer; the surface was regenerated with 100 mM HCl. Con A = *Canavalia ensiformis*, RCA = *Ricinus communis*, LCA = *Lens culinaris*, WGA = *Triticum vulgare*, VVL = *Vicia villosa*, TPL = *Lotus tetragonolobus*, BS II = *Griffonia simplifolia*.

3.5.6.4 DNA:Protein Interactions

The interaction of a nuclear oncoprotein (ETS1) and an ETS1-derived peptide with specific and mutant DNA sequences was investigated on the BIAcore™.[70] Streptavidin was conjugated to the sensor chip using EDC/NHS chemistry and biotinylated oligonucleotide sequences were captured followed by investigation of the association and dissociation of both the peptide and intact protein (see Figure 3.13). The oligonucleotide surface could be regenerated using 0.05% SDS.

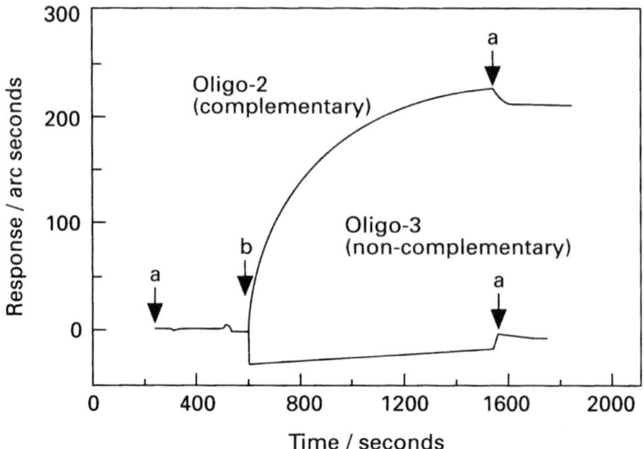

FIGURE 3.12 DNA:DNA interaction sensogram. Specific hybridisation of oligonucleotides complementary to the captured biotinylated oligonucleotide (Oligo-2) and noncomplementary (Oligo-3); a = addition of hybridisation buffer, b = addition of oligonucleotides.

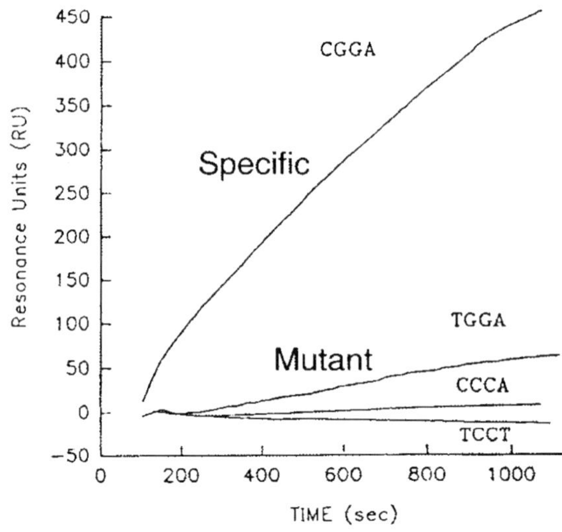

FIGURE 3.13 DNA:protein interaction sensogram. Interaction between the nuclear oncoprotein ETS1 and specific/mutant DNA. The DNA surface was regenerated using 0.05% SDS. CGGA is a specific DNA sequence and TGCA, CCCA, and TCCT are mutant DNA sequences.

3.5.6.5 Cellular Interactions

Binding of L cells bearing the CEA antigen to an immobilised anti-CEA antibody. A specific monoclonal antibody was immobilised onto an aminosilane-modified IASys™ cuvette at pH 7.4; the remaining active groups were then blocked using bovine serum albumin. Surface regeneration required 20 mM HCl and the binding of approximately 5×10^4 L cells per millilitre could be easily monitored and distinguished from nonexpressing cells (see Figure 3.14).[71]

3.5.6.6 sFv to an Antigen

Numerous examples exist in the literature to demonstrate the use of biosensors for comparisons of the binding parameters of antibody fragments with that of intact antibody. Our

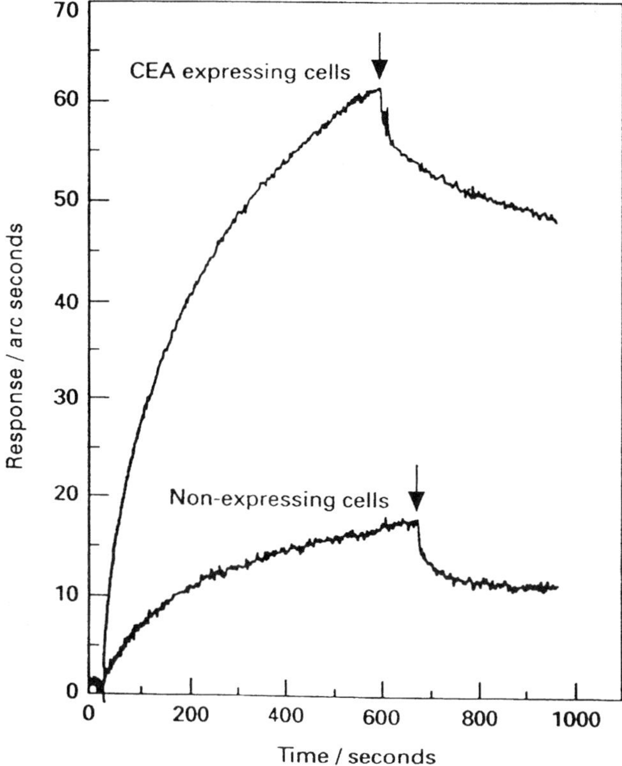

FIGURE 3.14 Binding of L cells to an anti-CEA antibody-derivatised surface. Cells were added and binding followed in about 10 min. The arrows indicate the washing out of unbound cells with phosphate-buffered saline.

experience is with sFv's derived from hybridomas producing anti-alkaline phosphatase antibodies which show varying degrees of cross reactivity with the bone and liver isoenzymes of this protein. Bone alkaline phosphatase extracted from the osteosarcoma cell line, Saos-2, was immobilised on the surface of a sensorchip using amine coupling chemistry.[63] Partially purified antibody or sFv were injected at a flow rate of 5 µl/min. Dissociation rates, which are independent of sample concentration, were determined by monitoring the decrease in signal following replacement of the sample with buffer (HEPES buffered saline). The dissociation kinetics (in real time) of the intact and sFv antibodies to immobilised antigen were 5×10^{-3} and 1.96×10^{-3} s^{-1}, respectively. Thus the off rate of the sFv was of a similar order to that of the intact antibody and is consistent with values published for sFv's against hen egg lysozyme.[72] An alternative approach to the use of purified antigen onto the sensorchip is to coat a second antibody, for example anti-mouse Fc-specific antibody, or an antibody against a peptide tag which can be incorporated into the DNA construct for the sFv. The antibody 9E10 which recognises the myctag peptide has been exploited for this purpose by many groups including ourselves. Using the model antigen lysozyme, and sFv contructs derived from the antibody D1.3, Prospero et al. demonstrated that good estimates of kinetic parameters of antibodies and genetically engineered fragments could be obtained using this approach.[73]

3.6 SUMMARY AND CONCLUSIONS

A wide range of bioaffinity ligands is available for use in sensor systems. The appropriate one for a particular molecule will depend upon the characteristics of the sensor device (detection technology, single vs. multiple usage) and on the molecular characteristics that are to be monitored. The practical difficulties of using sensor devices in biological matrices are less due to the bioaffinity agents chosen than to the nature of the sensor surface and the detection system used. In comparison with existing high-sensitivity immunoassay technologies using the same bioaffinity agents, sensor devices have still to realize their potential and seem unlikely to exceed the detection limits already obtained, even with signal enhancement techniques. The advantages of sensing systems are likely to be in their uses in real-time monitoring situations, in multiple analyte measurements using microfabrication technologies, or in single-use devices for near-patient or field-based testing.

REFERENCES

1. Gally, J. A. (1973), Structure of immunoglobulins. In *The Antigens*, Sela, M., Ed., Academic Press, New York, Vol. 1, p. 162.
2. Edelman, G. M. (1970), The covalent structure of a human λG-immunoglobulin X1. Functional implications, *Biochemistry*, 9, 3197-3205.
3. Nissonoff, A., Hopper, J. E., and Spring, S. B. (1975), *The Antibody Molecule*, Academic Press, New York, chap. 3.
4. Kabat, E. A. (1982), Antibody diversity versus antibody complementary, *Pharmacol. Rev.*, 34, 23-38.
5. Maki, R., Kearney, J. F., Paige, C., and Tongewa, S. (1980), Immunoglobulin gene rearrangements in immature B cells, *Science*, 209, 1366.
6. Perry, R. P., Kelley, D. E., Coleclough, C., and Kearney, J. F. (1981), Organization and expression of immunoglobulin genes in fetal liver hybridomas, *Proc. Natl. Acad. Sci. U.S.A.*, 78, 247-251.
7. Jeske, D. J., Jarvis, J., Milstein, C., and Capra, D. (1984), Functional diversity is essential to antibody diversity, *J. Immunol.*, 133, 1090-1092.
8. Bernard, O., Hozumi, N., and Tongewa, S. (1978), Sequences of mouse immunoglobulin light chain genes before and after somatic mutation, *Cell*, 15, 1133.
9. Berek, C. and Milstein, C. (1987), Mutation drift and repertoire shift in the maturation of the immune response, *Immunol. Rev.*, 96, 23-41.
10. Steward-Tull, D. E. S. and Rowe, R. E. C. (1975), Procedures for large-scale antiserum production in sheep, *J. Immunol. Methods*, 8, 37-45.
11. Hurn, B. A. L. and Chantler, S. M. (1980), Production of reagent antibodies. In: *Methods in Enzymology*, Vol. 70, Immunochemical Techniques, Part A, Academic Press, London.
12. Burrin, J. M. and Newman, D. J. (1991), Production and assessment of antibodies. In: *Principles and Practice of Immunoassay*, Price, C. P. and Newman, D. J., Eds., Macmillan, London, p. 19.
13. Benecerraf, B. and Germoin, R. N. (1978), The immune response genes of the major histocompatibility complex, *Immunol. Rev.*, 38, 70.
14. Vaitukaitis, J., Robbins, J. B., Nieschlag, E., and Ross, G. T. (1971), A method for producing specific antisera with small doses of immunogen, *J. Clin. Endocrinol. Metab.*, 33, 988-91.
15. Harlow, E. and Lowe, D., Eds., (1988), Immunisations: In *Antibodies: A Laboratory Manual*, Cold Spring Harbor Laboratory, Cold Spring Harbor, New York, p. 53-138.
16. Kohler, G. and Milstein, C. (1975), Continuous cultures of fused cells secreting antibody of pre-defined specificity, *Nature*, 256, 495-7.
17. Galfre, G. and Milstein, C. (1981), Preparation of monoclonal antibodies: strategies and procedures, *Methods Enzymol.*, 73, 3-46.
18. Gefter, M. L., Margulies, D. H., and Scharf, M. D. (1977), A simple method for polyethylene glycol promoted hybridisation of mouse myeloma cells, *Somat. Cell. Genet.*, 3, 231-236.
19. Chambers, R. E., Whicher, J. T., Perry, D. E., and Milford-Ward, A. (1987), Overestimation of immunoglobulins in the presence of rheumatoid factor by kinetic immunonephelometry, *Ann. Clin. Biochem.*, 24, 520-524.
20. Lamoyi, E. and Nisonoff, A. (1983), Preparation of $F(ab')_2$ fragments from mouse IgG of various subclasses, *J. Immunol. Methods*, 56, 235-243.

21. Rousseaux, J., Rousseaux-Provost, R., and Bazin, H. (1983), Optimal conditions for the preparation of Fab and F(ab')$_2$ fragments from monoclonal IgG of different rat IgG subclasses, *J. Immunol. Methods,* 64, 141-146.
22. Eng, R. H. K. and Person, A. (1981), Serum cryptococcal antigen determination in the presence of rheumatoid factor, *J. Clin. Microbiol.,* 14,700-702.
23. Winter, G. and Milstein, C. (1991), Man-made antibodies, *Nature,* 349, 293-299.
24. Marks, J. D., Griffiths, A. D., Malmqrist, M., Clackson, T. P., Bye, J. M., and Winter, G. (1992), By-passing immunization: binding high affinity human antibodies by chain shuffling, *Bio/Technology,* 10, 779-783.
25. Saiki, R. K., Scharf, S., Faloona, F., Mullis, K. B., Horn, G. T., Erlich, H. A., and Arheim, N. (1985), Enzymatic amplification of beta-globulin genomic sequences and restriction site analysis for diagnosis of sickle-cell anaemia, *Science,* 230, 1350-1354.
26. Bird, R. E., Hardman, K. D., Jacobson, J. W., Johnson, S., Kaufman, B. M., Lee, S. M., Lee, T., Pope, S. H., Riordan, G. S., and Whitlow, M. (1988), Single chain antigen-binding proteins, *Science,* 242, 423-426.
27. Huston, J. S., Levinson, D., Mudgett-Hunter, M., Tai, M. S., Novotny, J., Margolies, M. N., Ridge, R. J., Bruccoleri, R., Haber, E., Crea, R., and Oppermann, H. (1988), Protein engineering of antibody binding sites. Recovery of specific activity in an anti-digoxin single-chain FV analogue produced in *E. coli, Proc. Natl. Acad. Sci. U.S.A.,* 85, 5879-5883.
28. Clackson, T., Hoogenboom, H. R., Griffiths A. D., and Winter, G. (1991), Making antibody fragments using phage display libraries, *Nature,* 352, 624-628.
29. Vlatakis, G., Andersson, L. I., Muller, R., and Mossbach, K. (1993), Drug assay using antibody mimics made by molecular imprinting, *Nature,* 361, 645-647.
30. Liener, I. E., Sharon, N., and Goldstein, I. J., Eds. (1986), *The Lectins: Properties, Functions, and Applications in Biology and Medicine,* Academic Press, New York
31. Sumner, J. B. and Howell, S. F. (1936), *J. Bacteriol.,* 32, 227-237.
32. Hutchinson, A.. M. (1994), Characterisation of glycoprotein oligosaccharides using surface plasmon resonance, Proc. 4th Eur. BIA Symp., 84-87.
33. Townsend, R. R., Alai, M., Hardy, M. R., and Fenselau, C. C. (1988), *Anal. Biochem.,* 171, 180-191.
34. Doods, H. N. and van Meel, J. C. A. (1991), *Receptor Data for Biological Experiments,* Ellis Horwood, Chichester, England.
35. Williams, R., Buckle, M., and Buc, H. (1994), Direct analysis of the kinetics of binding of cAMP and DNA to the cyclic AMP receptor protein of Escherichia coli, Proc. 4th Eur. BIA Symp., 132-133.
36. Boyle, M. D. P., Ed. (1990), *Bacterial Immunoglobulin-Binding Proteins,* Vol. I, Microbiology, chemistry and biology, Academic Press, New York.
37. Boyle, M. D. P., Ed. (1990), *Bacterial Immunoglobulin-Binding Proteins,* Vol, II, Applications in Immunotechnology, Academic Press, New York.
38. Langone, J. J. (1978), ^{125}I-Protein A: a tracer for general use in immunoassay, *J. Immunol. Methods,* 24, 269-285.
39. Cruss, B. (1986), Structure of the IgG-binding regions of streptococcal protein G, *Embo. J.,* 5, 1567-1575.
40. Bayer, E. A. and Wilcheck, M. (1978), The avidin-biotin complex as a tool in molecular biology, *Trends Biochem. Sci.,* 3, N257-259.
41. Green, N. M. (1975), Avidin, *Adv. Protein Chem.,* 29. 85-133.
42. Bondeson, K., Frostell-Karlsson, A., Fagerstam, L., and Magnusson, G. (1993), Lactose repressor-operator DNA interactions: kinetic analysis by a surface plasmon resonance biosensor, *Anal. Biochem.,* 214, 245-251.
43. **Anon.,** Kinetic Characterisation of DNA Hybridisation Using Real Time BIA, *Short Communication 306,* Biosensor, Uppsala, Sweden.
44. Felder, S., Zhou, M., Hu, P., Urena, J., Ulrich, A., Chaudhuri, M., White, M., Shoelson, S. D., and Schlessinger, J. (1993), SH2 domains exhibit high-affinity binding to tyrosine-phosphorylated peptides yet also exhibit rapid dissociation and exchange, *Mol. Cell. Biol.,* 13, 1449-1455.

45. Zhang, Z., Frears, E., Blake, D. R., and Winyard, P. G. (1994), Observation of both proteinase and proteinase inhibitor activities by surface plasmon resonance, Proc. 4th Eur. BIA Symp., 94-99.
46. Gosling, J. P. (1990), A decade of development in immunoassay methodology, *Clin. Chem.,* 36, 1048-27.
47. Price, C. P. and Newman, D. J., Eds., (1991), *Principles and Practice of Immunoassay,* Macmillan, London.
48. Ekins, R. P., Chu, R., and Biggart, E. (1990), The development of microspot, multi-analyte ratiometric immunoassay using dual fluorescent-labelled antibodies, *Anal. Chim. Acta,* 227, 73-96.
49. Karlsson, R., Michaelson, A., and Mattsson, I. (1991), Kinetic analysis of monoclonal antibody-antigen interactions with a new biosensor based analytical system, *J. Immunol. Methods,* 145, 229-240.
50. Cush, R., Cronin, J. M., Stewart, W. J., Maule, C. H., Molloy, J., and Goddard, N. J. (1993), *Biosens. Bioelectron.,* 8, 347-393.
51. Scatchard, G. (1949), The attractions of proteins for small molecules and ions, *Ann. N. Y. Acad. Sci.,* 51, 660-672.
52. Altschuh, D., Dubs, M.-C., Weis, E., Zeder-Lutz, G., and van Regenmortel, M. H. C. (1992), Determination of kinetic rate constants for the interaction between a monoclonal antibody and peptides using surface plasmon resonance, *Biochemistry,* 31, 6298-6304.
53. Malmborg, A. C., Michaelsson, A., Ohlin, M., Jansson, B., and Borreaeck, C. A. K. (1992), Real time analysis of antibody-antigen reaction kinetics, *Scand. J. Immunol.,* 35, 643-650.
54. Matsuda, H. (1967), Theory of the steady-state current potential curves of redox electrode reactions in hydrodynamic voltammetry. II. Laminar pipe and channel flows, *J. Electroanal. Chem.,* 15, 325-36.
55. Gutfreund, H. (1971), *Enzymes: Physical Principles,* John Wiley & Sons, London, p. 157-174
56. Johnstone, R. W., Andrew, S. M., Hogarth, M. P., Pietersz, G. A., and McKenzie, I. F. C. (1990), The effects of temperature on the binding kinetics and equilibrium constants of monoclonal antibodies to cell surface antigens, *Mol. Immunol.,* 27, 327-333.
57. Thakkar, H., Davey, C. L., Medcalf, E. A., Skingle, L., Craig, A. R., Newman, D. J., and Price, C. P. (1991), Stabilisation of turbidimetric immunoassay by covalent coupling of antibody to latex particles, *Clin. Chem.,* 37, 1248-1251.
58. Butler, J. A. (1991), The behaviour of antigens and antibodies immobilised on a solid phase. In: *Structure of Antigens,* Van Regenmortel, M. H. V., Ed., CRC Press, Boca Raton, FL.
59. Monsan, P. and Combes, D.. (1988), Enzyme stabilisation by immobilisation. Immobilised enzymes and cells, Part D, *Methods Enzymol.,* 137, 584-598.
60. Hodgkinson, S. C. and Lowry, P. J. (1982), Selective elution of immunoadsorbed anti- (human prolactin) immunoglobulins with enhanced immunochemical properties, *Biochem. J.,* 205, 535-541.
61. Fulop, M. J., Webber, T., and Manchee, R. J. (1993), Use of a zwitterionic detergent for the restoration of the antibody binding capacity of immunoblotted *Francisella tubarensis* lipopolysaccharide, *Anal. Biochem.,* 203, 141-145.
62. Al-Abdulla, I. H., Mellor, G. W., Childerstone, M. S., Sidki, A. M., and Smith, D. S. (1989), Comparison of three different activation methods for coupling antibodies to magnetisable cellulose particles, *J. Immunol. Methods,* 122, 253-258.
63. O'Shannessy, D. J., Brigham-Burke, M., and Peck, K. (1992), Immobilisation chemistries suitable for use in the BIAcore surface plasmon resonance detector, *Anal. Biochem.,* 205, 132-136.
64. Spitznagel, T. M. and Clark, D. S. (1993), Surface density and orientation effects on immobilised antibodies and antibody fragments, *Biotechnology,* 11, 825-829.
65. Morgan, C. L., Newman, D. J., Burrin, J. M., and Price, C. P. (1995), The matrix effects on kinetic rate constants of antibody-antigen interactions are caused by viscosity, submitted.
66. Van Oss, C. J. (1991), Antigen-antibody reactions. In: *Structure of Antigens,* Van Regenmortel, M. H. V., Ed., CRC Press, Boca Raton, FL.
67. Jefferis, R. and Deverill, I. (1991), The antigen antibody reaction. In: *Principles and Practice of Immunoassay,* Price, C. P. and Newman, D. J., Eds., Macmillan, London.

68. Bhikhabhai, R., *Short Communication 407,* Biosensor, Uppsala, Sweden.
69. Watts, H. and Parkes, H., *IASys™ Application Note 3.3,* Fisons Applied Sensor Technology, Cambridge, U.K.
70. Fisher, R. J., Baxevanis, A. D., Fivash, M. J., Mavrothalassitis, G., Bladen, S. V., Moudrianakis, E. N., and Papas, T. S. (1992), *Short Communication 403,* Biosensor, Uppsala, Sweden.
71. Snary, D., IASys™ Application Note 5.2, Fisons Applied Sensor Technology, Cambridge, U.K.
72. Holliger, P., Prospero, T. D., and Winter, G. (1993), Diabodies, small bivalent and bispecific antibody fragments, *Proc. Natl. Acad. Sci. U.S.A.,* 90, 6444-6448.
73. Prospero, T. D., Holliger, P., and Winter, G. (1993), Rapid kinetics on surface captured antibody fragments, Third BIA Symp., London.

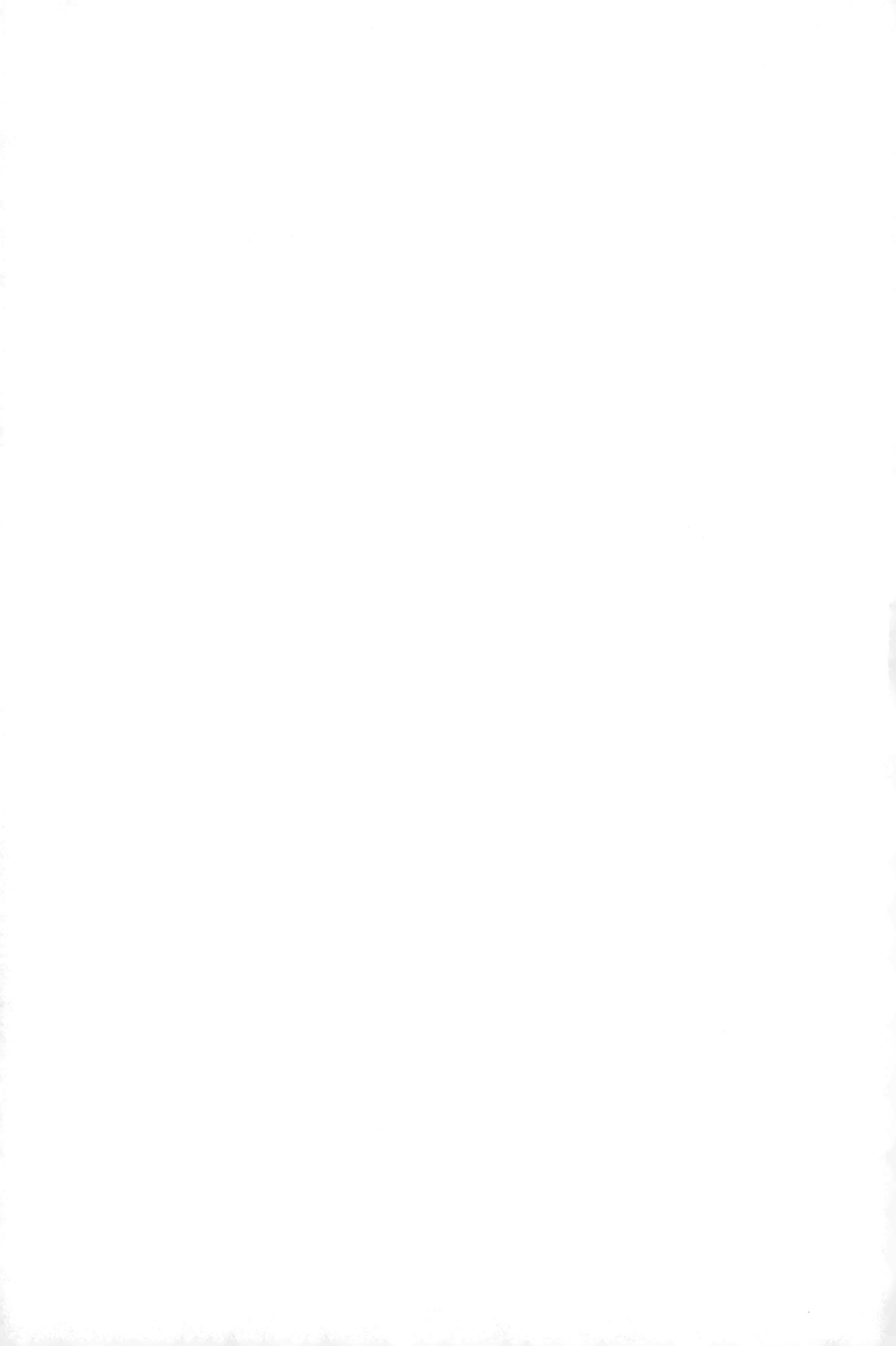

4 Probes for Nucleic Acids and Biosensors

Richard W. Titball and David J. Squirrell

CONTENTS

4.1 INTRODUCTION

The elucidation of the structure of the DNA duplex was heralded as a great breakthrough in understanding the way in which biological systems were controlled. However, few scientists could have fully appreciated the signficance of this finding nor could they have predicted the way in which this discovery would transform almost all aspects of our understanding of the biological sciences.

The sequence of nucleotides within a gene coding segment of DNA determines the unique properties of the product of that gene. If two strands of DNA with complementary sequences are aligned they will bind together, or "hybridise", to form a duplex.[1] It is the specificity of this pairing process which is exploited for the design and use of gene probes.

Gene probes have many applications. They can be used to examine the genetic makeup of an individual and can therefore reveal the presence of genes or mutant genes associated with genetically determined diseases.[2] Several of these, including phenylketonuria, Lesch-Nyhan syndrome, and factor IX deficiency, can now be diagnosed prenatally.[2] Progress with

0-8493-8905-4/97/$0.00+$.50
© 1997 by CRC Press, Inc.

the human genome organisation project over the next decade will facilitate further applications of gene probes — not only for prenatal diagnosis, but also for the identification of genes associated with diseases in later life such as cancer and heart disease.[2] In the longer term, the development of such powerful genetic characterisation techniques will permit therapies designed to alter the genes associated with these diseases.

Another application of gene probes will be for determining the presence of an organism in various environments. An obvious use will be for the detection of disease-causing microorganisms in water supplies, foodstuffs, or in plant, animal, or human tissues. Gene probes are already finding applications in such tests.[3-5] As the biotechnology revolution gains pace and plants, animals, and microorganisms are genetically engineered to modify their properties to meet our requirements, the regulatory systems for controlling and monitoring them will require the development of systems for their identification.

Gene probes are certain to play an increasingly important role in health care, agriculture, and environmental monitoring. However, at present, the use of gene probes requires relatively complex and time-consuming procedures which limit their full potential.[6,7] Biosensors (either in the strictest sense with direct linkage of binding events to signal transduction or, maybe in the nearer future with looser coupling between the hybridisation event and output generation) could be used to relieve current limitations of gene probe assays by making them faster and easier to perform. The aim of this chapter is to review the properties of gene probes and to examine whether gene probe biosensors are a realistic and realisable prospect which will find a place in society over the next decade.

4.2 PROPERTIES OF NUCLEIC ACID PROBES

4.2.1 Recognition of Nucleic Acid Sequences

The term nucleic acid **probe** describes a segment of nucleic acid which specifically recognises, and binds to, a nucleic acid **target**. The recognition is dependent upon the formation of stable hydrogen bonds between the two nucleic acid strands. This contrasts with interactions of antibody with antigen where hydrophobic, ionic, and hydrogen bonds play a role. The bonding between nucleic acids takes place at regular (nucleotide) intervals along the length of the nucleic acid duplex, whereas antibody-protein bonds occur only at a few specific sites. The frequency of bonding is reflected in the higher association constant for a nucleic acid duplex in comparison with an antibody-protein complex and indicates that, in principle, highly specific and sensitive detection systems can be developed using nucleic acid probes.[3,8] The specificity of nucleic acid probes relies on the ability of different nucleotides to form bonds only with an appropriate counterpart. Thus cytosine nucleotides form triple hydrogen bonds with guanine nucleotides and adenine nucleotides form double hydrogen bonds with thymidine nucleotides (see Figure 4.1). These considerations are important since the stability of the duplex will be influenced by the composition such that G/C rich sequences are more stable than A/T duplexes. In reality, the pairing of nucleotides may be more complex than that described above since uracil (as found in RNA) may also form stable bonds with adenine residues. In addition, several nucleotide analogues with modified pairing properties have been described. For example, the nucleotide analogue 2-aminoadenine[9] forms triple hydrogen bonds with thymidine. Other workers have used inosine, which forms a double hydrogen bond with cytosine, in place of guanine to increase the specificity of a probe.[10] The overall influence of the nucleotides within the probe is to alter the number of hydrogen bonds formed and so affect the temperature at which the hybrid dissociates and reassociates (the melting temperature: T_m). Any mismatch between probe and target causes a degree of destabilisation of the hybrid, which can be compensated for by lowering the temperature of the reaction. This property is obviously of significance in biosensors which can be temperature controlled, since the temperature must be set at a level permitting specific hybridisation to the target sequence whilst minimising nonspecific hybridisations.[11]

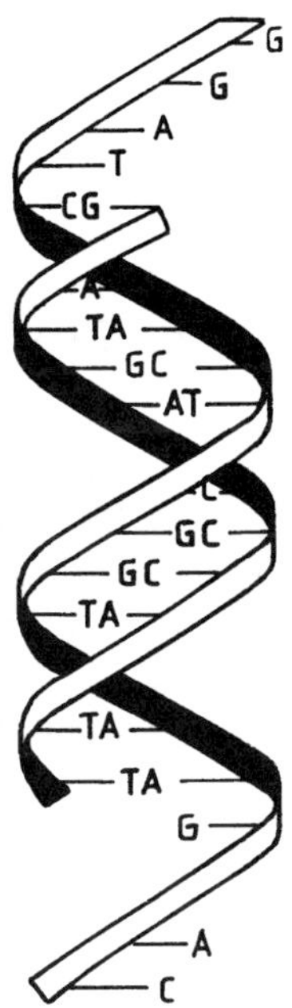

FIGURE 4.1 The recognition of a single-stranded nucleic acid fragment by a nucleic acid probe. The binding of a nucleic acid probe to a fragment of single-stranded DNA is shown. Triple hydrogen bonds form between paired G-C nucleotides whilst A-T nucleotide pairs are bonded by double hydrogen bonds. In the example shown, the probe and target sequences are complementary. The mismatching of nucleotides in the probe and target sequence would lead to destabilisation of the hybrid.

4.2.2 Design and Specificity of Nucleic Acid Probes

Gene probes can vary in length from tens to several hundred or even thousands of nucleotides. Generally, in recent years, the trend has been towards the design of short oligonucleotides — often fewer than 30 nucleotides in length. This trend has been facilitated by the development of efficient automated equipment for the synthesis of oligonucleotides. The design of short oligonucleotides without the loss of specificity is governed by several factors; specificity ultimately being a function of the frequency with which the target sequence might be encountered as a random event. This can be calculated using the equation:[12]

$$P_o = (1/4)^L \cdot 2C \tag{4.1}$$

where: P_o = probability of a sequence occurring randomly
L = length of the oligonucleotide (number of nucleotides)
C = complexity of target genome (nucleotide pairs)

When $4^L = 2C$ the chance of a sequence occurring randomly in the target genome is 1. With the *E. coli* genome of 4×10^6 base pairs a probe 15 nucleotides in length would be expected to react, on a random basis, with a probability of less than 1:1000. In practice, a minimum probe length of 20 to 25 nucleotides would be used to ensure specificity.

Other workers have devised additional "rules" for the design of oligonucleotide probes which enhance their specificity: the probe should not be able to anneal with itself to form hairpin structures, and should not contain tracts of three or more similar nucleotides. Since G-C bonds are stronger than A-T bonds it is also desirable to pick target regions with a G+C content of close to 50%, so that the probe-target hybrid will be most stable and most specific. For some target sequences it may be useful to know how the target DNA is folded such that accessible regions of the NA are targetted for probe design. Finally, in some laboratories, selected probe sequences are screened against one of the databases containing all reported DNA sequences to date, to gain a theoretical appraisal of the specificity of the probe. Together, these strategies have considerably enhanced our capability to design specific probes, but the final assessment of the utility of a probe can only be made by performing laboratory tests.

4.2.3 The Kinetics of Hybridisation of Gene Probes

The process by which the probe hybridises to target NA has been examined in detail by many workers.[13,14] The kinetics of this process are obviously of great significance when considering the performance of a biosensor based on NA probe technology. The most rapid hybridisation reactions occur when both probe and target are in solution, and under these conditions the reaction shows second-order kinetics.[14] In systems where the target nucleic acid is immobilised on a solid phase the hybridisation rate is 5 to 10 times slower.[15] In a solid phase hybridisation with the probe in excess, the kinetics of hybridisation will approximate to first order. Under these conditions, the rate of hybridisation can be increased by decreasing the probe length or increasing the probe concentration, as can be calculated from the equations of Meinkoth and Wahl[16] and Wetmur and Davidson.[17]

$$t_{1/2} = \frac{N \ln 2}{K_n\left(L^{0.5}\right)C} \tag{4.2}$$

where: N = probe complexity (N = probe length in nucleotides (L) for a probe with no repeated sequences).

K_n = nucleation constant = 3.5×10^5 for Na^+ concentrations in the range 0.4 to 1.0 M, pH 5 to 9, and hybridisation at 25°C below the T_m of the probe-target hybrid.

C = probe concentration (moles probe/litre).

L = probe length (number of nucleotides).

$t_{1/2}$ = time (s) for 50% hybridisation of probe to target.

The effect of probe length on the rate of hybridisation can be marked; under similar conditions, a 2-kb (kilobases) probe will take 161 h to reach an equivalent degree of hybridisation to the target as a 20-mer probe would reach in 10 min. In many of the nucleic acid biosensors currently under development the probe is immobilised onto a solid phase and the target is captured. Since the target DNA may be several hundred thousand kilobases in the case of chromosomal DNA, the biosensor configured in this way would appear to be at a marked disadvantage in terms of sensitivity. This limitation could be overcome in a number of ways. Hybridisation accelerators such as dextran sulphate,[18] polyethylene glycol (PEG),[19] and polyacrylic acid[20] can increase the hybridisation rate up to 100-fold for double-stranded probes (or target, in the case of biosensors). However, the simplest solution is to reduce the size of the target nucleic acid captured, to select short target molecules, or to configure the biosensor in a format which allows hybridisation to proceed in solution (see Figure 4.2). The target nucleic acid could be mechanically or enzymatically sheared to reduce the size or a short nucleic acid fragment could be generated using, for example, the polymerase chain reaction (PCR). In some cases short target molecules, such as plasmids or rRNA, are naturally present, eliminating any processing stage.

Other factors in addition to fragment length may have a significant influence on hybridisation reactions. These have been reviewed extensively by other workers.[13,14,18] Hybridisation of probe with target is optimal at a temperature 25°C below the T_m of the hybrid and is also affected by the ionic strength and viscosity of the solution. The effect of increasing NaCl

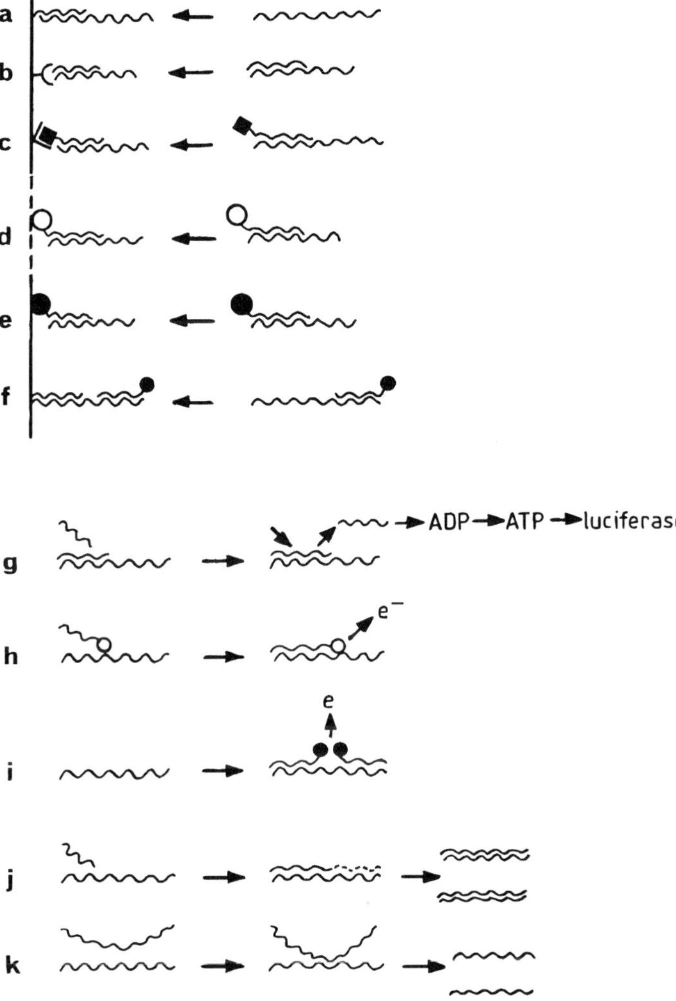

FIGURE 4.2 Formats for the configuration of gene probes in biosensors. Solid phase capture formats for gene probe biosensors are shown in panels **a** to **f** and solution-phase reactions with gene probes are shown in panels **g** to **k**. The target nucleic acid could be captured using a probe immobilised on a solid phase (**a**). If the probe is first reacted with target nucleic acid in solution then antibodies or other molecules which reacted with double-stranded DNA could be used to capture the probe-target hybrid (**b**). Solution-phase reaction of the target nucleic acid with a probe which had been labelled with a ligand would permit capture of the hybrid using a molecule (e.g., an antibody) with high affinity for the ligand (**c**). The labelling of the probe with a large ligand could permit capture of the hybrid using filtration (**d**), or labelling with a magnetic bead would permit capture of the hybrid using a magnetic field (**e**). In any of these formats, a second probe, labelled with a reporter group, could also be reacted with the target nucleic acid in solution (**f**) and the hybrid captured using the methods outlined in (**a**) to (**e**). In solution-phase reactions a number of methods have been proposed for detecting reaction of the probe with the target. A specific probe could be used to displace a prebound probe, which would then serve as a substrate in a chemiluminescent reaction (**g**). The use of a probe label, which is excited on binding to double-stranded DNA, would lead to the emission of detectable energy (**h**) as would the adjacent binding of two probes labelled, respectively, with exciter and emitter molecules (**i**). Several techniques have been described for the amplification of nucleic acid in solution including the polymerase chain reaction (**j**) and Q-beta replicase amplification of the nucleic acid target (**k**).

concentration, up to 3.2 M, can be marked[17,21] with a 5- to 6-fold increase in the rate of hybridisation of RNA with DNA on increasing the NaCl concentration from 0.2 to 1.5 M, it has been reported.[22] Control of these parameters is necessary in gene probe biosensors to allow reproducibility between tests. This situation contrasts with antibody-based biosensors where considerable latitude in temperature and ionic strength can be tolerated without significantly compromising the performance of the system.

4.3 EXTRACTION, IMMOBILISATION, AND AMPLIFICATION OF NUCLEIC ACIDS

4.3.1 Rapid Methods of Nucleic Acid Extraction

Since nucleic acids are almost invariably contained within a cell or virus particle, it is apparent that access of the probe to the target molecule is limited without a sample treatment stage. In many cases the sample can be treated with detergents and NaOH to lyse cells and denature proteins.[18] Treatment with NaOH would also denature double-stranded nucleic acids so that on neutralisation the single-stranded target molecules would be available for hybridisation. The presence of detergent would not significantly affect hybridisations, but would limit the effectiveness of some enzyme-based target amplification systems. This methodology may be suitable for samples containing relatively high concentrations of the target nucleic acid, and clinical samples for analysis using the Gen-Probe PACE™* system do not require anything other than an initial cell lysis step before reaction with the probe. Simple lysis steps with direct analysis of the released NA have also been proposed for microorganism detection in water samples.[23] Rapid sample preparation in this manner is less well suited to other environmental samples (such as soil samples) where cleanup and purification of the nucleic acid may be required before analysis.[24]

4.3.2 Amplification of Nucleic Acid Sequences

In principle, nucleic acid probes can detect picogram quantities of nucleic acid. For some applications this detection limit may be acceptable. However, for others, such as the detection of pathogens in the environment, this detection limit is not sufficiently sensitive. To improve the performance of a gene probe assay, it may be necessary to amplify the target. One approach may be to detect a target sequence which is naturally present in an amplified form. For the detection of bacteria an approach which has attracted particular attention over the past decade has been based on ribosomal RNA target molecules.[25,26] In the typical bacterial cell 10^3 to 10^4 copies of rRNA are present, providing a naturally amplified target. The utility of rRNA-based detection systems has been significantly enhanced by the finding that the rRNA is often unique to a bacterial species,[25] providing the opportunity to develop specific gene probes. Additional benefits from the selection of rRNA as the target molecule arise from the relatively small size of the molecule (which aids extraction and rapid diffusion in solution). Limitations of this approach occur mainly because of the similarity of rRNA from some related bacterial species, making specific detection impossible, and the highly folded nature of the rRNA molecule which can limit accessibility of the target sequence to the probe.

Alternative approaches to the amplification of the target molecule rely on the enzymatic amplification of a fragment of the nucleic acid to which the probe is able to bind. PCR is the best-developed amplification system.[27-29] Amplification of the target molecule is achieved using a thermostable DNA polymerase with repeated cycles of heating (to denature the duplex), cooling (to allow hybridisation of the probe with the target), and an intermediate temperature cycle which allows the DNA polymerase to replicate a fragment of the target molecule (Figure 4.2j). Laboratory PCR systems typically take several hours for an amplification of the target molecule by 10^6-fold, but in principle the time taken for cycling could

* Registered trademark of the Gen-Probe Corporation.

be reduced. Rapid PCR systems, taking 15 min, have been reported,[30] but it is not clear whether the time required for the PCR can be reduced to a few minutes, which would be desirable in a biosensor system. In addition, the enzymes involved in these amplification systems may be sensitive to inactivation by other materials present in the sample. For example, the PCR system cannot be used directly on samples rich in humic acid.[31]

Other systems using the ligase chain reaction or Q-beta-replicase amplification[32,33] have been developed over the past five years. The Q-beta-replicase system relies on the hybridisation of the probe sequence, flanked by 223 nucleotides from the MDV-1 phage (a derivative of phage Qβ). Unhybridised probe is removed by washing and the bound probe can then be eluted and serves as the substrate for Q-beta-replicase amplification (Figure 4.2k). The advantages of this system — the reaction may take less than 30 min for a billionfold amplification — are offset by the high background signal obtained in many systems.

Notwithstanding these problems, the amplification systems described above could be used in conjunction with a biosensor to detect low levels of target nucleic acid in the sample. Indeed, advantage could be taken of the amplification process to introduce labels into the amplified target molecules. These could be small ligands such as biotin to facilitate separation steps and/or labels such as fluorophores to aid detection.

4.3.3 Immobilisation of Nucleic Acid Probes on Solid Phases

It is conceivable that future biosensor systems will rely on solution hybridisation of probe with target nucleic acid. However, most of the reported applications rely on the immobilisation of one component (often the probe) onto a solid phase: the sensor surface. The immobilisation of nucleic acid on a solid phase has been used extensively in laboratories over the past decade, but the precise chemical interactions are relatively poorly understood. Nitrocellulose has frequently been used for the immobilisation of nucleic acid in hybridisation assays. Nitrocellulose membrane is convenient to use and results in high signal-to-noise ratios. Noncovalent forces are thought to be involved in the initial binding of nucleic acid[16] and baking at 80°C results in firm attachment of the nucleic acid to the solid phase. More recently, other solid phases have been favoured over nitrocellulose. The binding of nucleic acid to nylon, and especially cationic derivatives of nylon, is highly efficient involving hydrophobic and ionic interactions.[18,34,35] Nucleic acid binding to these membranes (350 to 500 mg/cm^2) is much higher than with nitrocellulose (80 to 100 mg/cm^2), but the signal-to-noise ratio may be lower.[36] Polyvinylidene difluoride (PVDF) solid phases are able to bind nucleic acid with even higher efficiencies than nylon, via hydrophobic and ionic forces. A variety of solid phases could therefore be used in biosensors and the selection of surfaces which promote hydrophobic interactions and ionic interactions (with the phosphate group of the nucleic acid) is essential. The configuration of the nucleic acid when bound to the membrane has not been investigated. Presumably the immobilisation of short fragments of nucleic acid may limit accessibility of the probe for hybridisation with target. Difficulties with immobilisation could be overcome by promoting binding of one end of the probe to a suitably modified solid surface. Synthesis of oligonucleotides with amino, thiol, or biotin groups at either the 5′ or 3′ end is now common practice and the authors envisage that probes with such modifications will become standard tools in the development of gene probe biosensors. Immobilisation of these modified probes will be controllable and will permit more efficient hybridisation reactions to take place.

4.4 HYBRIDISATION FORMATS FOR GENE PROBES

Many of the research applications of gene probes have relied on a simple, well-proven, and sensitive format in which the target DNA is first immobilised on a solid phase and then allowed to hybridise with a probe under closely controlled conditions. The probe may be labelled with a radioisotope, an enzyme, or a hapten. Such tests may be highly sensitive, detecting less than 1 pg of target DNA. However, they may take several hours or days to perform. When the requirement for rapid or real-time detection is considered it is apparent that these conventional laboratory techniques are not suited to development in biosensors.

A variety of methods, limited only by the ingenuity of the inventor, have been described for detecting probe binding to target nucleic acid. Figure 4.2 illustrates some of these configurations which may be suitable for biosensors. Capture of the target nucleic acid may be by direct hybridisation with an immobilised probe (Figure 4.2a). Equally possible is the use of a capture antibody which recognises the double-stranded hybrid (Figure 4.2b). In some formats the probe may be labelled with a hapten and the hapten can react with a suitable immobilised antibody or ligand[37,38] (Figure 4.2c). A possible disadvantage of any solid phase capture reaction is the time taken for the reaction to proceed to equilibrium. To some extent these problems can be overcome by coating the capture probe onto beaded particles and then collecting the hybrid complex attached to the bead. If latex beads are used the complex can be captured by filtration[20] (Figure 4.2d), but a much more rapid configuration relies on the use of magnetic beads which are rapidly captured onto a solid phase in an applied magnetic field[39] (Figure 4.2e). Any of these formats could be modified by the use of a second probe, labelled with a reporter group such as an enzyme, which reacts with the target at a different site[40-42] (Figure 4.2f). The advantage of such "sandwich" hybridisation formats resides in the increased specificity arising from two separate probe-target hybridisations.

The elusive goal of workers in the area of hybridisation formats has been the development of an efficient homogeneous assay, where all stages of the assay take place in solution with resultant gains in sensitivity and reductions in the time taken for the assay. Several workers have devised homogeneous assays, but in all cases the sensitivity of the systems has been disappointing. In the system described by Vary et al.[43] the target molecule displaced a prebound RNA probe (Figure 4.2g). The displaced probe was degraded into the constituent nucleotides, and the ADP generated after conversion to ATP by pyruvate kinase served as a substrate in a luciferase reaction. Not surprisingly, the level of background signal is high in this system and it is difficult to envisage how the system could be used in a biosensor where the target may be contained in a sample rich in ATP and ADP (e.g., from bacterial cells or tissues). An alternative approach to developing a homogeneous assay was described by Nelson et al.[44] The probe is labelled with an acridinium ester which can be cleaved from free probe but not from hybridised probe (Figure 4.2h). Since the acridinium ester emits chemiluminescence only when in the context of nucleic acid, any signal should arise from bound probe. This system has proven to be reasonably sensitive (about 1 ng of target) and has been used to detect an amplified target (rRNA). In another system proposed by Heller and Morrison,[45] two probes are allowed to hybridise to adjacent locations on the target DNA strand. One probe is labelled with a chemiluminescent exciter group (Figure 4.2i). This is able to excite a fluorescent reporter group attached to the second probe only when the two groups are in close proximity: when both probes have hybridised. Although this concept is elegant in principle, in practice the signal-to-noise ratio of the assay is low. Gene probe assays for the detection of some species of bacteria have been developed and marketed by the Gen-Probe Corporation, but have yet to receive wide acceptance. All of these examples do show that homogeneous assays can be developed and that some would be suitable for use in true biosensor systems.

4.5 BIOSENSORS

The development of gene probe biosensors is very much in a state of infancy. Direct monitoring of hybridisation reactions has been demonstrated with piezoelectric acoustic wave devices and the evanescent wave methods of total internal reflection fluorescence (TIRF) and surface plasmon resonance (SPR). These techniques, and studies with them concerning gene probes, are therefore described in detail below.

In addition, although involving procedures that are rather too indirect and slow to be qualified unreservedly as "biosensor" assays, details on the light-addressable potentiometric sensor (LAPS) are given since this has been used to provide sensitive quantitation of PCR reactions. Mention is also made of other approaches described in the literature.

4.5.1 Evanescent Wave Biosensors

4.5.1.1 Total Internal Reflection Fluorescence (TIRF)

The evanescent wave generated by totally internally reflected light at the surface of a waveguide penetrates a short distance into the surrounding medium (see Chapters 8 and 17). Fluorophores within the evanescent zone absorb light from the waveguide and light emitted from them is coupled back into the waveguide. A simple optical setup as shown in Figure 4.3a, in which emitted light travelling in the reverse direction to the excitation beam is measured, allows binding of fluorophores at subnanomolar concentrations to be observed.[46,47] Only fluorophores within about 100 nm of the waveguide surface are detected.[48] Unbound material further away than this does not interfere so assays can be performed without the need for wash steps, with great benefit in terms of reducing assay time. A review of TIRF can be found in Place et al.[49]

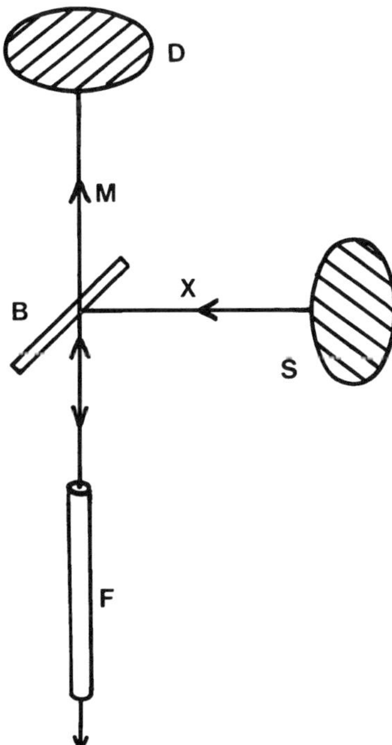

FIGURE 4.3a Diagrammatic representation of instrumentation required for total internal reflection fluorescence using a fibre optic waveguide. A light beam (X) at the excitation wavelength of the fluorophore is launched from a source (S) and enters the fibre optic waveguide (F) after reflection from a beam splitter (B). Fluorescence from labelled target nucleic acid bound to the surface is coupled into the fibre. Back-propagated emitted light (M) passes through the beam-splitter to the detector (D). Note: the excitation beam actually enters the fibre as a cone of light and a dichroic mirror can be used instead of a beam-splitter. See Glass et al.[75] for a detailed description.

The fluorescent reporter molecule required for gene probe TIRF assays can either be introduced as an intercalating dye,[50,51] or be covalently attached to an oligonucleotide. In the latter case the fluorescent tag may be directly linked to the target; for example, when the target is in the form of a PCR product in which a labelled primer has been used, it may be indirectly attached to the target in a "sandwich assay" or, as suggested by Hirschfeld and Block,[50] a "competition assay" format can be used where binding of a labelled oligomer is titrated against the target. These formats are illustrated in Figure 4.3b.

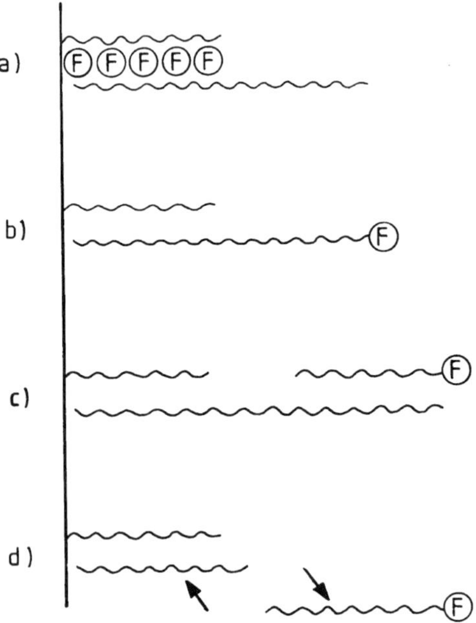

FIGURE 4.3b Formats for gene probe assays using a TIRF biosensor. In (**a**) formation of a nucleic acid duplex by binding of probe and target is signalled by the binding of an intercalating dye which preferably exhibits fluorescence enhancement so as to reduce the background from unbound dye. In (**b**) and (**c**) the target itself is tagged: as the product of an amplification reaction with a fluorophore-labelled primer in (**b**), and by a second probe in a sandwich assay in (**c**). A competition assay format is shown in (**d**) where target nucleic acid competes with a labelled oligonucleotide for binding to the probe.

Graham et al.[11] showed that it is possible to monitor specific hybridisation of labelled oligonucleotides using TIRF. Amino-ended 16- or 20-base DNA probes were covalently coupled to the surface of optic fibres and hybridisation to complementary fluorescein-ended oligonucleotides was monitored. Hybridisation was observable within seconds, and the initial rate of binding was shown to be proportional to the solution concentration of the target with a nanogram per millilitre of target being detectable. Hybridised target could be removed by heating, thereby allowing the optic fibres to be reused many times. The endpoint measurements made in conventional hybridisation assays take hours or days to perform[52] compared with a minute or so needed for the kinetic measurements that are possible with this technique (Figure 4.3c).

4.5.1.2 Surface Plasmon Resonance (SPR)

In SPR biosensors,[53,54] polarised light is totally internally reflected from the surface of a waveguide which is coated with a thin (e.g., 60 nm) film of a metal such as gold or silver. At a sharply defined angle of incidence the reflected beam is strongly attenuated (Figure 4.4a), its energy being transferred to the surface electrons with the generation of an intense,

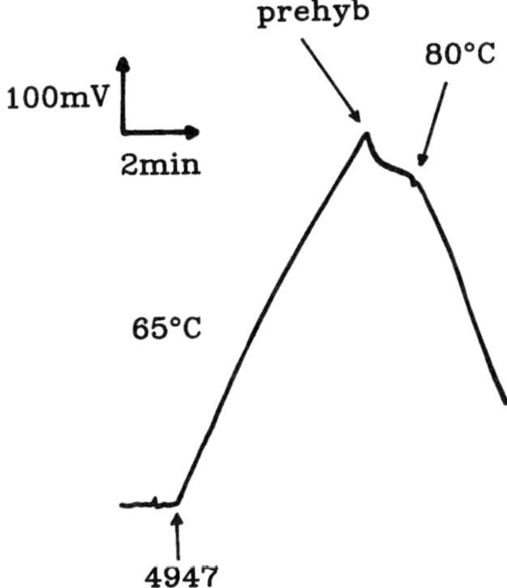

FIGURE 4.3c Binding of a fluorescein-labelled target to a probe immobilised on the surface of an optic fibre. Hybridisation, indicated as a rise in detector voltage, occurs immediately on introduction of the target (designated 4947). When target solution is replaced by buffer ("prehyb"), there is a small, rapid fall in output as unbound target within the evanescent zone is flushed away followed by slow dissociation at 65°C. As the temperature is raised to 80°C, rapid dissociation of target is observed.

evanescent electric field. The angle at which this resonance happens depends upon the wavelength of the light and the refractive indices of the waveguide and of the external medium. Material binding to the waveguide surface changes the refractive index there, and so changes the angle of resonance. The resultant angle shift is proportional to the amount of analyte bound. (For a detailed description of SPR biosensors, see Chapters 7 and 16.)

Because the signal is generated by an intrinsic property of the analyte — its refractive index or rather its difference from the solvent, which in the case of nucleic acids is relatively high at 1.66 compared to about 1.48 for proteins, the refractive index of water being 1.33 — no labels are required for SPR assays. In addition, no wash steps are required because separation of bound analyte from that in solution is provided by the evanescent field. This makes SPR assays very simple and rapid to perform.

Various instrument configurations are available for SPR. The simplest, conceptually, is the Kretschmann format[55] shown in (Figure 4.4b). This can be reconfigured as a solid-state device with a fan beam providing the incident light and an array detector measuring the reflectance over a range of angles simultaneously (Figure 4.5a). In a further development of this arrangement (Figure 4.5b) the fan beam is extended to give a wedge-shaped beam, and by use of a two-dimensional array detector several spots on the waveguide surface can be monitored simultaneously and independently.

Measurement of nucleic acid hybridisation by SPR was demonstrated by Charles and co-workers at Amersham:[56,57] 17- or 50-base oligonucleotide probes were attached to silver-coated waveguides at concentrations of around 100 femtomole/mm^2 (about 1 ng).* Allowing 30 min for hybridisation to occur, a 97-base target sequence could be detected with a sensitivity of approximately 1 femtomole/mm^2 (30 pg).

Extending this work to real-time analysis, Schwarz et al.[58] were able to detect 320 fg of a 97-base target and 24 fg of a 7.2-kb target within 5 min. These were captured by the 50-base probe immobilised on a 100-µm^2 sensing spot.

* The detection limits in these reports were given as amounts bound as determined through radiolabelling of the probes and targets. Solution concentrations were not stated.

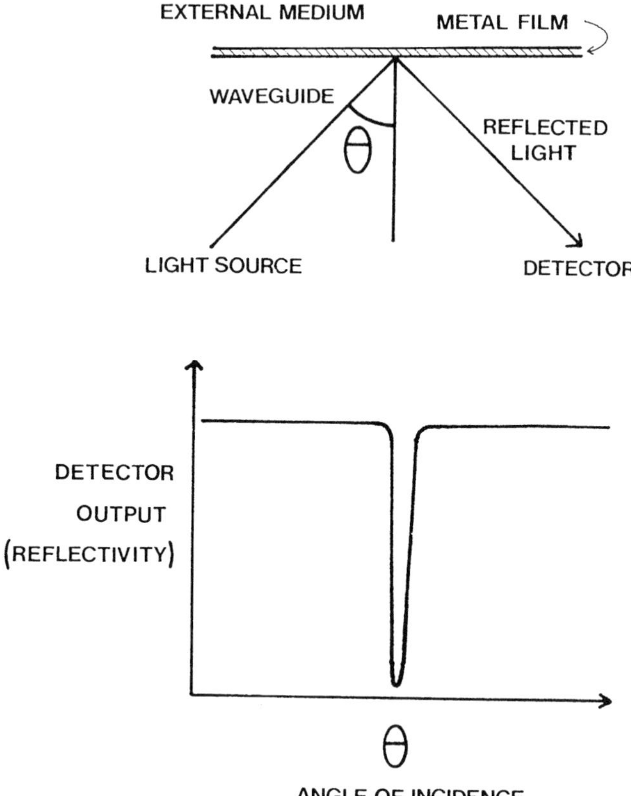

FIGURE 4.4a Surface plasmon resonance. Surface plasmon resonance occurs at a precisely defined angle of incidence (Θ) when light is totally internally reflected from the surface of a waveguide coated with a thin layer of an appropriate metal. The occurrence of resonance is signalled by a large reduction in the amplitude of the reflected light beam.

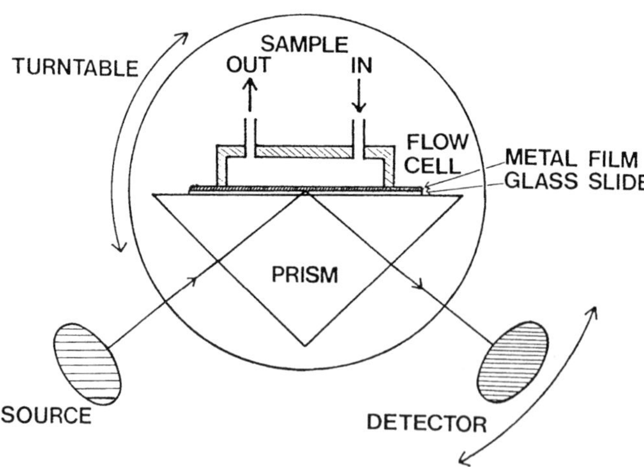

FIGURE 4.4b Diagrammatic representation of SPR apparatus using the Kretschmann format. The metal-coated glass slide is attached to the waveguide, a prism, held on a turntable such that the light from the source meets the surface at the axis of rotation. A flow cell clamped over the slide allows for sample introduction. The angle of incidence (Θ) is scanned by rotating the turntable. The detector is mounted coaxially and must move through 2Θ to track the reflected light beam.

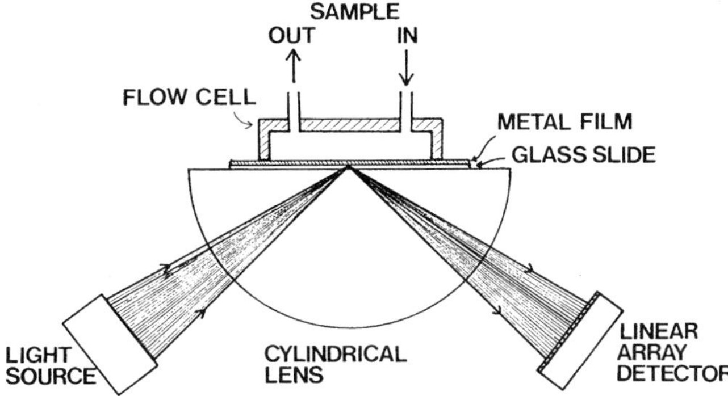

FIGURE 4.5a SPR using a fan beam configuration. By using a fan of light and a linear array detector no moving parts are required to carry out SPR assays.

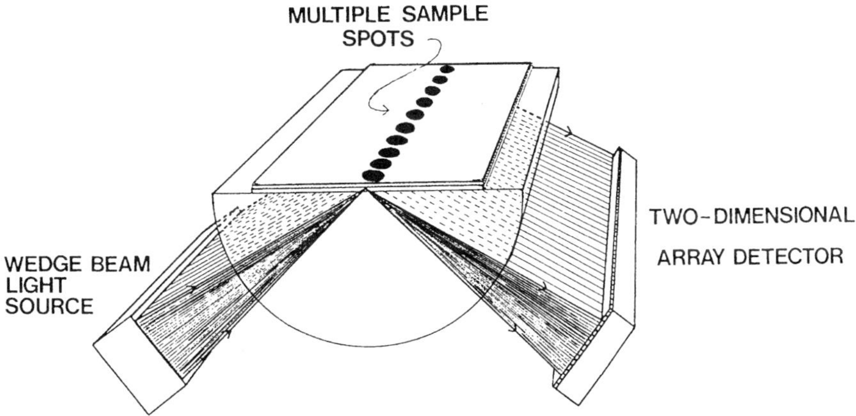

FIGURE 4.5b Multiple analyte SPR using a wedge beam configuration. Extending the fan of light into a wedge and using a two-dimensional detector allows SPR to be monitored along a line on the detector surface. With different probes immobilised at defined spots on this line simultaneous independent measurement of several hybridisation reactions should be feasible.

4.5.2 Acoustic Wave Devices

The shift in frequency of acoustic waves in piezoelectric crystals as the mass loading on the surface changes has generally been used for gas phase analyses. (On acoustic devices for biosensing, see Chapter 9.) Wu et al.[59] showed that nucleic acid hybridisation could be measured with these devices, but after hybridisation the crystals had to be dried before measurements were carried out. To monitor hybridisation *in situ*, a sensor must operate in solution and energy losses from oscillations perpendicular to the surface in a bulk acoustic wave device make this impractical. However, piezoelectric devices can be made which give oscillations only in the plane parallel to the surface, and these are usable in aqueous solution.

Such acoustic plate mode devices have been constructed by Andle and co-workers.[60,61] They covalently attached a 20-base poly T probe to the quartz sensor surface and could detect the hybridisation of 0.1 ng of a 900-base poly A target in 1 ml of solution held in the sample cell of the biosensor. Binding took place relatively slowly over several minutes, but conditions were unfavourable for hybridisation with the assays carried out at room temperature in phosphate-buffered saline. The sensor output was complex. An increase in frequency was observed at low target concentrations between 0.1 and 1 ng/ml. Conversely, a saturating concentration of target of 100 ng/ml caused a decrease in frequency. The increase was ascribed to elastic stiffening of the sensor surface caused by cross-linking of poly T probe oligonucleotides by the much longer target molecules, with the decrease being caused by mass loading with saturating target levels preventing cross-linking. Responses of the sensor were strongly temperature dependent. This was controlled by use of a dual line sensor, only one channel of which was coated with target.

4.5.3 Light-Addressable Potentiometric Sensor (LAPS)

LAPS is marketed as the Threshold* system. It was originally developed for the determination of nucleic acid contamination of genetically engineered pharmaceutical products with assays using DNA binding proteins.[62] The device comprises a silicon sensor with nine pH-sensitive spots. The spots are sequentially addressed through a single set of electrodes using an array of light emitting diodes, with the signal from each spot being read as it is illuminated. The signals needed to link the pH sensor to the biological assay are provided by the enzyme urease. Assays are carried out by filtration of sample and reagents through a nitrocellulose membrane with the filtration device defining spots on the membrane that correspond to the spots on the LAPS.

Olson et al.[63] have developed a gene probe assay for the LAPS and applied it to the measurement of PCR products. A biotin-labelled probe and a fluorescein-labelled probe are hybridised to internal sequences of one strand of the target. After addition of streptavidin, the solution is filtered through the nitrocellulose membrane which is coated with biotinylated BSA. Urease-labelled anti-fluorescein antibody is then drawn through the membrane, and after a further wash step bound urease levels are measured with the LAPS device. The assay is shown in Figure 4.6. Olson et al. could detect around 10^{-16} mol of target with their assay which, although complex and taking over an hour to perform, is comparatively rapid and gives good quantitation.

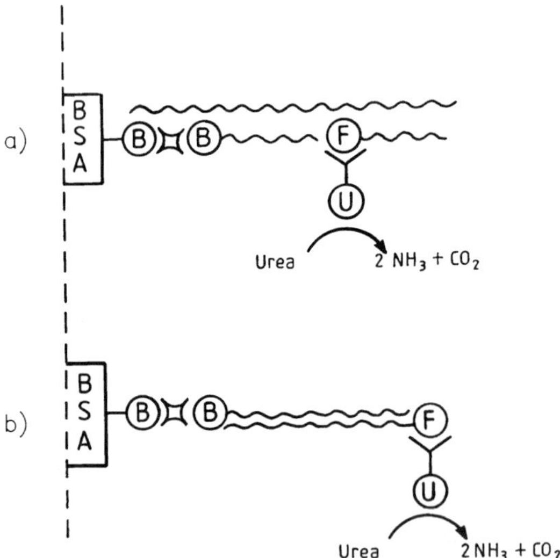

FIGURE 4.6 Gene probe assays using LAPS. Assays with the LAPS require a biotinylated nucleic acid for capture through streptavidin to a membrane coated with biotinylated bovine serum albumin (BSA). Attachment of a pH-change generating label is also required. This is achieved by using an anti-fluorescein antibody coupled to urease for binding to fluorescein-labelled nucleic acid. In (**a**), biotin- and fluorescein-labelled oligonucleotides are hybridised internally to one strand of a PCR-generated target nucleic acid strand. In (**b**), the product of a PCR reaction, in which one primer was 5'-biotinylated and the other was 5′-fluorescein labelled, is captured on the membrane.

* Trademark of Molecular Denier Corporation.

A more direct assay scheme for using the LAPS to measure product from PCR is also shown in Figure 4.6. Here, one PCR primer is labelled with biotin and the other with fluorescein, for capture and detection, respectively.

4.5.4 Liquid Crystals

Double-stranded nucleic acid has been shown to have liquid crystalline properties which could form the basis of biosensing devices. Yevdokimov et al.[64] have proposed that hybridisation of probe and target nucleic acids could be detected by liquid crystal-based biosensors, but so far have only reported experiments showing measurable changes with DNA-binding dyes, proteolysis of DNA-binding proteins (stellins), and the relaxation of supercoiled DNA by the action of a nuclease.[65]

4.6 CONCLUSION

At present only LAPS in the form of Threshold is commercially available as a device shown to be applicable to gene probe assays, but given the great gains to be had over conventional assays in terms of rapidity and quantitation, it can only be a matter of time before other, more direct, approaches come into general use. SPR in the form of the BIACore[66] from Pharmacia and the resonant mirror biosensor[67,68] (similar in practice to SPR and marketed as IASys from Fisons) are now available. These could be used for gene probe assays, but are not currently configured for this application especially in terms of temperature control of the reaction cells. Other versions of these and emerging evanescent wave technologies such as the fluorescent capillary fill device[69] could readily be applied to gene probe biosensing.

A crucial aspect in the future development of gene probe sensors will be sensitivity in comparison with methods using radiolabels. Inherently sensitive luminescent techniques such as enhanced chemiluminescence[70] come nearest to supplanting radiolabelling in conventional assays, and it may be that biosensors based on bio- or chemiluminescence will be developed that can rival radiolabelling in terms of detection limits, but supersede it in terms of speed.

If sensitivity comparable to that found with radiolabels is not achieved, amplification of the target will be essential, and we expect one of the main application areas of biosensors in gene probe assays will be in the *in situ* monitoring of amplification techniques such as PCR.[71] This will not only allow for the speeding up of analyses (only sufficient cycles to provide enough target to be detected will be required), but quantitation will be improved through the provision of data whilst, in the exponential phase, product and target concentrations are still related.[72]

Gene probes are chemically simpler than antibodies, but are informationally more complex and as a consequence gene probe biosensors should offer advantages over immunosensors. The simple repeating structure of polynucleotides makes them very robust and so they can, for example, be recycled through many assays by using high temperatures to achieve regeneration of the sensor surface, a process which would denature antibodies. The information encoded in gene probes can be designed for a particular use, whereas antibodies, especially monoclonal antibodies, are obtained essentially at random. Thus the specificity of gene probes can be tuned, for example, to give fine distinctions between strains of an organism or to recognise a whole genus. Gene probes may be synthesised with ease and it is a simple matter to add modifications during the process and thus facilitate labelling and immobilisation.

What will the future hold? Improvements in biosensor technology, methods of nucleic acid amplification, and assay formats are to be expected. Perhaps polypeptide nucleic acids (PNAs)[73,74] will prove to have greater flexibility than nucleic acids as gene probes. Could transfer RNAs prove to be suitable high copy number targets in assays for microorganisms? Perhaps nanotechnology and microelectronics will find application: the cross-linking of probe oligonucleotides by target, thought to have occurred in the experiments by Andle et al., suggests possibilities in this area. Whatever direction is taken it is certain that gene probe biosensors will eventually become indispensible.

REFERENCES

1. Watson, J. D. and Crick, F. H. C., Molecular structure of nucleic acids, *Nature*, 171, 737, 1953.
2. Lowe, J. B., Clinical applications of gene probes in human genetic disease, malignancy and infectious disease, *Clin. Chim. Acta*, 157, 1, 1986.
3. Edberg, S. C., Principles of nucleic acid hybridisation and comparison with monoclonal antibody technology for the diagnosis of infectious diseases, *Yale J. Biol. Med.*, 58, 425, 1985.
4. Tenover, F. C., Diagnostic deoxyribonucleic acid probes for infectious diseases, *Clin. Microbiol. Rev.*, 1, 82, 1988.
5. Highfield, P. E. and Dougan, G., DNA probes for microbial diagnosis, *Br. J. Biomed. Sci.*, 42, 352, 1988.
6. Van Brunt, J. and Klausner, A., Pushing probes to market, *Biotechnology*, 5, 211, 1987.
7. Siegler, N., DNA-based testing: a progress report, *Am. Soc. Microbiol. News,* 55, 308, 1989.
8. Noel, J. K., DNA probes vs. monoclonal antibodies, *Am. Clin. Prod. Rev.*, 5, 10, 1986.
9. Chollet, A. and Kawashima, E., DNA containing the base analogue 2-aminoadenine. Preparation, use as hybridisation probes and cleavage by restriction endonucleases, *Nucleic Acids Res.*, 11, 6513, 1988.
10. Varshey, U., Jahroudi, N., van de Sande, J. H., and Gedamu, L., Inosine incorporation in GC rich RNA probes increases hybridisation sequence specificity, *Nucleic Acids Res.*, 16, 4162, 1988.
11. Graham, C., Leslie, D. L., and Squirrell, D. J., Gene probe assays on a fibre-optic evanescent wave biosensor, *Biosens. Bioelectron.*, 7, 487, 1992.
12. Sambrook, J., Fritsch, E. F., and Maniatis, T., *Molecular Cloning: A Laboratory Manual*, 2nd ed., Cold Spring Harbor Laboratory, Cold Spring Harbor, New York, 1989.
13. Britten, R. J. and Davidson, E. H., Hybridisation strategy, in *Nucleic Acid Hybridsation, A Practical Approach*, Hames, B. D. and Higgins, S. J., Eds., IRL Press, Oxford. 1985.
14. Young, B. D. and Anderson, M. L., Quantitative analysis of solution hybridisation, in *Nucleic Acid Hybridsation, A Practical Approach*, Hames, B. D and Higgins, S. J., Eds., IRL Press, Oxford, 1985, chap. 3.
15. Bryan, R. N., Ruth, J. L., Smith, R. D., and LeBon, J. M., Diagnosis of clinical samples with synthetic oligonucleotide hybridisation probes, in *Microbiology, 1986*, Levine, L., Ed., American Society for Microbiology, Washington, D.C., 1986, 113.
16. Meinkoth, J. and Wahl, G., Hybridisation of nucleic acids immobilised on solid supports, *Anal. Biochem.*, 138, 267, 1984.
17. Wetmur, J. G. and Davidson, N., Kinetics of renaturation of DNA, *J. Mol. Biol.*, 31, 349, 1968.
18. Keller, G. H. and Manak, M. M., *DNA Probes,* Stockton Press, New York, 1989, 259 pp.
19. Amasino, R. M., Acceleration of nucleic acid hybridisation rate by polyethylene glycol, *Anal. Biochem.*, 152, 304, 1986.
20. Miller, C. A., Patterson, W. L., Johnson, P. K., Swartzell, C. T., Wogoman, F., Albarella, J. P., and Carrico, R.J., Detection of bacteria by hybridisation of rRNA with DNA-latex and immunodetection of hybrids, *J. Clin. Microbiol.*, 26, 1271, 1988.
21. Britten, R. J. and Kohne, D. E., Repeated sequences in DNA, *Science,* 161, 529, 1968.
22. Nygaard, A. P and Hall, B. D., Formation and properties of RNA-DNA complexes, *J. Mol. Biol.*, 9, 125, 1964.
23. Richardson, K. J., Stewart, M. H., and Wolfe, R. L., Application of gene probe technology to the water industry, *J. Am. Water Works Assoc.*, 83, 71, 1991.
24. Atlas, R. M., Bej, A. K., Steffan, R. J., and Perlin, M. H., Approaches for monitoring and containing genetically engineered microorgansims released into the environment, *Hazardous Waste Hazardous Mater.*, 6, 135, 1989.

25. Fox, G. E., Stackebrandt, E., Hespell, R. B., Gibson, J., Maniloff, J., Dyer, T. A., Wolfe, R. S., Balch, W. E., Tanner, R., Magrum, L., Zablen, L. B., Blakemore, R., Gupta, R., Bonen, L., Lewis, B. J., Stahl, D. A., Luehrsen, K. R., Chen, K. N., and Woese, C. R., The phylogeny of prokaryotes, *Science*, 209, 457, 1990.
26. Woese, C. R., Bacterial Evolution, *Microbiol. Rev.*, 47, 221, 1987.
27. Mullis, K. B., Process for Amplifying Nucleic Acid Sequences, U.S. Patent No. 4,683,202, 1987.
28. Mullis, K. B., Erlich, H. A., Arnheim, N., Horn, G. T., Saiki, R. K., and Scharf, S. J., Process for Amplifying, Detecting and/or Cloning Nucleic Acid Sequences, U.S. Patent No. 4,683,195, 1987.
29. Mullis, K. B. and Faloona, F. A., Specific synthesis of DNA *in vitro* via a polymerase catalysed chain reaction, *Methods Enzymol.*, 155, 335, 1987.
30. Wittwer, C. T., Fillmore, C. G., and Garling, D. J., Minimising the time required for DNA amplification by efficient heat transfer to small samples, *Anal. Biochem.*, 186, 328, 1990.
31. Smalla, K., Cresswell, N., Mendonca-Hagler, C., Wolters, A., and van Elsas, J. D., Rapid DNA extraction protocol from soil for polymerase chain reaction-mediated amplification, *J. App. Bacteriol.*, 74, 78, 1993.
32. Lizardi, P. M., Guerra, C. E., Lomeli, H., Tussie-Luna, I., and Kramer, F. R., Exponential amplification of recombinant RNA hybridisation probes, *Biotechnology*, 6, 1197, 1988.
33. Lizardi, P. M. and Kramer, F. R., Exponential amplification of nucleic acids: new diagnostics using DNA polymerases and RNA replicases, *Trends Biotechnol.*, 9, 53, 1991.
34. Cannon, G., Heinhorst, S., and Weissbach, A., Quantitative molecular hybridisation on nylon membranes, *Anal. Biochem.*, 149, 229, 1985.
35. Reed, K. C. and Mann, D. A., Rapid transfer of DNA from agarose gels to nylon membranes, *Nucleic Acids Res.*, 13, 7207, 1985.
36. Johnson, D., Gautsch, J., Sportsman, R., and Elder, J., Improved technique: utilizing nonfat dry milk for analysis of proteins and nucelic acids transferred to nitrocellulose, *Genet. Anal. Tech.*, 1, 3, 1984.
37. Yehle, C. O., Patterson, W. L., Boguslawski, S. J., Albarella, J. P., Yip, K. F., and Carrico, R. J., A solution hybridisation assay for ribosomal RNA from bacteria using biotinylated probes and enzyme-labelled antibody to DNA:RNA, *Mol. Cell. Probes,* 1, 177, 1987.
38. Viscidi, R. P., O'Meara, C., Farzadegan, H., and Yolken, R., Monoclonal antibody solution hybridisation assay for detection of human immunodeficiency virus nucleic acids, *J. Clin. Microbiol.*, 27, 120, 1989.
39. Dekker, S., Logan, K., Aswell, J., and Lawrie, J., Hybridisation assay for quantitative detection of viral nucleic acids: application to human immunodeficiency virus 1 and cytomegaolvirus, *Am. Soc. Microbiol. Abstr.,* C46, 1989.
40. Dunn, A. R. and Hassell, J. A., A novel method to map transcripts: evidence for homology between an adenovirus mRNA and discrete multiple regions of the viral genome, *Cell*, 12, 23, 1977.
41. Ranki, M., Palva, A., Virtanen, M., Laaksonen, M., and Soderlund, H., Sandwich hybridisation as a convenient method for the detection of nucleic acids in crude samples, *Gene*, 21, 77, 1983.
42. Ranki, M. and Soderlund, H. E., Detection of Microbial Nucleic Acids by a One-Step Sandwich Hybridisation Test, U.S. Patent No. 4,486,539, 1984.
43. Vary, C. P. H., A homogeneous nucleic acid hybridisation assay based on strand displacement, *Nucleic Acids Res.*, 15, 6883, 1987.
44. Nelson, N. C., Hammond, P. W., Wiese, W. A., and Arnold, L. J., Novel assay formats employing acridinium ester-labelled DNA probes, in Abstr. Third San Diego Conf., Practical Aspects of Molecular Probes, 1988.
45. Heller, M. J. and Morrison, L. E., Chemiluminescent and fluorescent probes for DNA hybridisation systems, in *Rapid Detection and Identification of Infectious Agents*, Kingsbury, D. and Falkow, S., Eds., Academic Press, San Diego, 1985, 245.
46. Anderson, G. P., Golden, J. P., and Ligler, F. S., Fiber optic biosensor: combination tapered fibers designed for improved signal acquisition, *Biosen. Bioelectron.*, 8, 249, 1993.
47. Walzcak, I. M., Love, W. F., Cook, T. A., and Slovacek, R. E., The application of evanescent wave sensing to a high-sensitivity fluoroimmunoassay, *Biosens. Bioelectron.*, 7, 39, 1992.

48. Lackie, S. J., Glass, T. R., and Block, M. J., Instrumentation for cylindrical waveguide evanescent fluorosensors, in *Biosensors with Fiber Optics*, Wise, D. L. and Wingard, L. B., Eds., Humana Press, Clifton, NJ, 1991, 225.
49. Place, J. F., Sutherland, R. M., and Dahne, C., Opto-electronic immunosensors: a review of optical immunoassay at continuous surfaces, *Biosensors*, 1, 321, 1985.
50. Hirschfeld, T. B. and Block, M. J., Cellule RTA, Appareil et Procede Pour Titrer un Polynucleotide dans un Liquid, Belgian Patent 1000572A4, 1987.
51. Sutherland, R. M., Analytical Method for Detecting and Measuring Specifically Sequenced Nucleic Acid, European Patent Appl. EP 86810201, 1987.
52. Anderson, M. L. M. and Young, B. D., Quantitative filter hybridisation, in *Nucleic Acid Hybridisation: A Practical Approach*, Hames, B. D. and Higgins, S. J., Eds., IRL Press, Oxford, 1985, chap. 4.
53. Liedberg, B., Nylander, C., and Lundstrom, I., Surface plasmon resonance for gas detection and biosensing, *Sensors Actuators,* 4, 299, 1983.
54. Daniels, P. B., Deacon, J. K., Eddowes, M. J., and Pedley, D. G., Surface plasmon resonance applied to immunosensing, *Sensors Actuators,* 15, 11, 1988.
55. Kretschmann, E., Die bestimmungen optischer konstanten von metallen durch anregung von oberflachen plasmashwingungen, *Z. Phys.*, 241, 313, 1971.
56. Pollard-Knight, D., Hawkins, E., Yeung, D., Pashby, D. P., Simpson, M., McDougall, A., Buckle, P., and Charles, S. A., Immunoassays and nucleic acid detection with a biosensor based on surface plasmon resonance, *Ann. Biol. Clin.*, 48, 642, 1990.
57. Evans, E. A. and Charles, S. C., The application of a rapid homogeneous biosensor based on surface plasmon resonance to chemistry, DNA probes and immunoassays, *Abstracts of 1st World Congress on Biosensors*, Elsevier Science, New York, 1990, 223.
58. Schwarz, T., Yeung, D., Hawkins, E., Heaney, P., and McDougall, A., Detection of nucleic acid hybridisation using surface plasmon resonance, *Trends Biotechnol.*, 9, 339, 1991.
59. Wu, T.-Z., Wang, H.-H., and Au, L.-C., Gene probe coated piezoelectric biosensors for biochemical analysis, *Chin. J. Microbiol. Immunol.*, 23, 147, 1990.
60. Andle, J. C., Vetelino, J. F., Lade, M. W., and McAllister, D. J., Detection of nucleic acid hybridisation with an acoustic plate mode biosensor, Proc. 1990 IEEE Ultrasonics Symp., Honolulu, HI, 1990, 291.
61. Andle, J. C., Vetelino, J. F., Lade, M. W., and McAllister, D. J., An acoustic plate mode biosensor, *Sensors Actuators,* B8, 191, 1992.
62. Hafeman, D. G., Parce, J. W., and McConnell, H. M., Light-addressable potentiometric sensor for biochemical systems, *Science*, 240, 1182, 1988.
63. Olson, J. D., Panfili, P. R., Zuk, R. F., and Sheldon, E. L., Quantitation of DNA hybridisation in a silicon sensor-based system: application to PCR, *Mol. Cell. Probes,* 5, 351, 1991.
64. Yevdokimov, Yu. M., Skuridin, S. G., and Lortkipanidze, G. B., Liquid-crystalline dispersions of nucleic acids, *Liquid Crystals*, 12, 1, 1992.
65. Yevdokimov, Yu. M., Skuridin, S. G., and Salyanov, V. I., General principles of creating biosensing units based on double-stranded nucleic acid liquid crystals, in *Molecular Electronics*, Lazarev, P. I., Ed., Kluwer Academic, The Netherlands, 1991, 317.
66. Jönsson, U. and Malmqvist, M., Real time biospecific interaction analysis (the integration of surface plasmon resonance detection, general biospecific interface chemistry and microfluidics into one analytical system), in Advanc*es in Biosensors*, Turner, A. P. F., Ed., JAI Press, London, 1992.
67. Cush, R., Cronin, J. M., Stewart, W. J., Maule, C. H., Molloy, J., and Goddard, N. J., The resonant mirror: a novel optical biosensor for direct sensing of biomolecular interactions. I. Principle of operation and associated instrumentation, *Biosens. Bioelectron.*, 8, 347, 1993.
68. Buckle, P. E., Davies, R. J., Kinning, T., Yeung, D., Edwards, P. R., Pollard-Knight, D., and Lowe, C. R., The resonant mirror: a novel optical biosensor for direct sensing of biomolecular interactions. II. Applications, *Biosens. Bioelectron.*, 8, 355, 1993.
69. Deacon, J. K., Thomson, A. M., Page, A. L., Stops, J. E., Roberts, P. R., Whitely, S. C., Attridge, J. W., Love C. A., Robinson, G. A., and Davidson, G. P., An assay for human chorionic gonadotropin using the capillary fill immunosensor, *Biosens. Bioelectron.*, 6, 193, 1992.

70. Kricka, L. J. and Thorpe, G. H. G., Bioluminescent and chemiluminescent detection of horseradish peroxidase labels in ligand binder assays, in *Luminescence Immunoassay and Molecular Applications*, van Dyke, K. and van Dyke, R., Eds., CRC Press, Boca Raton, FL, 1990, chap. 6.
71. Squirrell, D. J., Gene Probe Biosensor Method, International Patent Appl. PCT/GB92/01698, 1992.
72. Wiesner, R. J., Beinbrech, B., and Ruegg, J. C., Quantitative PCR, *Nature*, 366, 416, 1993.
73. Egholm, N., Buchardt, O., Christensen, L., Behrens, C., Freier, S. M., Driver, D. A., Berg, R. H., Kim, S. K., Norden, B., and Nielsen, P. E., PNA hybridizes to complementary oligonucleotides obeying the Watson-Crick hydrogen-bonding rules, *Nature*, 365, 566, 1993.
74. Patel, D. J., Marriage of convenience (nucleic acid recognition), *Nature*, 365, 490, 1993.
75. Glass, T. R., Lackie, S., and Hirschfeld, T., Effect of numerical aperture on signal level in cylindrical waveguide evanescent fluorosensors, *Appl. Opt.*, 26, 2181, 1987.

5 Membranes to Improve Amperometric Sensor Characteristics

Subrayal M. Reddy and Pankaj M. Vadgama

CONTENTS

5.1 INTRODUCTION

The past 20 years have seen the steady introduction of potentiometric and amperometric chemical sensors into clinical and biomedical areas. Biosensors can extend the analytical capability of such devices by combining the molecular specificity of a biological recognition entity with an operationally simple transducer. The biorecognition here may be based on catalytic conversion with, say, an enzyme or organelle acting as a catalytic agent transforming

0-8493-8905-4/97/$0.00+$.50
© 1997 by CRC Press, Inc.

a substrate into a measurable product. Alternatively, the analyte may only take part in a binding event as occurs with biorecognition based on an antibody or receptor. The transducer is required to follow the biochemical interaction, most typically a catalytic conversion, through registering the production or depletion of a species involved in the reaction. (Alternatively, the associated small temperature change due to heat evolved or consumed in the reaction can be measured — see Chapter 13.) The mode of detection may be "locked in" by the biochemical interaction to be followed, but beyond the actual optimised integration of these two components there is a key requirement to adopt an inherently effective mode of solute recognition (supplementary to that offered by the bioreagent) for practical application in complex biological matrices (viz., blood, blood subcomponents, environmental waters, bioreactors, and foodstuffs). These environments are essentially hostile to the device, and if extensive sample preparation is not to be required, one convenient route to controlling the exposure of any biosensor is to exploit solute gating membranes to enclose the transduction sequence (Figure 5.1).

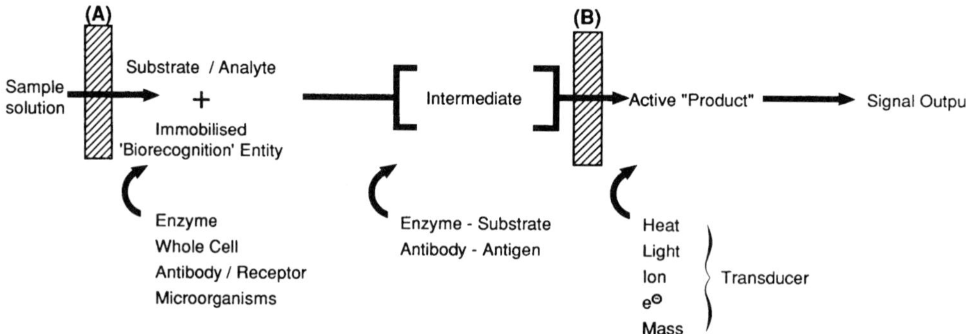

FIGURE 5.1 Schematic depicting various biosensing pathways. (A) An external interfacing membrane protecting the overall device and controlling access to the bioreaction phase. (B) An internal interfacing membrane creating a second control point for protecting the inner transducer element. For electron transfer this may be a redox active layer.

The use of membranes to localise and stabilise a bioreagent layer in a biosensor was first reported by Clark and Lyons,[1] who proposed entrapment of the enzyme glucose oxidase (GOD) between two microsolute permeable dialysis membranes. It was suggested that a pH change could be followed by the reaction:

$$\text{Glucose} + O_2 \xrightarrow{\text{GOD}} \text{Gluconic acid} + H_2O_2 \tag{5.1}$$

Alternatively, Updike and Hicks[2] reported use of an inner O_2-permeable membrane as part of an amperometric oxygen sensor to follow the local fall in pO_2; the glucose concentration in a test solution was then shown to be inversely related to the measured pO_2. While this marked the birth of a reagentless method of substrate analysis using a biosensor, it also exemplified the way in which membranes can serve to compartmentalise individual biosensor components. As with the original O_2 electrode, of course, a gas-permeable membrane not only allowed near-total elimination of interference, but all danger of mixing between the electrolyte of the inner O_2 electrode and the bioreagent layer. The drawback of requiring a background correction for the variability in sample pO_2 in this context might be regarded as a minor deficiency given the notable functional success demonstrated by Updike and Hicks through the use of membranes.

In much early work, dialysis membranes offered a highly convenient means of compartmentalising a macromolecule, notably the enzyme, while allowing microsolute substrates ready access. However, there was little in the way of transport control of relevant substrates, cosubstrates, and interferents, and the membrane was able to achieve little with regards to protecting the device from extremes of pH, ionic strength, passivating agents, or bioreagent poisons (viz., heavy metals).

This chapter discusses the development of membrane strategies for optimising electrochemical enzyme-based sensors of the amperometric type. However it needs to be borne in mind that the general use of membranes regardless of particular biosensor type can have significant functional benefits beyond the basic enzyme electrode. Tailored membranes are beginning to be used with other types of biorecognition (antibodies and receptors) as well as for other modes of transduction.

An alternative example of the role of a membrane providing an interface between the detecting and detected phase is that in the fibre-optic chemical sensor.[3] Here, the sensed species reacts with an immobilised reagent only after traversing an external, restricting boundary membrane, to produce an optically measurable change at a more controlled inner phase of the fibre surface. However, the membrane here and elsewhere has tended to provide a physically protective environment only, with little consideration given to the engineering aspects such as solute transport and surface chemistry.

There is therefore a need to highlight potential adaptation of polymeric and biomembranes to electrochemical biosensing, based on some knowledge of their physicochemical properties. Selectivity and general permeability properties will be presented, followed by a description of suitable sensor applications for a particular membrane construct.

5.2 STRUCTURE AND FUNCTION OF SYNTHETIC MEMBRANES

A membrane can be defined as a thin barrier separating two phases (typically liquid) across which controlled solute transport may be effected in a variably selective manner. Such solute separation may be directly related to the membrane's physical properties[4] (typically porosity) as well as its intrinsic chemical nature. Synthetic membranes may ideally be segregated into two well-defined groups, heterogeneous and homogeneous (Figure 5.2). With the latter, intrinsic polymer chemistry can be a more precise basis for solute discrimination; they do not possess structure at the colloidal level (5 to 50 nm) and therefore may be regarded as a symmetrical, continuous single phase without any identifiable structural irregularity.

The mode of solute transport, however, is fundamentally more intricate.[5,6] In order to traverse such a homogeneous membrane, the solute species must first be soluble in the polymeric phase. This is a function of the chemical potential of the diffusing species compared to those of the membrane and solutions on either side of the membrane. If the species is more soluble in the membrane phase than in the solvent then the solute concentration in the membrane increases. If the solute is less soluble in the membrane then its concentration drops. Transmembrane diffusion is then a consequence of solute-polymer interactions within the membrane, typically against a concentration or pressure gradient between the solutions on either side of the thin membrane (typically 5 to 40 μm thickness). The inevitable close contact between the solute and mobile polymer chains may allow for further selectivity in solute transport (permselectivity). Alternatively, a polymer such as poly(vinyl chloride) (PVC) by retaining a high level of plasticiser may also impart selectivity. Membrane plasticisation increases polymer chain mobility and molecular spacing within the membrane. Typical plasticisers include dioctylphthalate and isopropylmyristate. The resulting membrane therefore becomes more permeable. A membrane so plasticised may serve as a mechanically

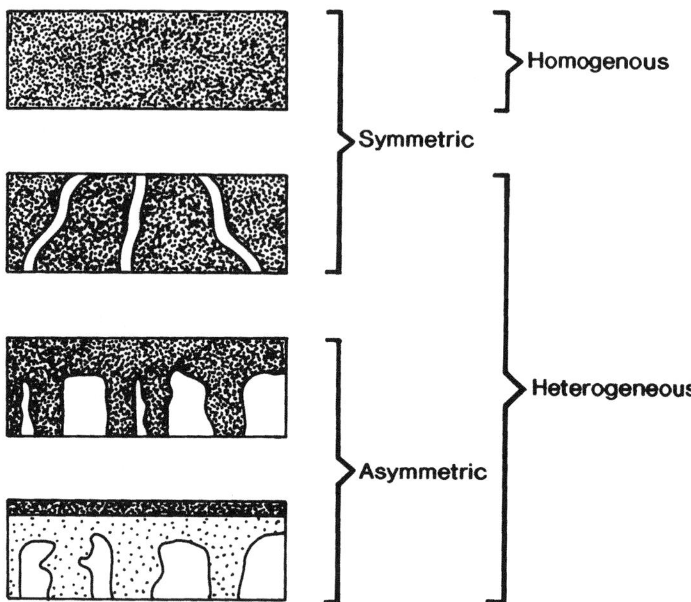

FIGURE 5.2 Diagrammatic cross sections through typical homogeneous and heterogeneous membranes emphasising symmetry and structure.

stabilised phase (Figure 5.3a) through which a lipophilic molecule may interact — an extension of the classic use of such membranes merely to retain affinity molecules as in the case of PVC-based ion selective electrodes.

Heterogeneous membranes possess a recognisable structure, and are essentially made up of a series of imperfections (at least at a microcrystalline level) retained in a functionally inert polymeric phase, notably glass frits and track-etched membranes. The latter are formed by selected site weakening with a collimated neutron beam, followed by local chemical etching to create defined pores. The result is a symmetric heterogeneous membrane with near-cylindrical pores which span the whole vertical cross section of the membrane (Figure 5.3b). Alternatively asymmetric membranes, usually formed by solvent casting, possess separate well-defined dense and porous layers. The dense "skin" layer is responsible for the basic permselective property, whereas the porous zone provides mechanical support. Examples of such structures are ion exchange membranes, such as sulphonated polysulfone membranes,[7] and hyperfiltration cellulose acetate membranes for desalination.[8]

Models for solute transport in coarsely porous membranes (with pore sizes in the micron range) assume a sieve-like behaviour with regard to particles discriminated on their radius relative to that of the pores. Koochaki et al.[9] did, however, demonstrate some inverse relation between the molecular weight (for subcolloidal-sized solutes) and the permeability coefficient for such membranes, suggesting some degree of resolution, possibly the result of solute/wall interactions. It must be recognised that with such coarse porous structures, at least in a stirred solution, transport via convection may arise and swamp any discrimination by chemical solute/membrane interactions.

Finely porous membranes (pore size 1 to 5 nm) show transport dominated by diffusion, with some molecules passing through the membrane imperfections and some through the polymer matrix itself.[10] Mode of solute transport (viz., permeability and permselectivity) is thus attributable as much to the method of fabrication and of the architecture of the membrane as to its constituent polymer.

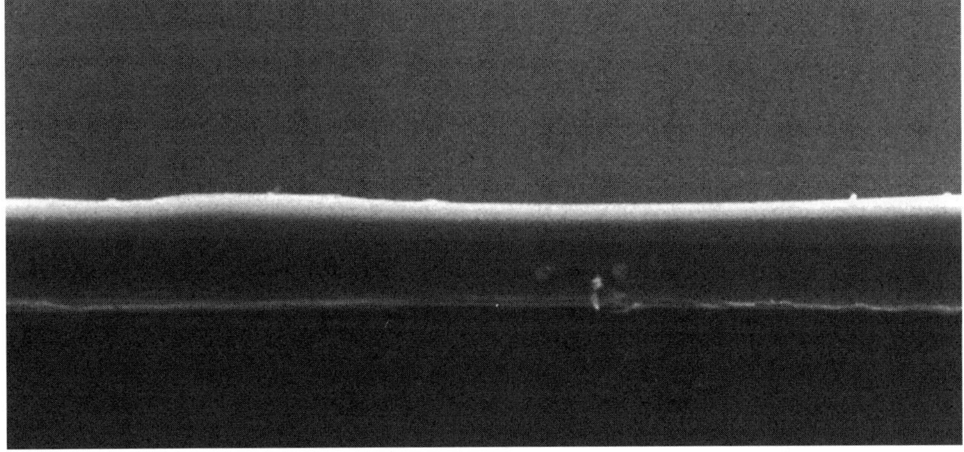

a

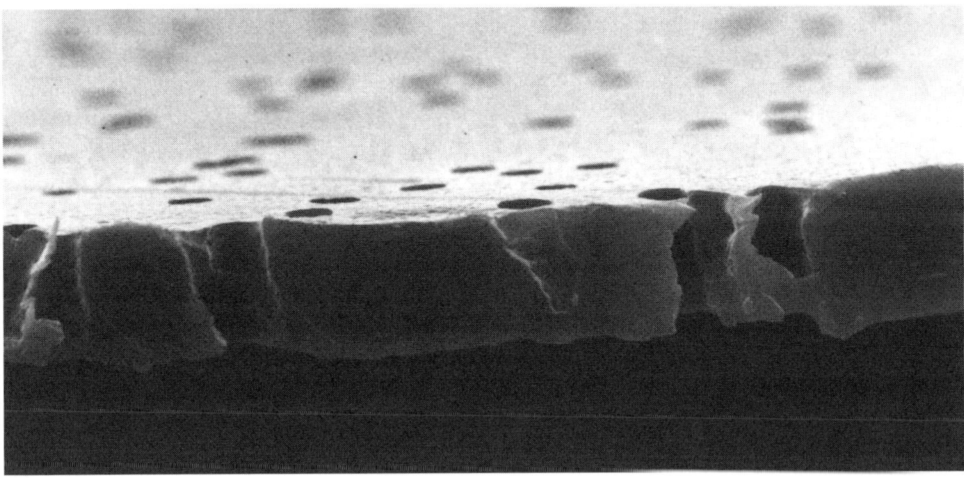

b

FIGURE 5.3 Scanning electron micrographs of synthetic membranes. An edge scan of (a) homogeneous PVC, and (b) heterogeneous (5 μm pore size) polycarbonate.

5.3 MEMBRANE FABRICATION AND SENSOR APPLICATIONS

5.3.1 Membrane Fabrication

Two general methods are used for fabricating polymeric membranes: by either quenching from a melt or by isolating from solution by evaporation of the solvent. The structure of membranes made by the former method depends upon the nature of the polymer (viz., intramolecular forces, chain rigidity, molecular weight, and branching) and, for a given polymer, upon the various kinetic factors involved in quenching. The latter of the two fabrication methods has been used almost exclusively to produce polymer membranes of the dense structure often demanded in biosensor applications; they furthermore have the advantage of being relatively easy to apply, create reproducible membranes, and demand relatively mild conditions.[11]

Dense cast films from a polymer solution can be obtained by complete dissolution of the polymer substrate in a solvent medium, with subsequent application of the polymer solution onto an inert surface, often of polytetrafluoroethylene (PTFE) or glass. Simple evaporation of the solvent (desolvation) then consummates the procedure, though the conditions of casting (viz., temperature, humidity, and rate of solvent loss) are known to have a significant effect on the permeability and permselective properties of the resultant membrane.[12] Derived fabrication procedures are frequently empirical, but permeability will be determined in part by the degree of close packing of the polymer chains which, in turn, is related to the degree of ordering achieved during various stages of membrane formation. Membranes may possess both ordered and disordered regions, respectively known as crystalline and amorphic, which can be varied to establish quite different permeability properties.

In a crystalline domain, the solute may be considered to be essentially insoluble in the matrix, and a low permeability can be regarded as being due to nonpartitioning (molecular exclusion) in the lattice structure. Transport therefore occurs in a selective manner through the more open structure of the amorphous phase. The crystalline/amorphous ratio for a given polymer membrane can be conveniently ascertained by electron microscopy and also by X-ray diffraction methods.[13] It is plausible to suggest that a range of properties such as mechanical strength, permeability, and interfacial characteristics may be controlled by merely determining a particular crystalline/amorphous ratio. However, little progress has actually been made in optimising the ability of fine tuning this parameter.

The degree of polymer chain close packing in an orderly, crystalline array is determined by the regularity of the repeating units of the precursor polymer chain coupled with the strength of interchain, intermolecular forces. Polystyrene, for example, may be prepared in two forms: atactic and isotactic; in the atactic form, the pendant phenyl is randomly distributed in the up/down position along the chain:

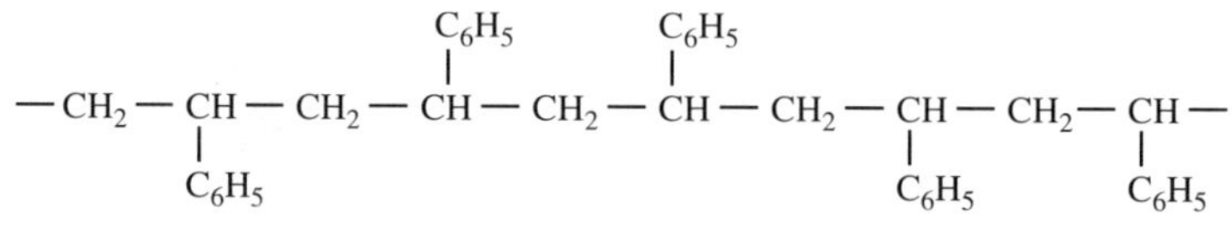

$$-CH_2-\underset{C_6H_5}{\underset{|}{CH}}-CH_2-\overset{C_6H_5}{\overset{|}{CH}}-CH_2-\overset{C_6H_5}{\overset{|}{CH}}-CH_2-\underset{C_6H_5}{\underset{|}{CH}}-CH_2-\underset{C_6H_5}{\underset{|}{CH}}-$$

The outcome is therefore an amorphous membrane structure. Other examples of random orientation are atactic polyvinyl chloride and polyacrylonitrile. By contrast, in an isotactic structure, all the phenyl groups are spatially ordered with the phenyls either entirely in the up or in the down position:

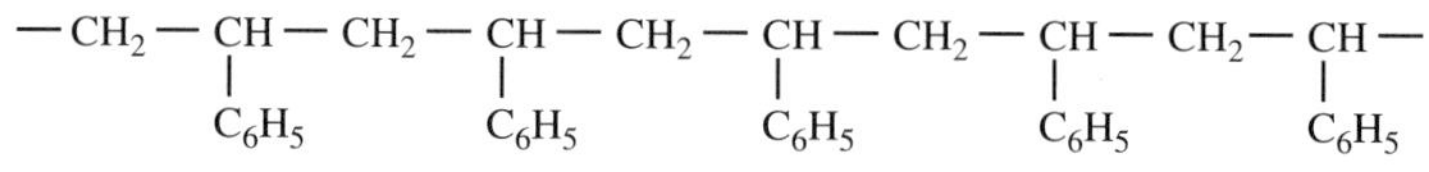

$$-CH_2-\underset{C_6H_5}{\underset{|}{CH}}-CH_2-\underset{C_6H_5}{\underset{|}{CH}}-CH_2-\underset{C_6H_5}{\underset{|}{CH}}-CH_2-\underset{C_6H_5}{\underset{|}{CH}}-CH_2-\underset{C_6H_5}{\underset{|}{CH}}-$$

This conformation drives the folding action of the polymer chains and therefore a degree of order (crystallinity) in packing of around 50% is achieved.

Efforts at controlling the degree of crystallinity have largely been based on increasing rates of desolvation from a polymer solution by using either higher boiling point solvents, swelling agents, or nonsolvents.[14] By incorporating a poor solvent for polymer dissolution the formation of molecular aggregates (a result of more favourable polymer-polymer interactions as compared with polymer-solvent interactions) is promoted. This effectively enforces structured regularity at the very early stages of membrane formation, leading to a finite degree of crystallinity in the subsequent polymer aggregation steps towards a final membrane. In nitrocellulose films, crystallinity increases, for example, in the solvent series methanol < ether-alcohol < acetone, an inverse relation to the solvating power of the solvent medium.[15]

Dense, solvent-cast homogeneous membranes may relatively easily be converted into porous structures to modify permeability. This can be accomplished by total immersion of a membrane into a swelling system followed by exchange of this system with a nonsolvent medium. Thus, immersion of nitrocellulose in ethanol (nonsolvent) and water (swelling medium), followed by subsequent washing in water, leads to a permeability change that is a direct consequence of membrane swelling. Incorporation of this swelling agent into a membrane causes the comparatively void-free structure to expand until the void fraction becomes comparable to that occupied by the polymer, thus imparting a significant overall porosity. Such treatment also affects the permselective skin layer of heterogeneous membranes which can thereby also be made more permeable.

5.3.2 Application to Electrochemical Sensing

High-porosity membrane structures have been attractive as external membranes in enzyme electrodes (Figure 5.4), since they allow controlled substrate flux to the subjacent enzyme layer without substrate levels being so depleted that a low sensitivity and long response time renders the device impractical. A membrane commonly used in this respect is the commercially available neutron track-etched polycarbonate;[9,16-18] the track-etching process, although expensive, adds little to the final sensor cost due to the small portion of membrane (about 1 cm^2) required per enzyme electrode. The defined (mainly nonconfluent) pores allow control over permeability while maintaining minimal diffusion distances, in contrast to the situation with tortuous pore membranes where distances for diffusion may be far greater than the geometric thickness of the membrane. Transmembrane solute flux is also more easily defined through control of membrane pore size and pore density.[10]

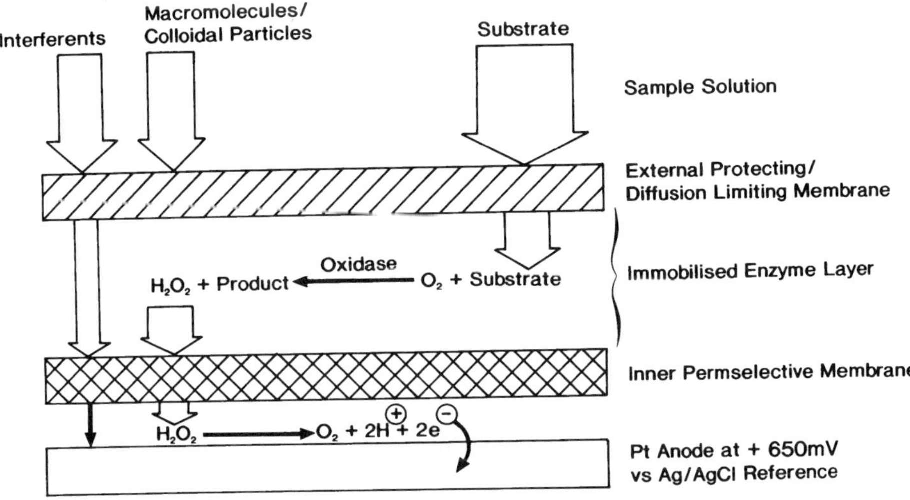

FIGURE 5.4 Schematic of a classical dual membrane amperometric oxidase electrode.

The incorporation of a specific lipophilic phase into the pores of the above microporous polycarbonate membranes[17] has created mosaic structures which allow further reduction of substrate access to the enzyme while, for example, ensuring adequate transport of O_2 (lipophilic) for more reliable operation of oxidase-based electrodes.

Lipophilic agents can be used as plasticisers for homogeneous membranes, for example, dioctylphthalate (DOP) and isopropylmyristate (IPM) incorporated into solvent-cast poly(vinyl chloride). Such membranes have been shown to achieve almost total rejection of ionic interferent species such as ascorbate and urate, which is a common problem in the assay of blood, especially for low-concentration substrates.

Ion exchange membranes are highly swollen polymer gels where the polymer possesses a fixed charge.[19] With a fixed positive charge (e.g., with quaternary ammonium and phosphonium ion groups), an anion exchange membrane results (Figure 5.5); with fixed negative charges (e.g., sulphate or carboxylate), a cation exchange membrane is produced. Selectivity is achieved on the basis of rejection of mobile ions of the same charge as those on the fixed group (co-ions) and the relatively unimpeded passage of ions of opposite charge (counterions). Nafion, a perfluorosulphonated hydrocarbon, has been shown to exhibit excellent selectivity for cationic species.[20] Transport occurs by both classical diffusion (down a concentration gradient) as well as by a charge transfer,[21] or an electron-hopping mechanism between adjacent redox centres, the Nafion matrix behaving as a catalytic support for this latter mode of transport. The selectivity properties of the membrane have ensured the almost complete rejection of anionic species, making it attractive as an inner permselective membrane for enzyme electrode use.

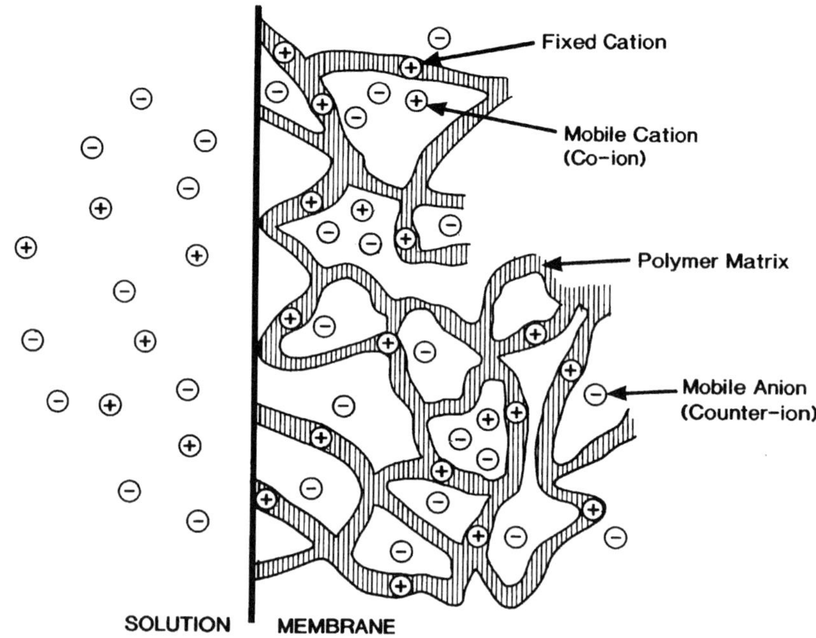

FIGURE 5.5 Representation of ion activity in the vicinity of an anion exchange membrane and solution interface.

In contrast to fixed groups bound covalently to the polymer backbone, a liquid ion exchanger can be incorporated into a polymer film during solvent casting. The ion exchanger can be held relatively strongly in the polymer matrix by noncovalent intermolecular forces. Poly(vinyl chloride) membranes plasticised with such agents have contributed to the advancement of ion-selective electrodes where interfacial ion binding is exploited;[22,23] however, their applicability to systems where solute flux is important has still to be established. Examples of liquid anion exchangers are quaternary ammonium salts of tricaprylmethyl ammonium ion (Aliquat® 336)[4] and phosphonium ion. Some basic studies of the selectivity of such species indicate that ion binding is determined by the energy of hydration of the putative transported ion, and as such the carrier properties will be essentially nonselective, showing a preference for all hydrophobic ions alike.[24] Interestingly, at least for ion-selective electrodes where a quaternary ammonium salt was used, these showed the greatest discrimination for large-size hydrophobic ions[25] where one might expect more specific intermolecular interaction to take place.

Permselectivity at anion-selective membranes has been achieved by rather more specific interactions between the mobile carriers and anions, through the formation of coordination complexes; reported carriers include porphyrins, corrins (e.g., vitamin B_{12}),[26] and organometallics.[23]

Knowledge of membrane fabrication and functioning is a prerequisite to the use of membrane structures as a means of finessing the construction and development of biosensors. In doing so, it is necessary to establish a much more methodical approach to membrane exploitation by taking into consideration end-user requirements, adaptability to the rigours of a biological environment, compliance to specific levels of sensitivity and linear dynamic range, and the imperatives of avoiding biofouling and interferent effects.

To date, membranes have been used most extensively for the optimization of electrochemical biosensors, including amperometric, potentiometric, and conductimetric modes of transduction. The operation of these devices is given below, in the context of membrane exploitation.

5.4 ELECTROCHEMICAL TRANSDUCTION

5.4.1 AMPEROMETRIC SENSORS

Amperometric enzyme/membrane electrodes (Figure 5.4) have received the most attention in the overall progression of biosensors. Here, the current generated when an electrochemically redox active species undergoes electron transfer at a reducing/oxidising electrode surface allows a particularly direct route to the generation of a convenient electrical signal. Oxidases, and to a lesser extent, dehydrogenases have of course been the ideal tandem systems to use because of their complementary redox behaviour to that of the electrochemical reaction. As regards glucose oxidase and most other oxidases, the end product in the presence of O_2 (Equation 5.1) is the electrochemically active hydrogen peroxide, which oxidises at a sufficiently anodic potential with the transfer of electrons to the electrode surface, subsequently translated into a current (Equation 5.2):

$$H_2O_2 \xrightarrow[\text{vs. Ag/AgCl}]{+650\text{ mV}} O_2 + 2H^+ + 2e^- \tag{5.2}$$

Commercial sensors have been realised based on this scheme, e.g., for the measurement of glucose in diabetic patients,[27] but in order to be sufficiently stable for direct use and handling it has become apparent that, at the very least, some form of mechanically robust structure, in the form of a membrane, is required as a closely opposed layer, typically as an outer barrier.[28-30]

While immobilisation of the relevant enzyme can be achieved in a variety of ways, e.g., chemical cross-linking,[31] gel entrapment,[32] and covalent binding to some chemically activated support,[33] it is a further attractive possibility to regard the membrane itself as an anchor for the weak, immobilised enzyme phase.

The above anchoring strategy can apply to an enzyme electrode whatever the inherent effect of the chemistry of the test solution to the enzyme layer. However, it is necessary to reconsider what role, if any, is to be played by any internal barrier layer between the enzyme and working electrode (Figure 5.4). Certainly, a working electrode exposed repeatedly to biological sample constituents may alter its surface properties, and dense membranes have often been utilised, at least in the case of H_2O_2 devices. However, instead of discriminating in favour of small readily resolvable molecules such as hydrogen peroxide, more demanding conditions have to be met when a dehydrogenase is exploited (viz., for substrates such as lactate, alcohol, and glycerol). The cofactor, nicotinamide adenine dinucleotide (NAD^+), is involved in the reaction, and its reduced form, NADH, has to be allowed to selectively traverse a membrane for either its direct or indirect (mediated) quantification; a tailored membrane selective for such a large polar molecule is much more difficult to achieve. The situation is potentially compounded by the membrane tending to retain any electrochemically generated by-products that might contribute to either distortion of surface electrochemistry or to the known passivating effect of the NADH at the electrode.[32] Table 5.1 briefly lists the classical functions of the outer and inner membranes of a dual membrane enzyme electrode.

TABLE 5.1
Functions of Outer and Inner Membranes of an Amperometric Biosensor

Membrane position in sensor	Benefits to amperometric sensor
Outer membrane	Tailors analytical range
	Mechanically protects enzyme layer
	Screens out unwanted macromolecular species (e.g., proteins)
	Offers a potentially compatible surface for contact with biological matrices (e.g., blood, tissue, fermentation broth, etc.)
Inner membrane	Screens out electrochemically active interferents
	Prevents electrode modification by interferents
	Controls product flow to electrode

When the system is "hard-wired" by the intervention of an immobilised mediator serving as an electron relay, as is the case for example when a ferrocene[35] (Fc) is used (Equations 5.3 to 5.5), then a physical (membrane) barrier of at least greater than atomic distances would be required to prevent interfering ions from reaching the electrode. However, this would also preclude mediated current flow, thereby closing the opportunity to afford environmental protection to the working electrode.

$$\text{Substrate} + \text{NAD}^+ \xrightarrow{\text{Dehydrogenase}} \text{Product} + \text{NADH} \tag{5.3}$$

$$\text{NADH} + 2\text{Fc}^+ \longrightarrow \text{NAD}^+ + \text{H}^+ + \text{Fc} \tag{5.4}$$

$$2\text{Fc} \longrightarrow 2\text{Fc}^+ + 2\text{e}^- \tag{5.5}$$

Of course a soluble, diffusible mediator could well be used instead, but unless retention in a mobile form is possible (behind a membrane), the mediator would be required to be added to the assay solution as a form of pretreatment.

5.4.2 Potentiometric Sensing

As with amperometric sensors, potentiometric electrodes have received considerable attention. Membrane technology has certainly been exploited in basic electrode fabrication, but since the principle of operation is that of a measured interfacial potential between the test sample and sensing membrane surface, the ground rules for membrane use have tended to be rather different from those of devices where quantitative transmembrane transport is required.

In the case of potentiometric enzyme electrodes, e.g., for analytes such as urea, amino acids, and penicillin, the outer membrane/enzyme construct is essentially the same as for amperometric devices. However, potentiometric sensors are so inherently robust and selective (viz., the NH_3 sensor for deaminases[36] and the pH sensor for hydrolases[37]), that it is usually not necessary to interpose yet another protective barrier between the enzyme and the transducer. Potentiometric sensors are also more amenable to utilisation with whole cell[38] (microbial and eukaryotic) as bioreagent, and here the retained packaging of the enzyme in the whole cell leads to the interposition of a host of biological membranes (plasma/organelle membrane, cell wall, etc.) that constitute diffusion barriers and which then extend response times. While potentiometric electrodes can be exquisitely selective where a gas-permeable membrane is used, the latter can further contribute significantly to extended response times.

One more-recent development has been the ion-selective field effect transistor (ISFET).[39-41] This device, not withstanding its intrinsic elegance, also requires to be protected via the agency of a covering barrier. While not a membrane in the classic sense, the encapsulating material also has an important function in protecting vulnerable components of the device from the consequences of hydration.

5.4.3 Conductimetric Sensing

Conductimetric enzyme electrodes operate by measuring a change in solution conductivity during an enzyme reaction as a consequence of the net change in the concentration of ionized species. Conductimetric methods show promise for particular analytes such as urea,[42] but suffer from practical problems of reproducibility in biological solution due to inter-sample variation in pH, ionic composition, and buffer capacity. The way in which membrane technology can overcome such difficulty has yet to be tackled, but it is possible that selective ion partitioning membranes may, in future, help to stabilise the conductivity transduction component in the face of sample variability. Table 5.2 lists the solute species present in a biological matrix (e.g., blood) which would be interfaced with the biosensing system, and exemplifies the roles played by the outer and inner membranes of a typical enzyme electrode (Figure 5.4).

5.5 SPECIFIC FUNCTIONAL MEMBRANES

The subsequent description is of specific membrane types as used for amperometric enzyme electrodes. These serve as a paradigm for other future practical biosensors (Figure 5.1), and furthermore is the area where biosensor membrane integration has brought clear advantages.

5.5.1 Track-Etched Polycarbonate Membranes

Microporous polycarbonate membranes are commonly available and have clear, defined pore sizes. Pore density and pore size can be independently controlled, though in practice exact control in the variability of these parameters is not easy during membrane manufacture.[43] The polymer used here, however, is mechanically robust and undergoes little or no swelling in aqueous media. Fine gradations in overall solute flux through the pores can be achieved and cellular, macromolecular, and colloidal material readily rejected; but inevitably there is little discrimination at a molecular level.[9] This lack of permselectivity has inherently defined their role as external membranes in conventional enzyme electrodes, in part to screen out particulates that would otherwise interfere with the function of the subjacent enzyme layer. However, they have been especially important in reducing substrate flux to the enzyme via the fine-tuning of membrane pore size. Though of only minor importance for any linear output system, this facility is of crucial relevance to the operation of a biotransducer where signal output is nonlinear due to the respective kinetic behaviour of the bioreagent; as with all other bioreceptors, this is the result of finite and limited ligand binding sites. In the case of most enzymes, saturation of binding occurs at quite low

TABLE 5.2
Relationship Between Key Solutes Present in Biological Test Solutions and Their Point of Selection of Essential Components (Table 5.2a) or Rejection of Interferents (Table 5.2b) in a Classical Dual (Inner/Outer) Membrane Amperometric Enzyme Electrode

A.

Solute	Average molecular weight (Da)	Point(s) of solute selection
O_2	32	Inner and outer
H_2O_2	34	Inner and outer
Oxalic acid	90	Outer only
Glucose	180	Outer only

B.

Solute	Average molecular weight (Da)	Point(s) of solute rejection
Ascorbic acid	176	Inner only
Fats (triacylglycerols	400	None
NADH	709	Inner only
Starch (amylose)	5,000	Outer and/or inner
Proteins (e.g., fibrinogen)	340,000	Outer only

concentrations, precluding direct use of enzyme electrodes in most undiluted biological fluids. The Michaelis constant K_m of most enzymes is therefore inappropriate for the analytical task. The extension of the analytical range is even more relevant for most food assay applications. The effect of the membranes (porosities $\leq 1\%$) is to reduce local substrate levels and thereby extend the apparent K_m of the enzyme to levels where undiluted samples can be processed. In the particular case of O_2 as an oxidase cosubstrate, depletion of oxygen in the enzyme layer is minimised by O_2 flux through the pores as well as by permeability of the gas through the polymer phase itself.

In the above situation, response is governed by rate limitation due to the transmembrane flux of solute (i.e., diffusion control); this is operationally much more advantageous than a system where response is governed by the vagaries of enzyme kinetics. Thus there is a much reduced impact of pH, ionic strength, background buffer, and inhibitors on the signal output. The analytical linear range increases with decreasing membrane pore size; typical linear ranges achieved for the glucose enzyme electrode (20 to 30 mM, with 0.01 μm pore size polycarbonate membranes) easily accommodate the range of interest for clinical measurement.[44] The range of a device governed by enzyme kinetics, on the other hand, would be 0.1 to 5 mM.

As the external membrane is inevitably the part of the device in direct contact with the bulk sample, interactions between the membrane surface itself and the biofluid are also an important factor as regards practical operation; this is really an area which has more in common with that of biomaterials than it does with sensor chemistry.

When blood is contacted with a foreign surface, protein adsorption occurs in seconds, followed by the arrival and deposition of subsequent quasipharmacological response organisms and cellular elements to the chemically "foreign" polymer surface. In parallel, there is the associated initiation of the clotting cascade. As a result the membrane surface is modified, and with such a deposited biolayer as an integral part of the enzyme electrode an alteration in analyte responsiveness results. This can be qualitatively attributed to a reduction in flux of substrate, but quantifying or predicting the rate at which this change will occur is not yet possible. This effect has been well documented in the case of polycarbonate membranes[45] and constitutes an important factor in enzyme electrode design, particularly for undiluted blood. A membrane laminate electrode comprising an outer polycarbonate membrane has been commercially exploited in an extracorporeal glucose sensor,[46] but here problems due to fouling were minimised with the aid of a specially formulated diluent buffer.

5.5.2 Hydrophobic Surface Modification

More recently, some increase in biocompatibility has been achieved through surface treatment of basic polycarbonate membrane structures. Such treatments include direct application of the lipid isopropylmyristate (IPM),[17] silanisation using organochlorosilanes,[16] and deposition of an amorphous hydrogen/carbon alloy, diamond-like carbon (DLC).[18] All such methods have not only imparted improved haemocompatibility, but by contracting membrane porosity they have radically enhanced the linear range of glucose sensors due firstly to reduced substrate flux and secondly to reduced glucose/O_2 flux ratios (Table 5.3).

TABLE 5.3
Effect of Outer Polycarbonate Membrane Modification on Resulting Glucose Sensor Characteristics

Mode of modification	Response to 0.04 mM ascorb. (μA)	Response to 0.04 mM urate (μA)	Upper linear limit (mM)	Correlation with routine method	Response time (min)
None	0.300	0.190	10	—	2.0
IPM[17]	0.025	0.015	100	0.969	2.0
Silane[16]	—	—	500	0.998	1.5
DLC[18]	0.001	0.001	80	0.999	3.0

Of the surface modification methods used, DLC coating is perhaps the most elegant. It involves sputtering, using a hydrocarbon source via fast atom bombardment onto a polycarbonate membrane surface.[47] The result is a dense amorphous hydrocarbon polymer coating. The process although expensive is cost effective considering the small amount of coated membrane (about 1 cm^2) used per sensor. DLC exhibits several useful properties including mechanical durability, chemical inertness, surface smoothness, and a level of bioinertness that appears to reduce surface fouling effects.[48]

DLC-coated polycarbonate membranes for use as external membranes showed, for example, that the permeability varied inversely with coating times (tested up to 7 min); linear characteristics of glucose enzyme electrodes with external DLC-coated membranes were correspondingly extended with increasing exposure time. Linearity achieved was inevitably greatest where very small (e.g., 0.01 μm)-diameter polycarbonate membranes had been used, though total pore blockage was also a problem here. There was evidence that with much reduced pore sizes, some degree of molecular selectivity could be conferred upon membranes. In future, inner permselective membranes may be eliminated (Figure 5.4) with both membrane functions residing in the outer membrane. Resistance to biofouling was also evident when unconditioned electrodes were used in blood, showing stabilised responses, which was improved with time of DLC coating (Figure 5.6). With an optimised system, a linear range of >80 mM was obtained with good comparison of the electrode method with that of a hospital laboratory assay of clinical samples ($r^2 = 0.99$)[18] (Figure 5.7).

Isopropylmyristate-treated polycarbonate membranes, though exhibiting glucose linear ranges up to 100 mM with relatively short response times (Table 5.3) and excellent rejection of interferents, do, however, suffer from lipid leaching effects, with sensor characteristics gradually deteriorating with time. This provisionally makes such membranes unsuitable for long-term use, though a means of stabilisation would appear to be feasible.

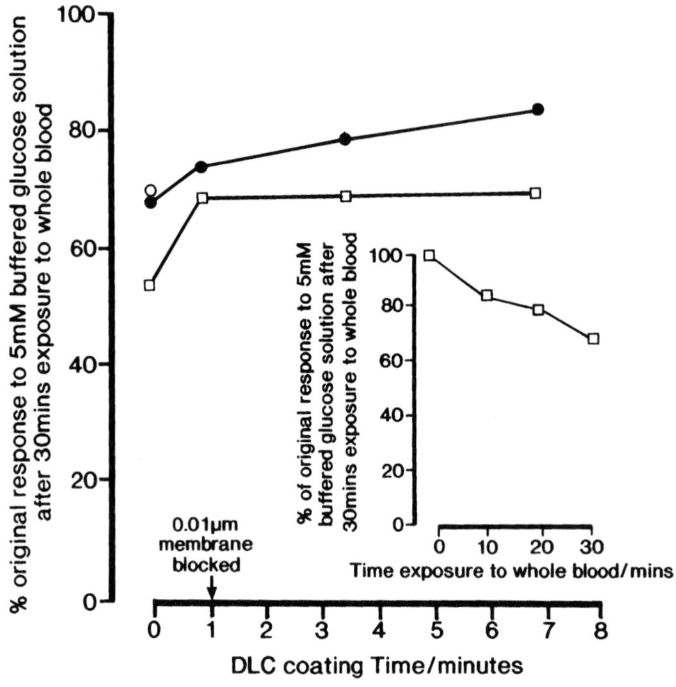

FIGURE 5.6 Relationship between percent original response of enzyme electrodes (after 30 min blood exposure) and DLC coating times with single-sided DLC-coated outer membranes and 0.05 μm pore radii uncoated lower polycarbonate membrane. (Insert: relationship between percent original response of enzyme electrode and time of whole blood exposure, with upper 0.1 μm pore radii compared 1 min single-sided DLC-coated upper membranes and lower 0.05 μm uncoated polycarbonate membrane. Upper polycarbonate pore radii: ○ 0.01; ● 0.05; □ 0.1 μm. Arrow indicates point at which the 0.01 μm membrane is blocked. (From Higson, S. P. J. and Vadgama, P., *Anal. Chim. Acta,* 271, 125, 1993. With permission.)

Silane-treated membranes[16] have conferred good stability over long-term use, and though the solvent-based coating procedure is less reproducible it may be possible to improve on this using a rigorously controlled environment for the coating process.

5.5.3 The Enzyme Layer

The enzyme layer needs to be regarded as a membrane structure in its own right. It is subject to the same types of fluxes as seen at the covering membranes. There is, therefore, likely to be some discrimination, at least of charged species; the enzyme layer has fixed negative as well as positive charges and, depending upon the overall net charge,[49] it is likely to influence the access of anionic interferents, some evidence for which has emerged from recent work.[50] Glucose oxidase, at about pH 7, operates well above its isoelectric point (pI = 5.6), resulting in an overall net negative charge at the enzyme. Accordingly, there could be screening of anionic interferents. This effect is not normally seen, but with very impermeable outer membranes where solute flux is already low, a further reduction of anion (ascorbate and urate) flux is observed. This effect is countered at high enzyme activity through the generation of gluconic acid product and lowering of local pH. Under a high solute flux, furthermore, protons

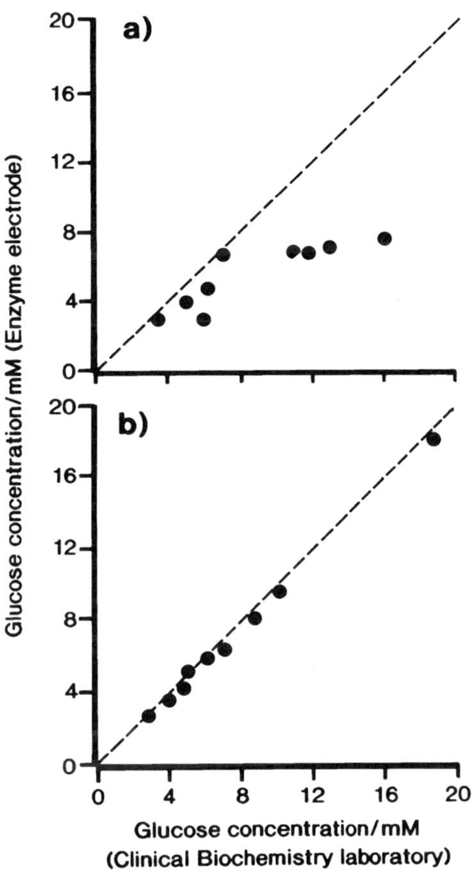

FIGURE 5.7 Correlation between whole blood glucose concentrations from clinical biochemistry laboratory analysis and enzyme electrode analysis. (a) Glucose enzyme electrode with upper 0.1 μm pore radii polycarbonate membrane with 1 min double-sided DLC coating, and lower 0.05 μm uncoated pore radii membrane; $r^2 = 0.74$. (b) Glucose enzyme electrode with upper 0.01 μm pore radii polycarbonate membrane with 1 min double-sided DLC coating, and lower 0.05 μm uncoated pore radii membrane; $r^2 = 0.99$. (From Higson, S. P. J. and Vadgama, P., *Anal. Chim. Acta,* 271, 125, 1993. With permission.)

formed as a result of electrochemical oxidation of H_2O_2 (Equation 5.2), may enter the enzyme layer, also contributing to the reduction of the net negative charge and therefore reducing the electrostatic repulsion of anionic interferents.

5.6 CELLULOSE ACETATE

5.6.1 Cellulose Acetate Membrane

Although surface-treated hydrophobic polycarbonate membranes exhibit some selectivity against common anionic interferents (Section 5.5.2), dense cellulose acetate membranes are directly suited to perform this function without pretreatment.[51] A membrane is prepared by simple solvent casting from a cellulose acetate solution in acetone,[12] typically on a glass plate or Petri dish.[52] As well as discrimination on the basis of charge,[53] high molecular weight solutes are also rejected. These factors have created a niche for cellulose acetate membranes as internal membranes in the classical enzyme electrode configuration (Figure 5.4). A whole variety of analytes have been assayed selectively including glucose,[16] urate,[54] lactate,[55] and oxalate.[56] Table 5.4 provides the characteristics of each of these sensors. The membrane also serves to eliminate the direct, nonenzyme-mediated interference due to the substrates urate and oxalate.[57]

TABLE 5.4
Characteristics of Glucose, Lactate, Urate, and Oxalate Sensors When Using an Inner Permselective Cellulose Acetate Membrane

Target analyte	Enzyme	Linear range (mM)	Steady state response time (min)	Biological matrix	Correlation with routine method	Outer membrane
Gluc.[16]	Glucose oxidase	1–50	0.5–1.5	Whole blood	r = 0.988 n = 44	Silane-treated PCM
Urate[54]	Uricase	<1.8	0.5–1.5	Whole blood	r = 0.975 n = 58	Silane-treated PCM
Lact.[55]	Lactate oxidase	1–15	1.0–3.0	Whole blood	r = 0.996 n = 46	Silane-treated PCM
Oxal.[56]	Oxalate oxidase	0.002–0.25	2.0–5.0	Diluted urine	r = 0.957 n = 10	Dialysis membrane

Note: Linear range also depends on the external membrane employed.

A less positive feature of employing an inner cellulose acetate membrane has been the reduction in linear range observed, compared with inner porous polycarbonate membranes.[56] This is probably due to the low permeability of the dense membrane structure to the transport of electrochemically generated O_2 (Equation 5.2) into the enzyme layer. The pO_2 in the enzyme layer would thus be too low to sustain the enzyme reaction at high glucose levels.[58]

5.6.2 Blood Compatibility

Signal drift of an H_2O_2-based glucose enzyme electrode after exposure to whole blood is not solely the result of external surface fouling, but partly due to ready access of diffusible passivating species to the working electrode.[59] The mechanism may be that adsorbed platelets and leukocytes may undergo degranulation on the surface, resulting in the release of low molecular weight solutes[60-62] such as adenosine diphosphate (ADP), serotonine, 5-hydroxytryptamine, and phosphoglycerides; these and other released solutes are candidates for electrode surface passivation. Importantly, such species appear not to generate an electrochemical "signature" and may create a barrier to H_2O_2 detection without evidence of their presence. Higson et al.[59] showed that by decreasing the pore size of an underlying polycarbonate membrane in a glucose enzyme electrode, it was possible to reduce the effects of such passivation. Indeed, a 0.01-μm polycarbonate membrane was shown to be a more effective barrier against (undefined) passivating low molecular weight solutes than even cellulose acetate. A loss of current output of up to 70% was observed over a 120-min exposure period. With increasing working electrode polarization (+200 to +800 mV vs. Ag/AgCl) at a cellulose acetate-mounted working electrode, the degree of passivation was shown to increase. This overpotential is tentatively attributed to the possible charged nature of the passivating species; accordingly, the dielectric properties[63] of any interposed membrane may be relevant to the electrode passivation process.

5.6.3 Surfactant-Modified Cellulose Acetate

A recent development in inner membrane technology has been the physical entrapment of surfactants into cellulose acetate during the solvent-casting procedure. To this end, the highly polar Triton X-100® and relatively nonpolar Tween 80® have been employed.[52] Both conferred enhanced selectivity for hydrogen peroxide over anionic solutes. It is possible here that the lipophilic surfactants coupled with the anionic cellulosic matrix were more effective in the rejecting of charged species. In addition to the improved selectivity, the dynamic response of modified cellulose acetate membrane electrodes was not prolonged.

As inner membranes of a glucose enzyme electrode, these modified membranes conferred improved haemocompatibility, although some electrode passivation did occur. This reinforces the idea that by cultivating internal membrane properties, it may be possible to improve operational biocompatibility, irrespective of external membrane fouling effects.

5.7 MEMBRANES FOR *IN VIVO* SENSORS

As well as *in vitro* glucose measurement, work has been directed to invasive glucose monitoring, especially for continuous glucose measurement. Needle-shaped electrodes have been devised in the main, with enzyme at the tip.[64] However, this provides a very small surface area over which to mount a covering membrane.

Deposition of membranes on the needle therefore requires more careful solvent-cast procedures, and in addition, use of a polymer which is strongly and reliably adherent to the needle structure. Polyurethane is an example of such a membrane. An adherent, protective polyurethane layer conferred many of the functional properties of microporous polycarbonate and other membranes to enable *in vivo* monitoring in subcutaneous tissue[65] and human diabetic subjects.[66] A key feature in this needle laminate system was a reduced O_2 dependence, thus allowing down to ~22 mmHg pO_2;[64] dynamic response was rapid (15 to 25 s) with a low signal drift (0.8 ± 1.3% per day) and a linear range to ~27.5 mM glucose. These characteristics are appropriate for monitoring of the hyperglycaemic diabetic patient.

An adaptation of this basic needle design by many researchers has confirmed the importance of polyurethane[67-69] as an ideal candidate for deposition over the tips of much finer needles (<0.4 mm o.d.), with stainless steel as the pseudoreference rather than silver[70,71] (Figure 5.8). A smaller implanted structure has distinct advantages as regards reducing the local inflammatory response.[72] The decrease in needle size would also reduce the dangers of an allergic (enzyme protein) response, local materials toxicity, and extent of local H_2O_2 generation, or any long-term carcinogenic effects.

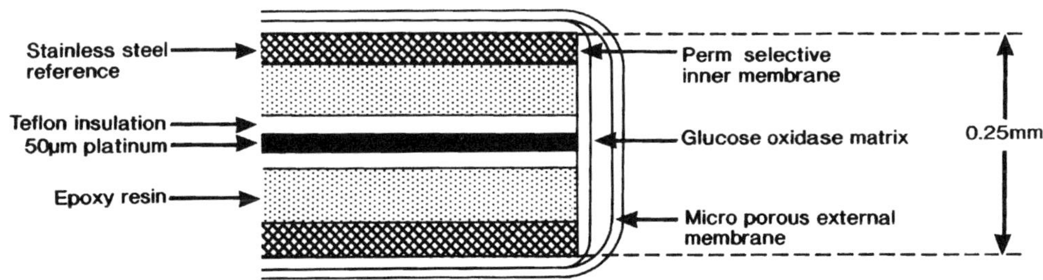

FIGURE 5.8 Schematic of a sheared-tip amperometric needle enzyme electrode.

Cellulose acetate is a prime candidate as an inner permselective membrane, and though used in earlier studies,[64] its ability to effectively screen against charged interferents was less than optimal, and it had an apparent detrimental effect on electrode linear range (<2 mM glucose); additionally, a tendency for the cellulose acetate to dissolve in solvents used to dip-coat the polyurethane layer was a distinct disadvantage. Polyethersulphone, an anionic membrane, dip-coated from a 4% dimethylsulphoxide solution, has proved not only to be more selective against interferents, but is mechanically more robust, solvent-resistant, and retains its structural integrity throughout sensor construction. Response to a mixture of electrochemical interferents, notably ascorbate (0.2 mM), cysteine (0.1 mM), glutathione (1.0 mM), and urate (1.0 mM) was found to be equivalent to <0.5 mM glucose, and resultant enzyme electrodes possessed stable linear outputs (>20 mM).

The enzyme membrane layer is dip-coated from a mixture of glutaraldehyde, albumin, and glucose oxidase. This is a particularly vulnerable layer on a small needle tip, and the covering polyurethane therefore is especially important in conferring mechanical integrity. In membrane studies, polyurethane has been found to exhibit favourable linearity and response size compared with other possible membrane materials including nylon. Indeed, by increasing the polyurethane depth and density by using successively dip-coated multiple polyurethane layers, improvements in linear range are observed (>70 mM glucose). This was additional to the reduced O_2 dependence of such coated sensors. The absolute requirement for oxygen cannot totally be eliminated for this type of system (Equation 5.1); but the dependence is sufficiently low to allow monitoring of glucose in venous blood and in hypoxic tissues. A key consideration, at least for continuous monitoring, is the need to increase the barrier membrane effect with a polymer of minimal residual thickness so as to avoid compromising response times. Also of importance for tissue use is the low substrate consumption of polyurethane-coated devices; the reduction in glucose flux allows reproducible sensing in an unstirred environment.

Sensor performance in whole blood is partly dependent on electrode tip geometry, but the uniformity of the deposited membranes is especially important. Electrodes with partially damaged or uneven membranes invoked exaggerated coagulation in blood, resulting in a rapid loss of response. Electrodes with smooth, intact membranes exhibited much better stability in whole blood, giving acceptable correlation with a standard laboratory spectrophotometric method ($y = 0.954x + 0.202$; $r = 0.991$, $n = 48$).[67] A 20% drift in calibrant response was also observed over a 6-week period, which included the analysis of 200 whole blood samples. The final system satisfied most of the requirements for an *in vivo* sensor of a typically sufficient linear range, short response time (<60 s), selectivity, stir independence, and stability in whole blood.

Current research into *in vivo* monitoring is geared towards nondestructive sterilisation protocols, improvement in electrode tip geometry to optimise the signal output in tissue,[68,69] and the development of more biocompatible masking membranes — not only to reduce surface fouling but also to ensure that contact between the antigenic enzyme layer and body tissues is avoided. Mechanical protection of the needle by a cannula mounting has also been considered in order to eliminate the risk of membrane detachment during sensor use.

5.8 POLY(VINYL CHLORIDE) (PVC) MEMBRANE

Among the most selective of membrane barriers thus far fabricated are those based on poly(vinyl chloride). Their application to amperometric sensing of neutral phenolic species (viz., paracetamol, catecholamines, etc.) contrasts distinctly with their use in ion-selective electrodes.[73,74] In the latter application, the PVC acts as a homogeneous phase, partitioning the test and internal reference solution. Selectivity is conferred by the relaxation of the ion impermeability properties of the membrane, made specific by the incorporation of a plasticiser, ion exchanger, or neutral carrier molecule. This leads to a transmembrane potential (Donnan potential) which counters any further ion penetration into the PVC. The measured potential may then be related directly to the activity of the target ions in the test solution. Electrodes constructed thus far have measured species such as H^+, K^+, Ca^{2+}, Cl^-, and organic anions such as formate, oxalate, and salicylate.[5] One drawback has been the nonspecific response to lipophilic ions, typically thiocyanate (SCN^-) and phenolics which occurs either in the presence or absence of a specific carrier. The effect is partially attributable to the species partitioning into the lipophilic polymeric PVC matrix.

Christie[75] has observed permeation of nonionized phenol through a phenolate-selective potentiometric device when using PVC plasticised with dioctylphthalate (DOP). It would therefore be valid to suggest that such transport of phenol through PVC could be followed using amperometric electrode strategies,[76] and the opportunity thus arises for creating PVC-mounted amperometric devices.

5.8.1 PVC Membranes for Amperometric Enzyme Electrodes

The lipids isopropylmyristate (IPM) and dioctylphthalate (DOP) were suitable candidates for PVC membrane plasticisation. Lipid incorporation was achieved by simply dissolving the respective plasticiser into the PVC casting solution.[77] Dioctylphthalate was found to be better incorporated than IPM into the polymer matrix. Both exhibited similar selectivity, but IPM-treated membranes exhibited superior sensitivity and faster responses (<3 min) with a range of electrochemically active species including ascorbate, urate, paracetamol, 4-aminophenol, and catechol. Due to the inherent lipophilic properties of the resulting membranes, their use on an amperometric electrode required consideration of the possible insulation of the Pt anode from the Ag/AgCl reference due to the absence of a retained internal electrolyte. This was avoided by the inclusion of an electrolyte-soaked hydrophillic dialysis membrane between the PVC and the electrode surface.

Plasticised PVC membranes exhibited excellent selectivity for phenolics over the more polar hydrogen peroxide and ionic species ascorbate, urate, and NADH. The selectivity was shown to be exceptionally superior to porous polycarbonate (0.05 μm) and cellulose acetate membranes (Figure 5.9); selectivity of PVC against cellulose acetate gave a greatly improved determinand:ascorbate interferent signal ratio of ×7 for hydrogen peroxide, ×180 for paracetamol, and ×230 for 4-aminophenol.[76]

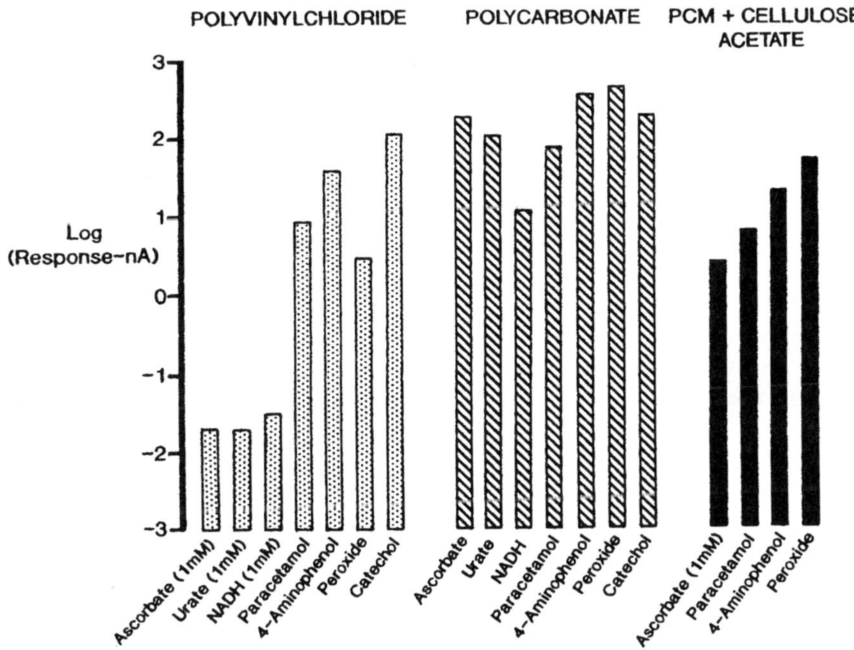

FIGURE 5.9 Responses to 0.1 mM solutions, except where shown, comparing PVC (0.06 g of PVC + 150 μl of IPM), polycarbonate (0.05 μm), and combined polycarbonate (0.03 μm)-cellulose acetate (2%) membranes. Phosphate buffer (pH 7.4), +0.65 V vs. Ag. (From Christie, I. M., Lloyd, S., and Vadgama, P., *Anal. Chim. Acta,* 269, 65, 1992. With permission.)

A multitude of sensor applications may be realised for the PVC/amperometric system provided the final signal species is PVC permeable (phenolic species). This includes the possibility of the direct electrochemical determination of paracetamol.

Substrate-specific dehydrogenases which are NAD cofactor dependent show promise for PVC-based biosensor adaptation. Gorton et al.[34] demonstrated that quinone mediators could be used to facilitate the electrochemistry of the NAD^+/NADH couple, reducing the normal overpotential (1.1 V vs. SCE) for the cofactor to the lower potentials of the quinone/hydroquinone couple. The reduced form of the quinone mediator, being a phenolic, would be readily able to permeate an inner selective PVC membrane whilst screening out charged interferents. Sensors based on such dehydrogenase enzymes may thus be realised for a range of corresponding substrates for anaerobic measurement, as required in, say, fermentation process control.

5.8.2 Blood Biocompatibility

A typical PVC membrane (0.06 g PVC, 150 μL IPM) placed over an anodic electrode, when treated with undiluted patient serum, exhibited no fouling either of the membrane or the electrode surface even after 90 min of continuous exposure. This apparent excellent biocompatible nature of the membrane may have been a consequence of the quasiliquid nature of the plasticised PVC membrane reducing the adsorption of serum proteins and the high selectivity of PVC reducing consequent permeation/passivation by low molecular weight solutes. Measurement of alkaline phosphatase (ALP) activity ($U\ l^{-1}$) (using 4-aminophenylphosphate as substrate) in serum was demonstrated to be an ideal application for PVC in the amperometric detection mode ($y = 1.3213 + 18.6295$; $r = 0.9931$, $n = 10$), since the 4-aminophenyl product of the enzyme reaction readily permeates the PVC.

The sensor haemocompatibility conferred by PVC membranes warrants further assessment of its wider applicability as a general interface between sensor and biological matrix. However, the lipophilic phase presented by the membrane, certainly of the dimensions used hitherto (~50 μm thickness) does rather limit the solute range to nonpolar species.

5.8.3 Unplasticised PVC

Unplasticised PVC, although also lipophilic in nature, has proved to have some ion permeability, particularly to organics. This is most likely due to residual void space in the polymer matrix available for ion residence. However, the discontinuous and nanoscale nature of the void space confers a high degree of diffusion restriction which renders them suitable only as outer membranes for selected enzyme electrodes. Organic ions such as lactate, ascorbate, urate, and oxalate thus appear to be measurable using such membranes. In the measurement of urine oxalate[65] (to assess the output of this ion in hyperoxaluraic stone formation), linearity was extended well above that for the more permeable polycarbonate and dialysis membranes to encompass the clinical relevant range for urine oxalate concentrations (0.1 to 0.5 mM).

Some preliminary efforts have also been directed towards substrate-selective outer membranes. This has been achieved via the incorporation of anion exchangers into the PVC membrane.[78] This has afforded membranes selective for anions over nonionic and cationic species (Figure 5.5). Sensors have subsequently been realised for the anionic substrates oxalate and lactate with much improved sensitivity as compared with unmodified PVC; though extended response times (8 to 12 min) have been observed, these can undoubtedly be decreased by reducing the membrane thickness of the plasticiser-containing structures; liquid exchanger incorporation has generally produced thicker membranes (Figure 5.10a) following solvent casting than has been achieved with, say, neutral plasticiser incorporation (Figure 5.10b).

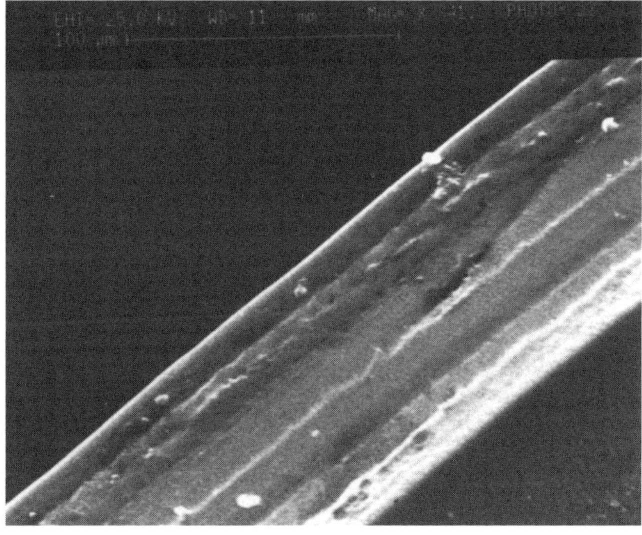

a

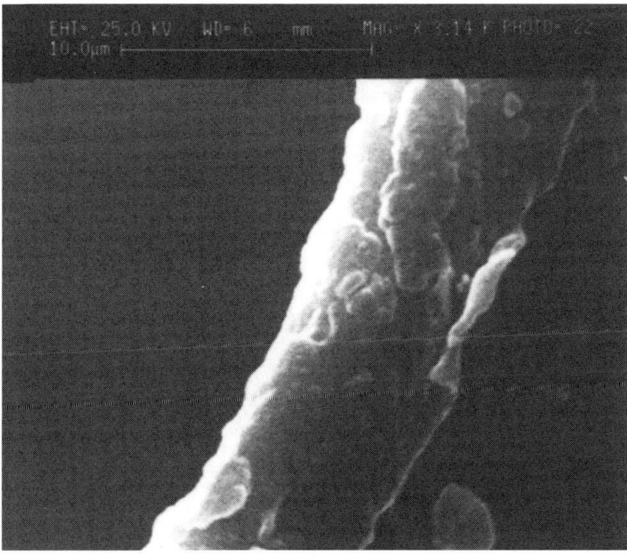

b

FIGURE 5.10 Scanning electron micrographs of PVC membrane edge. PVC plasticised with (a) liquid ion exchanger and (b) neutral lipid. (Note difference in micrograph scales emphasising the thicker nature of membrane (a).)

5.9 CONCLUSIONS

The majority of the membrane-based sensors discussed here meet key operational requirements such as response time, sensitivity, stability, ease of handling, and where evaluated, correlation with routine methods. Commercialization of these laboratory systems as alternative, perhaps more attractive, means of analysis requires a further perspective of recognizing the practical needs of potential users not versed in sensor technology.

There will be inevitable developments in effective signal processing techniques using IC technology, but this isolated advancement is prone to failure unless there is also an effort made at improving the materials aspects of sensors, especially through the use of membrane modifiers. While functional improvements have been obtained with membranes, very much greater attention is necessary in the enhancement of biocompatibility for both *in vitro* and *in vivo* sensing. For the latter, especially, a continued stable performance of the sensor is a necessity, and intermittent calibration is not a practical option.

Future improvements in membrane-based sensor design may well also be centred upon reducing the number of individual sensor and membrane components to the complexity of construction and manufacture. As envisaged with PVC membranes, designing selective properties into the external membrane phase could obviate the need for an inner permselective barrier, and ultimately the bioreagent layer could also be incorporated in this single structure.

The integration of the individual sensor components could reach an ultimate fabrication simplification with a single-step construct as has been reported in the case of film formation.[79] Ultimately, the nontransducing elements of both chemical and biological sensors warrant as much attention as has been given for the transduction chemistry alone.

REFERENCES

1. Clark, L. C. and Lyons, C., Electrode systems for continuous monitoring in cardiovascular surgery, *Ann. N.Y. Acad. Sci.,* 102, 29, 1962.
2. Updike, S. J. and Hicks, G. P., The enzyme electrode, *Nature,* 214, 986, 1967.
3. Coulet, P. R., Electrochemical and fiber optic biosensors for highly selective molecular targetting, *Anal. Lett.,* 24 (8), 1333, 1991.
4. Pusch, W. and Walch, A., Membrane structure and its correlation with membrane permeability, *J. Mem. Sci.,* 10, 325, 1982.
5. Lakshminarayanaiah, N., *Transport Phenomena in Membranes*, Academic Press, New York, 1969, 254.
6. Noble, R. D. and Way, J. D., *Liquid Membranes: Theory and Applications*, ACS Symposium, Series 347, American Chemical Society, Washington D.C., 1987.
7. Kinzer, K. E., Lloyd, D. R., Gay M. S., Wightman, J. P., Johnson, B. C., and McGrath, J. E., Phase inversion sulfonated polysulfone membranes, *J. Membr. Sci.,* 22, 1, 1985.
8. Cotton, C. K., Smith, K. A., Merill, E. W., and Farrell, P. C., Permeability studies with cellulosic membranes, *J. Biomed. Mater. Res.,* 5, 459, 1971.
9. Koochaki, Z., Higson, S. P. J., Mutlu, M., and Vadgama P., The diffusion limited oxidase-based glucose enzyme electrode: relation between covering membrane permeability and substrate response, *J. Membr. Sci.,* 76, 261, 1993.
10. Hwang, S. T. and Strong, S. D., Transport of dissolved carbon monoxide through silicon rubber membranes, *J. Poly. Sci. Poly. Symp.,* 41, 17, 1973.
11. Davies, M. L., Hamilton, C. J., Murphy, S. M., and Tighe, B. J., Polymer membranes in clinical sensor applications, *Biomaterials,* 13(14), 971, 1992.
12. Kesting R. E., Phase inversion membranes, *Am. Chem. Soc. Symp. Ser.,* 269, 131, 1985.
13. Bark, M. and Zachmann, H. G., Simultaneous measurements of small angle X-ray scattering, wide-angle X-ray scattering and heat exchange during crystallisation and melting of polymers, *Acta Poly.,* 44(6), 259, 1993.
14. Schnell, H., *Chemistry and Physics of Polycarbonates*, Interscience, New York, 1964, p. 131.
15. Kesting, R. E., *Synthetic Polymeric Membranes*, 1st ed., McGraw-Hill, New York, 1971, chap. 2.
16. Mullen, W. H., Keedy, F. H., Churchouse, S. J., and Vadgama, P. M., Glucose enzyme electrode with extended linearity; application to undiluted blood measurements, *Anal. Chim. Acta,* 183, 59, 1986.
17. Tang, L. X., Koochaki, Z. B., and Vadgama, P. M., Composite liquid membrane for enzyme electrode construction, *Anal. Chim. Acta,* 232, 357, 1990.
18. Higson, S. P. J. and Vadgama, P. M., Diamond-like carbon coated microporous polycarbonate as a composite barrier for a glucose enzyme electrode, *Anal. Chim. Acta,* 271, 125, 1992.
19. Helfferich, F., *Ion Exchange*, McGraw-Hill, New York, 1962.
20. Whitely, L. D. and Martin, C. R., Perfluorosulfonate ionomer film coated electrodes as electrochemical sensors: fundamental investigations, *Anal. Chem.,* 59, 1746, 1987.

21. Buttry, D. A. and Anson, F. C., Effects of electron exchange and single file diffusion on charge propagation in Nafion film containing redox couples, *J. Am. Chem. Soc.,* 105 (4), 685, 1983.
22. McDowell, W., Crown ethers as solvent extraction reagents — where do we stand, *J. Sep. Sci. Technol.,* 23, 1251, 1988.
23. Wotring, V. J., Johnson, D. M., Daunert, S., and Bachas, L.G., in *Immunochemical Assay and Biosensor Technology for the 1990's,* Nakamura, R. M., Kahasara, Y., and Rechnitz, G. A., Eds., American Society of Microbiology, Washington, D.C., 1992, p. 355.
24. Nagy, G., Gerhardt, G. A., Oke, A. F., Rice, M. E., Adams, R. N., Szentirmay, M. N., and Martin, C. R., Ion exchange and transport of neurotransmitters in Nafion films on conventional and microelectrode surfaces, *J. Electroanal. Chem.,* 188, 85, 1985.
25. Meyerhoff, M. E. and Opdycke, W. N., Ion selective electrodes, *Adv. Clin. Chem.,* 25, 1, 1986.
26. Palet, C., Munoz, M., Daunert, S., Bachas, L. G., and Valentine, M., Vitamin B_{12} derivatives as anion carriers in transport through supported liquid membranes and correlation with their behaviour in ion-selective electrodes, *Anal. Chem.,* 65, 1533, 1993.
27. Brunsman, A. R., New enzyme probe for glucose analysis, Pitts. Conf., Analytical Chemistry, YSI, Yellow Springs, Ohio, 1973.
28. Lonsdale, H. K., The growth of membrane technology, *J. Membr. Sci.,* 10, 81, 1982.
29. McDonnell, M. B. and Vadgama, P. M., Membranes: separation principles and sensing, *Sel. Electrode Rev.,* 11, 17-67, 1989.
30. Kurochkin, V. E., Raevskii, K. K., and Terovskii, V. B., Experimental verification of a response model of a membrane electrode, *J. Anal. Chem.,* 48 (4), 479, 1993.
31. Bradley, C. R. and Rechnitz, G. A., Immobilization barrier effects on the dynamic response characteristics of potentiometric adenosine deaminase enzyme electrode, membrane thickness effect, *Anal. Chem.,* 57, 1401, 1985.
32. Romette, J. L., Yang, J. S., Kusakabe, H., and Thomas, D., Enzyme electrode for specific determination of L-lysine, *Biotechnol. Bioeng.,* 25, 2557, 1983.
33. Amini, M. A. S., Vallon, J. J., and Bichon, C., Oxalate measured by oxalate oxidase electrode immobilized on a collagen membrane, *Anal. Lett.,* 22(1), 43, 1989.
34. Gorton, L., Csoregi, E., Dominguez, E., Emneus, J., Jonsson-Pettersson, G., and Marko-Varga, G., Selective detection in flow analysis based on the combination of immobilized enzymes and chemically modified electrodes, *Anal. Chim. Acta,* 250, 203, 1991.
35. Cass, A. E. G., Davis, G., Francis, G. D., Hill, H. A. O., Aston, W. J., Higgins, I., Plotkin, E. N., Scott, L. D. L., and Turner, A. P. F., Ferrocene mediated enzyme electrode for amperometric determination of glucose, *Anal. Chem.,* 56, 667, 1984.
36. Kawabe, T., Iida, T., Iijima, N., Mitamura, T., Hara, M., and Katsube, T., ISFET type threonine sensor using threonine deaminase from thermophilic bacterium, *Denki Kagaku,* 53(7), 514, 1985.
37. Nilsson, H., Akerlund, A., and Moabach, K., Determination of glucose, urea and penicillin using pH electrodes, *Biochim. Biophys. Acta,* 320, 529, 1973.
38. Hikuma, M., Obana, H., Yasuda, T., Karube, I., and Suzuki, S., A potentiometric microbial sensor based on immobilised *Escherichia coli* for glutamic acid, *Anal. Chim. Acta,* 116, 61, 1980.
39. Bergveld, P., Development of an ion-sensitive solid-state device for neurophysiological measurements, *IEEE Trans. Biomed. Eng.,* BME-17, 70, 1970.
40. Buck, R. P. and Hackleman, D. E., Field effect potentiometric sensors, *Anal. Chem.,* 49, 2315, 1977.
41. Moss, S. D., Janata, J., and Johnson, C. C., Potassium ion sensitive field effect transistor, *Anal. Chem.,* 47, 2238, 1978.
42. Lawton, B. A., Lu, Z. H., Pethig, R., and Wei, Y., Physicochemical studies of the activity of urease and the development of a conductimetric urea sensor, *J. Mol. Liquids,* 42, 83, 1989.
43. Alnajjar, S. A. R., Oliveira, A., and Piesch, E., Extension of the alpha-particle energy range in polycarbonate using multi step chemical or electrochemical etching, *Radiat. Prot. Dosimetry,* 27(1), 5, 1989.
44. Vadgama, P., Spoors, J., Tang L. X., and Battersby, C., The needle glucose electrode: in vitro peformance and optimisation for implantation, *Biomed. Biochim. Acta,* 48 (11/12), 935, 1989.

45. Tang, L. X. and Vadgama, P., Optimisation of enzyme electrodes, *Med. Biol. Eng. Comp.*, 28(3), B14, 1990.
46. Fogt, E. J., Dodd, L. M., Jenning, E. M., and Clemens, A. H., Development and evaluation of a glucose analyzer for glucose-controlled insulin infusion (Biostator), *Clin. Chem.*, 24, 1366, 1978.
47. Wild, C., Koidl, P., and Wagner, J., in *EMRS Symposia Proc.*, European Materials Research Society, Les Ulis, Koidl, P., and Oelhafer, P. (Eds.), 17, 1374, 1987.
48. Thomson, L. A., Law, F. C., Franks, J., and Rushton, N., Biocompatibility of diamond-like carbon coating, *Biomaterials,* 12, 37, 1991.
49. Ivnitskii, P. M. and Rishpon, J., Biosensor based on direct detection of membrane potential induced by immobilised hydrolytic enzymes, *Anal. Chim. Acta,* 282, 517, 1993.
50. Treloar, P. H., Higson, S. P. J., Desai, M. A., Christie, I. M., Ghosh, S., Rosenberg, M. F., Reddy, S. M., Jones, M. N., and Vadgama, P M., Ex-vivo sensors, in Uses of Immobilised Biological Compounds, NATO Proc., Brixen, Italy, 1993.
51. Koochaki, Z., Christie, I., and Vadgama, P., Electrode response to phenolic species through cellulosic membranes, *J. Membr. Sci.,* 57, 83, 1991.
52. Desai, M. A., Ghosh, S., Crump, P. W., Benmakroha, Y., and Vadgama, P. M., Internal membranes and laminates for adaptation of amperometric enzyme electrodes to direct biofluid analysis, *Scand. J. Clin. Lab. Invest.,* 214, 53, 1993.
53. Morita, Z., Ishida, H., and Shimamoto, H., Anion permeability of cellulosic membranes. 1. porosity of water swollen membranes, *J. Membr. Sci.,* 46, 283, 1989.
54. Keedy F. H. and Vadgama, P., Determination of urate in undiluted whole blood by enzyme electrode, *Biosens. Bioelectron.,* 6, 491, 1991.
55. Mullen, W. H., Churchouse, S. J., Keedy, F. H., and Vadgama, P. M., Enzyme electrode for measurement of lactate in undiluted blood, *Clin. Chim. Acta,* 157 (2), 191, 1986.
56. Reddy S. M., Higson, S. P. J., Christie, I., and Vadgama, P. M., Selective membranes for the construction and optimisation of an amperometric oxalate enzyme electrode, *Analyst,* 119, 949, 1994.
57. Beden, C., Cetin, I., Kahyaoglu, A., Takky, D., and Lamy, C., Electrocatalytic oxidation of saturated oxygenated compounds on gold electrodes, *J. Catal.,* 104, 37, 1987.
58. Puleo, A. C., Paul, D. R., and Kelley, S. S., The effect of degree of acetylation on gas sorption and transport behaviour in cellulose acetate, *J. Membr. Sci.,* 47(3), 301, 1989.
59. Higson S. P. J., Desai, M. A., Ghosh, S., Christie, I., and Vadgama, P., Amperometric enzyme electrode biofouling and passivation in blood: characterisation of working electrode polarisation and inner membrane effects, *J. Chem. Soc. Faraday Trans.,* 89 (15), 2847, 1993.
60. Mills, D. C. B., Robb, I. A., and Roberts, G. C. K., The release of nucleotides, 5-hydroxytryptamine and enzymes from human blood platelets during aggregation, *J. Physiol.,* 195, 715, 1968.
61. Zucker, M. B. and Borrelli, J., Relationship of clotting factors to serotonin release from washed platelets, *J. Appl. Physiol.,* 7, 432, 1955.
62. Haycox, C. L. and Ratner, B. D., Fourth World Biomaterials Congress, Berlin, 183, 1992.
63. Seanor, D. A., Electrical conduction in polymers, in *Electrical Properties of Polymers,* Seanor, D. A., Ed., Academic Press, New York, 1982, chap. 1.
64. Schichiri, M., Kawamori, R., Hakui, N., and Abe, H., Wearable artificial endocrine pancreas with needle type sensor, *Lancet,* 2, 1129, 1982.
65. Schichiri, M. Kawamori, R., Goriya, Y., Yamasaki, Y., Nomura, M., Hakui, N., and Abe, H., Glycemic control in pancreatomised dogs with a wearable artificial endocrine pancreas, *Diabetologia,* 24, 179, 1983.
66. Schichiri, M., Kawamori, R., Hakui, N., Yamasaki, Y., and Abe, H., Closed loop glycemic control with a wearable artificial pancreas, *Diabetes,* 33, 1200, 1984.
67. Churchouse, S. J., Battersby, C. M., Mullen, W. H., and Vadgama, P. M., Needle enzyme electrodes for biological studies, *Biosensors,* 2, 325, 1986.
68. Churchouse, S. J., Mullen, W. H., Keedy, F. H., Battersby, C. M., and Vadgama, P. M., Studies on needle glucose electrodes, *Anal. Proc.,* 23, 146, 1986.
69. Vadgama, P. and Desai, M. A., In vivo biosensors, in *Biosensor Principles and Applications,* Blum, L. J. and Coulet, P. R., Eds., Marcel Dekker, New York, 1990, Chap. 13.

70. Dymond, A. M., Kaechele, L. E., Jurist, J. M., and Crandall, P. H., Brain tissue reaction to some chronically implanted metals, *J. Neurosurg.,* 33, 574, 1970.
71. Jackson, W. F. and Duling, B. R., Toxic effects of silver-silver chloride electrodes on vascular smooth muscle, *Circ. Res.,* 53, 105, 1983.
72. Aderson, J. M., In vivo biocompatibility, in *Polymeric Biomaterials*, NATO ASI Series E: Applied Sciences, 106, Piskin, E. and Hoffman, A. S., Eds., Martinus Nijhoff, Boston, 1986.
73. Moody, G. J., Oke R. B., and Thomas, J. D. R., A calcium-sensitive electrode based on a liquid ion exchanger in a poly (vinyl chloride) matrix, *Analyst,* 95, 910, 1970.
74. Bailey, P. L., Electrodes based on ion exchangers and neutral carriers, in *Analysis with Ion Selective Electrodes*, 2nd ed., Heyden, Philadelphia, 1980, chap. 6.
75. Christie, I. M., Ph.D. Thesis, University of Wales, 1988.
76. Christie, I. M., Lloyd, S., and Vadgama, P., Plasticised poly(vinyl chloride) as a permselective barrier membrane for high selectivity amperometric sensors and biosensors, *Anal. Chim. Acta,* 269, 65, 1992.
77. Moody, G. J. and Thomas, J. D. R., Poly (vinyl chloride) matrix membrane ion-selective electrodes in *Ion Selective Electrodes in Analytical Chemistry*, Freiser, H., Ed., Plenum Press, New York, 1978, chap. 4.
78. Imperial Chemical Industries, Sensor Devices, Br. Patent Appl. 910 5406.4, 1991.
79. Christie, I. M., Lloyd, S., and Vadgama, P., Modification of electrode sufaces with oxidised phenols to confer selectivity to amperometric biosensors for glucose determination, *Anal. Chim. Acta,* 274, 191, 1993.

6 Microelectronic Devices

Alain Grisel

CONTENTS

6.1 INTRODUCTION

Biosensors are analytical devices based on the combination of a biological component and a suitable transducer. The concept of immobilizing a biochemical layer onto a transducer was introduced more than 30 years ago by Clark and Lyons.[1] Many different combinations of biological components and transducers were investigated. So far, the most advanced development has been achieved in the case of enzyme electrodes, i.e., biosensors based on the combination of an enzyme and an electrochemical transducer. Depending on the transducer used the enzyme electrodes can be classified as amperometric, potentiometric, or conductimetric, with the first two being the most commonly used.[2-4]

On the other hand, by taking advantage of the frequency shift of a quartz resonator surface with molecular mass changes of absorbed biomolecules, some research groups have suggested the use of transducers based on surface acoustic wave devices for biosensor realization.[41,42] Recent developments of optical devices have also shown the possible use of different techniques, such as light absorption measurement, surface plasmon resonance with input grating couplers, and difference interferometry for direct biosensing.[5]

Because of the interest in miniaturized sensors and in the development of disposable devices, the microelectronic technology appears to be the most convenient for transducer fabrication. Indeed, it allows mass production of miniaturized sensors which are of increasing interest for many potential analytical applications. For amperometric devices, two approaches can be used — thick film or thin film technology — both resulting in most cases in planar structures onto which enzymes or receptor molecules are immobilized.[6,7]

Several potentiometric devices, such as ISE (ion selective electrodes) or ISFET (ion sensitive field effect transistors) can also be used with suitable membranes when the biological reaction induces an ion concentration change or an enzymatic pH change.[8-10] Integrated optics, on the other hand, have recently shown that microoptoelectronics is an improving technology which may well be used in the near future for the manufacture of optical biosensors.[11-13]

0-8493-8905-4/97/$0.00+$.50
© 1997 by CRC Press, Inc.

The use of microelectronics technology can address not only the production of transducers, but it also offers the possibility of integrating on-chip electronics for signal processing and measurement system interfacing, thus resulting in the so-called "smart" sensors.[14] Among the different types of biosensors currently being investigated, the integrated immunosensor would drastically reduce the disadvantages of classical immunoassay techniques. Recently, antigen antibody pairs have been detected using either covalently immobilized receptors on ligands[5,15] or by receptor molecules combined in self-assembled lipid monolayers.[16] The methods used for the detection of ligands-receptors binding are impedance spectroscopy, surface plasmon resonance (SPR)[17] (Chapters 7 and 16), fluorescence, or absorption interferometry (Chapter 8) using input grating coupling (IGC).[12] Integrated electrochemical structures and integrated optics can be combined for demonstrating the evidence of direct immunosensing and selective detection of biological molecules.

6.2 ELECTROCHEMICAL DEVICES

The major investigations in the field of integrated biosensors have led to the feasibility of miniaturized electrochemical elements based on silicon technology, such as ISFET (ion sensitive field effect transistors) and thin-film noble metal electrodes. Both amperometric and potentiometric sensors have been developed using enzyme membranes (Chapter 2), immobilized antigens in lipid membranes, and other biospecific molecules (Chapter 3).

6.2.1 Integrated Amperometric Biosensors and Manufacturing Processes

Among amperometric enzyme electrodes, the most widely investigated is the glucose electrode due to its potential interest, especially in the field of human health care and bioprocess control. It is based on an amperometric transducer with two or three electrodes coupled with an enzymatic layer.

The advantage of the use of microelectronic technology in this case consists of well-defined metallic electrodes surrounded by insulating materials, such as Si_3N_4, covering their electrical contacts made in conducting material, here doped polysilicon. The sensitive layer consists of an enzymatic membrane containing the immobilized enzyme glucose oxidase on the working electrode. The detection principle is the electrochemical oxidation of peroxide generated in the following enzymatic reaction: glucose + O_2 + $H_2O \xrightarrow{\text{GOD}}$ gluconolactone + H_2O_2. Figure 6.1 shows a schematic drawing of planar electrodes integrated on silicon and two examples of microelectrodes for amperometric biosensors including an integrated glucose sensor.[7,25]

Amperometric measurements require two or three different electrodes: a working electrode, a counter electrode, and a reference electrode. The most suitable electrode materials are noble metals and different forms of carbon. The reference electrode is usually the conventional but miniaturized Ag/AgCl electrode. The deposition of these materials is performed either by thick-film or thin-film technology. The thick-film approach is usually presented as cheaper compared to the thin-film one. However, it suffers from a rather limited resolution (typically 100 μm) which can be prohibitive for some applications where critically small electrode dimensions are required. Thick-film technology is based on screen printing and firing of suitable pastes, usually onto a ceramic substrate.[3,6] (See Chapter 10 for a detailed description.)

Using Pt, Au, or Ag pastes, different electrodes can be made which after firing have a typical thickness of 10 to 50 μm. The commercial "Exactech" blood glucose sensor for diabetics is an example of a biosensor device based on thick-film technology. It uses a two-electrode planar geometry; a carbon paste impregnated with a mediator for the working electrode and an Ag/AgCl reference electrode.[18]

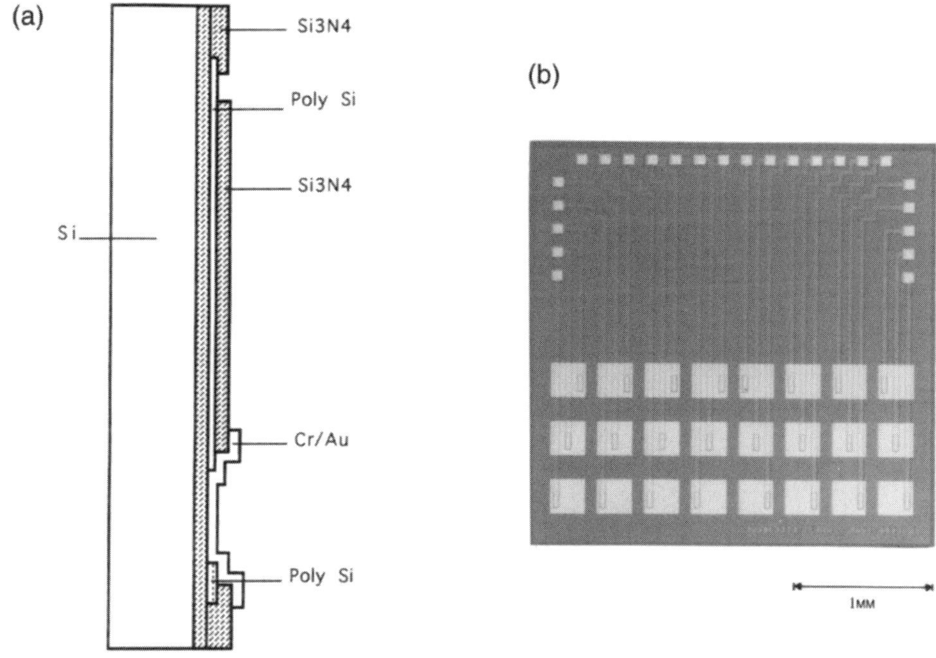

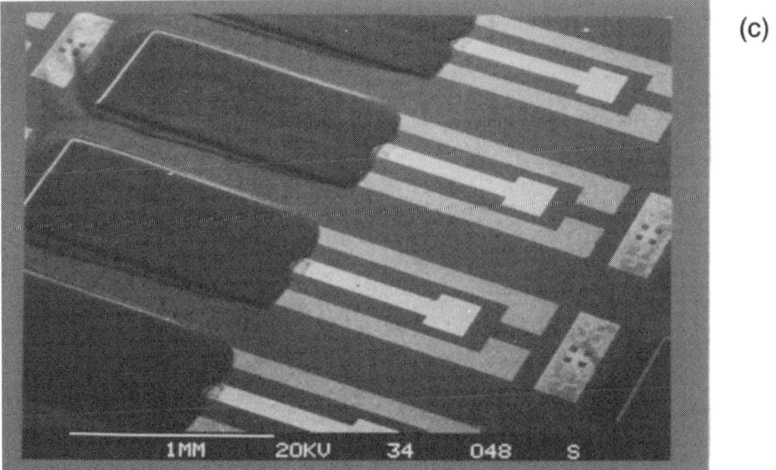

FIGURE 6.1 (a) Schematic drawing of planar electrodes integrated on silicon. (b) Array of 8 isolated planar electrodes of dimensions 300 μm × 300 μm. (c) Three-electrode structures covered with an enzymatic glucose oxidase membrane.

Thin-film technology is based on the photolithographic patterning of evaporated or sputtered metallic films onto silicon, glass, or polymeric substrates.[7,19-23] The advantage of this approach is its high resolution (down to 2 to 3 μm) and good control of patterned geometries. When Pt is used, the patterning is performed by lift-off instead of the commonly used chemical etching techniques. For thin-film noble metals, an intermediate adhesion layer (usually Ti) is required. Care has to be taken that this layer does not result in electrochemical

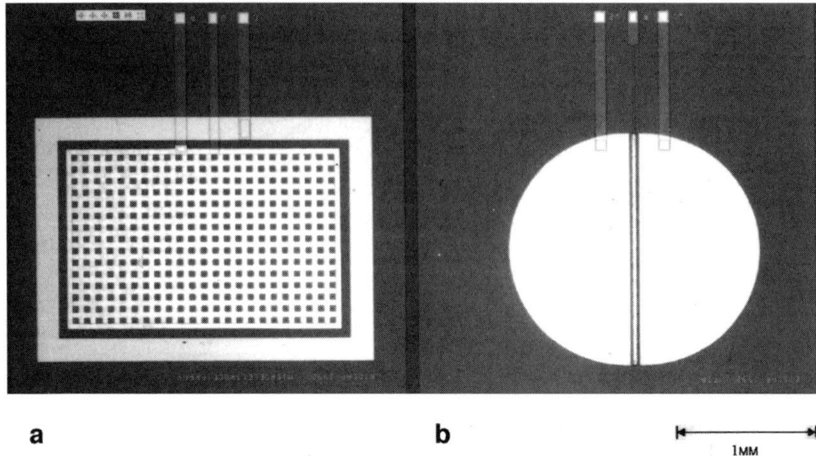

FIGURE 6.2 Microphotograph of two geometries of three-electrode structures. (a) Three-electrode structure consisting of, • An array of 5 µm × 5 µm working electrodes; • A reference electrode grid; • A surrounding counter electrode. (b) Two symmetrical half-circle electrodes. Working and counter electrodes separated by a thin reference electrode. The surface dimensions of the electrode chips are 3 mm × 3 mm.

interferences when utilizing the behavior of electrodes in solution.[24] Figure 6.2 shows different geometries of integrated electrode structures.

6.2.2 Immobilization Techniques and Polymeric Membrane Deposition

Optimization of the enzymatic membrane deposition is currently the most critical issue of biosensor manufacturing. Many different strategies for immobilizing enzymes onto various electrode materials have been described in the literature. The most commonly used is still the chemical method of enzyme entrapment within a membrane formed by a carrier protein, such as bovine serum albumin and the enzyme of interest (glucose oxidase). Glutaraldehyde has been the most extensively used cross-linking agent.[25,26] This enzyme immobilization can be performed on-chip or at the "on-wafer" level. Among other methods, covalent binding,[27] entrapment in a matrix,[28] and enzyme mixing within the carbon paste in the case of thick-film sensors should also be mentioned.[26] More recently, enzyme immobilization by electrochemical depositions, using either electrochemical polymerization to incorporate the enzyme within a polypyrrole matrix[25,29] or electrochemically aided adsorption,[25,30] have illustrated the interest of these geometrically well-controlled techniques.

Frequently, a mass transfer control regime such as diffusion limitation is an advantage for the functional characteristics of biosensors. The deposition of an additional outer polymeric membrane is thus often required, and its final characteristics, which depend on physical parameters like thickness and porosity, are of critical importance for sensor performance.

For the realization of an integrated biosensor, the biologically active material has to be immobilized on the electrochemical sensor. In most cases, an appropriate membrane is necessary to cover the active region in order to minimize fouling, prevent degradation of the sensor, or limit cross-sensitivity (Chapter 5).[25] An example of such a membrane is the pHEMA (hydroxyethyl methacrylate) hydrogel layer which can be structured by photolithography.[31]

The best up-to-date technique for depositing a hydrogel layer consists of photopolymerizing the membrane through a photolithographic mask by UV-initiated free-radical cross-linking of the polymer directly on the substrate.

6.2.3 ISFET-Based Biosensors

In 1976 Janata suggested the use of an enzyme-modified ISFET (ion sensitive field effect transistor), the ENFET (enzyme field effect transistor), as a base device for new microelectronic biosensors development. The first preliminary results were published in 1980,[32] with a pH-sensitive ISFET described as a penicillin-sensitive device. In order to achieve such a biosensor, Caras and Janata used a double pH-sensitive ISFET, the gate of one ISFET being covered by a membrane containing cross-linked albumin-penicillinase and the other having a membrane of only cross-linked albumin.

It has been demonstrated that the penicillinase present in the active gate membrane was sufficient to catalyze the hydrolysis of penicillin in the analyte, producing penicilloic acid on the pH-sensitive ISFET gate. This reaction creates a local decrease in the pH near the active ISFET gate, while the pH of the other inactive membrane on the second ISFET gate remains unchanged. A schematic drawing of the measurement setup is shown in Figure 6.3. The advantages of the differential measurement mode with such double ISFETs were reported to be the relative insensitivity to thermal or pH variations of the analyte.

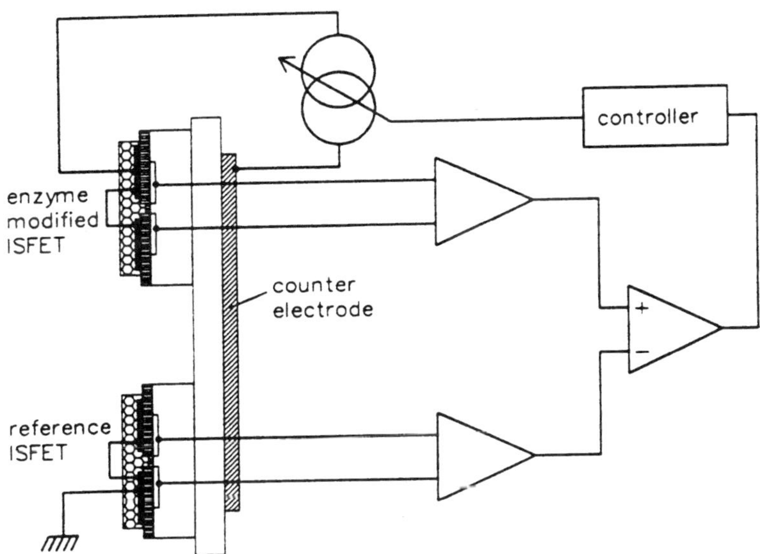

FIGURE 6.3 Differential measurement using one ISFET with an active enzyme-loaded membrane and one ISFET with an inactive membrane. (From van der Schoot, B. H., Voorthuyzen, H., and Bergveld, P., *Sensors Actuators,* B1, 546, 1990. With permission.)

The ISFET is operated as a MOSFET (metal oxide silicon field effect transistor) with the metal gate being replaced by the liquid analyte and the reference electrode usually being an Ag/AgCl electrode in equilibrium with a KCl solution. The released protons in the enzymatic reaction on ISFET 1 are responsible for the local pH decrease and the H^+ ions at the interface of the Al_2O_3 isolating gate create the field effect inducing a current I_{DS} in the channel of transistor 1. The output circuit is designed to keep the current I_{DS} constant by changing the output potential U_{1out}. In this configuration, the comparison of U_{1out} with U_{2out} coming from the inactive ISFET 2 gives a signal proportional to the penicillin present in the analyte.

The reported results, however, have shown that the buffer capacity of the analyte has a relevant influence on the ENFET sensitivity, linearity, and concentration range. A buffer concentration of 5 mM phosphate at pH 7 results in a linear response to penicillin in the range of 0.2 to 6 mM with a sensitivity of 16 mV $mmol^{-1}$, while an increase of phosphate concentration causes a proportional decrease of sensitivity, but increases the linear range. The upper limit of the response curve increases with higher buffer capacity, which induces a decrease of the pH value in the active membrane. The penicillinase activity, however, is greatly reduced when the pH is moving away from pH 7.

It was also noted that the device response was sensitive to solution stirring, which is not surprising because of the complex influences of distance and diffusion rates that always occur in biological thick membranes. Figure 6.4 shows a microscopic view of photopolymerized membranes on ISFET insulating gates, which can be used for enzyme immobilization. Using a double ISFET chip, the differential measurement described before can be realized.

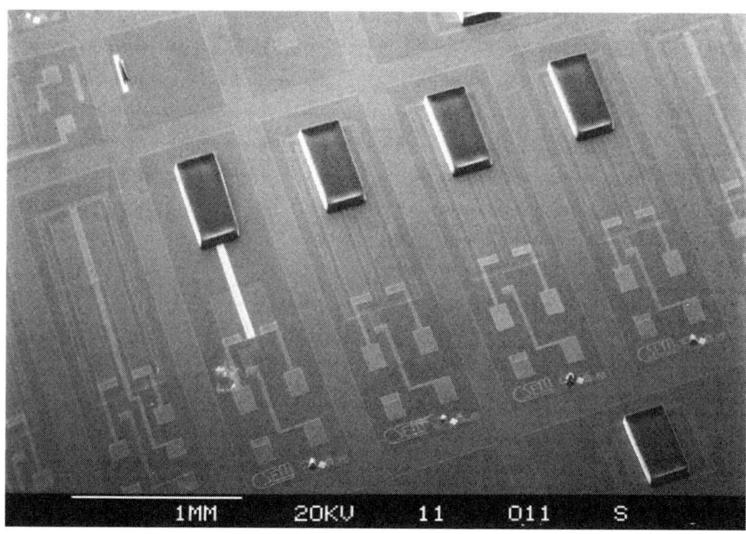

FIGURE 6.4 Microscopic view of photopolymerized membranes on ISFET insulating gates.

The first reported results on ENFETs have shown that these devices have the advantages of the small size, the membrane fixation techniques, and the dual sensor design for differential measurements; however, the various problems already known from conventional enzyme electrodes, such as buffer dependence of the sensitivity and pH dependence of the enzyme activity have not been solved.

These results have been confirmed for other enzymatic reactions for detecting glucose urea and acetylcholine with immobilized enzymes on ISFET gates such as glucose oxidase, urease, and acetylcholinesterase.[8,9,33,34] Using these results, the ENFET measurement techniques have been improved by systems such as pH-static enzyme sensors.[3] This method overcomes some of the difficulties of these enzyme-based biosensors. With such an improvement, the sensor response becomes independent of the buffer capacity in the sample solution.

6.3 SURFACE ACOUSTIC WAVE DEVICES

Piezoelectric crystals as transducer devices for chemical analysis were suggested by Sauerbrey in 1959.[43] Many applications, such as absorption hygrometers or sensitive detectors for gaseous components, have since been reported using piezoelectric sensors in the gas phase. The development of piezoelectric sensors that work continuously in the liquid phase has long been inhibited by the high energy losses at the solid/liquid interface of common acoustic transducers (see also Chapters 9 and 25).

Depending on the wave modes used as transducer mechanisms, three types of piezoelectric sensors can be distinguished. Bulk acoustic wave (BAW) devices commonly use thickness shear oscillations of piezoelectric crystals, while surface acoustic wave (SAW) devices use wavemodes propagating on the surface of piezoelectric materials. Furthermore, thin free membranes can be used in order to take advantage of the so-called lamb waves (LW), which are flexure acoustic waves of a thin piezoelectric free layer.

As the sensitivity of a piezoelectric detector is directly proportional to the square of the resonant frequency and inversely proportional to the surface area, the miniaturized surface acoustic wave (SAW) devices working at higher resonant frequencies are considered to be more sensitive transducers for chemical species, particularly in the gas phase.[44,45] However, common SAW devices would suffer from severe attenuation when used for measurements in liquids.

Most SAW devices in use are based on delay line oscillators, while direct resonator oscillators offer some advantages, particularly at high oscillator frequencies between 100 and 500 MHz. The more widely experimented SAW oscillators are realized on SiO_2 y-cut quartz with interdigital aluminum electrodes and are manufactured using standard microelectronic photolithographic techniques. Figure 6.5 shows a typical configuration of a delay line device with interdigital aluminum electrodes.

Recent development work focusing on immunosensing in aqueous media noticed that substrate materials like $LiTaO_3$ with high dielectric constant E and high piezoelectric efficiency would be improved by using horizontally polarized surface transverse waves (STW).[46] It has been found that these requirements can be fulfilled by commercially available low-loss devices designed for telecommunication applications. Such devices, operating between 200 and 500 MHz, have been tested in water immersion studies with an attenuation as low as 6 dB.

The key problem of such devices remains the immobilization of the selective bioreceptor onto the surface of the device in a way that preserves its actual properties. Because of their small mass loading on the sensing surface, in this case lipid monolayers are also thought to be the best membrane materials for biosensing. Selectivity would then be sought by integrating specific bioreceptors.

6.4 INTEGRATED OPTICS FOR BIOSENSOR MANUFACTURING

The availability of immunoassay techniques has been essential for recent progress in medical diagnostics. The improvement of the techniques through reliable and simple optical methods has suggested the use of planar optical devices, possibly manufactured with basic integrated optic techniques.[13,35-37]

The main interest of such new technologies is the possible "*in situ*" or "real time" investigation of molecular biological interactions and molecular recognition processes. Furthermore, direct optical absorption spectra,[38] solid/liquid interfacial refractometry,[5,39] and surface plasmon resonance (SPR)[11,35] have been successfully studied for direct biomolecular interaction investigations.

In diagnostics, as well as in pharmaceutical developments, label-free *in situ* monitoring of molecular recognition processes such as antibody-antigen reactions are of highest interest. Optical methods which can avoid the need for radioactive agents will obviously be preferred over conventional label techniques when comparable reliability can be obtained.[40]

In order to achieve such optical biosensor systems, the basic sensor device should consist of the following elements:

- An optical coupling element for driving a light beam to a thin-film optical waveguide with a controlled polarity and minimum intensity loss.
- A sensing element consisting of a thin-film optical waveguide having a suitable refractive index. The surface of the waveguide film interfaces the sample solution;

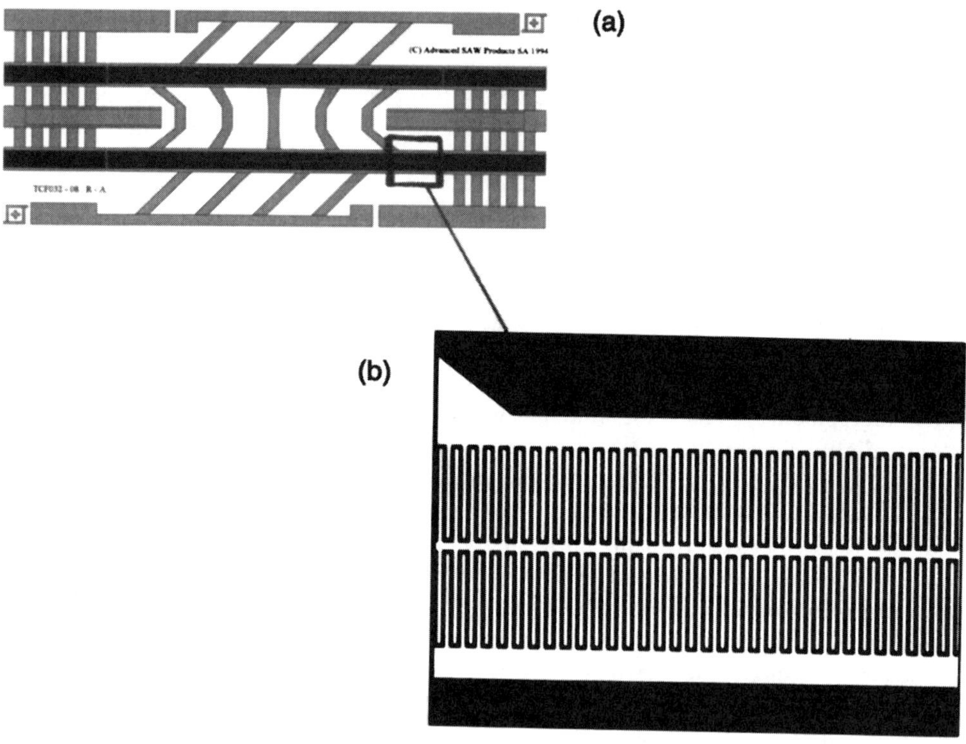

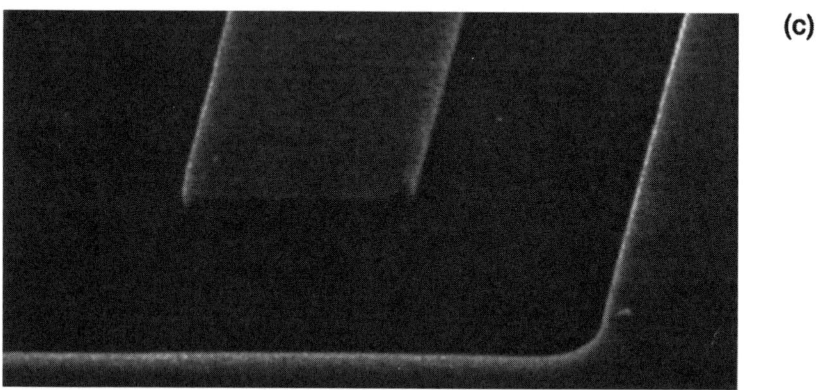

FIGURE 6.5 Typical configuration of a delay line device with interdigital aluminum electrodes. (a) Typical commercial SAW device from Advanced SAW Product, S.A. (b) Detail of the interdigitated electrodes. The active part of the transducer has a width of 221 μm and a length of 3.684 mm. (c) The dimension of the gap between the electrodes is 3.2 μm. With a pitch of 6.4 μm, the central frequency of the device is 254 MHz.

it carries the receptor molecules immobilized within a very thin covalently bound organic membrane.

- An optical component for analyzing the output light, as well as photodetectors, will then be necessary to measure phase deviations and absorbed intensity of the light induced by biological interactions, either in the reflected beam or in the evanescent field of the transmitted light.

As an example of optical measurement, it is possible to consider a polarized transmitted light through the thin-film waveguide; the sensing element will then respond to changes of refractive index within the penetration depth of the evanescent field.

The adsorption or binding of molecules to the surface of the waveguide film induces a distinctive change in the effective refractive indices of both transversal electric (TE) and transversal magnetic (TM) modes.

In the surface plasmon resonance (SPR) technology, the optical technique uses the same physical parameter, that is, the change in refractive index in the vicinity of the surface. In this case, however, the polarized light is reflected onto a metal surface on the reverse side of which specific receptors are immobilized. The typical SPR spectrum is observed by the intensity of the reflected light with the angle of the incident light beam. Any change in the refractive index at the surface will then be sensitively detected by modifying the value of the angle of incidence at the minimum reflected intensity.

As these optical sensing methods are complementary to electrochemical measurements, they are potential candidates for improving direct molecular recognition systems.

The state of the art of microsystem technology can now provide microstructures and integrated optics components in order to allow the integration of optical couplers, thin-film waveguides, optical components, and light detectors integrated either on the same silicon substrate or using microassembling techniques in a single-microsystem arrangement.

REFERENCES

1. Clark, L. C. and Lyons, C. L., *Ann. N.Y. Acad. Sci.,* 102, 29, 1962; *Methods in Enzymology,* Vol. 44, Mosbach, K., Ed., Academic Press, New York, 1976, 263-270.
2. Gernet, S., Koudelka, M., and de Rooij, N. F., Fabrication and characterization of a planar electrochemical cell and its application as a glucose sensor, *Sensors Actuators,* 18, 59-70, 1989.
3. van der Schoot, B. H. and Bergveld, P., ISFET based enzyme sensors, *Biosensors,* 3, 161-186, 1987/88.
4. Jacobs, P., Suls, J., and Sansen, W., Design and performance of a planar differential-conductivity sensor for urea, 7th Int. Conf. Solid-State Sensors and Actuators, 518-521, 1993.
5. Huber, W., Barner, R., Fattinger, Ch., Hübscher, J., Koller, H., Müller, F., Schlatter, D., and Lukosz, W., Direct optical immunosensing, *Sensor Actuators,* B6, 122-126, 1992.
6. Bilitewski, U., Rüger, P., and Schmid, R. D., Glucose biosensors based on thick film technology, *Biosens. Bioelectron.,* 6, 369-373, 1991.
7. Koudelka, M., Gernet, S., and de Rooij, N. F., Planar amperometric enzyme-based glucose microelectrode, *Sensors Actuators,* 18, 157-165, 1989.
8. Saito, A., Ito, N., Kimura, J., and Kuriyama, T., An ISFET glucose sensor having a silicone rubber membrane for undiluted serum monitoring, 7th Int. Conf. on Solid-State Sensors and Actuators, 575-578, 1993.
9. Kimura, J., Ito, N., and Kuriyama, T., A novel blood glucose monitoring method, an ISFET biosensor applied to transcutaneous effusion fluid, *J. Electrochem. Soc.,* 136, (6), 1989.
10. Shul'ga, A. A., Sandrovsky, A. C., Strikha, V. I., Soldatkin, A. P., Starodub, N. F., and El'skaya, A. V, Overall characterization of ISFET-based glucose biosensor, *Sensors Actuators,* B10, 41-46, 1992.
11. Lukosz, W., Principles and sensitivities of integrated optical and surface plasmon sensors for direct affinity sensing and immunosensing, *Biosen. Bioelectron.,* 6, 215-225, 1991.
12. Fattinger, Ch., The bidiffractive grating coupler, *Appl. Phys. Lett.,* 62(13), 1993.
13. Schlatter, D., Barner, R., Fattinger, Ch., Huber, W., Hübscher, J., Hurst, J., Koller, H., Mangold, C., and Müller, F., The difference interferometer: application as a direct affinity sensor, *Biosens. Bioelectron.,* 8, 109-116, 1993.
14. Sansen, W., de Wachter, D., Callewaert, L., Lambrechts, M., and Claes, A., A smart sensor for the voltammetric measurement of oxygen or glucose concentrations, *Sensors Actuators,* B1, 298-302, 1990.

15. Fattinger, Ch., Koller, H., Schlatter, D., and Wehrli, P., The difference interferometer: a highly sensitive optical probe for quantification of molecular surface concentration, *Biosens. Bioelectron.,* 8, 99-107, 1993.
16. Land, H., Duschl, C., Grätzel, M., and Vogel, H., Self-assembly of thiolipid molecular layers on gold surfaces: optical and electrochemical characterization, *Thin Solid Films,* 210/211, 818-821, 1992.
17. Terrettaz, S., Stora, T., Duschl, C., and Vogel, H., *LANGMUIR,* 1993, Vol. 9, No. 5, 1993, American Chemical Society, 0743-7463/93/2409, 1361-1369.
18. Aston, W. J., Product design and development, *Biosens. Bioelectron.,* 7, 85-89, 1992.
19. Yokoyama, K., Tamiya, E., and Karube, I., Amperometric glucose sensor using silicon oxide deposited gold electrodes, *Electroanalysis,* 3, 469-475, 1991.
20. Hintsche, R., Neumann, G., Dransfeld, I., Kampfrath, G., Hoffmann, B., and Scheller, F., Polyurethane enzyme membranes for chip biosensors, *Anal. Lett.*, 22(9), 2175-2190, 1984.
21. Yokoyama, K., Tamiya, E., and Karube, I., Performance of an integrated biosensor composed of a mediated and an oxygen-based glucose sensor under unknown oxygen tension, *Anal. Lett.,* 22(15), 2949-2959, 1989.
22. Urban, G., Jobst, G., Keplinger, F., Aschauer, E., Tilado, O., Fasching, R., and Kohl, F., Miniaturized multi-enzyme biosensors integrated with pH sensors on flexible polymer carriers for in vivo applications, *Biosens. Bioelectron.,* 7, 733-739, 1992.
23. Johnson, K. W., Mastrototaro, J. J., Howey, D. C., Brunelle, R. L., Burden-Brady, P. L., Bryan, N. A., Andrew, C. C., Rowe, H. M., Allen, D. J., Noffke, B. W., McMahan, W. C., Morff, R. J., Lipson, D., and Nevin, R. S., In vivo evaluation of an electroenzymatic glucose sensor implanted in subcutaneous tissue, *Biosens. Bioelectron.,* 7, 709-714, 1992.
24. Gernet, S., Koudelka, M., and de Rooij, N. F., Fabrication and characterization of a planar electrochemical cell and its application as a glucose sensor, *Sensors Actuators,* 18, 59-70, 1989.
25. Koudelka-Hep, M., Strike, D. J., and de Rooij, N. F., Miniature electrochemical glucose biosensors, *Anal. Chim. Acta,* 281, 461-466, 1993.
26. Bilitewski, U., Chemnitius, G. C., Rüger, P., and Schmid, R. D., Miniaturized disposable biosensors, *Sensors Actuators,* B7, 351-355, 1992.
27. Mann-Buxbaum, E., Pittner, F., Schalkhammer, T., Jachimowicz, A., Jobst, G., Olcaytug, F., and Urban, G., New microminiaturized glucose sensors using covalent immobilization techniques, *Sensors Actuators,* B1, 518-522, 1990.
28. Heineman, W. R., Hajizadeh, K., Tieman, R. S., Rauen, K. L., and Coury, L. A., Jr., Sensors based on polymer networks formed by gamma radiation cross-linking, Proc. 3rd Int. Meeting on Chemical Sensors, Cleveland, OH, 369-371, 1990.
29. Yon Hin, B. F. Y., Sethi, R. S., and Lowe, C. R., *Sensors Actuators,* B1, 550, 1990.
30. Johnson, K. W., *Sensors Actuators,* B5 (1-4), 85, 1992.
31. Van den Berg, A., Koudelka, M., van der Schoot, B. H., and Grisel, A., A universal on-wafer fabrication technique for diffusion limiting membranes for use in microelectrochemical amperometric sensor, Proc. 3rd Int. Meeting on Chemical Sensors, Cleveland, OH, 140-143, 1990.
32. Caras, S. D. and Janata, J., Field effect transistor sensitive to penicillin, *Anal. Chem.,* 52, 1935-1937, 1980.
33. Miyahara, Y., Moriizumi, T., and Idrimura, K., Integrated enzyme FETs for simultaneous detection of urea and glucose, *Sensors Actuators,* 7, 1-10, 1985.
34. Nakako, M., Hanazaito, Y., Maeda, M., and Shiono, S., Neutral lipid enzyme sensor based on Ion Senstive Field Effect Transistor, *Anal. Chem. Acta,* 185, 179-185, 1986.
35. Dubs, M. C., Altschuh, D., et al., Interaction between viruses and monoclonal antibodies studied by surface plasmon resonance, *Immunol. Lett.,* 31, 59-64, 1991.
36. Jönsson, U., et al., *Biotechniques,* 11, 620-627, 1991.
37. Karlsson R., et al. Measurement of antibody affinity, *Structure of Antigens,* CRC Press, Boca Raton, FL, 1992, 127.
38. Godman, D. S., White, P. L., and Anheier, N. C., *Appl. Opt.,* 29, 4583, 1990.
39. Tiefenthaler, K. and Kukosz, W., *J. Opt. Soc. Am.,* B6, 209, 1989.
40. Fägerstam L., A non-label technology for real time biospecific interaction anaylsis, *Techniques in Protein Chemistry,* II, Academic Press, New York, 1991.

41. Thompson, M., Arthur, C. L., and Dhaliwal, G. K., Liquid-phase piezoelectric and acoustic transmission studies of interfacial immunochemistry, *Anal. Chem.,* 58 120b, 1986.
42. Muramatsu, H., Tamiya, E., and Karube, I., Determination of microbes and immunoglobulins using a piezoelectric biosensor, *J. Membr. Sci.,* 41, 281-290, 1989.
43. Sauerbrey, G. Z., The use of oscillators for weighing thin layers and for microweighing, *Z. Phys.,* 155, 209-212, 1959.
44. Ash, E. A., Fundamentals of signal processing devices in *Acoustic Surface Waves,* Oliner, A. A., Ed., Springer-Verlag New York, pp 115-123, 1978.
45. Chang, S. M., Ebert, B., Tamiya, E., and Karube I., Development of chemical vapour sensor using SAW resonator oscillator incorporating odorant receptive LB films, *Biosens. Bioelectron.,* 6, 293-298, 1991.
46. Rapp. M., Moss, D. A., Wessa, T., and Ache, H. J., Immunosensing with commercially available low-loss surface acoustic wave devices, Biosensors '94, New Orleans, June 1994, 3.41.
47. van der Schoot, B. H., Voorthuyzen, H., and Bergveld, P., The pH-static enzyme sensor: design of the pH control system, *Sensors Actuators,* B1, 546-549, 1990.

7 Surface Plasmon Resonance (SPR) for Biosensing

Chris R. Lawrence and Norman J. Geddes

CONTENTS

7.1 INTRODUCTION

The development of a sensor capable of detecting the presence of very low levels of chemical and biological contaminants is of interest to a wide range of workers in fields as diverse as medical diagnostics, industrial process control, and environmental research. The exact requirements of each application vary, but it is generally desirable that the sensor be made compact and remote (to make *in situ* measurements, perhaps in hostile environments, e.g., detection of poisonous gases), that the response time be as short as possible (to enable "real-time" studies), and that the measurements be made in a nondestructive manner. Further, many situations involve the more exacting requirement that the sensor must be *material specific* (i.e., it must only be sensitive to the presence of one particular contaminant or analyte), an important stipulation if the device is to be used outside of a controlled environment.

Several possible techniques for real-time detection have been suggested, including the use of quartz crystal microbalances (QCM),[1] optic fiber coupling,[2] MOSFETs,[3] and surface acoustic wave devices.[4] Each method has its merits, but at present it appears that one of the most promising optical approaches to this problem involves the utilization of surface plasmons, that is, coupled electromagnetic field/charge density oscillations at a metal/dielectric interface. These may be used as extremely sensitive probes of the environment in their immediate vicinity.

This approach was first suggested by Nylander et al.[5] who described how a gas sensor could be constructed from a silver-coated prism, the outer surface of the metal being covered with an overlayer of silicon oil. When monochromatic p-polarized (TM) light was internally made incident upon the silver film, a plot of incident angle vs. reflectivity exhibited a "dip" at angles at which the surface plasmon resonance (SPR) was excited. The exact shape and

0-8493-8905-4/97/$0.00+$.50
© 1997 by CRC Press, Inc.

position of this dip was characteristic of the refractive index of the oil. When a mixture of halothane gas and nitrogen was passed over the oil's surface, halothane was absorbed and the refractive index of the overlayer altered, changing the form of the reflectivity plot and indicating the presence of the gas. A linear relationship between the angle of minimum reflectivity and the concentration of halothane was found.

This work generated considerable interest in the use of SPR techniques, for several reasons. Since the method was optical in nature, it could theoretically meet all of the aforementioned requirements of an ideal sensor: the specificity could be controlled by the choice of overlayer material, the technique was nondestructive and passive (no electronics were based at the sensor head), and it could probe hazardous environments (e.g., high pressure or temperature). Further, the sensitivity of the technique was considerable; the SPR probes the media to either side of the metal/dielectric interface through the optical electric (E) field which extends to distances comparable to the wavelength of the light utilized (i.e., over distances so small that the influence of individual monolayers of material may be significant).

In this chapter we will discuss SPR-based sensing techniques that could be used to study biological systems (i.e., to fabricate *biosensors*), giving a basic summary of the principles of SPR excitation before reviewing the various biosensor designs that have been proposed. A highly efficient surface plasmon-based biosensor designed by Pharmacia[6] is commercially available, but there still exists a gap in the market for a cheap, disposable, and portable biosensing device, and such factors will be discussed in this chapter. The choice and immobilization of the receptor layer is presented in Chapter 16.

7.2 THE TRANSDUCER:SPR TECHNIQUES

In Section 7.2.1 we examine which materials can advantageously be used in the construction of an SPR device and which wavelengths are suitable for the incident light used within the system.

In Section 7.2.2 we present possible geometries for SPR-based immunosensors and layouts for the measurement systems. The compactness and cost of the devices and instruments is discussed here, as are the basic properties of the thin layers — such as immobilized antibody layers with bound antigen — that can be analyzed. Techniques for an enhancement of the biocompatibility and sensitivity of the device are presented.

7.2.1 BASIC THEORY OF SPR EXCITATION

SPR excitation occurs when photons are made incident upon a metal/dielectric interface and induce a resonant charge density oscillation at that surface, creating a propagating wave. This wave, consisting of a perturbation of the almost-free electron plasma, is defined to be a surface plasmon resonance (SPR) or, to be more precise, a surface plasmon-polariton (SPP) (a polariton being a propagating wave created in a medium via interactions with photons). It will propagate over distances of approximately a few microns in the visible range, exhibiting exponentially decaying optical E-fields perpendicular to the interface which penetrate the adjacent media to a distance comparable to the wavelength of the incident light. It is these E-fields which make the behavior of the SPP so sensitive to its surroundings. The conditions under which such waves can be supported will now be discussed, but for a more detailed study the reader is referred to the work of Raether,[7] Sambles et al.[8] or Welford.[9]

Figure 7.1 illustrates the behavior of plane parallel monochromatic radiation made incident upon a smooth, planar interface between two media, both of which are chosen to be lossless (nonabsorbing) and nonmagnetic (i.e., the magnetic permeability, μ, is equal to μ_0). The light strikes the interface at some arbitrary angle θ, and is partially transmitted into the second medium, the remainder of the photons being specularly reflected. The angles involved

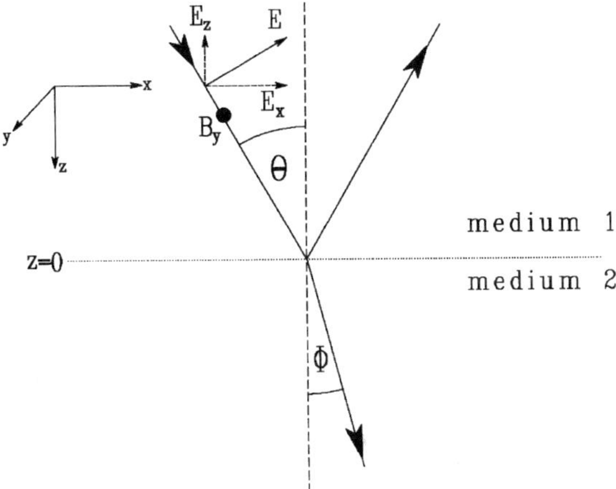

FIGURE 7.1 Representation of p-polarised (TM) light made incident upon a planar interface at an incident angle θ, producing a transmitted and a reflected beam. For a typical SPR device, medium 1 is a dielectric material such as glass or plastic, whilst medium 2 is a metal when visible-range incident light is chosen.

are related to the refractive indices of the media (n_1 and n_2), and the transmission angle Φ can be calculated from Snell's law

$$n_1 \cdot \sin(\theta) = n_2 \cdot \sin(\Phi) \tag{7.1}$$

further ramifications of which will be discussed in Subsection 2.2.1.

The light is chosen to be linearly polarized, with its electric (E) field vector either parallel (as in Figure 7.1) or perpendicular to the plane of incidence (the z-x plane in which both the incident and reflected beams are to be found). Light polarized in such a fashion is said to be p- (TM) or s- (TE) polarized, respectively, and any linearly polarized radiation can be described as a sum of the two cases. For the p-polarized case illustrated in Figure 7.1 there is an E-field component perpendicular to the interface such that $E_z = |E| \cdot \cos(\theta)$.

Associated with the differing refractive indices n_1 and n_2 of the media on either side of the interface are their differing dielectric permittivities values $\varepsilon_1 = (n_1)^2$ and $\varepsilon_2 = (n_2)^2$. We assume that the media do not absorb light, that is we take them to be lossless. (Permittivity will be more familiar to many readers as governing the capacitance of a dielectric-filled capacitor. Moving up in frequency from AC currents via microwaves to optics, the permittivity of a material continues to play an important role in its interaction with electromagnetic waves.)

Due to the change in permittivity across the interface, whilst the displacement field D_z is continuous (since it is presumed that no free charge is present), E_z changes in value from one medium to the other since

$$D_z = \varepsilon_0 \cdot \varepsilon_1 \cdot E_{z1} = \varepsilon_0 \cdot \varepsilon_2 \cdot E_{z2} \tag{7.2}$$

where ε_0 is the permittivity of free space. This change in E_z means that the polarization charge distribution across the interface is discontinuous, and that p-polarized light will necessarily give rise to the creation of charge at the boundary. On the other hand, s-polarized light has no component of E_z. Therefore, it will not produce such charges at the interface, and cannot be used to excite a surface charge oscillation such as an SPP. All further discussion will hence pertain to p-polarized light.

Extending this argument a little further, an SPP is a *surface-bound* mode involving a charge density that is actively trapped at the boundary. This requires that the dielectric permittivities of the two media are oppositely signed, so that the D_z components within the two media oppose each other to bind the charge at the surface. **This explains why SPR occurs at a metal-dielectric interface.**

The opaqueness of metals when exposed to visible light or to microwaves and their partial transparency to gamma radiation are well known. These properties are related to a given metal's permittivity which changes with the frequency of the incident electromagnetic waves. The change of permittivity with frequency is referred to as dispersive behavior. For an ideal metal consisting of undamped free-electrons, the optical permittivity of the material is dictated by a parameter known as the plasma frequency, ω_p, the value of which is characteristic of a given metal, representing the highest frequency at which its electrons can oscillate. The relationship can be expressed as

$$\varepsilon_{metal} = 1 - (\omega_p/\omega)^2 \tag{7.3}$$

where ω is the frequency of the incident radiation. At frequencies greater than ω_p, ε_{metal} is real and positive, and the metal is transparent to radiation, acting in a similar manner to a simple dielectric. If $\omega < \omega_p$, however, the electrons respond readily to the applied field and the material acts as a metal, canceling out the applied field, and ε_{metal} is negative. Thus p-polarized light can create charges at a metal-dielectric interface if its frequency is suited to the given metal.

It should be noted that, in real metals, factors such as resistive damping of the electrons' movement by defects and vibrations (phonons) will introduce an imaginary component of permittivity which represents absorptive effects. The choice of metal is not purely based upon the value of ω_p: this will be discussed later. Also, **it is possible to use certain semiconducting materials in place of the metal** since they can act in a metallic fashion (i.e., have negative ε) **when infrared light is utilized.**[10]

Medium 2 will now be treated as an ideal metal such that ε is real and negative, whilst medium 1 is still a lossless dielectric. In order to describe SPP excitation in more detail, it is necessary to apply Maxwell's electromagnetic wave equations to the behavior of the light at the interface. For SPP propagation in the x-direction, the waves can be described by the equations

$$E_1 = (E_{x1},0,E_{z1}) \cdot \exp[i(k_x \cdot x - \omega t)]\exp(ik_{z1} \cdot z) \tag{7.4}$$

$$H_1 = (0,H_{y1},0) \cdot \exp[i(k_x \cdot x - \omega t)]\exp(ik_{z1} \cdot z) \tag{7.5}$$

$$E_2 = (E_{x2},0,E_{z2}) \cdot \exp[i(k_x \cdot x - \omega t)]\exp(ik_{z2} \cdot z) \tag{7.6}$$

$$H_2 = (0,H_{y2},0) \cdot \exp[i(k_x \cdot x - \omega t)]\exp(ik_{z2} \cdot z) \tag{7.7}$$

where k_x is the x-component of the wavevector $k = 2\pi/\lambda$, and the fact that the light is p-polarized is specified by the choice of field components. Relationships between the various components of E and H can be determined via the equations $\nabla \cdot E = 0$ (Gauss' Theorem) and $\nabla \times E = -\mu.(dH/dt)$ (Faraday's law of electromagnetic induction, where $\nabla \times E$ is the curl of the electric field, expressing its vorticity, and ∇ is a vector operator of partial spatial differentiation). Boundary conditions at the interface further require that tangential E and H are continuous, meaning that $E_{x1} = E_{x2}$ and $H_{y1} = H_{y2}$. When all these conditions are combined they result in the expression

$$(\varepsilon_1/k_{z1}) = (\varepsilon_2/k_{z2}) \tag{7.8}$$

Further information can be gleaned from Figure 7.1. Since the wavevector lies in the direction of propagation of the light, it may be split into separate x- and z- components such that, for instance,

$$k_{x1} = (\varepsilon_1)^{1/2} \cdot k \cdot \sin(\theta) = k_x \quad (7.9)$$

and

$$k_{z1} = (-k_x{}^2 + \varepsilon_1 \cdot k^2)^{1/2} \quad (7.10)$$

$$k_{z2} = (-k_x{}^2 + \varepsilon_2 \cdot k^2)^{1/2} \quad (7.11)$$

Since the SPP exponentially decays into the adjacent media it is mathematically necessary that $ik_{z1} > 0$ and $ik_{z2} < 0$ (see earlier wave equations: z is positive in medium 2). Thus it is required that $(k_x)^2 > \varepsilon_1 \cdot (k)^2$, i.e., that *the wavevector in the x-direction must be greater than the maximum that can be supported in the dielectric*. Since the momentum (or more precisely, *pseudo* momentum) of a photon is expressed as the product $\hbar k_x$ (where $\hbar = h/2\pi$, and h is Planck's constant) it is generally stated that there is a momentum mismatch between the incident light and the SPP mode. The importance of this will be discussed later.

Substituting Equation 7.10 into Equation 7.8 gives the expression

$$k_x = k\ ((\varepsilon_1 \cdot \varepsilon_2)/(\varepsilon_1 + \varepsilon_2))^{1/2} \quad (7.12)$$

This shows that if k_x is real, representing a propagating mode, then $|\varepsilon_2| > \varepsilon_1$ (since ε_2 is negative). As previously mentioned, however, a real metal possesses an imaginary (loss-bearing) component of permittivity, and this makes k a complex quantity ($k_x = k_{xr} + i \cdot k_{xi}$). Substituting $\varepsilon_2 = \varepsilon_{2r} + i \cdot \varepsilon_{2i}$ into the above equation, whilst assuming that $|\varepsilon_{2r}|$ is much greater than either ε_1 or ε_{2i} , gives

$$k_{xr}\ \text{Å}\ k\ (\varepsilon_1)^{1/2} \cdot [1 - (\varepsilon_1)/(2 \cdot \varepsilon_{2r})] \quad (7.13)$$

and

$$k_{xi} = (1/2) \cdot k \cdot ((\varepsilon_{2i} \cdot \varepsilon_1{}^{3/2})/(\varepsilon_{2r}{}^2)) \quad (7.14)$$

The imaginary component of the wavevector dictates the width of the resonance, and the above shows that this is proportional to $(\varepsilon_{2i}/(\varepsilon_{2r}))^2$. Ideally then, we choose a metal with $|\varepsilon_{2r}| \cdot >> \varepsilon_{2i}$. When optical dispersion data (that is the variation of the permittivity with frequency) for various real metals are examined it becomes apparent that **only a few metals (e.g., Au, Ag, Al) can support sharp, well-defined SPP resonance in the visible region of the spectrum**, the region which is probably of most use when a sensor is being designed, although more are available at longer (infrared) wavelengths. The relative merits of the most commonly used metals are summarized in Table 7.1.

These equations also show a strong dependence of k_i and k_r upon ε_1. This implies that any change in the refractive indices of medium 1 will perturb the mode. Hence coating the surface of the metal with a dielectric overlayer (e.g., a Langmuir-Blodgett film[11] or protein coating[12]) will give rise to an observable change in the mode properties. Such changes would also occur if the refractive index of such an overlayer is altered, perhaps (as used in the example of Nylander et al.[5]) due to a gas being absorbed by the dielectric. **Thus an SPP-based device can sense either the *presence* or the *alteration* of a dielectric overlayer.**

TABLE 7.1
Metals Commonly Used to Support SPPs

Metal	Wavelength range	Comment
Silver	Visible and infrared	Degrades (sulfidizes)
Gold	Visible (not blue) and infrared	Stable, but broader SPPs than with silver
Platinum	Infrared	Stable
Aluminum	Ultraviolet through to near infrared	Very unstable (oxidizes)

To summarize, the excitation of an SPP can occur when p-polarized light is made incident upon a planar boundary between two media where ε_1 is real and positive, and $\varepsilon_2 = \varepsilon_{2r} + i \cdot \varepsilon_{2i}$, for which ε_{2r} is a negative quantity whose magnitude exceeds both ε_1 and ε_{2i}. However, the excitation of the mode requires momentum in excess of the maximum which may be supported in medium 1, and it is therefore impossible for incident light to couple directly to the SPP. The methods by which this extra momentum can be obtained will be discussed in the next section.

7.2.2 Coupling to the SPP Mode

7.2.2.1 Prism Coupling

One method by which light can be coupled to the surface plasmon utilizes a prism. As mentioned earlier, Snell's law describes the path taken by a beam striking an interface between media of differing refractive indices, using the incident angle θ and the values of n_1 and n_2 to determine the angle of refraction Φ (see Figure 7.1). The law can be thought of as an expression of the conservation of in-surface-plane momentum for the system, with the maximum possible component available in medium 2 existing when $\theta_2 = 90°$, i.e., when the light beam is *parallel* to the interface. This is achieved at an angle of incidence in medium 1 known as the critical angle, θ_c, for which

$$\sin(\theta_c) = (\varepsilon_2/\varepsilon_1)^{1/2} \tag{7.15}$$

Beyond θ_c there can be no propagating wave in medium 2, as the radiation possesses too great a momentum for the environment to support. Of course, the light beam still causes the oscillation of charges at the interface, producing evanescent fields which decay into medium 2 in a direction normal to the interface. (Evanescent waves persist only over a distance of the order of the wavelength. This spatial confinement is used in many optical devices to avoid interference from sample properties such as turbidity.) The momentum of these fields is given by $n \cdot \hbar \cdot k \cdot \sin(\theta_1)$, and lies in the x-direction. If $\sin(\theta_1) > \sin(\theta_c)$ (i.e., $\sin(\theta_i) > (n_2/n_1)$) then it is obvious that $n \cdot \hbar \cdot k \cdot \sin(\theta_1)$ must be greater than $n_2 \cdot \hbar \cdot k$, and that there is an enhancement of the x-component of momentum in the second medium.

This enhancement can be used to make coupling to the SPP possible, presuming that the metal/dielectric interface can be placed near enough to the interface at which total reflection is occurring. If the separation of the two boundaries is not optimized, then the mode may be either over- or undercoupled. For overcoupling (too small a separation) the resonance becomes broader and less intense, whilst for undercoupling it changes but also weakens. Hence it is important to set this distance correctly. In 1968, Otto[13] suggested the prism/air-gap/metal geometry shown in Figure 7.2a, a perfectly valid arrangement, but not the most commonly used due to the difficulty of maintaining a small (for visible light, less than 2 μm) and precise separation between prism and metal. Instead, a method proposed by Kretschmann and Raether[14] is favored (Figure 7.2b), in which the air gap is replaced by the metal itself. The

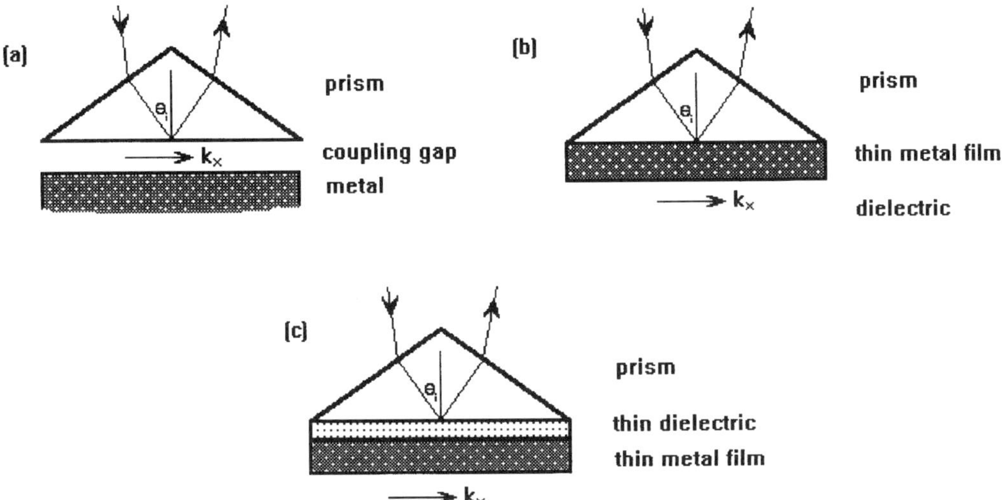

FIGURE 7.2 Prism-coupling geometries: (a) Otto, (b) Kretschmann-Raether, and (c) a mixed hybrid geometry.

prism is coated with a metal film such that the prism/metal and metal/dielectric interfaces are an optimum distance apart. This arrangement is far more mechanically stable, and is a more convenient basis for a biosensor design.

It is worth pointing out that some workers (e.g., Morgan and Taylor,[15] Pollard-Knight et al.[16]) use semicylindrical prisms in preference to the more conventional form which are triangular in cross section. The curved surface ensures that the incoming light is always normal to the surface of the prism, preventing beam-walkoff (the movement of the beam spot across the sample as θ varies) and minimizing the changes in reflectivity at the entrance and exit faces due to the angle change. Such prisms are expensive, however, due to the difficulty in polishing a surface to a perfect semicircular cross section, whereas it is relatively easy to produce high-quality planar faces. Further, data obtained from a plane-surfaced prism can be corrected mathematically so as to account for angle-dependent reflectivity variations, and although a certain degree of beam-walkoff is unavoidable, metal or dielectric overlayers can generally be considered uniform over the area of the beam-spot. Therefore the use of either type of prism is acceptable under all but exceptional circumstances. (A further geometry, illustrated in Figure 7.2c, will be discussed further on in this section).

In both prism-based geometries the SPP can be observed via reflectivity measurements. As previously explained, the momentum of the incoming light varies with the incident angle θ (namely, as $k_x = n \cdot k \cdot \sin(\theta)$), making a range of k_x-values accessible. Further, when momentum coupling occurs, energy is absorbed by the SPP and the component of reflected light is reduced in intensity, the reduction in the reflectivity giving a measure of the degree of coupling. Thus it is possible to derive a qualitative picture of the SPP from plots of reflectivity vs. incident angle, as illustrated in Figure 7.3. The most common method by which such data are obtained uses a θ/2θ stage, as illustrated in Figure 7.4. The metal-coated prism is placed upon a rotating table and illuminated with p-polarized, monochromatic light. The reflected beam is directed onto a detector which is set upon the outer section of the table. When the prism is rotated by θ degrees, this outer section rotates by 2θ, ensuring that the reflected beam remains centered upon the detector. The variation of reflectivity with incident angle is recorded. A reference beam is taken to account for any fluctuations in the light source's intensity, and phase-sensitive detection is employed to remove interference from background sources.

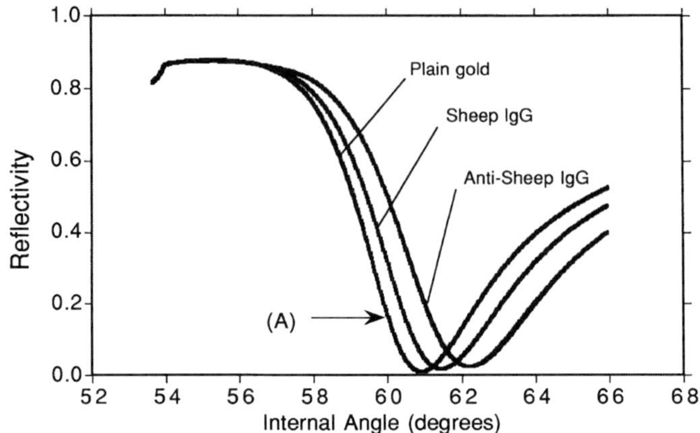

FIGURE 7.3 Reflectivity curves as a function of the incident angle of the laser beam, for plain gold, immobilized sheep IgG, and binding of anti-sheep IgG to the sheep IgG layer.

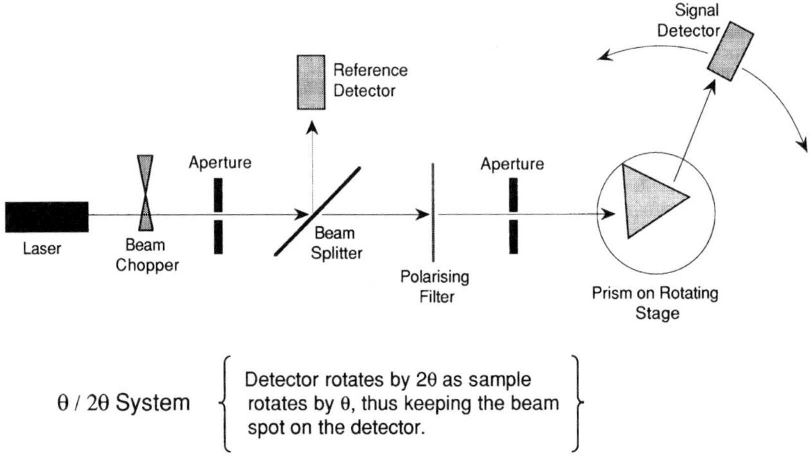

FIGURE 7.4 A diagram of a typical θ/2θ system.

An alternative method by which such reflectivity vs. angle plots can be obtained involves the simultaneous illumination of the prism across a range of incident angles. Light is focused onto the prism with a converging lens, and the reflected rays are measured with a diode array device (essentially a line of detectors) — see Figure 7.5, and the work by Matsubara et al.[17] This method gleans the entire angle spectrum at once, as well as making it possible to monitor fast processes by taking successive datasets over relatively short time-spans. The angular resolution of such devices is generally far less than that of a θ/2θ stage. A CCD (charge coupled device) camera is a more sensitive version of this apparatus (used, for instance, in the patent by Batchelder and Willson[18]), but is probably rather too expensive for a mass-produced biosensor.

Comparison between reflectivity vs. incident angle data and theoretical models allows the optical dielectric constants ε_r and ε_i of the metal (where $\varepsilon = \varepsilon_r + i \cdot \varepsilon_i$) and, in the case of the Kretschmann geometry (Figure 7.2b), the film's thickness to be determined. If the sample is then coated with a dielectric overlayer, these metal film parameters can be used in fitting subsequent reflectivity data, producing the **optical parameters of the overlayer**. This will be discussed in more detail later when specific biosensors will be dealt with.

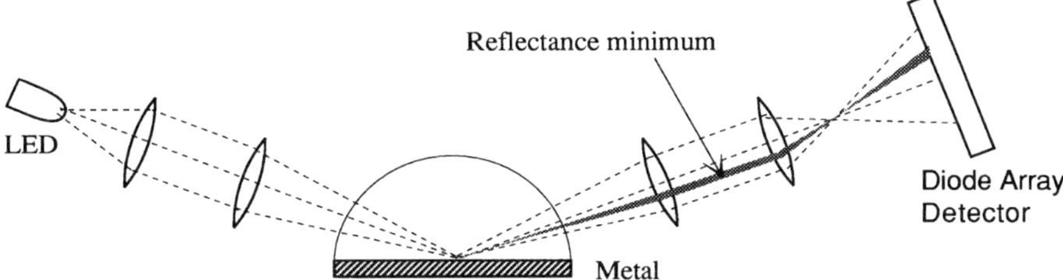

FIGURE 7.5 Representation of SPP detection via a diode array device.

Whilst a full plot of reflectivity vs. incident angle can provide a great deal of information, it would be difficult to integrate a θ/2θ stage into a portable biosensor, and it may be rather expensive to utilize a diode array. However, once the shape of the plot is known it is possible to design a device in which the incident angle is held constant. Several workers (e.g., Liedberg et al.[12] and Fontana et al.[19]) have studied the real-time deposition of biological molecules onto SPP-supporting surfaces by measuring the corresponding change in reflectivity at a specific angle. Looking at Figure 7.6, it can be seen that the gradient dR/dθ is approximately linear to the side of the minimum nearest the critical angle. When (in this case) proteins bind onto the metal's surface, the plasmon shifts away from θ_c. If the reflectivity is measured at approximately 1° to the left of the plasmon minimum, it will decrease linearly with respect to the shift in θ. Whilst this does not provide information pertaining to the optical constants of the metal, it gives an arbitrary measure of **film deposition speed.** Since it can subsequently be used to detect the binding of antigens to the proteins, a process dependent upon the affinity of the two species, it can be designed to act as a **molecule-specific biosensor**.

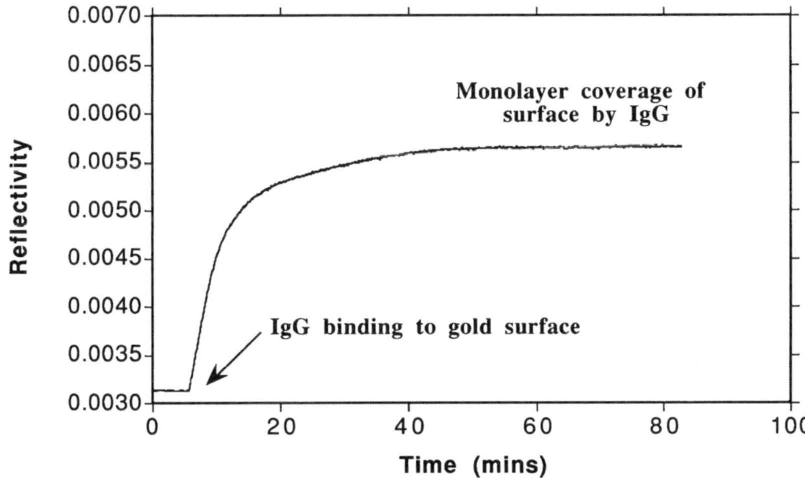

FIGURE 7.6 The change in reflectivity as a function of time during the immobilization of IgG to the gold surface. The angle of incidence was held constant (see point (A) shown in Figure 7.3).

Publications by Kooyman et al.[20] and de Brujin et al.[21] have discussed the sensitivity of such devices. They considered both the slope of the reflectivity plot dR/dk_x and the shift of the position of the SPP minimum with overlayer thickness dk_x/dt. They concluded that the most sensitive sensor in the visible light range would utilize a silver film. Given certain assumptions (such as that lineshape is invariant with overlayer thickness) this information is of interest, but other considerations, such as the tendency of silver to degrade (see Kovacs' work on sulfidization[22]) may prevail. A more fundamental method to improve sensitivity is proposed by Matsubara et al.[23] who suggest the use of *long-range* surface plasmons or LRSPs (first discussed by Sarid[24]). By inserting a dielectric layer between the prism and the metal film, *two* metal/dielectric interfaces (see Figure 7.2c) are made available, and two plasmons can be supported. Their E-fields in the z-direction (perpendicular to the interfaces) interact such that they are said to be *coupled* plasmon modes. When a reflectivity plot is examined, two modes are observed: a sharp resonance which represents a plasmon with a long propagation length (the LRSP), and a broader resonance which represents a case in which more energy is lost to the metal film, restricting its propagation length, and defining it to be a *short-range* surface plasmon (SRSP). Whilst the SRSP is of little relevance to this review, the LRSP is of interest, since it is far narrower than an ordinary SPP and may thus exhibit a greater value of dR/dk_x. Hence an LRSP-based sensor may theoretically be more sensitive to changes in organic overlayers than one which utilizes SPPs. This is especially important when it is considered that most biosensing involves the immersion of the active metal/dielectric surface in solution, a process which causes a broadening of the plasmon's reflectivity profile relative to the unimmersed case. This broadening can severely restrict the efficiency of a sensing device. For a more detailed discussion of coupled plasmons, the reader is referred to the paper by Welford and Sambles.[26]

Kooyman et al.[26] have shown that plasmon shifts can be recorded by sweeping across the angle of minimum reflectivity by means of a vibrating mirror. Suppose that the plasmon is at 5°, and the mirror sweeps out angles of incidence from 0° to 10°. If the reflectivity is recorded over one cycle (from 0° to 10° and back again) there will be two dips in the trace. The time between dips (t_d) over that single cycle will be half of the total sweep time. If the plasmon is perturbed so that its minimum moves to a higher angle (as would be the case if proteins bound to the surface of the metal) then the dips on the trace will move towards each other, and t_d decreases. Thus, by recording t_d it is possible to monitor even relatively fast biomolecular binding processes with good angular resolution in a time-averaged manner, although there will necessarily be a degree of beam-walkoff induced by this method (between 0.1 and 1 mm in the experiments discussed).

One other advantage of this method concerns the silver films deposited onto the prisms — whilst metal degradation shifts SPP modes, making it impossible to fit full angle-scans to theory, Kooyman et al.[26] suggested a method by which this could be corrected for. By using a second cell containing only pure buffer solution it is possible to monitor the shift of the SPPs that is solely due to the degradation of the metal, and this can be subtracted from the signal obtained from the active cell to produce an accurate measurement of the protein binding.

Oda and Fukui[27] have also incorporated mirrors into their sensors, but with a different aim in mind. Light is reflected from a mirror's surface and focused onto a prism by two converging lenses so as to be made internally incident upon its metal-coated face. The reflected light is collected by two similar lenses and focused onto a detector. By rotating the mirror it is possible to obtain a full angle-scan without any movement of the prism, and all of the information produced by a $\theta/2\theta$ device is obtained without mechanical complexity. Scans can be taken at great speed, the scan rate being determined by the rate of rotation of the mirror. The prism itself does not need to be rotated and can be clamped to the side of a vacuum chamber, by which means the designers have been able to study relatively fast vacuum deposition of silver films.[28] The relative simplicity and speed of this device may make it an attractive prospect for use as a biosensor.

Whilst all of the previously mentioned techniques rely upon optical measurements at a fixed wavelength, it is possible to obtain further information by varying this parameter. For example, it is advantageous to perform full angle-scans of reflectivity at a variety of wavelengths since, when these are matched to theory, the resultant values of overlayer thickness can be compared (and, if necessary, averaged) to ensure that accuracy is maintained — see, for instance, the work of Lawrence et al.[29] However, wavelength variations can be used in a more fundamental manner, and workers such as Kötz et al.[30] and Lopez-Rios and Vuye[31] have published work in which reflectivity has been measured for different light frequencies at a fixed angle. At a given angle there is only one frequency that will excite an SPP with maximum coupling efficiency. Other frequencies will be less efficient, producing broader and shallower modes. The reflectivity at a given angle will be minimized at a critical frequency, as already discussed. This approach is of limited usefulness since it cannot reveal as much information as a plot of reflectivity vs. incident angle (due to the optical parameters of the system being dependent upon the frequency of the incident light). Indeed, the use of a polychromatic light source in a prism-based biosensor has not yet offered any significant advantages over monochromatic devices, although — as will be described in the next section — a polychromatic grating-based biosensor has recently been developed.

The use of optic fibers in the design of a biosensor is of particular interest when it is desired that the sensing surface should be remote from the signal processing equipment (e.g., when a hostile or otherwise inaccessible environment is to be investigated). Whilst they can merely be used to transmit the light to a separate device, they can also act as an integral part of the sensing head, effectively *replacing* the prism. For instance, in recent work by De Maria et al.[32] the tip of a monomode optic fiber was cleaved at a specific angle such that, when it was coated with a silver film of a preset thickness, p-polarized (TM) light that was transmitted along the fiber could excite a surface plasmon at this surface (the angle of incidence being constant since the light in a monomode fiber travels along its axis of symmetry). By rotating the plane of polarization of the incident light with a half-wave plate (linear polarization being preserved in a monomode fiber) the intensity of the light reflected back along the fiber from the silvered surface could be varied, producing quasisinusoidal plots of reflectivity against the rotation angle that exhibited minima when the light was p-polarized (full coupling) and maxima when it was s-polarized (no coupling). Theoretically, such plots could be compared to those obtained when the surface is coated with protein overlayers; the presence of a film would perturb the angle at which optimal plasmon coupling occurred, meaning that the light was no longer coupling to the surface mode with maximum efficiency, and resulting in an increase in the minimum reflectivity observed. Whilst the results given are preliminary, the sensor's compactness and remote capability make it an attractive prospect.

An alternative approach by Jorgenson and Yee[33] involves the removal of cladding from an area of a multimode fiber, producing an active surface at the fiber's circumference. When this surface was coated with silver, light transmitted along the fiber could couple to surface plasmons at the silver/air interface. Since white (polychromatic) light was used, a plot of reflectivity vs. wavelength could be obtained by measuring the output at the fiber's end, showing a decrease in intensity as coupling efficiency varied. Because the light could be incident upon the glass/silver interface at a discrete variety of angles (due to the fiber's multimode nature), and since multiple absorptions are possible if the light strikes the interface more than once (exciting more than one plasmon), some care is needed in interpreting the data, but Jorgenson and Yee have found good agreement between experiment and theory when the fiber is immersed in fructose solutions of differing concentration (and thus refractive index). Hence, another possible biosensor configuration is illustrated in the following section, with similar advantages to the aforementioned fiber-based design.

7.2.2.2 Grating Coupling

All previous discussion has concerned systems in which the active metal/dielectric interface has been smooth and planar, and a prism has been required to enable momentum matching to occur. However, it is possible to couple incident light directly to the SPP mode by distorting the surface, and thereby introducing diffraction effects.

When light is made incident upon a planar surface it possesses a component of wavevector in the plane of that surface which is given by $k_x = n \cdot k \cdot \sin(\theta)$, in both the incident and the single reflected beam (since in-plane momentum is conserved). A surface that is distorted in

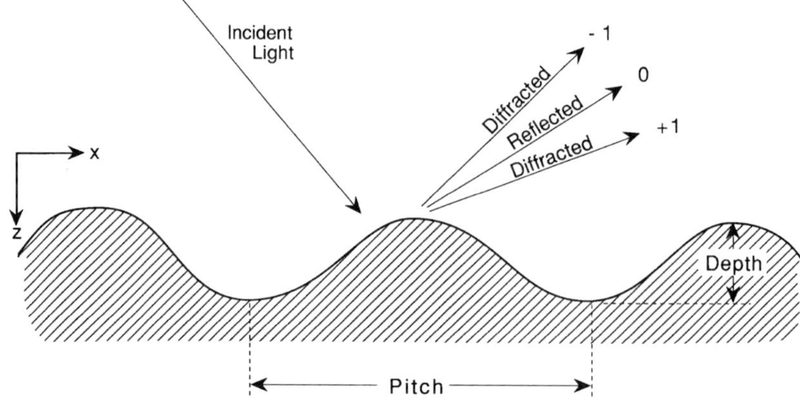

FIGURE 7.7 Diagrammatic representation of the diffraction of light at a grating's surface. Numbers indicate the "orders" of exiting beams.

a periodic fashion, however, can act as a diffraction grating. The light will be split into a series of diffracted beams at different diffraction angles α; these are known as orders, with the undiffracted beam being the zeroth order, and others being labeled with integer values as shown in Figure 7.7. As stated in de Broglie's relationship, the wavevector of a photon is given by the expression

$$p = h/\lambda = \hbar \cdot k \tag{7.16}$$

The wavelength of a photon is unchanged after diffraction, and therefore the total momentum of the photon must be constant. However, if α does not equal θ then the value k_x must have altered, as shown in Figure 7.8. It is clear that the diffraction grating is altering k_x in discrete steps, and this can be expressed by the equation

$$k \cdot \sin(\alpha) = k \cdot \sin(\theta) + N \cdot G \tag{7.17}$$

where N is an integer indicating the *order* of the diffraction, and G is a parameter known as the grating wavevector. The value of G is dependent upon the *pitch* λg of the grating (the distance which specifies the periodicity of the surface profile — see Figure 7.7) according to the expression $G = 2 \cdot \pi/\lambda_g$. Hence, if a metallic grating is used to provide a metal/dielectric interface, a plasmon mode can be observed if the condition

$$k_{spp} = k \cdot \sin(\theta) + N \cdot G \tag{7.18}$$

is met (see Figure 7.8), i.e., *an SPP can be directly excited at a grating's surface*. The resultant reflectivity minima are sometimes referred to as "Wood's anomalies" after R. W. Wood,[34] who first observed them in 1902.

This method of generating SPR affords one immediate advantage over prism-based techniques: there are no complications regarding the thickness of the metal film or dielectric spacers since the coupling gap is no longer required. Instead, coupling strength is now determined by the groove depth of the grating (see Figure 7.7) and this parameter is dictated in manufacture. It is, however, rather more difficult to model reflectivity data obtained from gratings. The mathematics used with prisms derives from Fresnel's equations,[35] all of which are based upon systems with planar interfaces, and which are unuseable in the case of corrugated interfaces. The grating-based data shown in Figure 7.9 has been fitted to a model by Chandezon et al.[36] who recast Maxwell's equations into a reference frame which treats

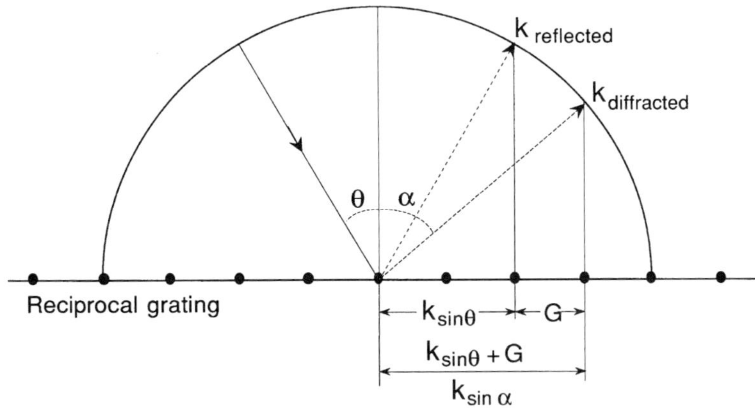

FIGURE 7.8 A representation in reciprocal space of the diffraction of light from a grating.

the sinusoidal surface of the grating as being planar. A couple of points are worth noting from the data. Whilst the feature at Å 14.5° is a simple SPP mode as expected, the reflectivity dip at Å 32.5° is due to a *second* SPP mode which travels in the opposite direction. Its shape is related to the distortion (nonsinusoidality) of the grating profile (see the work of Bryan-Brown et al.[37]). Also, the "critical angles" at ≃12° and ≃32.5° which *resemble* those seen in prism-based data are angles at which diffracted orders "disappear" below the horizon of the grating.

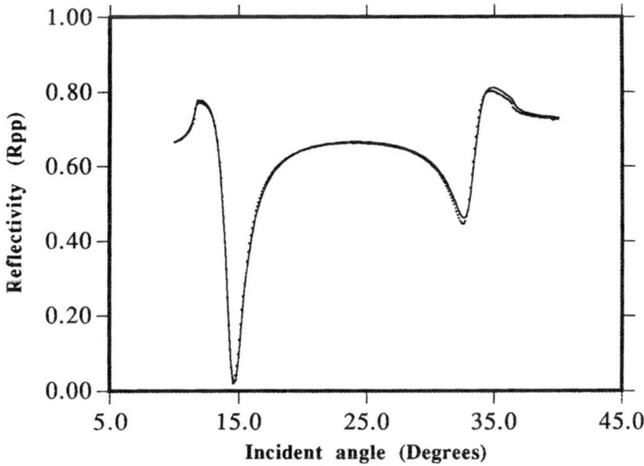

FIGURE 7.9 Reflectivity data obtained from a diffraction grating (points), with a corresponding theoretical fit (line) — see text.

As an aside, the gratings used by Bryan-Brown were manufactured by heating a silica glass holographic grating and taking an impression of its profile by pressing it against a sheet of Perspex. Once the resultant replica grating has been given a metal coating it can be used as the active surface of a biosensor. Since the production costs are so low once the master grating has been obtained, the replicas can be used as disposable active surfaces in a biosensor, an important advantage if a cheap and portable device is to be produced.

Compared to the use of prism-based SPR methods in biosensing, little attention appears to have been paid to grating-based techniques (since disclosure of the idea in a patent by Pettigrew in 1984[38]), despite their increasing use in chemical and gas sensors. Cullen et al.[39] have studied immuno-reactions via SPP reflectivity data obtained from gold-coated gratings.

In addition to full angle-scans of the SPR, constant-angle reflectivity changes during protein deposition were measured. The grating had to be immersed into a buffer solution, and this is where a major disadvantage in the use of gratings becomes apparent. With gratings the light must propagate through the solution before it can excite the SPP. Thus the sample solution must be optically transparent at the wavelength of the probing light. In the work of Cullen et al.[39] this requirement was met. Data were obtained both in air and solution. The optically denser solution shifted the mode to higher incident angles. Moreover, the reflectivity was less across the entire angle range because the reflected light is distributed among more orders (the number that can be supported being greater in a medium of higher refractive index). Similar data, obtained by Lawrence and Geddes (previously unpublished), are shown in Figure 7.10. A second report by Cullen and Lowe[40] involved the use of gratings in the study of nonspecific absorption. In this work, silver coatings with their narrower modes gave greater sensitivity.

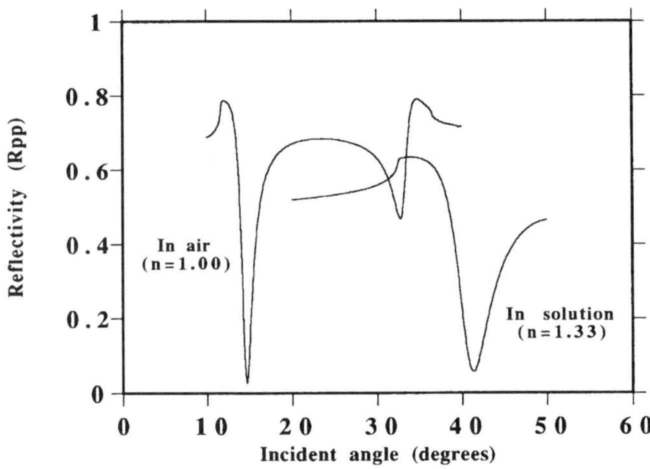

FIGURE 7.10 Comparison of reflectivity data obtained from a grating in an air ambient to that obtained from the same grating when immersed in water — see text.

In a patent by Drake et al.[41] two gratings are used in tandem as the basis of a polychromatic biosensor (detecting the presence of influenza A virus in the given example). A collimated beam of white light is made incident upon an antibody-coated grating. The reflected and diffracted light is directed (via a mirror) onto a blazed grating (one with a sawtooth profile) which splits the light into its component wavelengths. The light is then focused onto a 256-pixel photodiode array, and the intensity is measured at chosen wavelengths. The positions of the reflectivity minima are noted. If the antibody is exposed to its corresponding antigen such that binding occurs, the change in film thickness and/or refractive index will cause a shift in these positions. Thus, with the appropriate choice of antibody, a species-specific biosensor can be obtained.

A patent by Sawyers[42] discusses a more fundamental detail, the material from which the grating is made. For SPR to occur this material must possess a negative real component of optical dielectric permittivity. Many molecular species do not bind well to the surface of a metal. Moreover, since many reusable biosensors require acids to remove antigen from antibody it would be preferable to avoid the use of metals. Sawyers proposes the use of certain dielectrics which exhibit negative values of ε_r over discrete wavelength ranges. The materials which act as metals in this fashion all do so within only the *microwave* region of the spectrum (e.g., silicon carbide at 12 μm and calcium fluoride at 35 μm). This limits their usefulness considerably. Other materials with negative ε_r may be found for visible wavelengths. Polyacetylenes are an example (the effect depends upon strong optical resonance — see work by Philpott and Swalen[43] and Pockrand et al.[44]) and may have future potential.

A feature unique to grating-based SPP apparatus becomes apparent when the grating is rotated about the z-axis. Until now this discussion has been restricted to the case where the grooves have been set perpendicular to the plane of incidence, i.e., in the y-direction (see Figure 7.7). Thus p-polarized light has been able to excite an SPP since it possesses a component of E that is perpendicular to the metal's surface, whilst the E-field of s-polarized light has been aligned with the grooves, parallel to the interface, and SPR cannot be induced. In this situation the azimuthal angle ϕ is said to be zero. However, if the grating is rotated about the z-axis then *neither* E-field polarization will lie parallel to the grooves, but *both* will have access to a sloping portion of the surface ensuring that their E-fields will lie normal to the metal in some region. Hence both polarizations can excite a plasmon mode when the grating is twisted. As a consequence of this symmetry breaking, it is found that p-to-s conversion occurs at the plasmon angle. The conversion reaches a maximum value when $\phi = 45$, and increases with groove depth. Typical data are presented in Figure 7.11, in which Rps indicates the reflectivity due to this effect.

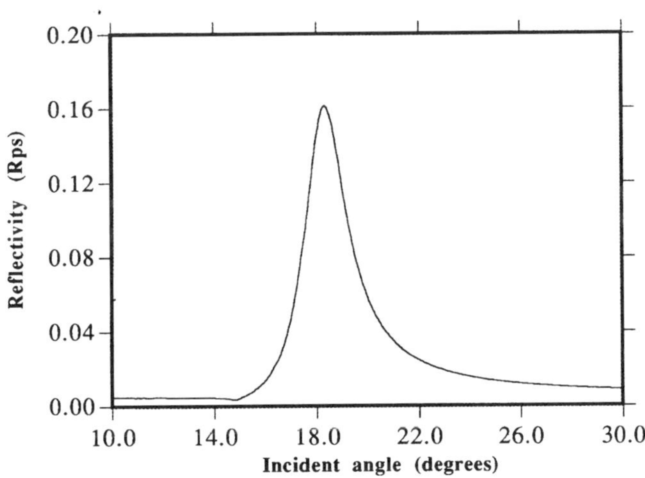

FIGURE 7.11 Reflectivity data obtained by measuring p-to-s polarization conversion due to a grating at an azimuthal angle of 45°, a peak value occurring at the plasmon angle.

The fact that it is now possible to look for a *maximum* value of reflectivity against a near-zero background presents a new range of possibilities that have yet to be fully explored. Work by Jory et al.[45] has involved the use of a twisted grating in a gas-sensing device. The prototype illuminates a silver-coated grating's surface with collimated polychromatic light from a broad-band red LED. The angle of incidence is held constant. Only one discrete wavelength of light can excite a plasmon at this set angle, and hence this wavelength is the most strongly reflected when the Rps signal is examined. However, if the surface of the grating is altered in some fashion (in the case of the prototype, by the condensation of alcohol vapor onto the metal) then a *different* wavelength is required to excite the mode. Thus, by integrating a wavelength detector into their device, Jory et al. demonstrated its use as a sensitive gas sensor; initial experiments show it to be capable of detecting a 0.9-nm overlayer of condensed vapor, and a tenfold improvement in sensitivity is anticipated once the kit has been optimized. Further, the device was constructed from relatively inexpensive components, contained no moving parts, and used fiber optic coupling to enable the sensing head to act remotely from both source and detector. It seems entirely plausible that this device could be used as an efficient biosensor. It is presently being investigated in a collaboration between Exeter University and C.S.I.R.O. (the Commonwealth Scientific and Industrial Research Organisation, Australia).

For a more detailed description of the use of gratings, including both their fabrication and spectral properties, the reader is referred to the book by Hutley.[46] Grating- and prism-based coupling techniques are summarized and compared in Table 7.2.

TABLE 7.2
Sample Geometries for SPR Excitation

Sample geometry	Comment
Prism: Otto	Small and precise gap must be maintained between prism's base and plasmon-supporting medium (metal), restricting access to sensing surface.
Prism: K-R (Kretschmann-Raether)	More practical than Otto since metal directly applied to prism's base.
Prism: hybrid	Dielectric medium between prism and metal enables two SPP to be supported, one of which (the LRSEP) is sharper than its equivalent in an Otto or K-R geometry.
Grating: general	Incident light must traverse analyte solution before striking grating.
Grating: "twisted"	Polarization conversion enables measurement of peak in reflectivity as opposed to usual minimum.
Optic fiber	Essentially as per "Prism: K-R". Compact and easily interfaced to other equipment.
General: constant angle	Allows monitoring of reaction sites *in situ*.
General: angle-scan	Determines ε_i and effective values of ε_r and thickness, but generally too slow a method for *in situ* measurement.
General: differential measurements	Increases sensitivity greatly, but equipment needs to be isolated from vibration and temperature changes.

7.2.2.3 Differential Measurements

Whilst very little work has yet been published, recent investigations have shown that the sensitivity of an SPR-based sensor can be greatly increased if differential measurements of reflectivity are obtained. The sensitivity of variable-angle SPR-based sensors depends upon the accuracy with which intensity changes, wavelength changes, or angular shifts can be measured, and in the case of a $\theta/2\theta$ rotating table the angular accuracy is typically 0.01°; a differential technique has been shown to improve this figure by at least two orders of magnitude, enabling the detection of far smaller perturbations of the SPR than has previously been possible.

This discussion will concern itself with a patent produced by Gass and Sambles[47] and the doctoral thesis of Gass,[48] in which an acousto-optic deflector (AOD) is used in a system taking differential measurements of an SPR. An AOD consists of a crystalline material in which an acoustic wave is generated via piezoelectric transducers: the acoustic wave interacts with light transmitted through the crystal and diffracts it, changing the angle at which it exits the crystal. This occurs because the acoustic wave produces a periodic density variation across the crystal, and hence diffracts the light in a manner analogous to Bragg reflection of X-rays from a crystal lattice. In the work of Gass, a TeO_2 crystal is used, with the transducers operating at a driving frequency of 80 MHz. By varying this frequency the period of the density oscillation could be changed, and hence the diffraction angle could be altered. Thus by varying the driving frequency at a "dither" frequency F_d the transmitted light beam could be made to oscillate between two diffraction angles, and when one discrete wavelength was used to excite an SPP it would oscillate across a small region of the reflectivity profile (e.g., in Gass' work, if the driving frequency was varied by 10 MHz then HeNe laser light (632.8 nm wavelength) was deflected by approximately 0.6°). If the angle of incidence θ_{av} about which the oscillations occurred was below the angle of the plasmon reflectivity minimum

θ_{SPP} then the reflectivity would oscillate sinusoidally at F_d and increase as the angle decreased. However, if the incident light oscillated about the SPP minimum then the reflectivity would increase whether the angle increased or decreased, and the reflectivity would vary with time at *twice* the dither frequency.

By using a phase-sensitive detector (PSD) that was locked to the dither frequency, *only signals that oscillate at the dither frequency were detected.* This meant that when $\theta_{av} = \theta_{SPP}$ there was zero output from the PSD, whereas there was a finite reading at angles just to either side of the minimum; when just below θ_{SPP} the reflectivity increases as the acousto-optical tunable filter's driving frequency is decreased, producing a negative output from the PSD, and vice versa. Figure 7.12 schematically illustrates the output from a PSD (lower graph) with reference to a typical SPP reflectivity profile (upper graph), showing that there is a very steep slope to the PSD profile in the region of the reflectivity minimum. It is this that makes the system highly sensitive to shifts of θ_{SPP}, since the signal is used to continually lock the AOTF driving frequency to the SPP minimum, and by measuring the driving frequency to within 1 kHz an angular sensitivity of around 5×10^{-5} can be obtained. This is an improvement of several orders of magnitude when compared to previous systems.

Modifications are possible, such as the use of polychromatic light so as to measure the change in reflectivity with wavelength at a constant angle (using an acousto-optic tunable filter (AOTF), a polychromatic device similar to the monochromatic AOD) since this allows fiber coupling without angle scans, and hence offers greater device potential.

However, it has to be said that the high sensitivity of an AOD can also inhibit the usefulness of this technique of measurement. It has been found that the system is easily perturbed by vibrations or slight temperature fluctuations (Gass stated that changes of more than 0.05°C caused appreciable thermal expansion or contraction of the apparatus), and hence the equipment must be protected from such effects if the quoted sensitivity is to be maintained. Despite this, the accuracy obtainable by such a method is extremely desirable if very low concentrations of low molecular weight analytes are to be detected, and it is likely that the technique will attract considerable interest in the near future.

7.3 CONCLUSIONS

SPR techniques are clearly well-suited to the detection and characterization of dielectric overlayers, and hence can be used to design extremely effective biosensors. Noninvasive measurements can be taken with great sensitivity, especially in the case of differential techniques, enabling the detection of gases or vapors that are absorbed into a dielectric overlayer, or the detection of antibodies if that overlayer consists of protein receptors. Direct measurements can be taken as the reaction progresses, enabling real-time monitoring of protein binding which, under certain circumstances, obviates the need for the stages of incubation and separation that are an integral part of most assay methods. This aspect also makes it possible to use SPR techniques as the basis of warning systems which will constantly sample a given environment until the concentration of a chosen contaminant reaches a preset level, triggering an alarm of some form.

As can easily be deduced from this review, there are a wide variety of SPR-based sensors, and most needs can be catered to simply by choosing the correct apparatus geometry. However, in the case of biosensors it is the receptor layer that will largely dictate the usefulness of the sensor since — whilst the choice of SPR technique is important — the final limit on the specificity and sensitivity of the device is set by the interaction between antibodies and antigens. This is discussed in Chapter 16 and details such further considerations as the chemical pretreatment of the transducer surface, the alignment of receptor sites to maximize binding efficiency, and the choice of receptor layer.

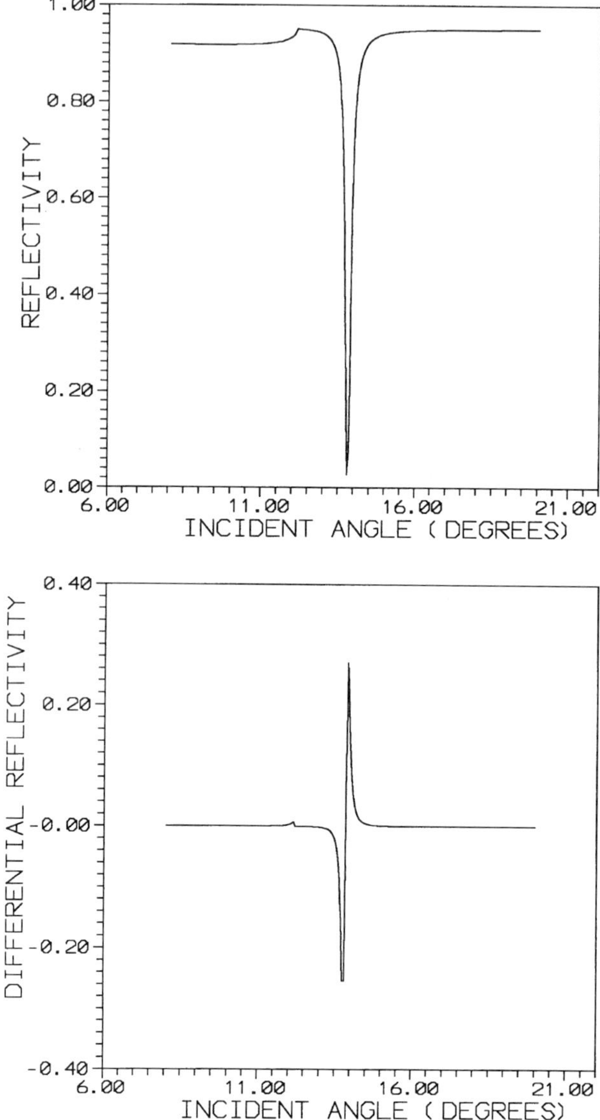

FIGURE 7.12 The differential technique of SPR measurement: a comparison of a typical SPP reflectivity profile (above) with its corresponding differential signal (below) — see text.

ACKNOWLEDGMENTS

The authors thank both Professor J. R. Sambles (Exeter University, U.K.) and Dr. N. Furlong (C.S.I.R.O., Melbourne) for many useful discussions during the preparation of this review, and are also grateful for the support of the Defence Research Agency at Malvern who helped support one of the authors (C.R.L.) at the beginning of this work.

REFERENCES

1. Ngeh-Ngwainbi, J., Suleiman, A. A., and Guilbault, G. G., Piezoelectric crystal biosensors, *Biosens. Bioelectron.*, 5, 13, 1990.
2. Seitz, W. R., Chemical sensors based on fiber optics, *Anal. Chem.*, 56/1, 16A, 1984.

3. Lundström, I., Shivaraman, S., Svensson, C., and Lundkvist, L., A hydrogen-sensitive MOS field-effect transistor, *Appl. Phys. Lett.*, 26, 55, 1975.
4. Roederer, J. E. and Bastiaans, G. J., Microgravimetric immunoassay with piezoelectric crystals, *Anal. Chem.*, 55, 2333, 1983.
5. Nylander, C., Liedberg, B., and Lind, T., Gas detection by means of surface plasmon resonance, *Sensors Actuators*, 3, 79, 1982/83.
6. Löfås, S. and Johnsson, B., A novel hydrogel matrix on gold surfaces in surface plasmon resonance sensors for fast and efficient covalent immobilization of ligands, *J. Chem. Soc. Chem. Commun.*, 21, 1526, 1990.
7. Raether, H., *Surface Plasmons on Smooth and Rough Surfaces and on Gratings*, Springer-Verlag, Berlin,1988.
8. Sambles, J. R., Bradbery, G. W., and Yang, F. Z., Optical excitation of surface plasmons: an introduction, *Contemp. Phys.*, 32/3, 173, 1991.
9. Welford, K. R., Optical Modes of Layered Structures Containing Nematic Liquid Crystals, Ph.D Thesis, University of Exeter, U.K., 1986.
10. Boardman, A. D., *Electromagnetic Surface Modes*, John Wiley & Sons, Chichester, 1982.
11. Pockrand, I., Swalen, J. D., Santo, R., Brillante, A., and Philpott, M. R., Optical properties of organic dye molecules by surface plasmon spectroscopy, *J. Chem. Phys.*, 69/9, 4001, 1978.
12. Liedberg, B., Nylander, C., and Lundström, I., Surface plasmon resonance for gas detection and biosensing, *Sensors Actuators*, 4, 299, 1983.
13. Otto, A., Excitation of nonradiative surface plasma waves in silver by the method of frustrated total reflection, *Z. Phys.*, 216, 398, 1968.
14. Kretschmann, E. and Raether, H., Radiative decay of non-radiative surface plasmons by light, *Z. Naturforsch.*, 23a, 2135, 1968.
15. Morgan, H. and Taylor, D. M., A surface plasmon resonance immunosensor based on the streptavidin-biotin complex, *Biosens. Bioelectron.*, 7, 405, 1992.
16. Pollard-Knight, D., Hawkins, E., Yeung, D., Pashby, D. P., Simpson, M., McDougall, A., Buckle, P., and Charles, S. A., Imunoassays and nucleic acid detection with a biosensor based on surface plasmon resonance, *Ann. Biol. Clin.*, 48, 642, 1990.
17. Matsubara, K., Kawata, S., and Minami, S., Optical chemical sensor based on surface plasmon measurement, *Appl. Opt.*, 27/6, 1160, 1988.
18. Batchelder, D. N. and Willson, J. P., U.K. Patent number, GB 2,197,065, 1988.
19. Fontana, E., Pantell, R. H., and Strober, S., Surface plasmon immunoassay, *Appl. Opt.*, 29, 4694, 1990.
20. Kooyman, R. P. H., Kolkman, H., Van Gent, J., and Greve, J., Surface plasmon resonance immunosensors: sensitivity considerations, *Anal. Chim. Acta*, 213, 35, 1988.
21. de Brujin, H. E., Kooyman, R. P. H., and Greve, J., Choice of metal and wavelength for surface-plasmon resonance sensors: some considerations, *Appl. Optics*, 31/4, 440, 1992.
22. Kovacs, G. J., Sulphide formation on evaporated silver films, *Surf. Sci.*, 78, L245, 1978.
23. Matsubara, K., Kawata, S., and Minami, S., Multilayer system for a high-precision surface plasmon resonance sensor, *Opt. Lett.*, 15/1, 75, 1990.
24. Sarid, D., Long-range surface-plasma waves on very thin metal-films, *Phys. Rev. Lett.*, 47, 1927, 1981.
25. Welford, K. R. and Sambles, J. R., Coupled surface plasmons in a symmetric system, *J. Mod. Opt.*, 35/9, 1467, 1988.
26. Kooyman, R. P. H., Lenferink, A. T. M., Eenink, R. G. and Greve, J., Vibrating mirror surface-plasmon resonance immunosensor, *Anal. Chem.*, 63, 83, 1991.
27. Oda, K. and Fukui, M., Instantaneous observation of angular scan-attenuated total reflection spectra, *Opt. Commun.*, 69(5,6), 361, 1986.
28. Fukui, M. and Oda, K., Studies on metal-film growth through instantaneously observed attenuated total reflection spectra, *Appl. Surf. Sci.*, 33/34, 82, 1988.
29. Lawrence, C. R., Martin, A. S., and Sambles, J. R., Surface plasmon polariton studies of highly absorbing Langmuir-Blodgett films, *Thin Solid Films*, 208, 269, 1992.
30. Kötz, R., Kolb, D. M., and Sass, J. K., Electron density effects in surface plasmon excitations on gold and silver electrodes, *Surf. Sci.*, 69, 365, 1977.

31. Lopez-Rios, T. and Vuye, G., Spectroscopy of very thin metal layers on metallic surfaces using optical excitation of surface plasmons, *Nuovo Cimento*, 39B/2, 823, 1977.
32. De Maria, L., Martinelli, M., and Vegetti, G., Fiber-optic sensor based on surface plasmon interrogation, *Sensors Actuators,* B12, 221, 1993.
33. Jorgenson, R. C. and Yee, S. S., A fiber-optic chemical sensor based on surface plasmon resonance, *Sensors Actuators,* B12, 213, 1993.
34. Wood, R. W., On a remarkable case of uneven distribution of light in a diffraction grating spectrum, *Proc. Phys. Soc.*, 18, 269, 1902.
35. Born, M. and Wolf E., *Principles of Optics*, Pergamon Press, Elmsford, NY, 1965, p 48.
36. Chandezon, J., Dupuis, M. T., Cornet, G., and Maystre D., Multicoated gratings — a differential formalism applicable in the entire optical region, *J. Opt. Soc. Am.*, 72, 839, 1982.
37. Bryan-Brown, G. P., Jory, M. C., Elston, S. J., and Sambles, J. R., Diffraction grating characterisation via the excitation of surface plasmon polaritons, *J. Mod. Opt.*, 40, 959, 1993.
38. Pettigrew, R. M., International Patent WO 84/02578, 1984.
39. Cullen, D. C., Brown, R. G. W., and Lowe, C. R., Detection of immuno-complex formation via surface plasmon resonance on gold-coated diffraction gratings, *Biosensors*, 3, 211, 1987/88.
40. Cullen, D. C. and Lowe, C. R., A direct surface plasmon-polariton immunosensor: preliminary investigations of the non-specific adsorption of serum components to the sensor interface, *Sensors Actuators*, B1, 576, 1990.
41. Drake, R. A. L., Sawyers, C. G., and Robinson, G. A., Australian Patent Number AU-A-10631/88, 1988.
42. Sawyers, C. G., U.K. Patent Number, GB 2,202,045, 1988.
43. Philpott M. R. and Swalen J. D., Exciton surface polaritons on organic crystals, *J. Chem. Phys.*, 69(6), 2912, 1978.
44. Pockrand I., Swalen J. D., Gordon J. G., and Philpott M. R., Exciton-surface plasmon interactions, *J. Chem.Phys.*, 70(7), 3401, 1979.
45. Jory, M. J., Vukusic, P. S., and Sambles, J. R., Development of a prototype gas sensor using surface plasmon resonance on gratings, *Sensors Actuators,* B17, 203, 1994.
46. Hutley, M. C., *Diffraction Gratings*, Academic Press, New York, 1982.
47. Gass, P. A. and Sambles J. R., U.K. Patent Number, GB 9208113.2, 1992.
48. Gass, P. A., Acousto-Optic Devices and Applications, Ph.D. Thesis, University of Exeter, U.K., 1991.

8 Immunosensors Based on Total Internal Reflectance

Rob P. H. Kooyman and Laura M. Lechuga

CONTENTS

0-8493-8905-4/97/$0.00+$.50
© 1997 by CRC Press, Inc.

8.1 INTRODUCTION

In the last decade the development of chemical sensors has become a very active research field both in university and in industrial laboratories. It has now become clear that technological innovations can result in sensor devices which allow for new, unprecedented applications. A striking example is the measurement of the pH within one single living cell.[1] More conventional, but nevertheless from a practical viewpoint very fascinating, are the large number of sensor devices that find their application in the biomedical and veterinary field, in the bioprocess (food) industry, and also in the monitoring of the biosphere.

All classes of chemical sensors have as a common, crucial element a selector function which should provide the necessary selectivity and sensitivity to one chemical species or one group of such species. For instance, for a potassium sensor, one ideally expects that the sensor only responds to changes in K^+ concentration and not, even indirectly, to variations in the concentration of other cations. Since the development of the hybridoma technique in the early 1970s[2] it was soon realized that antibodies, with their high specificity and affinity towards prespecified analyte molecules (*the antigens*), could become practical selector molecules in a chemical sensor system. An important advantage of the use of antibodies is that these can be prepared, using biotechnological methods, against virtually any molecule with a molecular mass >300. Examples of the use of antibodies are now found in a large variety of *immunoassays* such as RIA, ELISA, EIA, SPIA, etc.[3]

However, each of these methods suffers from one or more of the following handicaps: these assays sometimes require expensive instrumentation, are time consuming, can be laborious, and demand skilled personnel. Furthermore, all these methods require some method of adding a reagent compound. In recent years much effort has been put into improving these assays both from a (bio-)chemical and a transducer viewpoint. When one focuses upon the transducer principles utilized, it is seen that amperometric, potentiometric, and acoustic methods all have undergone significant improvements. Particularly, this holds for the optical transducer principles based upon the use of *optical wave guides*. In this chapter it will be outlined how from this technology a new generation of "immunosensors" emerges where many of the above-mentioned shortcomings have been overcome. Following a short discussion of antigen-antibody reactions relevant to the operation of an optical immunosensor, the physical mechanisms underlying the various principles will be reviewed. We will also be concerned with practical aspects concerning the manufacturing and the use of immunosensor systems. Finally some selected examples of applications will be discussed, together with an outlook on possible future directions. For reference in reading the following sections, a list of symbols and some typical values are given in lists A.1 and A.2 at the end of this chapter.

8.2 EXPLOITING ANTIBODIES IN A WAVE GUIDE SENSOR

8.2.1 BASIC CHARACTERISTICS

A generalized chemical sensor scheme can be visualized as depicted in Figure 8.1. A receptor layer, capable of specific recognition of analyte A in the presence of other molecules X is immobilized to a transducer device. The transducer, interrogated by some input stimulus I, produces a response R (electrical current or voltage) as a result of a binding event in this layer. The overall sensitivity of such a device will be determined by two separate factors, the rate of change of the nature of the receptor layer, denoted by S_{chem}, and the efficiency of transduction of S_{chem} to the response R, denoted by S_{trans}.

We will now limit our discussion to the case where the receptor layer consists of antibodies. It is well known that the immunoreaction between a (monoclonal) antibody (receptor Ab) and its corresponding antigen (analyte) is an affinity reaction:

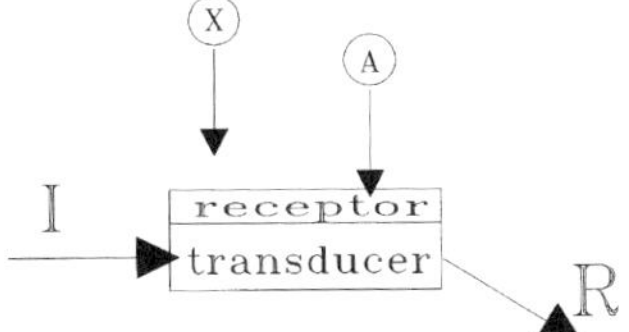

FIGURE 8.1 Chemical sensor: as a result of interaction of analyte A with a receptor layer the response R of the transducer to a stimulus I changes.

$$Ab + A \overset{K_a}{\Leftrightarrow} Ab \cdot A \tag{8.1}$$

Here K_a is the affinity constant, which for this type of reactions is in the range 10^7 to 10^{15} M^{-1}. It can easily be calculated (see, e.g., Reference 4) that in a solution containing a concentration [A] of analyte, the fraction of bound receptor molecules, Γ, is given by Equation 8.2:

$$\Gamma = \frac{K_a \cdot [A]}{1 + K_a[A]} \tag{8.2}$$

Although the immunoreaction described by Equations 8.1 and 8.2, strictly speaking, is an equilibrium reaction, in practice this condition is hardly met. The reason for this is that the rate constant for binding is extremely high for the immunoreaction.[5] Together with a high affinity constant this results in very low dissociation rate constants and, thus, generally a decreasing analyte concentration cannot be measured in a reasonable span of time. Therefore in a strict sense "immunosensors" should be rather denoted by "immunoassays".

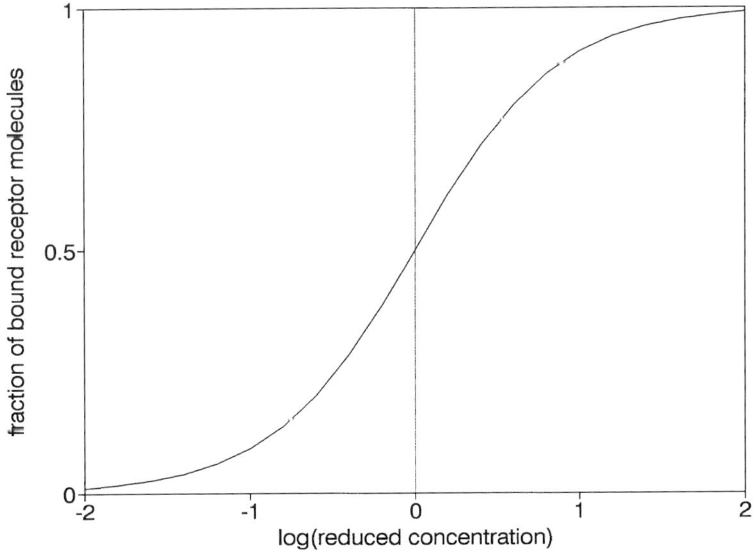

FIGURE 8.2 Fraction of bound receptors at the sensor surface as a function of $K_a \cdot [A]$.

In Figure 8.2, Γ is plotted as a function of the reduced analyte concentration $C = K_a \cdot [A]$. Now let us assume that we have a sensor device that measures the amount of bound receptor molecules, which is the case we will deal with in the following sections. For reasons of simplicity we take the sensor response R, which could be an output voltage, linear in Γ:

$$R = S_{trans} \cdot \Gamma \tag{8.3}$$

From the figure, several observations relevant to optimum sensor design can be made:

1. It is seen that at C = 1 the slope is a maximum, and for a sensor device the differential sensitivity, and thus the accuracy in measuring an analyte concentration, is a maximum at $[A] = 1/K_a$.
2. At high concentrations, C » 1, the sensor hardly responds to changes in concentration, whereas at low concentrations the sensor response is linear in the analyte concentration (cf. Equation 8.2). The minimum Γ that can be measured is determined by the accuracy of the R determination and, particularly, by the sensitivity factor S_{trans}.

Hence in order to completely specify a sensor performance, it is appropriate to define a chemical sensitivity S_{chem} relating the analyte concentration to Γ, and a transducer sensitivity S_{trans} describing the transducer response to a changing Γ. Of equal importance is the specificity of the antibody towards the analyte A. Ideally, the receptor should have an affinity constant K_x close to zero for interaction with other molecules X that can be present in the solution to be analyzed (cf. Figure 8.1). This is particularly important when the analyte of interest is present in a large excess of similar molecules. Inspection of Equation 8.2 indicates that for $K_a/K_x = 1000$ the transducer will only respond adequately when $[A]/[X] > \sim 0.01$.

Thus the design of a successful sensor system depends crucially on two elements:

1. Transduction of the biochemical to the physical domain: design of a biochemical interface with maximum S_{chem}. This implies preparation of antibodies with high K_a and a minimum cross-reactivity, and optimization of the surface concentration of antibodies in the receptor layer;
2. Transduction of the physical to the electrical domain: design of a transducer system with a maximum S_{trans}.

We will now outline how optical wave guides can be exploited to obtain very sensitive transduction schemes to the electrical domain.

8.2.2 Optical Wave Guides

8.2.2.1 Theory

The theory describing the propagation of light in optical wave guides has been described many times before;[6-10] therefore only a very short description will be given here. Conventionally, an electromagnetic plane wave propagating in a medium with refractive index n can be described by the electric field **E**:

$$\mathbf{E} = \mathbf{E}_0 \cdot \exp\{i(\omega t - \mathbf{k} \cdot \mathbf{r})\} \equiv \mathbf{E}_0 \cdot \exp\{i(\omega t - k_x \cdot x - k_y \cdot y)\} \tag{8.4a}$$

where ω is the angular frequency, t is the time, and **r** = (x,y) is the position vector. Note that $\mathbf{E}_0$ is a vector; the square of its absolute value corresponds to the intensity, whereas the components denote the polarization direction of the electric field. The wave vector **k,** whose direction is parallel to that of the wave propagation, will play a central role in the following. Additionally, it is important to note that the wave represented by Equation 8.4a is only propagating if both ω and k are (at least partly) real numbers.

The relation between **k**, ω, and n is given by:

$$|\mathbf{k}| = \left(k_x^2 + k_y^2\right)^{1/2} = \mathrm{n} \cdot 2\pi/\lambda = \mathrm{n} \cdot \omega/\mathrm{c} \tag{8.5}$$

with λ and c the wavelength and propagation velocity in vacuum, respectively.

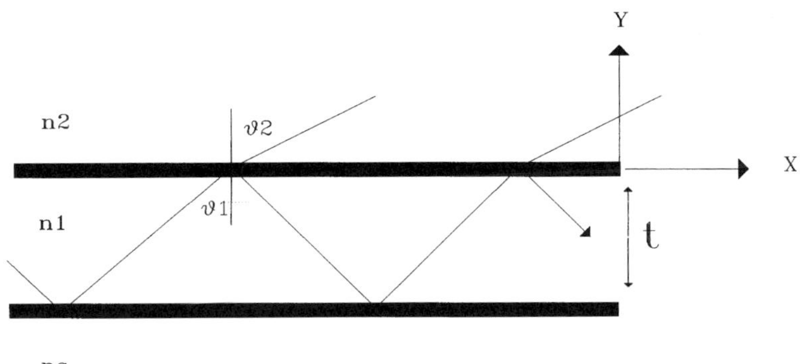

FIGURE 8.3 A light ray propagating in an optical wave guide. For definition of symbols, see text.

Consider a situation as in Figure 8.3, where a simple wave guide structure is depicted. A material with high refractive index n_1 and a certain thickness t is embedded between two materials with low refractive index n_2 and n_s, respectively. A light beam traveling in such a material under an angle ϑ with the direction normal to the surface will partly reflect at the interfaces. If ϑ is larger than the critical angle ϑ_c then all light will reflect at the interface. However, this does *not* imply that there is no optical power in the low index parts of the wave guide structure. This can be readily seen on the basis of Snell's law which states that the components of the wave vector parallel to the interface are equal on both sides of the interface:

$$k_{x1} = k_{x2} \tag{8.6}$$

Combination of Equations 8.5 and 8.6 yields an expression for the perpendicular component of the wave vector k_2 in medium 2:

$$k_{y2}^2 = \mathrm{n}_1^2 \cdot \left(\frac{2\pi}{\lambda}\right)^2 \cdot \left(\mathrm{n}_2^2/\mathrm{n}_1^2 - \sin^2\vartheta\right) \tag{8.7}$$

From this equation the physical meaning of ϑ_c can be appreciated: it is seen that for $\sin\vartheta > \sin\vartheta_c \equiv n_2/n_1$ the right-hand side is negative, and thus k_{y2} is purely imaginary. This implies that for $\vartheta > \vartheta_c$ in the direction y in medium 2 no traveling wave exists; instead a wave results that travels along the interface, and decays (is "*evanescent*") in the y-direction. The penetration depth of this field can be found by substituting $\kappa \equiv i.k_{y2}$ into Equation 8.7:

$$\mathbf{E} = \mathbf{E}_0 \cdot e^{-\kappa \cdot y} \cdot \exp\{i(\omega t - k_x \cdot x)\} \tag{8.4b}$$

Using Equation 8.7, it is found that for visible light the penetration depth κ^{-1} is in the range of 50 to 500 nm.

From Equation 8.4b it is now clear that in the immediate vicinity, at the low index side of the interface, an electric field is present, even in the case of total internal reflection. Returning to Figure 8.3, we see that the light beam after the first reflection event travels to the interface 1-s and reflects in a similar way. If $\vartheta > \vartheta_c$ then the light beam travels in a zigzag way through the structure with no loss of optical power. The electromagnetic field distribution within the wave guide is determined by the resulting interference pattern of the downward and upward traveling plane waves. Now, a net energy transport along the wave guide will only occur if this interference pattern is stationary over the complete length of the wave guide. This is the case if in one round trip of the light beam the phase changes by a multiple of 2π. Applying this to the wave guide of Figure 8.3 we find the wave guiding condition:[7-10]

$$2k_1 \cdot t \cdot \cos\vartheta_m - \phi_{1S}^{(i)} - \phi_{12}^{(i)} = m \cdot 2\pi; \qquad m = 0,1,\ldots \tag{8.8}$$

where we have taken into account that upon reflection at the interfaces 1-2 and 1-s phase jumps occur, dependent on the polarization state i = TM (p polarized) or TE (s polarized) of the light. Expressions for these phase jumps can be found, for example, in Reference 9. From Equation 8.8 it also follows that for a given wave guide structure, generally a so-called *cut-off* angle ϑ_0 exists above which no propagation is possible; only if $n_2 = n_s$ does this cut-off value not exist.[9] Thus only a discrete set of angles allows for unattenuated light propagation. With each of these propagation angles an electromagnetic field distribution (*mode*) across the wave guide is associated.[8,9] For a given wave guide structure each mode has a certain part of the total optical power stored in the evanescent field; generally, for increasing $\vartheta > \vartheta_c$, this part decreases. As we will see in the next section, this will have consequences for the design of a sensitive wave guide immunosensor.

Snell's law permits us to characterize the propagation of the various modes by a propagation constant β which is identical to the x-component of the wave vector:

$$\beta_m = n_1 \cdot k \cdot \sin\vartheta_m \tag{8.9}$$

This propagation constant plays a central role in the discussion of the sensitivity of the various wave guide sensors, because any change of the wave guide structure (refractive index profile, thickness) or nature of the light employed (wavelength, polarization state) will be reflected in β.

8.2.2.2 Optical Excitation of a Wave Guide Structure

Because in a wave guide light propagates via the process of total internal reflection, a light beam directed under a certain angle with the wave guide generally will not be able to excite a guided wave. In order to obtain energy transfer between the external light beam and the guided modes, it is necessary that both electromagnetic waves match. Commonly three different methods are used to excite a guided wave in a dielectric layer structure (see Figure 8.4):[9]

- *Endface coupling:* the intensity profile of a laser beam focused on the end face of a wave guide can be tailored to match that of a selected mode in the wave guide. As generally the thickness of a wave guide is fairly small (0.1 to 10 μm), this is only a practical option in a laboratory environment with stable optical setups.
- *Prism coupling:* an evanescent field is produced when the light beam strikes the prism base in the total internal reflection regime. By changing the angle θ the component of the wave vector parallel to the interface can be matched to that of a wave guide mode. If the feeding (prism) evanescent field and the receiving (wave guide) evanescent field overlap, then energy transfer from the external light beam to the guided mode occurs. Thus, it is necessary that prism base and wave guide interface are at very small distance (order of microns).

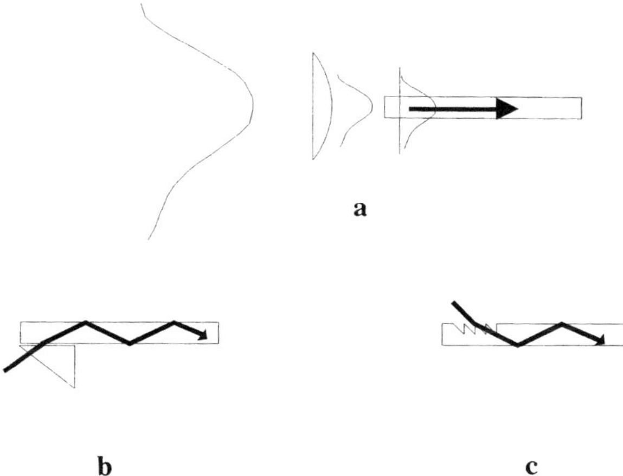

FIGURE 8.4 Common ways of coupling light into a planar wave guide: (a) endface coupling; (b) prism coupling; (c) grating coupling.

- *Grating coupling:* when a corrugated structure on top of a wave guide is irradiated by a light beam under a certain angle, as a result of diffraction a propagation constant can be produced matching that of a guided mode in the wave guide. Generally, the efficiency of this conversion is fairly low.

In view of the small lateral dimensions of the wave guide and in order to obtain a reasonable optical power in the wave guide the use of a laser light source with its high brightness and its very high degree of collimation is almost mandatory in these coupling methods.

8.2.3 Evanescent Wave Immunosensors

Consider Figure 8.5 where a wave guide structure is utilized as a substrate for an immobilized receptor layer. Such a layer can have a thickness of about 4 to 500 nm. Depending on the affinity of the receptor layer and the bulk concentration of analytes, a certain fraction of the receptor molecules will be involved in binding. From an optical viewpoint (cf. Figure 8.5) this results in a changed wave guide configuration; in particular, the refractive index profile n(y) will change. *A surface binding process probed by the evanescent field thus results in a changed propagation constant* β. This is the basic principle of all evanescent wave chemical sensors. Note that this principle provides an inherent *surface* sensitivity: any changes in the bulk solution will hardly affect the sensor response.

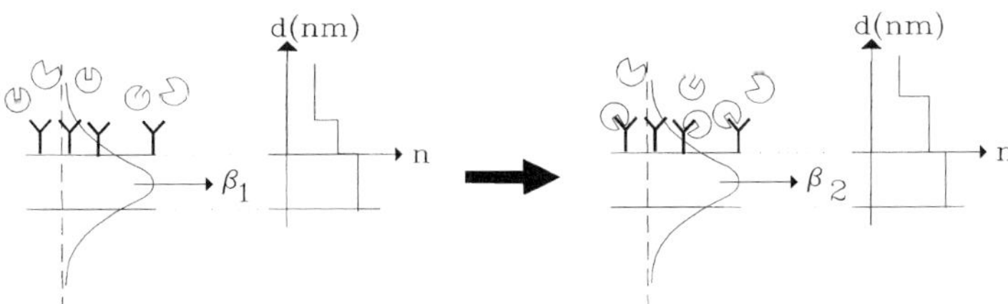

FIGURE 8.5 An immunoreaction at the surface of an optical wave guide modeled as a change of the refractive index profile; as a result β changes.

If Δn(y) contains an appreciable imaginary component, which is the case if the binding analyte is a colored species, the changing propagation constant will also have an imaginary character which is equivalent to a decreasing intensity of the guided mode. In such a case the wave guide acts as an extended light source for selective excitation of analyte molecules in the evanescent volume. The extinction of these molecules is directly related to the attenuation of the mode intensity. The operation of such an evanescent wave absorption sensor has been demonstrated before;[11] however, from an engineer's point of view this sensor concept is less attractive because at low absorbance one has to detect very small changes in the intensity of the propagating light against a very high background. Furthermore, a specific absorption band in the analyte of interest is required and this can cause a problem, particularly when one is interested in proteins as analyte which often only have nonspecific absorption bands in the UV. If one still would prefer to use such a method, then one should label the proteins with some suitable dye as a reporter molecule. In such a case the assay would consist of some competition or inhibition method, similar to that used in ELISA kits. Fluorescent evanescent wave sensors suffer from this same drawback, but their potentially enormous sensitivity could turn the scale in some applications. We will return to this in Section 8.3.6.

The big advantage of monitoring a real $\Delta\beta$ is that no external label molecules are required; only *intrinsic* parameters of the analyte of interest are determined. This approach allows for a general scheme of immunosensing based on direct detection. Thus only dielectric changes within the evanescent volume result in a measurable $\Delta\beta$. From Figure 8.5 it can be inferred that for a given number of receptor molecules per unit of area a fraction of the evanescent volume proportional to the molecular mass Mp of the analyte molecule will be populated by analytes: for a given affinity constant and a given bulk concentration of analytes the change $\Delta\beta$ will be larger for large molecules. Furthermore, it is expected that the refractive index difference between bulk solution, n_b, and analyte, n_p, will play an equally important role in establishing the overall transducer sensitivity: after all, in the binding process analyte molecules replace solvent molecules.

These statements can be quantified in the following expression:[12,13]

$$\Delta\beta = F \cdot \frac{n_p^2 - n_b^2}{n_b} \cdot \kappa \cdot \frac{\Delta\gamma}{\rho_p} \tag{8.10}$$

γ is the adsorbed mass per unit surface, and ρ_p is the density of the adsorbing analyte. The other symbols have been defined before.

The factor F in this equation is dependent only on the geometry of the wave guide used and on the nature of the mode that is excited. A knowledge of the behavior of F thus provides us with clues on how to design a wave guide sensor with maximum sensitivity. F can be calculated[13] by solving Equation 8.8. Figure 8.6 provides some representative results from such a calculation: here it was assumed that a protein with refractive index $n_p = 1.45$ adsorbs to the wave guide. The refractive index of the bulk solution — in most practical immunosensor applications it is water — is kept constant at $n_b = 1.33$. The figure illustrates a number of general conclusions[12,13] on the factors that affect sensor sensitivity:

- Because the lower-order modes as well as TM modes turn out to have a larger part of their optical power in the evanescent field compared to higher-order modes and TE modes, respectively, they exhibit better sensitivity.
- There is an optimum wave guide thickness. At this thickness the power in the evanescent field and the penetration depth that are both increasing with decreasing wave guide thickness, are balanced for maximum evanescent wave power density.
- Increase of the index contrast $n_l - n_p$ improves sensitivity.

To these points it can be added that surface sensitivity decreases with increasing wavelength.[12] It can thus be concluded that a high index material should be used that has very small

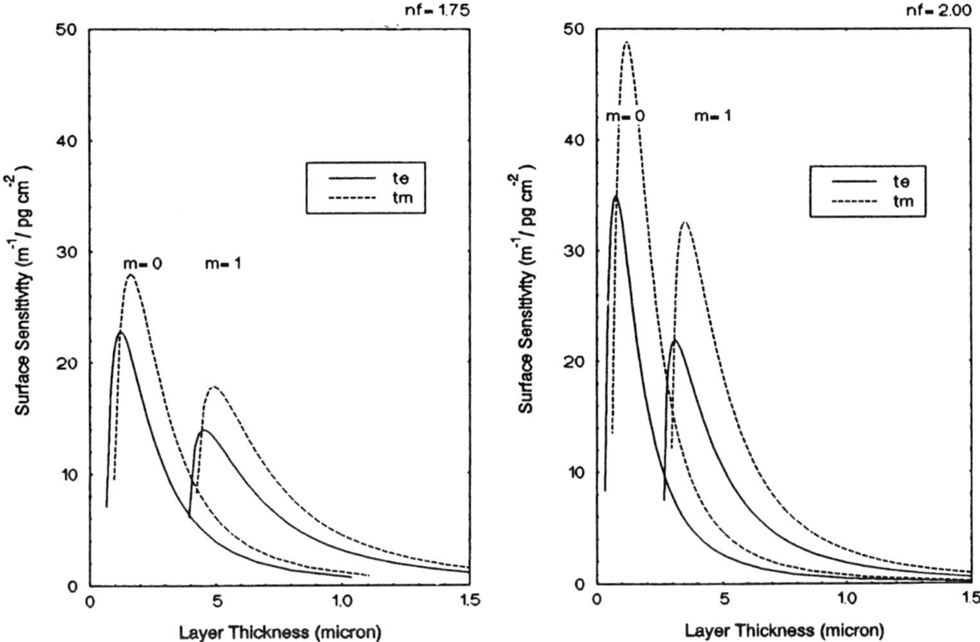

FIGURE 8.6 Surface sensitivity S_{trans} as a function of wave guide layer thickness; λ = 633 nm; n_s = 1.46. Parameters are the core refractive index, polarization state, and the mode number.

dimensions in the vertical direction. In practice, thicknesses down to ~100 nm and n_1 as high as 2.00 can be realized. Manufacturing techniques are described in Section 8.4.1.

In the foregoing, the only situation discussed was where a single species of protein binds to the surface. In an immunosensor the wave guide is precoated with an antibody receptor layer with refractive index n_{ab} ~1.45, that is, close to that of the analyte. In most cases it is therefore a good approximation to model the immunoreaction as a further growing of the layer (refer to Figure 8.5). Alternatively, it is numerically a simple matter to extend the optical model to a five-layer system where n_p and n_{ab} can be chosen independently.

8.3 TRANSDUCTION PRINCIPLES OF WAVE GUIDE IMMUNOSENSORS

Before proceeding to a discussion of the various principles that have been explored until now to detect a $\Delta\beta$ as a result of a layer growth, it is appropriate at this point to indicate how sensitivities of the different sensor principles should be compared. In the literature, quoted sensitivities can be found expressed in moles, molar, parts per million, grams per liter, and grams per unit of surface. It should be realized, however, that only an adsorbed amount of mass per unit of surface is a proper measure for estimating the optical transducer sensitivity (refer to Section 8.2.1). Although the other quantities may be relevant from a number of different points of view, they all assume some value of K_a, or of the surface density of immobilized receptors, or some value of the surface of interaction of the sensor interface.

To date a number of evanescent wave transduction schemes have been proposed. Except for surface plasmon resonance, which also is a member of this family and which is the subject of another chapter in this book, these will now be discussed. Their sensitivity performances will be expressed in the detectivity D_{trans},which can be seen (from Equations 8.3 or 8.10) to be composed of the ratio of minimum measurable response and the transducer sensitivity.

Practical aspects dealing with the manufacturing of the different types of wave guides will be postponed until Section 8.4.

8.3.1 Grating Coupler

The fact that a grating on either side of a wave guide can be used to couple light into the structure (cf. Section 8.2.2.2) has been exploited by Lukosz' group[14,15] to construct an immunosensor. An external light beam will excite a guided mode if the following condition is fulfilled:

$$\beta = k_0 \cdot n \sin \alpha + m \cdot 2\pi/\Lambda, \quad m = 0,1,2,... \tag{8.11}$$

Here, Λ is the grating period, and α is the angle under which the light beam enters the wave guide (see Figure 8.7). The same equation holds for the case where a guided mode is coupled out of the wave guide. Here α denotes the angle under which the light beam leaves the wave guide. A changing β as a result of binding thus results in a changing α. The efficiency of light-coupling into the wave guide structure is measured by a photodiode at the end of the slab. Alternatively,[16,17] the wave guide is excited by endface coupling (refer to Section 8.2.2.2), and by determining the position of the outcoupled beam on a photodiode array the outcoupling angle α is measured. The experimental angular resolution is about 5 millidegrees. The wave guide is manufactured of SiO_2–TiO_2 (n ~1.77), with a thickness around 100 to 200 nm. A He-Ne laser (λ = 633 nm) is used as a light source. For the obtained sensitivity with this configuration see Table 8.1.

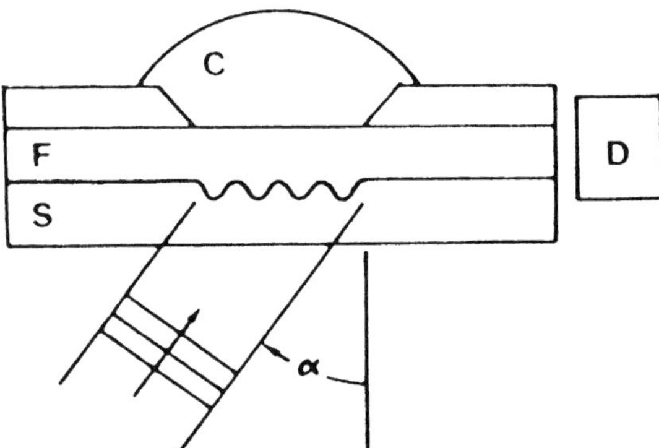

FIGURE 8.7 Grating coupler sensor: S, substrate; F, wave guiding film; C, measuring solution; D, detector. The angle α is defined in the text.

The wave guide has sufficient thickness for supporting both the lowest order TE and TM modes. Consequently, the incoupling angles for TE and TM can be separately determined, allowing for a determination of both the refractive index and thickness of the adsorbed layer. However, it should be added that with such thickness one sacrifices some sensitivity.[13]

8.3.2 Wave Guide Interferometer

In Figure 8.8a the operating principle of a Mach-Zehnder (MZ) wave guide interferometer is illustrated. Light from a source S is split in beamsplitter B1 and directed into a wave guide with two separate arms s and r, that can have different propagation constants β_r and β_s. After traveling a certain distance L, the two light beams recombine in a beamsplitter B2. If the difference in optical pathlengths is smaller than the coherence length of the light source, a

TABLE 8.1
Transducer Sensitivities of Various TIR Sensors

Transducing concept	S_{trans} (pg/mm²)	Ref.[a]
Grating coupler	6	17
Planar polarimeter	2	25
Fiber polarimeter	200	27
Planar interferometer	0.6	21
Resonant mirror	~6	30
Deflection sensor	5	13
Fiber fluorimeter[b]	~0.01	37
SPR[c] sensor	6	40, 41

[a] S_{trans} calculated, based on experimental data, obtained from quoted references.
[b] Calculation based on 600-μm-diameter fiber with 5 cm interaction length, ~5 dye molecules per protein molecule with M = 50 kDa.
[c] SPR: surface plasmon resonance; assumed angular resolution 2.10^{-3} degrees.

stationary interference pattern in the form of a series of fringes will be observed at location D. For one position in the fringe pattern the intensity can then be written as:[18]

$$I = I_0[1 + \cos(\varphi_r - \varphi_s)] \quad (8.12a)$$

with φ_r and φ_s the phase retardations accumulated from the position of B1 to the location in the fringe pattern monitored.

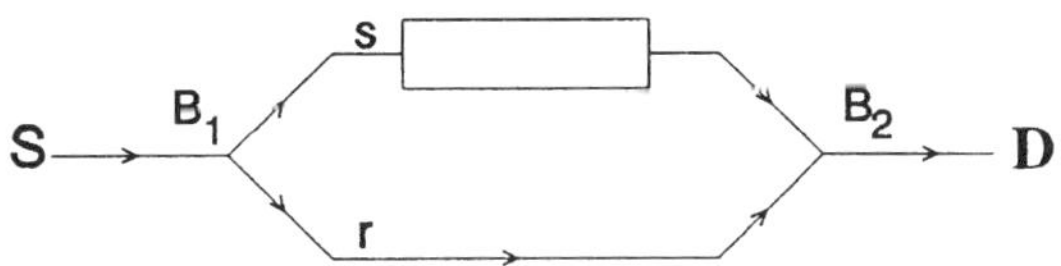

a

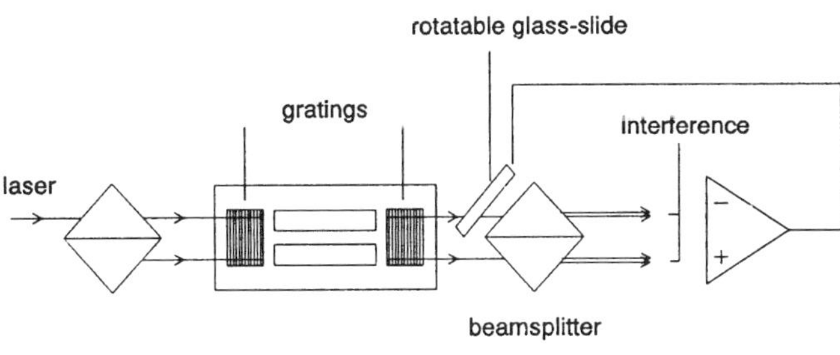

b

FIGURE 8.8 (a) Principle of Mach-Zehnder immunosensor; in the signal-arm **s** the immunoreaction takes place, arm **r** provides a reference; both beams are combined in beamsplitter B2. (b) Practical MZ wave guide immunosensor; only the arms **r** and **s** are contained in a wave guide. The rotatable glass slide serves as phase retarder in a feedback loop (cf. text).

As the phase retardation is given by $\varphi = \beta \cdot L$, we see that a changed difference $(\beta_r - \beta_s)$ results in a changed intensity at the monitored position:

$$I = I_0[1 + \cos\{L\cdot(\beta_r - \beta_s)\}] \tag{8.12b}$$

The transformation of this to a wave guide immunosensor is now conceptually very simple: if in arm s an adsorption process occurs, β_s will change and an intensity change will result. From Equations 12a and b the following key characteristics of this type of immunosensor can be inferred:

- The sensitivity can be increased by choosing a longer interaction length L.
- The intensity change is periodic in $\Delta\beta$; as a consequence it is impossible to determine absolute amounts of adsorbed mass; and one has to follow the complete adsorption process to quantify the adsorbed amount of material. However, dual wavelength detection schemes are available[19] to overcome this.
- The presence of two separate arms provides a very effective means to suppress common mode effects such as variation in composition of bulk solution or variation in temperature. However, this feature can turn into a disadvantage if both arms are not carefully matched to the same interaction length L; in that case the interferometer will exhibit a significant response to, e.g., temperature variations.

Heideman et al.[20-22] experimentally demonstrated the feasibility of such an MZ wave guide interferometer. A hybrid approach was followed, where the light splitting and recombining was done in bulk optics and only the paths s and r were running through a wave guide (see Figure 8.8b). The light in- and outcoupling was realized through gratings on top of the wave guide. In an active feedback setup,[23] where the intensity in a certain fringe is kept constant by adding a controlled additional phase retardation, a phase resolution of $10^{-4}.2\pi$ was obtained when using a He-Ne laser. With an optimized wave guide consisting of a 100-nm layer Si_3N_4 ($n = 2.00$) on top of SiO_2 and having an interaction length of 1 cm, a very high transducer sensitivity could be obtained (see Table 8.1). In this setup the main factor determining the sensitivity was the phase drift of $10^{-2}.2\pi$ per hour.

8.3.3 Wave Guide Polarimeter

As already mentioned, TE and TM modes exhibit different propagation constants for a given adsorbed layer, and a difference in phase retardation $(\varphi_{TE} - \varphi_{TM})$ develops. Thus, linearly polarized light entering a wave guide and exciting both TE and TM light modes, will transform to elliptically polarized light after exiting the wave guide, and it is the measure of ellipticity containing the information on the adsorbed amount of material. This principle is similar to that of the MZ interferometer: also in this concept two differently labeled light beams are mixed and the effect of the coherent addition of the two light beams is monitored. Most of the properties mentioned in Section 8.3.2 hold equally well for a polarimeter concept. However, an important advantage of the polarimeter concept is that the two optically traversed paths are now essentially confined within the same arm, and the design is expected to exhibit better inherent stability than the MZ device.

The concept of a planar wave guide polarimeter chemical sensor[24] has been experimentally demonstrated by Schlatter et al. (see Figure 8.9).[25] With a TiO_2–SiO_2 wave guide (thickness 230 nm, interaction length 12 mm) they obtained a sensitivity slightly worse than that of the MZ immunosensor (see Table 8.1). The limiting factor for this sensitivity proved to be a drift in response originating from wave guide microporosity.

The same concept, but implemented in a single mode fiber, was investigated by Heideman et al.[26,27] A special type of polarization-maintaining fiber was used, where the elliptically

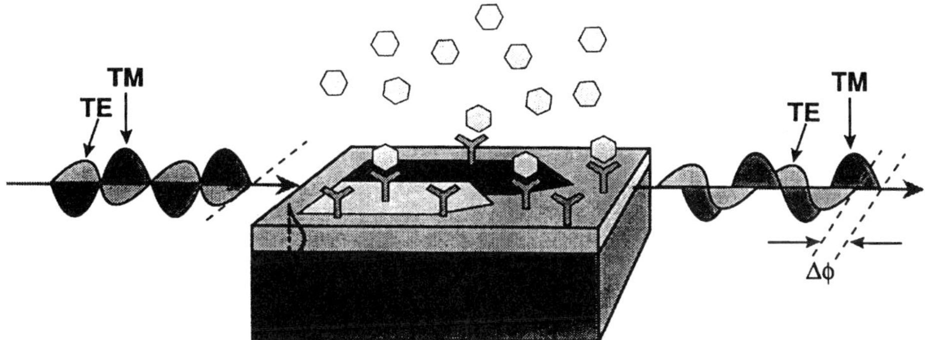

FIGURE 8.9 Principle of polarimeter immunosensor: TE and TM modes respond differently to a change in refractive index profile. (Reproduced from Fattinger, Ch., Koller, H., Schlatter, D., and Wehrli, P. et al., *Biosens. Bioelectron.*, 8, 99, 1993. With permission.)

shaped core is embedded in a D-shaped cladding. This cladding was etched such that the evanescent field around the core extended into the measuring solution. For a decladded fiber length of 5 cm this sensor system could measure an adsorbed protein mass down to approximately 200 pg/mm^2, a factor of 100 worse than proved to be possible with the planar polarimeter system. The main reason for this is that it is not possible in the fiber polarimeter to optimize wave guide thickness and refractive index profile. Thus the intrinsic sensitivity will be worse, resulting in a relatively larger influence of other factors such as temperature: it was found that a temperature instability of 0.1 K already produced a phase change equivalent to the above-mentioned S_{trans}.

8.3.4 Immunosensors Based on Light Deflection

Consider a situation as displayed in Figure 8.10a. A light ray enters a dielectric structure at position P and crosses the interface A/B, after which it leaves the structure at position P′. Given the dimensions of this plate, the angle φ, and the refractive indices of the regions A and B, the position of P′ can be calculated using Snell's law (Equation 8.6). Of course this same description holds equally well if the plate consists of a planar wave guide; the role of k_x will then be taken over by the propagation constant β. Thus, if a mode propagation difference exists between the two waveguiding regions A and B, then the guided mode will deflect at the interface. Kunz[28] has demonstrated this in a sensor where a water-porous wave guide film exhibited a thickness gradient changing as a function of relative humidity. In another approach, Heideman[13] covered the evanescent region above A with a hydrophilic material, and the region B with a hydrophobic material. On the thus coated wave guide chip antibodies were immobilized. An immunoreaction takes place only in region B, in view of the experimental finding[22] that there is an appreciable difference in binding capacity for antibodies immobilized on hydrophilic or hydrophobic surfaces. The envisioned advantage was that prior to the immunoreaction events the A and B coated regions exhibited almost identical β′s, thus providing an almost complete immunity against changes in the bulk solution. Preliminary experiments pointed to a sensitivity comparable to that of the planar polarimeter sensor (Table 8.1). The main problem was the chemical drift of the regions, probably caused by the microporosity of the hydrophilic and hydrophobic substrates.

The attractive aspect of this type of sensors is the very simple design, both in wave guide configuration and in opto-electronic instrumentation. An example of such a design is given in Figure 8.10b: here a divergent light beam enters the wave guide, consisting of region A, where the Si_3N_4 wave guide is covered by a thick SiO_2 layer, and region B that is covered with antibodies. The angle of incidence is chosen such that half of the beam strikes the A/B interface at an angle larger than the critical angle, whereas the other half of the beam transmits

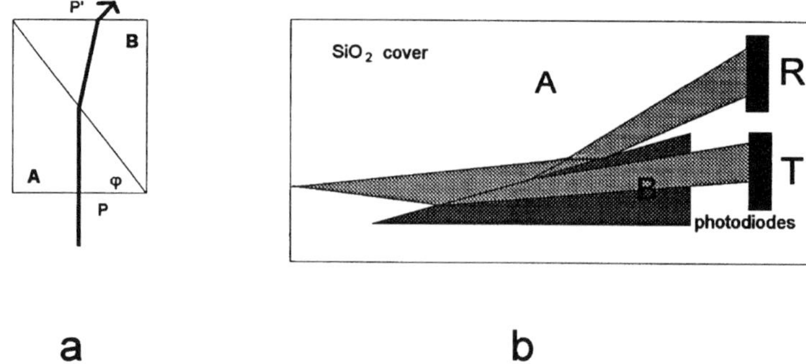

FIGURE 8.10 (a) Light deflection as sensing principle; for definition of symbols see text. (b) Practical example: as a result of surface binding the light reflectance/transmission ratio changes.

through region B. As a result of binding, β in region B changes and as a consequence the critical angle changes. The transmittance/reflectance ratio, measured by the two photodiodes R and T, respectively, will change, and can be used as a monitor for the immunoreaction. All the technology required to turn this concept[29] into a one-chip device is available, and thus a really simple device comes within reach.

8.3.5 Resonant Mirror

An interesting transduction scheme was recently demonstrated (see Figure 8.11);[30] use is made of the fact that in the displayed setup, where the prism-incoupled light immediately couples out, the reflected light undergoes a phase jump of π if the k_x of the incoming light matches the propagation constant of the wave guide structure on top of the prism. The angle ϕ under which this is the case is different for the TE and TM mode. Hence, if the wave guide is interrogated simultaneously with TE and TM light, the outcoming reflected light will generally have the same polarization state; only if the TE or TM mode is excited, the outcoming polarization state will rotate over 90°. By placing an analyzer in the output beam with its direction perpendicular to the original incoming polarization direction, the detector measures only an intensity if either the TE or TM mode is excited. By varying in some way the angle ϕ and imaging the outcoming light on a detector array, a change in β is transduced to a position on the detector array. The sensor assembly consists of a high index support on which a 1-μm SiO_2 layer and a titanium oxide layer (~100 nm) are deposited. The SiO_2 layer serves as an evanescent coupling gap for excitation of the TiO_2 wave guide. From the available data the obtained sensitivity appears slightly better than that of the surface plasmon resonance sensor (see Table 8.1), but it is expected that with an improved layer system this sensitivity will increase. Note that this device does not gain advantage from an increased interaction length, as is the case with the interferometric and polarimetric devices. Except for the sensitivity this device seems to accommodate all aspects that could attract potential users.

8.3.6 TIR Fluorescence Sensors

Common to all previously discussed sensor concepts is that the propagation properties of the guided light change as a consequence of a binding process. In the TIR fluorescence sensors (for an early review see Reference 31) the wave guide, that can consist of a slab[32,33] or a multimode fiber,[34-37] is merely used as a very effective light source for evanescent wave excitation of dye molecules in the immediate vicinity of the wave guide; simultaneously, emitted light from these molecules can be collected very efficiently. In Figure 8.12 an example of such a sensor is given. The guided mode with wavelength λ_1 excites within its evanescent field molecules that have an absorption cross-section for this wavelength. If the molecules

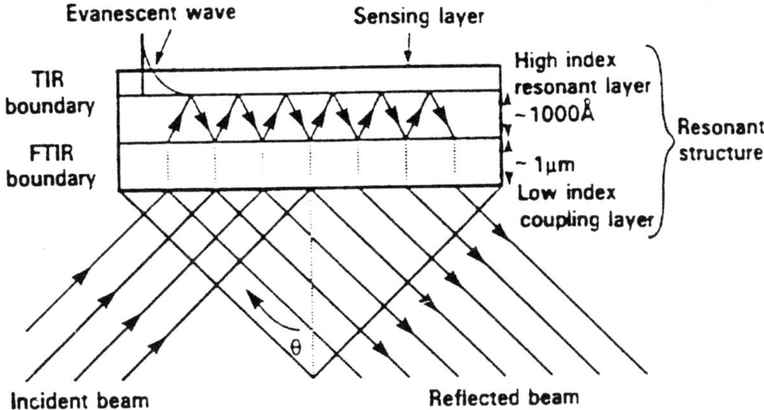

FIGURE 8.11 Resonant mirror: the relative phases of the reflected TE and TM components change if the TE or TM mode is excited; as a consequence the polarization state of the reflected light changes upon light incoupling. (Reproduced from Cush, R., Cronin, J. M., Stewart, W. J., et al., *Biosens. Bioelectron.*, 8, 347, 1993. With permission.)

emit fluorescence at λ_2, part of it will radiate away from the wave guide, but also a part of the total λ_2 radiation has an evanescent wave character. Consequently, by reciprocity, this fluorescence can excite a guided λ_2 mode within the wave guide which is very near to the cut-off value[38] (cf. Section 8.2.2.1). This detection scheme, where both the excitation and the monitored emission are evanescent waves in nature, has been definitely shown to be the most sensitive one in terms of net fluorescence collection efficiency of those molecules that are very near to the surface. The sensitivity that can be obtained for a dye molecule with a relatively high fluorescence quantum efficiency (fluorescein) is in the order of 10^7 molecules,[37] provided great care is taken to maintain the same light propagation characteristics over the complete length of the wave guide. In the design of Figure 8.12, this was realized by mounting a piece of completely decladded fiber within a low refractive index (PTFE: n ~1.35) holder. Immunosensors based on TIR fluorescence, where labeled analyte proteins are measured such as is usual in a competition assay,[3] have a sensitivity significantly better than that of any of the label-free concepts (see Table 8.1).

As already mentioned, this type of sensors has the disadvantage, as opposed to the direct-type sensors, that the detection scheme requires external reagents such as fluorescently labeled molecules. However, their prospects as to potential sensitivity remain very promising: it has been recently demonstrated that the background emission, which is the limiting factor for fluorescence detection, could be reduced to almost zero by further diminishing the measuring volume emission. This approach, accomplished in a near-field microscope setup, resulted in an emission sensitivity of one single dye molecule.[39] Although these experiments are not yet conducted in an aqueous solution, it is expected that within the near future the development of immunosensors will benefit from this innovation.

8.4 PRACTICAL ASPECTS

In this section we give an overview of the current fabrication technologies of the optical wave guide and the immobilization techniques for the receptor layer most often used. Practical details such as the use of different materials and techniques and ease of manufacture will be discussed as well as the performance of the different immobilization procedures of receptor molecules. Other characteristics of the sensor system such as assay time and calibration will be discussed in following subsections.

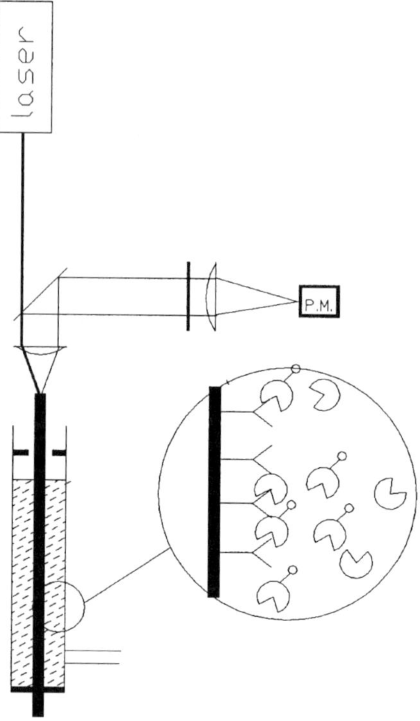

FIGURE 8.12 Layout of fiber fluorescence immunosensor. Excitation source: HeNe laser with λ = 543 nm. The fiber is decladded over the complete length; the optics are designed such that the full numerical aperture of the fiber is exploited. (Reproduced from Eenink, R. G., De Bruijn, H. E., Kooyman, R. P. H., et al., *Anal. Chim. Acta,* 238, 317, 1990. With permission.)

8.4.1 Wave Guide Technology

Although optical wave guides were originally developed for applications in the telecommunication field,[8] it was soon realized that their small size, mechanical stability, flexible geometry, noise immunity, and efficient light-conducting over long distances make them well-suited for implementation in sensor applications.[10]

Contrary to most optical fibers, the structure of a planar wave guide sensor can be tailored to a specific measuring situation by selecting appropriate materials, geometries, and manufacturing techniques. In this way it is possible to control the evanescent wave penetration depth and the refractive index profile, which are both important for the optimum performance of evanescent wave immunosensors. The fact that planar wave guides generally have a larger damping as compared to fibers is irrelevant for their use as chemical sensors. Moreover, planar wave guide structures are in principle well suited for integration of multiple functions (optical and electrical) on one substrate.

In the fabrication of a planar wave guide a thin dielectric film (usually, 0.1 to 10 μm) is deposited on a planar substrate. The methods usually employed for the fabrication of wave guides can be divided in two main types, viz., diffusion (ion-exchange) and deposition techniques (spin-coating, chemical vapor deposition [CVD], dipping, or plasma polymerization). The substrate materials can be glass, Si, III-V semiconductor compounds (GaAs, InP, ...), polymers, and electro-optic materials (ZnO, $LiNbO_3$).

Until now, mainly glass[12,16,25] and silicon[15,21] have been used as substrate materials in the fabrication of evanescent wave immunosensors. Glass has been widely used because it is very inexpensive and allows for application of a simple ion-exchange technique[42] that results in a low-loss optical wave guide. Silicon is an unique material as substrate owing to its abundance, low cost, high purity, chemical stability, and mechanical strength.

The chosen technique and substrate material depend mainly on the available laboratory facilities. If one has decided to use Si as substrate material and microelectronic technologies for the device fabrication, clean-room facilities and specialized personnel are required. For other, simpler technologies (ion-exchange, polymers) no expensive installations are needed.

Both in the grating coupler sensor[14] and in the planar polarimeter[43] the wave guide is made of amorphous SiO_2–TiO_2 produced by dip coating (sol-gel process). By pyrolysis at 550°C the gel-like organometallic coating is transformed into a hard inorganic SiO_2–TiO_2 film. The wave guiding films obtained in this way have a refractive index of $n_l = 1.79$ (determined by the ratio of SiO_2 to TiO_2 in the material) and a thickness between 160 and 190 nm. As substrates Pyrex® glass ($n = 1.47$) or Si wafers with SiO_2 buffer layers are used. For the grating coupler sensor the gratings are fabricated by an embossing technique.

However, an important drawback of the use of this technique is a slow but persistent change of the signal with time when SiO_2–TiO_2 wave guides are immersed in solution. This drift effect limits the performance of the sensor and is associated with the porosity of the wave guide material. The authors have proposed[15] that an additional heat treatment of the wave guide results in denser, less microporous films. With glass substrates, firing temperatures of up to 650°C were used. With Si/SiO_2 substrates temperatures above 850°C were possible, resulting in more compact wave guides with a drift effect greatly diminished ($\Delta\beta/\Delta t = 2.10^{-8}$ nm^{-1} h^{-1}). As the resolution of the sensor is $\Delta\beta_{min} = 2.10^{-8}$ nm^{-1}, the drift is only noticeable in an experiment lasting several hours.

The grating coupler sensor concept is now commercially available (BIOS-1 system, developed by ASI Instruments AG, Switzerland).

In the resonant mirror,[30] glass technology and material deposition techniques such as sputtering and ion-beam-assisted evaporation are employed for its fabrication. The sensor is fabricated by electron beam deposition of a high index material (HfO_2 or TiO_2) onto optically polished SiO_2 wafers. With this technology, the sensor chips can be made in large quantities and with manufacturing tolerances achievable in commercial coating setups at reasonable cost. This sensor concept has been recently introduced in the market (IAsys system, developed by Fisons Applied Sensor Technology, England).

In the silicon-based integrated optoelectronic technology the fabrication of the wave guide is mainly based on microelectronic standard techniques, such as wet and dry etching, photolithography, and chemical vapor deposition (CVD). The CVD techniques allow a high control of the wave guide layer homogeneity, both in thickness and refractive index profile. Several materials can be used as core and cladding, such as silicon nitride, phosphor-doped silicon dioxide, or silicon oxynitride for the core and silicon dioxide for the cladding. Silicon technology also offers the possibility of integrating detectors and electronics devices on the same chip (*hybrid integration*). Another interesting feature is the possibility of batch-wise mass-production at low cost.

The Mach-Zehnder interferometer immunosensor[21] seems to be one of the more promising concepts. An attractive aspect of this sensor is the possibility of using long interaction lengths. This is only possible if a technology is available to make homogeneous wave guiding layers (length in the order of centimeters) without appreciable losses. A practical option is the use of silicon microtechnology. The Mach-Zehnder interferometer is fabricated using standard techniques (Si/SiO_2/Si_3N_4/SiO_2). The high refractive index of the wave guiding layer (Si_3N_4, $n_l = 2.00$) in contrast with the aqueous cladding gives rise to a spatial electric field distribution with a relatively large evanescent wave intensity.

The sequence of steps required for manufacture of a Mach-Zehnder interferometer immunosensor is depicted in Figure 8.13. The SiO_2 buffer layer is grown by thermal oxidation. The Si_3N_4 layer is deposited by low pressure chemical vapor deposition giving a homogeneous layer with low losses (typically, 0.1 dB/cm). A protective layer of SiO_2 on top of the wave guide layer is deposited by plasma enhanced chemical vapor deposition (1.6 μm). The sensor area and reference area are defined by photolithography, followed by etching of the SiO_2 protective layer to have biochemical access to the wave guide surface.

Obviously, the overall procedure is rather laborious but it gives reproducible and stable sensor chips. Currently, this technology seems too expensive to be employed in the manufacturing of commercially attractive systems.

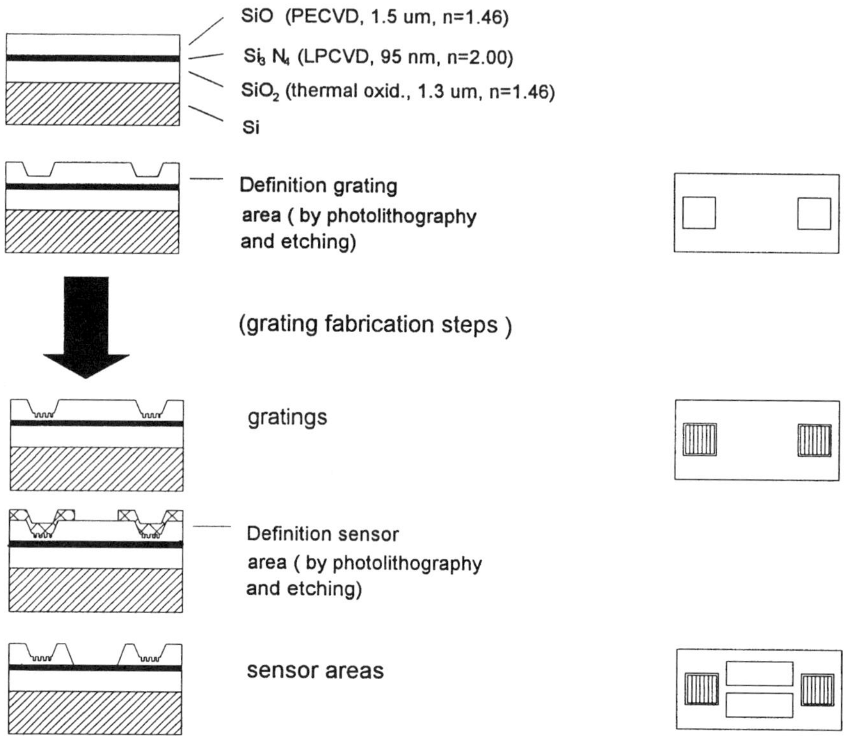

FIGURE 8.13 Fabrication steps for manufacture of MZI immunosensor. Only main steps are shown (right: top view; left: cross section).

8.4.2 Receptor Immobilization

As already mentioned in Section 8.2.1 an adequate preparation of the receptor layer is crucial for optimum performance of the sensor, through the term S_{chem}. In view of the complex structures of Abs[44] the design of a successful immobilization procedure is not straightforward. In the structure of an Ab, two differents parts, denoted as F_{ab} (antigen-binding fragment) and F_c (crystallizable fragment), can be distinguished. The F_{ab} fragments are situated at the end of the two arms of the Ab (represented as "Y"). As these binding sites are a small part of the protein, the rest could be involved in aspecific interactions with the molecules in solution and thus could degrade the specificity of the receptor layer.

Another complication arises from the fact that in many immobilization procedures reactive groups ($-NH_2$, –COOH, –SH, aromatic groups) in the Ab are randomly used for coupling. Generally this results in a receptor layer with random orientation of the Abs, with a partial obstruction of antigen binding sites.

The immobilization procedure should result in a receptor interface which ideally must fulfill the following requirements:

1. The surface density should have an optimal value in order to avoid steric hindrance[45] of analytes.
2. A highly ordered and aligned layer. In this way, the orientation of the protein permits a good accessibility of the F_{ab} fragments to the analyte.
3. A stable layer, i.e., with a long shelf lifetime and with no appreciable desorption.

In order to fulfill these demands several strategies have been used.[46] These include direct protein attachment to the substrate, and methods where the protein is attached to an intermediate layer previously immobilized to the substrate. A short description of the most common methods, visualized in Figure 8.14, is given in the following sections. In Table 8.2, the characteristics of these different immobilization methods are summarized.

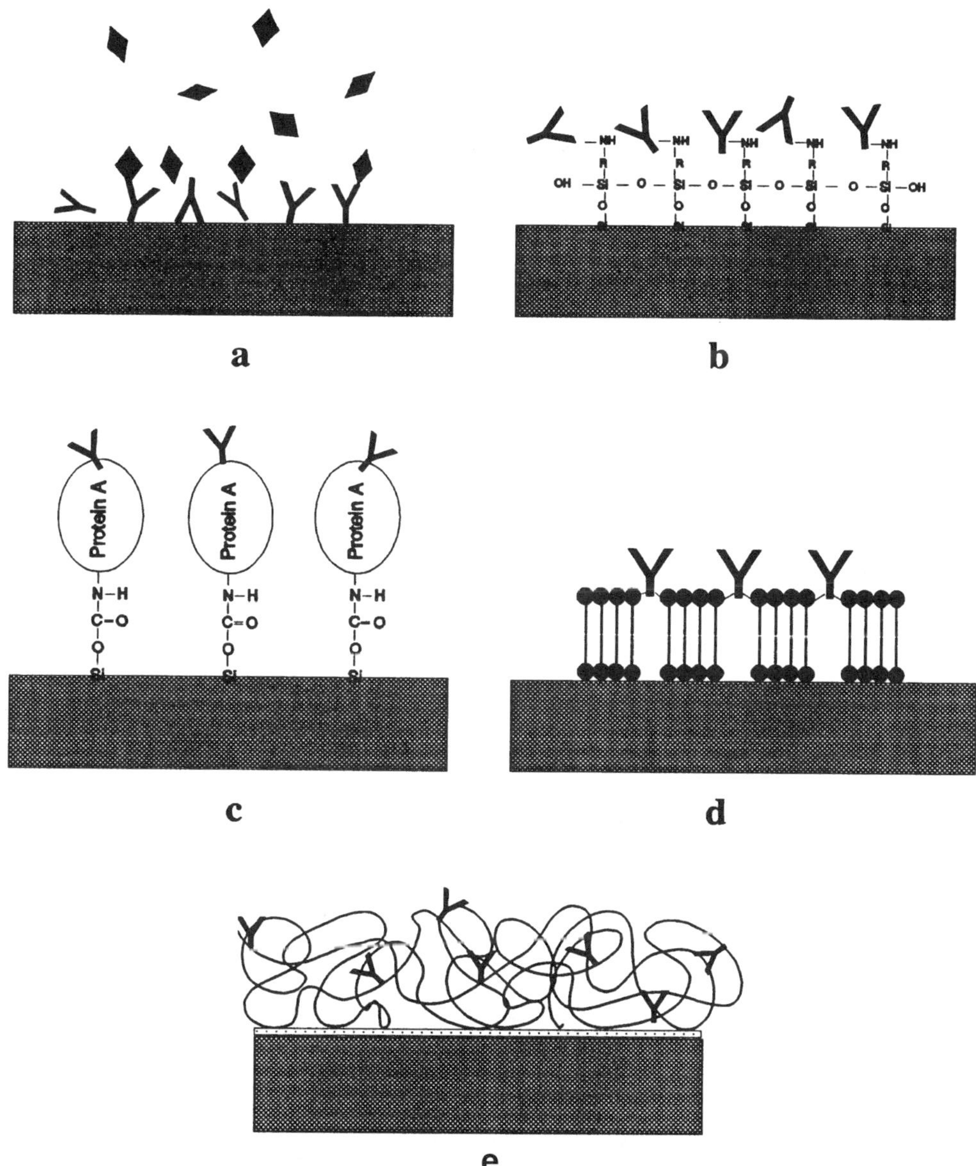

FIGURE 8.14 Different protein immobilization methods: (a) physical adsorption, (b) immobilization via silanization, (c) immobilization via protein A layer, (d) protein-LB film assembly, (e) antibody network.

TABLE 8.2
Characteristics of Different Ab Immobilization Methods

Immobilization method	Active Ab (ng/mm^2)	Ref.	Order	Stability
Physical adsorption				
Hydrophilic	0.41	46	—	±
Hydrophobic	2	46	—	±
BrCN method	1	49	—	+
Silanization				
Aminosilane	1.5	56	—	+
Phenethylsilane	2	56	—	+
Protein A	5	43	+	+
L-B film (silanization)				
1 Monolayer	3	53	+	—
4 Monolayers	30	53	+	—
Antibody network	~40	56	—	+

8.4.2.1 Physical Adsorption

For certain purposes (disposable sensors) it is sufficient to immobilize the protein by direct physical adsorption to the substrate. Binding results from weak electrostatic or van der Waals interaction. Although this simple procedure can give high yields at low costs, the binding strength to the substrate is not very high[47] and desorption can occur after some time. Moreover, protein adsorption generally results in an immobilization with random Ab orientation (see Figure 8.14a).

The nature of the protein immobilization on surfaces is to some extent determined by the surface properties, such as electric charge and hydrophobicity of the substrate employed. It has been demonstrated[22] that hydrophobic substrates result in receptor layers with higher activities than those found in hydrophilic ones.

8.4.2.2 Covalent Binding

Here we give only a very short description; for a much more detailed report we refer to the comprehensive review by Weetall and Lee.[48] A covalent binding is defined as a formation of a chemical bond between the antibody and the solid substrate. We will limit here to substrates that have as their main component SiO_2. Usually, prior to immobilization the substrate surface must be activated. Two different routes can be used: a direct one and the classical method of silanization.

The first includes the use of cyanogen bromide (BrCN) or aldehyde derivatives as active reagents to modify the surface, followed by a covalent attachment of the protein.[48] This procedure results in a surface density of immobilized IgG of 1 ng/mm^2 without any loss of antigen binding capacity after immobilization.[49] However, the method has the important disadvantage that the agent employed (BrCN) is highly toxic.

In the silanization procedure,[48] the surface is treated with an organosilane containing an organic functional group at one end and an alkoxysilyl group at the other end of the molecule. Coupling of the silane to the surface is via the alkoxysilyl group of the coupling agent and the metal oxide or silanol group on the support. Typical organosilanes commercially available include epoxy-, vinyl-, aminoalkyl-, sulfhydryl-, haloalkyl-, and aminoarylsilanes. After this first step, a bifunctional "linker" agent (glutaraldehyde, disuccinimidyl suberate,...) is attached, followed by coupling of the protein via its functional groups ($-NH_2$, $-SH$,...) to the group of the bifunctional agent that is not attached to the surface (cf. Figure 8.14b). Alternatively, the linker can be attached first to the protein.

Both methods result in a random immobilization of Abs. Introduction of a covalently coupled intermediate layer of protein A, which is known[47] to exhibit a high affinity to the F_c moiety of the Ab, results in an ordered receptor layer as depicted in Figure 8.14c. A surface density of immobilized IgG of 5 ng/mm^2 is obtained in this way.[43]

8.4.2.3 Langmuir-Blodgett Techniques

Owing to their uniform thickness, molecular orientation, and electrical and dielectrical properties, the implementation of Langmuir-Blodgett (LB) films has also been studied for the immobilization of proteins.[50,51] The LB film acts as an inert matrix in which the antibody can be incorporated. LB technology would make it possible to prepare, characterize, and modify well-ordered monolayers and multilayers of proteins with known thicknesses and chemical compositions and with a control of the binding site density.

However, the deposition of protein LB films suffers from numerous technical difficulties such as poor adhesion, fragility, impurities, and defects. The immobilized proteins tend to leave the surface, leading to weak stability and irreproducible binding sites density. Attempts to covalently couple the layer have been made,[52] and relatively high surface densities of active Abs have been reported,[53] but also in these cases the layer lacks sufficient stability. Until now, only laboratory developments have been described and no real use of a protein LB film in any device is known.[54]

8.4.2.4 Antibody Networks

A different approach (Figure 8.14e) is used in the BiaCore[55] sensor system and in the resonant mirror.[56] No attempt is made to bind a monolayer of receptors to the substrate; rather, a receptor *volume* is created. The receptor volume is formed by a hydrogel matrix that allows fast and simple *in situ* covalent binding of proteins in a reproducible way. With such a matrix (1) the complete evanescent volume is used, and (2) it is possible to immobilize more protein than on the surface directly. The sensitivity of the sensor is expected to increase as the effective surface density of active immobilized Abs is increased.

The matrix is formed by a flexible carboxy-methyl-modified dextran hydrogel covalently bound to the sensor surface. Subsequently, the antibodies are covalently attached to the gel via their nucleophilic groups, after an activation step of the gel with *N*-hydroxysuccinimide (NHS) and *N*-ethyl-*N*-(dimethylaminopropyl)carbodiimide (EDC). The thickness of the hydrogel layer is limited to 100 to 200 nm in order to avoid diffusional and binding problems with thicker layers. The dextran provides a hydrophilic and flexible matrix suitable for efficient immobilization, even at low concentrations. Activation-coupling-deactivation protocols have been developed[55] to perform repeated analysis. Model calculations[55] point to a maximum Ab surface concentration of approximately 40 ng/mm^2. It has been stated[56] that this type of immobilization method is superior to all other methods mentioned above (cf. Table 8.2).

This method can be used with a wide range of chemistries for immobilization of molecules where amino groups are lacking or are essential for biological functioning.

8.4.3 Assay Time

It has already been mentioned that the immunoreaction intrinsically is very fast; in most cases any rate-limiting circumstance will be due to the finite diffusion constant of the molecules involved. This can be appreciated from inspection of the following relation:[57]

$$\Delta = (D \cdot 2t)^{1/2} \tag{8.13a}$$

and the Einstein relation:[57]

$$D = \frac{R \cdot T}{N \cdot 6\pi\eta \cdot r} \quad (8.13b)$$

Here, R is the gas constant, T the absolute temperature, N is Avogadro's number, η is the solution's viscosity, and r is the (gyration) radius of the molecule under consideration. From Equation 8.13a it can be calculated what root-mean-square distance Δ a molecule with diffusion coefficient D will travel in a given time t, whereas Equation 8.13b serves to estimate the diffusion constant for a globular molecule with given radius r. Thus a 3-nm-radius protein (molecular mass approximately 50 kDa), in a water solution at room temperature, travels in 1 min only 100 μm. This time is even slower for larger proteins as can be seen from Equation 8.13b. As a consequence, in an initially homogeneous solution where a receptor interface capable of binding analytes is present, a depletion region near the interface will develop in the binding process, making the binding rate diffusion limited. A rather long incubation time to reach chemical equilibrium will be the result. To overcome this limitation one has to design the sample cell such that all analytes present in the measuring volume can reach the sensor interface within a reasonable span of time. This can be accomplished by employing a flow system in a sample cell, with its walls very close to the sensor surface. Eddowes[58] has made a detailed analysis of the overall kinetics of the antibody-antigen binding process in such a sensor assembly. It is found that a sample cell geometry where the maximum diffusion travel distance is approximately 100 μm is adequate for most purposes. This can be realized with a dedicated flow system. Additionally, in the same report a method is outlined where the analyte concentration is determined by measuring the rate of analyte binding to the sensor surface, rather than determining the equilibrium sensor response. Although this strategy might decrease the total assay time substantially, it should be noted that now heavier demands are placed upon the overall sensitivity of the sensor; moreover, a correct interpretation of the sensor response relies more on a detailed knowledge of the dynamic binding behavior in the cell assembly, which appears to be missing in a number of situations.[59]

8.4.4 Calibration

Surprisingly, in recent literature on optical immunosensors the problem of calibration is hardly addressed; to our knowledge only one report[60] deals explicitly with this question. Wave guide structures can be manufactured with sufficient reproducibility to characterize them beforehand with a certain sensitivity S_{trans}. For a prepared receptor layer it is much more difficult to mention an S_{chem} without actually measuring it, all the more when one takes into account the different conditions (measuring solution, presence of cross-reacting molecules, elapsed shelf time) under which such a receptor layer can be used. The fact that the immunoreaction is practically irreversible is also in this respect a complicating factor because this rules out a calibration with a standard analyte concentration; it is known that regeneration[61] of the sensor surface after use generally results in a decreased receptor binding capacity.

It seems that with the present state of the art of receptor layer preparation a direct dose-response measurement without a reference measurement is out of reach. Fortunately, most of the planar wave guide sensor concepts described in Section 8.3 can be relatively easily adapted such that one chip accommodates several independent channels. These channels can be covered by the same receptor layer, and one channel can then be employed to determine the actual S_{chem}, preferably by measuring a complete binding curve of the type depicted in Figure 8.2. A more sophisticated possibility, where no standard solutions are required, will be mentioned in Section 8.6.

8.5 APPLICATIONS

Until now, most experimental results obtained with evanescent wave immunosensors were aimed at demonstrating the sensitivity and/or ease of operation of the various devices. However, there are a few examples that are now beginning to enter the user's realm, although it should be added that to our knowledge none of the devices is currently utilized in routine large-throughput assays, as is customary in, e.g., ELISA kits.

It is fair to mention that the BIAcore SPR system, developed by Pharmacia Biosensor AB, in a number of respects is paving the way for acceptance of evanescent wave immunosensor technology, and the majority of reported applications were carried out with this system. As SPR immunosensors are the subject of two other chapters (Chapters 7 and 16) in this book we will not further discuss this, apart from mentioning that all reported SPR applications are equally possible with most of the devices described in this chapter.

A number of reports are devoted to the determination of affinity constants[21,25] of antibodies or the investigation of surface binding characteristics of proteins.[22] Generally, these studies are directly related to improvement of sensor performance, or they have a fundamental scientific purpose.

Other examples can be found in the biomedical field: both with the grating coupler[62] and with the planar polarimeter[25] an immunoassay was set up for detection of the (large) HbsAg antigen which is a marker for a hepatitis B infection. These measurements were done in human serum. The planar polarimeter device demonstrated a surface sensitivity (in serum) of 11 pg/mm^2, corresponding to 2.10^{-13} M of antigen, close to the clinically relevant concentration. In another biomedical assay, based upon TIR fluorescence[33] and aimed at detection of prostate specific antigen, a sensitivity of $\sim 3.10^{-12}$ M of antigen could be obtained[63] for whole blood samples — again, almost adequate for clinical use.

An example from another field is the detection of pesticides in an immunoassay utilizing the grating coupler device.[64] In view of the fact that pesticides are small molecules (M ~0.3 kDa) and thus are difficult to detect with sufficient sensitivity in a direct evanescent wave immunosensor, an assay was set up where immobilized derivatives of the pesticide atrazine and solution pesticide analytes competed for binding to antibodies added to the solution. A concentration of 10 nM of pesticide could be detected, which is nearly two orders of magnitude worse than is relevant for purposes of environmental monitoring.

Although these assays usually have not yet been optimized, the results illustrate the general concern that evanescent wave immunosensors still lack sufficient sensitivity; in the last discussed example even the direct sensing strategy, one of the more attractive features of this type of sensor, had to be abolished. There are some reports that describe an improvement of the sensitivity of approximately one order of magnitude by utilizing the complete evanescent volume.[55,56] In another recent study[45] it was demonstrated that a net ordering of immobilized receptors with controlled surface density could substantially improve the sensitivity. A different approach was followed by Buckle et al.,[56] who sacrificed the direct sensing strategy by using mass labels consisting of 30-nm colloidal gold particles. In a demonstration immunoassay gold-labeled albumin protein could be detected at a thousandfold better sensitivity compared to the unlabeled albumin.

8.6 PROSPECTS

We have seen that as a result of ten years of development of optical immunoassays a range of completely new devices has become available that in a number of aspects overcome the shortcomings of the more conventional ones. Not surprisingly, until now the main effort has been put into obtaining sufficient sensitivity, at least rivaling those belonging to previous generations. Obtaining a sensitivity similar to that of well-designed ELISA assays with their enzyme-amplification detection schemes appears to be only a matter of time.

Apart from the ongoing quest for sensitivity, obtained by increasing transducer sensitivity and receptor layer binding capacity, there are a number of additional lines of research that could result in really new immunosensor applications. Some of these will now be discussed.

8.6.1 Integrated Sensor Systems; Other Materials

All sensor systems discussed in this chapter are assembled from discrete components, where only the manufacturing of the planar wave guide benefits from clean-room techniques. However, these devices could gain much in stability and compactness, as well as in ease of operation, if the light source and the photodetectors could also be integrated on the same chip; moreover, the problem of efficient, stable, and easy light-coupling to the wave guide would be definitively solved. This technology is now becoming available.[65] Together with the micromachined microflow systems that were recently demonstrated[66] and whose manufacturing procedure can be made fully compatible with the silicon technology required for fabricating wave guide sensors, this could result in single-sensor blocks. Particularly, the sensor concepts realized in planar wave guide technology seem good candidates for such merging of technologies.

Apart from the well-developed silicon technology, there are two other technologies that might become important in the design of evanescent wave immunosensors:

1. Wave guide structures manufactured from III-V semiconductor compounds are potentially attractive because these materials are suitable for integration of wave guide structures, light sources, photodetectors, and high-speed electronics circuitry on one and the same chip (*monolithic integration*). This technology, applied to the development of optical sensors, is at an early stage of development.[67]
2. The use of electro-optic materials such as lithium niobate, zinc oxide, and certain polymers, could be of interest because their optical properties can be modulated by a low-frequency electric field. Apart from the outlook on novel sensor principles that these materials provide, their use is almost mandatory in fully integrated versions of interferometer sensors, where some way of controlling the optical pathlength within the wave guide is required. The use of electro-optic polymers has the additional advantage that they can to a large extent be tailored such that receptors can be optimally covalently immobilized; furthermore, polymers can be very easily deposited on a variety of substrates by using spin-coating or plasma deposition techniques. Research on the use of polymers as waveguiding material is a very active field.[68]

8.6.2 Reversible Immunosensors

It has previously been mentioned that owing to the very low dissociation rate constant of an antigen-antibody reaction it is generally not possible to monitor decreasing concentrations of the analyte. It has been demonstrated that binding can be broken by applying chaotropic solvents or pH steps,[61] or by a light-induced conformational change of a specialized polymer in the immediate vicinity of the antibody.[69] Although such procedures are certainly valuable to regenerate sensors after use, a more direct way towards a reversible immunosensor could be to increase the dissociation rate of the immunoreaction. One approach could be to use relatively small synthetically prepared polypeptides as receptors that have only a few binding sites with the analyte of interest.[70] The probability that in a receptor-target chemical equilibrium these few binding sites are simultaneously in a dissociated state will be significantly larger than is the case for an intact, complete antibody with its many binding sites. Preliminary experiments pointing to the feasibility of such a strategy have recently been published[71] for a system consisting of 13 residues containing polypeptide specific to lysozyme. In this context also the availability of random polypeptide banks[72] becomes increasingly important, because this allows for a selection procedure of peptides without relying on the availability of antibodies or, even more difficult, a detailed knowledge of the primary structure of the antibody binding site.

8.6.3 Multisensor Arrays

Some of the planar wave guide sensor geometries discussed in Section 8.3 are ideally suited to be implemented in a system where, on one single sensor chip, many different chemical reactions simultaneously can be monitored. The techniques for local immobilization of receptor molecules on such a surface have been developed.[73] Such arrays could be used in a number of ways, such as the option to perform multiple analyte measurements or the availability of internal calibration standards. Still more promising is the prospect of using the array in a pattern recognition scheme, where each immobilized receptor patch has its own range of affinities and specificities towards a predefined series of analytes. (Compare Chapters 23 to 27.) Calibration of these devices could be accomplished by neural network analysis. In such an approach the demands on specific binding capacity of the receptor molecules could be relaxed somewhat, which might be important in the development of reversible sensors along the above-mentioned lines.

A.1 LIST OF SYMBOLS

K_a : affinity constant
Γ : fraction of bound receptor molecules
κ^{-1} : penetration depth
β : wave guide propagation constant
TM : p-polarized mode
TE : s-polarized mode
t : waveguide thickness
t_r : immobilized receptor film thickness
n_b : refractive index of bulk solution
n_p : refractive index of analyte protein
n_l : refractive index of wave guiding film
n_r : refractive index of receptor layer
n_s : refractive index of wave guide substrate
S_{trans} : sensitivity factor, for example, change in propagation constant per bound analyte surface density
D_{trans} : detectivity (lowest detectable bound analyte surface density)

A.2 SOME TYPICAL VALUES

K_a : 10^7 to 10^{15} M^{-1}
Γ : 0 to 0.9
κ^{-1} : 50 to 500 nm for visible light
λ : 633 nm wavelength for He-Ne laser
l : 12 nm, example for interaction length
t : 100 nm to 10 μm
t_r : 4 to 500 nm
r_p : 3 nm: protein radius for 50 kDa
n_b : 1.33 for water
n_p : 1.45 for analyte protein
n_l : 1.79 for SiO_2–TiO_2, 2.00 for Si_3N_4

n_r : 1.45
n_s : 1.47 for Pyrex glass, 1.35 for PTFE
D_{trans} : 0.6 pg/mm^2 label-free (calc. for a current device)
D_{trans} : 0.01 pg/mm^2 with label (calc. for a current device)

REFERENCES

1. Tan, W., Shi, Z. Y., Smith, D., and Kopelman, R., Submicrometer intracellular chemical optical fiber sensors, *Science,* 258, 778, 1992.
2. Köhler, G. and Milstein, C., Continuous cultures of fused cells secreting antibody of predefined specificity, *Nature,* 256, 495, 1975.
3. Langone, J. J. and Van Vunakis, H., Eds., *Methods in Enzymology,* Vol. 73, Immunochemical Techniques Part D, Academic Press, New York, 1982.
4. Andrade, J. D., *Surface and Interfacial Aspects of Biomedical Polymers,* Vol. 2, Plenum Press, New York, 1987.
5. Absolom, D. R. and Van Oss, C. J., The nature of the antigen-antibody bond and the factors affecting its association and dissociation, *CRC Crit. Rev. Immunol.,* 6, 1, 1986.
6. Snijder, A. W. and Love, J. D., *Optical Waveguide Theory,* Chapman and Hall, New York, 1983.
7. Tien, P. K., Light waves in thin films and integrated optics, *Appl. Opt.,* 10, 2395, 1971.
8. Hunsperger, R. G., Integrated optics: theory and technology, *Springer Series in Optical Sciences,* Vol. 33, Springer-Verlag, Berlin, 1985.
9. Tamir, T., Ed., *Topics in Applied Physics,* Vol. 7: Integrated Optics, Springer-Verlag, Berlin, 1985.
10. Parriaux, O., Guided wave electromagnetism and opto-chemical sensors, in *Fiber Optic Chemical Sensors and Biosensors*, Wolfbeis, O. S., Ed., CRC Press, Boca Raton, FL, 1991.
11. Villarruel, C. A., Dominguez, D. D., and Dandridge, A., Evanescent wave fiber optic chemical sensor, *SPIE Proc.* 798, 225, 1987.
12. Lukosz, W., Principles and sensitivities of integrated optrical and SPR sensors for direct affinity sensing and immunosensing, *Biosens. Bioelectron.,* 6, 215, 1991.
13. Heideman, R. G., Optical Waveguide-Based Evanescent Field Immunosensors, Thesis, University of Twente, Enschede, 1993.
14. Tiefenthaler, K. and Lukosz, W., Sensitivity of grating couplers as integrated-optical chemical sensors, *J. Opt. Soc. Am. B.,* 6, 209, 1989.
15. Nellen, Ph. M. and Lukosz, W., Integrated optical input grating couplers as direct affinity sensors, *Biosens. Bioelectron.,* 8, 129, 1993.
16. Lukosz, W., Nellen, Ph. M., Stamm, Ch., and Weiss, P., Output grating couplers on planar waveguides as integrated optical chemical sensors, *Sensors Actuators,* B1, 585, 1990.
17. Clerc, D. and Lukosz, W., Integrated optical output grating coupler as refractometer and (bio-)-chemical sensor, *Sensors Actuators*, B11, 461, 1993.
18. Hecht, E. and Zajac, A., *Optics,* Addison-Wesley, London, 1974.
19. Williams, C. C. and Wickramasinghe, H. K., Optical ranging by wavelength multiplexed interferometry, *J. Appl. Phys.,* 60, 1900, 1986.
20. Heideman, R. G., Kooyman, R. P. H., Altenburg, B. S. F., and Greve, J., Simple interferometer for evanescent field refractive index sensing as a feasibility study for an immunosensor, *Appl. Opt.,* 30, 1474, 1991.
21. Heideman, R. G., Kooyman, R. P. H., and Greve, J., Performance of a highly sensitive optical wave guide Mach-Zehnder interferometer immunosensor, *Sensors Actuators,* B10, 209, 1992.
22. Heideman, R. G., Kooyman, R. P. H., and Greve, J., Immunoreactivity of adsorbed anti-human chorionic gonadotropin studied with an optical wave guide interferometric sensor, *Biosens. Bioelectron.,* 9, 33, 1994.
23. Vilkomerson, D., Measuring pulsed picometer displacement vibrations by optical interferometry, *Appl. Phys. Lett.,* 29, 183, 1976.
24. Lukosz, W. and Stamm, Ch., Integrated optical interferometer as relative humidity sensor and differential refractometer, *Sensors Actuators,* A25-27, 185, 1991.

25. Schlatter, D., Barner, R., Fattinger, Ch., Huber, W., Hübscher, J., Hurst, J., Koller, J., Mangold, C., and Müller, F., The difference interferometer: application as a direct affinity sensor, *Biosens. Bioelectron.,* 8, 109, 1993.
26. Heideman, R. G., Blikman, A., Kooyman, R. P. H., and Greve, J., Polarimetric optical fiber sensor for biochemical measurements, *SPIE Proc.,* 1510, 131, 1991.
27. Heideman, R. G., Kooyman, R. P. H., and Greve, J., Performance of an optical fiber polarimeter for biochemical measurements, *Sensors Actuators,* B12, 205, 1993.
28. Kunz, R. E., Gradient effective index waveguide sensors, *Sensors Actuators,* B11, 167, 1993.
29. Schipper, E. F., Kooyman, R. P. H., Borreman, A., Heideman, R. G., and Greve, J., Feasibility of highly sensitive optical wave guide immunosensors for pesticide detection: physical aspects, Proc. 5th Int. Meet. Chemical Sensors, Rome, 1994.
30. Cush, R., Cronin, J. M., Stewart, W. J., Maule, C. H., Molloy, J., and Goddard, N. J., The resonant mirror: a novel optical biosensor for direct sensing of biomolecular interactions. I. Principle of operation and associated instrumentation, *Biosens. Bioelectron.,* 8, 347, 1993.
31. Place, J. F., Sutherland, R. M., and Dähne, C., Opto-electronic immunosensors: a review of optical immunoassay at continuous surfaces, *Biosensors,* 1, 321, 1985.
32. Sutherland, R. M., Dähne, C., Place, J. F., and Ringrose, A. S., Optical detection of antibody-antigen reactions at a glass-liquid interface, *Clin. Chem.,* 30, 1533, 1984.
33. Smith, A. M., Optical waveguide immunosensors, *SPIE Proc.* 798, 206, 1987.
34. Glass, T. R., Lackie, S., and Hirschfeld, T., Effect of numerical aperture on signal level in cylindrical wave guide evanescent fluorosensors, *Appl. Opt.,* 26, 2181, 1987.
35. Newby, K., Reichert, W. M., Andrade, J. D., and Benner, R. E., Remote spectroscopic sensing of chemical adsorption using a single multimode optical fiber, *Appl. Opt.*, 23, 1812, 1984.
36. Kooyman, R. P. H., De Bruijn, H. E., and Greve, J., A fiber-optic fluorescence immunosensor, *SPIE Proc.,* 798, 290, 1987.
37. Eenink, R. G., De Bruijn, H. E., Kooyman, R. P. H., and Greve, J., Fibre-fluorescence immunosensor based on evanescent wave detection, *Anal. Chim. Acta*, 238, 317, 1990.
38. Lee, E. H., Benner, R. E., and Chang, R. K., Angular distibution of fluorescence from liquids and monodispersed spheres by evanescent wave excitation, *Appl. Opt.*, 18, 862, 1979.
39. Betzig, E. and Chicester, R. J., Single molecules observed by near-field scanning optical microscopy, *Science,* 262, 1422, 1993.
40. Liedberg, B., Lundström, I., and Stenberg, E., Principles of biosensing with an extended coupling matrix and surface plasmon resonance, *Sensors Actuators,* B11, 63, 1993.
41. Kooyman, R. P. H., Lenferink, A. T. M., Eenink, R. G., and Greve, J., Vibrating mirror surface plasmon resonance immunosensor, *Anal. Chem.,* 63, 83, 1991.
42. Giallorenzi, T. G., West, E. J., Ginther, R., and Andrews, R. A., Optical waveguides formed by thermal migration of ions in glass, *Appl. Opt.*, 12, 1240, 1973.
43. Fattinger, Ch., Koller, H., Schlatter, D., and Wehrli, P., The difference interferometer: a highly sensitive optical probe for quantification of molecular surface concentration, *Biosens. Bioelectron.,* 8, 99, 1993.
44. Alzari, P. M., Lascombe, M. B., and Polja, K. R. J., Three-dimensional structure of antibodies, *Annu. Rev. Immunol.,* 6, 555, 1988.
45. van den Heuvel, D. J., Kooyman, R. P. H., Drijfhout, J. W., and Welling, G. W., Synthetic peptides as receptors in affinity sensors: a feasibility study, *Anal. Biochem.*, 215, 223, 1993.
46. Ahluwalia, A., De Rossi, D., Ristori, C., Schirone, A., and Serra, G., A comparative study of protein immobilization techniques for optical immunosensors, *Biosens. Bioelectron.*, 7, 207, 1992.
47. Koller, E. and Wolfbeis, O. S., Sensor chemistry in *Fiber Optic Chemical Sensors and Biosensors,* Wolfbeis, O. S., Ed., CRC Press, Boca Raton, FL, 1991.
48. Weetall, H. H. and Lee, M. J., Antibodies immobilized on inorganic supports, *Appl. Biochem. Biotechnol.,* 22, 311, 1989.
49. Krapivinskaya, L. D., Krapivinsky, G. B., and Ratner, V. L., Immobilization of immunoglobulins on a quartz surface by BrCN without loss of antigen binding capability, *Biosens. Bioelectron.,* 7, 509, 1992.
50. Reichert, W. M., Bruclener, C. J., and Joseph, J., Langmuir-Blodgett films and black lipid membranes in biospecific surface-selective sensors, *Thin Solid Films,* 152, 345, 1988.

51. Lvov, Yu. M., Erokhin, V. V., and Zaitsev, S. Yu., Protein Langmuir-Blodgett films, *Biolog. Membr.*, 7, 917, 1990.
52. Kallury, K. M. R., Ghaemmaghami, V., Krull, U. J., and Thompson, M., Immobilization of phospholipids on silicon, platinum, indium/tin oxide and gold surfaces with characterization by X-ray photoelectron spectroscopy and time-of-flight secondary-ion mass spectrometry, *Anal. Chim. Acta*, 25, 369, 1989.
53. Dubrovsky, T. B., Demcheva, M. V., Savitsky, A. P., Mantrova, E. Yu., Yaropolov, A. I., Savransky, V. V., and Belovolova, L. V., Fluorescent and phosphorescent study of Langmuir-Blodgett antibody films for application to immunosensors, *Biosens. Bioelectron.*, 8, 377, 1993.
54. Turko, I. V., Lepesheva, G. I., and Chashchin, V. L., Stability and stabilization of IgG Langmuir-Blodgett films, *Thin Solid Films*, 230, 70, 1993.
55. Löfås, S., Malmqvist, M., Rönnberg, I., Stenberg, E., Liedberg, B., and Lundström, I., Bioanalysis with surface plasmon resonance, *Sensors Actuators*, B5, 79, 1991.
56. Buckle, P. E., Davies, R. J., Kinning, T., Yeung, D., Edwuards, P. R., and Pollard-Knight, D., The resonant mirror: a novel optical sensor for direct sensing of biomolecular interactions. II. Applications, *Biosens. Bioelectron.*, 8, 355, 1993.
57. Moore, W. J., *Physical Chemistry*, 5th ed., Longman, London, 1972.
58. Eddowes, M. J., Direct immunochemical sensing: basic chemical principles and fundamental limitations, *Biosensors*, 3, 1, 1987/88.
59. Sadana, A. and Sii, D., Binding kinetics of antigen by immobilized antibody: influence of reaction order and external diffusional limitations, *Biosens. Bioelectron.*,7, 559, 1992.
60. Robinson, G. A., Attridge, J. W., Deacon, J. K., Thomson, A. M., Love, C. A., Whiteley, S., Pugh, M., and Daniels, P. B., The calibration of an optical immunosensor—the FCFD, *Biosens. Bioelectron.*, 8, 371, 1993.
61. Vo-Dinh, T., Griffin, G. D., Ambrose, K. R., Sepaniak, M. J., and Tromberg, B. J., in *Polyaromatic Hydrocarbons: A Decade of Progress*, Cooke, M. and Dennis, A. J., Eds., Battelle Press, Columbus, 1988.
62. Tiefenthaler, K., in *Advances in Biosensors*, Turner, A. P. F., Ed., JAI Press, London, 1992, 261.
63. Bacarese-Hamilton, T., Daniels, P., Fletcher, J., O'Neill, P., and Stafford, C., Determination of PSA in whole blood using a rapid, biosensor-based assay, *Clinical Chemistry*, 40, 992, 1994.
64. Bier, F. F. and Schmid, R. D., Grating coupler immunosensors for pesticide detection, Proc. 2nd. World Congr. Biosensors, Geneva, 395, 1992.
65. Soref, R. A. and Lorenzo, J. P., All silicon active and passive guided wave components for $\lambda = 1.3$ and 1.6 μm, *IEEE J. Quantum Electron.*, 22, 873, 1986.
66. Lammerink, T. S. J., Elwenspoek, M., and Fluitman, J. H. J., Integrated micro-liquid dosing system, Proc. IEEE MEMS, Fort Lauderdale, 1993.
67. Zappe, H. P., Arnot, H. E. G., and Kunz, R., Technology and devices for hybrid and monolithic integrated optical sensors, Proc. Eurosensors VII, October 1993, Budapest (Hungary).
68. Stegeman, G. I., Seaton, C. T., and Zanoni, R., Organic films in non-linear integrated optics structures, *Thin Solid Films*, 152, 231, 1987.
69. Andrade, J. D., Liu, J. N., Herron, J., Reichert, M., and Kopeck, K., Fiber optic immunosensors: sensors or dosimeters, fiber optic and laser sensors, *SPIE Proc.*, 718, 280, 1986.
70. Welling, G. W., Van Gorkum, J., Damhof, R. A., Drijfhout, J. W., Bloemhoff, W., and Welling-Wester, S., A ten-residue fragment of an antibody directed against lysozyme as ligand in immunoaffinity chromatography, *J. Chromatogr.*, 548, 235, 1991.
71. Kooyman, R. P. H., Van den Heuvel, D. J., Drijfhout, J. W., and Welling, G. W., The use of self-assembled receptor layers in immunosensors, *Thin Solid Films*, 244, 913, 1994.
72. Devlin, J. J., Panganiban, L. C., and Devlin, P. E., Random peptide libraries: a source of specific protein binding molecules, *Science*, 249, 404, 1990.
73. Fodor, S. P. A., Leighton Read, J., Pirrung, M. C., Stryer, L., Tsai Lu, A., and Solas, D., Light-directed, spatially addressable parallel chemical synthesis, *Science*, 251, 767, 1991.

9 Acoustic Devices

Arnaldo D'Amico, Corrado Di Natale, and Enrico Verona

CONTENTS

9.1 INTRODUCTION

Electroacoustic devices can be successfully exploited to implement chemical sensors. In this context both bulk acoustic wave (BAW) and surface acoustic wave (SAW) propagation are suitable for sensor applications. The operation of acoustic-type chemical sensors is based on the changes produced by the measurand on the physical properties of suitable membranes made of chemically interactive materials (CIM). The material physical properties whose changes can be detected using acoustic probe techniques include mass density as well as both linear and non-linear elastic and viscoelastic properties. Because of the presence in the sensor of piezoelectric materials used for acoustic transduction, electric and dielectric properties of the membrane can also enter into the device response.

0-8493-8905-4/97/$0.00+$.50
© 1997 by CRC Press, Inc.

9.1.1 BAW Sensors

The schematic diagram of a BAW chemical sensor is shown in Figure 9.1. It consists of a BAW piezoelectric resonator with one or both surfaces covered by the membrane. The BAW structure is connected to a suitable amplifier to form an oscillator whose resonant frequency is related to both the physical and geometrical characteristics of the device. Any change in the physical properties of the membrane due to adsorption or absorption of chemical species from either the gas or liquid phase affects the resonant frequency of the structure. These can be detected with a high accuracy by checking the frequency shift of the oscillator. The resonator is usually made of quartz, and both longitudinal and shear modes can be used. As to the quartz, crystallographic cuts showing a highly stable temperature operation are carefully chosen in order to improve the possibility of obtaining satisfactory resolution values.

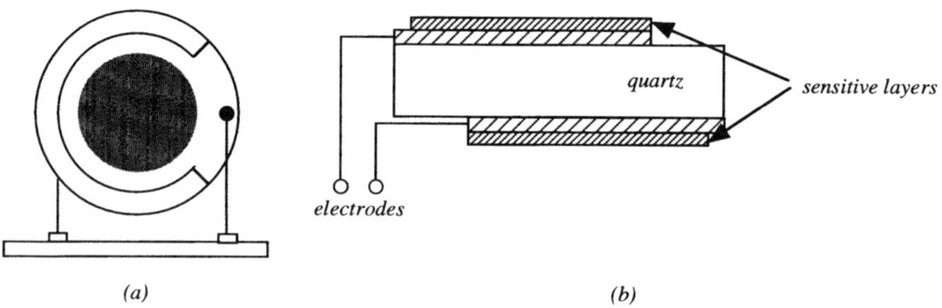

FIGURE 9.1 Schematic diagram of a BAW sensor (a) and its cross-section (b).

9.1.2 SAW Sensors

SAW-type chemical sensors exploit the propagation of surface acoustic waves along layered structures consisting at least of a substrate covered by the CIM (see Figure 9.2).

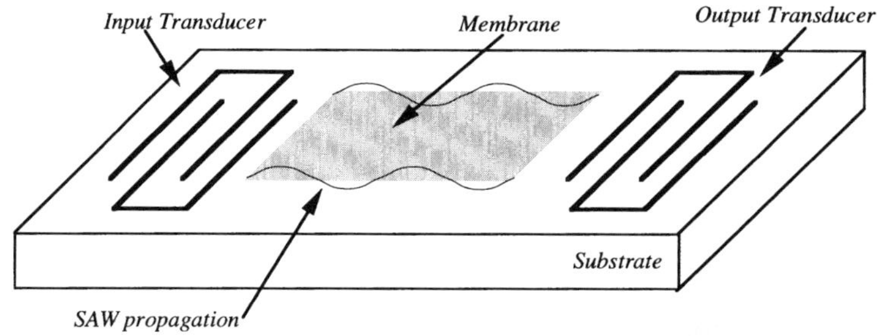

FIGURE 9.2 Basic structure of a SAW chemical sensor.

Changes produced by the measurand on the properties of the CIM can affect both the phase velocity and the propagation loss of the acoustic wave. Even though there are examples of SAW sensors based on the measurements of the acoustic loss, most of them, however, are based on the measurement of the changes in the phase velocity. These can be easily converted into frequency shifts, provided the device is configured like a SAW oscillator (SAW delay line oscillator, single- or two-port SAW resonator).

9.2 SAW PROPAGATION

SAW propagation can take place according to different modes, depending on the geometry of the acoustic structure and on the frequency scaling; Rayleigh waves, Sezawa waves, surface transverse waves (STW), and Bleustein-Gulyaev waves can propagate under different conditions on the plane surface of a semi-infinite structure; Lamb and Love waves propagate in acoustic structures defined by two plane and parallel free surfaces (plates). Most of these modes have been used to implement chemical sensors, the choice being influenced by the characteristics of the membrane and by the operation in gaseous or liquid environments. SAW-type chemical sensors are suitable for operation with many different kinds of membranes made of both organic and inorganic materials.

The possibility of using long acoustic propagation paths containing many acoustic wavelengths, together with the presence of many different possible mechanisms of interaction between SAWs and the measurand, gives to this kind of sensor the capacity of reaching high sensitivity values together with high versatility.

From the acoustic point of view the structure of a SAW chemical sensor can be schematized as a substrate covered by one or more layers made of different materials. One of the layers, usually the one abutting the environment under test, is made with the chemically interactive membrane. For the next considerations it is convenient to normalize all the thicknesses to the acoustic wavelength (λ). The substrate can be modeled as a plate or it can be approximated as a semi-infinite half-space depending on whether its thickness is less than a few wavelengths or larger than many wavelengths (Figures 9.3a,b). The normalized thicknesses of the layers are usually in the range between a small fraction ($10^{-2}/10^{-3}$) of a unit to a maximum of a few units.

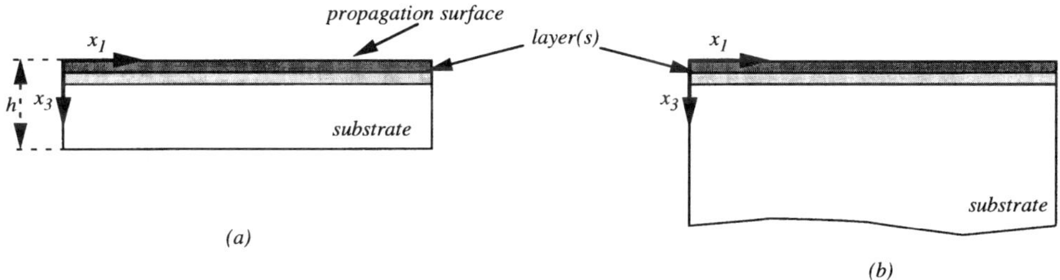

FIGURE 9.3 SAW propagation medium (a); and semi-infinite half space (b).

A complete theoretical analysis of SAW propagation in chemical sensors is outside the scope of this work as it would require the investigation of a variety of different experimental conditions that can take place. In fact, chemical sensing may require the use of membranes of varying nature showing different physical properties; the adjacent environment that can be both in liquid and gaseous phase can also enter into the acoustic propagation characteristics. Moreover, the presence of a piezoelectric medium, required for the electromechanical transduction of the wave, causes the acoustic propagation to be affected by both mechanical and electrical properties of the materials sharing the acoustic structure of the device. The use of linear elastic materials is widely preferred in SAW device technology.

Chemical sensing, however, may require that materials showing nonlinear elastic effects or viscous and viscoelastic behaviour are involved in SAW propagation. From the electrical transport point of view the materials used can be conductors showing a wide range of resistivities; they can be dielectrics or semiconductors.

SAW solutions for plane waves propagating along the x direction in the layered structures shown in Figure 9.3 are given in each medium by the superposition of n partial waves.[1] The components (u_i) of the particle displacement vector are given by:

$$u_i = \sum_{p=1}^{n} A_p a_i^{(p)} e^{ikb^{(p)}x_3} e^{j(kx_1 - \omega t)} \tag{9.1a}$$

with i = 1…3; while, for the electric potential Φ we have:

$$\phi = \sum_{p=1}^{n} A_p a_4^{(p)} e^{ikb^{(p)}x_3} e^{j(kx_1 - \omega t)} \tag{9.1b}$$

where k is the acoustic wavenumber and ω the angular frequency of the acoustic wave. For each partial wave p, A_p is the amplitude, $a_i^{(p)}$ are the mechanical displacement components, $a_4^{(p)}$ the electric potential amplitude, and finally $b^{(p)}$ the propagation constant along the x_3-direction, which gives the electroacoustic field profile with the depth.

The number n of partial waves depends on the characteristics of the medium; it is six for nonpiezoelectric materials, eight in piezoelectric materials, and ten in piezoelectric semiconductors. Here the charge density is the fifth component of the electroacoustic field which has to be included in Equations 9.1a and b.[2,3]

The solutions must satisfy both the mechanical motion equations and electric charge equations together with the proper boundary conditions at the free surfaces and at the interfaces between different media; the motion equation is given by:

$$\rho \frac{\partial^2 u_i}{\partial t^2} = \frac{\partial^2 T_{ij}}{\partial x_j^2} \tag{9.2}$$

where ρ is the mass density of the medium and T_{ij} represents the components of the stress tensor. The mechanical boundary conditions require the continuity of the particle displacement and of the stresses at the free surfaces and at the interfaces between different layers.

$$\begin{aligned} &T_{i3} = 0 \quad \text{at the free surfaces} \\ &\begin{cases} T_{i3} = T'_{i3} \\ \quad\quad\quad \text{at the interfaces} \\ u_i = u'_i \end{cases} \end{aligned} \tag{9.3}$$

where primed and unprimed quantities refer to adjacent media. In semi-infinite media, the boundary conditions require that the amplitude of the wave decays with the depth. This implies that only half of the partial waves (those showing the proper value of $b^{(p)}$) are considered. The electric components of the acoustic field must satisfy Maxwell's equations in the quasistatic regime or the charge transport equations, depending on the nature of the medium. This also determines the proper boundary conditions that have to be considered from time to time and that can assign the continuity at each interface of the electrical potential, of the normal component of the electric displacement and current, of the Fermi level (when two semiconductors are placed in contact), and so on. Sets of material constitutive equations link mechanical and electrical quantities in each medium. As an example, the constitutive equations of a piezoelectric medium are given by:

$$\begin{aligned} T_{ij} &= c_{ijkl} \frac{\partial u_k}{\partial x_l} + e_{nij} \frac{\partial \phi}{\partial x_n} \\ D_m &= c_{mkl} \frac{\partial u_k}{\partial x_l} + \varepsilon_{nm} \frac{\partial \phi}{\partial x_n} \end{aligned} \tag{9.4}$$

where both mechanical and electric magnitudes are linked by matrices of elastic constants c_{ijkl}, dielectric constants ε_{nm}, and piezoelectric constants e_{nij}. If the medium is not piezoelectric, the e's vanish so that the mechanical quantities are uncoupled to the electrical ones; the first half of Equation 9.4 gives the Hook's law of elasticity, while the second one applies to dielectric media. The evaluation of SAWs phase velocity $v_{ph} = \omega/\beta$, as well the amplitude of the electroacoustic field profile, requires the use of numerical computation techniques following the procedures outlined in the literature[1] once the material physical constants of all the media are known.

SAW propagation can take place according to different modes, depending on the structure under test and on the characteristics and crystallographic orientation of the substrate and of the layers. In isotropic materials or for higher symmetry directions of crystals, the u_1 and u_3 components of the displacement can be uncoupled from the u_2 one. The corresponding propagation modes are called sagittal or straight-crested in the former case and shear horizontal (SH) in the latter. In the presence of the piezoelectric effect the electric potential, depending on the propagation conditions considered, can couple either with sagittal or SH modes.

In the following, we briefly analyze the possible modes of SAW propagation that can take place under different experimental conditions.

9.2.1 Semi-Infinite Substrate

The simplest structure that can be considered for the propagation of the SAWs is the plane-free surface of a semi-infinite medium. Here only the Rayleigh mode propagates, consisting of two or three displacement components according to the remarks outlined in the previous section. The Rayleigh waves are not dispersive (their phase velocity does not depend on the acoustic frequency) and are widely used for SAW device applications. In chemical sensors their use is limited by the consideration that this structure has no practical application because of the necessity of using a CIM along the propagation path of the SAW.

9.2.2 Thin Layer on a Semi-Infinite Substrate

This is the common structure of SAW chemical sensors. It consists of a semi-infinite substrate covered by a thin layer (not thicker than a few wavelengths) of a different material (the chemical membrane). Here, depending on the properties of the layer and of the substrate materials, several different propagation conditions can take place:

The Rayleigh wave velocity in the layer is lower than that in the substrate — On limiting, for simplicity, our attention to the isotropic case, or to higher symmetry directions in crystals, the Rayleigh wave propagation takes place according to different modes as in the dispersion phase velocity curves shown in Figure 9.4a. The first Rayleigh mode shows a phase velocity that decreases from the value in the substrate to that in the film as the normalized thickness h/λ increases. At the same time, higher order modes appear whose velocity ranges between the values of the shear vertical (SV) wave in the substrate (cut-off velocity) and in the film. A similar behaviour is observed for SH modes. Here the requirement is that the SH velocity in the film is lower than that in the substrate (this condition in the case under analysis is usually satisfied). The corresponding phase velocity dispersion curves are shown in Figure 9.4b. In anisotropic conditions SAW propagation also takes place according to modes. All the modes show all the three components of the partial displacement vector. Nevertheless, usually some of the modes show a prevailing sagittal polarization (quasisagittal) while others show a prevailing SH polarization (quasi-SH). Under particular conditions of an SH mode, the Bleustein-Gulyaev wave can propagate along the surface of a piezoelectric plate covered by an infinitely thin massless conductor.

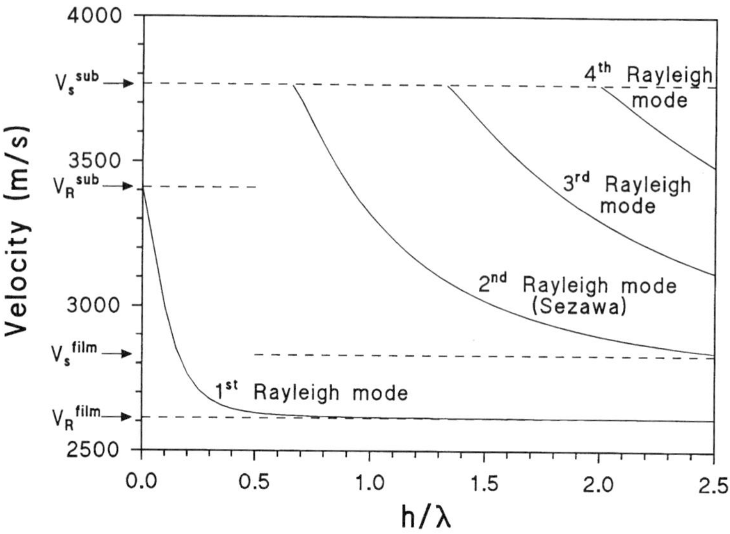

FIGURE 9.4a Dispersion curves for Rayleigh wave propagation along ZnO/SiO_2 layered structure — h/λ: normalized thickness; V_S and V_R are the velocities of the sheer and the Rayleigh waves, respectively.

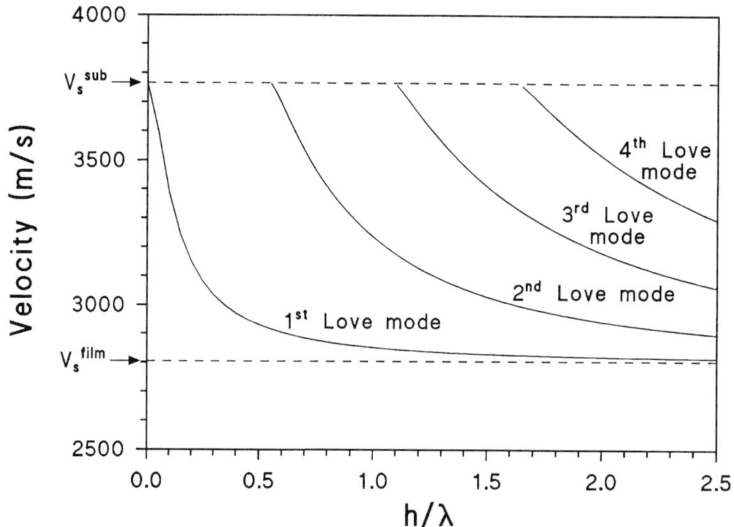

FIGURE 9.4b SH waves dispersion curves for propagation along ZnO/SiO_2 layered structure.

The Rayleigh wave velocity in the film is higher than that in the substrate — In this condition only one mode exists with saggital or quasisagittal polarization. The phase velocity of the mode increases with the normalized thickness of the film up to the cut-off value given by the SV wave velocity in the substrate. At higher h/λ values the mode is lossy as it radiates acoustic energy into the bulk of the substrate (see Figure 9.5). In a finite thickness plate the propagation of sagittal or quasisagittal modes (Lamb waves) and of SH or quasi-SH modes (Love waves) takes place. The corresponding phase velocity dispersion curves are shown in Figures 9.6a and b, respectively. The "a" and "s" in the Lamb wave dispersion curves stand for antisymmetric or symmetric and refer to the conditions where the displacements of the particles at the surfaces are symmetric or antisymmetric. It is worth noting how the phase velocity of the first antisymmetric mode vanishes at $h/\lambda = 0$. This behaviour, as we will examine in the following, can be exploited for SAW sensors operating in liquid environments. The eventual possible presence of thin layers at one or both the free surfaces of the plate modifies the dispersion curve.

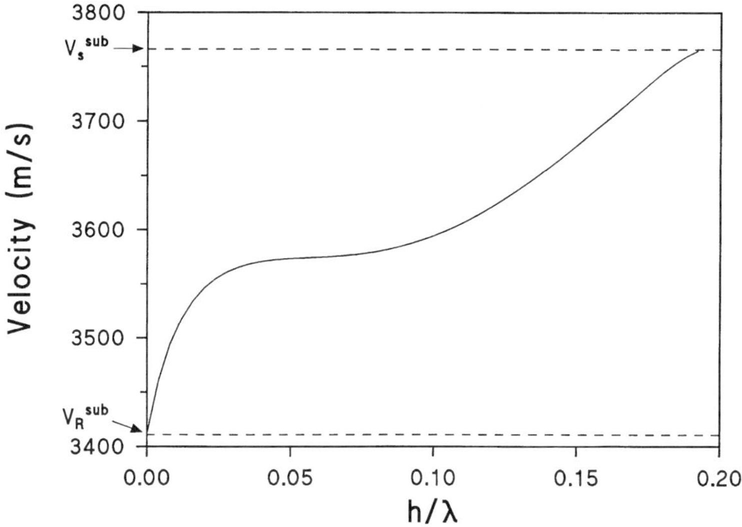

FIGURE 9.5 Rayleigh wave propagation along AlN/SiO_2 layered structure; h/λ: normalized thickness.

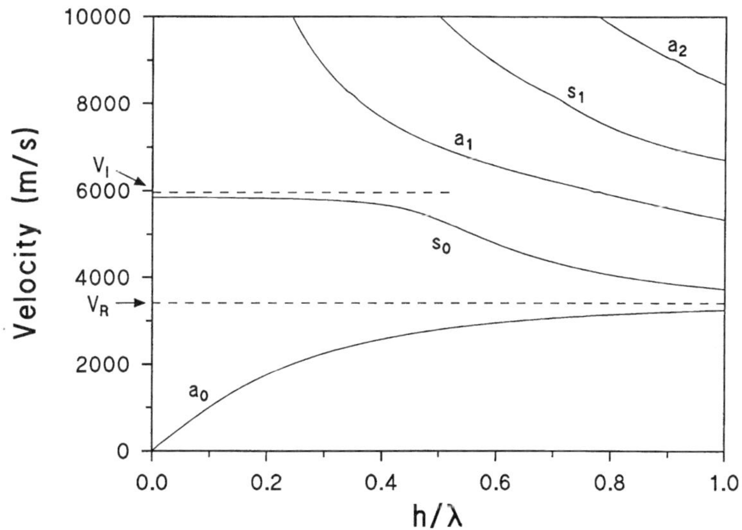

FIGURE 9.6a Lamb mode propagation along an SiO_2 plate; h/λ: normalized thickness.

9.3 SAW TRANSDUCERS

SAWs are usually generated and detected by interdigital transducers (IDTs). These consist of metal electrodes deposited on the free surface of a piezoelectric material as shown in Figure 9.7a. When a radio frequency r.f. signal is applied to the electrodes, a time-varying electric field is produced in the piezoelectric material as shown in the cross-section of Figure 9.7b. The two space periodic field components E_1 and E_3, depending on the piezoelectric

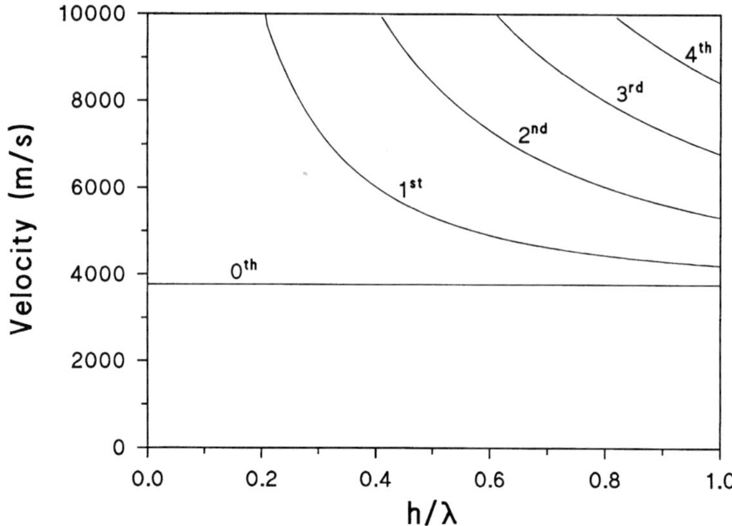

FIGURE 9.6b Love wave propagation along an SiO_2 plate.

properties and on the crystallographic orientations of the substrate, can couple with sagittal and/or SH acoustic modes.

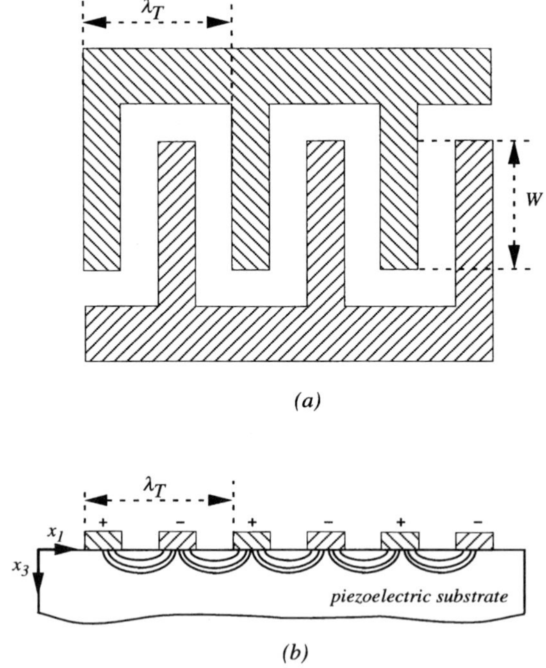

FIGURE 9.7 Schematic diagram of an interdigital transducer (a); cross-section (b) showing the electric field distribution in the piezoelectric substrate.

The spatial periodicity λ_T of the transducers determines the operation frequency f_o through the relation:

$$f_0 = \frac{v}{\lambda_T} \tag{9.5}$$

v being the phase velocity of the acoustic wave. The two other geometrical parameters of the electrodes: (finger-overlapping, W, and number, N, of finger pairs) give the geometrical aperture of the acoustic beam and the frequency bandwidth of operation, respectively. The frequency response of the transducers is of the type:

$$\operatorname{sinc}\left(N\pi\frac{f - f_0}{f_0}\right) \tag{9.6}$$

with a –3 dB relative bandwidth equal to 0.9/N.

The parallel and series equivalent circuits of the electrical port of the IDT are shown in Figures 9.8a and b, respectively. It consists of three different contributions: a static capacitance C_0, a radiation resistance R(f) (conductance G(f)), and a radiation reactance X(f) (susceptance B(f)). The reactance is zero at the center frequency f_o and it is usually ignored in calculations as its effect is small if compared to that of the static capacitance.

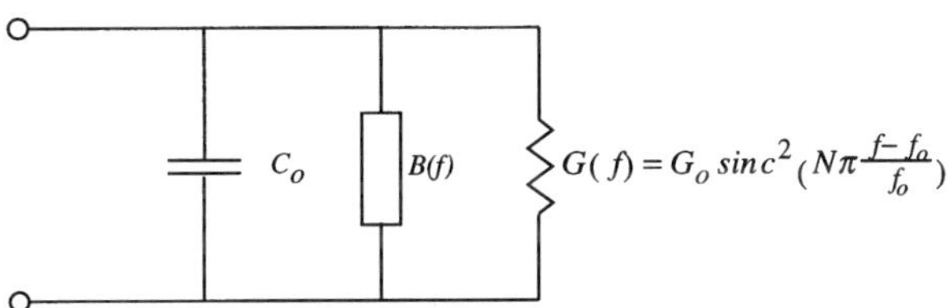

(a)

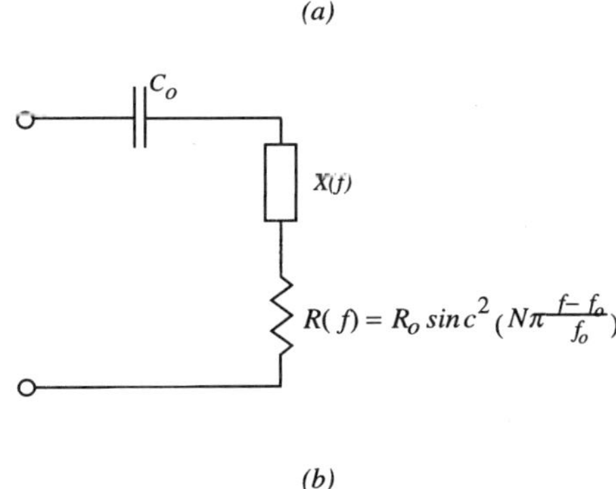

(b)

FIGURE 9.8a,b

The expressions for the elements of the equivalent circuits are[4,5]

$$\begin{aligned} \omega_0 C_0 &= 2\pi C_s vNd \\ G_0 &= 8k^2 C_s vN^2 d \\ R_0 &= \frac{1}{C_s v\left(\frac{\pi^2}{2K^2} + 8k^2 N\right)d} \end{aligned} \tag{9.7}$$

where C_s is the capacitance for fingers pair, K^2 is the electrochemical coupling coefficient and $d = W/\lambda_T$ is the directivity of the transducer. Values of C_s and K^2 for several substrates of common use are reported in Table 9.1. The electroacoustic transduction on nonpiezoelectric materials requires the use of the technology of thin piezoelectric films (such as zinc oxide — ZnO, aluminum nitride — AlN, cadmium sulfide — CdS,...). These can be deposited on a variety of substrates using sputtering techniques. They show a polycrystalline structure with a preferred orientation of the optical axis of the crystallites. Because of that the films exhibit a piezoelectric behaviour.

TABLE 9.1
SAW Characteristics for Substrates of Common Use

Materials	Cut	Prop.	Coupling coefficient K^2 (%)	Velocity m/s	Capacitance pair C_s (pF/m)
Quartz	HC	x	0.25	3209	55
Quartz	ST	x	0.16	3157	55
$LiNbO_3$	z	x	4.5	3488	460
$Bi_{13}GeO_{20}$	110	001	0.85	1620	—

The IDTs here can show four different configurations with the interdigital electrodes at one of the interfaces of the film and with or without a floating electrode at the opposite one (see Figure 9.9).[9] For these transducers it is necessary to take into account the presence of an additional geometrical parameter (the thickness h of the piezoelectric film) affecting the transducers performances. As an example, the plot of the electrochemical coefficient K^2 vs. normalized film thickness (h/λ_T) for the four IDT configurations in the case of ZnO, and AlN piezoelectric films on a (111) cut and (121) propagation Si substrate is shown in Figures 9.10a and b, respectively. As it can be seen, the configuration including the floating electrode shows a relative peak of K^2 at $h/\lambda_T = 0.05$, while the configurations with the interdigital electrodes at the interface show a second larger peak of K^2 at $h/\lambda_T = 0.5$.

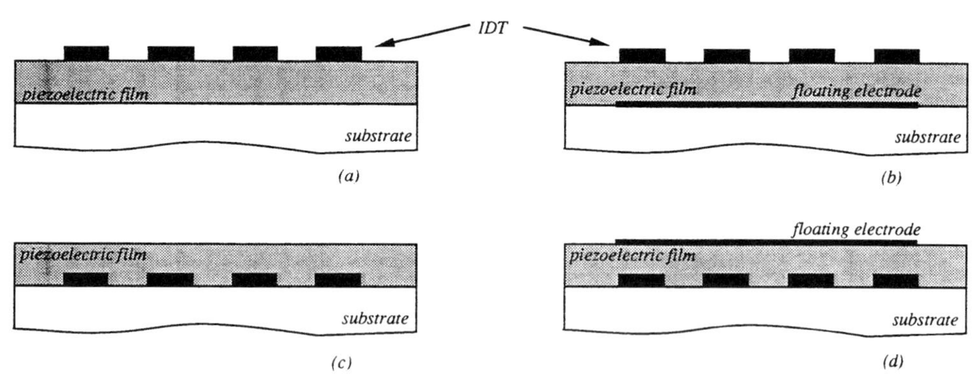

FIGURE 9.9 Four different configurations for IDTs on a piezoelectric film.

9.4 PIEZOELECTRIC MATERIALS FOR SAW APPLICATIONS

Following is a brief summary of the most commonly used piezoelectric materials for SAW applications.

Lithium niobate ($LINbO_3$) — Widely used in SAW technology because of its high electromechanical coupling coefficient and low acoustic propagation losses. It is used according

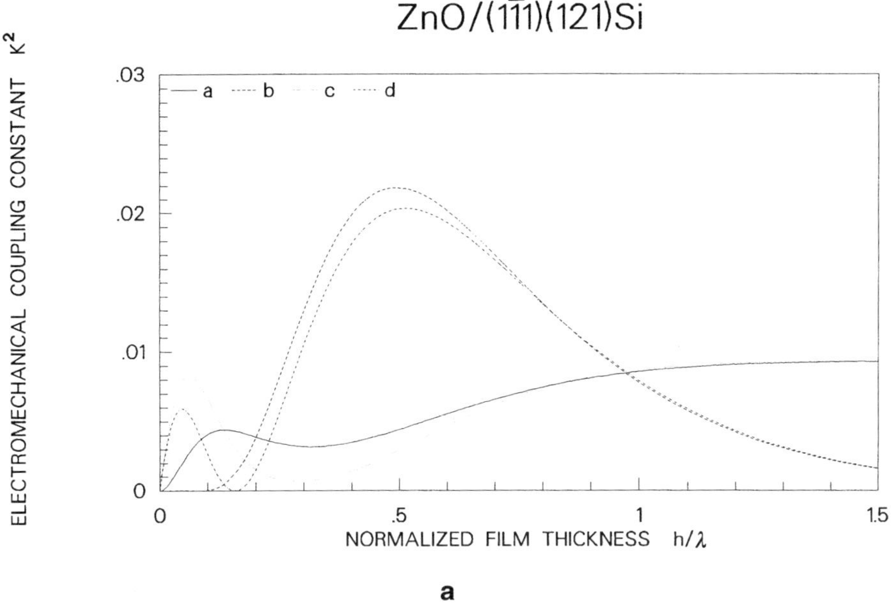

a

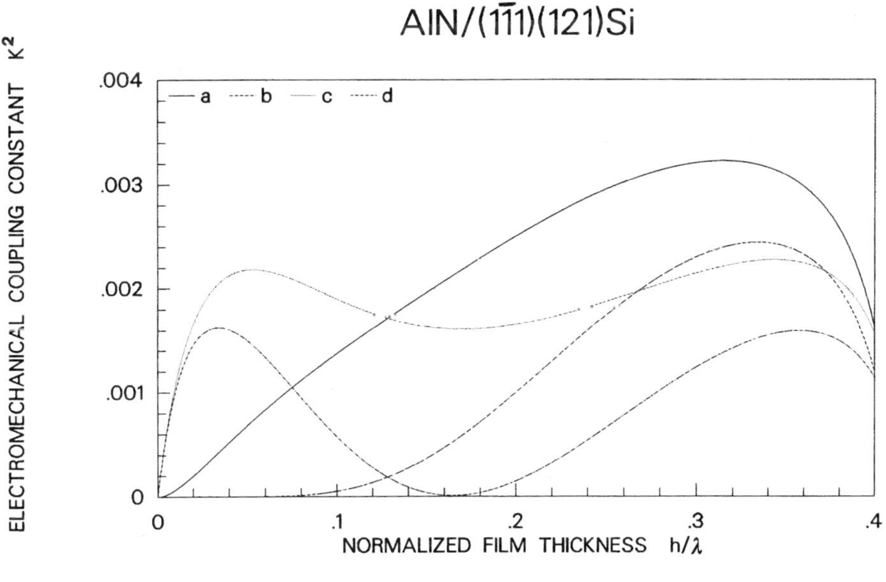

b

FIGURE 9.10 Electrochemical coupling coefficient k^2 vs. normalized piezoelectric film thickness h/λ for the four IDT configurations in the case of ZnO (a), and AlN (b) piezoelectric films on (111) (121) Si.

to different crystal, cut, propagation directions, the most known being (cut, propagation): y, x; 128 rot. y, x; 41.5 rot. y, x; with Rayleigh wave phase velocities ranging approximately from 3500 to 4000 m/s.

Lithium tantalate ($LiTaO_3$) — Not as widely used as $LiNbO_3$. It shows low propagation losses and an electromechanical coefficient approximately one order of magnitude lower. With respect to $LiNbO_3$, however, it shows a better stability with the temperature and a lower temperature coefficient of delay. The Rayleigh wave velocity, depending on the crystallographic orientation, is in the range 3200 to 3400 m/s.

Quartz (α-SiO_2) — Widely used for SAW applications (oscillators, filters, resonators) where a high temperature stability is required. For this reason it is highly recommended also for SAW sensors applications. Special crystallographic cuts, like the one called ST (132,75 rot. y in the yz plane, x propagation), show a zero temperature coefficient of delay at room temperature. It is interesting to note that for this cut (or other y-rotated cuts), when the propagation along the perpendicular to the x-axis is considered, IDTs generate SH waves instead of sagittal modes. The same substrate can thus be used to implement both Rayleigh and SH wave devices, depending on whether the x or the x-perpendicular direction is utilized. The electromechanical coupling in quartz is approximately two orders of magnitude lower than that in $LiNbO_3$.

Bismuth germanium oxide ($Bi_{12}GeO_{20}$) — Sometimes used in SAW applications when a low phase velocity is convenient. Phase velocities of the most common orientations of BGO ((001), (100), (111), (110), and (110), (001)) range between 1600 and 1800 m/s.

Piezoelectric films (ZnO, AlN) — The importance of these films for the implementation of SAWs devices on nonpiezoelectric substrates has been discussed before. They, for instance, make possible the integration of SAW devices with the electronic conditioning circuits on Si or on GaAs substrates. Piezoelectric films have been widely used for the transduction of Rayleigh-type waves. These films show a preferred orientation of the c-axis along the normal to the substrate surface. More recently it has been proved that piezoelectric films, when grown with the c-axis inclined with respect to the normal or lying on the substrate surface, are effective for the transduction of SH modes[7] (see Figure 9.11) and, as it will be shown in the following, SH modes are suitable for SAW sensing in liquid environments.

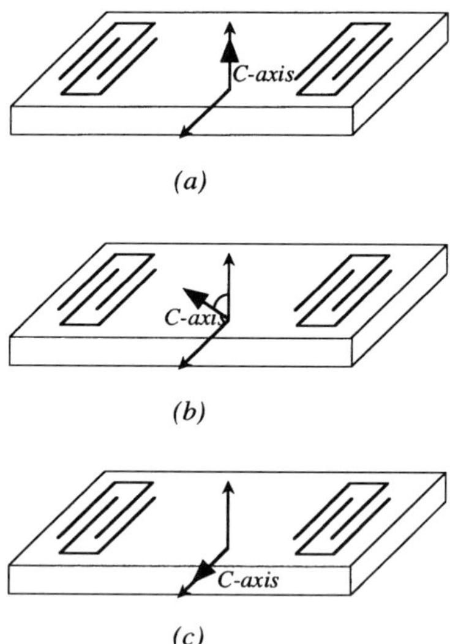

FIGURE 9.11 Different preferred orientations of the c-axis of crystallinity in the piezoelectric film: coupling of sagittal modes (a), sagittal and SH modes (b), and SH modes (c).

9.5 SAW SENSORS FOR OPERATION IN LIQUIDS

SAW chemical sensors were designed at first for operation in gaseous environments. Most of them have utilized, as acoustic mode, the first Rayleigh wave in the layered structure made by the substrate (usually piezoelectric) and the membrane shaped in the form of a thin film whose thickness is a small fraction of an acoustic wavelength. The structure is highly sensitive to any physical and chemical change in the surface characteristics of the membrane, and gives rise to strong responses of the device. After that, experiments were extended to sensors exploiting the propagation of STWs, Lamb waves in thin layered structures, etc.[8-10] These devices usually are not suitable for operation in liquid environments because of the strong mechanical coupling between the propagation medium and the adjacent liquid under test that gives rise to prohibitive acoustic propagation losses.

In order to investigate the possible operation of SAW-type sensors in liquids, it is necessary to take into account that ideal liquids can support only compressional stresses. Shear stresses can be coupled in real liquids only through the presence of viscoelastic constants; moreover the phase velocity of compressional waves in liquids is lower than that of SAW modes in solids. There are two possible conditions for SAW sensors operation in liquids.

9.5.1 Acoustic Modes With Mechanical Polarization in the Sagittal Plane (Rayleigh and Lamb Waves)

Here the SV component of the surface wave in the solid phase couples with the longitudinal one in the liquid phase (Figure 9.12a). Two different conditions can take place depending on whether the longitudinal wave velocity (v_l) in the liquid is lower or higher than that (v) of the SAW. When the first condition is satisfied, the acoustic energy of the surface wave is radiated into the liquid (compressional wave) at an angle $\vartheta = \arcsin\left(\frac{v}{v_l}\right)$, according to the wavevector diagram shown in Figure 9.12b. In the second case (Figure 9.12c) the angle ϑ and the wave vector in the liquid (k_l) become imaginary. This means that the acoustic wave is totally reflected into the solid and that only an exponential tail of the acoustic field penetrates the liquid. The required condition of low phase velocity can be satisfied by the lowest order flexural Lamb wave in plates (first antisymmetric mode a_o, see Figure 9.7a). The phase velocity of this mode drops to zero with the parameter h/λ. Devices based on this operation condition have been successfully exploited using the technology of chemically thinning Si membranes together with that of ZnO piezoelectric films[11,12] (see Figure 9.13).

9.5.2 SH Modes

Due to the fact that liquids do not support shear stresses, SAW devices using the propagation of SH modes (STWs, Love waves) are suitable for operation in liquid environments. The possible presence of viscoelastic terms in the liquid gives rise also for this propagation to an exponential tail of the acoustic field profile into the liquid, without excessive acoustic propagation losses. Liquid phase sensors exploiting the propagation of SH modes have also been successfully studied for the detection of ion concentrations and for the analysis of the viscoelastic properties of the liquids[13,14] (see Figure 9.14).

For both structures of liquid phase sensors, it is necessary to take into account that the presence of the exponential tail in the liquid makes the device more sensitive to the physical properties of the liquid itself with respect to the operation of the same device in a gaseous environment. For this reason, the use of efficient compensation techniques based on differential structures is strongly recommended.

9.6 SAW Sensor Response

The response of a SAW chemical sensor is produced by the superposition of many different contributions related to changes, induced by the analyte, of the physical properties of the membrane. The most important properties that enter into the propagation are the mass density

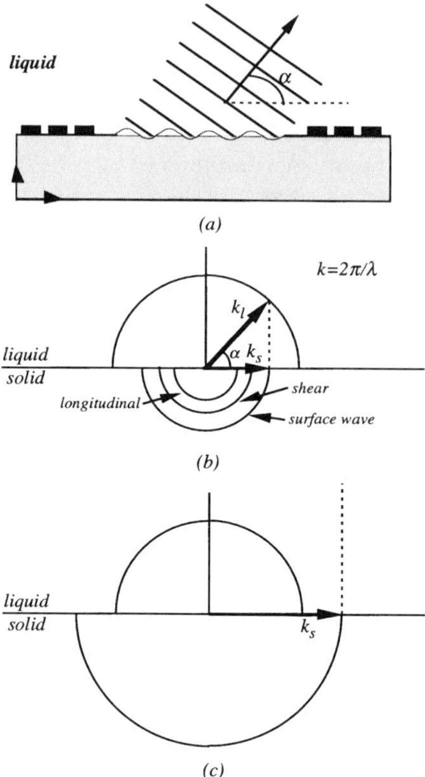

FIGURE 9.12 Mode conversion of a SAW onto a compressional wave in the liquid (a) and corresponding wavevector diagram (b); wavevector diagram for total SAW energy reflection into the solid (c).

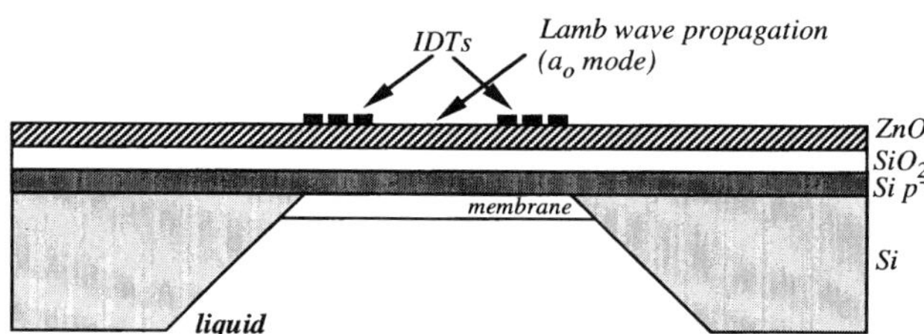

FIGURE 9.13 Cross section of a SAW sensor for operation in liquid, showing the silicon micromachining technology.

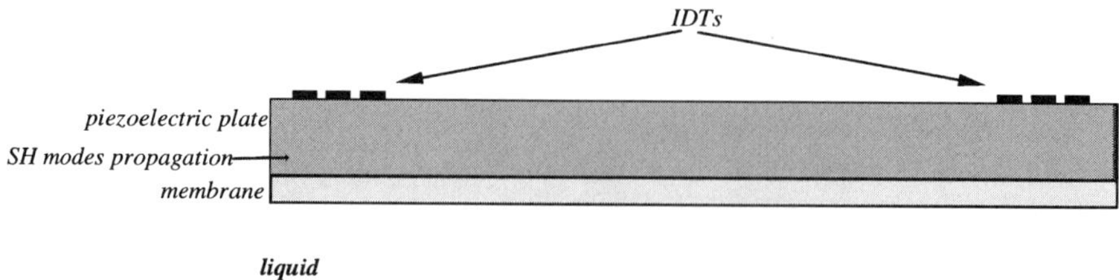

FIGURE 9.14 Schematic diagram of a SAW sensor operating in a liquid environment using the propagation of SH modes.

and the elastic constants. The electric properties of the membrane can also affect the SAW propagation through the piezoelectric coupling.

The response of a device upon exposure to the measurand can be evaluated, in principle, by analyzing the propagation in the specific structure in the two conditions of unmodified and modified membrane, provided that all the required material constants are known together with the changes produced by the analyte. As these changes are usually small, the response can be evaluated using the more simple perturbative approach.[15] Unfortunately, the changes in the membrane material are usually not known. The procedure can be utilized to solve the inverse problem of evaluating these modifications starting from experimental data obtained in a suitable number of different experimental conditions. The values so obtained can be used to optimize the performances of a device by a proper design of the electroacoustic structure of the sensor.[16]

Changes in the electrical resistance of the membrane can also strongly affect the propagation of SAWs for specific ranges of sheet resistivity of the film[17] (see Figure 9.15).

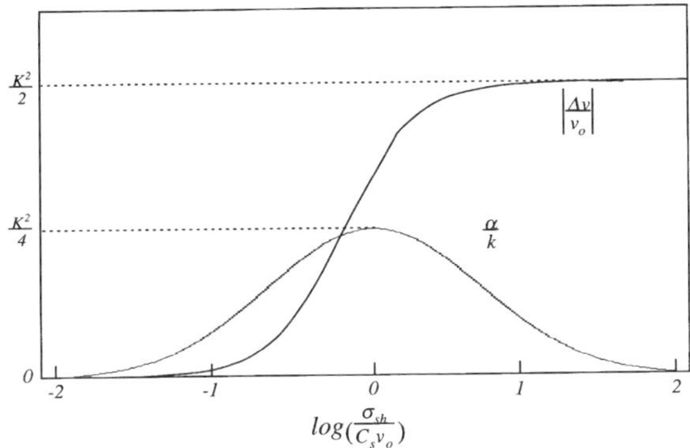

FIGURE 9.15 Fractional wave velocity shift Δ v/v and propagation loss $\frac{\alpha}{k}$ for SAW propagation on piezo-substrate (electromechanical coupling constant k^2) vs. sheet conductivity (σ) of the film overlay.

9.7 DETECTION TECHNIQUES

Depending on the specific SAW sensor, the acoustic parameter giving the device response can be either the phase velocity or the acoustic propagation loss. Most SAW chemical sensors operate on the phase velocity. The readout scheme for velocity changes can be based on two different detection techniques: the phase shift or the frequency shift.

9.7.1 PHASE SHIFT DETECTION

The operation of the phase shift technique is described in Figure 9.16. The SAW device is configured as a delay line and fed by a radio frequency r.f. signal. The phase of the signals at the input and at the output of the line are compared by a phase detector that gives a voltage proportional to their difference φ equal the phase delay of the acoustic line:

$$\varphi = 2\pi \frac{l}{\lambda} = 2\pi \frac{lf}{v} \tag{9.8}$$

Here l is the length of the line corresponding to the center-to-center distance of the IDTs, λ is the acoustic wavelength at the operating frequency f, and v is the acoustic phase velocity. Any change Δv in the velocity is detected as a change $\Delta\varphi$ in the phase delay φ_o of the wave.

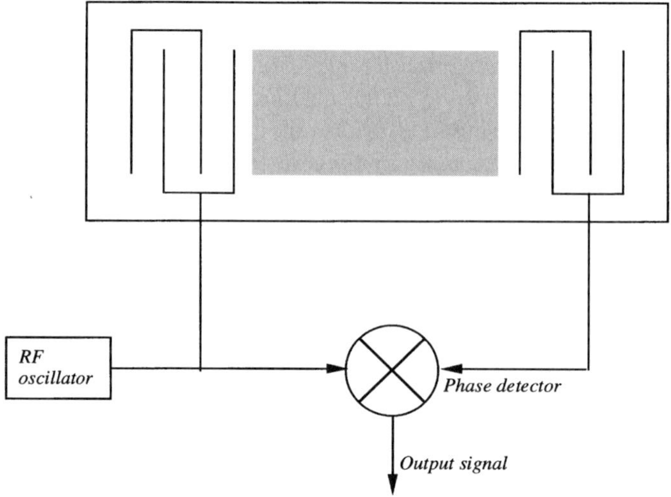

FIGURE 9.16 Schematic diagram of the phase shift detection technique.

$$\Delta\varphi = -2\pi \frac{lf}{v} \frac{\Delta v}{v} = -\varphi_0 \frac{\Delta v}{v} \tag{9.9}$$

The expression shows how the output signal, proportional to $\Delta\varphi$, can be magnified by increasing the phase delay. On the other hand, it is necessary to take into account the 2π period in the response of the phase detector, which gives a limit at high levels in the dynamic range of the device. The technique is rather simple in the operation and requires the use of an r.f. oscillator showing a higher frequency stability. The basis structure can be modified to operate using pulse-modulated r.f. bursts, in order to cancel the effect of electric feedthrough in high insertion loss delay lines as shown in Figure 9.17.

9.7.2 Frequency Shift Detection

The device is configured as a SAW-controlled r.f. oscillator. The structure can be that of a delay line or that of a single- or two-port resonator (see Figure 9.18). For all the structures, the frequency of the signal at the output is determined by the characteristics of the SAW element. The most widely used configuration for chemical sensors applications is that of the delay line oscillator. As shown for this structure, oscillation takes place when both phase and gain loop conditions are satisfied:

$$\varphi_{loop} = \varphi_a + \varphi_e = 2\,n\pi$$

$$G_{loop} = G_a + G_e \geq 1 \tag{9.10}$$

where n is an integer, φ and G stand for phase and gain respectively, while the subscripts a and e are quantities related to the acoustic line and to the electronic amplifier and electric connections, respectively. As $\varphi_a \gg \varphi_e$, from the first step of Equation 9.10, taking into account Equation 9.8, it follows that:

$$f = n\frac{v}{l} = n\frac{1}{\tau} \tag{9.11}$$

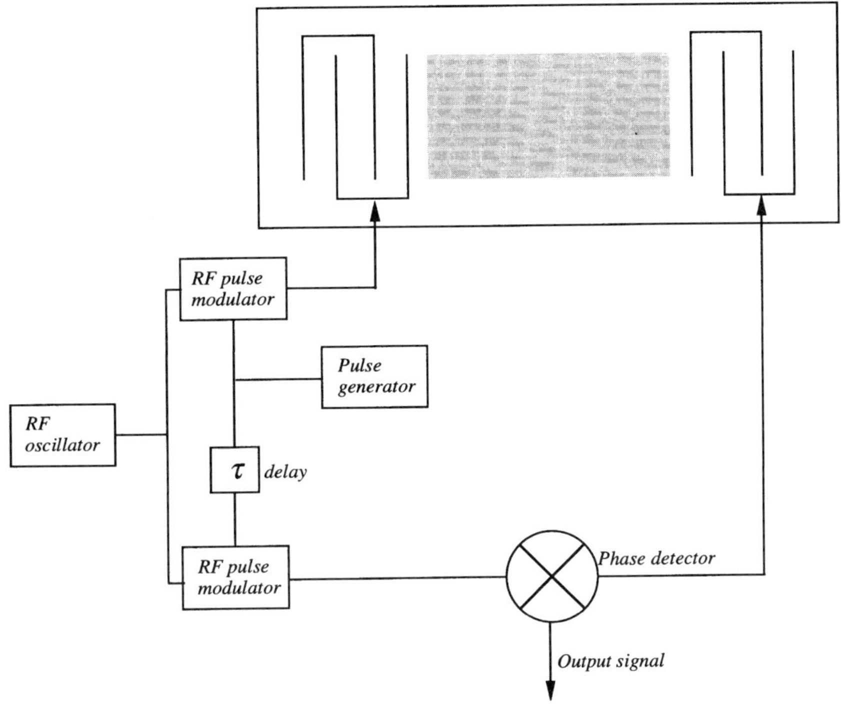

FIGURE 9.17 Schematic diagram of the phase shift detection technique in pulsed operation mode.

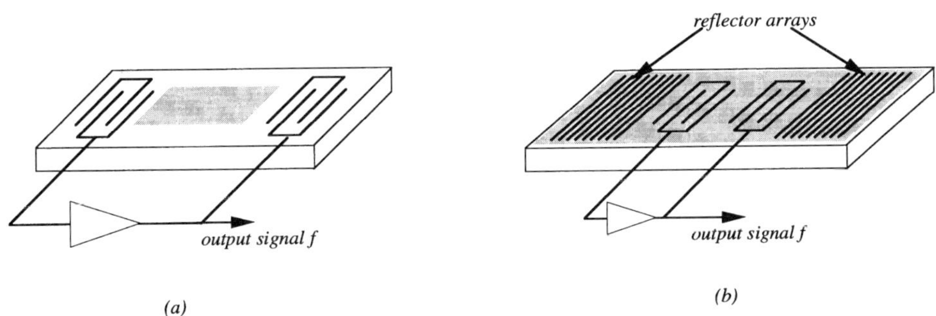

FIGURE 9.18 Frequency shift detection technique using a SAW delay line oscillator (a) or a two-port SAW resonator (b).

τ being the time delay of the line. Equation 9.11 gives the "comb" of frequency modes of the electroacoustic structure; the oscillation frequency is determined by the transfer function of the transducers and amplifiers, through the gain condition. Any change Δv in the phase velocity gives rise to a frequency shift Δf in the oscillation frequency f, given by:

$$\frac{\Delta f}{f} = \frac{\Delta v}{v} \tag{9.12}$$

The frequency shift technique is an accurate method of detection as frequencies can be measured with high precision (1 Hz or even better). In the frequency range used for SAW sensors applications (100 MHz) this means that relative velocity shifts as low as 10^{-8} can be detected. In addition, it is at low cost as only an unsophisticated amplifier is required, and finally the specific output signal (frequency) is a natural input for digital signal processing systems.

9.8 DIFFERENTIAL STRUCTURES AND COMPENSATION TECHNIQUES

As most sensors, SAW devices show a limited selectivity for the measurand. This means that other magnitudes can affect the sensor response giving rise to errors in the detection or, in any case, producing a noise that limits the resolution of the system. A typical error source for SAW sensors is due to temperature changes that affect the acoustic phase velocity. Temperature can in fact affect the sensor response in two ways: causing a drift in the reference value that can be detected as a signal and changing the device response to the analyte that modifies the calibration. The effect of the drift in the reference is even more severe for SAW devices operating in liquids, where the strong interaction of the acoustic propagation with the liquid under test makes the device sensitive to the physical characteristics (density, viscosity, etc.) of the liquid itself.

Zero-level drift is usually strongly reduced by using the so-called differential structure as shown in Figures 9.19a and b. It consists of two SAW structures of which only one is made sensitive to the measurand. The output signal is represented by the difference between those of the two devices. In this way common mode error sources such as temperature act almost the same way on the two parts and the corresponding signals are cancelled. Only the measurand, giving rise to different effects on the two arms, produces a detectable signal at the output. Changes in the calibration curve of the device could, in principle, be connected using the "sum" signal that gives a measure of the perturbing parameter (see Figure 9.20).

A further improvement in the selectivity of the device by analysis of the multimeasurands environment can be obtained through pattern recognition techniques performed using matrices of nxn different sensors and multiple deconvolution. See the more detailed discussion later in the chapter. All this can, in perspective, be done using the SAW technology on silicon in order to integrate the electroacoustic device, the amplifier, and signal processing circuits on the same substrate, to produce complex and compact devices at a competitive price.

9.9 QUARTZ RESONATOR STRUCTURES AS BASIC SENSORS

Most sensors, in the presence of a given measurand change, exhibit a voltage or current output and in this circumstance in order to obtain a digital output signal or even an output frequency, a voltage to frequency converter must be used. This adds some complication in these sensors in terms of postprocessing circuits. However, in addition to the SAW devices described above, there are other sensors based on piezomaterials that give an output ac signal at a certain frequency (see Reference 18). A detailed description of the physics and operating principles of BAW-based chemical sensors can be found in Reference 19. Quartz piezoelectric crystals characterized by a high Q-factor and a relatively small temperature sensitivity of the resonant properties, have been used for many years as mass detectors (see Reference 20). Sauerbrey[21] in 1954 showed that the relative change of the resonant frequency $\Delta f/f$ of a quartz (of thickness t) coated by a thin film (of thickness Δt) of any kind is almost equivalent to that of a quartz of a thickness $t + \Delta t$, and is given by:

$$\Delta f = \frac{\Delta m \, f_o}{S \, \rho \, N} \tag{9.13}$$

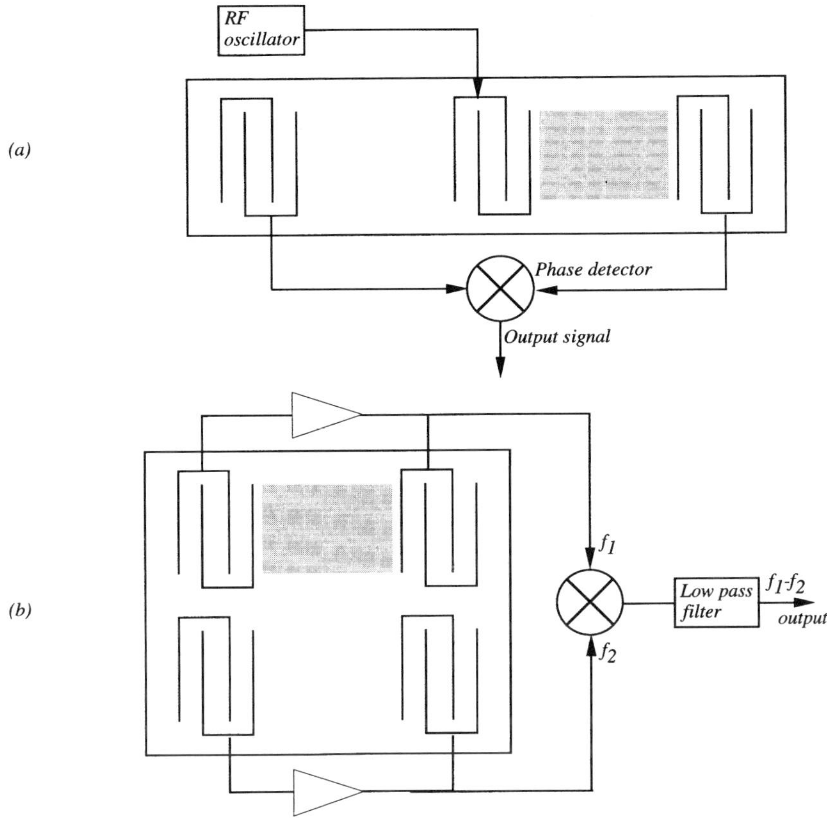

FIGURE 9.19 Differential structure for phase shift detection (a), and frequency shift detection (b).

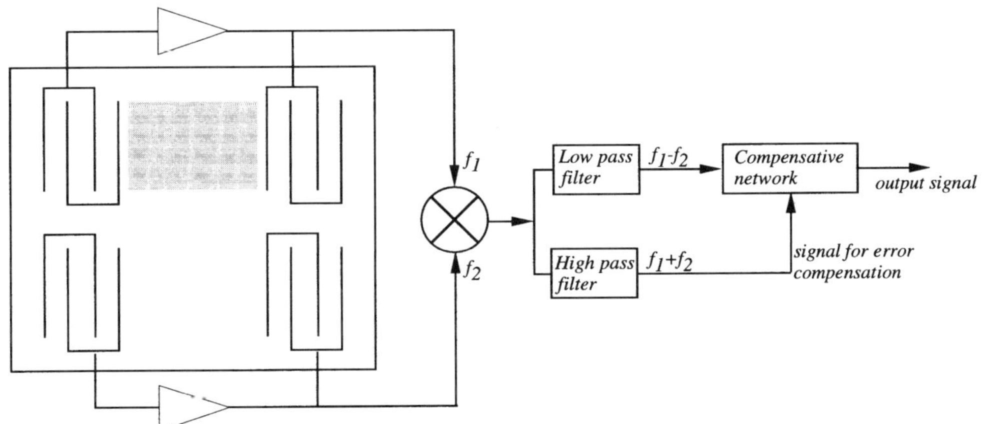

FIGURE 9.20 Differential structure allowing compensation for zero drift and calibration correction.

Δf is the frequency change due to the coated mass, Δm is the mass of the film, S (cm^2) is the area of the quartz, ρ is the quartz density, N is a constant related to the crystal, and f_o is the fundamental frequency of the piezoelectric crystal.

The Sauerbrey equation is based on the assumption that quartz and membrane have similar physical properties. In practice this is not the case and each new system (quartz plate plus membrane) should be studied and calibrated separately. In fact a membrane usually has intrinsic physical characteristics that could be very much different from those related to the quartz material. Different materials in series, with different densities, induce dissipation energy paths in relation to the propagation of elastic waves. Another source of energy dissipation is the incomplete adhesion of the membrane to the quartz surface. In any case the acoustic impedance of the two materials, Z_q (for the quartz) and Z_m (for the membrane), should be taken into account in order to try to have their ratio as close as possible to unity. As an example, aluminum on quartz offers a satisfactory impedance matching, and this circumstance justifies its use in contacting quartz plates in oscillator applications. When the quartz is used as a sensor with multilayered sensitive coating structures it may be necessary to pay attention to the above-mentioned problem especially in view of considerations dealing with medium- and long-term stability of the overall system.

The resonant frequency change Δf can also be expressed as follows:

$$\Delta f = -2.3\ 10^6\ f_0^2\ \frac{\Delta m}{S} \tag{9.14}$$

where Δm is the mass (g) of the coating deposited on one surface, f_o is expressed in MHz and represents the fundamental frequency of the piezoelectric crystal, S is the crystal area in cm^2, the constant being inversely proportional to the root of both the quartz density and the shear modulus. From Equation 9.14 it is possible to infer that for a crystal able to oscillate at about 10 MHz a mass sensitivity $\Delta f/\Delta m$ of the order of 0.5 $Hz/ng/cm^2$ can be considered possible. This demonstrates the extremely high sensitivity of this piezo device when utilized as a weight-measuring system.

The resolution limit has been estimated to be around 10^{-11} g and the possibility of using a coated quartz as a promising sensor for gas detection through a sorption process was proposed by King[22] in 1964. This kind of sensor is frequently called a quartz microbalance sensor. Equation 9.14 has been proved to be sufficiently accurate for mass changes that give rise to a frequency shift of about 10%. Advances in crystal and oscillator design have allowed continued oscillating even with frequency shifts of 20% of the unloaded quartz resonant frequency. Above this value nonlinearities can become prohibitive.

Figure 9.21 shows the electrical equivalent circuit of the quartz crystal including the mass-sensitive part. Figure 9.22 shows a typical chemical sensor structure based on quartz resonators. The quartz n 1 has incorporated a chemically interactive material, while the quartz n 2 represents the reference.

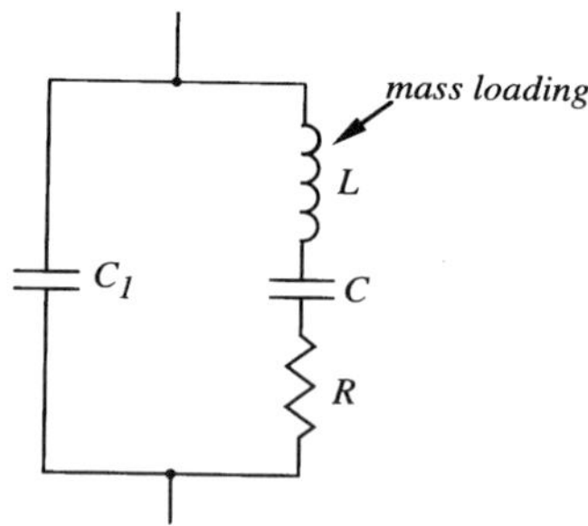

FIGURE 9.21 Electric equivalent circuit of a quartz resonator operating in air.

This structure, called differential, is suitable for reducing an undesired common mode source of errors such as temperature and pressure variations which could occur during the measurement. After the mixer and the low pass filter only the frequency difference Δf remains, containing the information related to the measurand through the interaction of the CIM (chemically interactive material).

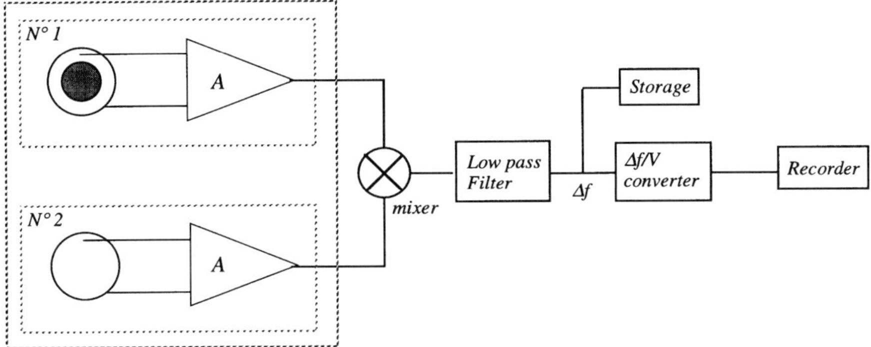

FIGURE 9.22 Schematic diagram of a differential piezo-oscillator configuration and read-out system.

9.9.1 Quartz Resonators in Liquids

In a suitable oscillator configuration piezocrystals also can oscillate in liquids.[23-25] In this case the frequency of oscillation is dependent on other parameters such as viscosity (η), density (ρ), and conductivity of the solution. It has been proved that in a solution of sucrose, glycerol, dimethylsulfoxide, ethyleneglycol, etc., the dependence of frequency changes on density and viscosity can, with a good approximation, be expressed as follows:

$$\Delta f = -f^{3/2} n \left[\frac{\eta_s \rho_s}{\pi \mu_q \rho_q} \right]^{1/2} \tag{9.15}$$

where n = 1 or 2 side coated crystal, η_s: solution viscosity, ρ_s: solution density, ρ_q: density of the quartz, and μ_q: share module of the quartz. When the conductivity of the solution is too high and the commonly used quartz systems are not able to oscillate, both contacts on the two quartz surfaces can be protected and isolated from the solution by using the configuration shown in Figure 9.23, where two thin films of Si_3N_4 are employed to improve the impedance between the two contacts and, as a consequence, to permit oscillations.

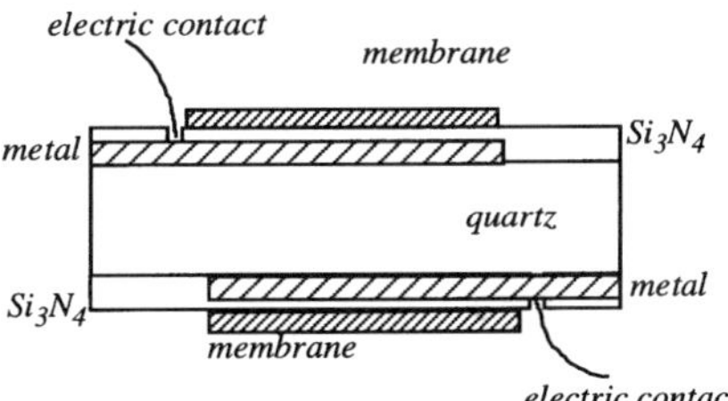

FIGURE 9.23 Cross-section of a quartz resonator for applications in liquids.

The behavior of the quartz sensors in liquids are of course more complex than those in air. To have an idea about the number of new interactions, Figure 9.24 shows, in this case, a possible equivalent electrical circuit of a quartz oscillator. The three different sections account for quartz, liquid loading, and mass loading.[24]

9.10 MULTICOMPONENT ANALYSIS APPLICATIONS

Multicomponent analysis is an experimental procedure consisting of the simultaneous measurement of several different quantities. Since the characterization of any kind of ambient medium

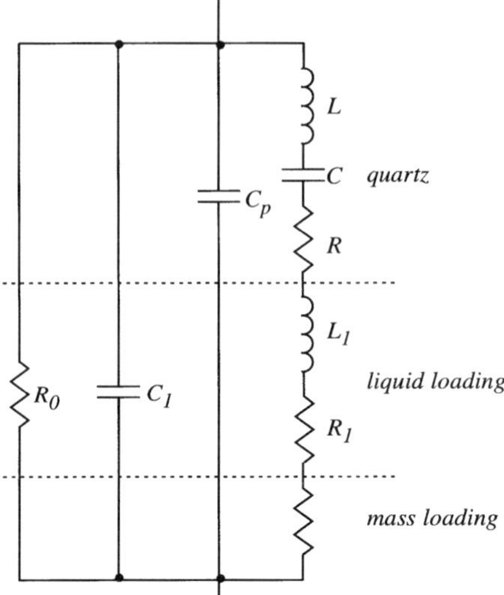

FIGURE 9.24 Electric equivalent circuit of a quartz resonator for operation in liquids.

is given by the simultaneous knowledge of different quantities, the multicomponent analysis is of great interest in any practical sensor application. In chemical sensing, multicomponent analysis can be classified in two main branches that can be called: *selectivity enhancement* and *electronic nose*.

The *selectivity enhancement* applications aim to overcome the intrinsic nonselectivity that chemical sensors show in order to allow the measurement of a set of different chemical quantities in mixed environments.

Under the denomination *electronic nose* are grouped all those applications aiming at the recognition of chemical patterns. A chemical pattern is defined as the simultaneous occurrence of a number of chemical species, each at a certain concentration level. The name electronic nose comes from the analogy of these systems with the natural olfaction, generalizing odors as chemical patterns. (See Part V of this book.)

Adopting the analytical chemistry language, the previously quoted applications can be named quantitative analysis and qualitative analysis — quantitative analysis answers to the question: *How much is present*? and qualitative analysis answers to: *What is it*?

From a mathematical point of view quantitative analysis is solved using the statistical regression methods[26] and qualitative analysis falls in the realm of the so-called pattern recognition (see Reference 27 and Chapter 27 in this book). In multicomponent analysis each sensor of the array must behave differently, so that in order to build up a sensor array it is necessary to have devices that can be easily differentiated from the chemical interface point of view. This requirement is met by BAW and SAW sensors. They can easily be coated with a large variety of different membranes that confer on them a large spectrum of selectivity characteristics. Also, the I/O characteristics of these sensors are approximately linear so that a simple linear method can be utilized for the array deconvolution when a limited range of concentrations is considered.

In addition to the previously quoted property, BAW sensors are also low cost and commercially available in a variety of configurations. For all these reasons BAW sensors have been the most utilized sensors for multicomponent applications.

An example of BAW sensors utilization in quantitative analysis can be found in Reference 28. In this application, BAW sensors coated with organic substances were used to measure component concentrations of mixtures of dichlorobenzene, trichloroethane, and dichloropropane. The concentrations of each component of the mixture were measured with an average relative error of less than 10%.

In qualitative analysis BAWs have been used for the recognition of five different whisky brands with an array of BAW sensors coated with different substances like lipids, sterols, and celluloses.[29] The deposition technique is very easy; the sensing material is firstly dissolved in a volatile organic material such as chloroform, then the solution is coated using a cotton swab; after the volatile vapor evaporates the BAW sensor is ready to operate.

Another application has been developed for the recognition of mixtures of organic solvents using polysiloxanes as coating materials[30] (see Chapter 25). Unlike the BAW sensors, the SAWs, due to the fact that they are not commercially available, have not been extensively utilized in array configuration. Nonetheless they have been proved to perform well when adopted[31] (see also Chapter 26).

9.11 APPLICATIONS OF ACOUSTIC-TYPE CHEMICAL SENSORS

It is worth pointing out that any kind of future development in acoustic-type chemical sensors is strongly related to the improvement of CIM (chemically interactive materials), which are responsible for the selective character of the sensors. The main problems in this area come from the CIM stability and their adhesion to the basic substrate of the device. Acoustic sensors for gases and those which are designed for operation in liquids require different CIM strategy, long studies, and many experimental data on reliability. When particular conditions have to be satisfied on both pressure and operating temperature values, this problem becomes even more difficult.

TABLE 9.2
SAW Chemical Sensors for Operation in Gas

Measurand	Membrane	Substrate propagation	Detection	Ref.
Gas chromatograph det.	Gas chromatographic partitioning liquid	$LiNbO_3$-SiO_2	Attenuation and velocity	32
SO_2	Triethanolamine	yz-$LiNbO_3$	Velocity	33,34,35,36
Acetone-methanol	Photoresist AZ-1350S	$ZnO/SiO_2/Si$	Velocity	37
Organic Vapors	PVC	(Lamb wave)	Velocity	38
	Isothermal meas.	STx-SiO_2	Velocity	139
H_2	Pd	yz-$LiNbO_3$ STx-SiO_2 $ZnO/SiO_2/Si$ (Rayleigh wave)	Velocity	8,40,41, 42, 43,44
NH_3	Pt	STx-SiO_2	Velocity	45
	Metal free phthalocyanine	STx-SiO_2	Velocity	46
NO_2	Lead phthalocyanine (PbPc)	yz-$LiNbO_3$	Velocity	17,47,48,49,50
	Langmuir-Blodgett film	yz-$LiNbO_3$	Velocity	51
CO	SnO_2	STx-SiO_2	Velocity	52
Vapors	Phosphatidylethanolamine	STx-SiO_2	Velocity	53
	Polymeric coating	STx-SiO_2	Velocity	54
Relative humidity	Polyethylmylfluorenol	STx-SiO_2	Velocity	55
(H_2O vap.)	Polyphenylacetylene	STx-SiO_2	Velocity	56
	Pt-DEBP	STx-SiO_2	Velocity	57

TABLE 9.3
SAW Chemical Sensors for Operation in Liquids

Measurand	Membrane	Substrate propagation	Detection	Ref.
Nucleic acid hybridization	Probe sequence of DNA	zx-$LiNbO_3$	Velocity	58
Cu_2^+ in H_2O		ST x ⊥ - SiO_2 SH waves in plates	Velocity	59
K^+ in H_2O	PVC valinomycin doped	ST x ⊥ - SiO_2 SH waves in plates	Velocity	60
Antigen - antibody reactions	Biological layer	z cut - $LiNbO_3$	Velocity	61
Viscosity	Biological layer	yx- $LiNbO_3$	Velocity	62
		Plate modes	Attenuation and/or velocity	12,13, 63,64
Viscoelastic constants of polymeric films		ST x ⊥ - SiO_2 SH waves in plates	Attenuation and velocity	65,66
Dielectric constants and conductivity of liquids		ST x ⊥ - SiO_2 SH waves in plates	Attenuation and velocity	67

TABLE 9.4
BAW Chemical Sensors

Measurand	Membrane	Ambient	Ref.
CO_2	Siloxane	Gas	68
	Polyphenolate	Gas	68
CO	α-cyclodextrine	Gas	68
CO_2, NO_2	Amine	Gas	68
SO_2	Tridodecylanine	Gas	69
Benzene	Carbowax 400	Gas	69
C_2C_4			
C_6H_{14}	Polymers	Gas	20
C_8H_{18}			
	Cholesterol		71
Odors	Ethylcellulose	Gas	70
	Lecithin		
	Perfluorinated by-layer		
Methanol	Polyvinylpyrrolidone	n-Hexane	24
Water	Various metals	Liquid	69

Of course all the possible combinations of sensing elements and CIM have not yet been explored, especially in the biosensors context. Many biological elements can be considered for activating the sensor action in biodevices: organisms, cells, organelles, enzymes, receptors, antibodies, nucleic acids, organic molecules, etc. Among them, or among new-generation materials, a satisfactory solution for the fabrication of almost ideal sensors could be found, in the near future.

In order to present an overview, certainly not exhaustive in depth, of the to-date applications three tables are presented here showing results and experiences of recent years. Table 9.2 shows a list of SAW applications for gas detection; Table 9.3 shows a list of SAW applications in liquids; and Table 9.4 shows some selected BAW applications for gases and liquids. (See also Chapters 25 and 26.)

ACKNOWLEDGMENTS

The authors wish to thank Professor E. L. Adler of McGill University, Montreal, Canada for having provided them with his PC Surface Acoustic Wave Program which has been used for the calculation of the SAW velocity dispersion curves and electromechanical coupling in piezoelectric films reported in the present work.

REFERENCES

1. Farnell, G. W. and Adler, E. L., Elastic wave propagation in thin layers, *Physical Acoustics,* Vol. 9, Mason, W. P. and Thurston, R. N., Eds., Academic Press, New York, 1972, pp. 35-128.
2. Swierkowski, S., van Duzer, T., and Turner, G. W., Amplification of acoustic surface waves in piezoelectric semiconductors, *IEEE Trans. Sonic Ultrasonics,* SU-20, 260, 1973.
3. Palma, F., Sacconi, I., and Das, P., Surface acoustic wave propagation and acoustoelectric interaction in multilayered piezoelectric semiconductors, *Superlattices Microstruct.,* 3, 181, 1987.
4. Hartman, C. S., Bell, D. T., and Rosenfeld, R. C., Impulse model design of acoustic surface wave filters, *IEEE Trans. Sonics Ultrasonics,* SU-20, 80, 1973.
5. Smith, W. R., Gerard, H. M., Collins, J. H., Reeder, T. M., and Shaw, H. J., Analysis of surface acoustic wave transducers by use of an equivalent circuit model, *IEEE Trans. Microwave Theory Tech.,* MTT17, 856, 1969.
6. Kino, G. S. and Wagers, R. S., Theory of interdigital couplers on nonpiezoelectric substrates, *J. Appl. Phys.,* 44, 1480 1973.
7. Carlotti, G., Fioretto, D., Palmieri, L., Petri, A., Socino, G., and Verona, E., Surface acoustic waves in c-axis inclined ZnO films, IEEE Ultrasonics Symp. Proc., Honolulu, HI, 4-7 Dec., 1990, p. 449.
8. Anisimkin, V. I., D'Amico, A., and Verona, E., Hydrogen detection with surface transverse acoustic waves, *Nuovo Cimento,* 11D, 503, 1989.
9. Rebiere, D., Pistré, J., Hoummady, M., Hauder, D., Cumin, P., and Planade, R., Sensitivity comparison between gas sensor using SAW and shear horizontal plate-mode oscillator, *Sensors Actuators,* B6, 174, 1992.
10. Wenzel, S. W. and White, R. M., A multisensor employing an ultrasonic Lamb wave oscillator, *IEEE Trans. Electron. Dev.,* ED 35, 735, 1988.
11. Wenzel, S. W., Martin, B. A., and White, R. M., Generalized Lamb wave multisensor, IEEE Ultrasonics Symp. Proc., Chicago, IL, 2-5 Oct. 1988, pp. 563-567.
12. Martin, B. A., Wenzel, S. W., and White, R. M., Viscosity and density sensing with ultrasonic plate waves, *Sensors Actuators,* A21-A23, 704, 1990.
13. Martin, S. J., Ricco, A. J., Nienczyk, T. M., and Frye, G. C., Characterization of S.H. acoustic plate mode liquid sensors, *Sensors Actuators,* 20, 253, 1989.
14. Caliendo, C., Amico, A. D., Mascini, M., Moscone, D., and Verona, E., Acoustic Love wave sensor for K^+ concentration in water solutions, *Sensors Actuators,* B7, 598, 1992.
15. Auld, B. A., *Acoustic Fields and Waves in Solids,* Vol. II, John Wiley & Sons, New York, 1973.
16. Anisimkin, V. I., Kotelyanskii, I. M., Verardi, P., and Verona, E., Elastic properties of thin film palladium for surface acoustic wave (SAW) sensor, *Sensors Actuators,* B23, 203, 1995.
17. Ricco, A. J., Martin, S. J., and Zipperian, T. E., Surface acoustic wave gas sensor based on film conductivity changes, *Sensors Actuators,* 8, 319, 1985.
18. Middelhoek, S., French, P. J., Huising, J. H., and Liau, W. J., Sensors with digital or frequency output, *Sensors Actuators,* 15, 119-133, 1988.
19. Mecca, V. M., Loaded vibrating quartz sensors, *Sensors Actuators,* A40, 1-27, 1994.
20. Schierbaum, K. D., Gerlach, A., Hang, M., and Gopel, W., Selective detection of organic molecules with polymers, and supramolecular compounds: application of capacitance, quartz microbalance and calorimetric transducers, *Sensors Actuators,* A31, 130-137, 1992.
21. Sauerbrey, G., Use of vibrating quartz for thin film weighing and microweighing (in German), *Z. Phys.,* 155, 206-222, 1959.
22. King, W. H., Piezoelectric sorption detector, *Anal. Chem.,* 36(9), 1735-1739, 1964.

23. Kanazawa, K. K. and Gordon J. G., The oscillation frequency of a quartz resonator in contact with a liquid, *Anal. Chim. Acta,* 175, 1295-1300, 1985.
24. Auge, J., Hauptmann, P., Hartmann, J., and Rosler, S., New design for QMC-sensors in liquids, Proc. 5th IMCS, Rome, 1994, July 11-14.
25. Muramatsu, H., Tamiya, E., and Karube, I., Computation of equivalent circuit parameters of quartz crystals in contact with liquids and study of liquid properties, *Anal. Chem.,* 60, 2142-2146, 1988.
26. Davide, F., Di Natale, C., and D'Amico, A., Sensor arrays figures of merit: definitions and properties, *Sensors Actuators,* B13-14, 327-332, 1993.
27. Gardner, J. and Bartlett, P., Eds., *Sensors and Sensory Systems for an Electronic Nose,* Kluwer Academic, Dordrecht, The Netherlands, 1992.
28. Carey, W. P., Beebe, K. R., and Kowalski, B. R., Multicomponent analysis using an array of piezoelectric crystal sensors, *Anal. Chem.,* 59, 1529-1534, 1987.
29. Nakamoto, T., Fukuda, A., Moriizumi, T., and Asakura, Y., Improvement of identification capability in an odor sensing system, *Sensors Actuators,* B3, 221-226, 1991.
30. Di Natale, C., Davide, F., D'Amico, A., Hierlemann, A., Schweizer, M., Mitrovics, I., Weimar, U., and Göpel, W., A hybrid neural network for the classification of binary mixtures, Technical Digest of the 5th Int. Meet. Chemical Sensors, Rome, 11-14 July, 1994.
31. Ballantine, D., Rose, S., Grate, J., and Wohltjen, H., Correlation of SAW device coating responses with solubility properties and chemical structure using pattern recognition, *Anal. Chem.,* 48, 3058-3066, 1986.
32. Wohltjen, H. and Dessy, R., Surface acoustic wave probe for chemical analysis. I. Introduction and instrument description. II. Gas chromatography detector, *Anal. Chem.,* 51, 1458, 1979.
33. Bryant, A., Lee, D. L., and Vetelino, J. F., A surface acoustic wave detector, IEEE Ultrasonics Symp. Proc., Chicago, IL, 14-16 Oct., 1981, p. 171.
34. Bryant, A., Poirier, M., Riley, G., Lee, D. L., and Vetelino, J. F., Gas detection using surface acoustic waves delay lines, *Sensors Actuators,* 4, 105, 1983.
35. Vetelino, J. F., Lade, R. K., and Falconer, R. S., Hydrogen sulfide surface acoustic wave gas detector, IEEE Ultrasonics Symp. Proc., Williamsburg, VA, 17-19 Nov., 1986, p. 549.
36. Thoma, R. and Kabitzsch, K., Sensors based on acoustic surface waves, *Radio Fernsehen Elektron.,* 34, 480, 1985.
37. Chuang, C. T. and White, R. M., Sensors utilizing thin membrane SAW oscillators, IEEE Ultrasonics Symp. Proc., Chicago, IL, 14-16 Oct., 1981, pp. 159-162.
38. Zellers, E. T., White, R. M., and Wenzel, S. W., Computer modeling of polymer-coated ZnO/Si surface acoustic wave chemical sensors, *Sensors Actuators,* 14, 35, 1988.
39. Martin, S. J., Ricco, A. J., Ginley, D. S., Zipperian, T. E., and Hanna, S., Isothermal measurements and thermal deposition of organic vapours using SAW devices, *IEEE Trans. Ultrason. Ferroelectrics Frequency Control,* UFFC-34, 142, 1987.
40. Caliendo, C., D'Amico, A., Verardi, P., and Verona, E., Surface acoustic wave hydrogen sensor on silicon substrate, IEEE Ultrasonics Symp. Proc., Chicago, IL, 2-5 Oct., 1988, p. 569.
41. D'Amico, A., Palma, A., and Verona, E., Surface acoustic wave hydrogen sensor, *Sensors Actuators,* 3, 31, 1982.
42. D'Amico, A., Palma, A., and Verona, E., Hydrogen sensor using a palladium coated surface acoustic wave delay-line, IEEE Ultrasonics Symp. Proc., San Diego, CA, 27-29 Oct., 1982, p. 308.
43. D'Amico, A., Gentili, M., Verardi, P., and Verona, E., Gas sensors based on improved SAW devices, Proc. 2nd Int. Meet Chemical Sensors, Bordeaux, France, 7-10 July, 1985, p. 743.
44. D'Amico, A., Palma, A., and Verona, E., Palladium surface acoustic wave interaction for hydrogen detection, *Appl. Phys. Lett.,* 41, 300 1982.
45. D'Amico, A., Petri, A., Verardi, P., and Verona, E., NH_3 surface acoustic wave gas sensor, IEEE Ultrasonic Symp. Proc., Denver, CO, 14-16, Oct., 1987, p. 633.
46. Barendesz, A. W., Vis, J. C., Nieuwenhnizen, M. S., Nieuwkoop, E., Wellekoop, M. J., Ghijsen, W. J., and Venema, A., A SAW chemosensor for NO_2 gas-concentration measurement, IEEE Ultrasonic Symp. Proc., San Francisco, CA, 16-18 Oct., 1985, p. 586.
47. Venema, A., Nieuwkoop, E., Wellekoop, M. J., Ghijsen, W. J., Barendesz, A. W., and Nieuwenhnizen, M. S., NO_2 gas-concentration measurement with a SAW chemisensor, IEEE Trans. Ultrason. Ferroelectrics Frequency Control, UFFC-34, 148, 1987.

48. Venema, A., Nieuwkoop, E., Wellekoop, M. J., Nieuwenhnizen, M. S., and Barendesz, A. W., Design aspect of SAW gas sensors, *Sensors Actuators,* 10 47, 1986.
49. Martin, S. J., Schweizer, K. S., Ricco, A. J., and Zipperian, T. E., Gas sensing with surface acoustic wave devices, Transucers '85 Philadelphia, PA, 11-14 June, 1985, pp. 71-73.
50. Rapp, M., Binz, D., Kabbe, I., Von Schickfus, M., Hunklinger, S., Fuks, H., Schrepp, W., and Fleishmann, B., A new high frequency high sensitivity SAW device for NO_2 gas detection in the sub-ppm range, *Sensors Actuators,* B4, 103, 1991.
51. Holcroft, B. and Roberts, G. G., Surface acoustic wave sensors incorporating Langmuir-Blodgett films, *Thin Solid Films,* 160, 445, 1988.
52. Nitta, M., Kanefusa, S., Ohtani, S., and Haradome, M., Oscillation waveforms of SnO_2-based thick CO sensors, *J. Electron. Mater.,* 13, 15, 1984.
53. Chang, S. M., Tamiya, E., and Karube, I., Chemical vapour sensor using a SAW resonator, *Biosens. Bioelectron.,* 6, 9, 1991.
54. Barger, W. R., Klusty, M. A., Snow, A. W., Grate, J. W., Ballantine, D. S., and Wohltjen, H., Surface acoustic wave sensors, chemiresistor sensors and hybrids using both techniques simultaneously to detect vapors, Symp. Sensor Science Technology, Cleveland, OH, 6-8 Apr., 11987, pp. 198-217.
55. Caliendo, C., D'Amico, A., Furlani, A., Iucci, G., Russo, M. V., and Verona, E., Surface acoustic wave humidity sensor, *Sensors Actuators,* B15-16, 288, 1993.
56. Caliendo, C., D'Amico, A., Furlani, A., Iucci, G., Russo, M. V., and Verona, E., A new surface acoustic wave humidity sensor based on a polyethynylfluorenol membrane, *Sensors Actuators,* B18, 82, 1994.
57. Caliendo, C., D'Amico, A., Furlani, A., Infante, G., Russo, M. V., and Verona, E., Organometallic polymer membrane for gas detection applied to a surface acoustic wave sensor, *Sensors Actuators,* B, 24-25, 670, 1995.
58. Andle, J., Vetelino, J., Lade, M., and McAllister, D., Detection of nucleic acid, hybridization with an acoustic plate mode microsensor, IEEE Ultrasonics Symp. Proc., Honolulu, HI, 4-7 Dec., 1980.
59. Martin, S. J., Ricco, A. J., and Frye, G. C., Sensing in liquids with SH plate mode devices, IEEE Ultrasonics Symp. Proc., Chicago, 2-5 Oct., 1988, p. 607.
60. Caliendo, C., D'Amico, A., Verardi, P., and Verona, E., K+ detection using shear horizontal acoustic modes, IEEE Ultrasonics Symp. Proc. Honolulu, HI, 4-7 Dec., 1990, p. 382.
61. Andle, J. C., Vetelino, J. F., and Lec., R., An acoustic mode immunosensor, IEEE Ultrasonics Symp. Proc., Montreal, 4-6 Oct., 1989, p. 579.
62. Nomura, T. and Yasuda, T., Measurement of velocity and viscosity in liquid using surface acoustic wave delay line, *Jpn. J. Appl. Phys.,* 29, 140, 1990.
63. Shana, Z. and Josse, F., Analysis of liquid phase based sensors utilizing SH waves on rotated y-cut quartz, IEEE Ultrasonics Symp. Proc., Chicago, 2-5 Oct., 1988, p. 549.
64. Ricco, A. J. and Martin, S. J., Acoustic wave viscosity sensor, *Appl. Phys. Lett.,* 50, 21, 1987.
65. Caliendo, C., Fioretto, D., Socino, G., and Verona, E., Determination of viscoelastic constants of thin films by acoustic plate modes, IEEE Ultrasonics Symp. Proc., Orlando, FL, 8-11 Dec., 1991, p. 387.
66. Caliendo, C., Carlotti, G., Fioretto, D., Palmieri, L., Socino, G., Verdini, L., and Verona, E., Absorption and velocity dispersion of acoustic waves in polyacrylate films, IEEE Ultrasonics Symp. Proc., Tucson, AZ, 20-23 Oct., 1992.
67. Niemczyk, T. M., Martin, S. J., Frye, G. C., and Ricco, A. J., Acoustoelectric interaction of plate modes with solutions, *J. Appl. Phys.,* 64, 5002, 1988.
68. Lucklum, R., Henning, B., Hauptmann, P., Schierbaum, K. D., and Vaihinger, S., Quartz microbalance sensors for gas detection, *Sensors Actuators,* A25-27, 705-710, 1991.
69. Hlavay, J. and Guibault, G. G., Applications of the piezoelectric crystals detector in analytical chemistry, *Anal. Chem.,* 49, 1890-1898, 1977.
70. Nakamoto, T., Fukuda, A., and Moriizumi, T., Improvement of identification capability in an odor-sensing system, *Sensors Actuators,* B3, 221-226, 1991.
71. Nakamoto, T., Fukuda, A., and Moriizumi, T., Perfume and flavour identification by odour-sensing system using quartz resonator sensor array and neural-network pattern recognition, *Sensors Actuators,* B10, 85-90, 1993.

Part III

Metabolism and Bioaffinity Sensors for Medicine, Food, and the Environment

10 Mediated Amperometric Biosensors

Stephen F. White and Anthony P. F. Turner

CONTENTS

10.1 INTRODUCTION

A realistic estimate of the worldwide market for biosensors is around $360 million by 1996, $700 million by the year 2000, and then rising sharply.[1] Probably the greatest impact from this burgeoning development will be felt in the field of medicine, particularly home diagnostic test kits. The current market for biosensors is dominated by mediated amperometric devices for glucose analysis. Undoubtedly, the introduction of the ExacTech glucose sensor, with annual sales of around $100 million, has helped to enhance the quality of life for many people suffering from diabetes. This is a rapid and reliable method for determining the concentration of blood glucose, carried out by means of a "user friendly" diagnostic tool. At the heart of this device lies a mediated biosensor. By adapting some of the methods of mass production used in the electronics industry, cheap disposable "one-shot" biosensors can be produced. Screen-printing (Figure 10.1) can be employed to produce a range of practical biosensor designs (Figure 10.2). In the near future the routine determination of a number of analytes may more readily be realized using mediated biosensor technology. A large European-wide research effort[2] is currently underway to develop *in vivo* sensors for a range of analytes

0-8493-8905-4/97/$0.00+$.50
© 1997 by CRC Press, Inc.

including glucose. For the glucose sensors the initial aim is to develop an implantable "hypoglycaemia alarm system"[3] capable of providing an early warning system, alerting the wearer to serious fluctuations in blood glucose. This may be based on a simple needle-type sensor, capable of being implanted in the subcutaneous tissue of the patient.

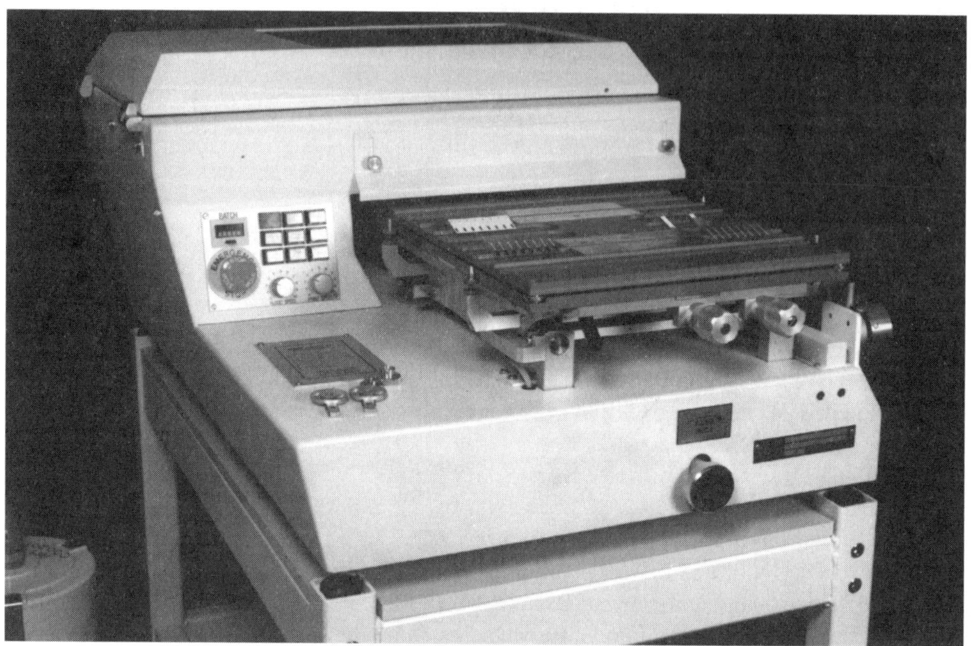

FIGURE 10.1 Screen printer used for the mass production of biosensors.

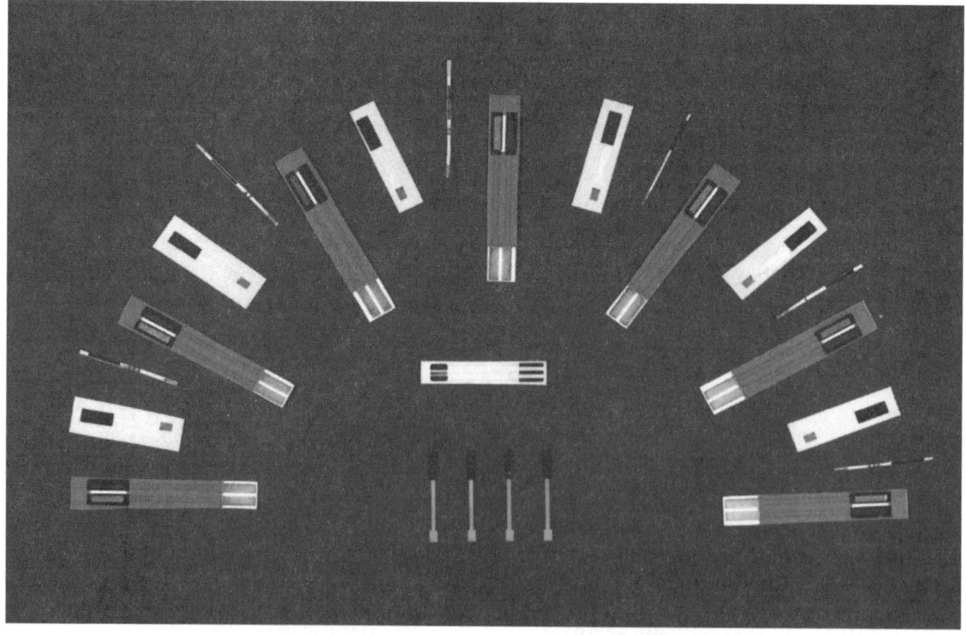

FIGURE 10.2 Range of biosensor designs fabricated using screen printing.

In other fields of activity, mediated biosensors are steadily being applied to a range of analytical tasks. Environmental monitoring is a task that is generally carried out at a site that can provide centralised laboratory facilities. In one scenario biosensor technology could provide small portable (perhaps hand-held) dedicated devices allowing rapid pollution detection in the field. Furthermore, operating "at-site" using on-line techniques, biosensors can monitor automatically both the presence and concentration of a known potential pollutant at remote sites. Water analysis has been the first area of environmental monitoring to be tackled by biosensors, because of the relative ease of using these devices in this medium (compared to air or soil sampling). The range of pollutants that could potentially be monitored in both freshwater supplies and seawater includes pesticides, herbicides, heavy metals, toxins, and other chemical residues.

Another potential growth area for biosensor use is the food industry. The demands for higher standards both in terms of quality and nutritional value seem set to increase. Government regulations (hygiene and consumer protection), and the needs of customers will have to be met in a highly competitive climate. The advent and continuing growth in demand for convenience foods, requiring specialised preservation and storage techniques, present an opportunity for biosensors where the detection of contamination (either deliberate or accidental) could be registered at an early stage. In addition, biosensors may be developed to monitor the quality of raw foodstuffs and their subsequent processing. Again, on-line monitoring with sensors may hold the key to maintaining the integrity of the food items being produced.

Overall, the range of biosensor research and development is truly on a global scale. Major conferences on biosensors are typically attended by people from over 60 countries and from every continent. Over a thousand papers and patents are published every year on the subject[4] and national programmes are in place throughout Europe and in as diverse locations as Russia, China, India, and Japan.

This chapter aims to outline the basic electrochemistry that underpins an important segment of current research: mediated amperometric biosensors. In addition, some of the recent applications (in the areas of medicine, food analysis, and environmental monitoring) of these devices will be reviewed.

10.2 BASIC ELECTROCHEMISTRY WITH MEDIATORS

The previous chapter presented a brief overview of the role of mediators in the successful operation of biosensors. A list of desirable characteristics was matched with a description of both the advantages and disadvantages of using these compounds. To understand fully how these compounds work and to appreciate any future contribution made by mediators to the continuing development of biosensors, it is necessary to explore further the parameters that control and influence their operation.

10.2.1 ELECTROCHEMISTRY

As a starting point it is worth remembering that amperometry is dominated by the presence of a heterogeneous system. An electrochemically active species can only be detected at the interface between the electrode and the electrolyte. When in operation, this will tend to have repercussions on the distribution of the analyte throughout the sample solution. The effect will be to encourage diffusion within the sample solution, in fact leading to the creation of a diffusion layer at the surface of the electrode. Furthermore, when the electrode is poised at a sufficient potential, an electronic double layer will be formed. This layer is formed by the distribution of mobile electrons on the electrode surface, paired with corresponding (opposite charge) ions on the solution side. This is an effect caused by the ability of conducting phases, such as electrolytes and metals, to concentrate excess charge on their boundaries. Overall, the dimensions of this layer can be measured in nanometres (tens of Angstroms).

A number of factors can affect the electrode reaction rate (or current) including:

1. The electron transfer at the electrode.
2. Mass transport; generally considered to be part of an overall mechanism involving diffusion (e.g., random molecular motion), convection (circulation flow, e.g., due to stirring), and migration (e.g., the movement of ions along an electric field).
3. Chemical reactions that either proceed or follow the electron transfer, e.g., protonations, dimerizations, or catalytic decompositions on the electrode surface.
4. Surface effects such as adsorption and desorption.

The majority of amperometric biosensors demonstrated to date have used a three-electrode system (although two-electrode systems are more common in commercial devices). One electrode is the "working electrode" where the biological sensing element is immobilised. When a positive potential is applied, any molecule that is oxidised will relinquish electrons to the electrode. If left unchecked, this would eventually lead to the generation of a large potential difference (because of the stoichiometric imbalance). To overcome this pitfall, a second "counter electrode" is included in the system. The function of this electrode is to complete the circuit, hence the electrons can pass (via the external circuit) back into solution under the pressure of the power supply. Obviously this leads to a reduction process occurring at the counter electrode, equal in magnitude to the oxidation occurring at the working electrode. This flow of electrons will be the current, generated by the biosensor, that is measured and correlated with the presence of a desired analyte. The third electrode in the system is the reference electrode. This electrode will be composed of a material of known chemical composition, containing both forms of a redox couple, e.g., $Hg/HgCl_2$ (saturated calomel electrode), Ag/AgCl (silver/silver chloride electrode). The internationally accepted primary reference couple has been designated the standard hydrogen electrode reaction (SHE). Reference potentials are usually quoted with respect to this reaction. For example, the potential of the saturated calomel electrode (SCE) is 0.242 V vs. the SHE. Because its potential is fixed, the reference electrode provides a stable reference point against which the working electrode can be measured. Therefore the potential of the working electrode is controlled with respect to the reference electrode. As a general rule of electrochemistry, both current and potential cannot be controlled simultaneously.

In practice, two types of reactions occur at an electrode. One category involves the process outlined above where electron charges are transferred across the electrode/solution interface, i.e., oxidation and reduction. Because they obey Faraday's law (the amount of chemical reaction caused by the flow of current is proportional to the amount of electricity passed) these events are termed faradic processes. In contrast, nonfaradic currents can occur when charge does not cross the electrode/solution interface. These external currents are generated by changes in the potential, electrode area, and solution composition initiated by processes such as adsorption and desorption. In addition, a capacitive charge will be generated at the electrode surface as a result of redistribution of charged and polar species. Generally, both faradic and nonfaradic currents will be generated when an electrode reaction takes place. In contrast, if a strongly oxidising or reducing potential is applied and the rate of electron transfer between the redox species and the electrode is fast, the faradic current will be controlled by the rate of diffusion to the electrode.

Closer examination of the double layer reveals an area, close to the electrode surface, where the electron transfer actually occurs. This area is made up of several layers and is known as the Helmholtz layer. The inner layer (or inner Helmholtz layer) closest to the electrode is composed of solvated ions arranged in an orderly manner, directly opposite the electrode. Immediately behind this layer is a diffuse band of ions, forming a discontinuous range of potentials (the outer Helmholtz layer, OHP), with the potential increasing linearly with distance from the electrode surface to the edge of the OHP. The interaction of the solvated ions with the electrode involves only long-distance electrostatic forces. Furthermore, the excess charge at the outer layer is taken to be equal and opposite to the excess charge on the surface of the electrode. The thickness of this diffuse band will be determined by the total ionic concentration in the solution.

Overall, the effect of the potential difference across the double layer will be to assist the transfer of an ion through the double layer in one direction, whilst impeding its passage in the opposite direction. In effect this will lead to an increase in the potential on an ion moving from the solution to the electrode surface. To get from the OHP to the electrode an ion must surmount an energy barrier. As a consequence of the discontinuity in the potential range, the distance of this transition state from the OHP is some fraction β (the symmetry factor) of the total distance. This leads to a general expression for the intrinsic charge transfer rate constant:

$$k = C \exp - [(G^{\#\#} + \beta nEF)/RT]$$

where C is a constant, $G^{\#\#}$ is the free Gibbs energy of activation, n the number of electrons transferred, E the potential, and F the Faraday constant.

Generally, the rate of an electrochemical reaction at an electrode (where the surface area can be determined accurately) is expressed as a rate per unit surface area. This is usually stated in terms of current density (i), where the current is divided by the area. Using this convention, the Butler-Volmer equation (one of the most important in electrochemistry) can be used to express the relationship between the rate of a reaction (*i*) and the potential difference across the electrode-solution interface. Overall, the size of the current at a given potential will be determined by the Butler-Volmer equation for both the forward and backward reactions:

$$i = i_e [\exp\{(1 - \beta)FE/RT\} - \exp\{-\beta FE/RT\}]$$

When the equilibrium potential is applied, there is no net reaction occurring and i_e (the exchange current density) is equal for both oxidation and reduction; in this case *i* is equal to zero. If the applied potential is changed from the equilibrium value (termed the overpotential) then the corresponding current (both in terms of magnitude and direction) will alter.

At large positive values for the overpotential, the first exponential term in the Butler-Volmer equation will tend to dominate and the second term can be disregarded. In contrast, at large reducing potentials the second term of the expression will dominate. At small (positive and negative) values for the overpotential both terms must be considered.

Increasing the overpotential beyond the equilibrium potential will result in an exponential rise in current until a point is reached where the diffusion of the electroactive species to the electrode (not the electrode kinetics) will become a limiting factor. If it is assumed that linear diffusion to a planar electrode is occurring, the current profile over this range can be described by adapting Fick's second law of diffusion in one dimension. This derivation is known as the Cottrell equation:

$$i_t = \frac{nFD^{1/2}C_o}{pi^{1/2}t^{1/2}}$$

where D is the diffusion coefficient and t the time. From this expression it can be seen that the current will decay with respect to $t^{1/2}$.

10.2.2 Cyclic Voltammetry

Cyclic voltammetry is an analytical technique that has proved to be a valuable tool for determining a range of electrochemical parameters. In particular, for deriving the characteristics of mediating compounds for use in biosensors. A range of factors including redox potential, electrochemical rate constant, and stability can be successfully determined using this approach. The technique is based on sweeping the potential (over a predetermined range) applied to a working electrode immersed in a quiescent solution between two limits at a fixed scan rate. From one of the fixed limits the potential is changed linearly with time; when the second limit is reached the potential direction is reversed. As the potential alters, the current output is recorded and a current-potential voltammogram is generated. An electrochemically active species displays a reversible reduction pathway such as:

$$O + ne^- \rightleftarrows R$$

where O is the oxidised form, R is the reduced form, and ne^- is the number of electrons transferred.

Under conditions of the application of a positive potential, the surface concentration of O will change according to the Nernst equation:

$$[O]/[R] = \exp\,[(nF/RT)\,(E - E^o)]$$

where E is the applied potential, E^o the redox potential, R is the gas constant, and T the temperature. When the reaction is under diffusional control, the concentration of oxidised species (under reducing conditions) will be related to the magnitude of the current observed. Characteristically, the current will increase with increasing potential. Eventually this will lead to a rapid depletion in the concentration of oxidised species in the region around the electrode surface. This event is shown by a reduction in the current and will be depicted by a peak in the cyclic voltammogram. As the potential sweep is reversed, reoxidation occurs and a second peak will be generated by the initial rise in the current followed by a decrease in the concentration of reduced species. For a reversible one-electron reaction, the peak-to-peak separation will be 57 mV and the anodic and cathodic currents will be the same. Furthermore, the peak potentials are independent of the scan rate. With planar diffusion, the magnitude of both currents can be described by the Randles-Sevik equation:

$$I = -2.69 \times 10^5\, n^{3/2} C_o D^{1/2} \nu^{1/2}$$

where $\nu^{1/2}$ is the square root of the scan speed and $D^{1/2}$ is a diffusion coefficient. The peak currents will be proportional to $v^{1/2}$ and the ratio of the anodic to cathodic peak currents is equal to unity.

Furthermore, with a perfectly reversible system the half-wave potential ($E_{1/2}$) will be equal to the equilibrium potential, i.e., the potential at which both the oxidised and reduced forms are present, in the same concentrations, at the electrode surface.

By coupling a reversible electron transfer step with a catalytic compound such as an enzyme, the reaction will proceed by the following pathway:

$$R + e^- \longrightarrow O; \quad \text{Enzyme} + O \xrightarrow{K_{cat}} R$$

where O and R represent the oxidised or reduced forms of the electrochemically active species, respectively, and K_{cat} is a pseudo first-order rate constant. With this system, the reduced form can be regenerated by the reaction of the enzyme. If the value of k_{cat} is small, then the enzymatic reaction will not have a dramatic effect on the shape of the voltammogram and a plot typical of the reversible system will be generated. In contrast, if a large value for k_{cat} is obtained and the reduced species is being rapidly regenerated by the enzyme, then the observed cyclic voltammogram will alter radically. The depletion of reduced species, through oxidation, will be complemented by the increased concentration of reduced species via the enzymatic reaction. The effect of this will be to generate a plateau response, instead of a peak. Furthermore, the catalytic removal of oxidised species will lead to the elimination of the cathodic peak. The plateau current is expressed by the following equation:

$$i = nFAC_o\ (D_o k_{cat})^{1/2}/1 + \exp[nF/RT(E - E_{1/2})]$$

where D_o is the diffusion coefficient of the electroactive species, A is the area of the electrode, C_o is the concentration of O in the bulk solution, and $E_{1/2}$ is the half-wave potential. The value of k_{cat} can be determined experimentally using the ratio between the diffusion controlled current (i_d) and the catalytic current (i_k).[5]

Using these data, it is possible to verify that a catalytically coupled reaction is occurring. By plotting the current function against the sweep rate of the voltammogram, a distinction can be made between the peak currents in the presence and absence of enzyme. When the current is controlled by the enzymatic coupled reaction, the kinetic current is related to the diffusional current by $(kRT/nFv)^{1/2}$. This can be termed as a kinetic parameter k_{cat}/a, where $a = nFV/RT$. A plot of i_k/i_d against the sweep rate can be used to determine the slope k_{cat}/a values. These results can be used to determine where the current is under kinetic, diffusional, or mixed control. Plotting values for (k_{cat}/a) against V^{-1} will, under pseudo first-order rate conditions, give a good estimate of the value for k_{cat}. Furthermore, a plot of k_{cat} against known concentrations of enzyme will be linear, from which the k_s (the homogeneous second-order rate constant for catalysis) value can be determined.

In effect, these experiments (involving cyclic voltammetry, mediators, and enzyme coupled systems) can be used to characterise the performance of a selected mediator for a particular biosensor application. Chiefly, this includes the electrochemically determined rate constants and the redox potential.

One drawback that has hampered the development of biosensors based on mediators concerns the stability of these devices. For many applications the mediator is adsorbed directly on to the surface of a suitable electrode. In fact, the overall mechanism of mediation relies on a certain degree of solubilisation occurring at the electrode-solution interface. As an example, ferrocene (or its derivatives) was originally[6] deposited in an organic phase onto the electrode surface. Hence, when the sensor was operated in an aqueous phase the insoluble mediator was held at the surface. When the working electrode is poised at an oxidising potential, ferricinium ions are produced. These ions are more readily soluble in the aqueous phase and a significant loss of mediator can occur. To overcome this disadvantage, stable, mediated, modified conducting polymers have been constructed and investigated. For example,[7] glucose sensors were constructed incorporating gold microelectrodes modified with a polypyrrole. The polymerisation of pyrrole has been used in the construction of numerous sensors. One attraction to using this polymer lies in the easily controlled manner of its deposition, e.g., it will only polymerise at an electroactive surface. Enzymes and other molecules such as mediators can be entrapped in the polymer. Furthermore, the chemical and physical properties of the film can be changed by altering experimental factors such as pH, the applied potential, or ionic concentration. Dicks et al.[7] deposited the polypyrrole film from a solution of acetonitrile, then ferrocenecarbonyl chloride was covalently coupled to the film. By optimising the sensor fabrication process, the authors were able to construct a biosensor that was stable in the presence of a saturating glucose solution for 5 days with only a 5% decline in response.

Another recent[8] approach to overcoming the problem of mediator washout was to embed the mediator and enzyme in a colloidal graphite emulsion matrix. In order to entrap the mediator, a cationic membrane was fixed over the immobilisation layer. Electrostatic repulsion, between the positively charged membrane and the positive ferricinium ions effectively trapped the mediator at the electrode surface. The electrodes were claimed to be easily fabricated and produced a rapid response over a significant linear range of glucose. Furthermore, the electrodes could be stored dry, losing 30% of their activity after 6 months.

Another important contribution has been the approach to modify the enzyme by covalent attachment of the mediator to the protein.[9] By the use of electron relay centres, electrical contact between the redox active centre of glucose oxidase and the bare electrode surface was achieved.

10.3 MEDIATED BIOSENSORS FOR CLINICAL USE

The following describes just a few of the numerous mediated amperometric biosensors that have recently been reported. With a rapidly developing and diversified field of research such as clinical sensing devices, it would be impossible to cover every facet of recent work. To obtain an in-depth understanding and to follow this evolving technology the reader is advised to consult dedicated journals (such as Biosensors & Bioelectronics, Elsevier, Oxford) and recent publications (such as Advances in Biosensors, JAI Press, London). The most widely used reaction involves glucose oxidase with a ferrocene derivative as mediator. Many variations on this approach have been published.[4,10] Despite the prevalence of glucose sensors, however, a range of other clinically important analytes has also been monitored using mediated biosensors.

10.3.1 Glucose

The evolution of amperometric glucose electrodes has been one of the cornerstones of biosensor development. An enormous number of these sensors have been described and it would be impossible in one short chapter to describe even a fraction of this work. Instead, we choose to mention one of the most important areas for glucose monitoring. Probably the greatest challenge for the clinical monitoring of blood glucose levels will be the development of in *vivo* sensors. The idea for in *vivo* monitoring of glucose, using an enzyme electrode incorporating glucose oxidase, was suggested by Clark[11] almost 30 years ago. Before this goal can be accomplished a number of hurdles will have to be overcome:[4] first and foremost, the sensor must not be detrimental to the health of the patient; calibration of the biosensor (*in situ*) may be difficult; electrochemical interferences (e.g., ascorbic acid and acetaminophen) susceptible to oxidation at the electrode surface may interfere with the signal; implantation of the sensor device will trigger an immune response that could alter the local levels of glucose, leading to an inaccurate signal (biocompatability and biostability are linked to this last point); and the sensor must operate for a significant period of time to avoid frequent replacement.

Several mediator-based sensors, for *in vivo* monitoring of glucose have been described. In one example, the sensor[3] used in an implantation experiment was based on the mediator dimethylferrocene. The enzyme glucose oxidase was immobilised on Sepharose® beads and retained (with the mediator) in a 22-G Teflon® cannula. A dialysis membrane was secured over the exposed surface of the electrode. The sensor was implanted in the subcutaneous tissue of a nondiabetic human and was used to monitor blood glucose levels during a 75-g oral glucose tolerance test.

A recent publication[12] listed 23 designs for glucose sensors; around half of these sensors have been tested in *vivo*. Almost all of these sensors were amperometric enzyme electrodes, two of which were mediator based (the ferrocene sensor previously described and a second sensor based on the conducting salt TTF^+TCNQ^-, operating at a potential of +250 mV).

One problem that could occur from using mediators for *in vivo* applications concerns their possible toxicity. The lethal dose (LD_{50}) and the maximum dose (MTD) of 7,7,8,8-tetracyanoquinodimethane (TCNQ) and TTF were recently experimentally assessed[13] by single dose administration to CBA-line mice. Blood constitution, accumulation, acute and subacute dermal and eye irritation, skin sensitization, and delayed type hypersensitivity were all investigated. The authors' findings indicated that both TCNQ and TTF were low toxicity compounds. Other reports have highlighted the leaching of ferricinium ions originating from 1,1-dimethylferrocene when the mediator was incorporated into a glucose sensor. In this instance, the mediator was simply adsorbed on the surface of a graphite electrode. This has obvious implications for any *in vivo* sensor fabricated using these compounds, where sensitivity to ferrocene and its derivatives may pose a problem. A retention mechanism must be a priority, to prevent possible poisoning from free ferricinium ions.

10.3.2 Cholesterol

Tentative links between the frequency of high concentrations of cholesterol, in human serum, and cardiovascular disease have been made. Hence a rapid, reliable, and cost effective way of either mass screening or individual home monitoring may assist in assessing the concentration of the analyte. Normal human serum is reported to contain from 1.29 to 2.07mM free cholesterol and 3.36 to 6.47mM total cholesterol.

A number of mediated amperometric biosensors for cholesterol determination have been described. Using ferrocene as the mediator and a selection of different enzymes, three different routes were recently outlined.[14] One scheme involved the enzymes cholesterol esterase, cholesterol dehydrogenase, and diaphorase (an enzyme known to react readily with ferrocene). The reaction was initiated by the liberation of cholesterol from cholesterol esters by cholesterol esterase. Cholesterol dehydrogenase catalysed the oxidation of cholesterol to cholesterone. As a result of this reaction NAD was reduced to NADH, which in turn led to the reduction of diaphorase. This enzyme reduced ferricinium to ferrocene. Finally, the ferrocene generated was oxidised at a suitable potential. Hence the current could be related to the concentration of cholesterol in the sample. Cholesterol concentrations up to 1 mM could be determined, but the sensor was sensitive to the surfactants used to extricate cholesterol esters from lipoprotein complexes in serum.

A second approach was to use the enzyme cholesterol oxidase purified from *Schizophylum commune*. Again, cholesterol esterase was used to isolate free cholesterol. Reduction of the cholesterol oxidase by the oxidation of cholesterol was followed by oxidation by ferricinium ions. The ferrocene produced was subsequently oxidised at the electrode.

A third approach was to use the two enzymes cholesterol oxidase and cholesterol esterase, with a third enzyme, peroxidase. The enzyme peroxidase can detect the presence of hydrogen peroxide, a product of the oxidase reaction. During the catalytic cycle, peroxidase is oxidised. Ferrocene can act as electron donor to the peroxidase; in doing so it is oxidised to ferricinium. By reducing the ferricinium ions back to ferrocene, using an electrode poised at a reducing current, accurate measurements of cholesterol measurements could be made. The authors state that the third approach was the most successful, with the other two methods suffering from inhibition effects and a narrow pH range (for cholesterol oxidase from *Schizophylum commune*).

Microelectrodes have several advantages over the use of traditional macroelectrodes. For *in vivo* use, the much smaller dimensions of microelectrodes will assist in the implantation of the sensor into tissue. Because these electrodes only draw a small current (sometimes as low as 10^{-17}A[8]) they may operate in the virtual absence of a supporting electrolyte. This may be an important consideration where the oxidation wave of an electrolyte may disguise the current-voltage profile of the analyte. Other important advantages include an enhanced signal-to-noise ratio (enabling lower limits of detection to be ascertained, again particularly of interest for *in vivo* applications), and the fact that the electrodes can operate easily in flow systems where their response is less flow dependent (compared to macroelectrodes).

One recent report[15] described the use of microelectrodes constructed from platinum to measure cholesterol. These sensors were prepared by etching a cavity in the tip of the electrode and packing this hole with a porous composite material. Contained within this packing material was the redox mediator $Os(bpy)_3(PFG)_2$ embedded in a Teflon® emulsion. The mediator was synthesised from osmium II chloride and loaded onto the electrode using cyclic voltammetry. The enzymes used to fabricate the sensors, cholesterol oxidase and cholesterol esterase, were immobilised by adsorption over the mediator surface. By using microelectrodes, the authors stated that reproducible steady, state currents could be obtained without forced convection because of the high mass transport rate per unit area of sensor surface. Furthermore, the limiting current was insensitive to fluctuations in natural convection in bulk solution. The cholesterol sensor produced constant values for up to 60 days and the cholesterol esterase-based sensor 20 days.

10.3.3 Lactate

The overproduction of lactate, resulting from a depletion of oxygen in tissue, has been recognised as a major factor in the development of metabolic acidosis. Increases in the concentration of blood lactate levels indicate a change to anaerobic metabolism in working skeletal muscles. By monitoring the anaerobic threshold (via lactate determination) of patients who have suffered a severe heart failure, it may be possible to ascertain the severity of the ailment.[26] Determining the concentration of lactate in blood can be used to assess the degree of acidosis that may occur after surgery.[17] Other areas of clinical interest include measurement of lactate in foetal blood[18] and in cerebrospinal fluid[19] for the diagnosis of meningitis. In the field of veterinary medicine, lactate determination has an important role to play, e.g., assessing the adequacy of training programmes for horses and lactate acidosis in ruminants.

A number of mediated biosensors for lactate determination have been described. The enzyme lactate oxidase has been shown to couple with a range of mediators, including ferrocene derivatives.[20,21] A bienzyme amperometric lactate-specific electrode, incorporating the enzymes lactate dehydrogenase and diaphorase, was recently reported.[22] The sensor operated by initially oxidising lactate by muscle lactate dehydrogenase, resulting in the reduction of NAD:

$$CH_3CHOHCOO^- + NAD^+ \rightarrow CH_3CHOHCOO^- + NADH + H^+$$

NADH was oxidised by the mediator hexacyanoferrate (II), catalysed by diaphorase:

$$NADH + 2Fe(CN)_6^{3-} \rightarrow NAD^+ + 2Fe(CN)_6^{4-} + H^+$$

The $Fe(CN)_6^{4-}$ was subsequently oxidised at a platinum electrode poised at a potential of +300 mV vs. a SCE reference electrode. By relating steady-state currents to lactate concentrations, the linear range of these sensors was from 0.2 to 8 mM.

The application of mediators with carbon paste electrodes has recently been described.[23] Mixed carbon paste electrodes were constructed by doping the paste with a biological element (e.g., enzyme or microorganism) and the mediator. This approach resulted in sensors that could provide a fast response, low cost, and the possibility of miniaturisation. The authors prepared the electrodes by mixing known concentrations of the enzyme lactate oxidase, graphite powder, and mediator (i.e., ferrocene; 1,1-dimethylferrocene; *N,N*-dimethylaminomethyl-ferrocene; Meldola blue) in paraffin oil. Following mixing, the paste was packed into Teflon® tubing and electrical contact was made via a platinum wire. Sensors based on ferrocene and its derivatives operated at a potential of between 200 and 400 mV (vs. SCE) and the electrodes incorporating Meldola blue at 50 to 250 mV. Variations in the dynamic ranges were observed between all the sensors. The ferrocene-based sensors were sensitive to ascorbic acid, a known electrochemically active species present in blood. This finding would inhibit the sensors' use in real samples. To overcome this problem it would be necessary to incorporate a selective membrane, a practice common in the fabrication of other biosensor systems, to screen out ascorbate and other possible interferents. In contrast, the response to ascorbate was significantly lower (5.3% compared to 83% for dimethylferrocene) and the sensitivity was higher for electrodes based on Meldola blue.

Another mediator that has been shown to couple successfully with lactate oxidase is tetrathiafulvalene[24] (TTF). Previously, TTF had been shown to be a good mediator for facilitating electron transfer from glucose oxidase to graphite electrodes. These sensors were constructed using carbon foil as the base electrode. The TTF was absorbed directly onto the electrode from a solution of mediator in acetone. Following enzyme immobilisation, the electrodes were tested over a range of lactate concentrations. The reaction profile was as follows:

$$\text{lactate} + 2\text{TTF}^{+} \rightarrow \text{pyruvate} + 2\text{TTF}^{+} + 2\text{H}^{+}$$

$$2\text{TTF}^{+} \rightarrow + 2\text{e} \ (200 \text{ mV vs. Ag/AgCl})$$

Lactate is catalysed to pyruvate by the enzyme. Subsequently, TTF oxidises the enzyme, i.e., it is a competitor with oxygen. Anodic oxidation of the reduced mediator is related to concentrations of lactate present in the sample. The authors suggest that this approach may be applicable to the mass production of one-shot disposable lactate sensors.

10.3.4 Theophylline

Apart from metabolites, mediated biosensors have also been developed to monitor other compounds of clinical interest. Theophylline (1,3-dimethylxanthine) is a widely prescribed drug for the treatment of asthma and other pulmonary conditions. It is a bronchodilator and respiratory stimulant. The drug requires strict therapeutic control within a narrow range (10 to 20 mg l^{-1}). Concentrations in excess can be toxic and dosage below the range is ineffective. Potential biosensors for monitoring theophylline were constructed,[25] based on the catalysed oxidation of theophylline oxidase, a haem-containing enzyme. Several mediated systems were investigated with NMP (phenazine methasulphate); TCNQ providing the most favourable response. Sensors based on this conducting salt (operating at an applied potential of +100 mV vs. Ag/AgCl) produced a linear response comparable to the clinically relevant range. In addition, no electrochemical interference was reported from caffeine, theobromine, or 3-methylxanthine at levels up to 100 mg l^{-1}.

10.3.5 Acetylcholine

Acetylcholine has been recognised as an important neurotransmitter, and choline is its metabolite. A recent report[26] described the fabrication and operation of a mediated biosensor, based on TTF, to determine acetylcholine concentrations. The sensors were constructed using carbon paste electrodes and prepared with a mixture of TTF, choline oxidase, and acetylcholinesterase in paraffin oil. Overall, the reaction scheme was as follows:

$$\text{acetylcholine} + H_2O \rightarrow \text{choline} + \text{acetic acid}$$

$$\text{choline oxidase (FAD)}$$

$$\text{choline} \rightarrow \text{betine aldehyde} + \text{choline oxidase } (FADH_2)$$

$$\text{choline oxidase } (FADH_2) + 2TTF^+ \rightarrow \text{choline oxidase (FAD)} + 2TTF + 2H^+$$

$$2TTF \rightarrow 2TTF^+ + 2e^- \text{ (at the electrode)}$$

Tetrathiafulvalene was found to act as an efficient mediator between the flavin redox centre of choline oxidase and the carbon electrode. The sensors were operated at an applied potential of +200 mV (vs. SCE), where the lower level of detection was 0.5 μM acetylcholine. Operating at this potential, the sensors had a linear range that extended up to 400 μM acetylcholine. Despite these results, the authors noted that for a practical sensor to monitor neurochemical applications the lower limit of detection must be reduced. Furthermore the response time must be reduced to no more then a few seconds, compared to the 30 s recorded for these sensors.

10.3.6 Electrochemical Immunoassays

The development of electrochemical immunoassays is another important area of clinical diagnostics that has been investigated using mediated amperometric sensors. Conventional immunoassays are based on detecting radioactivity, which has obvious disadvantages in terms of complex measuring instruments, long assay times, and potential health hazards. Electrochemically based immunoassays, incorporating mediators have recently been demonstrated and point the way to a faster, more sensitive approach.

Using an enzyme amplification system, based on the enzymes alcohol dehydrogenase and diaphorase, a number of selected antigens have been successfully determined using this approach. One investigation involved the detection of the thyroid stimulating hormone[27] thyrotropin. The method was based on a two-site immunoassay involving two monoclonal antibodies directed against nonoverlapping epitopes. One antibody, labelled with the enzyme alkaline phosphatase, was mixed with sample solution and added to a microtitre plate coated with the second antibody. Following an immunoincubation and washing period, the activity of the dual antibody-antigen "sandwich" was determined using the enzyme amplification system. The initial step involves the dephosphorylation of $NADP^+$ to NAD by the enzyme alkaline phosphatase, in proportion to the bound label. Alcohol dehydrogenase then catalyses the oxidation of ethanol to acetylaldehyde, utilising the NAD produced by the first reaction. Diaphorase then acts to oxidise NAD back to $NADH^+$, which in turn leads to the reduction of two molecules of hexacyanoferrate III to hexacynanoferrate II. This compound is subsequently oxidised at a graphite electrode. The current produced by this oxidation was integrated for 10 s and the charge consumed was used to construct a calibration graph related to the concentration of antigen. Published results showed that the lower limit of detection was 0.046 mIU/L and the sensor system had a dynamic range between 0 and 2.5 mIU/L. This approach had earlier been used to fabricate a system for determining prostatic acid phosphatase.[28]

10.4 MEDIATED BIOSENSORS FOR FOOD ANALYSIS

Mediated biosensors have the potential to play a significant role in the food industry. A number of biosensor systems, principally aimed at this sector, have been described. Again, only a few selected systems are described here.

10.4.1 Glucose

Glucose determination, particularly in fermentation processes, can form an important part of process monitoring. For this particular application the sensor must be robust, simple to operate, and have a significantly long lifetime. Generally, there are two approaches to using biosensors for process monitoring (not including off-line analysis): *in situ* and on-line. The use of *in situ* sensors provides advantages in terms of a rapid real time measurement and reduced problems from sample-taking, i.e., risks of contamination when extracting samples from the fermenter. However, the sensor must be sterilizable and not prone to contamination from cells or cell debris (present in the process vessel). In addition, it must be free from reagents that could leach out and contaminate the fermenting liquid. Furthermore, calibration of the sensor must be possible during the fermentation.

An improved mediated glucose enzyme electrode for the *in situ* monitoring of glucose during a baker's yeast fermentation, has been described.[29] A two-part fermenter probe, based on a design described by Bradley et al.,[30] was constructed (Figure 10.3). The inner part contained the enzyme electrode, composed of four working electrodes, modified with the mediator 1,1-dimethylferrocene. Glucose oxidase was immobilised on three of the electrodes; the fourth mediated electrode was used to provide a stable baseline signal. Sterility was maintained by the use of polycarbonate (of 0.015 μm pore size) and metal membranes (of 2 μm pore size), enclosing the outer housing. The sensor could be calibrated *in situ* by the use of a continuous stream of buffer that flowed between the outer housing and the enzyme electrode. Operating at a potential of +220 mV vs. a centrally located Ag/AgCl reference electrode, the sensor was used to monitor glucose pulses introduced into the fermenter. After 4 days of continuous use the sensor recorded a 15% loss in response. The authors state that the linear range of the sensor was up to 10 g l^{-1} and the correlation with off-line analysis was acceptable.

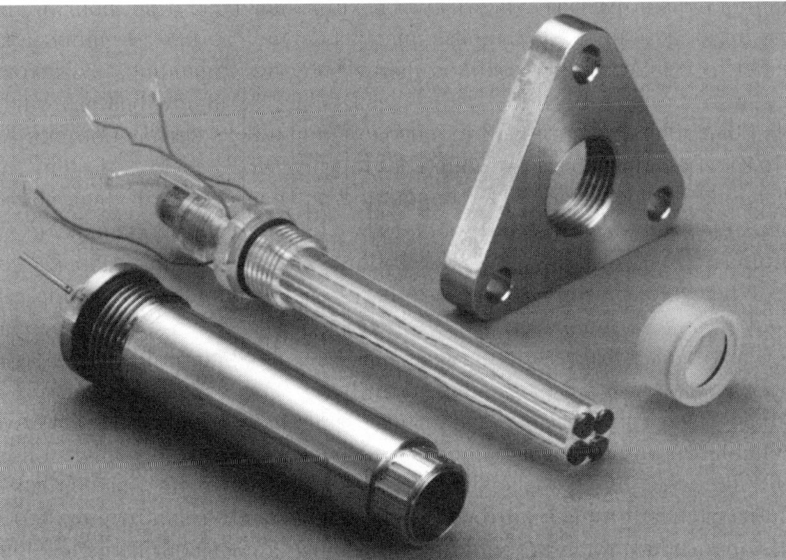

FIGURE 10.3 Mediated biosensors used for *in situ* fermentation broth monitoring (clearly shown are the four sensing heads of the device).

10.4.2 Glutamate

Apart from its role as a neurotransmitter, glutamate is an important compound in the food industry. Added to many foodstuffs as a flavour enhancer, the amount of glutamate present can be used to evaluate an aspect of food quality. The following describes three different approaches that have been used to construct mediated biosensors for glutamate determination.

The use of a flexible redox polymer to enhance electrical communication between L-glutamate oxidase and a conventional carbon electrode was recently described.[31] Glutamate oxidase catalysed the following reaction:

$$\text{L-glutamate} + O_2 + H_2O \rightarrow \text{2-ketoglutarate} + NH_3 + H_2O_2$$

Preparation of the ferrocene-ethylene-siloxane redox polymer was carried out by the hydrosilylation of the terminal vinyl group of the appropriate ferrocene containing ethylene oxide oligomer with a respective copolymer (methylhydrosiloxane-dimethylsiloxane) in a ratio of 1:2. The sensors were prepared by coating the electrode surface with the polymer, followed by adsorption of the enzyme onto the polymer. Cyclic voltammograms depicted a large increase in the oxidation current (with no increase in the reduction current) when glutamate was added to electrodes cycling in phosphate buffer, hence confirming an efficient electron transfer from enzyme to electrode. Operating at a potential of +400 mV (vs. Ag/AgCl), the lower limit of detection was 0.01 mM with a response time of less than 10 s to reach a steady state.

Carbon paste electrodes were used to construct a glutamate sensor based on the mediator TTF and glutamate oxidase.[32] This mediator was chosen because of its extremely low solubility in aqueous solutions (a point of particular importance for a potential *in situ* sensor operating in a fermenter) and the low potential required to regenerate the mediator at the electrode.

The electrode was fabricated by mixing the mediator with graphite powder to form the basis of the electrode, followed by immobilization of the enzyme (using glutaraldehyde) over the modified electrode surface. In order to enhance the stability of the sensor and reduce the effects of possible electrochemical interferents, an outer membrane (composed of resorcinol and 1,3-phenylenediamine) was electrochemically deposited over the electrode surface. Experiments involving cyclic voltammetry confirmed the efficiency of TTF as an efficient electron transfer mediator between glutamate oxidase and the carbon paste electrode. Operating at an applied potential of +150 mV (vs. Ag/AgCl) the sensors had a lower limit of detection at 2.6 μM glutamate. The linear range extended up to 0.8 mM glutamate and the response time was 2 min, to reach a steady state. The sensor was used to determine the concentration of glutamate in a range of foodstuffs including soy sauce, chicken soup mix, seasoning, and party dip. Comparisons were made to results obtained using a standard spectrophotometric assay for L-glutamate with the biosensor. A good correlation was obtained between both sets of results, indicating the reliability of the biosensor. Furthermore, the sensors were reported to be highly stable, giving reproducible results.

A third approach[33] used a modified version of the glucose sensor, described earlier for *in situ* glucose monitoring. The mediator 1,1-dimethylferrocene was again used, this time in conjunction with glutamate oxidase. A potential of +220 mV (vs. Ag/AgCl) was applied between the working and reference electrode. Following calibration the sensor was used to determine the glutamate concentration in a number of foodstuffs. These sensors had a linear range of between 0.2 and 2 mM glutamate and a response time of 60 s (to reach 95% of the steady-state current). Again, a good calibration was obtained between the glutamate biosensor and a conventional assay procedure.

These three examples demonstrate the potential advantages of using biosensors for these applications. In particular the reduced analysis time required is an asset; for the last example, a single foodstuff sample required 5 to 7 min of preparation and analysis time. In contrast, preparation and analysis time using a conventional test kit required 45 min.

10.4.3 Lysine

Lysine is one of the essential amino acids required by humans and many other mammals. Furthermore, L-lysine is a limiting amino acid in a number of basic foods, such as cereals, and its concentration essentially controls the nutritional quality of the food. The production of L-lysine is therefore an important goal for food industries.

A mediated amperometric biosensor for determining lysine was recently reported[34] that was based on the enzyme lysine dehydrogenase. The enzyme was entrapped within a gelatin support on a cellulose membrane. Anodic detection at 400 mV (vs. Ag/AgCl) was facilitated by the presence of ferricyanide ions. A detection limit of 7×10^{-8} M and linearity up to 7×10^{-4} was reported. Using a flow injection analysis system, a sample throughput of 40 h^{-1} was achieved. A wide range of compounds commonly found in fermentation broths, mammalian cell cultures, and biological fluids were investigated to ascertain their possible electrochemical interference. No significant interference was reported for this sensor. The sensor was reported to be useful for up to 25 days.

Further potential food monitoring applications for biosensors are listed in Table 10.1.

TABLE 10.1
Potential Food Monitoring Applications for Enzyme-Based Biosensors Beyond Those (for Glucose, Glutamate, and Lysine) Discussed in Section 10.4

Substrate	Food	Enzyme(s)
Alcohol	Beer and wines	Alcohol oxidase
Sucrose	Fruit drinks	Invertase/mutarotase/glucose oxidase
Hypoxanthine	Fish freshness	Xanthine oxidase/peroxidase
Cholesterol	Butter and other edible fats	Cholesterol oxidase
Lactate	Yogurt	Lactate oxidase
Lactose	Milk	Galactosidase/glucose oxidase

10.5 MEDIATED BIOSENSORS FOR ENVIRONMENTAL CONTROL

Mediated biosensors based on the use of whole cells have been used for a number of applications where the detection of a pollutant in an aqueous media was the desired aim. Biosensors based on microbial cells possess a number of advantages compared to (isolated) enzyme-based sensors; these include:

1. Microbial cells are cheaper to isolate, i.e., there is no requirement for costly extraction and purification steps, unlike enzymes.
2. Cells can display a high degree of stability.
3. Cells are less vulnerable to fluctuations in the operating environmental conditions.
4. Intact cells offer the possibility of carrying out complex reaction sequences involving a range of enzymes and cofactors.

Disadvantages include:

1. Lower specificity, compared to (isolated) enzymes.
2. Longer response and recovery times.

Microbial cell-based sensors utilising soluble mediators have been developed to monitor a number of pollutants in water. Advances in this area of monitoring include the development of the Biocheck,[35] a purpose-built instrument designed to detect microbial contamination in fluids. This device is based on the ability of mediator(s) such as *p*-benzoquinone to abstract electrons from the respiratory chain of the microorganism. Reoxidation of the mediator at an electrode gives a direct indication of the microbial activity found in a sample solution. A device based on this design is now available commercially (Midas Pro, Biosensore, Italy). Another approach was based on monitoring, electrochemically, the photosynthetic activity of the cyanobacterium *Synechococcus* using the mediators ferricyanide and *p*-benzoquinone.[36] When the organism was illuminated with light (660 nm) the action of the photosynthetic pathway resulted in the reduction of the mediators. The mediators diffused to the electrode and were subsequently oxidised, the resultant current was correlated to the steady-state photosynthetic activity. In the presence of a range of potential pollutants (herbicides such as linuron, dichlorichloro-phenyl-methyl urea, and atrazine) the current response altered significantly.

Enzyme-based sensors have been developed to monitor potential pollutants, including the fabrication of biosensors for the detection of cholinesterase activity.[37] Many insecticides can act as inhibitors to the enzyme cholinesterase. For this application screen-printed sensors incorporating the redox mediator TCNQ were used. Butylthiocholine was used as the substrate and this compound was used to calibrate the sensor. In the presence of several known cholinesterase inhibitors, the response from the sensors was depressed. The authors note that the sensors were cheap to produce and demonstrated good reproducibility and stability. Furthermore, the sensors could be developed to monitor the presence of cholinesterase inhibitors in aqueous environments.

10.6 CONCLUSIONS

The examples discussed here are only a very small part of the work that has been carried out using mediated biosensors. The increasing use of biosensors, particularly in the areas of application outlined above, seems certain. Obviously, the full details of development and production costs of biosensors are not public knowledge, but a good deal of rewarding information can be gleaned by examination of published accounts and various public statements. It is clear that the single-product company, Medisense, required on the order of \$12 million to reach the marketplace with their glucose sensor and a further \$13 million to consolidate this position. Much of this was spent on marketing rather than R&D. However, target production costs for a glucose sensor would be around 10 cents. Pharmacia Biosensor appears to have spent a similar total sum to reach the marketplace with its SPR device. The medical market is considerably more demanding than some process and environmental applications in terms of regulatory requirements. In addition, much of the unknown territory has now been charted. It is now conceivable to develop new mediated biosensors at a very small fraction of the above costs, although the economies of scale will always be a dominant factor in production costs. Hence small, niche markets can be served with a modest investment in development — but they must support a relatively high cost per sensor — an order of magnitude or so higher than sensors intended for a mass market.

REFERENCES

1. Anon., *Biosensors: A New Realism,* CBL Publishing, Cranfield, U.K., 1991.
2. Turner, A. P. F., *Advances in Biosensors Supplement 1*, JAI Press, London, 1993.

3. Pickup, J. C., Claremont, D. J., and Shaw, G. W., *In vivo* biosensors for use in clinical medicine. In, *In-Vivo Chemical Sensors*, Alcock, S. J. and Turner, A. P. F., Eds., Cranfield Press, Cranfield, U.K., 1993, 9.
4. Turner, A. P. F., Biosensors, *Curr. Opinion Biotechnol.,* 5, 49, 1994.
5. Davis, G., Electrochemical techniques for the development of amperometric biosensors, *Biosensors,* 1, 161, 1985.
6. Cass, A. E. G., Davis, G., Francis, G. D., Hill, H. A. O., Aston, W. G., Higgins, I. J., Plotkin, E. V., Scott, L. D. L., and Turner, A. P. F., Ferrocene mediated enzyme electrode for amperometric determination of glucose, *Anal. Chem.,* 56, 667, 1984.
7. Dicks, J. M., Hattori, S., Karube, I., Turner, A. P. F., and Yokozawa, T., Ferrocene modified polypyrrole with immobilised glucose oxidase and its application in amperometric glucose microsensors. *Ann. Biol. Clin.*, 47, 607, 1987.
8. Rosen-Margalit, I. and Rishpon, J., Novel approaches for the use of mediators in enzyme electrodes, *Biosens. Bioelectron.*, 8, 315, 1993.
9. Degani, Y. and Heller, A., Direct electrical communication between chemically modified enzymes and metal electrodes. 1. Electron transfer from glucose oxidase to metal electrodes via electron relays, bound covalently to the enzyme, *J. Phys. Chem.*, 91, 1285, 1987.
10. Cardosi, M. F. and Turner, A. P. F., Mediated electrochemistry. In *Advances in Biosensors I,* Turner, A. P. F., Ed., JAI Press, London, 1991, 125.
11. Clark, L. C., The enzyme electrode. In *Biosensors Fundamentals and Applications,* Turner, A. P. F., Karube, I., and Wilson, G. S., Eds., Oxford University Press, New York, 1987.
12. Pickup, J. C. and Thevenot, D. R., European achievements in sensor research dedicated to *in vivo* monitoring. In *Advances in Biosensors Supplement I*, Turner, A. P. F., Ed., JAI Press, London, 1993, 201.
13. Kulys, J., Simkevicienev, V., and Higgins, I. J., Concerning the toxicity of two components as mediators in biosensor devices: 7,7,8,8-tetracyanoquinodimethane (TCNQ) and tetrathiafulvalene (TTF), *Biosens. Bioelectron.*, 7, 495, 1992.
14. Hill, H. A. O. and Sanghera, G. S., Mediated amperometric enzyme electrodes, In *Biosensors A Practical Approach,* Cass, A. E. G., Ed., Oxford University Press, Oxford, 1990, 19.
15. Motonaka, J. and Faulkner, L. R., Determination of cholesterol and cholesterol ester with novel enzyme microsensors, *Anal. Chem.,* 65, 3258, 1993.
16. Berqvist, Y., Hed, K., and Kalberg, B., An improved flow injection method for determination of lactate during excercise studies, *Int. J. Sports Med.,* 9, 73, 1988.
17. Aravena, G., Reinbach, R., and Rios, F. G., Surgery associated impairments of lactate and acid-base parameters. *Cell. Mol. Biol.,* 29, 279, 1983.
18. Eguilez, A., Lopez-Bernal, A., McPherson, K., Parrilla, J. J., and Abad, L., The use of intrapartum fetal blood lactate measurements for early diagnosis of fetal distress, *Am. J. Obstet. Gynaecol.*, 147949, 1983.
19. Dwivendi, C. and Reddy, C. M., Diagnostic use of cerebospinal fluid lactic acid levels in meningitis, *J. Med.,* 14, 395, 1983.
20. Preneta, A. Z., Studies on Lactate Oxidising Enzymes and Their Application to Ferrocene Based Enzyme Electrodes for Lactate, PhD thesis, Cranfield University, Cranfield, U.K., 1987.
21. White, S. F., Higgins, I. J., D'Costa, E., Bradley, J., and Schmid, R. D., Amperometric detection of lactate: a comparison between mediated and platinised carbon electrodes. In *Biosensors: Fundamentals Technologies and Applications,* Scheller, F. and Schmid, R. D., Eds., VCH Publishers, Weinheim, 1992, 403.
22. Durliat, H., Causserand, C., and Comtat, M., Bienzyme amperometric lactate-specific electrode, *Anal. Chim. Acta,* 231, 309, 1990.
23. Kulys, J., Schuhmann, W., and Schmidt, H.-L., Carbon paste electrodes with incorporated lactate oxidase and mediators. *Anal. Lett.*, 26(6), 1011, 1992.
24. Palleschi, G. and Turner, A. P. F., Amperometric tetrathiafulvalene-mediated lactate electrodes using lactate oxidase adsorbed on carbon foil, *Anal. Chim. Acta,* 234, 459, 1990.
25. McNeil, C. J., Cooper, J. M., and Spoors, J. A., Amperometric enzyme electrodes for determination of theophylline in serum, *Biosens. Bioelectron.,* 7, 375, 1992.
26. Hale, P. D., Lie, L.-F., and Skotheim, T. A., Enzyme modified carbon paste tetrathiafulvalene electrodes for the determination of acetylcholine, *Electroanalysis,* 3, 751, 1991.

27. Cardosi, M. F., Birch, S. W., Smith, B. M., and Johannsson, A., An enzyme-amplified electrochemical immunoassay for thyrotropin, *Electroanalysis,* 1, 297, 1989.
28. Cardosi, M. F., Birch, S. W., Stanley, C. J., Johannsson, A., and Turner, A. P. F., An electrochemical immunoassay for prostatic acid phosphatase incorporating enzyme amplification. *Am. Biotechnol. Lab.,* 7(5), 50, 1989.
29. Bradley, J. and Schmid, R. D., Optimisation of a biosensor for *in situ* fermentation monitoring of glucose concentration, *Biosens. Bioelectron.,* 6, 669, 1991.
30. Bradley, J., Anderson, P. A., Dear, A. M., Ashby, R. E., and Turner, A. P. F., Glucose biosensors for the study and control of bakers yeast fermentation. In *Computer Applications in Fermentation Technology: Modelling and Control of Biotechnical Processes,* Fish, N. M., Fox, R. I., and Thornhill, N. F., Eds., Elsevier, London, 1989, 47.
31. Hale, P. D., Hung, S.-L., Okamoto, Y., and Skotheim, T. A., Glutamate biosensors based on electrical communication between L-glutamate oxidase and a flexible redox polymer, *Anal. Lett.,* 24(3), 345, 1991.
32. Almedia, N. F. and Mulchandani, A. K., A mediated amperometric enzyme electrode using tetrathiafulvalene and L-glutamate oxidase for the determination of L-glutamic acid, *Anal. Chim. Acta,* 282, 353, 1993.
33. Vahjen, W., Bradley, J., Bilitewski, U., and Schmid, R. D., Mediated enzyme electrode for the determination of L-glutamate, *Anal. Lett.*, 24(8), 1445, 1991.
34. Dempsey, E., Wang, J., Wollenberger, U., and Ozsoz, M., A lysine dehydrogenase-based electrode for biosensing of L-lysine, *Biosens. Bioelectron.,* 7, 323, 1992.
35. Turner, A. P. F., Allen, M., Schneider, B. H., Swain, A., and Taylor, F., An inexpensive method for ultra rapid detection of microbial contamination in industrial fluids, *Int. Biodeterioration,* 25, 137, 1989.
36. Rawson, D., Willmer, A. J., and Turner, A. P. F., Whole cell biosensors for environmental monitoring, *Biosensors,* 4, 299, 1988.
37. Kulys, J. and D'Costa, E., Printed amperometric sensor based on TCNQ and cholinesterase, *Biosens. Bioelectron.,* 6, 109, 1991.

11 Commercial Devices Based on Amperometric Biosensors

Frieder W. Scheller and Dorothea Pfeiffer

CONTENTS

11.1 INTRODUCTION

Traditionally, enzymes have been used as analytical reagents to measure substrate molecules by catalyzing the turnover of these species to detectable products. Not only the substrates of enzyme-catalyzed reactions but also activators such as heavy metals, prosthetic groups such as flavins (e.g., flavin adenine dinucleotide: FAD), inhibitors (including carbamates, organophosphorus compounds), and also the enzymes themselves (for example, acetylcholine esterase, alkaline phosphatase, transaminases, amylases, cellulases) are accessible to measurement.

Based on the progress achieved in immobilizing techniques, analytical enzyme reactors have been applied in flow analyzers in combination with electrochemical detectors. This concept was pioneered in the form of the Technicon Analyzers and is still current as reflected by new devices of this type. The direct spatial integration of a "mini" reactor with a suitable transducer is the characteristic feature of *biosensors*.

The development of this field was initiated by Clark, who created the first enzyme electrode in 1962.[1] He simply placed a glucose oxidase solution on the sensing surface of the "Clark-type" oxygen electrode and held it in place with an additional (semipermeable) membrane facing the measuring solution. The next stage was reached in 1967 by Updike and Hicks,[2] using gel entrapment of the enzyme. In this way, the operating stability of the enzyme electrode has been increased and the sensor preparation has been simplified. This combination of an exchangeable enzyme membrane and a pencil-like electrode body has proven very successful and it is still used in the majority of commercial analyzers.

0-8493-8905-4/97/$0.00+$.50
© 1997 by CRC Press, Inc.

In the 1970s, carbon electrodes were introduced as base transducers in enzyme electrodes[3-5] and the natural cosubstrates of oxidoreductases, e.g., oxygen, cytochrome c, or NAD^+, were substituted by artificial electron transferring substances — the mediators.[5-7] This was followed by the production of amperometric electrodes using thick-film and thin-film metal deposition on different substrate materials.[8] The planar shape of the electrode requires the fixation of the biocomponent on the metal surface (Figure 11.1).

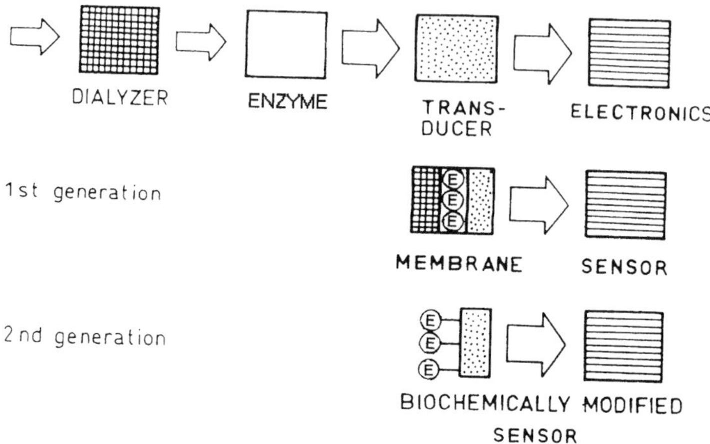

FIGURE 11.1 Generations of enzyme electrodes (E: enzyme). According to their level of integration, the enzyme electrodes described in the literature can be subdivided into two generations. In the simplest approach (first generation), the biocatalyst is entrapped between or bound to the membranes and this arrangement is fixed at the surface of the transducer. The direct adsorption or covalent binding of the biocatalyst at the electrode surface permits the elimination of semipermeable membranes (second generation). Further miniaturization is achieved by direct binding of the biocatalyst to an electronic device transducing and amplifying the signal.

Whereas spectrophotometric methods dominate in traditional enzymatic analysis, amperometric enzyme electrodes are at the leading edge in the application of immobilized enzymes. This may be expected to continue at least until the end of the 1990s.

11.2 PRINCIPLES OF COUPLING BIOCATALYTIC REACTIONS AND AMPEROMETRIC ELECTRODES

The following modes of signal transfer have been described in the literature for biospecific electrodes (see also Table 11.1).

Enzyme electrodes based on oxidases combined with amperometric H_20_2 measurement have become the most common design in biosensors. However, electroactive substances being converted at the electrode contribute to the total current.

The natural electron acceptors of many NAD-independent dehydrogenases, as for example those of glucose, oligosaccharides, methylamines, cytochrome b_2, and the oxidases of glucose, lactate, pyruvate, glycolate, sarcosine, and galactose can be replaced by redox-active mediators.[5] With these mediators an applied electrode potential of around +200 mV is sufficient; this decreases the interferences by reducing substances and enables one to couple such enzymes to electrodes in an oxygen-free solution. The mediators can be added to the measuring solution or they are integrated in the electrode body. In the simplest approach the solid mediator is introduced in crevices of the carbon electrode body[9] and a dialysis membrane prevents it from leaching out. In the next developmental stage, the mediator is adsorbed onto the electrode surface or it is admixed to the carbon paste of the electrode body.[4] Finally, in

TABLE 11.1
Coupling of Biocatalytic Reactions to Amperometric Electrodes

Biocomponent	Transferring substances	Mode of indication
Oxidases	O_2, H_2O_2	Steady state current
Microorganisms	Redox mediators	First or second derivative of i-t curves
Dehydrogenases	Conducting polymers, electrons (direct e-transfer) $NAD(P)^+/NAD(P)H$	Peak height or area of cyclic voltammograms or i-t curves
Hydrolases	Conducting polymers (indirect amperometry)	

the most recent devices, all reagents — enzyme, mediator, and cosubstrate — have been integrated into the electrode surface. Figure 11.2 provides a schematic illustration of the different types of amperometric enzyme electrodes applied in a range of different commercial devices.

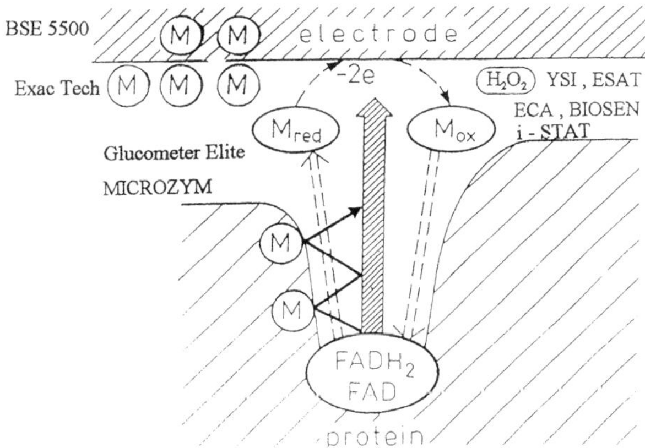

FIGURE 11.2 Scheme of signal transfer used in enzyme electrode-based glucose analyzers — M: mediator, FAD: flavin adenine dinucleotide of the glucose oxidase. See Tables 11.2 and 11.3 for a key to the analyzer codes. Anodic oxidation of the peroxide formed by the enzymatic reduction of the cosubstrate oxygen generates the concentration-dependent signal in the analyzers YSI, ESAT, ECA, BIOSEN, and i-STAT (right side). Ferricyanide, a soluble mediator, is applied for transferring the chemical signal from the glucose-converting enzyme — the glucose oxidase — to the amperometric electrode in the Glucometer Elite and the analyzer MICROZYM. Ferrocene adsorbed at the indicator electrode is oxidized to the ferrocinium species which acts as the cosubstrate of glucose oxidation. This reaction is exploited in the ExacTech "Pen sensor". The carbon paste electrode of the BSE 5500 contains both the enzyme and the mediator within the electrode body resulting in a reagent-less operation. Finally the hopping of electrons from the $FADH_2$ group of the enzyme via artificial "relays" to the electrode (lower left side) may be applied in coming devices.

Adsorption of redox polymers containing benzoquinone or heavy metal ion complexes at carbon electrodes results in the catalysis of the electron transfer by "wiring" the enzyme molecules to the electrode.[10] When enzymes and mediators are coimmobilized at the surface or within the electrode, addition of auxiliary substances during the measuring process can be avoided, thus a *reagent-less* regime becomes feasible.

An alternative to the application of mediators is the direct electron transfer between the prosthetic (non-amino acid) group of the enzyme and the redox electrode. Heterogeneous electron transfer reactions have been realized with more than 30 different proteins, mainly electron transferases, but also substrate-converting oxidoreductases.[11] Adsorption of modifiers which promote an appropriate orientation of the protein results in a facilitated direct electron transfer with different redox enzymes, e.g., cytochromes and ferrodoxins. The mediator-free electron transfer within bulk-modified carbon paste electrodes has been used for sensor application. Peroxidase[12] and the PQQ-containing dehydrogenases[13] have been applied in reagent-less sensor arrangements for hydroperoxides, gluconates, and fructose, respectively.

11.3 PERFORMANCE AND APPLICATION

The most relevant fields of practical application of enzyme electrodes are medical diagnostics, process control in bioreactors, food analysis, and environmental monitoring.

Most clinical laboratory analyses concern metabolites in body fluids in the micro- and millimolar concentration range. Status determination and continuous *in vivo* monitoring of these substances are particulary important in intensive care, surgery, and life-threatening situations.

A better understanding of several diseases requires the measurement of steroids, drugs and their metabolites, and protein factors. Since they lie in the concentration range of 10^{-11} to 10^{-9} mol/l, the concentration of these substances can only be determined by immunoassays at present.

11.3.1 AUTOANALYZERS FOR CENTRALIZED LABORATORIES

The prevalence of diabetes in industrialized countries amounts to approximately 4%. Therefore the selective determination of blood glucose is of the utmost importance for the screening and treatment of diabetes. The normal concentration of glucose in blood serum ranges between 4.2 and 5.5 mmol/l, pathological situations may cause an increase up to more than 30 mmol/l.

Clinical chemists are interested in autoanalyzers characterized by high measuring frequency as well as in portable bedside-type analytical devices with short lag time between sample withdrawal and availability of the result. Therefore, enzyme electrode-based analytical systems for the application of highly diluted as well as undiluted media have been developed and commercialized. In order to cover the relevant analyte concentrations in both types of samples, the measuring range of the respective enzyme electrodes has to be shifted by almost two decades (Figure 11.3). Glucose analyzers based on enzyme electrodes have been brought onto the market in the United States, Japan, France, Lithuania, and Germany (Table 11.2). As compared with conventional enzymatic analysis, the main advantages of such analyzers are the extremely low enzyme demand (a few milliunits per sample), the simplicity of operation, and the high analytical quality.

The majority of enzyme electrode-based analyzers developed to date operate on *diluted* samples. Development began with the measurement of discrete blood or serum samples using stirred measuring cells and internal dilution. Because of the good analytical performance of the most prominent representatives (YSI, Glucoprocesseur, Industrial Modul), this type of device is still used and its applicability has been expanded for the determination of saccharides, lactate, alcohol, uric acid, amylases, amino acids, and ascorbic acid, especially in the smaller medical laboratories (see Table 11.2). Using a sample volume of about 50 µl, the serial imprecision (that is, the coefficient of variation) is below 2% with a sample throughput of more than 40/h.

An enhancement of sample frequency of up to 180/h has been achieved by the integration of segmented continuous-flow systems. The resulting analyzers have been on the market since the early 1980s for metabolites like glucose and lactate. They process prediluted samples and

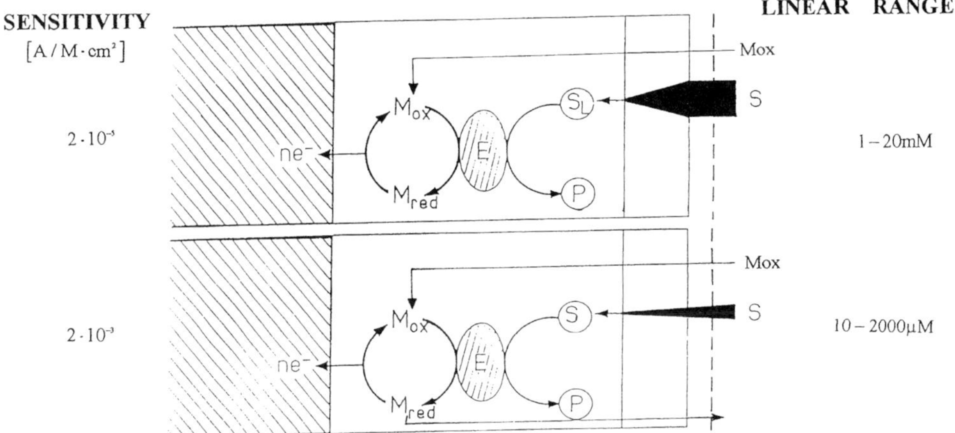

FIGURE 11.3 Schematic representation of the variation in membrane permeability for shifting the linear measurement range. To adapt the measuring range, the permeability of the sensor's covering layer is decreased for the substrate in order to decrease its influx from the undiluted medium (upper scheme). The permeation of the cosubstrate M_{OX} (e.g., oxygen), on the other hand, should not be reduced as compared with the membrane arrangement for diluted samples (lower scheme). M: mediator, e.g., oxygen; S: substrate of the enzyme, i.e., glucose; P: product of the enzyme-catalyzed reaction; E: enzyme.

are especially well suited for centralized medical laboratories. Representatives are ESAT (PGW Prüfgeräte-Werk Medingen, Dresden, Germany), EBIO (Eppendorf-Netheler-Hinz, Hamburg, Germany), BIOSEN 5030L and 5030G (EKF Industrial Electronics, Magdeburg, Germany), and Auto-Stat GA-112 (Daiichi, Japan).

Since uric acid is a risk factor for gout and other diseases, diagnosis of hyperuricemia is increasingly important. Normal levels of uric acid in serum are 200 to 400 μmol/l. The UA-300 analyzer of Fuji Electric (Japan) uses a uricase membrane fixed on a hydrogen peroxide selective layer;[14] 20 μl of blood serum is required and a sample throughput of 50 to 60/h at a CV (coefficient of variation) of 3% is achieved.

The ESAT (PGW Prüfgeräte Werk Medingen GmbH, Germany) has been equipped with a uricase membrane and employed for uric acid assay in serum. Satisfactory agreement with the uricase-catalase reference method was obtained; the deviation of the mean value was as low as +2.4 μmol/l. The reagent costs of the method amount to only one tenth of those required for the manual photometric method.

At present the determination of lactate does not belong in the list of most frequently performed analyses in clinical chemistry, yet its popularity in the diagnosis of shock and myocardial infarction and in neonatology and sports medicine is increasing. Therefore, strong efforts have been made to develop sensor-based lactate analyzers which may be readily used at the bedside. The normal lactate concentration in blood is below 2.7 mmol/l. For accurate lactate determination in diluted whole blood, hemolysis of the sample is required to take account of the (low) lactate content of erythrocytes. On the other hand, the glycolytic reactions in the sample have to be efficiently and rapidly inhibited in order to avoid lactate formation.

The first enzyme electrode-based lactate analyzer was developed in 1976 by La Roche (Switzerland). It uses cytochrome b_2 and (soluble) ferricyanide in a tiny reaction chamber on top of a platinum electrode polarized at +0.25 V. A good correlation with the spectrophotometric method using deproteinized blood was found. The same principle is applied in the MICROZYME-L (SGI, France) (see Table 11.2). Other lactate analyzers use lactate oxidase (LOD). This enzyme is immobilized between a cellulose acetate membrane and a polycarbonate membrane in the YSI 23L Instrument (U.S.).

TABLE 11.2
Enzyme Electrode-Based Autoanalyzer

Model	Company	Analyte	Measuring range (mM)	Sample through-put (1/h)	Functional stability
YSI 2300 G	Yellow Springs Instr. (U.S.)	Glucose	0.0–27.8	45	7 d
YSI 2300 L		Lactate	0.0–15.0	45	7 d
YSI 2700		Lactose	0.0–58.4	45	10 d
		Ethanol	0.0–70.0	45	5 d
		Sucrose	0.0–55.5	45	10 d
ESAT 6660	PGW Medingen, Dresden	Glucose	0.6–45.0	120	15 d
ESAT 6661	(Germany)	Lactate	0.5–30.0	120	10 d
ECA 180		Glucose	0.6–45.0	180	15 d
INDUSTRIAL MODUL		Lactose	0.5–100.0	60	15 d
		Ascorbate	0.5–45.0	60	15 d
		Lysine	1.0–100.0	60	15 d
SUPER G	Dr. Müller GmbH Dresden RLT Arnsberg (Germany)	Glucose	0.6–50.0	150	15 d
EBIO 6666	Eppendorf-Netheler-Hinz,	Glucose	0.6–50.0	120	15 d
	Hamburg (Germany)	Lactate	0.5–30.0	120	10 d
BIOSEN 5030 L	EKF Industrial Electronics,	Lactate	0.5–30.0	80	10 d
BIOSEN 6030 G	Magdeburg (Germany)	Glucose	0.6–50.0	80	15 d
GLUCO 20	Fuji Electric Corp. (Japan)	Glucose	0.0–27.0	90	> 500 samples
UA-300 A		Uric acid	5.0–60.0	3	
AUTO-STAT GA112	Daiichi (Japan)	Glucose	1.0–40.0	120	
STAT Analyzer S80	Analyt. Instr. Corp.(Japan)	Glucose	0.0–50.0	120	
AMPEROMET-RIC	Universal Sensors, Inc	Glucose	0.003–3.0	30–60	> 500 samples
BIOSENSOR	New Orleans (U.S.)	Lactate	0.01–2.5	30–60	> 500 samples
DETECTOR		Urea	0.1–10.0	6	> 500 samples
		Uric acid	0.006–0.6	20–60	> 500 samples
		Sucrose	0.006–2.0	30–60	> 500 samples
		Ethanol	0.0–10.0	30–60	> 500 samples
		Ascorbate	0.001–0.5	30–60	> 500 samples
		Glutamate	0.01–1.0	30–60	> 500 samples
		Lactose	0.01–3.0	20–60	> 500 samples
		Lysine	0.01–20.0	3–15	> 500 samples
EXSAN	Acad. Sci. Lithuania,	Glucose	2.0–30.0	45	
	Inst. Biochem. Vilnius	Lactate	0.1–15.0	45	
	(Lithuania)	Urea	2.0–40.0	30	
		Cholest.	0.5–10.0	20	
ENZYMAT	Seres (France)	Glucose	0.3–22.0	60	
		Lysine	0.1–2.0	60	
		Choline	1.0–29.0	60	
TOA-GLU 11	TOA Electronics Ltd.	Glucose	0.0–55.5	60	
GLUCOPRO-CESSEUR	Tacussel (France)	Glucose	0.05–5.0	90	> 2000 samples
MICROZYM-L	SGI, Toulouse (France)	Lactate	0.05–15.0	60	> 200 samples
		Glucose	0.25–27.0	60	> 400 samples

TABLE 11.2 (CONTINUED)
Enzyme Electrode-Based Autoanalyzer

Model	Company	Analyte	Measuring range (mM)	Sample through-put (1/h)	Functional stability
OLGA	Biometra (Germany)	Glucose	0.6–50.0	120	15 d
		Lactate	0.5–30.0	120	10 d
NOVA-CRT	NOVA Biomedical (U.S.)	Glucose	1.1–30.0	50	7 d
TAT-Profile 5		Lactate	0.0–15.0	50	7 d
		Urea	0.7–35.0	50	7 d
SENSOMAT	Gonotec Berlin (Germany)	Ethanol	0.0–0.32	15	50 samples
IONOMETER EG-HK	Fresenius AG (Germany)	Glucose	2.0–50.0	60	> 2 months

The lactate-analyzing ESAT 6661 (Prüfgeräte-Werk Medingen GmbH, Dresden, Germany) and EBIO 6666 (Eppendorf, Hamburg, Germany) are based on lactate oxidase immobilized in polyurethane and covered on both sides by cellulose membranes. Both analyzers are characterized by a sample throughput of 120/h and high functional stability of the enzyme sensors (see Table 11.2).

The concentration of urea in blood (blood urea nitrogen, BUN) is an important parameter in clinical chemistry in the assessment of kidney failure. The normal levels of urea in serum are 3.6 to 8.9 mmol/l.

Kulys et al.[15] studied urea determination by difference measurement between two antimony electrodes covered with exchangeable membranes. Urease was attached in the pores of a macroporous membrane by glutaraldehyde. This layer was covered with a monoacetylcellulose membrane. The membrane for the auxiliary electrode was prepared in the same manner, but using BSA instead of urease. The assay of urea was carried out with a differential amplifier which simultaneously differentiated the time course of the potential difference between enzyme and auxiliary electrode (kinetic method). Thus, a response time of only 20 s was possible. The calibration graph was linear between 0.2 and 2 mmol/l urea.

An amperometric urea sensor based on the pH dependence of the anodic oxidation of hydrazine[16] has been utilized in the ESAT (PGW Prüfgeräte Werk Medingen GmbH, Dresden, Germany) for hemodialysis monitoring. Measurement of serum urea with the device yielded only a poor correlation because variations of the pH and buffer capacity of the biological sample caused by proteins and bicarbonate gave rise to random deviations. The assay was improved by subtracting the signal of an enzyme-free electrode connected to a second analyzer.

The Lipid Analyzer ICA-LG 400 from the Japanese company Toyo Jozo is capable of measuring a whole group of analytes, namely cholesterol, triglycerides, and phospholipids by using enzyme electrodes. Serum samples have to be preincubated with the appropriate hydrolases, i.e., cholesterol esterase, lipoprotein lipase, and phospholipase D. The measurement is performed by using enzyme electrodes involving cholesterol oxidase, glycerokinase, glycerophosphate oxidase, and choline oxidase immobilized on an oxygen probe. Using a sample volume of 30 μl, a measuring frequency of 40/h is obtained. Although the prospects for this method appear exciting, the analyzer has not yet reached the market.

11.3.2 Point-of-Care Testing

To assure rapid results immediately after sample withdrawal, some companies have achieved *undiluted* whole blood analysis eliminating any preanalytical procedure (see Table 11.3). A rapid determination is important, especially with respect to metabolic substances that exhibit fast changes in concentration.

The first commercial second-generation glucose sensor has been introduced by Genetic International (now MediSense) in the U.K.[17] The sensor is based on a ferrocene-modified glucose oxidase electrode strip. For glucose determination a drop of blood is transferred to a disposable enzyme electrode strip which is then inserted into a pen-sized readout instrument. The response time is only 30 s, more rapid than that of photometric test strips. Venous as well as capillary blood may be used as sample material. The CV is 3.9% for the normal concentration range. Significantly lower precision has been found in the hypoglycemic range.

TABLE 11.3
Enzyme Electrode-Based Portable Devices

Model	Company	Analyte	Measuring range	Functional stability
ExacTech	MediSense (U.S.)	Glucose	1.1–33.3 mM	Disposables
Satelite G		Glucose	2.0–33.3 mM	Disposables
Glucometer Elite	Bayer Diagnostics (Germany)	Glucose		Disposables
i-STAT PCA	i-STAT Corp. Princeton (U.S.)	Glucose	2.9–23.6 mM	Disposables
		Urea	1.0–43.0 mM	Disposables
Medisensor 2001	MedTest Systems (U.S.)	Glucose		Disposables
		Uric acid		Disposables
BSE 5500	ORION Anal. Technol. Inc. (U.S.)/ DOSIVIT (France)	Glucose	1.6–16.0 mM	Disposables
		Sucrose	1.6–16.0 mM	Disposables
		Lactose	1.6–16.0 mM	Disposables
BIOSEN 6020 G	EKF Industrial Electronics (Germany)	Glucose	0.5–20.0 mM	24 d
BIOSEN 5020 L		Lactate	0.5–20.0 mM	10 d

The Glucometer Elite which has been distributed by Bayer Diagnostik combines the principle of "capillary fill device" with the electrochemical detection of a soluble mediator — ferricyanide. This approach allows simple handling that makes it well suited for use in the physician's consulting room and for home care. However, the spontaneous reactions of the ferricyanide with reducing substances, e.g., ascorbic acid or uric acid, influence the measured value, and the cost of U.S. $1 per measurement is rather high.

I-Stat Corp. (U.S.) has commercialized a pocket device useful for the analysis of glucose and urea as well as that of electrolytes. The base transducers are microfabricated thin-film metal sensors for H_2O_2 and ammonium ion-sensitive electrodes.

In the design of portable enzyme electrodes, the performance goals are quite different from those for laboratory autoanalyzers. Enzyme membrane-based devices are working with a biological component that can be designed for repeated use for thousands of measurements for analytes such as blood glucose, lactate, or urea. The functional stability depends on the quality of the enzyme membrane material used. Designed for long-term operation, for example, are the autoanalyzer STAT-Profile 5 (NOVA Biomedical, U.S.) and the Ionometer (Fresenius, Germany), which permit the analysis of metabolites like glucose and lactate in addition to electrolytes and blood gases.

The *portable* enzyme membrane electrode-based BIOSEN 5020L and BIOSEN 6020G (EKF Industrial Electronics, Magdeburg, Germany) on the other hand, besides good analytical performance, are characterized by an extremely short lag time between sample withdrawal and measuring the result. Therefore, and because of their mobility, these systems are particularly well suited for application to different sports facilities and intensive care away from centralized laboratories.

11.3.3 On-Line Measurement in Health Care

The invasive application of biospecific electrodes for direct analysis of substances like metabolites or enzymes is one of the most important challenges of biosensor designers. However, on-line analysis in humans has a critical demand for hemocompatibility and must not cause any cytotoxic, carcinogenic, or genotoxic reactions, or inflammation, irritation, or sensitization.

While a few chemical catheter sensors analyzing blood gases based on electrochemical as well as optical detectors are already on the market (Puritan-Bennett/Carlsbad, U.S.; Optex/Houston, U.S.; Optical Sensors for Medicine/U.S.; Pfizer/New York, U.S.; VIA Medical/San Diego, U.S.; Abbott/Minneapolis, U.S.; Biomedical Sensors/England), no biosensor for invasive application is commercially available as yet.

However, encouraging results concerning invasive analysis have been obtained by a few groups. Wilson et al.[18] succeeded with a 21-gauge needle-shaped glucose oxidase sensor (based on a Clark-type probe) implanted subcutaneously. After an *in vivo* equilibration period of 2 to 4 h, more than 60 glucose sensors were working after 24 h and 7 sensors after 4 days. Potentially interfering substances such as ascorbate are retarded by a negatively charged inner membrane. Subcutaneous tissue has been used as the sampling site because of the lower risk of infection and blood clotting as compared to that after intravascular implantation. Metabolic monitoring is accomplished by an exterior monitor.

Abel et al.[19] were successful in the subcutaneous implantation of a needle-shaped glucose electrode (based on a Clark-type probe) in dogs. The special modified two-electrode system needs only 30 min for equilibration after implantation.[20]

Armour et al.[21] proposed the application of two three-electrode systems to detect the oxygen consumption during glucose oxidation. Catalase was used to improve the half-life time of glucose oxidase. From their point of view, risk of clotting seems minimal using an intravascular implantation site. Implanted into the superior vena cava of various dogs, the sensor sensitivity is decreased by only 26% after 1 to 15 weeks.

Koudelka et al.[22,23] implanted more than 22 thin-film metal glucose oxidase electrodes subcutaneously in normal rats; 30% of the sensors applied were stable for 8 days after the equilibration period of 90 min.

Urban et al.[24] described glucose oxidase thin-film metal electrodes for invasive application that were characterized by high analytical performance, combined with an integrated pH sensor and suited to *in vivo* application as well.

Nevertheless, no truly reliable implantable sensor has yet reached the market. In the meantime, bedside-type discrete analyzers seem to offer the most economic and reliable means for critical care. In addition, an *ex vivo* on-line analysis based, for instance, on microdialysis sampling, seems to be helpful.

The first on-line glucose monitoring system "BIOSTATOR" has been brought onto the market by Miles Laboratories (Elkhart, IN, U.S.). This system needs external circulation of blood (through a double-lumen catheter; volume near 30 ml/24 h). Before measurement, the whole blood-heparin mixture has to be diluted. Because of these reasons the BIOSTATOR is suited only for clinical application.

Moscone and Mascini[25] demonstrated a portable glucose monitor based on microdialysis sampling. The GLUCODAY (Ampliscientifica, Milano, Italy) contains a hollow fiber placed into the bloodstream or subcutaneously in the left arm. It is combined with an *ex vivo* biosensor flow cell to monitor the blood glucose level over a period of 24 h. The placement of the microdialysis in the human body is followed by a 30-min period of equilibration. Sometimes the authors observed nonmetabolic signals, probably caused by nervous contractions of the muscle close to the sampling site.

A similar system is described by Meyerhoff et al.[26] The combination of a commercial needle-type dialysis probe (CMA/Microdialysis AB, Stockholm, Sweden) with glucose sensor (Unitec, Ulm, Germany) resulted in a reliable method for continuous glucose monitoring in dialysate for up to 21 h.

Thus, there are a few on-line control systems commercially available consisting of adequate sampling and external sensor analysis. All these systems have been successfully applied to diabetic monitoring over several hours, resulting in the improvement of the assessment of labile diabetic patients.

11.3.4 Bioprocess and Environmental Control

Bioreactor process control and food industry quality assurance require enzyme electrodes for *in situ* analysis. However, direct application in bioreactors is associated with significant difficulties:

1. The sensor has to be sterilized,
2. Calibration has to be performed by discrete measurements or *in situ*,
3. Often the analyte concentration exceeds the linear range of the sensor,
4. Various interfering compounds have to be dealt with, and
5. Thermal and mechanical stress may cause inactivation of the sensor.

Therefore, no *in situ* system is commercially available as yet.

An appropriate approach for on-line process monitoring is the combination of enzyme electrodes with flow injection analysis. For the determination of glucose and lactate this is incorporated in the OLGA system (Biometra, Göttingen, Germany). Carbon paste electrodes containing both the enzyme and mediator substance are the key components of the analyzer BSE 5500 commercialized by DOVISIT (France) and ORION (U.S.). The low electrode potential reduces the influence of potentially interfering substances.

A mechanical sampling system automatically leading the sample through a sterilized chamber before dilution has been designed at the Massachusetts Institute of Technology (U.S.). The equipment has been combined with the Enzymat analyzer (Seres, France) in order to monitor the production of monoclonal antibodies against fibronectin by hybridoma cells.[27] Every 30 min the concentrations of glucose, lactate, and glutamine were measured in parallel. The enzymes were contained in glutaraldehyde-crosslinked gelatin membranes mounted on oxygen electrodes. The sensor for glutamine determination comprised coimmobilized glutaminase from *Escherichia coli* and glutamate oxidase from *Streptomyces* sp. The measured data permit the derivation of a relationship between the substrate concentrations, ATP flux, and cell growth.

Microbial sensors are being routinely used for the analysis of effluent water in Japan.[28] They indicate the wastewater constituents that can be assimilated by microbes, i.e., a parameter similar to the biological oxygen demand (BOD). A conventional BOD determination requires 5 days and is thus unsuitable for process control. Sensors for rapid BOD estimation have been developed by using immobilized cells of *Bacillus subtilis* and *Trichosporon cutaneum*,[29] measuring the acceleration of respiration resulting from nutrient supply, i.e., no steady state has to be reached. The sensor is calibrated in a solution containing equimolar concentrations of glucose and glutamic acid. The signal depends linearly on concentration up to 100 mg/l. The smallest detectable concentration is 4 mg/l. The short measuring time makes the sensor highly suitable for the monitoring of wastewater treatment.

A limitation to this approach is the difference in conversion velocities of various organic wastewater components by the microbial cells. Macromolecules such as starch and proteins are not indicated at all. This might be overcome by enzymatic sample pretreatment or by the use of hybrid sensors.

REFERENCES

1. Clark, L. C. and Lyons, C., Electrode systems for continuous monitoring in cardiovascular surgery, *Ann. N.Y. Acad. Sci.*, 102, 29, 1962.
2. Updike, S. J. and Hicks, G. P., Immobilized enzyme electrode, *Nature,* 214, 986, 1967.
3. Shu, F. R. and Wilson, G. S., Rotating ring-disk enzyme electrode for surface catalysis, *Anal. Chem.*, 48 1679, 1976.
4. Ikeda, T., Katasho, I., Kamei, M., and Senda, M., Electrocatalysis with a glucose-oxidase-immobilized graphite electrode, *Agric. Biol. Chem.*, 48(8), 1969, 1984.
5. Razumas, V. J., Jasaitis, J. J., and Kulys, J. J., Electrocatalysis on enzyme-modified carbon materials, *Bioelectrochem. Bioenerg.,* 12, 297, 1984.
6. Cass, A. E. G., Davis, G., Francis, G. D., Hill, H. A. O., Aston, W. J., Higgins, I. J., Plotkin, E. V., Scott, L. D. L., and Turner, A. P. F., Ferrocene-mediated enzyme electrode for amperometric determination of glucose, *Anal. Chem.*, 56, 667, 1984.
7. Ikeda, T., Miki, K., and Senda, M., Theory of catalytic current at the biocatalyst electrode with entrapped mediator, *Anal. Sci.*, 4, 133, 1988.
8. Karube, I., Sode, K., and Tamiya, E., Microbiosensors, *J. Biotechnol.*, 15, 267, 1990.
9. Mindt, W., Racine, P., and Schläpfer P., Enzyme electrode, U.S. Patent 3,838,033, 1974.
10. Cenas, N. K., Pocius, A. K., and Kulys, J. J., Biosensors based on redox polymers, *Bioelectrochem. Bioenerg.,* 11, 61, 1983.
11. Armstrong, F. A., Probing metalloproteins by voltammetry, *Struct. Bonding,* 72, 137, 1990.
12. Gorton, L., Jönsson-Pettersson, G., Csöregi, E., Johansson, K., Domiguez, E., and Marko-Varga, G., Amperometric biosensors based on an apparent direct electron transfer between electrodes and immobilized peroxidases, *Analyst*, 117, 1235, 1992.
13. Ikeda, T., Matsushita, F., and Senda, M., Amperometric fructose sensor based on direct bioelectrocatalysis, *Biosens. Bioelectron.*, 6, 299, 1991.
14. Pfeiffer, D., Scheller, F. W., Setz, K., and Schubert, F., Amperometric enzyme electrodes for lactate and glucose determinations in highly diluted and undiluted media, *Anal. Chim. Acta,* 281, 489, 1993.
15. Kulys, J. J., Gureviciene, V. V., Laurinavicius, V. A., and Jonuska, A. V., Urease sensors based on differential antimony electrodes, *Biosensors*, 2, 286, 1986.
16. Scheller, F. W., Kirstein, D., Kirstein, L., Schubert, F., Wollenberger, U., Olsson, B. Gorton, L., and Johansson, G., Enzyme electrodes and their application, *Philos. Trans. R. Soc. London, Ser.*, B, 316, 85, 1987.
17. Spinas, G. A., Andres, U. R., Heinzinger, T., and Berger, W., Evaluation des Pen-Meters zur Blutzuckerbestimmung bei ambulanten Diabetikern, *Schweiz. Med. Wochenschr.,* 120, 125, 1990.
18. Wilson, G., Zhang, Y., Reach, G., Moatti-Sirat, D., Poitout, V., Thevenot, D. R., Lemonnier, F., and Klein, J.-C., Progress toward the development of an implantable sensor for glucose, *Clin. Chem.,* 38, 1613, 1992.
19. Abel, P., von Woedtke, T., Reprin, K., Schlosser, M., and Fischer, U., Glucose biosensor for in vivo application, in *In Vivo Chemical Sensors — Recent Developments*, Alcock, S. J. and Turner, A. P. F., Eds., Cranfield Press, Cranfield, U.K., 1993, 16.
20. Schwock, A. and Abel, P., Verfahren zur kontinuierlichen Analyse von Bestandteilen einer Flüssigkeit. German Patent 43 352 413, 1993.
21. Armour, J. C., Lucisano, J. Y., McKean, B. D., and Gough, D. A., Application of chronic intravascular blood glucose sensor in dogs, *Diabetes*, 39, 1519, 1990.
22. Koudelka, M., Rohner-Jeanrenaud, F., Terrettaz, J., Bobbioni-Harsch, E., de Rooij, N. F., and Jeanrenaud, B., In vivo behaviour of hypodermically implanted microfabricated glucose sensors, *Biosen. Bioelectron.* 6, 31, 1991.
23. Koudelka-Hep, M., Strike, M. J., and de Rooij, N. F., Miniature electrochemical glucose biosensors, *Anal. Chim. Acta,* 281, 461, 1993.

24. Urban, G., Jobst, G., Keplinger, F., Aschauer, E., Tilado, O., Fasching, R., and Kohl, F., Miniaturized multi-enzyme biosensors integrated with pH sensors on flexible polymer carriers for in vivo applications, *Biosens. Bioelectron.*, 7, 7, 1992.
25. Moscone, D. and Mascini, M., Microdialysis and glucose biosensor for in vivo monitoring, *Ann. Biol. Clin.*, 50, 323, 1992.
26. Meyerhoff, C., Bischof, F., Sternberg, F., Zier, H., and Pfeiffer, E. F., On line continuous monitoring of subcutaneous tissue glucose in men by combining portable glucosensor with microdialysis, *Diabetologia*, 35, 1087, 1992.
27. Romette, J. L., Mammalian cell culture process control: sampling and sensing, in *Biosensors International Workshop 1987, GBF Monographs, 10,* Schmid, R. D., Ed., VCH Publishers, New York, 1987, 81.
28. Hikuma, M. and Yasuda, T., Microbial sensors for estimation of biochemical oxygen demand and determination of glutamate, in *Methods in Enzymology,* Vol. 137, Immobilized Enzymes and Cells, Part D, Mosbach, K., Ed., Academic Press, San Diego, 1988, 124.
29. Riedel, K., Neumann, B., and Scheller, F. W., Mikrobielle Sensoren auf Basis von Respirationsmessungen, *Chem.-Ing.-Tech.*, 64, 518, 1992.

12 Microelectronic Biosensors for Clinical Applications

Gerald Urban

CONTENTS

12.1 INTRODUCTION

The rapid progress in medical sciences in the last decades of the 20th century is attributed to advanced pharmacological and biochemical developments and the rise of microelectronic technology. The successful advance of this technology is inherently connected to the completely new production methods which enable the production of a large quantity of identical devices in one batch.

This cheap and reliable production technology has changed the way of life, primarily in the developed countries, including especially the medical sciences. Starting with discrete assembled printed circuit boards, this technology now covers integrated circuits incorporating computers on chips. These technologies became state of the art and have recently been extended to peripheral devices, particularly sensors.

The benefits of the mentioned technology such as inexpensive mass production, high reproducibility, and the capability of integrating various functions on a miniaturised scale raised the expectation of a great abundance of microelectronic sensors. Up to now this expectation has not been entirely fulfilled; primarily, only physical sensors such as pressure or temperature sensors and CCD imaging and measuring chips in cameras have been successfully introduced into the market.

Microelectronics play a great role in medical imaging techniques and data acquisition and processing but are less prominent in medical sensors. The reasons will be explained in more detail in the next sections. Although a large number of microelectronic biosensors have

0-8493-8905-4/97/$0.00+$.50
© 1997 by CRC Press, Inc.

been designed for clinical applications up to now, most of them are at an early stage of research.

12.2 BIOMEDICAL INSTRUMENTATION FOR CLINICAL DIAGNOSTICS

Clinical diagnostics still has a high priority in medical practice. The microelectronic revolution has played an important role in establishing noninvasive diagnostic tools (Table 12.1).

TABLE 12.1
Overview of Noninvasive Diagnostic Tools[1-6]

Diagnostic tool	Spatial resolution	Temporal resolution	Monitoring capability	Metabolic parameter
X-ray diagnosis	0.1 mm	0.1 s	Limited	No
Computer tomograph (CT), X-ray	<1 mm	Seconds	Discrete	No
Positron emission tomography	3–5 mm	Minutes	No	Tracer
Ultrasound (US) imaging	>0.1 mm	Real time	Yes	No
Nuclear magnetic resonance (NMR) imaging	<1 mm	0.5–2 h	Discrete	H^+, (P,C)

It can be seen that clinically important metabolic parameters can be measured only by using radioactive tracers or NMR. Continuous measurements of metabolic parameters such as are required for monitoring in the intensive care unit (ICU) will not be performed with imaging technologies in the near future. Metabolic parameters are accessible only by standard clinical laboratory methods. In recent years, clinical laboratory instrumentation has achieved a high degree of sophistication, with the ability to process hundreds to thousands of samples routinely in a day. Several different instruments are available, ranging from parallel to sequential sample processing. Urgent, acute samples can be processed in a specific way. Additionally, haematological and serological instruments and test kits have shown rapid growth in the market place.

However, modern clinical practice urgently requires decentralised monitoring tools, especially for tasks in intensive care and acute medicine and point-of-care systems which cannot be performed by standard clinical laboratory methods.[7]

Today, instruments for physical parameters such as temperature, pressure, respiration, electrophysiological parameters, or cardiac output are standard monitoring tools. The monitoring of oxygen saturation, transcutaneous measurement of pO_2 for children, and extracorporal blood gas monitoring are now entering the ICU.

For a generalised metabolic monitoring and, more generally, for decentralised laboratories, small and reliable sensing and measuring elements are necessary, but have not been available on a broader scale till now. Such required devices can be realised in the form of "sensors", elements which receive physicochemical information and transform such information into an electrical signal. To measure metabolic parameters selectively, especially a single specific substance out of the variety of biochemical substances present in a biological sample, "biosensors" are required.

A biosensor is a device incorporating a biological sensing agent either intimately connected to or integrated into a transducer[8] able to perform a variety of clinical analyses in principle. For clinical analysers different parameters have to be measured simultaneously.[7,9,10] Therefore, miniaturised *and* integrated multianalyte biosensors are required which is, in principle, the domain of microelectronic technology. The parameters of greatest interest are glucose, lactate, urea, creatinine, blood gases, and electrolytes which have to be measured for whole-blood testing in the emergency case and for satellite laboratories. For monitoring purposes the measurement of the same parameters is required, with glucose topping the list of analytes that clinicians would like to measure continuously *in vivo*.[11] Also the discrete measurement of glucose for diabetics is of outstanding interest with a market volume of more than U.S. $\$10^9$ in 1994.[7]

In all cases miniaturisation and integration are expected to decrease the overall production price by using large-scale integration techniques or to minimise geometrical dimensions for *in vivo* applications.

In the last few years an increasing number of papers were published dealing with biosensors utilising immobilised enzymes, antibodies, cells, tissue slices, or receptors integrated on different transducer elements. To get a general overview about biosensors some excellent reviews are available in References 8, 12, and 13 as well as in chapters in this book.

A variety of electrochemical, calorimetric, optical, and mechanical transducing elements can be used and therefore one has to pay attention to these basic transducing elements, which are of outstanding importance for realising microelectronic biosensors.

12.3 MICROELECTRONIC BIOSENSORS

The role of microelectronic technology has been highlighted in the introduction, now we have to ask: What is a microelectronic biosensor? The term "microelectronic" is usually reserved for semiconductor technology and related technologies such as thin-film technology. The ultimate goal for producing microelectronic biosensors is the realisation of a complete microanalysis system and therefore the definition has been extended to include thick-film, hybrid, and microsystem technology. All cited technologies exhibit their own typical features; important examples are shown in Table 12.2.

TABLE 12.2
Overview of Important Production Technologies

	Si-technology	Thin-film technology	Thick-film technology
Plant price (rel.)	100	10–50	1
Degree of miniaturization	Sub-0.5 μm	Sub-μm	0.1 mm
Flexibility in developing special processes	Very low	Very high	Medium
Minimum pieces per year (approx.)	10^5	10^3	10^2
Cost per piece			
High production numbers	Very low	Low	Low
Low production numbers	Very high	High	Low
Reproducibility, reliability	Very high	High	Medium

All cited technologies are able to produce millions of devices per year in a typical fabrication site. The detailed price per device is related to the size of the device, number of processed devices per batch, overall production volume, equipment investment, and automation of production. On the other hand, automation with inherently higher investment costs makes sense only with high production volumes or by using standard processes. High-volume and automated processing of devices using micrometer structures is the domain of Si technology and thin-film technology. If there is no need for extreme miniaturisation and no advantage gained from a special high technology (e.g., monolithic integration), a low-tech production such as screen printing is recommended.

By choosing the right production technology one has to bear in mind that the main reason for developing microelectronic biosensors is the expectation to obtain a preferably decentralised, portable analytical device for unskilled personnel, with high reproducibility and reliability and low production costs. Therefore one has to check the intended application and the market to choose the right production technology in terms of the expected production volume and the required technological processes which should be the standard ones.

One of the often-cited arguments is the benefit of using standard silicon technology for sensor production. However, there are not too many biosensor applications with a high-volume market, which is required to make use of the benefits of silicon technology, and also very few biosensors need the integration of microelectronic components in the near vicinity of the transducer. Additionally, in a CMOS line it is rarely possible to use materials that are required for the best-suited transducers needed in biosensors, and the immobilisation techniques for biological components are usually quite incompatible to CMOS device production. Therefore already marketed microelectronic biosensors make use of thin-film and screen printing technology!

Another problem related to microelectronic biosensor production is testing. On a wafer level only optical inspection can be performed, and the reproducibility of biosensor performance has to be very high for random sampling testing if calibration of the biosensor at the measuring site is not possible. Therefore it is very important in developing biosensors to have a look at the needs of customers, companies manufacturing analytical devices, and markets, and not be fascinated by a "technology driven" sensor realisation only.

In the design of microelectronic biosensors, first of all the transducing element as the base device of the microelectronic biosensor is of importance. Of all transducing devices developed, the electrochemical and thermal elements are most readily accomplished as biosensor base devices using microelectronic technology. Acoustic transducers such as piezoelectric, micro balance, and SAW devices are being developed primarily for volatile analytes and more recently for antibody detection and are mostly at the research stage;[14-16] optical devices for antibody detection are in an evaluation phase.

Despite the required miniaturisation of the transducer the sensor performance should be stable for a sufficiently long time period, exhibiting full response in undiluted biological fluids such as serum, blood, or fermentation broth. Therefore, designers of a microelectronic biosensor have to overcome several problems, namely, to choose the right transducer for the measuring problem and the appropriate technology for producing them.

Secondly, one has to immobilise biological sensing agents on a large-scale level compatible with microelectronic production techniques and to retain full sensor response in undiluted media. In most of the sensor achievements presented in the literature, simple immobilisation procedures are chosen which are not favourable either for enzyme stability or for the required production technology.

Thirdly, it is necessary to get the right membranes and production technologies for them, so as to create the interface between the surface of the sensor and analyte, a topic treated more stringently in recent years.[17] (See Chapter 5 in this book.)

12.4 INTEGRATED OPTICAL DEVICES

Optical sensors are interesting analytical tools capable of performing a variety of different measurements.[18] Most of the work has been done on measuring pH, O_2, and CO_2, but biosensing devices have also been investigated and marketed.[18-21]

Integrated optical devices combine microelectronic production technology with the inherent advantages of optical sensing. Many of these developments are at an early state of research but a variety of optical biosensors can be realised in principle. Integrated optical device manufacturing is nowadays commercially available (IOT) and nearly all optical elements can be integrated and miniaturised on a chip.[22]

The biosensing devices are mainly focusing on affinity principles such as, e.g., antibody-antigen reactions, and are based on surface plasmon resonance,[23] grating couplers,[24] or interferometers.[25] It seems possible to produce stable and highly sensitive devices based on these principles[26] and further investigations can lead to miniaturised sensor modules with reduced cost, size, and complexity (see Chapters 7, 8, and 16 in this book).

12.5 MICROELECTRONIC BIOSENSORS BASED ON CALORIMETRIC TRANSDUCERS

Calorimetric biosensors are based on the detection of the heat of biological reactions which is caused by enthalpy changes. The microcalorimetric sensing principle is very versatile because of the exothermic nature of nearly all enzymatic reactions[27] and was introduced as conventionally constructed device very early.[28] If a reaction is occurring in an adiabatically isolated mass, as defined by a calorimeter, then the temperature of the mass will change according to the expression

$$\Delta T = \frac{\Delta Q}{MC_c} \quad (12.1)$$

where ΔT is the temperature change, ΔQ is the energy difference, M the total mass of the calorimeter, and C_c is the total thermal capacity of the calorimeter.

Calorimetric biosensors with conventional thermistors as transducers were invented early by proposing a thermal biosensor in a flow stream.[29] So far, the design of enzyme thermistors does not entirely match the market demand, but it seems well suited for special applications.[29,30] A number of devices have utilised discrete pairs of thermistors for differential measurements with immobilised enzymes or with separate enzyme columns.[28-30]

As a second transducer type, thermopile sensors are well suited for performing differential measurements because of the underlying physical principle and reproducibility. With conventional designs there are some difficulties related to size, sensitivity, and mechanical stability of thermocouples.

If silicon technology is involved, thermal sensors are liable to suffer from the high thermal conductivity of silicon, which can dramatically decrease their sensitivity.[31] However, by use of micromachining and integrated silicon technology, a powerful thermal biosensor can be realised. Using a thermopile integrated on a thin micromachined silicon membrane reduces thermal loss due to the Si substrate and so excellent performance can be accomplished.[32] The thermopile is dependent on basic physical principles with the inherent ability to measure temperature differences directly with high common-mode rejection.[32] Furthermore, the compatibility with silicon technology enables size reduction and direct immobilisation of the biochemical sensing part onto the chip.

Thermopiles made according to standard bipolar or CMOS processes can be purchased from XENSOR Integration (Delft, The Netherlands).

An array of p-type silicon/Al thermocouples is connected to form a thermopile and integrated in an n-type silicon epitaxial layer. By standard micromachining techniques a membrane is formed comprising the sensing junctions (Figure 12.1). Enzyme immobilisation was performed in a simple way by dropping enzyme solution within the cavity formed during the micromachining process on the reverse side of the thermopile.

To examine glucose, urea, and penicillin sensors in a flow injection mode (FIA) appropriate enzymes can be immobilised.[32] The measuring range is very limited in all reported cases due to enzyme kinetics, and a more sophisticated setup is required.

To perform calorimetric measurements in a conventional way the lack of well-matched thermistors is a drawback. Recently a thin-film thermistor based on amorphous germanium has closed this gap.[33] The temperature resolution is 0.1 mK and the time resolution in the millisecond range. By placing such an integrated miniaturised thermistor (Figure 12.2) into an enzyme column, urea or glucose can be measured, but of course with the same drawback

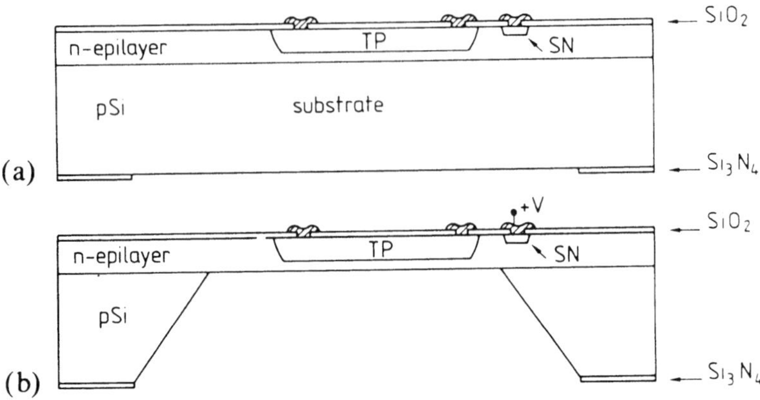

FIGURE 12.1 Schematic cross section of the thermopile summarizing the different processing steps of fabrication. (a) Wafer thick sensor with 500 μm substrate thermally short-circuiting the thermopile (TP). Shaded areas: Al (aluminum). (b) Micromachined sensor with a 5 μm-thick membrane giving 100 times higher thermal resistance and sensitivity. TP = p-type diffusion in the epilayer, designed for a low sheet resistance and a high Seebeck coefficient. SN = p-type diffusion region for contacting the epilayer; contact metal Al. After completion of the electrochemically controlled etch process, only the 5 μm-thick silicon epilayer remains underneath the thermopile. (From Van Herwaarden, A. W., Duyn, D. C., Oudheusden, B. W., Sarro, P. M., *Sensors Actuators,* A21-A23, 621, 1993. With permission.)

of a limited measuring range due to enzyme kinetics and oxygen deficiency problems. For clinical applications the calorimetric method was extended for whole-blood measurements of glucose.[34]

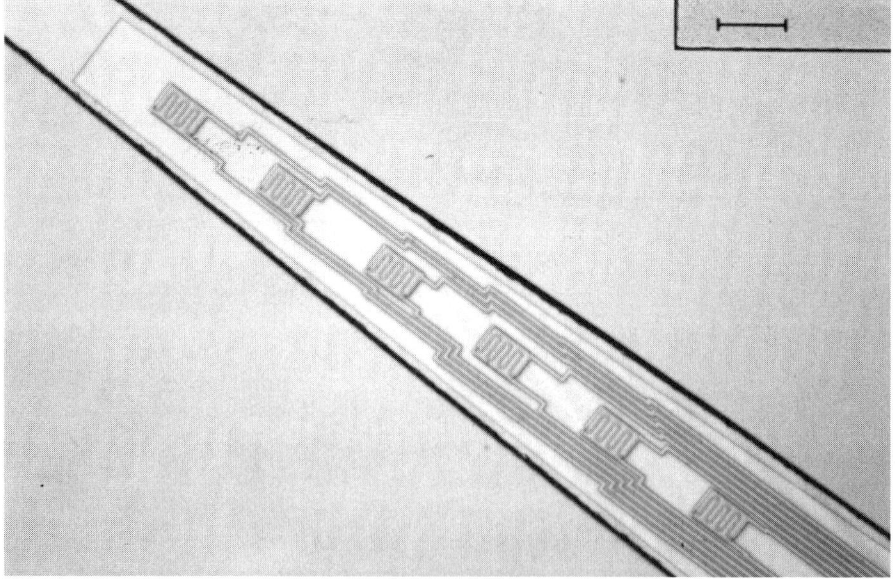

FIGURE 12.2 Thermistor array with six single thin-film thermistors integrated on a needle-shaped glass substrate. The bar represents 100 μm.

Using microelectronic and micromachining tools an array of thermistors covered by different enzymes can be easily produced leading to multianalyte detection using the same transducing principle.[35] Using such technologies the sample volume can be reduced to 1 µl, and the response time is well below 1 min. Even for an *in vivo* approach such a measurement method can be used.[36]

Calorimetric biosensors applications beyond the clinical sector are described in more detail in this volume in Chapter 13.

12.6 ELECTROCHEMICAL BIOSENSORS

Electrochemical biosensors based on well-known and therefore the most common transducing principles have been investigated intensively during the last 30 years. Electrochemical transducers can be divided into conductometric, potentiometric, and amperometric measuring principles.

12.6.1 Conductometric Biosensors

A simple transducing principle is the measurement of impedance between planar electrodes which is changed by altering the ionic content of the measuring system. If biological sensing elements are immobilised on such electrodes biosensors can be produced using changes of the conductivity in the electrolyte solution caused by biological reactions or changes of the double layer capacitance by binding or affinity reactions of the biological molecules immobilised on the electrode surface. Planar interdigitated electrodes for impedimetric measurements can be produced by means of microelectronic technology[37] (Figure 12.3).

Although this measuring principle has been known for a long time more investigations have to be done to understand the transduction principle in more detail for use in biosensing.[38] One obstacle is the high concentration of the ionic background which is always present in biological samples,[39] and a second one is associated with electrode fouling.

One advantage of this general transducing principle is the ease in creating biosensing arrays sensitive to urea, L-asparagin, and creatinine.[37] Such arrays gives a fast response, but are responding with nonlinear characteristics and are limited in the measuring range. For practical applications and commercialisation many more investigations still remain to be done in future.

12.6.2 Potentiometric Transducers

Potentiometric measurements involve the determination of the electrical potential between two electrodes at zero current flow. A standard three-electrode electrochemical cell is built with a reference electrode, a working electrode, a counter electrode, and an electrolyte. The reference electrode has to establish a constant potential independent of the electrolyte used. This is not easily performed even in a conventional measuring setup, and therefore various constructions were investigated using different electrolyte chambers and porous plugs.[40] For microelectronic realisation this problem becomes very severe.[41] The working electrode has to respond directly to the analyte to be measured. The most common potentiometric device is the pH electrode and related ion-selective electrodes. Such devices respond to changes in the analyte concentration by varying the electrical potential as described by the Nernst equation:

$$E = E_o + RT/zF^* \ln a_1/a_2 \tag{12.2}$$

E is the electromotive force, E_o the standard potential, R the gas constant, T the absolute temperature, z the number of the exchanged electrons, F the faradic constant, and a_1 is the activity of the species to be detected; a_2 is usually set as $a_2 = 1\ mol^{-1}$.

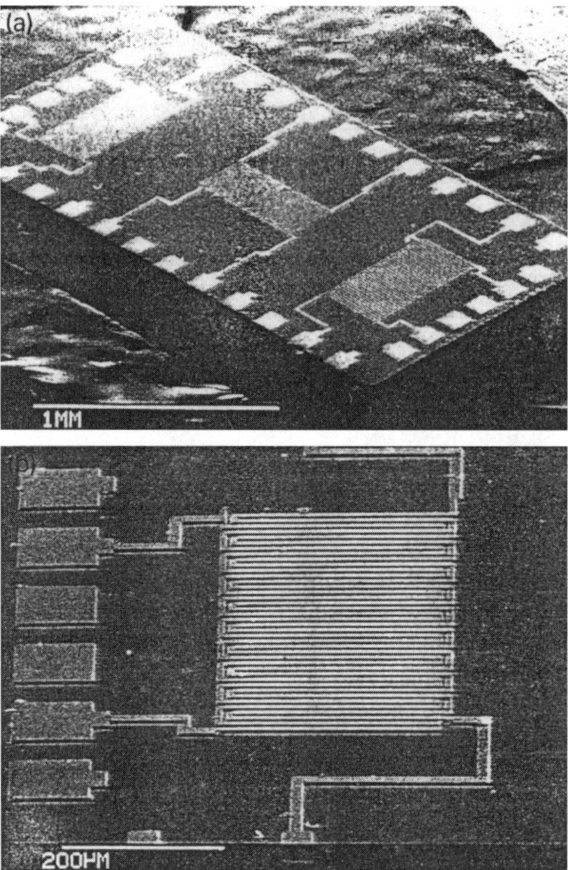

FIGURE 12.3 Scanning electron micrograph of (a) a miniature conductance device before wire bonding and encapsulation, and (b) the electrode configuration of a miniature conductance cell showing the two serpentined and interdigitated electrodes. (From Cullen, D. C., Sethi, R. S., Lowe, C. R., *Anal. Chim. Acta*, 231, 33, 1990. With permission.)

The first representative of a potentiometric sensor was the pH-glass electrode invented in 1906.[42] Decades of development resulted in the invention of many more ion-selective electrodes including more recently those based on neutral carrier membranes[43] and of the microelectronic ion selective field effect transistor (ISFET).[44] Such an ISFET was originally used for pH detection, but by casting with ion-selective membranes many different ion-selective sensors can be obtained in principle.[45,46] Even a multiparameter electrolyte-sensitive chip for clinical applications was constructed.[46] To obtain a microelectronic biosensor, a biological substance has to be immobilised onto the sensing surface of the ISFET.

The enzyme-containing FET, called ENFET, is fabricated from an ISFET by casting a thin membrane containing the enzyme over an ion-selective membrane or an inorganic gate insulator. The underlying mechanism of ISFETs is described in References 8 and 47 and the enzyme reactions in References 8, 12, and 13. An example of an ENFET is shown in Figure 12.4 where the enzyme is immobilised in a thin gel layer over an ion-selective membrane.

Local changes in the ion concentration as a result of substrate conversion by the immobilised enzymes have been measured using pH[8] or fluoride-sensitive field effect transistors (pF-ISFET),[48] or ammonia-sensitive FETs.[49]

Immunosensing with the FET gate by the direct detection of protein interaction has been described in the literature, but it seems that a direct detection of protein interaction with a pH-sensitive gate of a FET is limited by fundamental principles.[50]

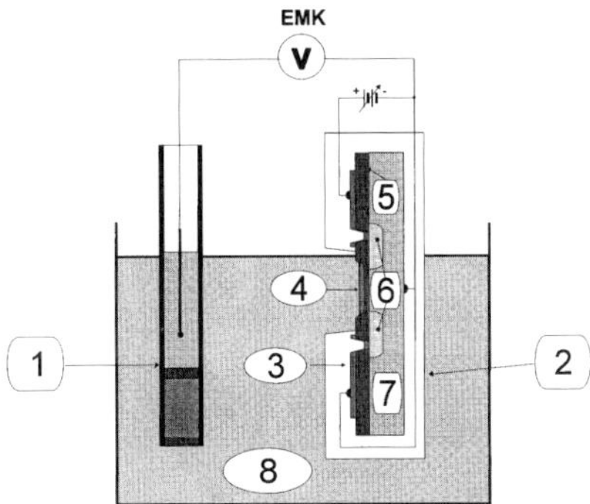

FIGURE 12.4 Schematic set up and cross section of an ENFET device. (1) Reference electrode, (2) encapsulated ENFET, (3) contact pad, (4) enzyme-containing membrane, (5) SiO_2, (6) n^+ -doped silicon, (7) p-doped silicon, and (8) analyte.

One of the great advantages of FET-type biosensors is the possibility of using a differential method which allows measurements with a pseudo-reference electrode[51] but with the drawback of weak stability. However, for a biosensor device one can circumvent the problem of nonspecific responses, for example, to the pH changes in the analyte by using pH-ISFET as reference devices.[48,52] Another advantage is the placement of a preamplifier in the near vicinity of the highly resistive electrode in the case of ISFETs.

Looking into the literature one wonders why FET-type biosensor devices have not conquered the market yet. First of all the ISFET device in itself exhibits some problems: drift, sensitivity to ambient light, dependence on buffer capacity in the sample, encapsulation problems, and sensitivity to contamination are the main problems for commercialisation.[47] The provisional gate materials for pH sensing, SiO_2 and Si_3N_4, exhibit a large drift and don't show the expected Nernstian response.[44,53] Using special gate materials such as Al_2O_3 or Ta_2O_5 an enhancement of slope and better drift properties have been achieved.[47,54] Interesting to note are the differences reported from different authors in sensor performance, which depend obviously on the chosen technological process, showing the lack of deep insight into the main physical processes and technological steps. This means that although the ISFET has a history of two decades (compared with eight decades for the pH-glass electrode), a lot of work still remains to be done.

Additionally, the expected advantage in using a standard silicon technology is lessened by the fact that it is not possible to use the described special gate materials in a standard CMOS foundry. Furthermore, the problems related to packaging are severe and it was tried to create suspended gates and sophisticated assembling procedures.[47,55] For certain applications, solutions could be found which satisfy the special needs, but up to now no general approach has been found that would suit a wide range of applications with a single design.

A further cited argument for ISFET technology is the price. Producing thousands of devices at once with high reproducibility yields low production prices, but the price is related to pieces per batch and that means area per sensor and yield. This works against the ISFET because of the relatively large area required for a device and the complicated encapsulating procedures which have to be carried out to protect this device against contamination. Therefore only a few ISFET pH sensors have entered the market in the last years.[56]

For biosensor devices these problems are enlarged because of the additional integration of a biological component on a planar device surface. A fundamental limitation of typical ENFET is the biochemical principle used because the sensing reactions have to be a pH change or a variation of surface potential. In the important case of glucose sensing one would have to use a double enzyme system to get optimum sensitivity, which increases the complexity of the system.[57]

Different approaches were reported for enzyme immobilisation and membrane deposition including drop-on techniques,[48,61] ink-jet printing,[58] and photolithographically patterned enzyme membranes.[59,60] Integrated multibiosensors based on ISFET can be produced by using a photosensitive polymer which incorporates the enzyme and is spun onto the gate[60] (Figure 12.5). This is in principle compatible with microelectronic technology. The major technological steps are shown in Figure 12.6.

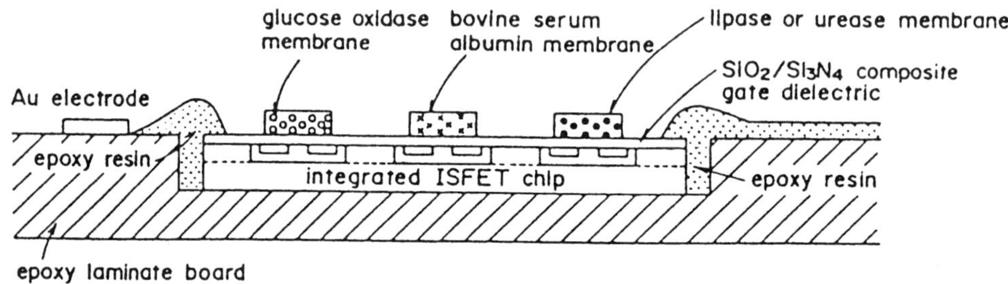

FIGURE 12.5 Schematic cross-section of a FET-based multibiosensor. (From Hanazato, Y., Nakako, M., Satorus, S., Mitsuo, M., *IEEE Trans. Electron. Dev.*, 36(7), 1303, 1989. ©1989 IEEE. With permission.)

The reported measuring range for glucose is 5 mM, which is rather weak, and some cross sensitivities due to problems regarded with buffer type and capacity were also reported. Another approach immobilises enzymes by printing with an ink jet nozzle.[58] To overcome problems with conducting silicon substrates a sapphire-based ISFET was produced. A photopolymer was used to create enzyme solution pools and to protect ISFET surface from mechanical damage. In these pools about 100 drops of enzyme solutions were emitted; an example of such a structure is shown in Figures 12.7 and 12.8. Using such a method an integrated glucose- and urea sensor can be produced. But again the measuring range is very limited.

A possibility to extend linear range and to perform measurements in whole blood is to use a further diffusion-limiting membrane.[62] Though such an approach will slow down the sensor response, nevertheless, measurements in serum and biological fluid are possible. Due to the fact that nearly all ENFET approaches lead to insufficient or unsatisfying sensor performance, no ISFET-based biosensor has been fully commercialised for wider applications to date.

Another approach is the use of the potentiometric principle with planar thin-film electrodes on a separate chip but in close vicinity to a FET input amplifier. Glucose and urea chips are now on the market commercialised by the i-STAT company. These sensors are based on ion-sensitive electrodes. The problems of stability are circumvented by a simple on-chip calibration procedure and by the use of such microelectronic electrodes as disposable single-shot probes.[63,64] Such microelectronic biosensor systems have reached the clinical market already. ISFET and ENFET manufacture are discussed in Chapter 6 in this book.

12.6.3 Amperometric Biosensors

The most investigated and discussed biosensors are based on amperometric principles. Using this principle the faradic current derived from a redox reaction at an electrode is measured. Applying a distinct potentiostatically controlled voltage between a working electrode and the electrolyte, whereas all redox species are electrochemically converted, results in a stationary

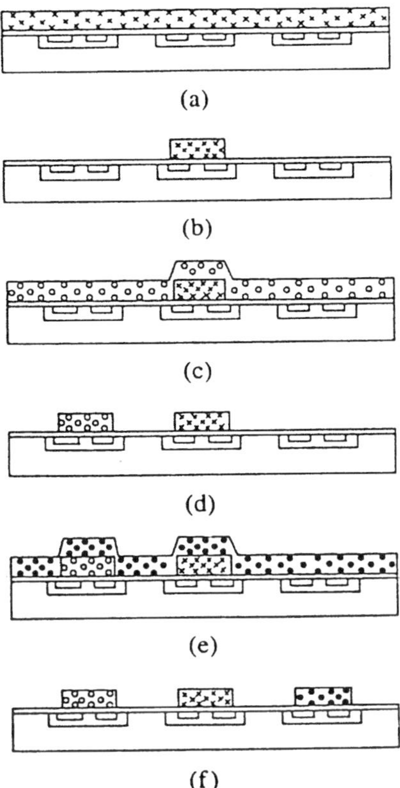

FIGURE 12.6 Major steps in the fabrication of a multibiosensor sensitive to glucose and triolein. Symbols representing enzyme membranes are the same as in Figure 12.5 (a) Coating of BSA photopolymer solution, (b) exposure to the light and development with water; (c) coating of GOD photopolymer solution; (d) exposure and development of coated GOD membrane; (e) coating of lipase-photopolymer solution; (f) patterning of lipase membrane. (From Hanazato, Y., Nakako, M., Satorus, S., Mitsuo, M., *IEEE Trans. Electron. Dev.*, 36(7), 1303, 1989. ©1989 IEEE. With permission.)

current following Equation 12.3. In this case a diffusion controlled measurement of redox species can be obtained:

$$I = nFADc_0/d \tag{12.3}$$

where I is the diffusion-limited current, n the number of the exchanged electrons per reaction, F the faradic equivalent, A the electrode area, D the diffusion constant of the analyte, c_0 the analyte concentration, and d the thickness of the diffusion layer.

In contrast to the potentiometric principle where nearly no transport of analyte to the sensor occurs, the amperometric measurement requires the control of faradic current at the electrodes and the diffusion of an analyte towards the electrode. This divides the problems related to amperometric sensing devices into transducer- and diffusion-related ones. Due to the long history of the principle it is not astonishing that miniaturised enzymatic amperometric biosensors produced by means of thin- and thick-film technology have been investigated extensively in recent years.[65,70] Amperometric biosensors combine the specificity and selectivity of biological sensing components with the analytical power of electrochemistry. Electrochemical analysis using planar thin-film metal electrodes as a transducer can be done with high performance *in vitro*.[71] Because of the use of metal electrodes which can be placed on nearly all substrates, thin- and thick-film technology is the method of first choice. The

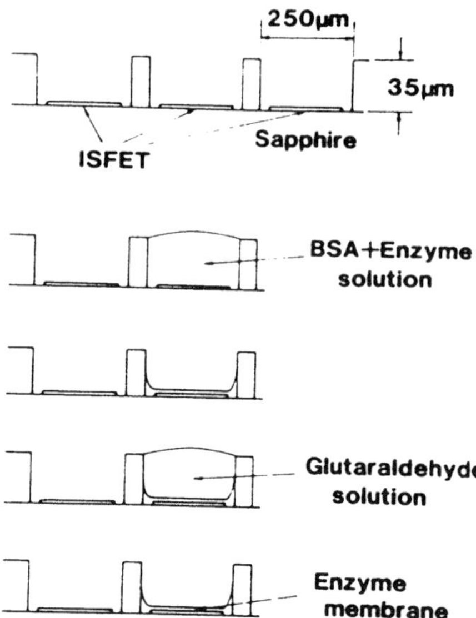

FIGURE 12.7 Immobilized enzyme membrane fabrication process. The enzyme-BSA solution was dropped into the 35-µm-deep microwell and allowed to dry; afterwards, the glutaraldehyde solution was dropped into the enzyme-containing well for cross-linking. After cross-linking and drying the solution, a membrane with a thickness well below 1 µm was formed. (From Kimura, J., Kawana, Y., Kuriyama, T., *Biosensors,* 4, 41, 1988. With permission.)

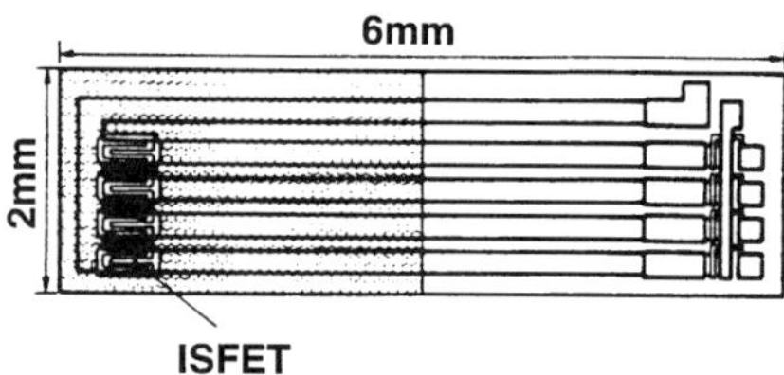

FIGURE 12.8 A multi-ISFET device coated by photopolymer (hexagonal shading) as described in Figure 12.7. (From Kimura, J., Kawana, Y., Kuriyama, T., *Biosensors,* 4, 41, 1988. With permission.)

limitation which occurs with silicon device technology no longer plays a role and biosensor production is not restricted to silicon production lines.

Placing an amperometric device in real samples, e.g., blood, a degradation of electrochemical performance over time occurs due to contamination of the electrode and thus reducing electrochemically accessible reaction sites.[72] Therefore, surface modifications or special electrode materials such as carbon are needed and the electrodes have to be covered with functional membranes to ensure full faradic current (see Chapter 5). This poses a problem in the production, even with special technologies. For microelectronic biosensors the immobilisation procedure of enzymes is a further problem. Again, different approaches were tried including drop-on techniques,[65] ink-jet printing,[73] spray techniques,[66] electropolymerisation,[68] lift-off techniques,[67,70] and photolithographically patterned enzyme membranes.[69]

At present, nearly all of the cited amperometric microelectronic sensors intended for long-term application are unable to work well in undiluted blood and even some few conventional sensor systems are able to measure glucose and lactate concentration in undiluted media for a longer time period.[74,75] Transducer- and biomembrane-related difficulties with electrochemical transducers have to be overcome for measurements in undiluted biological media.

Transducer-related problems — Using common electrochemical techniques, the poisoning of the electrodes is a well-known problem.[72] Additionally, electrochemical interference from substances such as paracetamol, ascorbic acid, or uric acid can disturb an accurate measurement if such devices are operated at high applied potentials as required with the commonly used H_2O_2 detection system.

Biosensing and membrane-related problems — Enzyme instability and consequently insufficient performance are main problems not only with microelectronic amperometric devices. Membrane fouling caused by protein adsorption is another problem occurring on all types of sensors, leading to a decrease in sensitivity. To overcome the described problems apart from the dilution method the solution is to utilise complex membrane systems.[74-76]

Solutions to transducer-related problems — The best investigated systems use H_2O_2 producing oxidases. The subsequent oxidation of H_2O_2 on the working electrodes at a potential of +400 to 650 mV vs. an Ag/AgCl reference electrode serves as transducing mechanism. The problem of interferences which are also oxidised at this potential can be overcome by difference methods using an enzyme-covered electrode and a blank electrode. Such systems are able to compensate for electrochemical interference but cannot hinder fouling of the electrodes.[76] A further method is the use of mediated devices allowing reduced working potentials down to +200 mV where most of the interfering substances are not oxidised.[77] The drawback of mediator-based devices in long-term applications is the leakage of mediators.[68] However, for short term measurements this is an excellent way to overcome the mentioned problems. The first miniaturised electrochemical device for measuring glucose in whole blood was a mediated system produced in thick-film technology by screen printing.[78] This disposable, single-shot system is produced and actually marketed widely by the Medisense company. Several other companies are now following with similar approaches.[79,80] For long-term operation other approaches have to be used. To protect the Pt working electrodes against fouling *and* to prevent erroneous reading due to electrochemical interference, an electropolymerised semipermeable membrane can be utilised.[81] The major advantage of electropolymerised semipermeable membranes for microelectronic devices compared with the conventionally used cellulose acetate membranes is the possibility to microstructure them by performing the electropolymerisation on a wafer by electrical interconnection of all working electrodes. The reported semipermeable membrane consists of an electropolymerised di-amino-benzene polymerised in phosphate buffer (pH = 7). The polymerisation was done by cycling the potential between 200 and +800 mV for a certain period. In principle, such an electrode modification hinders fouling in an excellent manner.[82]

Solutions to biosensing and membrane-related problems — To overcome problems regarding immobilisation of biological substances and to establish diffusion limitation a variety of technologies were applied. In the case of the cited mediated disposable glucose sensor, screen printing of free enzymes and mediator was used. Due to the solubility of both substances only single-shot applications can be performed. For long-term applications more sophisticated methods have to be used. A miniaturised planar amperometric glucose sensor was created on sapphire substrates. Thin-film titanium-gold electrodes are covered with an enzyme layer which was patterned by a lift-off technique.[70] An example is shown in Figure 12.9. This sensor exhibits a fast response time of 30 s but the linear measuring range is poor.

The continuous *in vivo* measurement of glucose by an implanted sensor in patients is of great importance. Such a monitoring can lead to a better control of normoglycaemia, a better quality of life, and a hypoglycaemic alarm which is of outstanding importance.[83] Therefore, another example of a planar glucose biosensor with Pt electrodes on a silicon substrate was developed for *in vivo* measurements[65] (Figure 12.10).

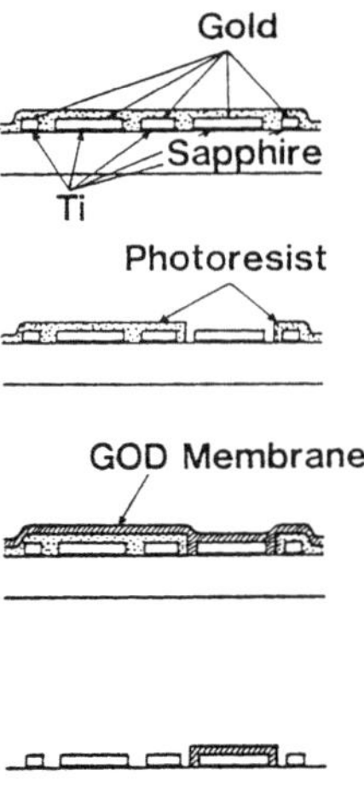

FIGURE 12.9 Glucose oxidase immobilized membrane patterning process. The photoresist is spun onto the substrate, exposed, and developed . Afterwards, the GOD membrane is spun on the photoresist and structured by a lift-off process. (From Murakami, T., Nakamoto, S., Kimura, J., Kuriyama, T., Karube, I., *Anal. Lett.*, 19 (19&20), 1973, 1986. With permission.)

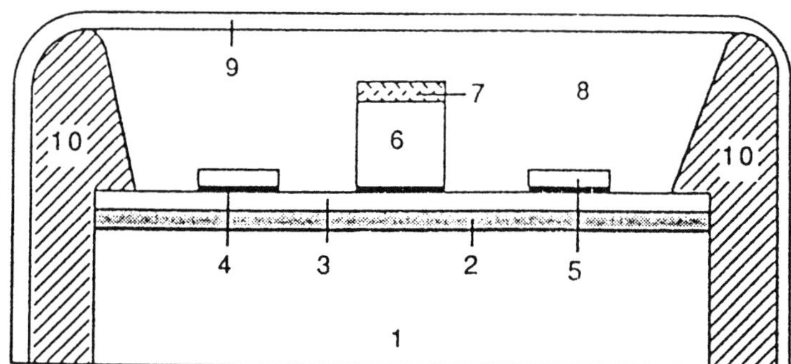

FIGURE 12.10 Schematic cross section of the glucose sensor. (1) Silicon substrate, (2) SiO_2, (3) Al_2O_3, (4) Ti, (5) Pt, (6) Ag, (7) AgCl, (8) enzyme membrane, (9) polyurethane membrane, (10) epoxy encapsulant. (From Koudelka, M., Gernet, S., DeRooij, N. F., *Sensors Actuators,* 18, 157, 1989. With permission.)

The enzyme glucose oxidase was immobilised by the well-known GDA-BSA method and the whole sensor was covered subsequently by a polyurethane membrane. This silicon chip had to be sawed and assembled on a flexible carrier for application as was the *in vivo* sensor; the assembled catheter is shown in Figure 12.11 and was successfully evaluated in rats.[84] This sensor gives encouraging results in aqueous solutions and subcutaneous applications. Drawbacks of this device are the complicated mounting and assembling procedures which are difficult and cumbersome.

Another approach places the Pt electrodes directly on a flexible polymer carrier.[85] The Eli Lilly company developed a three-electrode transducing system based on a polyimide carrier with electroadsorbed enzyme and a highly oxygen permeable membrane covering the sensor. Such a system was tested *in vivo* and published results seems encouraging. Due to the problems related to implanted sensors, company policies cancelled this project.

For microelectronic production and for getting clinically reliable sensors, the UV-initiated free radical cross-linking of the polymer directly on the substrate is a big advantage in designing the physical-chemical properties of the membrane.

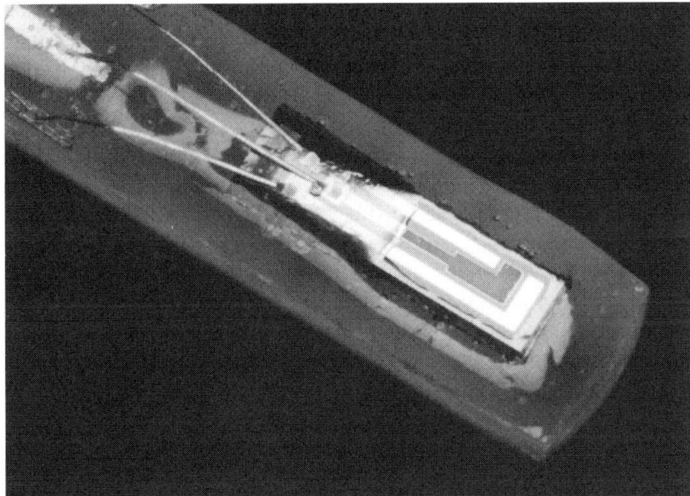

FIGURE 12.11 Photograph of the encapsulated sensor. The width is 0.8 mm, the length of the whole sensor is 3 mm, and that of the active part is 1 mm. (From Koudelka, M., Gernet, S., DeRooij, N. F., *Sensors Actuators* 18,157, 1989. With permission.)

An interesting development is the use of planar biosensors with immobilised enzymes incorporated in the photopatterned hydrogel PVA-SBQ.[69] To suppress interferences a difference measurement was introduced with an active and a deactivated enzyme membrane. Deactivation of GOD was performed in an oven at 95°C for 6 min. This also leads to a convenient production process which is compatible with microelectronic technology (Figure 12.12).

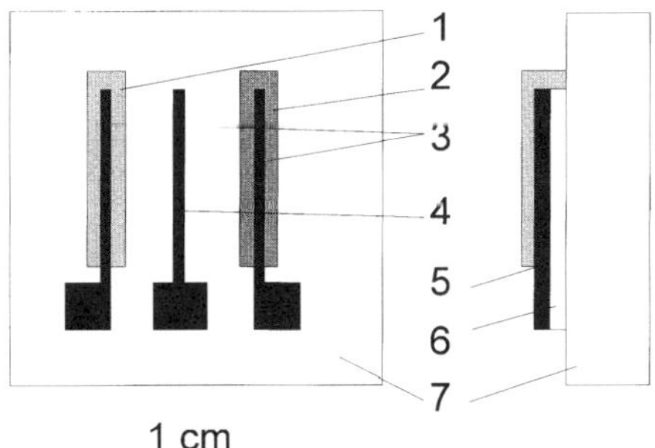

FIGURE 12.12 Schematic setup and cross section of the glucose sensing device. (1) PVA photopolymer with active GOD, (2) PVA with deactivated GOD, (3) anode (working electrodes), (4) common cathode, (5) Au layer (150 nm), (6) Cr layer (10–30 nm), (7) glass substrate.[69]

Such sensor devices are encouraging and interesting, showing the possibility for creating microelectronic amperometric biosensors, but suffer from an insufficient measuring range and were not tested in whole blood, which is required for clinical applications.

A combination of different technologies such as electropolymerisation and photopatternable enzyme membranes can lead to reliable sensor systems. An easy to handle thin-film process was developed for immobilising different H_2O_2-producing enzymes.[82] The hydrogel layer containing, e.g., the enzyme GOD, can be patterned by photolithography and could be placed selectively on the individual working electrode.[76] An uppermost photopatternable membrane was introduced containing the enzyme catalase which decomposes excess H_2O_2 into O_2 and water in order to prevent the release of the cytotoxic agent H_2O_2 into the biological environment. This membrane also prevents electrode fouling by blood components because of the low protein deposition characteristics of pHEMA.[86] To increase the diffusion pathway and to separate the H_2O_2 source (GOD) and the H_2O_2 sink (catalase), an additional pHEMA membrane was placed between the GOD and catalase membrane. This device is shown in Figure 12.13.

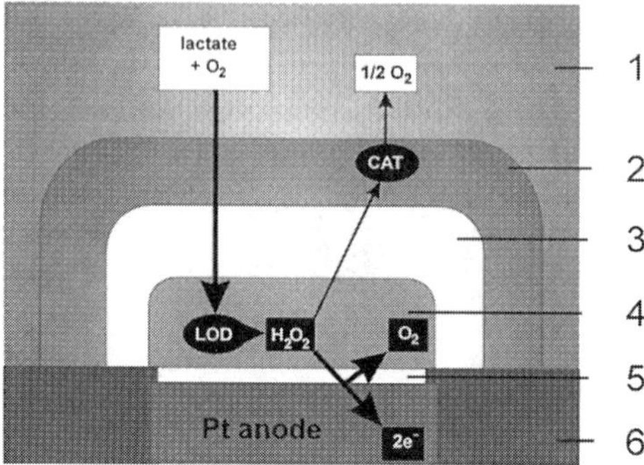

FIGURE 12.13 Schematic cross section and reaction pathways for a lactate sensor. (1) Analyte, (2) catalase-containing photopolymer, (3) spacer membrane, (4) lactate oxidase photopolymer, (5) modified Pt-electrode, (6) substrate.

The electropolymerisation of the semipermeable membrane can be performed on the Pt electrodes on a wafer as well as the photopatternable enzyme membranes. Subsequently, the additional diffusion barrier and the catalase layer were placed over all working and counter electrodes in the same manner. Multianalyte chips can be produced in this way using microelectronic technology. The sensors do not show any dependence on interferences.[82] They exhibit extended linear ranges with high sensitivities and low residual currents. Due to the wafer processing a high reproducibility can be obtained.[82] The thin hydrogel membranes exhibit a fast response time of 25 s to 98% equilibrated signal and a fast hydration time of several minutes. The sensor chips can be stored dry for at least 3 months at 4°C without changes in performance. The long-term operational stability in undiluted bovine serum spiked with analyte is more than 1 week at 37°C.

This is an example that multienzyme sensor devices can be designed to obtain precise, reliable, integrated biosensors with an extended measuring range for clinical use. They can be produced by means of microelectronic technology. Such multi-enzyme sensors were accomplished by immobilising different enzymes into stacked membranes which were structured by photolithography. This is an important step towards commercialisation, and an additional feature is the possibility to integrate additional electrochemical sensors for measuring O_2, CO_2, and pH on one substrate. Such an integrated lab on a chip seems to be a realistic vision and can revolutionise the point-of-care testing. Additionally, the technology of photopatterned multienzyme sensors can be used for the creation of *in vivo* devices on a flexible polyimide strip[87] (Figure 12.14).

12.7 MICROANALYTICAL SYSTEMS

The technology for integrating different biosensors on a chip is the basis for the lab on-chip which will require additional liquid handling and optionally active liquid treatment. Different approaches for a microanalytical system (μTAS) are published[88,89] and are now an emerging field of research. A liquid-handling system with integrated miniaturised biosensors was constructed and is able to perform continuous monitoring in undiluted human blood[90] (Figure 12.15).

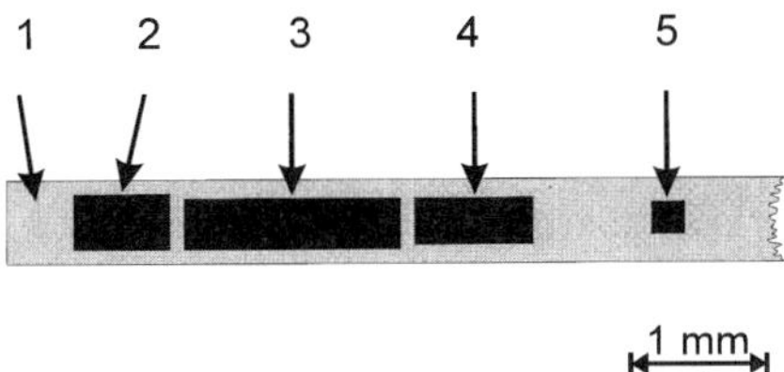

FIGURE 12.14 Schematic setup of the flexible integrated glucose and lactate sensor with a thickness of 0.13 mm. (1) Polyimide carrier, (2) lactate sensor, (3) counter electrode, (4) glucose sensor, (5) Ag/AgCl reference electrode.

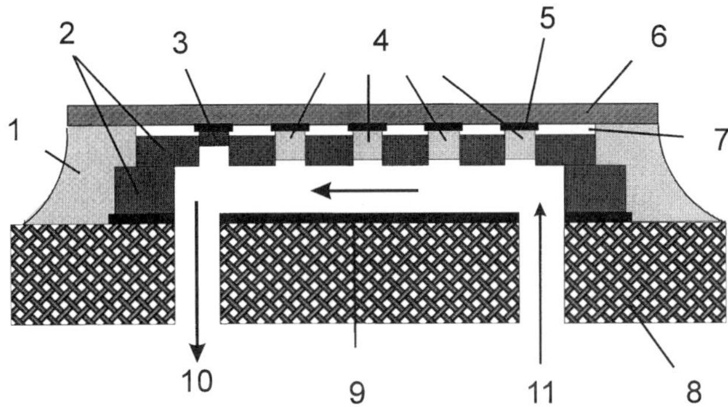

FIGURE 12.15 Integrated multienzyme sensor implemented into a microflow cell. (1) Glue, (2) spacer membranes (0.3 mm thick), (3) Ag/AgCl reference electrode, (4) individual enzyme sensors for measurement of glucose, lactate, glutamate, and glutamine, (5) Pt-working electrodes, (6) glass substrate, (7) SiN_x insulation layer, (8) printed circuit board, (9) Au counter electrode, (10) outlet, (11) inlet.

Also, different companies are now entering the market with microphysiometers[91] based on light-modulated potentiometric measurement techniques. Microchip arrays for parallel binding and detection of DNA or proteins for drug discovery and different clinical microsystems are under development.[92]

12.8 CONCLUSIONS AND OUTLOOK

As a conclusion it can be stated that the enthusiasm and the high expectations in microelectronic biosensors have not yet been fulfilled and that technological breakthroughs and further work are still needed to fulfill them in the long run. Up to now only niche markets can be covered by microelectronic biosensor devices for remote locations with the exception of the widely marketed disposable glucose sensing devices.

Increasing production volumes resulting in lower prices of devices will push the whole market and open additional markets. The expectations of using small samples as well as small reagent volumes, minimisation of time expenditure by skilled clinical people, and minimisation of calibration fluids consumption and waste are still key advantages of such a microtechnology.

If it is possible to obtain highly reliable devices to process thousands of samples immediately with an appropriate production technology to supply portable devices, a breakthrough of microelectronic biosensor systems is still to be expected.

Perhaps one has to be aware that the technological realisation of microelectronic biosensors will not necessarily be in a way which is now the common expectation, but for such market-driven applications as bedside and satellite laboratories a distinct solution can still be expected in the near future.

REFERENCES

1. Michaelis, T., Merboldt, K., Hänicke, W., Gyngell, M., Bruhn, H., and Frahm, J., On the identification of cerebral metabolites in localized ^{1}H NMR Spectra of human brain in vivo, *NMR Biomed.*, 4, 90, 1991.
2. Chira, I., Wach, P., Hönig, H., and Zeichen, R., Glukosebestimmung mittels NMR-Spektrometrie, *Biomed. Technik,* 34, 210, 1989.
3. Johnson, G., MR microscopy pushes limits of spatial resolution. *MR,* Spring, 38, 1991.
4. Millner, R., Richter, K. P., Jenderka, K. V., and Heynemann, H., Gewebedifferenzierung mit Ultra-schall, *Biomed. Technik Band 36,* Erg.Bd.1, 35, 1991.
5. Krestel, D., Bildgebende Systeme für die medizinische Diagnostik, Siemens, 1988.
6. Yamamoto, L. Y., Thompson, C. J., Diksic, M., Meyer, E., and Feindl, W., Positron Emission Tomography, *Radiat. Phys. Chem.,* 24(3-4), 385, 1985.
7. *MedPro Month*, 3 March, 44, 1995.
8. Turner, A. P. F., Karube, I., and Wilson, G., *Biosensors: Fundamentals and Applications*, Oxford University Press, Oxford, 1987.
9. Astrup, J., Symon, L., Branston, N., and Lassen, Na., *Stroke,* 8, 51 1977.
10. Strang, R. H. C. and Bachelard, H. S., *J. Neurochem.,* 20, 987 1973.
11. Pickup, J. C., In vivo glucose monitoring: sense and sensorbility, *Diabetes Care,* 16(2), 535, 1993.
12. Hall, E. A. H., *Biosensors*, Redwood Press (Open University Press Biotechnology Series), Melsham, U.K., 1990.
13. Scheller, F. and Schubert, F., *Biosensoren, Beiträge zur Forschungstechnologie*, Akademie Verlag, Berlin 1989, chap. 18.
14. Grate, J. W., *Biosensoren, Beiträge zur Forschungstechnologie,* Akademie Verlag, Berlin, 1989, chap. 25.
15. D´Amico, A., Di Natale, C., and Verona, E., *Biosensoren, Beiträge zur Forschungstechnologie,* Akademie Verlag, Berlin, 1989, chap. 9.
16. Karube, I., Chang, Sasaki, and Yokoyama, K., *Biosensoren, Beiträge zur Forschungstechnologie,* Akademie Verlag, Berlin, 1989, chap. 26.
17. Turner, A. P. F., Newman, J. D., and White, S. F., Fabrication technology for membranes, in conference proceedings, Sensor 95, Nürnberg, Germany, 1995, 619.
18. Wolfbeis, O. S., Ed., Fiber Optical Chemical Sensors and Biosensors, Vols. 1 and 2, CRC Press, Boca Raton, FL, 1991.
19. Gehrich, J., Lübbers, D., Opitz, N., Hansmann, D., Mikker, W., Tusa, J., and Yafuso, M., Optical fluorescence and its application to an intravascular blood gas monitoring system, *IEEE Trans. Biomed. Eng.* BME-33(2), 117, 1986.
20. Weigl, B., Trettnak, W., Holobar, A., Klimant, I., Gruber, W., Hager, R., Benes, R., and O´Leary, P. , Determination of pH, oxygen, and carbon dioxide in microgravity bioreactors with emphasis on application in BIOST (Bioprocessing space technology). Proc. 5th Eur. Symp. Life Sciences Research in Space, Arcachon, France, 1993 (ESA SP-366, August 1994).
21. **Anon.,** BIA gets set for the next century, *BIA J.,* 2(1), 5, 1995.
22. Roß, L., Integrated optical components in substrate glasses, *Glastechnol. Berlin,* 62(8), 285, 1989.
23. Karlsson, R., Michaelson, A., and Mattson, L., Kinetic analysis of monoclonal antibody-antigen interactions with a new biosensor based system, *J. Immunol. Methods.,* 145, 229, 1991.
24. Nellen, Ph. M. and Lukosz, W., Integrated optical input grating couplers as direct affinity sensors, *Biosens. Bioelectron.,* 8, 129, 1993.
25. Stamm, Ch. and Lukosz, W., Integrated optical difference interferometer as biochemical sensor, *Sensors Actuators,* B18-19, 183, 1994.
26. Kunz, R. E., Duveneck, G., and Ehrat, M., Sensing pads for hybrid and monolithic integrated optical immunosensors, *Proc. SPIE*, 2331, 1994.

27. Spink, C. H., Analytical calorimetry in biochemical and clinical applications, *CRC Crit. Rev. Anal. Chem.,* May 1, 1980.
28. Mosbach, K. D. and Danielsson, B., An enzyme thermistor, *Biochim. Biophys. Acta,* 364, 140, 1974.
29. Danielsson, B. and Mosbach K., Theory and application of calorimetric sensors, in *Biosensors Fundamentals and Applications,* Oxford University Press, Oxford, 1987.
30. Wehnert, G., Sauerbrei, A., Bayer, Th., Scheper, Th., Schügerl, K., and Herold, Th., Application of an enzyme thermistor for the determination of glucose in complex fermentation media, *Anal. Chim. Acta,* 200, 73, 1987.
31. Muramatsu, H., Dicks, J. M., and Karube, I., Integrated-circuit bio-calorimetric sensor for glucose, *Anal. Chim. Acta,* 197, 347, 1987.
32. Bataillard, P., Steffgen, E., Haemmerli, S., Manz, A., and Widmer, H., An integrated silicon thermopile as biosensor for the thermal monitoring of glucose, urea and penicillin. *Biosen. Bioelectron.,* 8, 89, 1993.
33. Urban, G., Kamper, H., Jachimowicz, A., Kohl, F., Kuttner, H., Olcaytug, F., Goiser, P., Pittner, F., Schalkhammer, T., and Mann-Buxbaum, E., The construction of microcalorimetric biosensors by use of high resolution thin-film thermistors, *Biosen. Bioelectron.,* 6, 275, 1991.
34. Xie, B., Hedberg, U., Mecklenburg, M., and Danielsson, B., Fast determination of whole blood glucose with a calorimetric micro-biosensor, *Sensors Actuators,* B15-16, 141, 1993.
35. Xie, B., Danielsson, B., and Winquist, F., Miniaturized thermal biosensors, *Sensors Actuators,* B15-16, 443, 1993.
36. Muehlbauer, M., Guilbeau, E., and Towe, B., Applications and stability of a thermoelectric enzyme sensor, *Sensors Actuators,* B2, 223, 1990.
37. Cullen, D. C., Sethi, R. S., and Lowe, C. R., Multi-analyte miniature conductance biosensor, *Anal. Chim. Acta,* 231, 33, 1990.
38. Jacobs, P., Suls, J., and Sansen, W., Performance of planar differential-conducitvity sensor for urea, *Sensor Actuator,* B20, 193, 1994.
39. Watson, L. D., Maynard, P., Cullen, D. C., Sethi, R. S., Brettle, J., and Lowe, C. R., A microelectronic conductimetric biosensor, *Biosensors,* 3, 101, 1987/88.
40. Ives, D. J. G. and Janz, G. J., Eds., *Reference Electrodes—Theory and Practice,* Academic Press, New York, 1961.
41. van den Berg, A., Grisel, A., van den Vlekkert, H. H., and De Rooij, N. F., A micro-volume open liquid-junction reference electrode for pH-ISFETs, *Sensors Actuators,* B1, 425-432, 1990.
42. Cremer, M., *Z. Biol.,* 47, 562, 1906.
43. Ammann, D., Morf, W. E., Anker, P., Meier, P. C., Pretsch, E., and Simon, W., Neutral carrier based ion-selective electrodes, *Ion-selective Electrode Rev.,* 5, 3, 1983.
44. Bergveld, P., Development, operation, and application of the ion-sensitive field-effect transistor as a tool for electrophysiology, *IEEE Trans. Biomed. Eng.,* BME-19(5), 342, 1972.
45. Thompson, J. M., Performance evaluation of ISFETs and other ISE sensors for whole blood ion assay, *Med. Biol. Eng. Comput.,* 28, B29-B33, 1990.
46. Sibbald, A., Covington, A. K., and Carter, R. F., Simultaneous on-line measurement of blood K+, Ca2+, Na+, and pH with a four-function ChemFET integrated-circuit sensor, *Clin. Chem.,* 30(1), 135, 1984.
47. Lundström, I., van den Berg, A., van der Schoot, B., and van den Vlekkert, H., Field effect chemical sensors in *Sensors,* Göpel, W., Hesse, J., and Zemel, J., Eds., VCH Publishers, Weinheim, Vol. 2, 469-523, 1991.
48. Hintsche, R., Dransfeld, I., Scheller, F., Pham, M., Hoffmann, W., Hueller, J., and Moritz, W., Integrated differential enzyme sensor using hydrogen and fluoride ion sensitive multigate FETs, *Biosens. Bioelectron.,* 5, 327, 1990.
49. Winquist F. and Danielsson B., *Semiconducting Field Effect Devices in Biosensors — A Practical Approach,* Cass, A. E. G., Ed., IRL Press, Oxford, 1990, 171.
50. Bergveld, P., A critical evaluation of direct electrical protein detection methods, *Biosens. Bioelectron.,* 6, 55, 1991.
51. Bergveld, P., van den Berg, A., van der Wal, P. D., Skowronska-Ptasinska, M., Sudhölter, E. J. R., and Reinhoudt, D. N., How electrical and chemical requirements for REFETs may coincide, *Sensors Actuators,* 18, 309, 1989.

52. Kuriyama, T., Kimura, J., and Kawana, Y., A single chip biosensor. *NEC Res. Dev.,* 78, 1, 1985.
53. Matsuo, T. and Esashi, M., *Sensors Actuators,* 1, 77, 1981.
54. Abe, H., Esashi, M., and Matsuo, M., *IEEE Trans. Electron. Devices,* ED-26, 1939, 1979.
55. van Hal, R. E. G., Bergveld, P., Engbersen, J. F. J., and Reinhoudt, D. N., Characterization and testing of polymer-oxide adhesion to improve the packaging reliability of ISFETs, *Sensors Actuators, B*23, 17, 1995.
56. **Anon.,** Technical digest, SENTRON.
57. Hanazato, Y., Inatomi, K., Nakako, M., Shiono, S., and Maeda, M., Glucose-sensitive field-effect transitor with a membrane containing co-immobilized gluconolactonase and glucose oxidase, *Anal. Chim. Acta,* 212, 49, 1988.
58. Kimura, J., Kawana, Y., and Kuriyama, T., An immobilized enzyme membrane fabrication method using an ink jet nozzle, *Biosensors,* 4, 41, 1988.
59. Shiono, S., Hanazato, Y., and Nakako, M., Urea and glucose sensors based on ion sensitive field effect transistor with photolithographically patterned enzyme membrane, *Anal. Sci.,* 2, 517-521, 1986.
60. Hanazato, Y., Nakako, M., Satorus, S., and Mitsuo, M., Integrated multi-biosensors based on ion-sensitive field-effect transitor using photolithographic techniques, *IEEE Trans. Electron. Dev.,* 36(7), 1303, 1989.
61. Anzai, J., Tezuka, S., Osa, T., Nakajima, H., and Matsuo, T., Urea sensor based on an ion-sensitive field effect transistor. IV. Determination of urea in human blood, *Chem. Pharm. Bull.,* 35(2), 693, 1987.
62. Saito, A., Ito, N., Kumura, J., and Kuriyama, T., An ISFET glucose sensor with a silicone rubber membrane for undiluted serum monitoring, *Sensors Actuators,* B20, 125, 1994.
63. Erickson, K. and Wilding, P., Evaluation of a novel point-of-care system, the i-STAT portable clinical analyzer, *Clin. Chem.,* 39/2, 283, 1993.
64. Jacobs, E., Vadasdi, E., Sarkozi, L., and Colman, N., Analytical evaluation of i-STAT portable clinical analyzer and use by nonlaboratory health-care professionals, *Clin. Chem.,* 39/6, 1069, 1993.
65. Koudelka, M., Gernet, S., and DeRooij, N. F., Planar amperometric enzyme-based glucose microelectrode, *Sensors Actuators,* 18, 157, 1989.
66. Yokoyama, K., Sode, K., Tamiya, E., and Karube, I., Integrated biosensor for glucose and galactose, *Anal. Chim. Acta,* 218, 137, 1989.
67. Murakami, T., Nakamoto, S., Kimura, J., Kuriyama, T., and Karube, I., A micro planar amperometric glucose sensor using an Isfet as a reference electrode, *Anal. Lett.,* 19 (19&20), 1973, 1986.
68. Tamiya, E., Karube, I., Hattori, S., Suzuki, M., and Yokoyama, K., Micro glucose sensor using electron mediators immobilized on a polypyrrole-modified electrode, *Sensors Actuators,* 18, 297, 1989.
69. Takatsu, I. and Moriizumi, T., Solid state biosensors using thin-film electrodes, *Sensors Actuators,* 11, 309, 1987.
70. Nakamoto, S., Ito, N., Kuriyama, T., and Kimura, J., A lift-off method for patterning enzyme-immobilized membranes in multi-biosensors, *Sensors Actuators,* 13, 165, 1988.
71. Pifl, C., Jachimowicz, A., Urban, G., Kohl, F., Goiser, P., Theiner, J., and Nauer, G., A new type of thin-layer microelectrode for in vivo voltammetry. Electro-oxidation of Dopamine, DOPAC, and ascorbic acid, *Sensors Actuators,* B1, 468, 1990.
72. Elbicki, J. M. and Stephen, W. G., Ultrafiltration of human serum to determine the size of species that poison voltammetric electrodes, *Biosensors,* 4, 251,1989.
73. Newman, J. D., Turner, A. P. F., and Marazza, G., *Anal. Chim. Acta,* 262, 13, 1992.
74. Pfeiffer, D., Scheller, F., and Setz, K., Amperometric enzyme electrodes for lactate and glucose determinations in highly diluted and undiluted media, *Anal. Chim. Acta,* 281(3), 489, 1993.
75. Kost, G., Wiese, D., and Bowen, T., New whole blood methods and instruments: glucose measurement and test menus for critical care, *JIFCC,* 3(4), 160, 1991.
76. Urban, G., Jobst, G., Keplinger, F., Aschauer, E., Tilado, O., Fasching, R., and Kohl, F., Miniaturized multi-enzyme biosensors integrated with pH-sensors on flexible polymer carriers for in vivo applications, *Biosens. Bioelectron.,* 7, 733, 1992.

77. Matthews, D., Holman, R., Brown, E., Sreemson, J., Watson, A., and Hughes, S., Pen sized digital 30-second blood glucose meter, *Lancet*, 778, 1987.
78. Cass, A. E. G., Davis, G., Francis, G. D., Hill, H. A. O., Aston, W. J., Higgins, I. J., Plotkin, E. V., Scott, L. D. L., and Turner, A. P. F., Ferrocene-mediated enzyme electrode for amperometric determination of glucose, *Anal. Chem.*, 56, 667, 1984.
79. Pollmann K. H., Gerber, M. T., Kost, K. M., Ochs, M. L., Walljng, P. D., Bateson, J. E., Kuhn, L. S., and Han, C. A., Enzyme electrode system, U.S. Patent 5,288,636, 1994.
80. Yoshioka, T., Biosensor utilizing enzyme and a method for producing them, U.S. Patent 5,192,415, 1993.
81. Geise, R., Adams, J. M., Barone, N. J., and Yacynych, A. M., Electropolymerized films to prevent interferences and electrode fouling in biosensors, *Biosens. Bioelectron.*, 6, 151, 1991.
82. Urban, G., Jobst, G., Aschauer, E., Tilado, O., Svasek, P., and Varahram, M., Performance of integrated glucose and lactate thin-film microbiosensors for clinical analyzers, *Sensors Actuators,* B19, (1-3), 592, 1994.
83. Fischer, U., Rebrin, K., Woedtke, T. V., and Abel, P., Clinical usefulness of the glucose concentration in the subcutaneous tissue — properties and pitfalls of electrochemical biosensors, *Horm. Metab. Res.*, 26, 515, 1994.
84. Bobbioni-Harsch, E., Rohner-Jeanrenaud, F., Koudelka, M., deRooij, N., and Jeanrenaud, B., Lifespan of subcutaneous glucose sensors and their performances during dynamic glycaemia changes in rats, *J. Biomed. Eng.,* 15, 457, 1993.
85. Mastrototaro, J., Johnson, K., Morff, R., Lipson, D., Andrew, C., and Allen, D., An electroenzymatic glucose sensor fabricated on a flexible substrate, *Sensors Actuators,* B5(1-4), 139, 1991.
86. Jeyanthi, R. and Rao, P. R., In vivo biocompatibility of collagen-poly(hydroxyethyl methacrylate) hydrogels, *Biomaterials*, 11, 238, 1990.
87. Urban, G., Jobst, G., Keplinger, F., Aschauer, E., Fasching, R., and Svasek, P., Miniaturized integrated biosensors, *Technol. Health Care,* 1, 215, 1994.
88. Manz, A., Graber, N., and Widme, H. M., Miniaturized total chemical analysis system: a novel concept for chemical sensing, *Sensors Actuators,* B1, 244, 1990.
89. van den Berg, A. and Bergveld, P., Eds., *Micrototal Analysis Systems,* Kluwer Academic, Norwell, MA, 1995.
90. Urban, G., Jobst, G., Svasek, P., Varahram, M., Moser, I., and Aschauer, E., Development of a micro flow system with integrated biosensor array, in *Micrototal Analysis Systems,* Kluwer Academic, Norwell, MA, 1995, 259.
91. Bousse, L., McReynolds, R. J., Kirks, G., Dawes, T., Lam, P., Bemiss, W. R., and Parce, J. W., Micromachined multichannel systems for the measurement of cellular metabolism, *Sensors Actuators,* B20(2-3), 145, 1994.
92. **Anon.,** Microminiature tools affecting lab products, source: biomedical business international, *Labmedica Int.,* 11/12, 1994.

13 Calorimetric Biosensors

Silke Kröger and Bengt Danielsson

CONTENTS

13.1 PRINCIPLE OF CALORIMETRIC BIOSENSORS

Calorimetry can be used for direct measurement of heat changes associated with thermochemical processes (Grime, 1985). The conversion of a substance by a biocatalyst is in general accompanied by heat release into the surroundings, since most bioreactions are exothermic and not 100% efficient. In classical calorimetry this fact is used for bioanalysis, measuring heat changes and calculating the corresponding amount of substrate conversion. In the past, studies required instrumentation with a high level of sophistication leading to relatively high costs and consequently a lack of applicability for routine analysis.

In the 1970s, investigations were carried out aiming to develop simpler calorimetric devices to bring the method to broader application. In the new instruments developed at this time, a sort of biosensor was created by bringing a biological component (enzymes, organelles, microorganisms, plant or animal cells, and even tissue) into close proximity to a physical transducer. The metabolic activity of the biocomponent causes an increase in temperature, which is transformed into a detectable electronic signal by the physical transducer. The signals are processed, amplified, and recorded. This group of instruments can be called calorimetric biosensors.

Especially in the early work, a broad range of different biocomponents, substances, measurement principles, and setup designs were investigated. As always in tool development, some combinations proved more useful than others, and in the following years research concentrated more and more on optimisation and application of the most promising devices. The following sections will give an overview of available equipment and the state

0-8493-8905-4/97/$0.00+$.50
© 1997 by CRC Press, Inc.

of the art in the field. We try to point out drawbacks as well as advantages of the different instruments to provide a guideline for the selection of an appropriate tool for a given analytical problem.

13.2 DIFFERENT DEVICES AND THEIR CHARACTERISTICS

The nomenclature used to describe different instrument types in the area of calorimetric biosensors differs from author to author and has always seemed to be a source of confusion. In Figure 13.1 the nomenclature according to Grime (1985) has been adopted, which constitutes a scheme wherein the devices described in the sections below can be inserted.

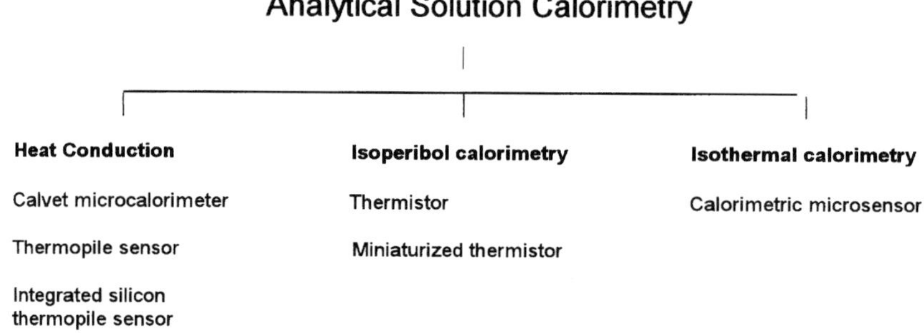

FIGURE 13.1 Classification and configurations for calorimetric sensors. The calorimetric sensors in the diagram are configured as calorimetric biosensors by immobilizing a sensing agent such as an enzyme onto the calorimetric device or by incorporating an enzyme microcolumn in the immediate vicinity of the device.

In this scheme calorimeters are classified according to the way heat transfer between the reaction vessel and its surroundings takes place (see also the overview in Chapter 1, Section 1.2.2.2). Heat conduction calorimeters provide a rapid heat exchange between the reaction vessel and an isothermal heat sink surrounding it. Temperature changes are measured as voltage output of a thermoelectric transducer between them. In isothermal calorimeters the temperature of the reaction vessel is kept constant by heat compensation, that is either Joule heating or Peltier cooling for compensation of the reaction enthalpy.

The most commonly used technique for calorimetric biosensors is isoperibol (isothermal jacket) calorimetry, which can be regarded as a variation of the adiabatic principle. Isoperibol instruments are devices which measure the temperature change in the reacting solution. The immediate environment enveloping the reaction cell remains at constant temperature. One reason why isoperibol devices have been so successful is the ease of combination with flow-injection analysis (FIA), which is a preferred technique in bioanalysis because of good precision, operational stability, and versatility.

The following paragraphs will give further information about the different types of calorimetric instrumentation and provide examples of biosensor devices.

13.2.1 HEAT-CONDUCTION CALORIMETRY

According to Wadsö (1987), the Calvet microcalorimeter (Figure 13.2) is one of the best-known types of heat conduction calorimeters. Its design is based on the early design by Tian (Calvet and Prat, 1956, 1963) and it consists of a large aluminium block which serves as the heat sink for two (or four) calorimetric units normally used as a differential system. Each unit contains a thin-walled metal cylinder defining the space for the calorimetric vessel which is surrounded by a wire-wound thermopile (with the reference junctions) in

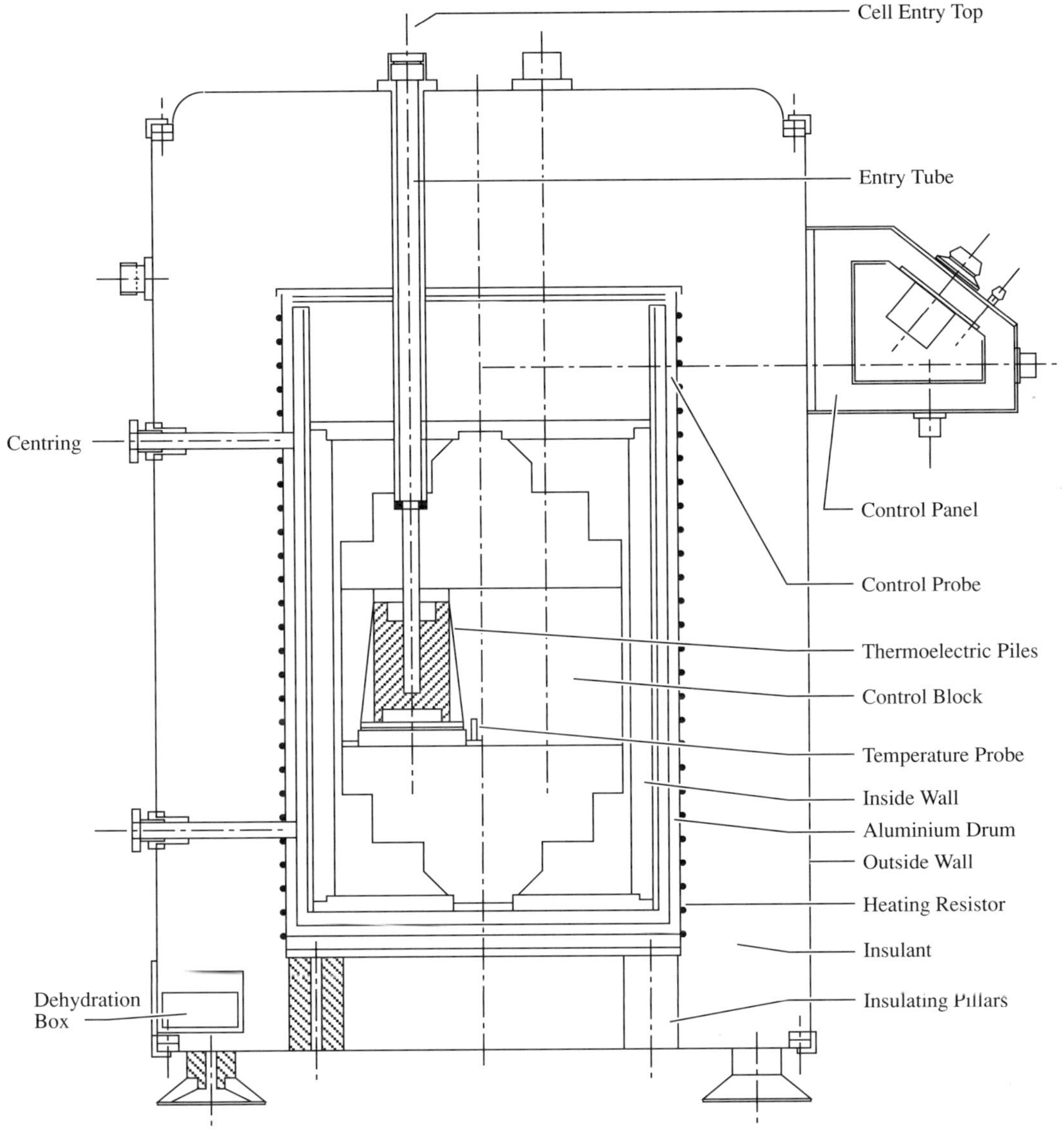

Cell Entry Top
Entry Tube
Centring
Control Panel
Control Probe
Thermoelectric Piles
Control Block
Temperature Probe
Inside Wall
Aluminium Drum
Outside Wall
Heating Resistor
Insulant
Dehydration Box
Insulating Pillars

a

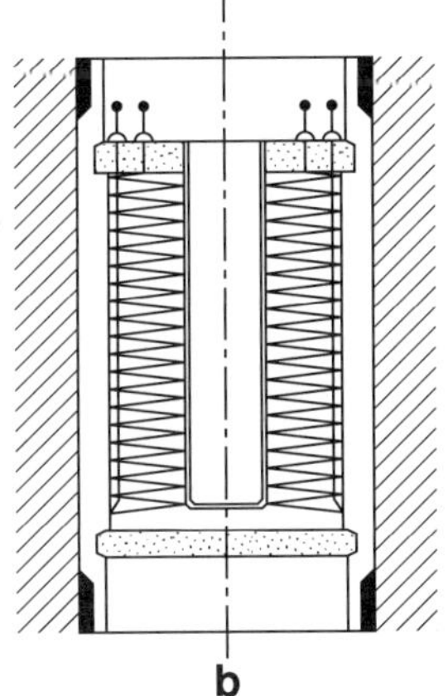

b

FIGURE 13.2 (a) Schematic diagram of a twin microcalorimeter of the Calvet type showing one of the calorimetric units. (b) Detector arrangement. (Courtesy of Setaram, France.)

contact with the heat sink. The design of the vessel can be different depending on the application. The reaction volume is usually 15 to 100 ml, the sensitivity is at the microwatt level, and the long-term stability is high. A separate thermopile for Peltier effect cooling can be used.

The Calvet microcalorimeter and similar types of heat conduction microcalorimeters as described in Wadsö (1987) have been used for thermal and energetic studies of cellular biological systems. In 1974 Pennington applied a small-volume microcalorimeter for the determination of peroxide with peroxidase using a Peltier device. More recently, a miniaturised device has been described (Muehlbauer, 1989, 1990) based on a thin-film thermopile, for the detection of glucose and urea. In this enzyme thermopile sensor, about 50 antimony-bismuth thermocouple pairs are evaporated onto a thin mylar sheet, which is then bent to form a cylinder and mounted at the tip of a polyethylene catheter of 3 mm in diameter. The enzyme is immobilised on this tip by dip-coating together with a cross-linking agent (Figure 13.3).

Bataillard et al. (1993b) applied an integrated silicon/thin film thermopile as biosensor for the thermal monitoring of glucose, urea, and penicillin. The high rejection of thermal noise, due to the working principle of thermopiles and due to the close contact between thermopile and enzyme, reduces the need to accurately control the ambient temperature (Bataillard, 1993a), and in combination with their small size makes them potentially implantable in order to perform *in situ* monitoring of blood parameters. The transducer does have an intrinsic sensitivity of 70 mV/K and a temperature resolution on the order of 0.01 mK. For more detail see Table 13.1 and Figure 13.4.

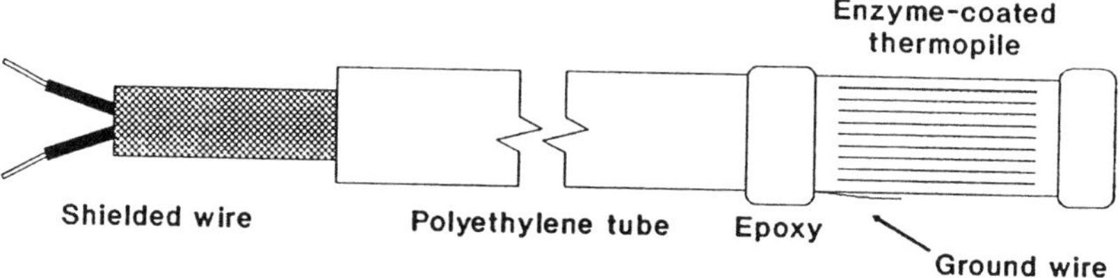

FIGURE 13.3 Thermoelectric enzyme sensor. (From Muehlbauer, M. J., Guilbeau, E. J., Towe, B. C., and Brandon, T. A., *Biosens. Bioelectron.*, 5, 1, 1990. With permission.)

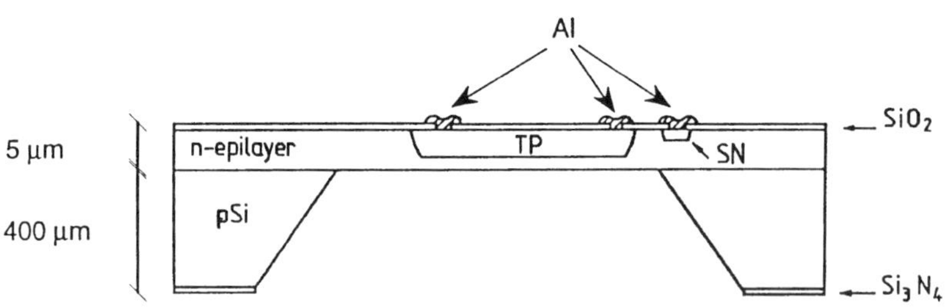

FIGURE 13.4 Schematic cross-sectional view of an integrated silicon thermopile. TP: p-type diffusion region in the epilayer with low sheet resistance and a high Seebeck coefficient; SN: p-type diffusion region for contacting the epilayer. The epilayer thickness is reduced to 5 µm underneath the thermopile by electrochemically controlled etching. (From Bataillard, P., Steffgen, E., Haemmerei, S., Manz, A., and Widmer, H. M., *Biosen. Bioelectron.*, 8, 89, 1993. With permission.)

13.2.2 Isothermal Calorimetry (Heat-Compensation)

In adiabatic-shield or isothermal calorimeters there is no net heat exchange with the surroundings. The temperature difference between the adiabatic shield and the vessel is kept at zero during the whole calorimetric measurement by automatically controlled heat evolution in the shield heater. Many important calorimeter constructions are based on the adiabatic shield principle and used in demanding measurements, especially when reactions of long durations are involved. Due to its comparatively complex design this calorimeter type has found rather limited use in the biosensor area to date. In modern miniaturised formats, however, it has been applied in relatively simple constructions to compensate for variations in the ambient temperature by utilising the heat of the effluent for thermostatting the adiabatic shield (Xie et al., 1993a) as shown in Figure 13.5.

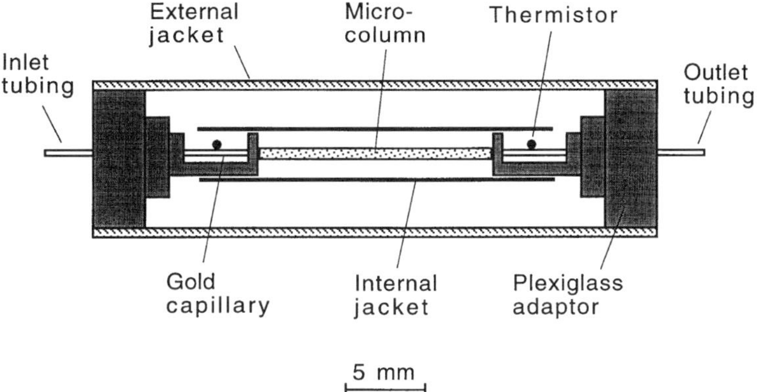

FIGURE 13.5 Miniaturized calorimetric biosensor with an adiabatic shield and a 0.6 mm (ID) × 15 mm microcolumn. (From Xie, B., Hedberg, U., Mecklenburg, M., and Danielsson, B., *Sensors Actuators,* B15-16, 141, 1993. With permission.)

13.2.3 Isoperibol Calorimetry

This is one of the most common and simplest types of calorimeters and the one that has been used most for constructing thermal biosensors. It can also be called an isothermal jacket calorimeter and has the calorimetric vessel thermally insulated from the surrounding thermostatic jacket or bath. It can be characterised as being nearly adiabatic.

The enzyme thermistor described by Mosbach et al. (1975) has been used in numerous applications, of which some are listed in Section 13.3. Using whole cells instead of enzymes as biocatalysts, the system can be applied as a "microbe thermistor" (Mattiasson et al., 1977). Performance details for the instrumentation are given in Table 13.1, schematic design diagrams in Figure 13.6, and a detailed construction drawing is shown in in Figure 13.7. One miniaturised system of this type of biosensor has been fabricated on a silicon chip (Xie et al., 1992) (see Figure 13.8).

Another isoperibol biosensor construction consists of a bead thermistor head with a silicone tube surrounding it and offering support for enzyme immobilisation (Shimohigoshi et al., 1995). Performance data for this miniaturized device (Figure 13.9) are also given in Table 13.1.

An integrated multienzyme thermistor device for the simultaneous assay of more than one analyte is shown in Figure 13.10.

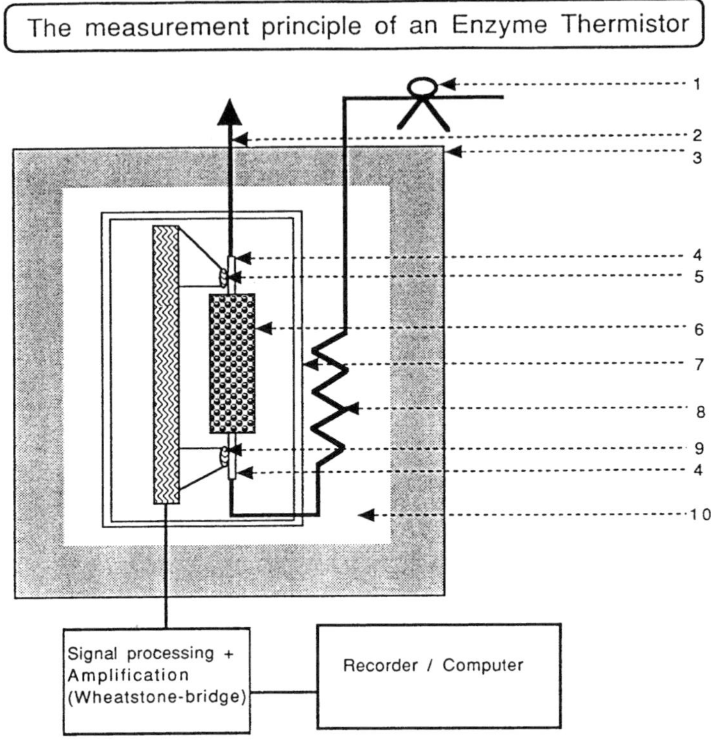

1. Sample injection valve + loop
2. Buffer stream (sample)
3. Polyurethane foam
4. Gold capillary
5. Measurement thermistor
6. Column (filled with biocomponent, exchangeable)
7. Heat-sink (inner aluminium block)
8. Heat exchanger
9. Reference thermistor
10. Outer aluminium block

FIGURE 13.6 Schematic design diagrams of the enzyme thermistor.

13.2.4 Overview of Instrumentation Characteristics

Table 1 will give an overview of important features of different devices described in the literature.

13.3 APPLICATIONS OF CALORIMETRIC BIOSENSORS

Of the different biosensor devices introduced above, instruments using heat-conduction and isoperibol calorimetry have been most frequently applied. In these groups, thermopiles and enzyme thermistors, respectively, have been most successful. Their usefulness will be demonstrated by describing a number of applications in different bioanalytical areas.

13.3.1 Industrial Processing

The area of industrial processing includes fermentations and application of microorganisms or enzymes for controlled substrate turnover to produce desired bioproducts or their precursors.

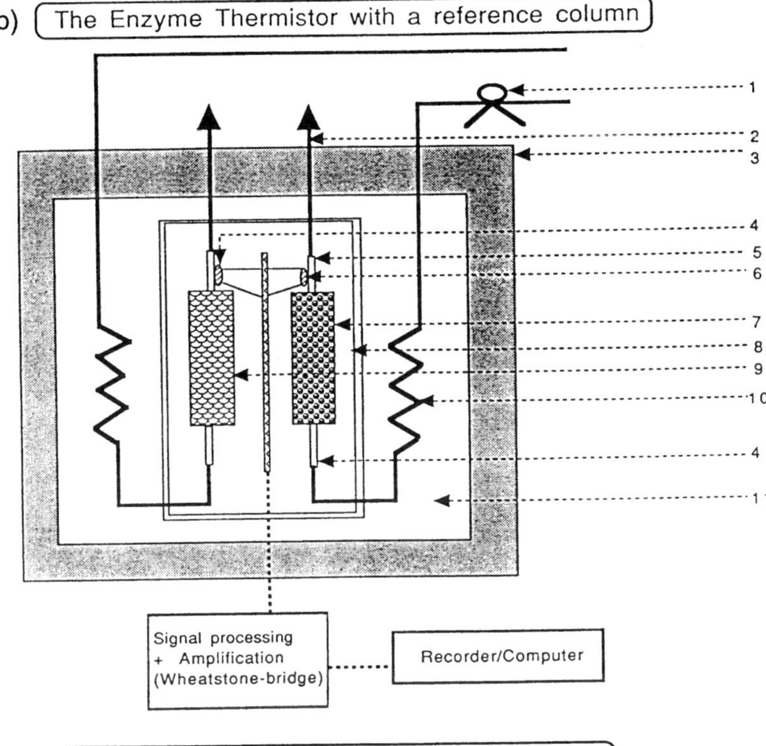

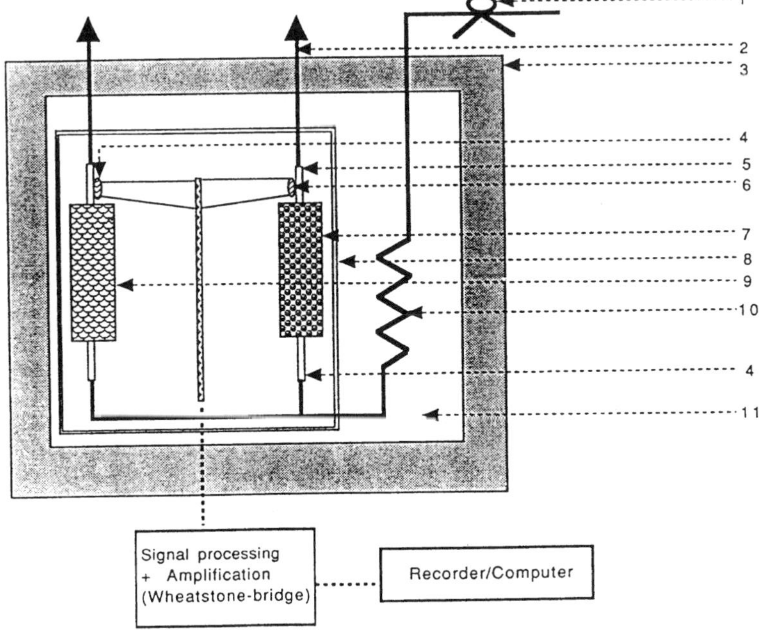

FIGURE 13.6 (continued) Key for b and c: 1. Sample injection valve + loop; 2. Buffer stream (sample); 3. Polyurethane foam; 4. Reference thermistor; 5. Gold capillary; 6. Measurement thermistor; 7. Measurement column (filled with biocomponent); 8. Heat-sink (inner aluminum block); 9. Reference column (inactive biocomponent); 10. Heat exchanger; 11. Outer aluminum block.

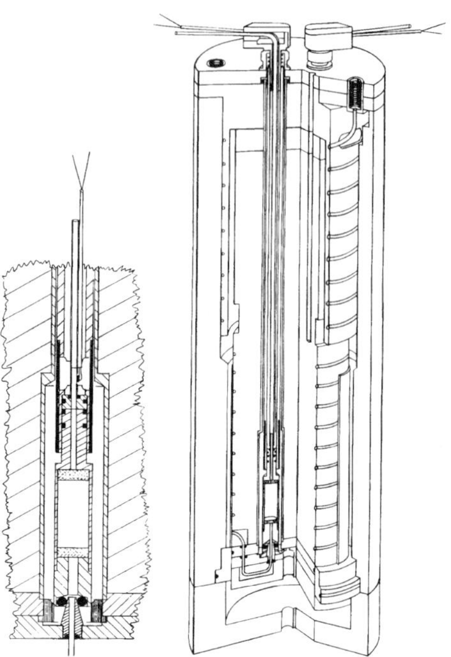

FIGURE 13.7 Detailed construction drawing of enzyme thermistor with aluminium constant temperature jacket and aluminium heat sink. The enlarged section shows the attachment of a column and the transducer arrangement. (Reproduced from Danielsson, B., *J. Biotechnol.,* 15, 187, 1990. With permission.)

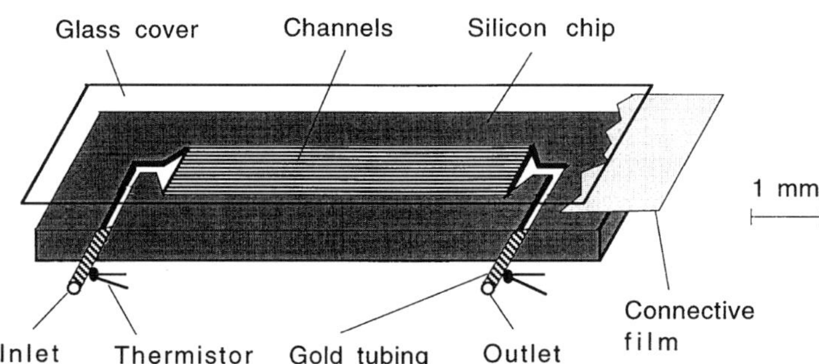

FIGURE 13.8 Schematic diagram of a thermal microbiosensor fabricated on a silicon chip. (Reproduced from Xie, B., Danielsson, B., Norberg, P., et al., *Sensors Actuators,* B6, 127, 1992. With permission.)

Monitoring and control of these fermentations and processes are essential for cost- and time-effective performance. In general, the fermentations are controlled by monitoring of secondary parameters such as pH, O_2, and CO_2. Biosensors are useful tools for monitoring (Danielsson, 1991) because they analyse directly a substrate, metabolite, or product concentration and thereby allow a more direct evaluation of the state of the process. The following examples show how monitoring and control can be performed.

Mandenius et al. (1985) have used an enzyme thermistor for on-line monitoring and control of enzymatic sucrose hydrolysis to glucose and fructose in a plug-flow reactor. Immobilised glucose oxidase/catalase were the biocomponents for determination of the glucose concentration and invertase for the sucrose. The setup was later extended by addition of a β-glucosidase precolumn in the flow prior to the enzyme thermistor to monitor cellobiose

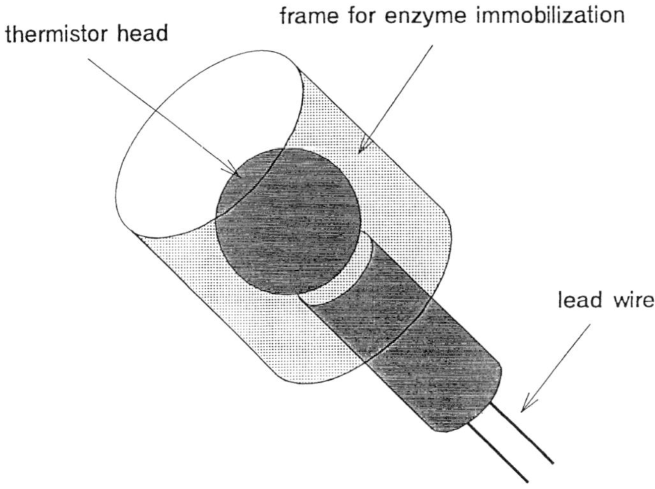

FIGURE 13.9 Miniaturized calorimetric device consisting of a bead thermistor head with silicone tube surrounding it and offering support for enzyme immobilisation. (From Shimohigoshi, M., Yokoyama, K., and Karube, I., *Anal. Chim. Acta,* 303, 295, 1995. With permission.)

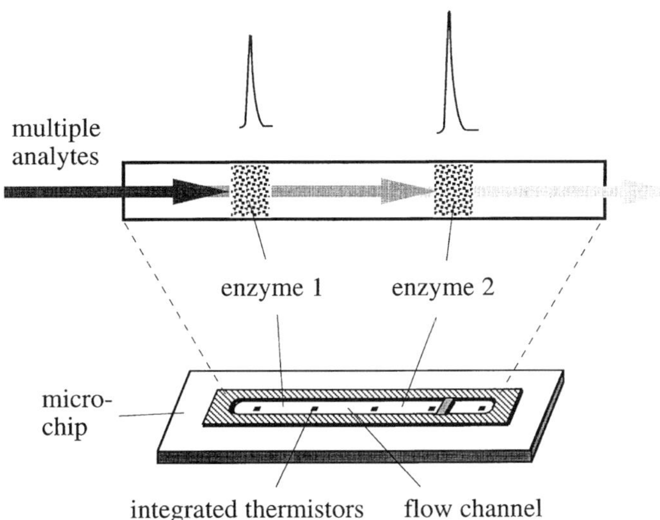

FIGURE 13.10 Integrated multienzyme thermistor device for the simultaneous assay of more than one analyte.

in a cellulose hydrolysate (Mandenius and Danielsson, 1988). The β-glucosidase converted the cellobiose to glucose, which was detected with glucose oxidase coimmobilised with catalase.

Using the same instrumentation with a continuous flow of microbial suspension from an *Escherichia coli* fermentation instead of a biocatalyst, Hörnsten et al. (1986) monitored metabolic activity during production of molecular hydrogen. Even though the apparatus used in this experiment, strictly speaking, is not a "biosensor", the possibility of measuring cellular activity in fermentations by metabolic heat production is an interesting application of an enzyme thermistor instrumentation. The principal use of calorimetric methods for the determination of biomass in fermentors using different instruments has been discussed by Reardon and Scheper (1991).

TABLE 13.1
Important Characteristics of Calorimetric Biosensors

Part A

No	Name	Measurement principle	Setup description	Biol. component(s)	Substances analyzed
1	Microcalorimeter based on an integrated silicon thermopile	Heat-conduction, flow injection analysis (FIA)	The thermopile is a silicon chip onto which 120 thermojunctions have been realized. The biological component is directly immobilized (or confined) onto the reverse side of the sensor. No thermostatting or special insulation is necessary. The biosensor is operated in a specially designed flow-through cell	Various immobilized enzymes and whole living cells (deposited onto the sensor and confined by means of an ultrafiltration membrane)	According to enzymes used Substrates and inhibitors of living cells
2	Enzyme microthermopile sensor	Heat-conduction, flow injection, or batch	An enzyme is immobilized on the sense junctions of a microthermopile while the reference junctions carry a deactivated enzyme. The thermopile sensor is placed either in a flow stream or is vibrated in solution	Glucose oxidase (catalase and urease have also been tested)	According to enzyme, glucose primarily
3	Enzyme thermistor (ET)/thermal assay probe (TAP)	Isoperibol Flow injection analysis (FIA)	The biological component is immobilized in a thermostatted column (25°C, 30°C, 37°C). Heat changes are detected with closely matched thermistors and transformed into electrical signals by a DC-type Wheatstone bridge. The instrument can be used with or without reference column (single- or split-flow)	Various enzymes (single or coupled), immobilized cells, immunoadsorbents (antibodies)	According to biocomponent used Substrates Inhibitors Antigens
4	Miniaturized enzyme thermistor	Isoperibol Batch injection analysis	Measurements are performed in a heat-insulated cell (Styrofoam box) at room temperature. Glucose oxidase is immobilized with PVA in the frame around the thermistor. Bovine serum albumin (BSA) is immobilized instead of GOD around the reference thermistor. The resistances of the thermistors are measured with digital multimeters and converted to temperature values with a PC. Nonspecific signals are eliminated by evaluating the difference between measurement and reference thermistor	Glucose oxidase and catalase	Glucose

Part B

No.	Sensitivity/range	Operational lifetime	Calibration (stability)	Reproducibility
1	Depends on the thermopile design. Transducer: standard 5 × 5 mm, 120 thermocouples, and 5 μm silicon membrane, Sensitivity: 10 V/W in air and 1.3 V/W in FIA conditions, temperature resolution: 10^{-5}, power resolution: 0.2–0.4 μW in FIA conditions Biosensor: 35 μV/mM glucose, 25 μV/mM urea, with peak-to-peak noise around 0.5 μV. With an approximately 60-fold dilution (for the elimination of unspecific matrix effects) the detection limit for above-mentioned analytes ranges from 2 to 5 mM.	Depends on the enzyme used, e.g., GOD + catalase 50% signal loss in 40 days, urease 50% signal loss in 15 days, lactamase 35% signal loss in 35 days, creatinine deaminase 35% signal loss in 60 days	Frequent recalibration necessary in FIA (1 every 10 to 30 injections)	Standard deviation of 3–5%
2	With antimony-bismuth pile coupled to a GOD enzyme, there is an ability to measure ±5.0 mg% and a thermal noise approximately 0.1 mK when in solution (~0.03 mM)	Depends on enzyme, immobilization method, loading, presence of antibacterial agents, and general handling: 3 days to 1 month	Frequent calibration required due to apparent enzyme gel activity decline. Sensors with replaceable enzyme (micro-flow system) are less sensitive but due to replenishment do not show decay	Within 5% for glucose
3	Theoretical 100 mV change in the recorder for a temperature change of 1 mK; practical useful range 10 mK change; linear range usually 10^{-5} to 10^{-1} mol/1 substance (~0.01–100 mM depending on substance and enzyme)	Depends on biocomponent used, several months or several hundreds of determinations	Daily calibration (one point) sufficient if excess of enzyme is used, frequent injection of standards for inhibition studies	Standard deviation down to 0.5–1% under optimized conditions
4	Depends on the resolution of the digital multiplier, e.g., 0.1 ohm resistivity change equal to 0.4 mK temperature change. The linear range is 1–4 mM for glucose	Depends on the durability of the polymer used for GOD immobilization, about 1 week	Daily calibration is needed to cancel the enzyme deactivation	—

TABLE 13.1 (CONTINUED)
Important Characteristics of Calorimetric Biosensors

No.	Time per measurement	Part C Automation	Disturbances	Ref.
1	When using a mixing chamber for the dilution of the samples in the FIA manifold, 1 injection every 3 min. Without mixing chamber, down to 1.5 to 2 min per analysis. A sensor is operational a few minutes after being mounted in the FIA-setup	Data acquisition and treatment and flow analysis manifold (pumps, valves) fully automated	Nonspecific heat effects: changes in ionic strength, viscosity, etc. can be overcome by active dilution of the sample in the mixing chamber. An alternative method consists of using a differential arrangement (two sensors on the same pin-grid array)	Bataillard (1993) Personal communication P. Bataillard and S. van Herwaarden
2	Several seconds (very fast), no warmup; sample volume depends on configuration of sensor, in the range of 20 ml	Possible; Automated insertion of probe into sample	The device is sensitive to the flow environment and to thermal eddies in solution if adequate stirring is not achieved. Vibrating probe sensors for immersion into open beakers of solution have good behavior	Muehlbauer (1990) Personal communication E. J. Guilbeau
3	Depending on flow rate (0.5–2 ml/min) and sample volume (0.02–1 ml) ca. 1–10 min; on-line measurements are possible; the warm-up time for a new column is 30 min to 2 h, the instrument takes ca. 2–4 h when newly started	Possible Computerization of different setups has been accomplished	Nonspecific heat-effects (not in split-flow), clogging of enzyme column (dialysis membrane or filtration can help)	Mosbach (1975) Danielsson (1990), personal experience
4	5 min after sample injection	Now impossible, but will be possible using FIA system	Sudden variation of room temperature	Shimohigoshi (1995) Personal communication I. Karube

The determination of the production and release of human proinsulin by genetically engineered *Escherichia coli* in batch cultivation has been performed with an automated thermometric enzyme immunoassay (TELISA) system (Birnbaum et al. 1986). The thermistor column in this case was filled with antibodies against beef insulin immobilised on Sepharose® B4. Horseradish peroxidase was conjugated to beef insulin. Centrifuged medium samples were mixed with known amounts of enzyme-labelled insulin and injected in the buffer flow through the ET. Consecutively injected substrate was converted in inverse proportion to the insulin content of the sample. The substrate conversion was detected thermometrically and the results correlated well with conventional radioimmunoassay determinations. One assay took 13 min and the detection range for insulin was 0.1 to 50 μg/ml.

A different "sandwich binding assay" was suggested by Brandes et al. (1993) for monitoring of IgG production from hybridoma cells that produce only one IgG. A small column is filled with protein A. The IgG sample and then a genetically fused protein conjugate of protein A and β-galactosidase are injected into the buffer stream. The β-galactosidase activity in the column therefore depended on the IgG concentration in the sample. The next step was the injection of lactose, which was converted to glucose and galactose. The final detection step was the measurement of glucose concentration by glucose oxidase and catalase in an enzyme thermistor. The assay took 16 min at a flow rate of 0.6 ml/min, the lower detection limit was 33 pmol per injection of rabbit IgG with a standard deviation of 4 to 5%, and the column could be used for more than 50 cycles.

In 1984, Decristoforo and Danielsson developed an automated calorimetric flow injection analysis (FT-FIA) method for β-lactams like the penicillins and cephalosporins. The enzymes they used were penicillinase P-0389, bactopenicillinase, and cephalosporinase immobilised on CPG. The analysis was performed off-line with centrifuged samples. This method proved very useful as a routine assay for penicillin.

Continuing the application of this method, Rank et al. (1992) realised the implementation of a computer controlled biosensor setup in a process environment for the on-line monitoring of penicillin V in production-scale fermentations (160 m^3) of *Penicillium chrysogenum* at Novo Nordisk A/S (Denmark). To avoid contamination problems, the samples were withdrawn via an appropriate sampling unit and a cell-free aliquot was preconditioned and analysed in the flow injection system. A new set of difficulties put upon the system by the harsh conditions in a real industrial environment had to be solved, but the correlation with the HPLC reference method was excellent. One approach to protection of the monitoring equipment was placing the complete instrumental setup in an insulated cupboard next to the monitored fermentor. The measurement concept was extended to industrial on-line monitoring of glucose, L-lactate, glycerol, acetaldehyde, and ethanol, as well as penicillin V (fermentation of *Penicillium chrysogenum* and *Saccharomyces cerevisiae*) and the signals were corrected for nonspecific heat by using the split-flow mode (Rank et al., 1995).

In order to monitor several compounds in parallel, Hundeck et al. (1992) developed a new model of the enzyme thermistor with four channels. The system is computer controlled and can be run as a stand-alone device. With this instrument glucose, maltose, sucrose, and lactose could be monitored for up to 300 h in the cultivation processes (*Bacillus licheniformis, Saccharomyces cerevisiae*). The information obtained from such on-line analyses provides a valuable basis for process optimisation from the point of view of economy as well as safety. The instrument was applied in the bioprocess control of industrial-scale cultivation of *Bacillus licheniformis* in order to produce proteases which are ingredients of washing powders. The nutrient dosage is of great importance for this fermentation, since substrate excess leads to increased biomass production without higher protease concentration, and substrate deficiency to a loss in cell activity. The biosensor delivered the data necessary for adjusting feed parameters to optimise productivity (Scheper et al., 1996).

Prestudies for industrial processing have been undertaken by Gemeiner et al. (1993). The evaluation of the catalytic properties of immobilised cells and enzymes is an important issue for successful large-scale biotransformation. To verify the mathematical model for the cephalosporin transforming activity of immobilised *Trigonopsis variabilis*, the activity of the cells was determined with an enzyme thermistor after different immobilisation procedures. Even though a number of simplifications are required for this approach, the ET proved suitable for rapid, simple estimation of the kinetic properties of particle-immobilised biocatalysts and the obtained data can be applied to biocatalyst design and bioreactor mathematical modelling.

13.3.2 Food Chemistry

Food chemistry is an area in which few industrial applications of calorimetric biosensors have been realised. Nevertheless, a number of substances of interest for food analysis can be determined by thermometric devices, e.g., L-ascorbic acid, cellobiose, ethanol, D-galactose, D-glucose, L-lactate, lactose, oxalate, sucrose, and urea. The concentration ranges for linear correlation between the substrate amount and measured heat development vary according to the substance under investigation from 5 μM to 200 mM (Danielsson, 1994).

Kiba et al. (1984) describe a flow enthalpimetric measurement method for D-glucose in soft drinks, wines, beers, and jam, using glucose oxidase and coimmobilised catalase with 1,4-benzoquinone as electron acceptor. Since the oxygen limitation was eliminated by the use of benzoquinone, a linear range from 0.02 to 75 mM glucose could be reached. In the case of food ingredients, the usual concentrations are comparatively high — a fact which facilitates sample treatment. Simply by dilution, disturbances due to complex sample matrices can often be eliminated. For analysis of beverages, 1 ml of sample was boiled for 3 min in a 10-ml evaporation tube and afterwards filled up to 10 ml with 50 mM quinone solution in pH 6.0 buffer. Jam (1 g) was boiled in hot water, diluted with buffer to 50 ml, the insoluble material was filtered off, and 1 ml of the filtrate was diluted to 10 ml with the quinone solution. The analysis results were in agreement with the certified glucose values of the food samples, the glucose oxidase column served for at least 3000 samples with a possible frequency of 40 samples per hour.

In contrast to food constituents, high sensitivity is required for the detection of food contaminants. Satoh (1993) described a flow-injection calorimetric system for urea in acid media with the use of acid urease, which made it possible to detect urea directly in alcoholic beverages (linear range up to 2 mM). In the presence of ethanol, urea is transformed to urethane, a carcinogenic, mutagenic, and teratogenic substance. To avoid health risks for the consumer it is important to be able to detect and eliminate the urea. Satoh suggested an enzyme reactor filled with immobilised urease as an elimination step after ethanol production, which could be controlled by an enzyme thermistor in split-flow mode. In his experiments a sample volume of 1 ml was analysed with 1.5% standard deviation ($n = 10$), an assay time of 5 min, and a long-term stability of more than 1800 samples in 4 months.

Another monitoring system for toxic compounds in food has been introduced by Mandenius et al. (1983). Their investigations focused on amygdalin and cyanide in industrial food samples of sweet and bitter almonds as well as apricots. The instrument was again an enzyme thermistor with immobilised β-glucosidase as biocomponent. An assay time of 5 min was achieved with a linear detection range of 0.1 to 20 mM.

13.3.3 Medical Field

Clinical biochemistry has traditionally been a very important area for biosensor development. Knowledge of the concentration of different metabolites in serum, whole blood, saliva, and sweat offers valuable information about the physiological state of a patient, possible diseases, and a possibility for controlling the success of medical treatment. The most common analytes are glucose and urea. Measurement methods for these substances have been described from the very beginning of instrument development. For example, Rich et al. (1979) developed a thermistor enzyme probe, an isoperibol batch system for urea using urease. The device consisted of a glass-encapsulated thermistor sealed in a U-shaped piece of glass tubing with epoxy cement and using a drop of mercury covering the thermistor for both heat conduction and enzyme immobilisation. A drawback in the design of this instrument was that it necessitated large sample volumes (100 ml).

Considerable progress in the field of glucose analysis, which is of special importance for diabetes patients, has been made with integrated silicon thermopiles, miniaturised enzyme thermistors, and new calorimetric microbiosensors. Some years ago, Xie and co-workers (1992) started development of microbiosensors that could be produced by micromachining. As an intermediary step, miniaturised enzyme thermistor models were produced which were found to give unexpectedly good performance in spite of a relatively simple design. With respect to sensitivity, precision, physical dimensions, and column longevity (cost per assay), these devices should be very competitive with instruments currently used for home measurements of blood glucose in diabeties provided a suitable pump and sample injection valve could be developed (Xie et al., 1993a). Carefully selected enzyme carrier materials make it possible to run untreated whole-blood samples directly through the immobilised enzyme column. Due to their general applicability these thermal biosensors are useful for clinical measurements of other metabolites as well, such as urea and lactate, as has been shown by Xie and co-workers (1994a). Multisensor chips permit simultaneous determination of more than one analyte in the sample (Xie et al., 1995). In order to increase the linear range of analysis based on oxidases, an electrochemical regeneration system based on the use of ferrocene mixed with immobilised enzyme in a conducting microcolumn was developed (Xie et al., 1993b). This hybrid biosensor is independent of the oxygen concentration in the medium and avoids some of the interferences commonly associated with electrochemical devices since the enzyme reaction is followed thermometrically. In addition, chips with an integrated thermopile construction have been tested as an alternative to the thermistors normally used. It appears that the thermopiles are somewhat less flow-sensitive than thermistors, but presently they possess lower sensitivity, although it is sufficient for blood glucose measurements (Xie et al., 1994b).

A logical extension of the work on miniaturised sensors is to combine this technology with experience from process monitoring to attempt to develop instrumentation for bedside monitoring of metabolites. Work is well in progress on a system for bedside monitoring of glucose in diabetic patients over shorter periods of time (hours to a few days). Future developments may even permit the construction of implantable devices. One factor that speaks strongly for thermal biosensors in this context is the good long-term stability of the transducer involved, because of the fact that it never comes in direct contact with the sample or any other fluid.

13.3.4 Environmental Monitoring

For environmental studies two different concepts are important: substance-specific analysis using enzymes (substrate or inhibition) and more general measurements applying whole cells.

Mattiasson et al. (1978) used an enzyme thermistor-urease system to detect heavy metal ions, in particular, copper and mercury in water solutions by enzyme inhibition. A typical assay cycle consisted of an injection of a urea standard, then an inhibitor pulse, and after a defined period (such as 30 s) one more urea standard. The inhibitory effect is evaluated by comparison of the response to the standard solution before and after the sample injection. The system is regenerated by rinsing with iodide-EDTA solution. The useful concentration range for the detection of the inhibitor can be selected by varying the amount of enzyme and the length of the sample pulse: as an example, a 5-min pulse of 0.2 ppb mercury chloride led to a 25% decrease in enzyme activity at a relatively low enzyme loading.

In addition, Satoh (1991, 1992) described flow injection microdeterminations using enzyme thermistors with different immobilised enzymes for the detection of heavy metal ions. The heavy metal ions were detected due to their reactivating effect on apoenzymes. A number of different ions, with the sensitivity range for their detection and the recognition element used, are listed in Table 13.2.

Another configuration was described by Mattiasson et al. (1979), who used two different approaches for pesticide analysis. They prepared a crude enzyme solution able to hydrolyse organophosphate insecticides. The enzyme was coupled with glutaraldehyde to controlled pore glass. The insecticides, e.g., parathion, cyanophos, and diazinon, were dissolved in the perfusion buffer (Tris pH 8.9, 1% Triton® X-100) and injected as a 10-min pulse into an enzyme thermistor in split-flow mode. The instrument measured a heat output due to insecticide hydrolysis and consecutive puffer protonization. For parathion, the detection limit was approximately 10 ppm.

TABLE 13.2
Detection of Heavy Metal Ions by Apoenzyme Reactivation Methods

Metal	Recognition element	Range [mMol]
Zinc II	Alkaline phosphatase	0.0010–1.0
Zinc II	Bovine carbonic anhydrase	0.025–0.25
Zinc II	Carboxypeptidase A	0.1–0.5
Copper II	Ascorbate oxidase	0.001–0.05
Copper II	Galactose oxidase	5.00–20.00
Cobalt II	Alkaline phosphatase	0.04–1.0
Cobalt II	Bovine carbonic anhydrase	0.005–0.2

From Satoh, I., *Netsu Sokutei,* 18(2), 89, 1991.

The second approach was based on inhibition of acetylcholine esterase. One unit of acetylcholine esterase was reversibly immobilised via lectin binding to Con A-Sepharose and could be rinsed off with a pulse of 0.2 M glycine-HCl, pH 2.2. Reversible immobilisation of enzymes and whole cells in the enzyme thermistor column, utilising specific lectin-glucoprotein interactions, had been introduced earlier (Mattiasson and Borrebäck, 1978) and is especially useful for inhibition studies where the enzyme has to be replaced very often. The enzyme activity was determined with 10 mM butyrylcholine as a substrate. A 5- to 10-min pulse of pesticide solution was introduced into the flow buffer, followed by a second substrate pulse. The decrease in activity was proportional to the amount of pesticide, with a detection limit below 1 ppm.

To adapt this system to on-line monitoring, for example, in wastewater control, the next step was to investigate the occurrence of the contaminant, e.g., a pesticide, in a substrate containing flow buffer. Kröger and Danielsson (unpublished) found that due to this change in setup it was even possible to differentiate between reversible and irreversible inhibition and quantify a reversible inhibitor. Since it is possible with the calorimetric method to use the natural substrate acetylcholine to assay a cholinesterase, instead of the commonly used thiocholines, this methodology might be useful in medical research as well.

Utilization of whole cells as the monitoring element has been realised by Thavarungkul et al. (1991). *Pseudomonas cepacia* capable of metabolising aromatic compounds were immobilised in Ca^{+}-alginate beads and their response to aromatic substances, e.g., salicylate, was monitored with an enzyme thermistor.

13.3.5 Miscellaneous Applications

Enzyme thermistors have also found some applications in more research-related topics such as the direct estimation of intrinsic kinetics of immobilised biocatalysts (Štefuca et al., 1990). Here the enzyme thermistor offered a rapid and direct method for the determination of kinetic constants (K_i, K_m, V_m) for immobilised enzymes. For the investigated system, saccharose and immobilised invertase, the correlation between the results obtained with the enzyme thermistor and an independent differential reactor system was very good within a range of 1.0 to 1.5 ml/min flow rate.

Determination of ADP and ATP by multiple enzymes in recycling systems: pyruvate kinase and hexokinase coimmobilised on aminopropyl CPG, was demonstrated by Kirstein et al. (1989). In addition, a second reactor with L-lactate dehydrogenase, lactate oxidase, and catalase was used to increase the sensitivity from 6×10^{-5} M without recycling at all, to 2×10^{-6} M in the kinase bienzyme reactor, and finally 1×10^{-8} M with the dual recycling system, corresponding to an overall amplification of 1700-fold.

The use of an enzyme thermistor as a specific detector for monitoring different enzymes in the eluents from chromatographic procedures (Danielsson et al., 1981; Danielsson et Larsson, 1990) has the advantage of being applicable in optically dense solutions where spectrophotometric methods fail, and of being able to operate on-line or for discrete samples.

In 1988 Flygare and Danielsson made use of the ability of enzymes to function as catalysts in organic solvents. Performing the biosensor analysis in these solvents gives improved solubility of certain substrates and products, sometimes changes the substrate specificity of the enzyme, or even leads to new enzymatic reactions. A specific advantage for thermal analysis in organic solvents is their lower heat capacity and higher thermal expansion coefficient, leading to a large gain in sensitivity (Danielsson and Flygare, 1989).

Flygare et al. (1990) used the enzyme thermistor for the control of an affinity purification. Here lactate dehydrogenase (LDH) was recovered from a solution by binding to a special Sepharose gel. The addition of the gel to the solution was controlled by a PID controller or a desktop computer according to the amount of unbound LDH detected with the enzyme thermistor. Both systems enabled rapid and accurate assessment of the correct addition of adsorbent.

13.4 FUTURE PERSPECTIVES

The number of possible applications listed above in Section 13.3 proves the apparently very high versatility of calorimetric biosensors. Unfortunately, their commercial success has been limited to date, as has been the case for most biosensors. Few have fulfilled the high expectations created in their early days. It is not easy to describe the reasons for this phenomenon, but certainly a number of factors did lead to this situation.

In order to be accepted on the analytical market, biosensors have to compete with the already accepted techniques such as HPLC analysis. It is not always easy to convince industries that a new technique might be as good as or even superior to the already established standard methods. To be successful, biosensors have to be considerably cheaper to buy or to run than other instruments. To achieve this goal, miniaturisation and mass production are important steps. Another possibility is niche application, trying to find situations where common analytical devices have failed so far. (See also Chapter 1, Section 1.4.)

A major advantage of calorimetric devices is their relative robustness. Especially in cases where on-line measurements for monitoring of concentrations are required, they have proved to be useful tools. Unlike most other chemical sensors, those based on thermal transducers can be mounted in a protected way that prevents fouling of the base transducer and thus a change in its response. This endows thermal biosensors with unmatched operational stability, restricted only by the stability characteristics of the enzyme layer. This stability is of particular importance in long-term concentration monitoring. Applications outside of research laboratories are thus expected to increase, especially for the more advanced miniaturised designs.

REFERENCES

Bataillard, P., Calorimetric sensing in bioanalytical chemistry: principles, applications and trends, *Trends Anal. Chem.*, 12(10), 387, 1993a.

Bataillard, P., Steffgen, E., Haemmerli, S., Manz, A., and Widmer, H. M., An integrated silicon thermopile as biosensor for the thermal monitoring of glucose, urea, and penicillin, *Biosens. Bioelectron.*, 8, 89, 1993b.

Birnbaum, S., Buelow, L., Hardy, K., Danielsson, B., and Mosbach, K., Automated thermometric enzyme immunoassay of human proinsulin produced by *Escherichia coli, Anal. Biochem.,* 158, 12, 1986.

Brandes, W., Maschke, H.-E., and Scheper, T., Specific flow injection binding assay for IgG using protein A and a fusion protein, *Anal. Chem.*, 65, 3368, 1993.

Calvet, E. and Prat, H., Microcalorimetrie, *Applications Physiochimique et Biologiques,* Manson, Paris, 1956.

Calvet, E. and Prat, H., *Recent Progress in Microcalorimetry,* Pergamon Press, London, 1963.

Danielsson, B., Bülow, L., Lowe, C. R., Satoh, I., and Mosbach, K., Evaluation of the enzyme thermistor as a specific detector for chromatographic procedures, *Anal. Biochem.,* 117, 84, 1981.

Danielsson, B., Calorimetric biosensors, *J. Biotechnol.,* 15, 187, 1990.

Danielsson, B. and Larsson, P.-O., Specific monitoring of chromatographic procedures, *Trends Anal. Chem.,* 9(7), 223, 1990.

Danielsson, B., Fermentation monitoring, *Curr. Opinion Biotechnol.*, 2, 17, 1991.

Danielsson, B., Enzyme thermistors for food analysis, in *Food Biosensor Analysis*, Wagner, G. and Guilbault, G. G., Eds., Marcel Dekker, New York, 1994, chap. 8.

Danielsson, B. and Flygare, L., Biothermal analysis performed in organic solvents, *Anal. Lett.,* 22(6), 1417, 1989.

Decristoforo, G. and Danielsson, B., Flow injection analysis with enzyme thermistor detector for automated determination of b-lactams, *Anal. Chem.*, 56, 263, 1984.

Flygare, L. and Danielsson, B., Advantages of organic solvents in thermometric and optoacoustic enzymic analysis, *Ann. N.Y. Acad. Sci.,* 542, 485, 1988.

Flygare, L., Larsson, P.-O., and Danielsson, B., Control of an affinity purification procedure using a thermal biosensor, *Biotechnol. Bioeng.*, 36, 723, 1990.

Gemeiner, P., Stefuca, V., Welwardova, A., Michalkova, E., Welward, L., Kurillova, L., and Danielsson B, Direct determination of the cephalosporin transforming activity of immobilized cells with use of an enzyme thermistor. 1. Verification of the mathematical model, *Enzyme Microb. Technol.*, 15, 50, 1993.

Grime, J. K., *Analytical Solution Calorimetry*, John Wiley & Sons, New York, 1985.

Hörnsten, E. G., Danielsson, B., Elwing, H., and Lundstroem, I., Sensorized on-line determination of molecular hydrogen in *Escherichia coli* fermentations, *Appl. Microbiol. Biotechnol.,* 24, 117, 1986.

Hundeck, H. G., Huebner, U., Luebbert, A., Scheper, T., Schmidt, J., and Weiss M., Development and applications of a four-channel enzyme thermistor system for bioprocess control, in *GBF Monographs Biosensors: Fundamentals, Technologies and Applications*, Vol. 17, Scheller, F. and Schmid, R. D., Eds., VCH Publishers, Weinheim, Germany, 1992, 321.

Hundeck, H. G., Weiß, M., Scheper, T., and Schubert, F., Calorimetric biosensor for the detection and determination of enentiomeric excess in aqueous and organic phases, *Biosens. Bioelectron.,* 8, 205, 1993.

Kiba, N., Tomiyasu, T., and Furusawa, M., Flow enthalpimetric determination of glucose, based on oxidation by 1,4-benzoquinone and use of an immobilized glucose oxidase column, *Talanta*, 31(2), 131, 1984.

Kirstein, D., Danielsson, B., Scheller, F., and Mosbach, K., Highly sensitive enzyme thermistor determination of ADP and ATP by multiple recycling enzyme systems, *Biosensors*, 4, 231, 1989.

Mandenius, C. F., Buelow, L., and Danielsson, B., Determination of amygdalin and cyanide in industrial food samples using enzymic methods, *Acta Chem. Scand.*, B37, 739, 1983.

Mandenius, C. F., Buelow, L., Danielsson, B., and Mosbach, K., Monitoring and control of enzymic sucrose hydrolysis using on-line biosensors, *Appl. Microbiol. Biotechnol.*, 21, 135, 1985.

Mattiasson, B. and Borrebäck, C., An analytical flow system based on reversible immobilization of enzymes and whole cells utilizing specific lectin-glucoprotein interactions, *FEBS Lett.*, 85(1), 119, 1978.

Mattiasson, B., Larsson, P.-O., and Mosbach, K., The microbe thermistor, *Nature*, 28(5620), 519, 1977.

Mattiasson, B., Rieke, E., Munneke, D., and Mosbach, K., Enzymic analysis of organophosphate insecticides using an enzyme thermistor, *J. Solid-Phase Biochem.*, 4(4), 263, 1979.

Mattiasson, B., Danielsson, B., Hermannsson, C., and Mosbach, K., Enzyme thermistor analysis of heavy metal ions with use of immobilized urease, *FEBS Lett.*, 85(2), 203, 1978.

Mosbach, K., Danielsson, B., Borgerud, A., and Scott, M., Determination of heat changes in the proximity of immobilized enzymes with an enzyme thermistor and its use for the assay of metabolites, *Biochim. Biophys. Acta,* 403, 256, 1975.

Muehlbauer, M. J., Guilbeau, E. J., and Towe, B. C., *Anal. Chem.,* 61, 77, 1989.

Muehlbauer, M. J., Guilbeau, E. J., Towe, B. C., and Brandon, T. A., Thermoelectric enzyme sensor for measuring blood glucose, *Biosens. Bioelectron.*, 5, 1, 1990.

Pennington, S. N., A small-volume microcalorimeter for analytical determinations, *Anal. Biochem.,* 72, 230, 1976.

Rank, M., Gram, J., and Danielsson, B., Implementation of a thermal biosensor in a process environment: on-line monitoring of penicillin V in production-scale fermentations, *Biosens. Bioelectron.*, 7, 631, 1992.

Rank, M., Gram, J., and Danielsson, B., Industrial on-line monitoring of penicillin V, glucose and ethanol using a split-flow modified thermal biosensor, *Anal. Chim. Acta,* 281, 521, 1993.

Rank, M., Gram, J., Stern-Nielsson, K., and Danielsson, B., On-line monitoring of ethanol, acetaldehyde and glycerol during industrial fermentations with *Saccharomyces cerevisiae, Applied Microbiol. Biotechnol.*, 42(6), 813, 1995.

Reardon, K. F. and Scheper, T., Determination of cell concentration and characterization of cells, in *Biotechnology*, Vol. 2., 4th ed., Rehm, H.-J., Reed, G., Pühler, A., and Stadler, P., Eds., VCH Publishers, Weinheim, Germany, 1992, 321.

Rich, S., Ianiello, R. M., and Jespersen, N. D., Development and application of a thermistor enzyme probe in the urea-urease system, *Anal. Chem.,* 51(2), 204, 1979.

Satoh, I., Flow-injection calorimetry of heavy metal ions using apoenzyme reactors, *Netsu Sokutei,* 18(2), 89, 1991.

Satoh, I., Use of immobilized alkaline phosphatase as an analytical tool for flow-injection biosensing of zinc (II) and cobalt (II) ions, *Ann. N.Y. Acad. Sci.*, 672, 240, 1992.

Satoh, I. and Takagi, D., Use of immobilized acid urease for photometric biosensing of urea in acid perfusion media, 7th Int. Conf. Solid-State Sensors and Actuators, Yokohama, Japan, 514, 1993.

Scheper, T. H., Hilme, J. M., Lammers, F., Muller, C., and Reinecke, M., Biosensors in Bioprocess Monitoring, *J. Chromatogr.,* 725(1), 3, 1996.

Shimohigoshi, M., Yokoyama, K., and Karube, I., Development of a bio-thermochip and its application for the detection of glucose in urine, *Anal. Chim. Acta,* 303, 295, 1995.

Štefuca, V., Gemeiner, P., Kurillová, L., Danielsson, B., and Báles, V., Application of the enzyme thermistor to the direct estimation of intrinsic kinetics using the saccharose-immobilized invertase system, *Enzyme Microb. Technol.,* 12, 830, 1990.

Thavarungkul, P., Hakanson, H., and Mattiasson, B., Comparative study of cell-based biosensors using *Pseudomonas cepacia* for monitoring aromatic compounds, *Anal. Chim. Acta*, 249, 17, 1991.

Wadsö, I., Calorimetric techniques, in *Thermal and Energetic Studies of Cellular Systems*, James, A. M., Ed., Wright, Bristol, 1987, chap. 3.

Xie, B., Danielsson, B., Norberg, P., Winquist, F., and Lundström, I., Development of a thermal micro-biosensor fabricated on a silicon chip, *Sensors Actuators,* B6, 127, 1992.

Xie, B., Hedberg, U., Mecklenburg, M., and Danielsson, B., Fast determination of whole blood glucose with a calorimetric micro-biosensor, *Sensors Actuators,* B15-16, 141, 1993a.

Xie, B., Khayyami, M., Nwosu, T., Larsson, P.-O., and Danielsson, B., Ferrocene mediated thermal biosensor, *Analyst*, 118, 845, 1993b.

Xie, B., Harborn, U., Mecklenburg, M., and Danielsson, B., Urea and lactate determined in 1 µl blood samples with a miniaturized thermal biosensor, *Clin. Chem.*, 40, 2282, 1994a.

Xie, B., Mecklenburg, M., Oehman, O., Danielsson, B., Norlin, P., and Winquist, F., Development of an integrated thermal biosensor for the simultaneous determination of multiple analytes, *Analyst,* 120(1), 155, 1995.

Xie, B., Mecklenburg, M., Oehman, O., Winquist, F., and Danielsson, B., Microbiosensor based on an integrated thermopile, *Anal. Chem. Acta*, 299(2), 165, 1994b.

Xie, B., Winquist, F., and Danielsson, B., Miniaturized thermal biosensor, *Sensors Actuators,* B15-16, 443, 1993.

14 Microbial and Enzyme Sensors for Environmental Monitoring

Christine Wittmann, Klaus Riedel, and Rolf D. Schmid

CONTENTS

14.1 INTRODUCTION

The complex composition of environmental samples usually demands highly sophisticated analytical methods, most of which are time-consuming because they require sample pretreatment procedures such as enrichment and cleanup to enable trace analysis. In addition, these methods are often quite expensive for reasons of demanding complicated equipment and

0-8493-8905-4/97/$0.00+$.50
© 1997 by CRC Press, Inc.

highly trained personnel. To give an example, the complete analysis of a drinking water sample consists of the determination of a series of different parameters such as anions (chloride, sulphate, phosphate, ammonia, nitrite, nitrate, etc.), cations (ions of Na, K, Ca, Mg, Fe, Cd, Pb, As, Cu, Ni, Zn, etc.), with some of them being heavy metals, and whole groups of compounds (e.g., pesticides, phenols, halogenated and polyaromatic hydrocarbons, polychlorinated biphenyls). The pesticide group alone consists of some hundred different substances. In the case of wastewater, the chemical oxygen demand (COD), the adsorbable fraction of organic halogenated compounds (AOX), and the biochemical oxygen demand (BOD) are some of the main sum parameters which have to be analyzed to gain knowledge about the degradation behaviour of these compounds if present in the wastewater sample.

Microbial sensors are perhaps best suited for a rapid determination of a sum parameter in a rather complex sample by exploiting the multiceptor behaviour of the microorganism for a broad range of degradation processes for several compounds of environmental concern. Microorganisms exhibiting a metabolic pathway for a compound of environmental interest can be screened from highly contaminated areas, or microorganisms used for special sanitation purposes can be applied to sensor development. The main advantage of most microbial sensors is that they work in a "reagent-free" mode and are low-cost devices for on-site use in monitoring and screening environmental samples very rapidly. One way to increase selectivity is the induction of single metabolic pathways in the respective microorganisms via growth in a medium containing a high amount of the compound to be degraded. Another way is the isolation of the appropriate enzyme system responsible for the catalysis of a single compound and the development of enzymatic sensors. Among the metabolism sensors the microbial sensors therefore provide a rapid first information about the composition of rather complex matrices, whereas the enzymatic sensors are more suitable for a fast response to more defined single compounds. In this chapter, the metabolism sensors for the determination of environmentally relevant compounds are described in detail and compared with the respective conventional analysis methods.

14.2 MICROBIAL SENSORS

In most cases, the ability of microbial sensors to recognize a group of substances is exploited for the determination of complex variables such as the sum of biodegradable compounds in wastewater (BOD) and the mutagenicity of compounds, the latter belonging to the group of sensors for toxicity monitoring. In some cases, defined metabolic pathways in the microorganisms were induced, leading to microbial sensors for a more selective analysis of compounds (e.g., phenol, nitrite, nitrate, ammonia). The most commonly measured electrochemical parameter is the consumption of oxygen with the classic Clark oxygen electrodes. Figure 14.1 shows the Clark oxygen sensor with the immobilized microbial cells.

14.2.1 Determination of Single Substances

14.2.1.1 Phenol

Phenolic compounds may occur naturally, arising mostly from the lignins of decaying wood. The most serious phenol pollution, however, derives from industrial waste produced by coke ovens, oil refineries, petrochemical production, aircraft maintenance, fibreglass manufacture, and the plastics industry. The highly toxic effects of phenols on humans are well documented. Phenols are also highly toxic to fish: 6 mg/l is the lethal dosis for trout with a 3-h incubation. Therefore, a maximum permissible concentration of 0.5 μg/l phenol is prescribed in the EC Directive for Drinking Water (the naturally occurring phenolic compounds which do not react with chlorine are excluded). The WHO (World Health Organisation) recommends a maximum phenol concentration of 1 μg/l as the highest allowed value for drinking water.

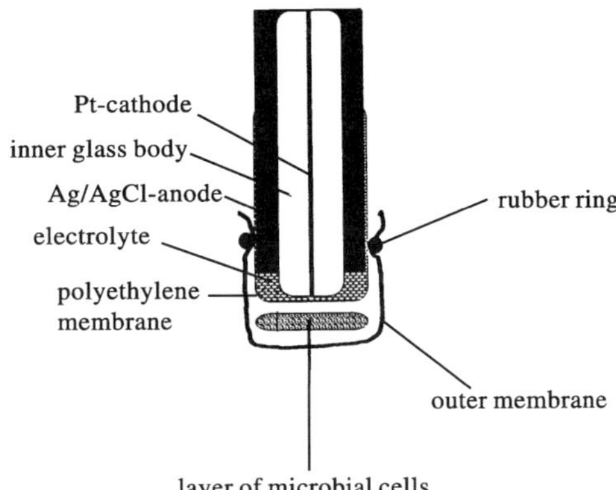

FIGURE 14.1 Schematic diagram of microbial Clark-oxygen electrode. (From Beyersdorf-Radeck, B. et al., *Analytical Letters,* 27(2), 285-298, 1994. With permission.)

The classic method of phenol analysis is the 4-aminoantipyrine (4-AAP) method which has the advantage of short analysis times (15 min to 1 h). It is based on the condensation of phenols with 4-AAP with subsequent alkaline oxidation and spectrophotometric detection. This method has generally been adopted for water and wastewater analysis. Another possibility is the use of liquid chromatography methods that employ direct amperometric detection of phenols, exploiting their tendency to polymerize upon anodic oxidation and thus form insulating films on the electrode. A disadvantage in this case is that electrode fouling has been reported when the injected sample contained more than 200 ng of a phenol.

Phenols can also be detected using microbial or enzyme sensors. Table 14.1 gives an overview of the characteristic parameters of microbial sensors for the analysis of phenol. The use of the following microorganisms in combination with oxygen electrodes is described: *Trichosporon cutaneum* (recently reclassified as *T. beigelii*), *Candida tropicalis*, *Bacillus subtilis*, *Rhodococcus* sp., *Pseudomonas* sp., *Alcaligenes* sp. Phenol is decomposed in two steps by the microorganisms (e.g., *Trichosporon cutaneum, Rhodotorula* species) as shown in Figure 14.2. In the first step, phenol is converted to catechol, an o-diol, via an o-hydroxylating flavin monooxygenase, and in a second step the catechol is cleaved to cis,cis-muconic acid by a catechol-1,2-oxygenase. The two steps consume two moles of oxygen per mole phenol. In moderate amounts, phenol derivatives scarcely interfere with phenol detection. Catechol and resorcinol are most likely to cause trouble whereas cresols and chlorophenols have very little effect. However, the detection limits reached with any of the microbial sensors were higher than the 0.5 μg/l prescribed as the maximum permissible concentration by the EC Directive for Drinking Water.

14.2.1.2 Halogenated Compounds

Haloaromatic compounds play an important role as industrial products and biocides. In addition, halogenated organic compounds can also be produced as a byproduct during drinking water preparation (raw water treatment/purification) via the chlorination step. Halogenated organic compounds cause considerable environmental problems because of their toxicity and persistence in the biosphere. One main reason is that the ability of animals to degrade haloaromatic compounds is extremely restricted. To give a current example, pentachlorophenol is used extensively as a wood preservative due to its fungicidal activity and until recently even as a preservative in household furniture, resulting in some severe health problems. Chlorophenols, in addition, are detectable by taste and smell at concentrations as low as 0.001 μg/l. The protection of drinking water in Europe has led to pertinent regulation by the EC Directive for Drinking Water and national legislation, e.g., the German

TABLE 14.1
Microbial Sensors for Phenol Detection With Oxygen Electrodes

Microorganism	Immobilization	Detection limit (µmol/l)	Standard deviation (SD, %)	Response time (min)	Stability (days)	Ref.
Trichosporon cutaneum (beigelii)	Teflon membrane of oxygen electrode coated with thin layer of cell paste	20 (= 2 mg/l phenol)	5	0.25 (3 min assay time)	At least 5 days at RT or >100 assays	Neujahr and Kjellen (1979)
Rhodococcus sp.	Immobilized with 10% polyvinyl alcohol to a polyethylene membrane	2 (= 0.2 mg/l) (measuring range — 80 µmol/l)	5	0.25	> 14 days (immobilized cells stored dry retain their activity for 2 years)	Riedel et al. (1991b)
	Cells entrapped in polyvinyl alcohol, immobilized on the polyethylene membrane of the oxygen electrode	4 (= 0.4 mg/l) phenol, 0.5 mg/l 2-, 3-, 4-chloro-phenol (measuring range—20 µmol/l)	5.5	1.5-2 (steady state), 5–10 s (kinetic mode)	> 21 days	Riedel et al. (1993)
Escherichia coli		>50 µg/l phenol, (>500 µmol/l) > 50 mg/l 2-chlorophenol 1.2 µmol/l 2,5-dichlorophenol 1.0 3,5-dichlorophenol 0.16 2,4,5-trichlorophenol 0.004 2,3,5,6-tetrachlorophenol 0.009 pentachlorophenol		30		Gaisford et al. (1991)
Rhodotorula sp.	Thin layer of cells immobilized to the Teflon membrane of the oxygen electrode and fixed by a dialysis membrane	1 mg/l (measuring range—7 mg/l) 1 mg/l (measuring range—9 mg/l)	2 1	5–10 s kinetic method 30 s steady state/endpoint method	The response slope of the sensor decreases in 12 days by about 90%	Ciucu et al. (1991)

Note: Legal limit 0.5 µg/l phenol in drinking water (5nmol/l).

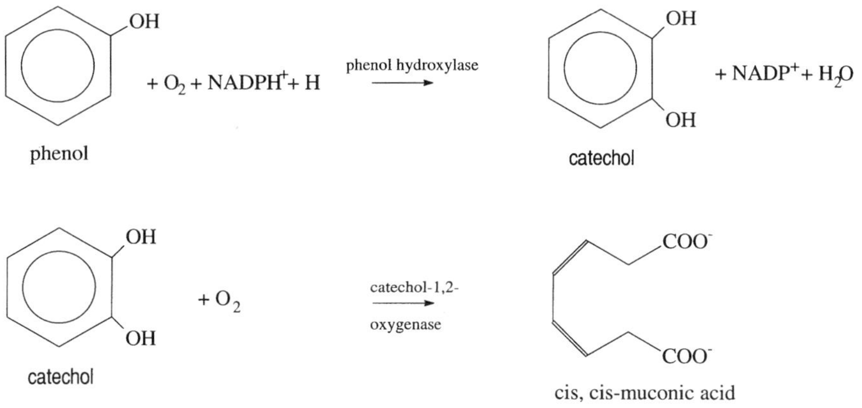

phenol + O_2 + $NADPH^+$ + H —phenol hydroxylase→ catechol + $NADP^+$ + H_2O

catechol + O_2 —catechol-1,2-oxygenase→ cis, cis-muconic acid

FIGURE 14.2 Microbial phenol degradation.

Drinking Water Ordinance, which set limits for polycyclic aromatic hydrocarbons (PAH) and other halogenated organic compounds. The upper limit for PAH (reference compounds: fluoranthene, benzo-3,4-fluoranthene, benzo-11,12-fluoranthene, benzo-3,4-pyrene, benzo-11,12-perylene, inde-(1,2,3-cd)-pyrene) concentrations in drinking water is prescribed to be 0.2 μg/l. For the sum of the following halogenated compounds: 1,1,1-trichloroethane, trichloroethylene, tetrachloroethylene, and dichloromethane, the upper limit is set at 0.025 mg/l and the maximum permissible concentration for carbon tetrachloride is 0.003 mg/l.

The classic methods for the determination of haloaromatic compounds are based mainly on chromatographic procedures such as gas chromatography (GC) with electron capture detection or coupled with mass spectrometric detection, or high-performance liquid chromatography (HPLC) with ultraviolet detection. Some methods, e.g., PAH analysis by a chromatographic method, have been standardized in Germany. The chromatography procedures are time-consuming, as enrichment and cleanup steps are required prior to analysis. In addition, expensive equipment is needed which confines the procedures to laboratory use because of the size and weight of the devices.

Various microorganisms exist that are capable of degrading aromatic and haloaromatic compounds. Table 14.2 gives an overview of the important assay characteristics of microbial sensors for the analysis of halogenated compounds. The most detailed knowledge of the degradative mechanism for halogenated compounds comes from studies with *Pseudomonas* sp. B13 (cf. Riedel et al., 1991a). *Pseudomonas* sp. B13 hydroxylates 3-chlorobenzoate via 3- and 5-chloro-3,5-cyclohexadiene-1,2-diol-1-carboxylic acid to 3- and 4-chlorocatechol, respectively, which are further degraded by ring cleavage to 2- and 3-chloro-cis,cis-muconic acid. The chloromuconic acid is converted to 4-carboxymethylene-2-buten-4-olides concomitant with dehalogenation. The degradation of 3-chlorobenzoate by *P. putida* 87 starts with decarboxylation producing 3-chlorophenol, which is transformed into chloropyrocatechol, which in turn is cleaved to chloromuconic acid and eventually dechlorinated. This strain was investigated for 3-chlorobenzoate determination by Riedel et al. (1991a). *Rhodococcus* sp. is able to metabolise phenols and chlorophenols. Chlorophenols are hydroxylated to chlorocatechols and 3- and 4-chlorocatechol further converted to cis-4-carboxymethylene-but-2-en-4-diole. The phenoxyhydroxylase of *Rhodococcus* has a broad substrate specificity and is capable of transforming phenols with up to three chlorine substituents. A *Rhodococcus* sp. sensor for the analysis of benzoate, phenol, and 2-, 3-, and 4-chlorophenol was described by Riedel et al. (1991b, 1993). Biosensors containing *Trichosporon beigelii (cutaneum)* strains represent a new approach to the rapid measurement of monochloro- and dichlorophenols (Riedel et al., 1995). The *T. beigelii (cutaneum)* E4 is especially suitable for the determination of chloroderivatives because this strain shows no reaction to benzoate (Table 14.3). It has a high specificity to 4-chloro-, 3-chloro-, 2,4-, and 2,5-chlorophenol. The signals for the mono- and dichlorinated phenols are higher than for the nonchlorinated compound phenol. In principle, the *T. beigelii (cutaneum)* E4 is more suitable for the determination of chlorophenols than *Rhodococcus* sp. P1. A linear relationship between the current range and the concentration of 4-chlorophenol can be observed up to 40 µmol/l and the detection limit for all studied substrates is 2 µmol/l. The attained detection limit of 50 µg/l of chlorophenols means it is not yet suitable for practical application because the permissible concentration in drinking water is 0.5 µg/l of phenols (EC Directives for Drinking Water, German Drinking Water Ordinance). Microorganisms capable of degrading polychlorinated biphenyls (PCB) have been isolated and found to vary considerably in the number and type of PCB congeners they oxidize. Three particularly interesting PCB-degrading organisms are *Alcaligenes eutrophus* H850, *Corynebacterium* MB1, and *Pseudomonas putida* LB400. These strains are exceptional in that they degrade an unusually wide range of PCB congeners. *Alcaligenes eutrophus* JMP134 grows on 2,4-dichlorophenoxyacetic acid (2,4-D) as the only carbon source. This strain was used by Beyersdorf-Radeck et al. (1991) for 2,4-D detection.

TABLE 14.2
Microbial Sensors for Halogenated Compounds With Oxygen Electrodes

Analyte	Microorganism	Measuring range (mmol/l)	Response time (min)	Precision (%)	Stability	Ref.
3-Chlorobenzoate	*Pseudomonas putida* 87	0.040–0.20 3-chlorobenzoate 0.004–0.16 benzoate d.l.: 0.4 mmol/l 4-chlorobenzoate, 0.8 mmol/l 2-chlorobenzoate	0.25	5.5		Riedel et al. (1991a)
4-Chlorophenol	*Rhodococcus* sp.	0.004–0.020	0.25	5.5	> 21 Days	Riedel et al. (1993)
2,4-Dichloro-phenoxyacetic acid	*Alcaligenes eutrophus*	0.2–1.0	0.25			Beyersdorf-Radeck (1991)
Chlorophenols	*Rhodococcus* sp.	0.004–0.020 phenol, 2-, 3-, 4-chloro-phenol	0.25	5.5	> 21 Days	Riedel et al. (1993)
	Trichosporon beigelii (cutaneum)	0.0002 2-, 3-, 4-chlorophenol	0.25	5.5	21 Days	Riedel et al. (1995)

Note: d. l.: detection limit.

However, it is obvious that the lower detection limits reached were too high for an application to monitoring drinking water in accordance with legislative requirements. In addition, in any case cross reactivities with related compounds were reported leading to overestimations of single compounds in complex matrices. Moreover, not for every compound of environmental concern are microorganisms available with the capability of degrading the respective substance.

TABLE 14.3
Selectivity of a *Trichosporon beigelii E4 (cutaneum)*[a] and *Rhodococcus* sp. *P1*[b] Sensor to Phenol and Benzoate and Their Chloroderivatives

Substrates	Activity (%)	
	Trichosporon	*Rhodococcus*
Phenol	100	100
2-Monochlorophenol	373	43
3-Monochlorophenol	875	45
4-Monochlorophenol	1167	53
2,3-Dichlorophenol	538	36
2,4-Dichlorophenol	725	20
2,5-Dichlorophenol	1077	15
Benzoate	0	14
2-Monochlorobenzoate	0	11
3-Monochlorobenzoate	42	8
4-Monochlorobenzoate	0	2

[a] Riedel et al., 1995.
[b] Riedel et al., 1993.

14.2.1.3 Determination of Other Compounds of Environmental Relevance: Nitrate, Nitrite, Nitrilotriacetic Acid, Phosphate, Sulfite, Ammonia, Methane, Formic Acid

The compounds treated in this section normally occur in nature and, indeed, in trace concentrations may be essential for the maintenance of "normal conditions" in the biosphere, but when accumulated in abnormal quantities they upset the established ecological equilibria and become an environmental risk. The nitrogen content (in the form of nitrate, nitrite, or ammonia) of lakes, rivers, and streams usually arises from the ground water, sewerage effluent, or drainage and leaching from agricultural land. The last is the most significant input and nitrate levels have increased substantially over the last 40 years because of the increased use of nitrogen-based fertilizers. Excessive ingestion of nitrate by mammals may, through possible metabolic conversion into nitrites, cause methaemoglobinaemia and, in the presence of high amine diets or amine-derived drugs, lead to the formation of alkyl nitrosamines, which have carcinogenic properties. Usually little more than half of the amount of fertilizer nitrogen applied is actually recovered in the crop, therefore the extensive use of artificial fertilizers in agriculture has been implicated as a major cause of the increasing nitrate concentrations in natural waters and as a factor in the growing problem of eutrophication. The EC Directive for Drinking Water and the German Drinking Water Ordinance, for instance, set limits of 0.5 mg/l for ammonia, 0.1 mg/l for nitrite, and 50 mg/l for nitrate. Several methods are available for the determination of the nitrogen compounds in water, mostly applying spectrophotometric methods.

The microbial sensors based on several microorganisms and investigating different transducers for detection of the analytes considered here are listed in Table 14.4. Compared to the classic spectrophotometric methods in the field, they obviously have no advantages with the exception of the ammonia and the methane sensor. For the classic analysis of ammonia, an ammonia gas electrode consisting of a combined glass electrode and a gas-permeable membrane is usually employed. In this case, the determination must be performed under highly alkaline conditions (above pH 11). However, volatile compounds such as amines often interfere. Therefore, an ammonia sensor with the nitrifying bacteria, *Nitrosomas* sp., utilizing ammonia as the sole source of energy, in combination with an oxygen electrode can be used to advantage.

Methane is a clean fuel and major component of city gas (88% methane), but forms an explosive mixture with air (5 to 14% methane). Most of the commercially available gas sensors use certain semiconductors based on the fact that the gases cause a change in the electrical conductivity of these semiconductors (see Chapter 23). In general, methane is detected via GC analysis. In the case of the microbial sensor, a methane-oxidizing bacterium isolated from a natural source and identified as *Methylomonas flagellata* was used with an oxygen electrode. *M. flagellata* utilizes methane as its sole source of energy. The sensitivity of the microbial sensor is described as being higher than that of gas chromatography. The minimum measurable concentration of methane is 148 μM with the gas chromatographic method compared to 13 μM with the microbial electrode method.

14.2.1.4 Metal Ions

Heavy metals are ubiquitous throughout the environment, though anthropogenic sources can frequently lead to increased concentrations of toxic metals which can cause deleterious effects due to their displacement of essential metal ions, blocking of essential functional groups, and/or their interactions with enzymes and biological membranes. For this reason, the following maximum heavy metal concentrations are defined in the EC Directives for Drinking Water and by the German Drinking Water Ordinance: 40 μg/l lead, 5 μg/l cadmium, and 1 μg/l mercury. In addition, the WHO recommendations set the following limits: 0.05 mg/l for copper and 5 mg/l for zinc. All the heavy metals exhibit a high fish toxicity. The classic detection methods used for trace analysis of heavy metals are atomic absorption spectrometry (AAS) and inductively coupled plasma emission spectrometry (ICP) with detection limits in the picogram range. Both methods are very sophisticated and require expensive equipment and highly trained personnel. An alternative in some cases is the use of anodic stripping voltammetry. One possibility for a whole-cell sensor is to use certain microorganisms such as bacteria, yeasts, fungi, lichens, mosses, and water plants because of their ability to accumulate metal. The ability of mosses from the species *Sphagnum* to accumulate cations from a solution was first observed in 1936. The moss has a modifying matrix consisting of nonesterified polyuronic acids. As a result, it exhibits a strong ability to exchange ions at polyuronic acid levels between 10 and 30% of the moss dry weight. Ions with a higher charge are more easily incorporated into the structure than those with less charge. The selected moss belongs to the species *Sphagnum* and allows selective preconcentration of lead coming from diluted solutions. The application of a carbon paste electrode modified by *Sphagnum* sp. for the determination of lead (II) in natural and drinking waters by anodic stripping differential pulse voltammetry was described by Ramos et al. (1993).

Another approach using *Escherichia coli* in combination with the luciferase reaction was described for the detection of aluminum by Guzzo et al. (1992). Aluminum is generally present in natural waters in concentrations ranging from 30 to 670 ng/ml; the mean concentration in rivers is 420 ng/ml. There is no limit given in drinking water regulations such as the EC Directives for Drinking Water although aluminum has been linked to the induction of Alzheimer's disease-like effects in mammals and to the damage of gill epithelia in fish. Guzzo et al. (1992) performed a transcriptional fusion of *Vibrio harveyi* luxAB genes (encoding bacterial luciferase) to the FliC gene of *Escherichia coli.* Luminescence was shown to be induced (in liquid media) in the presence of 1 to 10 μg/ml aluminum, but not copper, iron, or nickel. Luminescence is markedly increased at pH 5.5, where aluminum is more soluble than at pH 7.0. However, aluminum also stimulates luciferase enzyme activity *in vivo.*

TABLE 14.4
Microbial Sensors for the Determination of Other Compounds of Environmental Relevance

Analyte	Microorganism	Indicated electrochemical species	Measuring range (mmol/l)	Response time (min)	Stability (days)	Ref.
Phosphate	*Chlorella vulgaris*	O_2	8–70	1		Matsunaga et al. (1984)
Sulphite	Hepatic microsome	O_2	0.06–0.34 SD: 7%	10	2 Days/20 assays	Karube and Tamiya (1987)
Lead	Moss: *Sphagnum* sp.	Carbon paste electrode, anodic stripping differential pulse voltammetry	d. l.: 2 ng/ml lead (15 min preconcentration time) SD: 4.8%			Ramos et al. (1993)
Ammonia	Nitrifying bacteria: *Nitrosomonas* sp.	O_2	0.005–2.5 SD: 4%	4 s	> 10 Days/ 200 assays	Karube et al. (1981a) Karube and Tamiya (1987)
Methane	*Methylomonas flagellata*	O_2	0.013–6.6 SD: 5%	1–2 s (assay time: 1 min) 3 (steady state)	> 20 Days/ 500 assays	Okada et al. (1981)
Nitrate	*Azotobacter vinelandii*	NH_3	0.01–0.8	7–8	> 2 Weeks	Kobos et al. (1979)
	Pseudomonas aeruginosa	CO_2	20–200 mg/l d. l.: 8 mg/l SD: 0.6%	10 min assay time (30 min cycle time)		Hikuma et al. (1993)
Nitrite	*Nitrobacter* sp.	O_2	0.01–0.6 SD: 5%	10 (12 for regeneration)	> 21 Days/400 assays	Karube et al. (1982a) Karube and Tamiya (1987) Okada et al. (1983)
	Nitrifying bacteria from activated sludge	O_2	0.15–5	3		
Nitrilotriacetic acid	*Pseudomonas* sp.	NH_3	0.1–0.7	5	Interference: serine, glycine, urea, ammonia	Kobos and Pyon (1981)
Formic acid	*Clostridium butyricum*	H_2 fuel cells	0.22–22	20		Matsunaga et al. (1980)
Benzoate	*Rhodococcus* sp.	O_2	0.002–0.08 SD: 5.5%	0.25	> 14 Days	Riedel et al. (1991b)

Note: d. l.: detection limit, SD: relative standard deviation.

These results are specific to *E. coli*, as no such aluminum stimulation was observed in the luminescent bacterium *V. harveyi*.

With an analogous system it is possible to determine Hg(II) at a concentration of 0.1 μmol/l and Cu(I/II) at a concentration of 0.1 μmol/l. These microbial sensors were constructed by using genetic engineering to fuse the lux or light-emitting genes from *Vibrio fischeri* with genetic regulatory genes from *E. coli* and *Serratia marcescens* which respond to copper and mercury ions (Holmes et al., 1993).

14.2.2 Determination of a Sum Parameter

14.2.2.1 Biochemical Oxygen Demand (BOD)

The biochemical oxygen demand (BOD_5) is one of the most important and widely used tests for the measurement of organic pollution. According to the "Abwasserabgabengesetz" (law on effluent levies) in Germany, the taxes a company has to pay to the government for the wastewater produced are still calculated as a measure of the chemical oxygen demand (COD) and the content of the adsorbable fraction of halogenated organic compounds (AOX), although the use of the BOD_5 as a third measure is still being discussed. The BOD_5 test measures biodegradable organic compounds in wastewaters. It requires, in practice, an incubation period of 5 days at 20°C. A rapid method to estimate the 5-day BOD based on immobilized whole cells and an oxygen electrode has been developed as a BOD sensor. The first BOD sensor was described by Karube et al. (1977a, b, c).

At the Research Centre for Advanced Science and Technology (RCAST, Tokyo, Japan) and at the Zentralinstitut für Molekularbiologie (ZIM, Berlin, Germany) BOD sensors were developed with a view to commercial exploitation. The cultivated microorganisms applied consisted of pure strains with a broad substrate range to improve the reproducibility of the assay and to allow a complete detection of the water load. The yeast *Trichosporon cutaneum*, which was recently reclassified as *T. beigelii*, turned out to be the most useful. Another way to reach a broad substrate range is to combine microorganisms with different substrate spectra. The sensor with the bacterium *Rhodococcus erythropolis* and the yeast *Issatchenkia orientalis* combines the complementary substrate specificity of both strains and made it possible to handle a wide range of different wastewater matrices, including not only municipal sewage treatment plants but also plants which treat wastewater mainly from industrial dischargers (Riedel et al., 1996). Another major advantage is that both species are nonpathogenic in contrast to *T. cutaneum/beigelii*. There are five instruments commercially available for BOD analysis based on a microbial sensor: the BOD 2000 from Central Kagaku Corp., Tokyo, the BODypoint from AUCOTEAM-Ingenieurgesellschaft mbH, Berlin, the BSB-Modul from Prüfgerätewerk Medingen GmbH, Dresden, the ARAS from Dr. Lange GmbH, Berlin, (cf. Figure 14.3), and the RODTOX from Kelma, Niel, Belgium (measuring BOD and toxicity). With these instruments a sample throughput of 2 to 20/h can be attained with a measuring range from 0 to 500 mg/l BOD. Other data about BOD sensors using various microorganisms (*Bacillus polymyxa*, *B. subtilis*, *B. licheniformis*, *Hansenula anomala*, *Clostridium butyricum*, *Pseudomonas* sp., *Escherichia coli*, *Trichosporon cutaneum*, *Rhodococcus erythropolis*, and *Issatchenkia orientalis*) combined with oxygen electrodes are listed in Table 14.5.

Many microorganisms have variants which show resistance to toxic substances. Ohki et al. (1990) studied the bioaccumulation of arsenic (As) by freshwater algae isolated from arsenic-polluted environments. Some bacteria contaminated with algae culture containing As(V) were isolated and one of the bacteria species was identified as *Pseudomonas putida*. This bacterium is an aerobic heterotroph which exhibits extreme resistance to As(V); it can even multiply at concentrations above 5000 mg/l of inorganic As(V). *P. putida* ingests carbohydrates and proteins. Therefore, if the bacterium is employed in microbial sensors, BOD biosensing can be conducted in the presence of high levels of As(V).

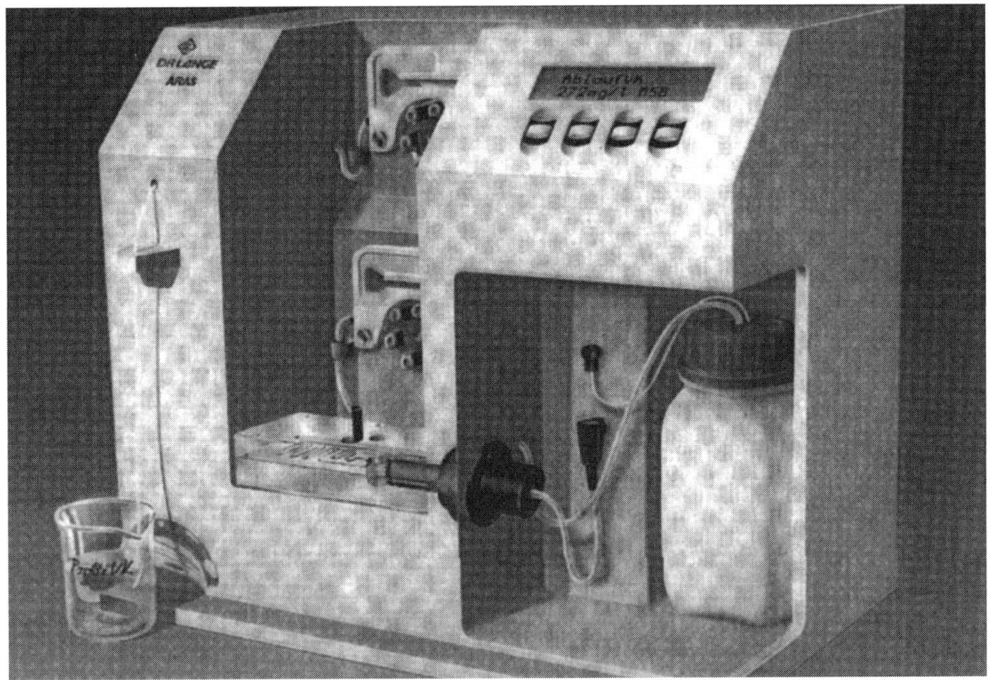

FIGURE 14.3 Commercial sensor BOD system ARAS (Dr. Lange GmbH, Berlin).

14.2.3 Determination of Toxicity: Inhibition of Metabolism

14.2.3.1 Total Toxicity

On the basis of bioassays, e.g., the assay investigating luminescent bacteria, there are several approaches using microbial sensors for the assessment of toxicity with a focus on mutagenesis testing. The ultimate goal is to replace the long-term carcinogenicity tests with laboratory mammals, which are not only time-consuming, but also demand laboratory animals for the experiments. One approach measuring the toxicity degree of a matrix (gaseous emission, wastewater, environment, atmosphere of a working room) is a test developed by Campanella et al. (1987). The assay is based on the measurement of the oxygen uptake and the carbon dioxide production or the redox potential following the breathing activity of an established number of cells of the yeast *Saccharomyces cerevisiae*. It requires only 15 min to complete. The steps in the test are: (1) determination of the consumed oxygen and of the produced carbon dioxide under reference conditions, (2) addition of the compound or matrix to be tested, (3) determination of the new breathing rate (consumption of O_2, production of CO_2), and (4) correlation between data in (1) and (3) and calculation of the toxicity degree or index of the tested compound or matrix. The toxicity degree $i = (1 - K_i/K_f)$ for several matrixes was calculated using the change in slope of the kinetic CO_2 formation by breathing cells when a toxic substance was added. Lethal effects corresponding to no production of CO_2 and no consumption of O_2 were reported at the following concentrations of toxic compounds: 100 ppm Hg, 100 ppm Cd, and 100 ppm naphthalene.

Another approach to assessing the toxicity of compounds with a mutagenic potential is a microbial sensing system utilizing a membrane mutant of *Escherichia coli* and recombinant DNA technology developed by Lee et al. (1992) for the determination of pesticides in the environment. The emission of light in *E. coli* was achieved by cloning the genes encoding firefly luciferase and by injecting the luminescent substrate, luciferin. ATP synthesis in *E. coli* is carried out in the cytoplasmic membrane through glycolysis, TCA cycle,

TABLE 14.5
Determination of Biochemical Oxygen Demand (BOD) With Microbial Sensors

Microorganism	Immobilization	Measuring range (mg/l BOD)	Response time (min)	Precision (%)	Stability (days)	Ref.
Bacillus polymyxa	K-carrageenan	1–12	15	6.0	60	Su et al. (1986)
Clostridium butyricum	Polyacrylamide	50–300	30–40 at 37°C	7.0	40	Karube et al. (1977 b,c)
	Collagen membrane	5–22	15 at 30°C 15	7.5	30	
Bacillus subtilis	Centrifugation on paper	2.2–22	0.13–0.25	5.0	40	Riedel et al. (1987)
	Polyvinylalcohol	2–20	0.25–0.5	5.0	30	Riedel et al. (1988)
Bacillus licheniformis 7B and *Bacillus subtilis*	Polyvinyl alcohol	5–80	0.25–0.5 (4 min baseline recovery)		> 200 Assays/ > 2 months	Tan et al. (1993)
Issatchenkia orientalis *Rhodococcus erythropolis*	Polyvinyl alcohol	6–800	0.5–1	<5	40	Riedel et al. (1996)
Hansenula anomala	Attached to nylon	0.01–0.4	15–20		7	Kulys and Kadzkiauskiene (1980)
	Sandwich between fluorinated ethylene propylene and acetylcellulose membrane	1–45	13–20	6.0	Storage life-time > 1 year	Li and Chu (1991)
Pseudomonas sp.	Sandwich between fluorinated ethylene propylene and acetylcellulose membrane	1–40	13–20	6.0	Storage life-time > 1 year	Li and Chu (1991)
Pseudomonas putida	Filtration on acetylcellulose membrane	1–66	8		7 (50 runs or > 1 week)	Ohki et al. (1990)
Thermophilic bacteria isolated from Japanese hot spring	Filtration on nitrocellulose membrane	1–12	7		>40	Karube et al. (1989)
Trichosporon cutaneum	Filtration on acetylcellulose	5–100	18	3.0–6.0	30	Hikuma et al. (1979) Harita et al. (1985)
	Centrifugation on paper	4.4–100	0.13–0.25	4.0	40	Riedel et al. (1987)
	Polyvinylalcohol	4–100	0.25-0.5	5.0	30	Riedel et al. (1988)
		4–100	< 0.5	3.3	48	Riedel et al. (1990)
	Filtration on acetylcellulose membrane	3–60	0.3	6	>17 Days/ 400 assays	Karube (1990)

TABLE 14.5 (CONTINUED)
Determination of Biochemical Oxygen Demand (BOD) With Microbial Sensors

Microorganism	Immobilization	Measuring range (mg/l BOD)	Response time (min)	Precision (%)	Stability (days)	Ref.
Activated sludge	Collagen	5–22	15	7.5	10	Karube et al. (1977a)
	Polyacrylamide	50–350	30	6.0	10	Karube et al. (1977b)
	Attached to nylon	2–22	20	9.0	20	Strand and Carlson (1984)

and oxidative phosphorylation, which is the pathway of electrons to oxygen. Accordingly, the emission of light in *E. coli* could be achieved by luciferase and ATP produced inside the cells and by addition of the luminescent substrate luciferin. A considerable increase in sensitivity to toxic substances was obtained by using the membrane mutant of *E. coli* instead of the wild type. Pesticides and herbicides (such as metoxuron, isoproturon, ioxinyl, and propanil) could be detected by the decrease of *in vivo* luminescence at concentrations down to 50 μg/l.

14.2.3.2 Mutagenesis Testing

Preliminary screening for mutagens has been achieved with a system containing two microbial sensors, one with a recombinant deficient strain of *B. subtilis* or *Salmonella typhimurium* (Rec^-) and the other with a wild strain (Rec^+) (Karube et al., 1981b, 1982b). The addition of mutagens damaged the DNA in both strains, but the wild-type strain (Rec^+) had the ability to repair the damaged DNA and the concentration of viable organisms remained constant, whereas the viability of the Rec^- strain decreased accompanied by a decrease in respiration (increase in current). The sensitivity of this sensor system was three to six times higher than that of conventional methods (e.g., minimum measurable concentration of mutagen AF-2 is 1.6 μg/ml). Finally, Karube et al. (1983) described a mutagen sensor based on the formation of phages in *E. coli* induced by mutagens. As a result of phage induction the cell respiration changed and this could be measured with an oxygen electrode.

14.3 ENZYME SENSORS

Enzyme sensors for the analysis of compounds of environmental concern can be divided into three groups based on the type of enzyme reaction. In the first and easiest case, the pollutant is directly converted by the enzyme and the reaction product can be determined electrochemically by optical methods or with the use of other transducers. An example presented in this chapter are phenol electrodes based on the immobilization of mushroom polyphenol oxidase on an oxygen or modified graphite electrode. Most enzyme sensors applied to environmental analysis belong to the group of enzyme inhibition assays, e.g., organophosphates and carbamates act as strong inhibitors for cholinesterase and can be detected via the degree of enzyme inhibition. A third approach is the use of apoenzymes, e.g., cofactor-free enzyme where a specific heavy metal is coordinated in the active site of the enzyme and functions as a cofactor in the catalytic reaction.

14.3.1 Analysis of Single Substances

14.3.1.1 Heavy Metal Ions

Table 14.6 shows some of the possibilities for using enzyme sensors in the determination of heavy metal traces. The majority of the enzyme sensors shown use apoenzymes. Metalloenzymes need heavy metal ions to maintain their catalytic activity, since these ions are generally coordinated in an active site of the metalloenzyme and function as a cofactor in the catalytic reaction. Removing the metal from the cofactor-bound enzyme (holoenzyme) with strong chelating agents forms the corresponding cofactor-free enzyme (apoenzyme) lacking enzyme activity. The apoenzyme can be reversibly activated by exposure to the metal-containing sample so that metal ions can be taken up and trapped in the active site. Thus the amount of metal coordinated in the catalytic centers of the enzyme molecules is related to the enzyme activity and, in turn, is proportional to the amount of metal added. Therefore, the trace metal content can be evaluated by measuring the enzyme activity of the reactivated apoenzyme. The biosensing method for microdetermination of heavy metals is applicable to the detection of any kind of metalloenzyme activity. Micromolar levels of Zn(II) and Cu(II) have been successfully assayed through activation of the immobilized apoenzyme (alkaline phosphatase and galactose oxidase or tyrosinase, respectively).

TABLE 14.6
Enzyme Sensors for Heavy Metal Determination

Analyte	Enzyme	Transducer	Measuring range (mmol/l)	Regeneration	Stability (days)	Ref.
Hg(II)	Urease inhibition: urease	Ammonia gas electrode	0–150 nmol/l	Thioacetamide + EDTA	Interference: silver, copper	Ögren and Johansson (1978)
Zn(II)	Apoenzyme: alkaline phosphatase	Planar pH-ISFET	0.01–1.0 SD: 2.3%	2,6-Pyridine-dicarboxylate	Assay time: 2 h >48 Assays/3 weeks Interference: Co(II)	Satoh and Aoki (1990)
Zn(II)	Apoenzyme: alkaline phosphatase	Thermistor for calorimetric detection	0.01–1.0	2,6-Pyridine-dicarboxylate	120 Assays/>2 months Interference: Co(II)	Satoh (1991)
Cu(II)	Apoenzyme: galactose oxidase	Polarographic oxygen electrode or membrane-covered Pt/Ag/AgCl electrode	0.1–10 SD: 7%	*N,N*-Dimethyl-dithiocarba-mate	Assay time 30 min, >30 assays/1 month	Satoh et al. (1991)
Cu (II)	Apoenzyme: tyrosinase	FIA with oxygen electrode	Up to 0.05	Cu(II) was stripped by NaCN	n. d.	Mattiasson et al. (1979)

Note: SD: relative standard deviation; FIA: flow injection analysis, n.d.: not determined.

Only a few reports have appeared concerning the determination of metals by enzyme inhibition. In most of the studies, urease has been used as a model enzyme. Mercury inhibited the splitting of urea into bicarbonate and ammonia, the concentration of the latter being measured by an ammonia gas electrode. Only silver and copper interfere.

14.3.1.2 Phenol Analysis

Table 14.7 gives an overview of the application of tyrosinase enzyme sensors for phenol analysis. Polyphenol oxidase from mushroom is a bifunctional catalyst with both phenol hydroxylase and polyphenol oxidase activities. Polyphenol oxidase catalyzes the oxidation of phenol by dissolved oxygen to yield 1,2-benzenediol and the subsequent oxidation of this product to o-benzoquinone. The reaction is shown in Figure 14.4. If the reactions are carried out in the presence of a mediator, hexacyanoferrate (II), then instead of detecting the oxygen consumption, the o-benzoquinone oxidizes the complex ion to hexacyanoferrate (III) with the concomitant regeneration of 1,2-benzenediol. Hexacyanoferrate (III) can be monitored spectrophotometrically at 420 nm or amperometrically by measuring the current resulting from the reduction to hexacyanoferrate (II). If catechol is formed it is oxidized like phenol. If tetracyanoquinodimethane (TCNQ) is used on a graphite electrode, the electrode reaction is a cathodic process of TCNQ reduction. However, even with the enzymatic sensors for phenol determination, the lower detection limits required by drinking water legislation could not be reached.

14.3.1.3 Determination of Other Compounds of Environmental Concern: Phosphate, Nitrite, Nitrate, Sulphate

The compounds treated in this segment are of environmental concern if present in increased amounts in environmental samples, especially in drinking waters. In addition to the nitrogen content, ortho-, pyro-, and tripolyphosphates lead to eutrophication if they are present in amounts high enough to tip the ecological equilibrium in natural waters. Therefore, the EC Directive for Drinking Water prescribes a maximum allowed concentration of 5 mg/l P_2O_5. In general, phosphate is determined by spectrophotometric methods based on the formation of binary and ternary heteropoly acids and ion associates. The reaction of phosphate with the molybdenum ion in acidic solutions is well known, producing phosphomolybdate, which is subsequently reduced to molybdenum blue.

Tables 14.8 and 14.9 show data of enzyme sensors for the detection of nitrite, nitrate, sulphate, and phosphate. It is obvious that these compounds can be measured using suitable enzymes for the catalysis of the respective substance and appropriate transducers. However, a disadvantage of the enzymatic sensors described was that they require sophisticated equipment, and overestimations due to cross-reactivities with related compounds and derived from matrix effects were possible.

A dual enzyme system for the electrochemical measurement of alkaline phosphatase catalytic reaction was used by Guilbault and Nanjo (1975). When the glucose formed from glucose-6-phosphate is sensed electrochemically, it is possible to follow the reaction in which phosphate inhibition decreases glucose formation, thus lowering the response to the dual enzyme electrode. The dual enzyme electrode exhibits cross-reactivities with other oxyacids such as arsenate, tungstate, molybdate, and borate ions as well as glucose-6-phosphate.

A phosphate sensor based on the phosphate dependence of pyruvate oxidase was reported by Kubo et al. (1991). Pyruvate oxidase derived from *Pediococcus* sp. catalyses the oxidation of pyruvate in the presence of phosphate and oxygen with the formation of acetylphosphate, hydrogen peroxide, and carbon dioxide. The consumption of oxygen was determined for phosphate calculation.

TABLE 14.7
Enzyme Sensors for Phenol Analysis With Tyrosinase (EC 1.14.18.1, Mushroom Polyphenol Oxidase)

Detection	Measuring range (μmol/l)	Precision (%)	Detection limits (μmol/l)	Response time	Stability (days)	Ref.
FIA with redox mediator: hexacyano-ferrate(II)	10^{-6}–10^{-4} M	2%	Photometric: 3 mg/l	10 min assay time		Zachariah and Mottola (1989)
Spectrophoto-metric (420 nm) or amperometric			Amperometric: 0.025 mg/l 0.018 mg/l	20 s contact time 30 s contact time		
Graphite elect-rode with tet-racyanoqui-nodimethane (TCNQ)	0.23–65		0.23 μmol/l phenol Interference: 100% phenol, 93% *p*-cresol, 330% catechol	12 or 35 s	1 Week (5–8% residual activity after 5 days)	Kulys and Schmid (1990)
Carbon paste electrode (reversible electrochemical reduction of the *o*-quinones formed from phenols in the tyrosinase reaction)	0.01–200 (the highest permissible conc. according to the Czechoslovak standard CSN 83061 is 0.05 mg/l (= 0.53 μmol/l)	<4%	10 nmol/l Catechol, 13 nmol/l phenol	40 s (*o*-diphe-nols) 2 min (mono-phenols)	85% enzyme activity after storage for 5 months/150 assays	Skladal (1991b)
Clark oxygen electrode	1–46 (in n-hexane) 5–190 (in aqueous buffer solution)	4.4% (in n-hexane) 7.2% (in aqueous phosphate buffer)	0.5 μmol/l (in n-hexane) 2.6 μmol/l (in aqueous phosphate buffer)	<2 min	>20 days Interference: 100% phenol, 25.2% *p*-Cl-phenol, 16% *m*-Cl-phenol, 1.5% *o*-Cl-phenol, 15.6% *p*-cresol, 15.6% *m*-cresol, 3% *o*-cresol, 12% *p*-Br-phenol, 0.1% guaiacol	Campanella et al. (1992)
Clark oxygen electrode	0.1–5 (in chloroform saturated with aqueous buffer)			3 min	15 Samples/h	Schubert et al. (1992)

Another method of determining phosphate ions is based upon the nucleoside phosphorylase catalyzed reaction for which the presence of inorganic phosphorus is indispensable. The two

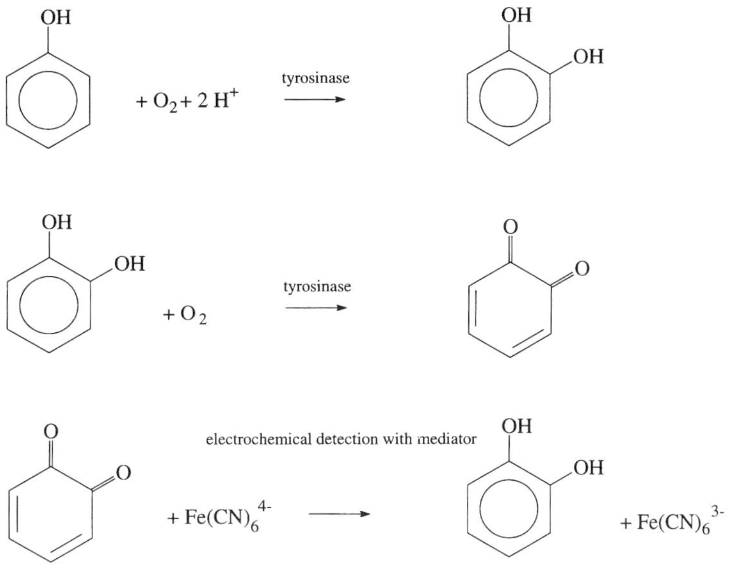

FIGURE 14.4 Phenol determination with tyrosinase.

enzymes, nucleoside phosphorylase and xanthine oxidase, can be used in a dual enzyme system. In dependence on the phosphate concentration, inosine is phosphorylated while hypoxanthine is formed. In the second reaction hypoxanthine is oxidized with the simultaneous consumption of oxygen and formation of hydrogen peroxide. Again, the depletion of oxygen, measured by an oxygen electrode, served as a measure of the phosphate concentration in the sample.

14.3.2 Determination of Toxicity: Enzyme Inhibition

14.3.2.1 Cholinesterase Inhibition Test

The organochlorine insecticides (DDT, aldrin, lindane, etc.) used in the past have been progressively replaced with organophosphorus compounds. The latter show low environmental persistence but have a high acute toxicity. Regulations are now being strictly enforced in Europe, with a maximum concentration of 0.1 μg/l for individual pesticide residues and 0.5 μg/l for the sum of pesticides in drinking water. In general, the group of organophosphate and carbamate insecticides is analysed via GC/MS and HPLC, which require sophisticated, expensive equipment and skilled personnel.

Cholinesterases are known to be inhibited by carbamates and organophosphates, the inhibitory effects being influenced by the type of compound and its concentration. Therefore, these compounds may be toxic for a whole organism. Determination of the enzyme activity after incubation of the enzyme with a water sample provides information both about the presence of these insecticides and at the same time on the toxic potential of the sample. Cholinesterases catalyse the hydrolysis of esters in choline and the corresponding acid. Depending on the substrate specificity acetyl- and butyrylcholinesterases can be distinguished. Acetylcholinesterase (AChE) is a hydrolase enzyme with rather narrow specificity for acetylcholine and related compounds. It is found in high concentrations in nerve tissue. Acetylcholine is an active neurotransmitter and a target for nerve gases and insecticides. The activity of cholinesterases can be determined using acetylthiocholine as enzyme substrate by measuring the thiocholine formed (cf. Figure 14.5). As early as 1974 a sensor was introduced by Goodson and Jacobs based on the electrochemical oxidation of thiocholine at platinum electrodes. The thiocholine was produced by the enzymatic reaction from butyrylthiocholine iodide. Since then, many sensors have been reported either exploiting the same principle,

TABLE 14.8
Enzyme Sensor for Phosphate Determination

Enzyme	Measuring range (μmol/l)	Precision (%)	Indicated electrochemical species	Assay time (min)	Stability	Ref.
Alkaline phosphatase (EC 3.1.3.1) and glucose oxidase (EC 1.1.3.4)	d. l.: 10^{-4} M	5.9	H_2O_2 Cross-reactivities: arsenate, tungstate, molybdate, borate	5–10	>100 Assays/3 months	Guilbault and Nanjo (1975)
Nucleoside phosphorylase and xanthine oxidase	0.3–1.0 mmol/l	10	O_2	3	>70 Assays/30 days	Watanabe et al. (1988)
Nucleoside phosphorylase (EC 2.4.2.1) and xanthine oxidase (EC 1.2.3.22)	10–250		H_2O_2	Response time: 2 min (baseline recovery: 5 min)	30 Assays	Haemmerli et al. (1990)
			O_2	Response time: 20 s (baseline recovery: 5 min)		
Pyruvate oxidase (EC 1.2.3.3)	12–80	5.9	O_2	7	7 Days (response decreased to 50% of the initial value)	Kubo et al. (1991)
Nucleoside phosphorylase (EC 2.4.2.1) and xanthine oxidase (EC 1.1.3.22)	0.5–100	5	O_2	1.5	>8 Days/300 assays	Wollenberger et al. (1992)

Note: d. l.: detection limit.

TABLE 14.9
Enzyme Sensors for Determination of Other Compounds of Environmental Relevance

Analyte	Enzyme	Indicated electrochemical species	Detection limit (mmol/l)	Ref.
Nitrite	Nitrite reductase	NH_3 gas sensor	50	Kiang et al. (1975)
Nitrate	Nitrate reductase and nitrite reductase	NH_4	50	Kiang et al. (1978a, b)
Sulphate	Arylsulphatase	Pt	100	Cserfalvi and Guilbault (1976)

i.e., the oxidation of thiocholine at platinum electrodes or modified graphite electrodes, or using acetylcholine or butyrylcholine, respectively, as the enzyme substrate. Parameters of several cholinesterase inhibition sensors are presented in Table 14.10. The detection can be performed either with a pH measurement or by coupling the cholinesterase reaction with another enzyme, choline oxidase, and subsequent hydrogen peroxide determination (cf. Figure 14.6). Optical detection systems have also been described (Wolfbeis and Koller, 1989). They are based on the colour reaction triggered by an artificial substrate of cholinesterase or the detection of thiocholine with Ellman's reagent (DTNB = 5,5′-dithiobis-2-nitrobenzoate) (cf. Figure 14.7).

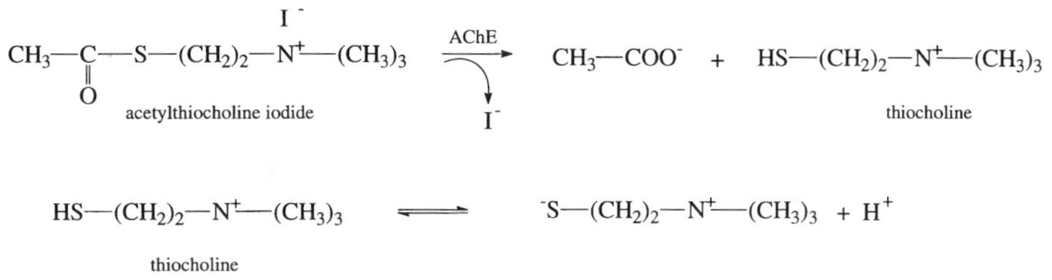

$$CH_3{-}\underset{\underset{O}{\|}}{C}{-}S{-}(CH_2)_2{-}\overset{I^-}{N^+}{-}(CH_3)_3 \xrightarrow[\ I^-]{AChE} CH_3{-}COO^- + HS{-}(CH_2)_2{-}N^+{-}(CH_3)_3$$

acetylthiocholine iodide — thiocholine

$$HS{-}(CH_2)_2{-}N^+{-}(CH_3)_3 \rightleftharpoons {}^-S{-}(CH_2)_2{-}N^+{-}(CH_3)_3 + H^+$$

thiocholine

FIGURE 14.5 Cholinesterase inhibition (AChE: acetylcholinesterase).

The reactivation of enzyme activity depends on the type of inhibition. The enzyme activity of cholinesterase is reversibly inhibited by carbamate insecticides and irreversibly inhibited by organophosphate and organothiophosphate insecticides (after replacement of S by O) by phosphorylating the serine OH group of the enzyme. The resulting enzyme-phosphorus bond cannot be broken by water, but more nucleophilic reagents such as quaternary pyridinium compounds (e.g., 2-pyridinealdoxime methiodide, PAM) are able to reactivate the inhibited enzyme (cf. Figure 14.8).

As a representative example a flow injection analysis (FIA) system suitable for the automated determination of enzyme inhibitors (Kindervater et al., 1990) is described here in more detail. The main component is a magnetic reactor containing the cholinesterase immobilized on magnetic particles, allowing the automated release of inactivated enzyme and its replacement by fresh enzyme by switching an electromagnet on and off (cf. Figure 14.9). The determination of enzyme activity was carried out using the method described by Ellman et al. (1961) prior to and after the incubation of the enzyme with the insecticide solution. The enzymes used were butyrylcholinesterase from horse serum and acetylcholinesterase from bovine erythrocytes. The enzyme substrate was acetylthiocholine. The whole pesticide determination procedure consisted of the following steps: (1) injection of acetylthiocholine without acetylcholinesterase into the magnetic reactor: basic absorption of the system, (2) filling the magnet reactor with the magnetic beads, (3) injection of acetylthiocholine: determination of the initial enzyme activity (difference between (3) and (1)), (4) addition of a constant volume of the water sample, (5) injection of acetylthiocholine: determination of the decrease in enzyme activity (difference between (3) and (5)), (6) compensation of the magnetic field and release of the magnetic beads from the system. The sensitivity of this system was dependent on the pesticide and the reaction time. Detection limits of 0.5 μg/l carbofuran and malaoxon could be reached. In Figure 14.10, standard inhibition curves in the concentration range of 0.80 to 60 μg/l are shown for malaoxon, carbofuran, paraoxon, and paraoxon-methyl.

Electrochemical detection was used for the development of disposable sensors made by thick-film technology. A working and an auxiliary electrode were printed on a ceramic substrate with a platinum paste and a printed silver electrode was used as the reference electrode. The layout was the same as described earlier for sensors for substrates of oxidases (Bilitewski et al., 1992). A paste containing graphite modified with tetracyanoquinodimethane (TCNQ) and butyrylcholinesterase was printed on the working electrode. Hence,

TABLE 14.10
Enzyme Sensors Based on Cholinesterase Inhibition

Detection	Enzyme	Substrate	Measuring ranges (μg/l)	Detection limits (μg/l)	Regeneration	Ref.
FIA with photometric detection of 5,5′-dithiobis(2-nitrobenzoic) acid (= DTNB)	Acetylcholinesterase (AChE) from electric eel	Acetylthiocholine iodide	6.5–120 μg/l Carbaryl 2–15 μg/l Propoxur 0.1–5 μg/l Carbofuran	6.5 Carbaryl 2 Propoxur 0.1 Carbofuran		Quintero et al. (1991)
FIA with photometric detection (enzyme bound to poly(maleinic anhydride) in Celite® 545 column)	AChE from electric eel (EC 3.1.1.7)	Acetylthiocholine iodide		10^{-3} M paraoxon 10^{-2} M carbamates (e.g., carbaryl)	Obidoxime	Battacharya et al. (1981)
Potentiometric: with a glass pH electrode via pH shift	AChE from electric eel (EC 3.1.1.7) Butyrylcholinesterase (BuChE) (EC 3.1.1.8)	Acetylcholine Butyrylcholine chloride	ppb-ppm Methylparathion, azinphosethyl, mevinphos	8 ppm Methylparaoxon (6 min incubation)		Durand et al. (1984)
pH electrode	AChE	Acetylcholine chloride	Reversible inhibition: 0.1 mg/l aldicarb Irreversible inhibition: 50 dichlorvos, 2.5 parathionethyl after oxidation	3.2 Parathion	Pyridine-2-aldoxime-methyliodide (PAM) Stability: >50 days at –4°C, >15 days/60 assays	Schwedt and Hauck (1988)

Glass electrode	BuChE from horse serum (EC 3.1.18)	Butrylcholine chloride		3 Ethylparaoxon 5 Methylparaoxon 4 Malathion 15 Fenitrothion 14 Ethylparathion 14 Methylparathion	PAM	El Yamani et al. (1988)
FIA with magnetic particles and photometric detection of DTNB or electrochemical detection by the oxidation of the thiocholines	AChE from bovine erythrocytes (EC 3.1.17) Choline oxidase (ChO) from *Alcaligenes* sp. (EC 1.1.3.17)	Acetylcholine Acetylthiocholine 5,5′-Dithiobis-2-nitrobenzoic acid (DTNB)	Electrochemical device: ceramic substrate Working electrode (paste containing graphite modified with tetracyanoquinodimethane (TCNQ)) Auxiliary electrode (platinum paste) Reference electrode (silver)	0.5 Carbofuran, 0.5 malaoxon	Assay time 20 min	Kindervater et al. (1990)
Glass electrode or Pd/PdO electrode Ir/IrO_2 electrode as pH sensor	AChE (EC 3.1.1.7)	Acetylcholine chloride		10^{-9} M paraoxon, methyl parathion 10^{-10} M malathion	PAM Response time: 5–7 min	Tran-Minh et al. (1990)
Amperometric hydrogen peroxide determination	AChE (EC 3.1.1.7) and ChO (EC 1.1.3.17)	Acetylcholine, choline	10–100 Paraoxon, aldicarb	2 Paraoxon, aldicarb	Assay time: 20 min	Bernabei et al. (1991)
ISFET with pH-sensitive gate area	AChE (EC 3.1.17)	Acetylcholine chloride	0.3–1.2 mg/l Dichlorvos	0.3 mg/l Dichlorvos	PAM Stability: 23 days	Dumschat et al. (1991)

TABLE 14.10 (CONTINUED)
Enzyme Sensors Based on Cholinesterase Inhibition

Detection	Enzyme	Substrate	Measuring ranges (μg/l)	Detection limits (μg/l)	Regeneration	Ref.
Cobalt phthalocyanine-modified carbon paste electrode for polarographic detection)	BuChE from horse serum (EC 3.1.1.8)	Butyrylthiocholine iodide	0.3–15 Hostaquick 0.3–64 Nogos 5–250 Metathion 4–61 Actellic 7–170 Decemtion 10–130 Zolone 7–270 Ekalux 40–820 Dimecron 10–310 Supracid 100–280 Marshal 80–980 Seedox	0.3 mg/l Hostaquick 80 mg/l Seedox 0.3 mg/l Nogos 5 mg/l Metathion 4 Actellic 7 Decemtion,Ekalux 10 Zolone Supracid 40 Dimecron 100 Marshal	20 Analyses with a single ChE membrane	Skladal (1991a)
pH glass electrode	BuChE from horse serum (EC 3.1.1.8)	Butyrylcholine chloride		1 ppm Carbofuran 4 ppm Carbaryl 0.2 ppm Paraoxon	Stability: 10 days, assay time: 30 min (disposable biosensor membranes maintain their original enzyme activities for 3 years when stored dry)	Kumaran and Tran-Minh (1992a)

Amperometric hydrogen peroxide determination	AChE from electric eel (EC 3.1.1.7) and ChO from *Alcaligenes* sp. (EC 1.1.3.1.7)	Choline chloride Acetylcholine iodide		10 nM paraoxon	Obidoxime 2 months stable when stored at 4°C in phosphate buffer and 1 year in a dry state	Marty et al. (1992)
Amperometric hydrogen peroxide determination	AChE from electric eel (EC 3.1.1.7) and ChO from *Alcaligenes* sp. (EC 1.1.3.1.7)	Acetylcholine chloride Acetylthiocholine chloride DTNB		10^{-10} M paraoxon and carbofuran 10^{-7} M aldicarb, phosphamidon 10^{-6} M parathion-methyl, fonofos	30 min incubation	Mionetto et al. (1992)
FIA with pH electrode	AChE (EC 3.1.1.7)	Acetylcholine chloride		8 ppb Azinphosmethyl 1 Azinphos-ethyl 275 Bromophosmethyl 50 Carbaryl 6 Carbofuran 50 Dichlorovos 45 Fenitrothion 0.5 Malathion 25 Paraoxon 10 Parathion-ethyl 15 Parathionm-ethyl	PAM 12 weeks stable when stored at 4°C without any loss of activity	Kumaran and Tran-Minh (1992b)

TABLE 14.10 (CONTINUED)
Enzyme Sensors Based on Cholinesterase Inhibition

Detection	Enzyme	Substrate	Measuring ranges (μg/l)	Detection limits (μg/l)	Regeneration	Ref.
Amperometric hydrogen peroxide determination	AChE (EC 3.1.1.7) BuChE (EC 3.1.1.8) ChO (EC 1.1.3.17)	Choline Acetylcholine Butyrylcholine		1 (120 min incubation) 2 (30 min incubation time) for organophosphorus pesticides		Palleschi et al. (1992)
pH-FET (ENFET with enzyme, REFET without enzyme)	AChE from electric eel (EC 3.1.1.7) BuChE from horse serum (EC 3.1.1.8)	Acetylcholine chloride Butyrylcholine chloride		0.0002 μg/l Diisopropyl-fluorophosphate 25 μg/l Paraoxon-methyl 24 μg/l Trichlorfon	PAM Assay time: 20 min	Nyamsi Hendji et al. (1993)
FIA with spectrophotometric detection	AChE from electric eel (EC 3.1.1.7)	Acetylthiocholine iodide DTNB	50–800 μmol/l Paraoxon 60–600 μmol/l carbamoylcholine	50 μmol/l paraoxon 60 μmol/l Carbamoyl-choline 5% SD	PAM	Takruni et al. (1993)
ENFET (enzyme-modified FET device)	AChE from electric eel	Acetylcholine		Few ppb paraoxon after 20 min of incubation Few hundreds ppb parathion, azinphos-methyl	PAM	Colapicchioni et al. (1992)

Note: FIA: flow injection analysis.

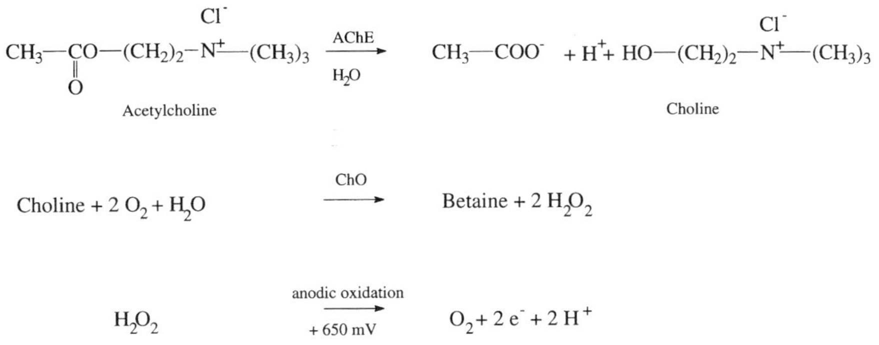

$$CH_3{-}CO{-}(CH_2)_2{-}N^{+}{-}(CH_3)_3\,Cl^- \xrightarrow[H_2O]{AChE} CH_3{-}COO^- + H^+ + HO{-}(CH_2)_2{-}N^{+}{-}(CH_3)_3\,Cl^-$$

Acetylcholine → Choline

$$\text{Choline} + 2\,O_2 + H_2O \xrightarrow{ChO} \text{Betaine} + 2\,H_2O_2$$

$$H_2O_2 \xrightarrow[+650\ mV]{\text{anodic oxidation}} O_2 + 2\,e^- + 2\,H^+$$

FIGURE 14.6 Cholinesterase inhibition with AChE and ChO (AChE: acetylcholinesterase, ChO: choline oxidase).

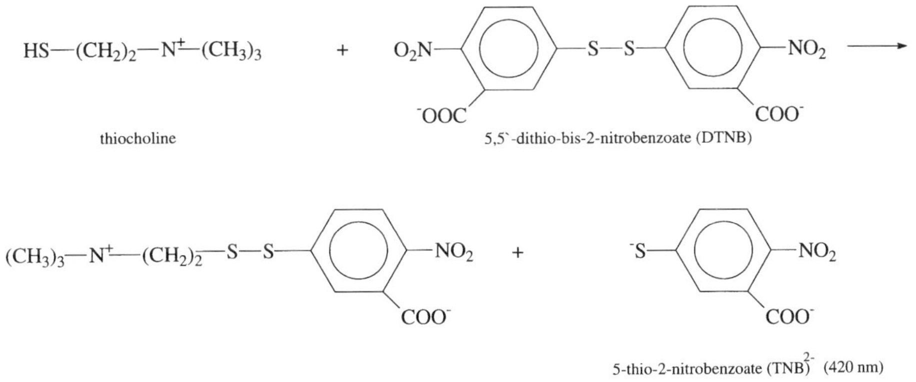

$$HS{-}(CH_2)_2{-}N^{+}{-}(CH_3)_3 + O_2N{-}C_6H_3(COO^-){-}S{-}S{-}C_6H_3(COO^-){-}NO_2 \longrightarrow$$

thiocholine + 5,5'-dithio-bis-2-nitrobenzoate (DTNB)

$$(CH_3)_3{-}N^{+}{-}(CH_2)_2{-}S{-}S{-}C_6H_3(COO^-){-}NO_2 + {}^-S{-}C_6H_3(COO^-){-}NO_2$$

5-thio-2-nitrobenzoate (TNB^{2-}) (420 nm)

FIGURE 14.7 Ellman reaction.

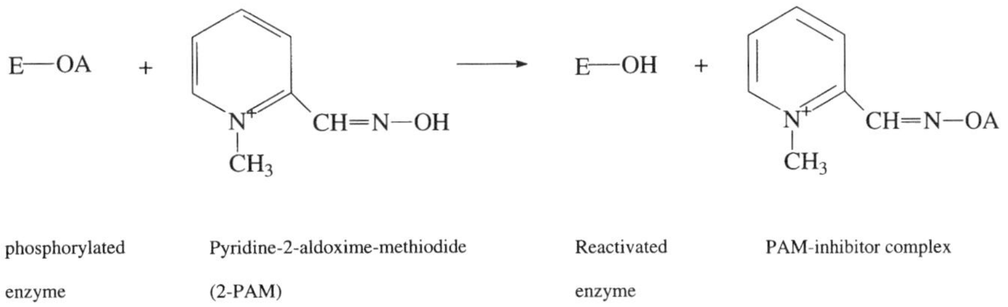

$$E{-}OA + \text{(N-methylpyridinium-2-CH=N-OH)} \longrightarrow E{-}OH + \text{(N-methylpyridinium-2-CH=N-OA)}$$

phosphorylated enzyme + Pyridine-2-aldoxime-methiodide (2-PAM) → Reactivated enzyme + PAM-inhibitor complex

FIGURE 14.8 Cholinesterase regeneration with pyridine-2-aldoxime methiodide (PAM).

the whole sensor was fabricated by thick-film technology. The enzyme activity was measured using butyrylthiocholine as the enzyme substrate and monitoring the current resulting from the oxidation of thiocholine at 100 mV. The concentration of the substrate was 3 mmol/l. The activity was measured prior and subsequent to incubation of the sensor in a solution containing the pesticide. The incubation time was 15 min. The sensitivity was again dependent on the inhibiting compound, but the limits of pesticide concentration in drinking water given by the European Drinking Water Act (0.1 μg/l for a single pesticide or 0.5 mg/l for the sum of all pesticides) could only be obtained after preconcentration procedures.

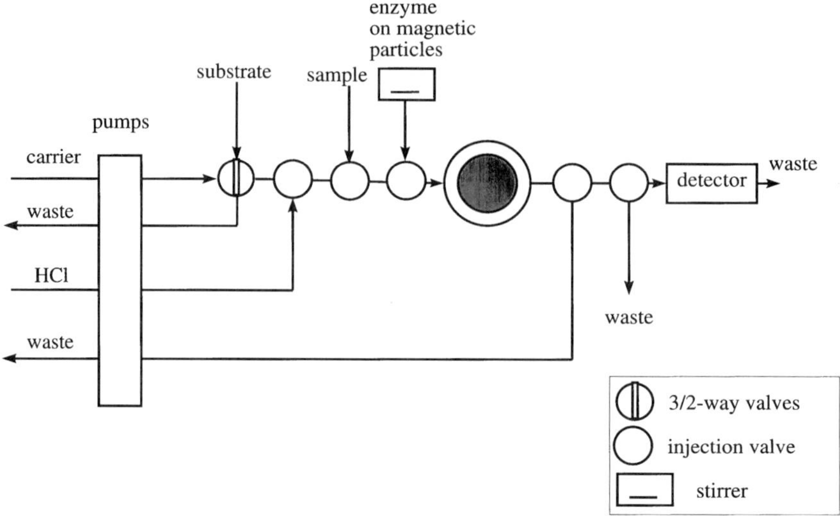

FIGURE 14.9 Instrumentation setup for cholinesterase inhibition FIA.

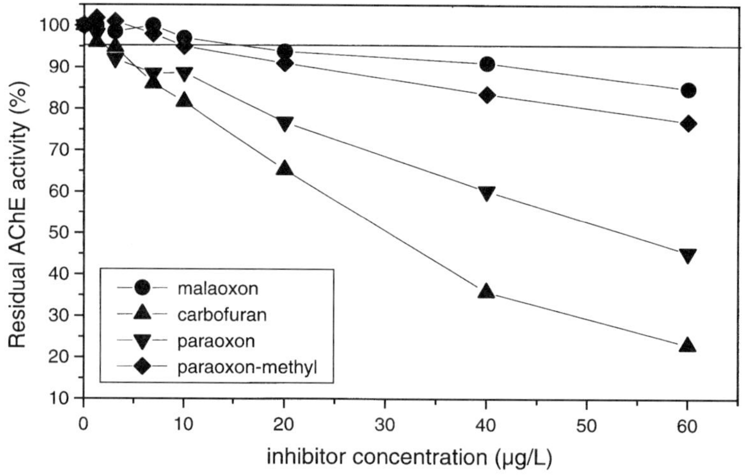

FIGURE 14.10 Standard curve for malaoxon determination with the photometric detection FIA.

14.4 CONCLUSIONS

In general, with the exception of the BOD sensor none of the other microbial and enzymatic sensors for environmental analysis described are ready for application yet with regard to legislative requirements and compared to the conventional analysis methods in the field, i.e., GC/MS, HPLC, AAS, ICP, and the spectrophotometric detection methods. For this reason, only the BOD sensor has been applied commercially. In general, the standardized BOD-5 test as the conventional analysis method requires a time period of 5 days until the result is available. For the operator of a wastewater plant and the companies which have to dispose of their industrial wastewater, it is important to be able to obtain knowledge about the amount of biodegradable compounds in their wastewater more quickly. As the BOD sensors already on the market have a sample throughput of 2 to 20/h, this yields results quickly enough to be able to decide how to proceed with the wastewater treatment.

However, there are some restrictions existing due to legislation. In most countries, including Germany, the BOD-5 test is the industrial standard and as such is recognized by the government even though the BOD-5 test does not allow the actual monitoring of wastewater and the constant regulation of a wastewater plant. Therefore, in most countries the respective actual industrial standards still preclude the application of the BOD sensor. One exception is Japan, where the basis for a broad application of the BOD sensor was already prepared in 1990 by its fixation as industrial standard. Therefore, in Japan the BOD sensor is described as a standardized JIS (Japanese Industrial Standard Committee) method (JISK 3602), whereas in Germany the BOD-5 test is the only method standardized. Since the introduction of the BOD sensor in Japan the market has grown to reach 2.5×10^8 Yen or approximately DM 4 million in 1993.

The main objection to the BOD sensor is that there are some principal differences existing between the BOD sensor and the BOD-5 test:

1. A fundamental distinction is that the biosensor uses a single species of microorganism whereas the conventional method uses many species of microorganisms obtained from the activated sludge of the respective wastewater plant.
2. The BOD sensor gives insight into the current process of metabolization of organic compounds in the wastewater by the sensor, providing a sort of snapshot. In contrast, the conventional BOD-5 measures the sum of various biochemical processes in a biosludge over a period of 5 days (hydrolysis of polymers, e.g., starch, changes in the composition of a population, etc.).
3. As a biochemical activity test, the microbial BOD sensor needs to be calibrated before a comparison with the conventional BOD-5 is possible.

The use of so-called GGA standards (150 mg/l glucose and 150 mg/l glutamic acid with a BOD-5 value of 220 mg/l) is not possible as they are contaminated by the microorganisms. Glucose or glycerol proved to be more suitable for this purpose (Riedel et al., 1996). With regard to the different measuring principles and the different compositions of wastewater, the sensor-BOD values are not identical to the BOD-5, but analogous (cf. Figures 14.11 and 14.12). With the aid of specific conversion factors it is possible to calculate the BOD-5 from the sensor-BOD values. These factors depend on the composition of the wastewater sample. Therefore, any given factor is applicable only to one particular stage of an individual sewage treatment plant (Table 14.11). The ratios sensor-BOD/BOD-5 were in the range of 0.4 to 2.0 for inflow to sewage plants and 0.3 to 1.0 for outflow. The sensor-BOD values for some wastewaters are higher than those determined by BOD-5. This means that the content of low molecular organic acids, ketones, and alcohols is responsible for an important part of the BOD value in a wastewater sample. These compounds give high signals with the BOD sensor (Table 14.12). The conversion factors show the possibility of using the sensor method to determine the BOD-5 of municipal and industrial wastewater.

Table 14.13 gives an overview of the maximum permissible concentrations of compounds in drinking water set by the EC Directives and the lowest detection limits of the respective microbial and enzymatic sensors reported in the literature presented in this chapter. In most cases, the detection limits obtained are obviously too high for application to monitoring drinking water samples according to the EC Directives. This is the main reason that there has been no breakthrough in building a prototype sensor for commercial use in the case of biosensors for the analysis of phenols and nitrite, the microbial sensors for the determination of phosphate, detergents, cadmium, mercury, and the herbicide 2,4-dichlorophenoxyacetic acid, and the enzymatic sensors for the analysis of copper, zinc, and the group of organophosphates and carbamates. The microbial sensors as a group have a major disadvantage in their insufficient sensitivities towards the analytes.

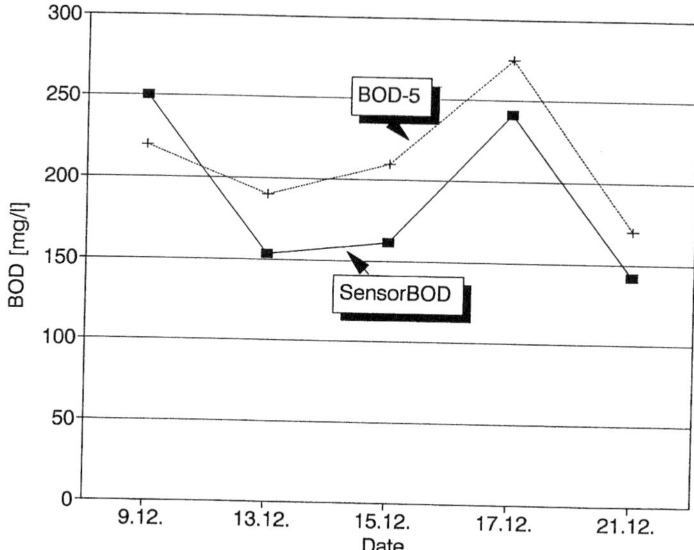

FIGURE 14.11 Comparison between BOD values estimated by the sensor and by the 5-day method, and COD of inflow of sewage treatment plant with 2.5 million population equivalent over several days. (From Riedel, K. et al., *Biosens. Bioelectron.*, 1996, in press. With permission.)

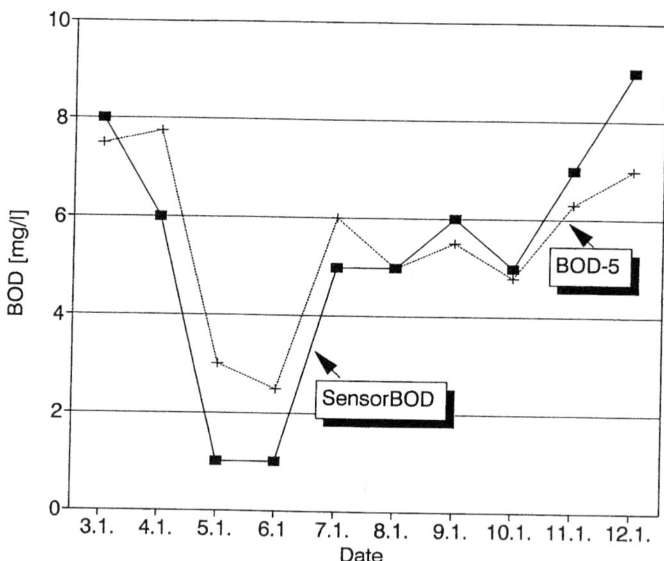

FIGURE 14.12 Comparison between BOD values estimated by the sensor and that determined with the 5-day method and COD of outflow of sewage treatment plants with 200,000 population equivalent in range of over several days. (From Riedel, K. et al., *Biosens. Bioelectron.*, 1996, in press. With permission.)

However, even if a sensitive measurement was possible (e.g., copper, lead, nitrate), the selectivities of these sensors are still not high enough as they usually show cross reactivities with related compounds. The determination of organophosphate and carbamate concentrations in a range around 0.1 μg/l was not possible on the basis of cholinesterase inhibition without prior enrichment or treatment of the water sample. When the two enzymes cholinesterase and choline oxidase were combined, some organophosphates and carbamates could be

TABLE 14.11
Correlation Factors BOD-5/Sensor BOD

Sewage treatment plant	Population equivalent	Inflow Outflow	Correlation factors BOD-5/sensor BOD
Municipal and industrial wastewater	2.5 million	Inflow	1.225
		Outflow	1.05
Wastewater	900,000	Inflow	2.01
		Outflow	0.299
Municipal wastewater	250,000	Inflow	0.411
		Outflow	0.799
Municipal and food industry wastewater	200,000	Outflow	1.05
Municipal wastewater	50,000	Outflow	0.88
Municipal wastewater	50,000	Inflow	0.965

From Riedel, K., Uthemann, R., Yang, X., and Renneberg, R., *Biosens. Bioelectron.*, 1996, in press. With permission.

TABLE 14.12
BOD-5/Sensor BOD Factors of Pure Substrates

		Sensor BOD (mg/mg)	
Substrate	BOD-5 (mg/mg)	*T. cutaneum (beigelii)* (Hikuma et al., 1979) GGA-standard	*I. orientalis* + *R. erythr.* (Riedel et al., 1996) Glycerol standard
Glucose	0.5–0.78	0.72	0.31
Fructose	0.71	0.54	0.9
Sucrose	0.49–0.76	0.36	0.06
Lactose	0.45–0.72	0.06	0.02
Acetate	0.34–0.88	1.77	3.65
Lactate	0.63–0.88	0.72	0.22
Ethanol	0.93–1.67	2.9	6.28
Glycerol	0.62–0.83	0.51	1.00
Glutamate	0.64	0.7	2.04
Glycine	0.52–0.55	0.45	0.29

detected at concentrations smaller than 0.1 μg/l. However, the main disadvantage of the cholinesterase inhibition sensors in general is that with all the devices, the insecticides exhibited various inhibition constants, so that the analysis of a real sum parameter can not be achieved.

As a result, in the case of the microbial sensors the sensitivities and selectivities have to be increased. This can be performed by using genetic engineering of specific metabolic pathways. Another possibility is to isolate the appropriate enzymatic system from the microorganisms and enhance sensitivity by protein design and molecular modelling techniques. On the other hand, enzymatic sensors often lack stability compared to the microbial

TABLE 14.13
Comparison of Maximum Permissible Concentrations (MPC) Set by the EC Directives for Drinking Water With the Lowest Detection Limits Reached by the Microbial and Enzymatic Sensors

Compound	MPC set by the EC Directives for drinking water	Lowest detection limit reached with microbial sensors	Lowest detection limit reached with enzymatic sensors
Phenols	0.5 μg/l	0.2 mg/l	1.3 μg/l
Ammonia	0.5 mg/l	0.09 mg/l	—
Nitrite	0.1 mg/l	0.5 mg/l	2.5 mg/l
Nitrate	50 mg/l	0.6 mg/l	3 mg/l
Phosphate	5 mg/l P_2O_5	890 mg/l P_2O_5	55 μg/l P_2O_5
Sulphate	250 mg/l	—	9.6 mg/l
Detergents	200 μg/l Laurylsulfate	0.1 mmol/l nitrilotriacetic acid	—
Copper	Recommended: 100 μg/l (astringent taste >3000 μg/l)	6.3 μg/l	3.2 mg/l
Zinc	Recommended: 100 μg/l (astringent taste >5000 μg/l)	—	0.65 mg/l
Cadmium	5 μg/l	100 mg/l	—
Mercury	1 μg/l	2 μg/l	—
Lead	50 μg/l	2 μg/l (Moss)	—
Sum of: 1,1,1-trichloroethane, trichloroethylene, tetrachloroethylene, dichloromethane	0.025 mg/l	—	—
Carbon tetrachloride	0.003 mg/l	—	—
Pesticides	0.1 μg/l Single substance 0.5 μg/l Sum of compounds		
2,4-Dichlorophenoxy-acetic acid		44 mg/l	—
Organophosphates and carbamates	0.5 μg/l		1 μg/l
Aldicarb	0.1 μg/l Single compound		2 μg/l
Azinphos ethyl			1 μg/l
Azinphos methyl			8 μg/l
Bromophos methyl			275 μg/l
Carbaryl			6.5 μg/l
Carbofuran			0.022 μg/l
Dichlorovos			50 μg/l
Diisopropylfluorophosphate			0.0002 μg/l
Fenitrothion			15 μg/l
Fonofos			246 μg/l
Malaoxon			0.5 μg/l
Malathion			0.033 μg/l
Paraoxon			0.028 μg/l
Paraoxon ethyl			3 μg/l
Paraoxon methyl			5 μg/l
Parathion			3.2 μg/l

TABLE 14.13 (CONTINUED)
Comparison of Maximum Permissible Concentrations (MPC) Set by the EC Directives for Drinking Water With the Lowest Detection Limits Reached by the Microbial and Enzymatic Sensors

Compound	MPC set by the EC Directives for drinking water	Lowest detection limit reached with microbial sensors	Lowest detection limit reached with enzymatic sensors
Parathion ethyl	0.1 μg/l Single compound		10 μg/l
Parathion methyl			0.263 μg/l
Phosphamidon			30 μg/l
Propoxur			2 μg/l
Trichlorfon			24 μg/l

sensors. However, the miniaturization of biosensors and the development of portable biosensor measuring systems is an attractive feature for environmental monitoring. This will lead to the development of economical sensor systems. It can be estimated that the average costs for laboratory analysis for an environmental sample could be reduced from \$130–\$200 to \$1–\$15.

REFERENCES

Battacharya, S., Alsen, C., Kruse, H., and Valentin, P., Detection of organophosphate insecticide by an immobilized enzyme system, *Environ. Sci. Technol.*, 15(11), 1352, 1981.

Bernabei, M., Cremisini, C., Mascini, M., and Palleschi, G., Determination of organophosphorus and carbamic pesticides with a choline and acetylcholine electrochemical biosensor, *Anal. Lett.*, 24 (8), 1317, 1991.

Beyersdorf-Radeck, B., Riedel, K., Neumann, B., Scheller, F., and Schmid, R. D., Microbial sensors for the determination of aromatics and their chloroderivatives, *Int. Symp. Environ. Biotechnol.*, Verachtert, H. and Verstraete, W., Eds., Oostende, The Netherlands, pp. 65-68, 1991.

Bilitewski, U., Chemnitius, G. C., Rüger, P., and Schmid, R. D., Miniaturized disposable biosensors, *Sensors Actuators*, B7, 351, 1992.

Campanella, L., Paoletti, A. M., and Tranchida, G., Biosensor of total toxicity, *Tossicol. Chim.*, 61-63, 1987.

Campanella, L., Sammartino, M. P., and Tomasetti, M., New enzyme sensor for phenol determination in non-aqueous and aqueous medium, *Sensors Actuators*, B7, 383, 1992.

Ciucu, A., Mageearu, V., Fleschin, S., Lucaciu, I., and David, F., Biocatalytical membrane electrode for phenol, *Anal. Lett.*, 24 (4), 567, 1991.

Colapicchioni, C., Barbaro, A., and Porcelli, F., Fabrication and characterization of ENFET devices for biomedical applications and environmental monitoring, *Sensors Actuators*, B6, 202, 1992.

Cserfalvi, T. and Guilbault, G. G., An enzyme electrode based on immobilized arylsulphatase for the selective assay of sulphate ion, *Anal. Chim. Acta*, 84, 259, 1976.

Dumschat, C., Müller, H., Stein, K., and Schwedt, G., Pesticide-sensitive ISFET based on enzyme inhibition, *Anal. Chim. Acta*, 252, 7, 1991.

Durand, P., Nicaud, J. M., and Malleviale, J., Detection of organophosphorus pesticides with an immobilized cholinesterase electrode, *J. Anal. Toxicol.*, 8, 112, 1984.

El Yamani, H., Tran-Minh, C., Abdul, M. A., and Chavanne, D., Automated system for pesticide detection, *Sensors Actuators*, 15, 193, 1988.

Ellman, G. L., Courtney, K. D., Andres, V., and Featherstone, R. M., A new rapid colorimetric determination of acetylcholinesterase activity, *Biochem. Pharmacol.*, 2, 88, 1961.

Gaisford, W. C., Richardson, N. J., Haggett, B. G. D., and Rawson, D. M., Microbial biosensors for environmental monitoring, *Biochem. Soc. Trans.,* 19, 15, 1991.

Goodson, L. H. and Jacobs, W. B., Use of immobilized enzyme product in water monitoring, Proc. Natl. Conf. Control of Hazardous Material Spills, AICHE and USEPA, San Francisco, CA, pp. 292-299, 1974.

Guilbault, G. G. and Nanjo, M., A phosphate-selective electrode based on immobilized alkaline phosphatase and glucose oxidase, *Anal. Chim. Acta*, 78, 69, 1975.

Guzzo, J., Guzzo, A., and DuBon, M. S., Characterization of the effects of aluminum on luciferase biosensors for the detection of ecotoxicity, *Toxicol. Lett.*, 64/65, 687, 1992.

Haemmerli, S. D., Suleiman, A. A., and Guilbault, G. G., Amperometric determination of phosphate by use of a nucleoside phosphorylase-xanthine oxidase enzyme sensor based on a Clark-type hydrogen peroxide or oxygen electrode, *Anal. Biochem.*, 191, 106, 1990.

Harita, K., Otani, Y., Hikuma, M., and Yasuda, T., BOD quick estimating system utilizing a microbial electrode, in: *Instrumental Control of Water and Wastewater Treatment in Transportation Systems,* Proc. IAWPRC Workshop, Drake, R. A. C., Ed., Pergamon Press, Oxford, 529-532, 1985.

Hikuma, M., Matsuko, H., Takeda, M., and Tonooka, Y., Microbial electrode for nitrate based on *Pseudomonas aeruginosa, Biotechnol. Tech.*, 7 (3), 231, 1993.

Hikuma, M., Suzuki, H., Yasuda, T., Karube, I., and Suzuki, S., Amperometric estimation of BOD by using living immobilized yeasts, *Eur. J. Appl. Microbiol. Biotechnol.*, 8, 289, 1979.

Holmes, D. S., Dubey, S. K., and Gangolli, S., Development of biosensors to measure metal ion. In: *Biohydrometallurgical Technologies,* Torma, L. A. E., Alpel, M. L., and Brierley, C. L., Eds., The Minerals, Metal, and Material Society, 659, 1993.

Japanese Industrial Standard, Apparatus for the estimation of biochemical oxygen demand (BOD_5) with microbial sensor, JIS K 3602, 1990.

Karube, I., Microbial sensor, *J. Biotechnol.*, 15, 255, 1990.

Karube, I., Matsunaga, T., Mitsuda, S., and Suzuki, S., Microbial electrode BOD sensors, *Biotechnol. Bioeng.*, 19, 1535, 1977b.

Karube, I., Matsunaga, T., and Suzuki, S., A new microbial electrode for BOD estimation, *J. Solid-Phase Biochem.*, 2, 97, 1977c.

Karube, I., Mitsuda, S., Matsunaga, T., and Suzuki, S., A rapid method for estimating BOD by using immobilized microbial cells, *J. Ferment. Technol.*, 55, 243, 1977a.

Karube, I., Nakahara, T., Matsunaga, T., and Suzuki, S., Salmonella electrode for screening mutagens, *Anal. Chem.*, 54, 1725, 1982b.

Karube, I., Nakahara, T., Matsuoka, M., and Suzuki, S., Measurement of mutagens by microbial sensor. *Denki Kagaku oyobi Kogyo Butsuri Kagaku*, 51, 103, 1983 (Japanese).

Karube, I., Okada, T., and Suzuki, S., Amperometric determination of ammonia gas with immobilized nitrifying bacteria, *Anal. Chem.,* 53, 1852, 1981a.

Karube, I., Okada, T., Suzuki, S., Suzuki, H., Hikuma, M., and Yasuda, T., Amperometric determination of sodium nitrite by a microbial sensor, *Eur. J. Appl. Microbiol. Biotechnol.*, 15, 127, 1982a.

Karube, I. and Tamiya, E., Biosensors for environmental control, *Pure Appl. Chem.*, 59 (4), 545, 1987.

Karube, I. and Suzuki, S., Preliminary screening of mutagens with a microbial sensor, *Anal. Chem.*, 53, 1024, 1981b.

Karube, I., Yokoyama, K., Sode, K., and Tamiya, E., Microbial BOD sensor utilizing thermophilic bacteria, *Anal. Lett.*, 22 (4), 791, 1989.

Kiang, C., Kuan, S., and Guilbault, G. G., A novel enzyme electrode method for the determination of nitrite based on nitrite reductase, *Anal. Chim. Acta*, 80, 209, 1975.

Kiang, C. H., Kuan, S. S., and Guilbault, G. G., Enzymatic determination of nitrate: electrochemical detection after reduction with nitrate reductase and nitrite reductase, *Anal. Chem.*, 50, 1319, 1978a.

Kiang, C. H., Kuan, S. S., and Guilbault, G. G., Enzymatic determination of nitrate: fluorimetric detection after reduction with nitrate reductase, *Anal. Chem.*, 50, 1323, 1978b.

Kindervater, R., Künnecke, W., and Schmid, R. D., Exchangeable immobilized enzyme reactor for enzyme inhibition tests in flow-injection analysis using a magnetic device. Determination of pesticides in drinking water, *Anal. Chim. Acta*, 234, 113, 1990.

Kobos, R. K. and Pyon, H. Y., Application of microbial cells as multistep catalysts in potentiometric biosensing electrodes, *Biotechnol. Bioeng.*, 23, 627, 1981.

Kobos, R. K., Rice, D. J., and Flournay, D. S., Bacterial membrane electrode for the determination of nitrate, *Anal. Chem.*, 51, 1122, 1979.

Kubo, I., Inagawa, M., Sugawara, T., Arikawa, Y., and Karube, I., Phosphate sensor composed from immobilized pyruvate oxidase and an oxygen electrode, *Anal. Lett.*, 24, 1711, 1991.

Kulys, J. and Kadziauskiene, K., Yeast BOD sensor, *Biotechnol. Bioeng.*, 22, 221, 1980.

Kulys, J. and Schmid, R. D., A sensitive enzyme electrode for phenol monitoring, *Anal. Lett.*, 23 (4), 589, 1990.

Kumaran, S. and Tran-Minh, C., Insecticide determination with enzyme electrodes using different enzyme immobilization techniques, *Electroanalysis*, 4, 949, 1992a.

Kumaran, S. and Tran-Minh, C., Determination of organophosphorus and carbamate insecticides by flow injection analysis, *Anal. Biochem.*, 200, 187, 1992b.

Lee, S., Suzuki, M., Tamiya, E., and Karube, I., Sensitive bioluminescent detection of pesticides utilizing a membrane mutant of *Escherichia coli* and recombinant DNA technology, *Anal. Chim. Acta*, 257, 183, 1992.

Li, Y.-R. and Chu, J., Study of BOD microbial sensors for waste water treatment control, *Appl. Biochem. Biotechnol.*, 28/29, 855, 1991.

Marty, J.-L., Sode, K., and Karube, I., Biosensor for detection of organophosphate and carbamate insecticides, *Electroanalysis*, 4, 249, 1992.

Matsunaga, T., Karube, I., and Suzuki, S., A specific microbial sensor for formic acid, *Eur. J. Appl. Microbiol. Biotechnol.,* 10, 235, 1980.

Matsunaga, T., Suzuki, S., and Tomoda, R., Photomicrobial sensors for selective determination of phosphate, *Enzyme Microb. Technol.*, 6, 355, 1984.

Mattiasson, B., Nilsson, H., and Olsson, B., An apoenzyme electrode, *J. App. Biochem.*, 1, 377, 1979.

Mionetto, N., Rouillon, R., and Marty, J.-L., Inhibition of acetylcholinesterase by organophosphorus and carbamates compounds. Studies on free and immobilized enzymes, *Z. Wasser Abwasser Forsch.*, 25, 171, 1992.

Neujahr, H. Y. and Kjellen, K. G., Bioprobe electrode for phenol, *Biotechnol. Bioeng.*, 21, 671, 1979.

Nyamsi Hendji, A. M., Jaffrezic-Renault, N., Martelet, C., Clechet, P., Shul'ga, A. A., Strikha, V. I., Netchiporuk, L. I., Soldatkin, A. P., and Wlodarski, W. B., Sensitive detection of pesticides using a differential ISFET-based system with immobilized cholinesterases, *Anal. Chim. Acta*, 281, 3, 1993.

Ögren, L. and Johansson, G., Determination of traces of mercury(II) by inhibition of an enzyme reactor electrode loaded with immobilized urease, *Anal. Chim. Acta*, 96, 1, 1978.

Ohki, A., Shinohara, K., and Maeda, S., Biological oxygen demand sensor using an arsenic resistant bacterium, *Anal. Sci.*, 6, 905, 1990.

Okada, T., Karube, I., and Suzuki, S., Microbial sensor system which uses *Methylomonas* sp. for the determination of methane, *Eur. J. Appl. Microbiol. Biotechnol.*, 12, 102, 1981.

Okada, T., Karube, I., and Suzuki, S., NO_2 sensor which uses immobilized nitrate oxidizing bacteria, *Biotechnol. Bioeng.,* 25, 1641, 1983.

Palleschi, G., Bernabei, M., Cremisini, C., and Mascini, M., Determination of organophosphorus insecticides with a choline electrochemical biosensor, *Sensors Actuators*, B7, 513, 1992.

Quintero, M.C., Silva, M., and Perez-Bendito, D., Enzymatic determination of n-methylcarbamate pesticides at the nanomolar level by the stopped-flow technique, *Talanta*, 38(11), 1273, 1991.

Ramos, J. A., Bermejo, E., Zapardiel, A., Perez, J. A., and Hernandez, L., Direct determination of lead by bioaccumulation at a moss-modified carbon paste electrode, *Anal. Chim. Acta*, 273, 219, 1993.

Riedel, K., Beyersdorf-Radeck, B., Neumann, B., and Scheller, F., Microbial sensors for determination of aromatics and their chloroderivatives. III. Determination of chlorinated phenols using *Trichosporon beigelii (cutaneum)* containing biosensors, *Appl. Microbiol. Biotechnol.*, 43, 7, 1995.

Riedel, K., Hensel, J., and Ebert, K., Biosensoren zur Bestimmung von Phenol und Benzoat auf der Basis von Rhodococcuszellen und Enzymextrakten, *Zentralbl. Mikrobiol.*, 146, 425, 1991b.

Riedel, K., Hensel, J., Rothe, S., Neumann, B., and Scheller, F., Microbial sensors for determination of aromatics and their chloroderivatives. II. Determination of chlorinated phenols using a *Rhodococcus*-containing biosensor, *Appl. Microbiol. Biotechnol.*, 38, 556, 1993.

Riedel, K., Lange, K.-P., Stein, H.-J., Kühn, M., Ott, P., and Scheller, F., A microbial sensor for BOD, *Water Res.*, 24 (7), 883, 1990.

Riedel, K., Naumov, A. V., Boronin, A. M., Golovleva, L. A., Stein, H. D., and Scheller, F., Microbial sensors for determination of aromatics and their chloroderivatives. I. Determination of 3-chlorobenzoate using a *Pseudomonas*-containing biosensor, *Appl. Microbiol. Biotechnol.*, 35, 559, 1991a.

Riedel, K., Renneberg, R., Kühn, M., and Scheller, F., A fast estimation of biochemical oxygen demand using microbial sensors, *Appl. Microbiol. Biotechnol.*, 28, 316, 1988.

Riedel, K., Renneberg, R., Liebs, P., and Kaiser, G., Microbial sensors, *Stud. Biophys.*, 119 (1-3), 163, 1987.

Riedel, K., Uthemann, R., and Renneberg, R., Determination of BOD with a combination-sensor containing *Rhodococcus erythropolis* and *Issatchenkia orientalis, Biosens. Bioelectron.*, 1996 (in press).

Satoh, I., An apoenzyme thermistor microanalysis for zinc(II) ions with use of an immobilized alkaline phosphatase reactor in a flow system, *Biosens. Bioelectron.*, 6, 375, 1991.

Satoh, I. and Aoki, Y., Biosensing of zinc(II) ions using an apoenzyme reactor and an ISFET detector in flow streams, *Denki Kagaku*, 58 (12), 1114, 1990.

Satoh, I., Kasahara, T., and Goi, N., Amperometric biosensing of copper(II) ions with an immobilized apoenzyme reactor, *Sensors Actuators*, B1, 499, 1991.

Schubert, F., Saini, S., Turner, A. P. F., and Scheller, F., Organic phase enzyme electrodes for the determination of hydrogen peroxide and phenol, *Sensors Actuators*, B7, 408, 1992.

Schwedt, G. and Hauck, M., Reaktivierbare Enzymelektrode mit Acetylcholinesterase zur differenzierten Erfassung von Insecticiden im Spurenbereich, *Fresenius Z. Anal. Chem.*, 331, 316, 1988.

Skladal, P., Determination of organophosphate and carbamate pesticides using a cobalt phthalocyanine-modified carbon paste electrode and a cholinesterase enzyme membrane, *Anal. Chim. Acta*, 252, 11, 1991a.

Skladal, P., Mushroom tyrosinase-modified carbon paste electrode as an amperometric biosensor for phenols, *Collect. Czech. Chem. Commun.*, 56, 1427, 1991b.

Strand, S. E. and Carlson, D. A., Rapid BOD measurement for municipal wastewater samples using a biofilm electrode, *J. Water Pollut. Control Fed.*, 56, 464, 1984.

Su, Y. C., Huang, J. H., and Liu, M. L., A new biosensor for rapid BOD estimation by using immobilized growing cell beads, *Proc. Natl. Sci. Council B. ROC*, 10, 105, 1986.

Takruni, I. A., Almuaibed, A. M., and Townshend, A., Flow injection study of inhibition and reactivation of immobilized acetylcholinesterase: determination of the pesticides paraoxon and carbamoylcholine, *Anal. Chim. Acta*, 282, 307, 1993.

Tan, T. C., Li, F., and Neoh, K. G., Measurement of BOD by initial rate of response of a microbial sensor, *Sensors Actuators*, B10, 137, 1993.

Tran-Minh, C., Pandey, P. C., and Kumaran, S., Studies on acetylcholine sensor and its analytical application based on the inhibition of cholinesterase, *Biosens. Bioelectron.*, 5, 461, 1990.

Watanabe, E., Endo, H., and Toyama, K., Determination of phosphate ions with an enzyme sensor system, *Biosensors*, 3, 297, 1988.

Wolfbeis, O. S. and Koller, E., Fiber optic detection of pesticides in drinking water, in: *GBF Monographs*, 13, 221, Schmid, R. D. and Scheller, F., Eds., VCH Publishers, Weinheim, 1989.

Wollenberger, U., Schubert, F., and Scheller F. W., Biosensor for sensitive phosphate detection, *Sensors Actuators*, B7, 412, 1992.

Zachariah, K. and Mottola, H. A., Continuous-flow determination of phenol with chemically immobilized polyphenol oxidase (tyrosinase), *Anal. Lett.*, 22 (5), 1145, 1989.

15 Bioaffinity Sensors for Environmental Monitoring

Christine Wittmann and Rolf D. Schmid

CONTENTS

15.1 INTRODUCTION

In this chapter antibody-based and receptor-based sensors are presented for application in the field of environmental analysis. Both types of biosensors belong to the group of bioaffinity sensors within which, in most cases, the antibody-antigen and receptor-ligand binding reaction is not directly observed but can be followed by a detection reaction. A disappointingly low number of references are found in the literature covering immunosensors and receptor-based sensors for environmental monitoring. Pesticides are the analytes most commonly targeted by those groups known to be actively investigating environmental immunosensors. The main reason is that due to intensive agriculture, with the associated use of a large number of different pesticides, there is a growing concern about the quality of drinking water and food, e.g., corn and vegetables, as both are directly involved in the nutrition chain. Therefore, in combination with food and drinking water quality legislation, there is a high demand for the availability of fast screening methods. To give an example of legislation, the protection of drinking water in Europe has led to pertinent regulations, in particular the European Drinking Water Act, which sets permissible limits for the amount of pesticide residues in drinking water. The upper limit for pesticide concentrations in drinking water is set at 0.1 μg/l for a single substance and 0.5 μg/l for the total of all pesticides, including metabolites. During the last 7 years, university research groups as well as several companies came up with a series

0-8493-8905-4/97/$0.00+$.50
© 1997 by CRC Press, Inc.

of highly sensitive immunoassays for the analysis of pesticides and other compounds of environmental interest (cf. Table 15.1). The main application for these immunoassays is still in the field of water analysis, but the determination of pesticides in plant and soil samples (Wittmann and Hock, 1990) as well as in food (Wittmann and Hock, 1993) has been reported.

With the availability of pesticide-selective antibodies for the very sensitive determination of pesticide residues the possibility of using these antibodies for immunosensor development opened up in the mid-1980s. Concerning the environmental air matrix, one approach to continuously monitor acute toxins was described utilizing the piezo effect in combination with parathion-specific antibodies for the analysis of this insecticide in air. The different immunosensor formats and their suitability for pesticide analysis are described in detail in this chapter.

TABLE 15.1
Immunoassays for the Analysis of Compounds of Environmental Concern

Herbicides	Fungicides	Insecticides	Other compounds of environmental interest
Alachlor	Benomyl and metabolites	Aldicarb	BTEX[a] (= benzene, toluene, ethyl benzene, xylene)
Atrazine[a] and other triazines[a]	Blasticidin S	Allethrin[a] and S-bioallethrin[a]	PCB (polychlorinated biphenyls): Arochlor 1232
Chlorsulfuron	Carbofuran	Benzoylphenylurea derivatives	TNT[a] (2,4,6-trinitro-toluene)
Cyanazine	Fenpropimorph	Carbamate	Long-chain hydrocarbons (e.g., kerosine, diesel fuel)
2,4-Dichlorophenoxyacetic acid[a] and 2,4,5-trichloro-phenoxyacetic acid	Metalaxyl	Chlordan	Pentachlorophenol
Diclofopmethyl	Sulfathiazol	DDA (2,2-bis(*p*-chloro-phenyl)acetic acid	
Dinitro aromates	Triadimefon	DDT	
Maleinhydrazide[a]		Dieldrin	
Metazachlor		Diflubezuron	
Metolachlor		Endosulfan and other chlorodienes	
Molinate		Fenitrothion[a]	
Norflurazon		Heptachlor[a]	
Paraquat[a]		Iprodion	
Picloram		Malathion	
Trifluralin		Paraoxon[a] and Parathion[a]	
		Permethrin[a] and other pyrethroids[a]	

[a] Monoclonal antibodies are available for these immunoassays.

The receptor-based sensors described so far use as the receptor either the photoreaction centres isolated from bacteria or work with an intact chemosensing structure. In the latter case, only a qualitative statement about the presence or absence of several pesticide compounds could be given. In the case of the photoreaction centres, the sum of photosystem-II herbicides acting as inhibitors in photosynthesis could be determined. As the biosensors applying whole cells (cyanobacteria) and organelles (thylakoids) are the basis for the development of the centre-based reaction biosensors they are treated in this chapter. Only a few papers dealing with receptor-based sensors can be found in the literature as mostly the mass production, isolation, and stabilization of the receptors is tedious.

15.2 IMMUNOSENSORS

Most of the immunosensors described and selectively presented in this chapter were developed for pesticide analysis, mainly in environmental water samples. The methods generally used to monitor pesticides in water supplies are high-performance liquid chromatography (HPLC) and gas chromatography with mass spectrometric detection (GC/MS). Usually these procedures are preceded by enrichment steps which can render analysis cumbersome, especially in the case of hydrophilic pesticides. As a result, these procedures are complex and often beyond the capabilities of the some 3000 drinking water suppliers in Germany. For this reason, in the last few years serological methods such as immunoassays for pesticide analysis have been developed and put onto the market. A number of pesticides, especially herbicides, can now be detected with commercially available immunoassay kits. A number of biosensor formats have also been proposed for pesticide analysis. Antibody-based flow injection analysis (FIA) is of significant interest, since it allows virtually continuous monitoring and is therefore a suitable concept for establishing "alarm systems".

Such very sensitive FIA systems for the analysis of pesticides have been under development for several years. Real time analysis of binding events is one step forward on the way from immunoassays to immunosensors. These direct methods are either based on optical formats such as grating couplers, surface plasmon resonance, interferometry, and fibre optics, or on electrochemical principles, especially on the piezoelectric effect. (More on these methods in Chapters 7, 8, 9, and 16.) None of these direct transducing principles are suitable yet for the detection of low molecular weight compounds such as most pesticides and other toxins of environmental interest, because a more sensitive measurement range for the analytes is required.

15.2.1 Flow Injection Immunoanalysis Assays (FIIA) for Pesticide Determination

Since the mid-1980s pesticide-specific antibodies have been developed along with competitive enzyme immunoassays which use them. Thus, the development of a flow injection analysis (FIA) system using these antibodies for the determination of a specific pesticide was rendered possible.

FIA represents a potentially useful measuring device for continuously monitoring the presence of pollutants — in nearly all cases, pesticides — especially in drinking water supplies. Based on an enzyme immunoassay for investigating polyclonal anti-atrazine antibodies (Wittmann and Hock, 1989), the first report of the suitability of the FIA format for pesticide analysis was made in 1989 (Stöcklein et al., 1989). The antibodies were immobilized on activated membranes (Fluorotrans transfer and Immunodyne, PALL) oriented by protein A precoating. The antibody-containing membranes were then mounted in a specially constructed reactor and removed after each assay; a new membrane strip was inserted for each new test. All reagents are pumped in a cross flow over the membrane reactor. The principle of this format is the same as for a sequential competitive enzyme immunoassay where the analyte competes with the corresponding enzyme-labelled analyte (in this case atrazine conjugated to peroxidase) for the limited binding sites of the anti-atrazine antibodies. The fluorescent enzyme-generated product is measured downstream in the flow-through cell of a fluorescence detector, where the peak height and area are registered with an integrator. The result is inversely proportional to the pesticide concentration, which means that the higher the peak the lower the pesticide concentration. The system is controlled by a time processor

(Alphotronic). One assay takes 15 min to complete. The detection limit reached for atrazine with the polyclonal antibody R14 was reported to be 10 µg/l.

The sensitivity of the FIA system could be improved by the use of another atrazine-specific antibody. In addition, Krämer and Schmid (1991a,b) developed a membrane reactor which allowed the automated removal of spent antibody, thus producing a fully automatic "alarm system". The use of the polyclonal antibody C193 yielded very low detection limits for atrazine (0.02 µg/l) and propazine (0.03 µg/l), although the standard deviation was somewhat increased (10 to 20%) compared to the average variation coefficient of 4% for the respective enzyme immunoassay. This membrane reactor-based FIA was successfully applied to the analysis of atrazine traces in environmental water samples of different origins and compositions, e.g., various kinds of surface waters, and validated by comparison with GC and HPLC data (Wittmann and Schmid, 1993).

A disadvantage of the membrane FIA was that monoclonal anti-atrazine antibodies (as described by Giersch and Hock, 1990; and Giersch, 1993) and other antibodies could not be used because the immobilization of these antibodies onto the membrane resulted in a very high background signal caused by an extremely large amount of unspecific binding.

To overcome this as well as problems with the membrane-exchange mechanism such as the higher detection limit of the membrane FIA (compared to enzyme immunoassay), the higher coefficients of variation, and the larger amounts of antibody needed per assay, we developed an antibody column reactor (Wittmann and Schmid, 1994). For this purpose, we investigated several support materials (e.g., diverse glasses, partly exhibiting active sites such as, for example, amino groups for cross-linking, nylon, latex, polyacrylamide, polystyrene) and various immobilization methods (adsorptive, covalent, via protein A, and via the avidin/biotin system). We finally decided to immobilize the antibodies via the avidin/biotin system on glass or polystyrene beads which were filled into a column reactor.

With this device the FIA system was regenerable with the aid of glycine/HCl buffer, pH 2.0. The final FIA format takes 15 min to complete, but it allows the regeneration of the immobilized antibody activity for a minimum of 500 measuring cycles. Thus, an automatic control of the status of water contamination by particular pesticides could be obtained depending, of course, on the availability of specific antibodies. Figure 15.1 shows the instrument setup of the FIA based on the column reactor, and Figure 15.2 depicts some typical standard curves for atrazine and simazine analysis. Table 15.2 compares data from the enzyme immunoassay with those from the two FIA systems based on the membrane and the column reactor. With the column reactor FIA, detection limits for atrazine of 0.001 µg/l using a polyclonal antibody and 0.03 µg/l with a monoclonal antibody could be reached in combination with an average standard deviation of only 4%. The successful validation of this FIA system was described by Wittmann and Schmid (1994).

15.2.2 Immunosensing Devices for Pesticide Analysis

Table 15.3 gives an overview of the literature dealing with the development of immunosensors for the analysis of environmental toxins, especially pesticides. There are only a few papers dealing with the analysis of pesticide traces with immunosensors. The optical devices dominate, especially the use of optical silica fibres combined with fluorescein-labelled antibodies (Bier et al., 1992; Betts et al., 1991; Anis et al., 1993; Jockers et al., 1993a). However, two direct measurement principles have also been described, namely the application of piezoelectric quartz crystals (Guilbault et al., 1992; Ngeh-Ngwainbi et al., 1986) and of grating couplers (Bier et al., 1991; Bier and Schmid, 1994). In general, the direct, nonlabelling observation of antibody-pesticide binding is unsatisfactory in terms of sensitivity since, in most cases, the detection limits are rather high compared to the immunosensing formats using enzymes, fluorescent dyes, or other labels to amplify and detect the antibody-antigen reaction.

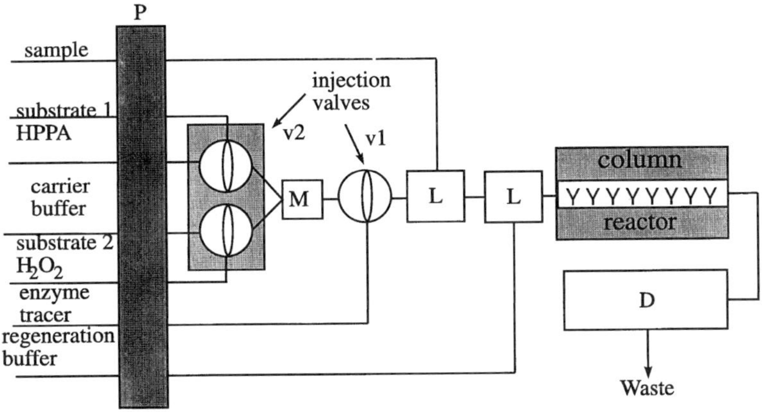

FIGURE 15.1 Instrument setup of FIIA. Five pumps with different reagents work in a time-controlled sequence. All reagents have to pass through the antibody reactor where the specific antibodies are located. These antibodies are immobilized after biotinylation on avidin-derivatized polystyrene or glass beads. The antibody-coated beads are filled in a specially constructed antibody column reactor which is regenerated within each measuring cycle. The fluorescence of the enzyme reaction product is measured with a fluorimeter and the peak level and/or area are registered with an integrator or by computer (Q-FIA program). P: pump, M: mixing chamber, L: Lee valve (3/2-way valve), D: detector (fluorimeter combined with an integrator and/or computer). (From Wittmann, C. and Schmid, R. D., *J. Agric. Food Chem.*, 42, 1041-1047, 1994. With permission.)

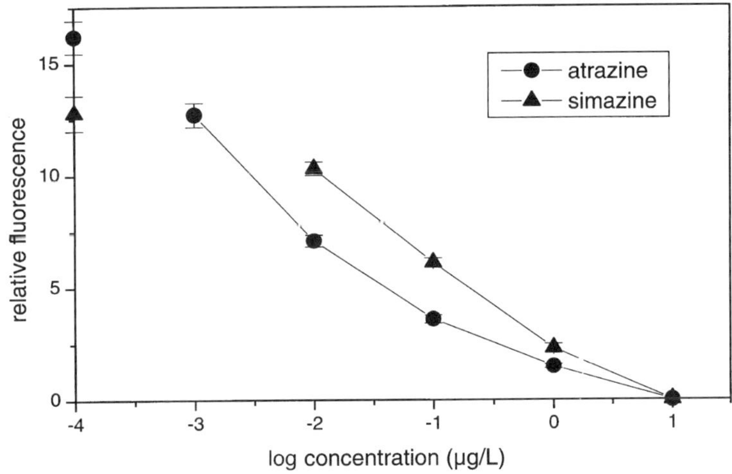

FIGURE 15.2 Representative standard curves for atrazine and simazine determination by FIIA with two different polyclonal antibodies.

In the case of the grating coupler used by Bier et al. (1991), a detection limit of 10 µg/l terbutryn was reached which could be pushed to 3.8 µg/l by the application of a kinetic measurement and calculation of the results (Bier and Schmid, 1994). This is due to the fact that, in the case of the grating coupler, antibody-pesticide binding is observed as the change in the adlayer thickness. As the molecular weights of most pesticides are in the range of 200 to 400 Da, the change in adlayer thickness caused by the pesticide binding to the pesticide-specific antibody is rather small. For sensitivity to be improved, either the affinity of the antibodies to their analyte has to be increased or the transducing element has to be improved in terms of reaching lower detection limits.

TABLE 15.2
Aspects of Assay Characteristics

Aspect	Enzyme immunoassay	Membrane FIA	Column FIA
Antibodies	Adsorbed to polystyrene wells of a microtitre plate	Covalently bound to a preactivated membrane oriented by protein A precoating	Biotinylated antibodies are reacted with avidin bound to polystyrene or glass beads
Amounts of reagents used:			
Antiserum	0.0006 μl C193/0.0015 μl K4E7 per microtitre plate with 96 cavities	0.21 μl C193	0.050 μl C193/K4E7 for 500 measuring cycles
Enzyme tracer	0.0001 μl Tracer (C193)/0.00025 μl (K4E7) per microtitre plate	0.043 μl Tracer	0.010 μl Tracer (C193/K4E7) for 500 measuring cycles
Number of samples	18 Samples on 1 plate (4 replicates of the samples and the 6 standards)	Samples are measured successively	Samples are measured successively
Time per assay	90 min	15 min	15 min
Time to analyze 26 samples (3 replicates) including 6 standards	90 min	24 h	24 h
Probability of experimental error	High	Low	Low
Use as a control unit	Not possible	Possible	Possible

For the same reasons, the usefulness of the piezo effect as a method of directly measuring pesticides is limited in terms of the sensitivities which can be reached and the lower detection limit for pesticides. The measurement principle behind the piezoelectric crystal immunosensor is the reduction in the oscillating frequency of a piezo element (usually a quartz crystal) when its mass is increased, e.g., when an antigen is bound to an antibody immobilized on the quartz surface. In this case, changes in mass are used as a measure for the pesticide concentration in a sample. In general, piezoelectric sensors are used to analyze samples in the gaseous phase, as was the case in the work of Ngeh-Ngwainbi et al. (1986). They worked on the detection of parathion in the gaseous phase using a parathion-specific antibody. A detection limit of 2 ppb parathion could be reached.

Guilbault et al. (1992) described a piezoelectric crystal immunosensor using a polyclonal antibody from sheep for atrazine analysis in water samples. The authors calculated a detection limit of only 0.03 μg/l, which was astonishingly low, and they stated in their paper that this stands in conflict with the theoretical data from the Sauerbrey equation. They assumed that the reason for the high sensitivity described was that they dried the quartz crystals after the immunoreaction and measured the oscillation changes before and after the immunoreaction in the gaseous phase. In addition to the piezoelectric crystal balance, surface acoustic wave (SAW) devices have been used as the basis of immunosensors and these are described in Chapter 9.

Another immunosensing format based on electroconductivity measurement was presented by Sandberg et al. (1992). They performed a special ELISA format using electroconductive polythiophene as a solid support. Utilizing analogous sequential coupled reactions, a dopant (such as iodine) can be quantitatively produced by the bound enzyme. Under the influence

TABLE 15.3
Immunosensors for Pesticide Analysis

Analyte	Antibodies used	Assay time	Detection limit (μg/l)	Regeneration	Transducer	Ref.
Atrazine	S84 (pab from sheep)	ca. 1 h	0.03–100 SD: 8%	Glycine/HCl, pH 2.5 Reusable for 8–9 assays	Piezoelectric quartz crystal	Guilbault et al., 1992
Terbutryn	K1F4 (mab)	ca. 1 h	10	Acid >50 Assays	Planar monomode waveguides with grating coupler	Bier et al., 1991
Model analytes: phenytoin, theophylline, phenobarbital, digoxin	Fab fragments		25 nmol/l	5–10 Days 10–20 Times reusable	Fibre optics	Betts et al., 1991
Terbutryn	K1F4 (mab)	ca. 1 h	0.1	Acidic buffer + proteinase 300 Assays	Hard-clad silica fibre	Bier et al., 1992
Pyrethroid derivative	mab				Silica fibre	Northrup et al., 1989
Pesticide	pab	ca. 15 min	0.025–250 SD: 15–30%		ELISA with electroconductive polythiophene as solid support	Sandberg et al., 1992
Imazethapyr	pab (from rabbits and sheep)		0.3	Reusable	Fibre optics	Anis et al., 1993
Atrazine	K1F4 (mab)	ca. 1 h	ca. 0.1 nmol/l SD: >20%	Reusable	Fibre optics	Jockers et al., 1993a
Terbutryn	K1F4 (mab)	50 min	15 nmol/l = ca. 3.8 μg/l	Reusable	Grating coupler	Bier and Schmid, 1994
Parathion (in the gaseous phase)		Response time 1–2 min	2-35 ppb Parathion, cross-reactivities with malathion, methyl parathion SD: 6%		Piezoelectric quartz crystals	Ngeh-Ngwainbi et al., 1986

Note: SD: relative standard deviation; pab: polyclonal antibodies; mab: monoclonal antibodies.

of a dopant, a suitable electroconductive polymer, e.g., polyacetylene or polythiophene, can simultaneously serve as the solid phase to support immobilized antibodies and, through conductivity modulation by the dopant, function as the measuring device. The electrical changes can be measured with a voltmeter. Preliminary results from this group showed that sensitivities in the low parts per billion range are reached (25 ng/l).

The optical method generally applied for exploiting the immunoreaction for the measurement of pesticide traces is fibre optics (cf. Table 15.3). This method is described in more detail in the work of Bier et al. (1992), for example. A derivative of the s-triazines, aminohexylatrazine, was immobilized on one end of a hard-clad silica fibre which had been stripped of cladding. The fibre was inserted into a flow-through cuvette. In Figure 15.3 the instrument setup, the principles behind fibre optics, and a typical recorder readout are depicted. Anti-triazine antibodies conjugated with fluorescein isothiocyanate (FITC) were detected after binding to the fibre via the evanescent field. In the presence of triazines, especially terbutryn, the fluorescence signal decreases due to the inhibition of antibody binding to the fibre. The detection limit of the sensor for terbutryn was calculated to be 0.1 μg/l. When a weak competitor was used, 11-(4-ethylamino-6-methyl-thio-s-triazine-2yl) undecanoic acid, the detection limit could be lowered 100-fold compared to when aminohexylatrazine was used (Jockers et al., 1993a). A disadvantage of the whole system was the high standard deviation (CV >20%). In general, the use of immunosensors based on fibre optics yielded acceptable detection limits although the time required for one assay amounted to nearly one hour.

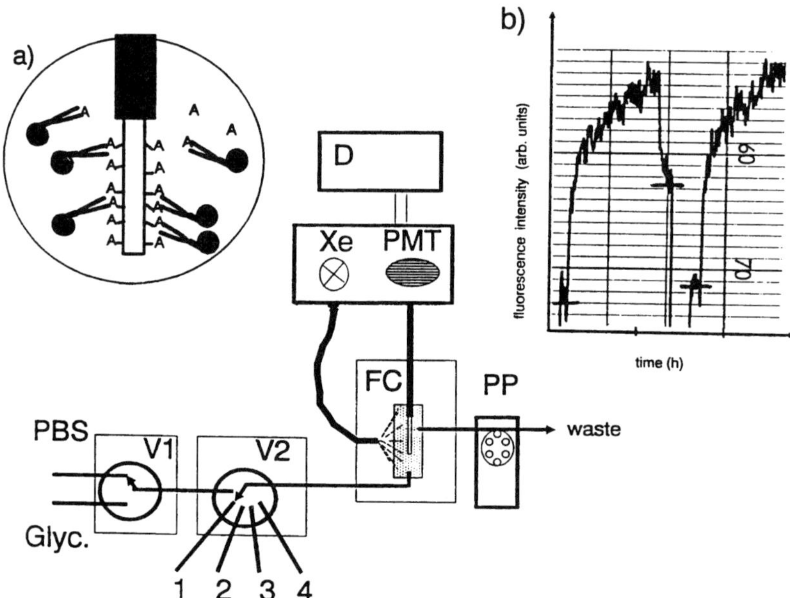

FIGURE 15.3 Experimental setup of fibre optic immunosensor. The fibre core with immobilized triazine (A-), visualized in insert (a), was introduced in a flow-through cell (FC). The samples (1-4) previously supplemented with fluorescence-labelled anti-atrazine antibody were assayed successively with a multichannel valve (V2). V1: 3/2-way valve, PP: peristaltic pump, Xe: xenon flash lamp, PMT: photomultiplier tube, D: data collection unit (recorder); a typical readout of the photomultiplier current out of a series of several consecutive measurements is shown in insert (b). (From Jodass, R. et al., *J. Immun. Methods*, 163, 161-167, 1993. With permission.)

15.3 RECEPTOR-BASED SENSORS

15.3.1 Determination of a Sum Parameter

15.3.1.1 Whole Cells (Algae, Phototrophic Bacteria, Cyanobacteria) for Herbicide Detection

The development of a relatively simple electrochemical test for the determination of photosystem-II herbicides and its application to the analysis of water samples has been described by Rawson and Willmer (1987), Rawson et al. (1989), Hansen (1990), Stein (1992), and Rawson (1988). Table 15.4 shows a comparison of some important assay parameters obtained with this method. Due to efforts in reducing the whole cell exhibiting photosynthetic activity to isolated photoreaction centres (a receptor protein), the whole-cell sensors for herbicide detection are treated in this chapter. The water industry's use of mediator-assisted amperometric whole-cell biosensors monitoring microbial photosynthetic electron transfer to screen for herbicides in intake protection is described.

TABLE 15.4
Whole-Cell Biosensors for Herbicide Detection

Organism used	Detection method	Analytes	Detection limit (μg/l)	Stability	Ref.
Synechococcus *Anabaena cylindrica* *Anabaena variabilis*	Mediator-assisted amperometry	Dichlorophenylmethylurea (DCMU) Chlortoluron Linuron	<200	6 Days Response time <10 min	Rawson and Willmer, 1987
Synechococcus	Mediated amperometry	Herbicides in the urea, nitrile and triazine family	20–50	7 Days	Rawson et al., 1989
Synechococcus	Graphite electrode	Atrazine Linuron Diuron Metoxuron	10 100 200 50	6 Days Assay time: 10 min	Hansen, 1990; Stein, 1992
Synechococcus leopoliensis Komarek ATCC 27144	Graphite electrode	Atrazine Diuron	20–50		Rawson, 1988

Carbon dioxide-specific electrodes have been used in conjunction with immobilized bacteria. The biocatalyst must incorporate complete photosystems capable of carrying out the Hill reaction. Isolated thylakoids, chloroplasts, and intact photosynthetic prokaryotic or eukaryotic cells are capable of acting as such biocatalysts. The complexity of preparation and poor stability of isolated membranes and organelles, though, reduce their attractiveness as biocatalysts. Cyanobacterial and algal cells are easily maintained in axenic culture and harvested to give uniform batches of material. The absence of membrane-bound organelles in the cyanobacteria makes these organisms particularly suitable for biosensor use. That their photosynthetic electron transport (PET) system can be accessed makes them superior to chloroplasts. Other advantages are that the use of whole cells in biosensors offers increased stability and ease of immobilization.

To facilitate the transfer of electrons from the PET chains of the organisms to the surface of the indicator electrode, mediators interact at sites along the ET chain and become reduced — in effect, acting like terminal electron acceptors. Subsequent reoxidation at the working electrode results in a steady flow of current which is measured by external circuitry. The magnitude of the current is proportional to the photosynthetic activity of the organisms and any perturbations in the ensuing current/time curve are used to indicate the presence of a pollutant. The cells are immobilized onto the surface of bacteriological filters which allow the diffusion of both toxicant and mediator molecules to the cells and the diffusion of reduced mediator to the electrode surface. A broad range of herbicides can be detected using the cyanobacterium *Synechococcus* although no identification of the pollutant is possible. Since the lowest detection limit described so far is 10 μg/l for atrazine (Hansen, 1990), these biosensors are unsuited for monitoring the contamination of drinking water by herbicides in the concentration range of relevance; according to the European Drinking Water Act the sum of all pesticides in a drinking water sample must be below 0.5 μg/l. For this reason, further work is required to produce mutants of *Synechococcus* which are inhibited by significantly lower levels of specific photosystem-II herbicides, thus allowing a better identification of the herbicides present in the water sample.

15.3.1.2 Isolated Photoreaction Centres from *Rhodobacter sphaeroides*

The tertiary structures of several bacterial photoreaction centres have been elucidated and several of these protein complexes have been cloned. As a result, protein engineering techniques were applied in order to understand the electron transport phenomena on a molecular level. In the last few years, several laboratories began work on procedures for the use of isolated photoreaction centres as herbicide-specific biosensors (Bylina et al., 1989; Carpentier et al., 1991; Katz and Solov'ev, 1992; Jockers et al., 1993b,c; Jockers and Schmid, 1993).

On the way to reducing the *Synechococcus* cell to isolated photoreaction centres, a photoelectrochemical cell using thylakoid membranes isolated from spinach leaves was used to develop a phytotoxicity biosensor (Carpentier et al., 1991). A simple, one-compartment photoelectrochemical cell that uses photosynthetic membranes to produce photocurrent was developed. In this cell, the light energy absorbed by the plant pigments is converted into reduced species which, in turn, exchange their electrons at a working electrode. Artificial electron acceptors can be used to mediate the transfer of electrons from the membranes to the electrode and consequently increase the magnitude of the photocurrent generated. A three-electrode system connected to a scanning potentiostat was used. When the preparation was illuminated a strong photocurrent was produced. Several pollutants or toxic compounds such as several herbicides, nitrite, and sulfite derivatives, can inhibit photosynthetic electron transport.

The photocurrent originates from the following electron transfer pathway. After light absorption by the thylakoid membranes, reduced species are formed in the photosynthetic electron transport chain at the level of photosystem II and I. The latter can reduce ambient dissolved oxygen to form superoxide ions, which dismute spontaneously into hydrogen peroxide. The degradation of hydrogen peroxide at the working platinum electrode produces the photocurrent. Measurements are performed rapidly (<5 min) and require only small volumes (80 μl).

Table 15.5 gives an overview of the few publications which have already studied detection methods using isolated photoreaction centres from *Rhodobacter sphaeroides* for herbicide analysis. In Figure 15.4, a scheme of the photochemistry and arrangement of the chromophores in the bacterial photoreaction centre is depicted. So far, no biosensing system working on the basis of bacterial photoreaction centres has been produced and validated.

15.3.2 Determination of Toxicity With Whole Cell Sensors

15.3.2.1 Antennules of Blue Crab Working as Chemoreceptors for Pesticides

The idea that receptors could be fitted with potentiometric electrodes to produce biosensors was presented as early as 1975. By 1985 the use of the highly specific chemoreceptors in the antennules of moths for gas analysis was proposed. In 1986 a biosensor, called a receptrode, using intact chemoreceptor structures was developed originally for the selective determination of amino acids (Barker et al., 1990; Belli and Rechnitz, 1986; Buch, 1992; Buch et al., 1991; Buch and Rechnitz, 1989 a,b; Zink and Rechnitz, 1989). After this technique was improved its potential application in pesticide detection was studied by Zink and Rechnitz

TABLE 15.5
Biosensors Based on Photoreaction Centres Isolated from *Rhodobacter sphaeroides*

Detection principle	Detection limit (µg/l)	Ref.
A photoelectrode was obtained by monolayer adsorption of bacterial reaction centres from *Rhodobacter sphaeroides* at a quinone-modified electrode.	—	Katz and Solov'ev, 1992
Herbicides are monitored by absorption changes at 860 nm after photobleaching for 2 s. The system consists of 3 components: sample cell, light source and detector for absorption measurements, and a computer data processing unit.	10 Terbutryn 650 Atrazine 2300 *o*-Phenanthroline 3960 Diuron	Jockers et al., 1993b
Artificial aldehydes (herbicides/quinones covalently linked to long-chain aldehydes) are bound to the Q site of bacterial reaction centres (RC) via its quinone/herbicide moiety. Added herbicides compete with the artificial aldehydes for available Q sites, resulting in the displacement of RC-bound artificial aldehydes. These aldehydes are then available as substrates for bacterial luciferase.	No displacement or competition was observed	Jockers and Schmid, 1993
The binding process of either ubiquinones or photosystem-II herbicides can be observed directly, immobilizing a herbicide derivative on a grating coupler surface. Free herbicide competes with the immobilized derivative for the RC incorporated in liposomes.	0.2 µmol/l Terbutryn	Jockers et al., 1993c

(1989). The receptrode circumvented the difficulties associated with isolating, stabilizing, and immobilizing receptors by utilizing an intact chemosensing structure (the antennule of *Callinectes sapidus*) as a chemical transducer attached to the tip of an inert pick-up electrode. The tip of the antennule is a biramous structure consisting of an endopod and exopod. A tuft of several hundred hair-like sensilla, known as aesthetascs, is located on the endopod, the larger of the two dactyl branches. The dendrites of many (usually more than 100) sensory neurons innervate these aesthetascs. The chemoreceptor proteins are contained within the cellular membranes of these dendritic structures. A concentration gradient of sodium and potassium ions is maintained across the neuromembrane by means of an ATP/ATP-ase driven "sodium pump" mechanism. This nonequilibrium condition results in a transmembrane potential of approximately –90 mV. When a stimulant molecule binds to a receptor protein the neuromembrane becomes more permeable to sodium ions, thus allowing the transmembrane potential to ground to zero. A potential of zero is established after approximately 6000 sodium ions have entered the cell. This relatively small number of ions can traverse the membrane quite rapidly; thus the mechanism responsible for generating the change in potential is not significantly impeded by long diffusion times. The sodium pump mechanism then quickly reverses the polarity of the membrane until the initial resting potential of –90 mV is restored. The entire sequence occurs in a few milliseconds.

If the series of events is monitored with electrodes whose output is displayed on an oscilloscope, a potential "spike" is observed for each depolarization. Furthermore, as stimulant concentrations increase, the number of binding events increase and the frequencies of the spike potential generations increase proportionally. Thus, the chemoreceptor cells rapidly convert chemical signals into electrical signals. Concerning pesticide analysis, so far this

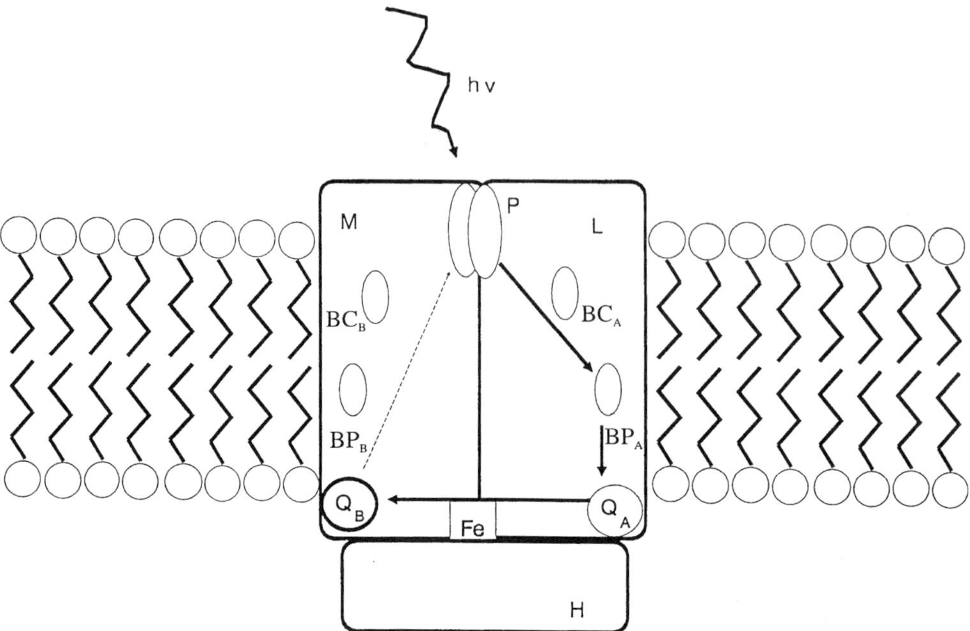

FIGURE 15.4 Schematic representation of the photochemistry and arrangement of the chromophores in the reaction centres of *Rhodobacter sphaeroides*. H, L, M: protein subunits; P: bacteriochlorophyll dimer; BC_A, BC_B: bacteriochlorophyll A, B; BP_A, BP_B: bacteriopheophytin A and B; Q_A: primary quinone; Q_B: secondary quinone; Fe: iron; 100 ms = half time of electron transfer from Q_A to P; 1s = half time of electron transfer from Q_B to P; 0.1 ms = electron transfer from Q_A to Q_B. (From Jockers, R., Bier, F. F., Schmid, R. D., et al., *Anal. Chim. Acta,* 274, 185, 1993. With permission.)

receptrode can only be used for the qualitative screening of water samples for the presence of environmental compounds toxic for the crab.

Zink and Rechnitz (1989) reported the following detection limits for several pesticides: 10^{-2} mol/l for amitrol, 10^{-6} mol/l for lindane, and 10^{-6} mol/l for fonofos. The chemoreceptor-based sensor did not react to metribuzin or diazinon.

15.4 CONCLUSIONS

As yet, only the immunoassay technique and its automated version, the flow injection immunoanalysis (FIIA), permit reaching the low detection limits demanded by the EC Directive for Drinking Water. This has resulted in the commercial availability of a series of enzyme immunoassays for pesticide analysis. Their main advantage as compared to the classical methods in residue analysis is that they allow for rapid, inexpensive monitoring in water samples without any prior enrichment or pretreatment step.

Several detection principles perused for the construction of immunosensors were described here. Looking at the direct immunosensors developed to date, one can clearly understand that by measuring changes in mass (piezocrystal balance) or in the adlayer thickness (optical sensors), small-molecule analytes such as pesticides can only be determined at higher concentrations unless enhancement techniques are used. The main aspect limiting the sensitivity is still the level of the antibody affinity constants rather than the sensitivity of the detection principle. This is especially obvious in the case of the highly sensitive optical devices. It is absolutely necessary to use a suitable label, e.g., an enzyme, to enhance the immunoreaction, thus always yielding lower detection limits for such an indirect format compared to the direct observation of the antibody-pesticide binding. In addition, due to the immunoassay performance at equilibrium the relative standard deviations (RSD) are always smaller than the ones reached with the immunosensors working in a kinetic mode.

Another hurdle for the direct immunosensors, especially in the case of the optical sensors is that the sophisticated equipment necessary is at present still quite expensive and, in its present form, can not yet be used for environmental field test applications. In our opinion, the immunosensors working with a label amplifying the immunoreaction are much more promising in environmental analysis applications. Until now, with the fibre optic sensors working with a fluorescence label and using electroconductive polymers, the detection limits are still higher than the ones achieved with the respective enzyme immunoassay or the FIIA. To come up with a real immunosensor exhibiting the same low measuring range as an immunoassay, we suggest a homogeneous assay format working with an enzyme, another fluorescence label, or a high amount of entrapped dye molecules.

Another parameter limiting a broad application of immunochemical methods in general is the necessity of a series of different pesticide-selective antibodies. The production of polyclonal and monoclonal antibodies targeted for small molecules such as pesticides always requires a time period of at least half a year to obtain antibodies with high affinities and selectivities. This depends mainly on the fact that for small analytes an immunoconjugate always has to be prepared by starting with a pesticide derivative and a high molecular weight compound, e.g., bovine serum albumin. To accelerate the procedure, the production of recombinant single-chain antibodies and Fab fragments expressed in various prokaryotic and eukaryotic hosts (e.g., *Escherichia coli*, Baculovirus transfecting insect cells) was started recently. This procedure opens up the possibility of providing tailor-made antibodies exhibiting high affinities and selectivities to the analyte via site-directed mutagenesis and molecular modelling.

In the case of the receptor-based sensors, further work has to be investigated to create a suitable detection system for the receptor-ligand interactions. The receptrode sensor applying the antennules of the blue crab can only serve as a qualitative measure of the presence or absence of a compound toxic for the crab. How far this toxicity to the blue crab is convertible in terms of risk assessment for a human being is another critical point of concern. To date, the cyanobacteria electrode working with whole cells is the only useful method for detecting photosystem-II herbicides in water samples. A great disadvantage of this electrode, however, is its low sensitivity and its poor selectivity. The lowest reported detection limit for the herbicide atrazine was 10 μg/l. Compared to the detection limits reached with the FIIA (1 ng/l for atrazine) this turned out to be more than three orders of magnitude higher.

So far, no biosensing system working on the basis of isolated reaction centres from bacteria has been realized. One problem resides in the stabilization of the isolated reaction centres in the assay system. Another reason is that so far no useful approach for the transducer design has been demonstrated. One future possibility in case of the receptor-based sensors is the design of the photoreaction centres by site-directed mutagenesis and molecular modelling thus increasing their selectivity to certain herbicides and their affinity to these substances at the same time. Once the mutants are prepared, a pattern indicative for an analyte mixture in a sample is conceivable and thus the information content after the measurement could be shifted dramatically (see Chapters 20 and 27). In the case of the immunosensors, the use of chemometrics for pattern recognition is the next goal and is a big challenge to the analyst.

REFERENCES

Anis, N. A., Eldefrawi, M., and Wong, R. B., Reusable fiber optic immunosensor for rapid detection of imazethapyr herbicide, *J. Agric. Food Chem.*, 41, 843, 1993.

Barker, T. Q., Buch, R. M., and Rechnitz, G. A., Intact chemoreceptor-based biosensors, *Biotechnol. Prog.*, 6, 498, 1990.

Belli, S. L. and Rechnitz, G. A., Prototype potentiometric biosensor using intact chemoreceptor structures, *Anal. Lett.*, 19 (3 &4), 403, 1986.

Betts, T. A., Catena, G. C., Huang, J., Litweiler, K. S., Zhang, J., Zafrobelny, J. A., and Bright, F. V., Fiber-optic-based immunosensor for haptens, *Anal. Chim. Acta,* 246, 55, 1991.

Bier, F. F., Stöcklein, W., and Schmid, R. D., Direct observation of anti-atrazine antibody binding using grating couplers, in: *GBF Monographs*, Vol. 17, Schmid, R. D. and Scheller, F., Eds., VCH Publishers, Weinheim, 1991, 205-208.

Bier, F. F., Stöcklein, W., Böcher, M., Bilitewski, U., and Schmid, R. D., Use of a fibre optic immunosensor for the detection of pesticides, *Sensors Actuators,* B7, 509, 1992.

Bier, F. F. and Schmid, R. D., Real time analysis of competitive binding using grating coupler immunosensors for pesticide detection, *Biosens. Bioelectron.*, 9, 125, 1994.

Buch, R. M., Intact chemoreceptor-based biosensors: antennular receptrodes, in: *ACS Symposium Series*, American Chemical Society, Washington, D.C., 1992, chap. 5.

Buch, R. M., Barker, T. Q., and Rechnitz, G. A., Intact chemoreceptor biosensors based on Hawaiian aquatic species, *Anal. Chim. Acta,* 243, 157, 1991.

Buch, R. M. and Rechnitz, G. A., Intact chemoreceptor based biosensors. Extreme sensitivity to some excitatory amino acids, *Anal. Lett.,* 22 (13 & 14), 2685, 1989a.

Buch, R. M. and Rechnitz, G. A., Intact chemoreceptor-based biosensors. Responses and analytical limits, *Biosensors*, 4, 215, 1989b.

Bylina, E. J., Jovine, R. V. M., and Youvan, D. C., A genetic system for rapidly assessing herbicides that compete for the quinone binding site of photosynthetic reaction centers, *Bio/Technology*, 7, 69, 1989.

Carpentier, R., Loranger, C., Chartrand, J., and Purcell, M., Photoelectrochemical cell containing chloroplast membranes as a biosensor for phytotoxicity measurements, *Anal. Chim. Acta,* 249, 55, 1991.

Giersch, T., A new monoclonal antibody for the sensitive detection of atrazine with immunoassay in microtiter plates and dipstick formate, *J. Agric. Food Chem.*, 41, 1006, 1993.

Giersch, T. and Hock, B., Production of monoclonal antibodies for the determination of s-triazines with enzyme immunoassays, *Food Agric. Immunol.*, 2, 85, 1990.

Guilbault, G. G., Hock, B., and Schmid, R., A piezoelectric immunobiosensor for atrazine in drinking water, *Biosens. Bioelectron.*, 7, 411, 1992.

Hansen, P. D., Biosensor with cyanobacteria for the detection of herbicides in water, *DECHEMA Biotechnology Conferences*, VCH Publishers, Weinheim, 1990.

Jockers, R., Bier, F. F., and Schmid, R. D., Enhancement of immunoassay sensitivity by molecular modification of competitors, *J. Immunol. Methods*, 163, 161, 1993a.

Jockers, R., Bier, F. F., Schmid, R. D., Wachtveitl, J., and Oesterhelt, D., Herbicide biosensor based on photobleaching of the reaction centre of *Rhodobacter sphaeroides, Anal. Chim. Acta*, 274, 185, 1993b.

Jockers, R. and Schmid, R. D., Detection of herbicides via a bacterial photoreaction centre and bacterial luciferase, *Biosens. Bioelectron.*, 8, 281, 1993.

Jockers, R., Bier, F. F., and Schmid, R. D., Specific binding of photosynthetic reaction centres to herbicide-modified grating couplers, *Anal. Chim. Acta,* 280, 53, 1993c.

Katz, E. Y. and Solov'ev, A. A., Photobioelectrodes on the basis of photosynthetic reaction centres. Study of exogenous quinones as possible electron transfer mediators, *Anal. Chim. Acta,* 266, 97, 1992.

Krämer, P. M. and Schmid, R. D., Automated quasi-continuous immunoanalysis of pesticides with a flow injection system, *Pestic. Sci.*, 32, 451, 1991a.

Krämer, P. and Schmid, R., Flow injection immunoanalysis (FIIA) — a new immunoassay format for the detection of pesticides in water, *Biosens. Bioelectron.*, 6, 239, 1991b.

Ngeh-Ngwainbi, J., Foley, P. H., Kuan, S. S., and Guilbault, G. G., Parathion antibodies on piezoelectric crystals, *J. Am. Chem. Soc.*, 108, 5444, 1986.

Northrup, M., Stanker, L. H., Vanderlaan, M., and Watkins, B. E., Development and characterization of a fibre optic immuno-biosensor, in: *Spectroscopy of Inorganic Bioactivators. Theory and Applications — Chemistry, Physics, Biology and Medicine*, Theophanides, T., Ed., Kluwer Academic, Dordrecht, 1989, 229-241.

Rawson, D. M. and Willmer, A. J., The development of whole cell biosensors for on-line screening of herbicide pollution of surface waters, *Toxicity Assessment*, 2, 325, 1987.

Rawson, D. M., Whole cell biosensors, *Int. Ind. Biotechnol.*, 8 (2), 18, 1988.

Rawson, D. M., Willmer, A. J., and Turner, A. P. F., Whole-cell biosensors for environmental monitoring, *Biosensors*, 4, 299, 1989.

Sandberg, R. G., van Houten, L. J., Schwartz, J. L., Bigliano, R. P., Dallas, S. M., Silvia, J. C., Cabelli, M. A., and Narayanswamy, V., A conductive polymer-based immunosensor for the analysis of pesticide residues, in: *ACS Symposium Series*, Vol. 511, Americal Chemical Society, Washington, D.C., 1992, chap. 8.

Stein, P., Bakterienelektroden mit Synechococcus und Escherichia coli. Ein kontinuierliches Testsystem zur Online-Überwachung von Oberflächengewässern, in: *Schr.-Reihe Verein WaBoLu*, Hansen, P. D. and Steinhäuser, K. G., Eds., Gustav Fischer, Stuttgart, 1992, 265-275.

Stöcklein, W., Krämer, P., and Schmid, R. D., Flow injection immunoanalysis (FIIA) for the determination of pesticides in water, in: *GBF Monographs*: *Biosensors: Applications in Medicine, Environmental Protection and Process Control*, Vol. 13, Schmid, R. D. and Scheller, F., Eds., VCH Publishers, Weinheim, 1989, 307-312.

Wittmann, C. and Hock, B., Improved enzyme immunoassay for the analysis of s-triazines in water samples, *Food Agric. Immunol.*, 1, 211, 1989.

Wittmann, C. and Hock, B., Evaluation and performance characteristics of a novel ELISA for the quantitative analysis of atrazine in water, plants and soil, *Food Agric. Immunol.*, 2, 65, 1990.

Wittmann, C. and Hock, B., Analysis of atrazine residues in food by an enzyme immunoassay, *J. Agric. Food Chem.*, 41, 1421, 1993.

Wittmann, C. and Schmid, R. D., Development and application of an automated quasi-continuous immunoflow injection system to the analysis of pesticide residues in water and soil, *J. Agric. Food Chem.*, 42, 1041, 1994.

Wittmann, C. and Schmid, R. D., Application of an automated quasi-continuous immuno flow injection system to the analysis of pesticide residues in environmental water samples, *Sensors Actuators*, B15-16, 119, 1993.

Zink, P. and Rechnitz, G. A., Intakter Chemorezeptor als Biosensor zur Pestiziderfassung, *Fresenius Z. Anal. Chem.*, 333, 645, 1989.

16 Monitoring Immunoreactions with SPR

Norman J. Geddes and Chris R. Lawrence

CONTENTS

16.1 INTRODUCTION

Surface plasmon resonance (SPR) occurs when light is made incident upon a metal/dielectric interface and couples to a charge-density oscillation, reducing the amount of light that is reflected. The efficiency of the coupling is angle dependent, and hence a plot of reflectivity vs. the incident angle of the light reveals a dip, the shape of which is characteristic of the optical constants of the materials at or very near the interface. An earlier chapter in this book (Chapter 7) has detailed the various ways by which this effect can be utilized to monitor the deposition or alteration of dielectric overlayers upon a metal surface, and it was shown that highly efficient biosensors could (and have) been constructed in such a fashion.

However, it was also stated that whilst the exact manner in which the SPR-based transducer operates is of great importance, it is the protein receptor layer upon the surface of the metal (i.e., the *biochemistry* of the situation) that will set the final limits upon sensitivity and selectivity. This chapter will discuss the choice of this receptor layer, the various published methods by which the efficiency of protein binding can be maximized, and the present achievements and future aims of workers in the field of SPR-based biosensing.

0-8493-8905-4/97/$0.00+$.50
© 1997 by CRC Press, Inc.

16.2 ATTACHMENT OF RECEPTORS TO THE TRANSDUCER SURFACE

16.2.1 The Antibody Receptor Layer

In terms of using SPR to transduce a signal between an antibody and antigen during interaction at the surface of a metal there are a number of approaches that can be used. We have discussed the plasmon coupling methods commonly performed as well as the means for detecting the reflectivity changes associated with such interactions, the particular choice being dependent on the user's specific requirements. However, in order to create a "sensor" it is necessary to combine the receptor chemistry with the transducer system as shown schematically in Figure 16.1. For the SPR transducer to act as a highly sensitive detector it requires a receptor layer which is both sensitive to the material requiring detection and also selective, so as to avoid false readings from the binding of nonspecific material. Antibodies (or antigens) have been chosen to form this receptor layer as they naturally have these properties, being specifically raised against the analyte of interest in a host animal.[1] In many cases their response to the analyte has already been demonstrated in other assay methodologies, e.g., enzyme-linked immunosorbent assay or ELISA,[2] where their activity, specificity, and selectivity can be determined. Antibodies are comprised of polypeptide chains, are globular in form, and are considered to have two main regions: the carbohydrate region (Fc) and the receptor site regions (Fab) (again, see Figure 16.1). There are only two specific receptor sites on the antibody on the Fab portion. The optimum situation for these to be available for interaction with the antigen is for the Fc portion to be bound to the metal surface. There are numerous ways in which antibody receptors can be immobilized onto metal surfaces, some involving quite complex procedures to enhance the alignment of the Fab receptor sites. The different immobilization procedures that have been investigated with SPR will now be discussed. The key aspect is their effectiveness in creating a sensing layer for the detection of analytes.

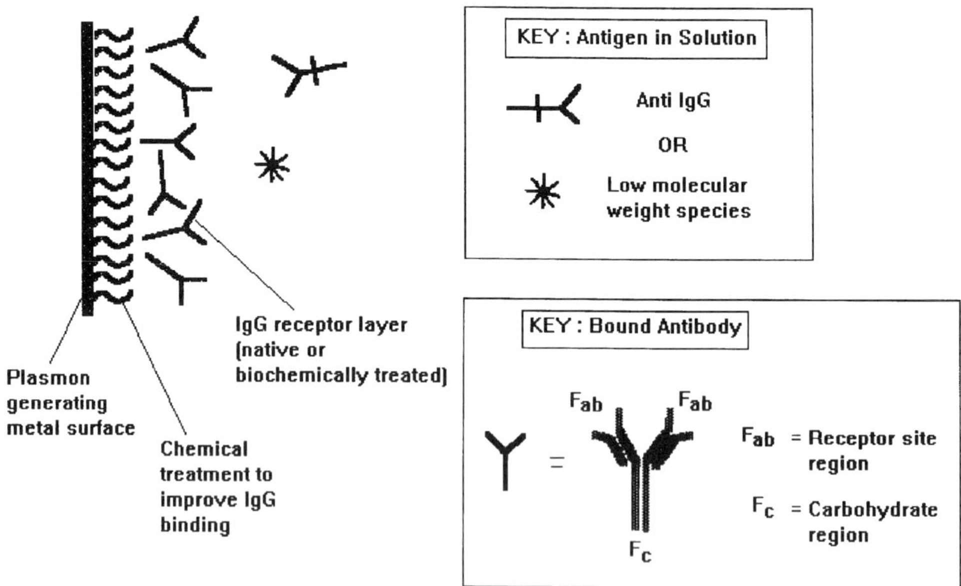

FIGURE 16.1 Schematic representation of antibody or IgG bound to the plasmon-generating surface. Binding of the antigen (in solution) to the antibody receptors occurs under appropriate conditions. To the lower right is a schematic representation of IgG showing the two main receptor sites and the carbohydrate regions.

16.2.2 Monitoring Immunoreactions With SPR

With the appropriate choice of coupling method for generating the surface plasmon mode and the experimental arrangement for detection, the binding of receptor layers to the metal and their subsequent interaction with their biospecific partners can be investigated. These immunoreactions invariably involve the binding of antibodies to the metal surface with the antigen in a solution to which the bound antibody layer is exposed. The reaction of analyte (antigen) with receptor (antibody) can be studied in two ways with SPR. With a "complete" plasmon scan of wavelengths or angles, the reflectivity data can be compared to Fresnel theory for optical multilayers. This allows an evaluation of the full dielectric properties, the real and imaginary parts of the dielectric permittivity, ε_r and ε_i, and the thickness, d, of both the antibody layer and subsequent binding of antigen.

Figure 16.2 shows plasmon curves taken from a $\theta/2\theta$ stage arrangement for plain gold, gold with an adsorbed IgG layer, and the change when anti-IgG binds to the IgG. It is clear that the "dip" in the reflectivity curve shifts to higher angles as protein binds to the metal. The solid line through the data points represents a fit to Fresnel theory (discussed later). These plasmon curves are usually measured after binding interactions between antibody and antigen have reached equilibrium. Comparison between experiment and theory yields the protein layer thickness associated with "final" bound amounts. It typically requires 2 to 3 minutes to determine a full reflectivity curve. Hence this method does not allow evaluation of faster immobilization/binding kinetics.

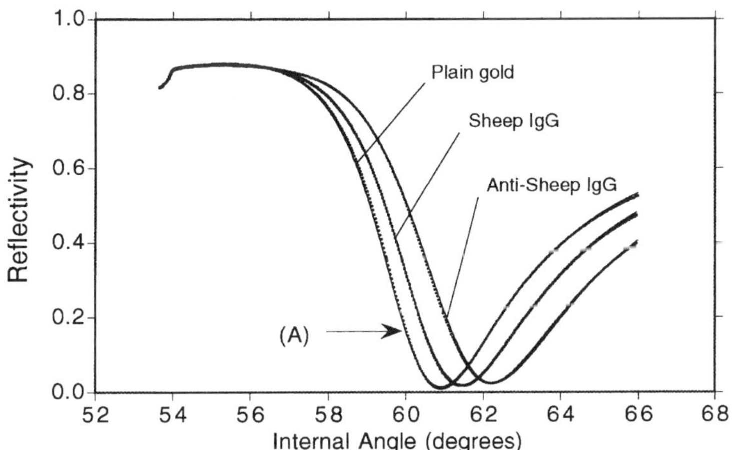

FIGURE 16.2 Reflectivity curves as a function of the incident angle of the laser beam, for plain gold, immobilized sheep IgG, and binding of anti-sheep IgG to the sheep IgG layer.

If real-time events are of interest then the plasmon technique is operated in the second mode. The prism is first rotated to an angle a few degrees off the plasmon minimum, where the curve is near-linear in shape. The reflectivity at that angle is then monitored as a function of time (if the reflectivity is monitored too close to the minimum angle shifts due to binding events will be nonlinear). An indication of appropriate choice of scanning angle is shown by the arrow (A) in Figure 16.2.

Binding events shift the plasmon minimum to larger angles as further momentum is required of the incoming light to achieve maximum coupling. As the angle shifts so the reflectivity increases. The change in reflectivity for IgG binding to gold is shown in Figure 16.3. The reflectivity changes rapidly as the sheep IgG is first introduced to the buffer solution adjacent to the gold surface. After a short time the response slows to reach a new equilibrium value. If sufficient IgG is added this value is associated with monolayer coverage of the metal.

At lower concentrations the final change in reflectivity is concentration dependent. However, equilibrium can take a prohibitively long time in this low-concentration regime. A faster method for determination of analyte concentration involves the initial rate of change of the reflectivity curve, which is also concentration dependent. A standard curve of the rate of change of reflectivity against concentration enables the concentration of unknown analyte solutions to be determined in a matter of a few minutes.

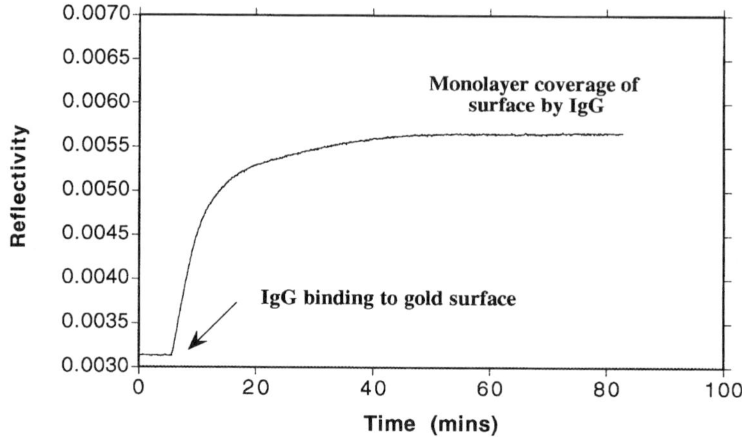

FIGURE 16.3 The change in reflectivity as a function of time during the immobilization of IgG to the gold surface. The angle of incidence was held constant (at point (A) shown in Figure 16.2).

16.2.2.1 Direct Adsorption of Antibodies to the Metal Surface

One of the simplest approaches for the immobilization of antibody receptor layers onto metals (i.e., the surface plasmon-supporting surface) is adsorption from solution. The attraction between antibody and metal involves hydrophobic forces.[3] The immunoreaction most often studied is that between proteins, i.e., an immunogamma globulin (IgG) and an anti-IgG protein raised against the IgG chosen. One such pair are human serum albumin (HSA). (mol wt 65,000) or HSA-IgG and anti-HSA (mol wt 150,000), the anti-HSA being raised in a different host animal to the HSA. The HSA can be immobilized directly onto the metal (either silver or gold) after injection into the buffer solution adjacent to the metal surface, shown schematically in Figure 16.4. Adsorption of the IgG causes a shift in the plasmon angle, similar to the shifts shown in Figure 16.2, (see work by Liedberg, et al.,[4] Kooyman et al.,[5] and Cullen et al.[6]), indicating coverage of the metal by HSA. Comparison of the reflectivity data (using the full plasmon curve) to a theoretical Fresnel fit enables the thickness of the bound HSA layer to be determined provided a value for ε_r is assumed. When ε_r is taken to be 2, then the thickness of the HSA layer is 4 nm;[5] this thickness changes to 5 nm for an ε_r of 1.47.[4] The HSA forms only a single receptor layer upon adsorption: attempts to bind more HSA to the surface have been unsuccessful.[4] Further, the IgG cannot be removed by rinsing with water, indicating strong binding to the surface.

The interaction of anti-HSA with the immobilized HSA layer (Figure 16.4) was investigated via the change in reflectivity at fixed angle, or more precisely the rate of change of reflectivity with time at fixed angle. In this way the concentration of anti-HSA in solution could be determined. In the range of 200 to 0.02 μg/ml the initial rate of reflectivity change was found to be directly proportional to the anti-HSA concentration.[4] There is some question, however, about depletion of anti-HSA from solution for the lowest concentrations, this causing the concentration of anti-HSA to vary during binding to the HSA. This may ultimately limit the measurable concentration range,[5] particularly where only small shifts in the plasmon angle occur.

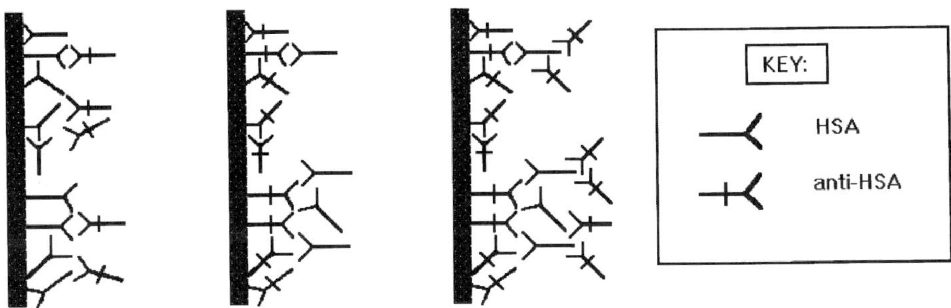

FIGURE 16.4 From left to right: HSA binding to the surface with anti-HSA binding to the HSA; anti-HSA binding to the surface with HSA binding to the anti-HSA; "sandwich-layer" binding of a second layer of anti-HSA.

When the reverse interaction is studied, i.e., anti-HSA is immobilized at the metal surface with HSA binding to it (Figure 16.4), changes in the plasmon angle on HSA binding are significantly lower.[5,6] The measured signal is about 40 times lower[5] for identical molar quantities of anti-HSA and HSA. Since HSA binding to anti-HSA gives only a small shift in the plasmon angle, a sandwiching method is sometimes used to enhance the shift. Another solution containing anti-HSA is added (see Figure 16.4). This second anti-HSA binds to the HSA/anti-HSA layer and a further shift is seen in the plasmon angle. This shift is larger than that on initial HSA addition because of the larger size of the anti-HSA. The plasmon shifts due to HSA binding to anti-HSA are much lower than in the reverse case. This has been related to the size difference between the two species, but it can also be attributed to fewer reaction sites available for interaction on the anti-HSA molecule compared with the HSA. In the case of anti-HSA binding to immobilized HSA, nonspecific binding occurs (i.e., not directed to the Fab portion of the HSA molecule), since the receptor sites are on the "free" or "in solution" protein and will bind to numerous sites on the HSA.[5,6] However, when the anti-HSA is immobilized to the surface its orientation controls the interaction between the two species. Binding will only occur if the Fab receptor sites are pointing away from the metal surface.

Attempts have been made to investigate the specificity of HSA/anti-HSA interactions. The HSA-immobilized layer is exchanged for bovine serum albumin (BSA), and exposed to anti-HSA in solution. The reflectivity shifts are halved compared to HSA layer,[6] indicating, in this case, a fairly high level of nonspecific binding (~50%). Nonspecific binding effects were much lower when the HSA-immobilized layer was exposed to solutions of ovalbumin. Only a 7% change in the plasmon angle was recorded compared to the HSA/anti-HSA reaction.[6]

Similar results were obtained for interactions of BSA (mol wt 68,000) with anti-BSA (mol wt 150,000)[7] and α-feto protein (mol wt 70,000) with anti-α-feto protein (mol wt 150,000).[8] In one case the anti-α-feto protein was immobilized via glutaeraldehyde rather than directly to the gold.[9] The shift in plasmon angle for the glutaeraldehyde-treated gold was found to be greater than for direct absorption, due to increased amounts of bound anti-α-feto protein. However, the experimental reproducibility was reduced since it was more difficult to control the amount of anti-α-feto protein immobilized to the sensor surface.

Although it is clear from these observations that SPR can be utilized to detect immunoreactions between IgG and anti-IgG, there are some points regarding the immobilization method that require further discussion. When a full plasmon curve is generated it is necessary to assume a value for ε_r, the real part of the dielectric permittivity,[4-6] in order to obtain the thickness d of bound IgG or anti-IgG layers. In fact, in order to attempt to obtain the thickness and dielectric parameters for the IgG layers it is first necessary to fully characterize the metal layer itself prior to protein adsorption. A unique solution for ε_r, ε_i, and d (for the metal) can be found by taking a complete plasmon curve which includes data before the critical angle.[10] Since the immobilization of the IgG to the gold only perturbs the plasmon mode, unique solutions are not possible for these subsequently adsorbed layers. Only the product "d.(n – 1)" is obtainable for a nonabsorbing layer. This of course limits the capacity of the technique unless one of the parameters can be determined by an independent method. Generally, the size of the protein molecules is known from other measurements, (for example Tanford's work on BSA molecules[11]), and values for ε_r are chosen such that a thickness close to the expected value is obtained. It is possible to determine effective "changes" in thickness relative to a complete monolayer coverage when independent data are not available. This can be useful when, for instance, a concentration of anti-IgG or IgG is of interest. The reduction from the thickness associated with monolayer coverage is proportional to the protein concentration at levels lower than those required for monolayer coverage.

A major assumption in fitting the reflectivity data with Fresnel theory is that the layers (gold/IgG/anti-IgG) are generally considered as having smooth interfaces between them. However, the effect of surface roughness between IgG and bound anti-IgG layers, for instance, has been analyzed.[12] In the case of anti-HSA/HSA bound to silver, the width of the measured reflectivity profile was found to be greater than that calculated for a smooth interface. Whilst this is believed to indicate surface roughness, the increased broadening was also observed for the plain silver film (the chosen metal) after immersion in the buffer solution. Hence the differences may also be indicative of degradation of the silver film due to the buffer. Indeed, although silver has the sharper resonance in both air and solution when compared with gold,[5] giving greater sensitivity (i.e., binding events cause greater shifts in angle or reflectivity change), silver suffers from degradation when immersed in buffer solutions.[4] Gold is more commonly chosen for the surface plasmon-supporting layer since it is inert in buffers, and any plasmon changes must be due to the IgG binding to the metal. Additionally, analysis of the data obtained from gold films is not complicated by conversion of the outer layer of the metal to a sulfide or oxide, a common occurrence in nonnoble metals.

The orientation of the IgG or anti-IgG on immobilization, and therefore the position of the receptor sites relative to the metal surface, can also be important. As mentioned above, the ordering is not so critical when IgG is immobilized for sensing anti-IgG, but it is when sensing a species to which it has been specifically raised against (i.e., similar to the case when anti-IgG is bound first to the metal for the detection of IgG). Since there are only two sites available for antibody/antigen interaction, it is necessary that the orientation is such that the sites can be accessed. This becomes particularly important when sensing small analytes (i.e., below a molecular weight of 10,000) and where the signal is weak. Specific alignment of the IgG receptor layer is not achieved when the IgG is simply adsorbed onto gold. Further chemical treatment of the gold prior to IgG immobilization is necessary.

Procedures for improving the orientation of the antibody receptors are now receiving attention. A number of different chemical coupling methods have been investigated via SPR (orientation is also important for other transducer technologies as well as more conventional assay techniques). The alignment methodologies lead to improved signal-to-noise ratios and reduced nonspecific binding. These methodologies are discussed in the remainder of this chapter. Also, the HSA/aHSA (anti-HSA sometimes being denoted as aHSA) immunoreactions discussed in this section are summarized in Table 16.1.

16.2.2.2 The Biotin-Avidin Immunoreaction

The biotin-avidin/streptavidin system has received much attention as a model system in immunoreaction studies (see work by Daniels et al.,[8] Wilchek and Bayer,[13] Bayer and Wilchek,[14] Morgan and Taylor,[15] and Morgan et al.[16]). Both avidin (mol wt 62,000), a protein component found in avian egg white, or its bacteria analogue streptavidin (mol wt 63,000) have a high binding affinity to biotin (or vitamin H, mol wt 250). The gold surface

TABLE 16.1
Immunoreactions Involving HSA and aHSA

Binding	Comment
HSA adsorbed to metal	Monolayer coverage[4] with HSA strongly bound (cannot remove by rinsing)
aHSA adsorbed to metal	As per HSA, but molecules larger so that shift in SPP is of greater magnitude
aHSA to bound HSA	A further shift in the SPP angle
	Initial rate of change of reflectivity is proportional to the concentration of aHSA present[4]
HSA to bound aHSA	Shift 40 times less than for aHSA to bound HSA due to the size difference between the molecule[5] and limitations upon binding site availability
Sandwiching	Blind aHSA to the HSA/aHSA/metal of the previous case to produce a larger angle shift, the magnitude of which is proportional to the amount of bound HSA
aHSA to bound BSA	Only a 50% shift[6] in comparison to that observed when bound HSA is exposed to aHSA
Ovalbumin to bound HSA	Only a 7% shift[6] in comparison to that observed when bound HSA is exposed to aHSA

Note: Similar results have been observed in studies of BSA/aBSA: Only a 50% shift[6] in comparison to that observed when bound HSA is exposed to aHSA[7] and α-fetoprotein/anti-α-fetoprotein[8] — see text for details.

is first silanized and biotin covalently bound via exposure to *N*-hydroxysuccinimide. The biotin is then reacted with avidin in solution. For concentrations greater than 10^{-5} M the avidin binds to produce single monolayer coverage. Selectivity of the biotin-avidin response was shown by exposing BSA to the biotin layer. Only a 20% shift in the plasmon angle occurred, compared with avidin exposure. The measurement of reflectivity at fixed angle showed a strong dependence on avidin concentration between 10^{-8} and 10^{-7} M (see Ref erence 8).

The high selectivity between avidin (or streptavidin) and biotin can be used to aid measurement of IgG/anti-IgG interactions. Biotin (or more specifically the nitrophenyl ester of D-biotin) is bound to gold via hydroxyl functionalities that are formed via the use of chromic acid.[16,15] Avidin or streptavidin then binds to the immobilized biotin layer after exposure in solution (see Figure 16.5). Streptavidin has four binding sites available for interaction with the biotin, and once bound has sites still available for interaction with biotin in solution. Biotinylation of IgG in fact allows the IgG to bind to the streptavidin layer through the biotin/streptavidin reaction. The IgG is then available itself for further interaction with its biospecific partner. This approach has been used to study a sex hormone binding globulin (SHBG). (mol wt 80,000–100,000).[15]

A receptive layer of monoclonal antibodies to SHBG is first prepared. They are then biotinylated and bound to the streptavidin layer (SHBG is a glycoprotein that binds strongly to testosterone; the antibody to this was chosen for study as it has a low cross-reactivity with other compounds in the serum containing the SHBG). From the shift observed in the plasmon angle it was established that 50% of the available surface was coated with anti-SHBG. Incomplete coverage was attributed to steric hindrance. The bound anti-SHBG antibody was used to monitor concentrations of SHBG in the 0.8 to 50 nmol/l range, although there was a large variation in SPR response for the lowest concentration studies. The surface was washed and dried after each treatment and before plasmons were measured

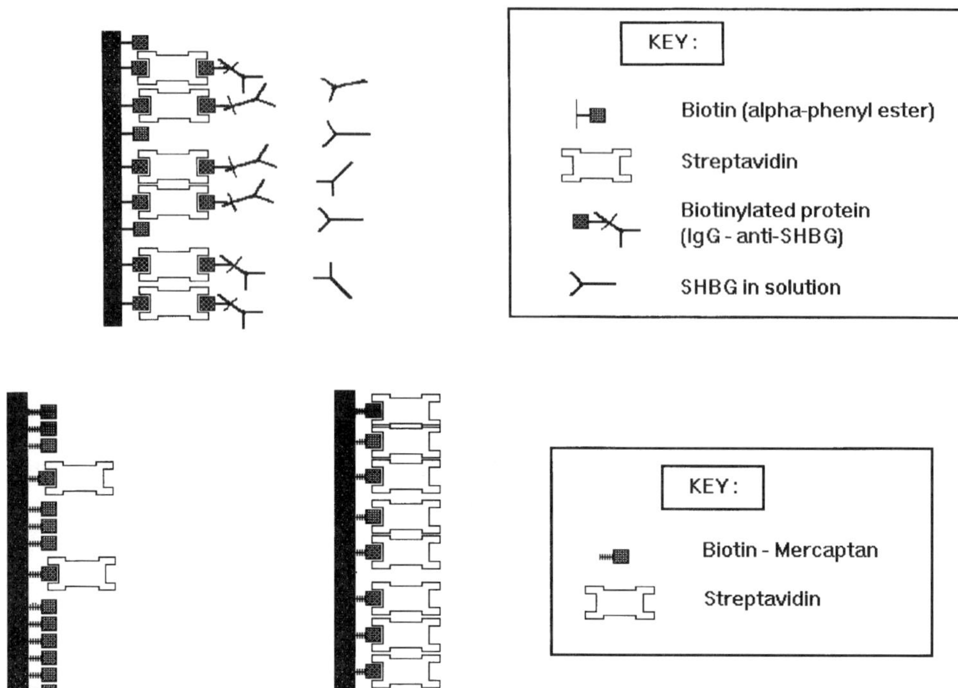

FIGURE 16.5 Above, the use of the biotin-streptavidin reaction to aid in biotinylated IgG binding to the metal surface is illustrated. Below, the thiolation of biotin to bind streptavidin to the surface is shown. If the biotin layer is too closly packed then streptavidin reaction is impaired.

(i.e., "in air" rather than "in solution" measurements[15]). This drying procedure is thought to aid in the removal of nonspecifically bound material, although it does preclude "real time" measurements of the interactions. An appropriate exposure time between anti-SHBG and the SHBG in solution must be used. No binding of the SHBG occurred, even for the highest concentrations of 410 nmol/l, if the anti-SHBG was not immobilized to the surface of the streptavidin. Sensor specificity is thus demonstrated.

The use of the biotin/streptavidin reaction provides a means of binding a receptor layer to the sensor surface. However, the biotinylation of the IgG is unlikely to significantly align the receptors on the surface since 25% of the available NH_2 groups on the IgG had been biotinylated. Biotinylation of a more specific region of the IgG, such as the Fc portion, might improve alignment.

16.2.2.3 Thiolation of the Metal Surface

The chemisorption of thiol monolayers on gold has recently become a well documented example of so-called "self assembly". In principle such layers are ideally suited for the study of molecular recognition.[17] The thiols (or in some cases disulfides) generally consist of a methylene chain (about 10 CH_2 units) and a second end-group functionality like OH. The influence of this end functionality on the absorption of proteins to surfaces has been studied, for it was found that self-assembled thiol layers with hydrophobic methyl end groups allow the binding of significantly more protein than similar layers with hydrophilic hydroxyl functionalities.[18] Through such functionalization of the metal surface considerable control over protein/antibody binding is envisaged. Thiolation methods will have impact on the biosensing fields, especially in the area of receptor alignment. Their use has now been studied with SPR (in work by Häussling et al.[19]).

As mentioned in the previous section, there is a very high affinity between biotin and avidin. Their interaction can be monitored using biotinylated mercaptans or disulfides chemisorbed onto gold via the sulfur moiety.[20] A self-assembled single layer is formed by exposing the gold to solutions (10^{-4} M) of the mercaptans/disulfides in trichloromethane/ethanol (1:1 ratio) for about 6 h. Biotin coating of the gold surface was confirmed by taking full SPR scans which yield thicknesses comparable with anticipated monolayer coverage. After biotin functionalization, the surface was exposed to streptavidin (10^{-7} M), and the interaction was followed in real time by monitoring the change in the reflectivity. Closely packed monolayers of the thiol gave poorer binding of the streptavidin compared with biotinylation, even though the latter generated fewer streptavidin binding sites on the gold surface (see Figure 16.5). This agrees with STM measurements showing that a more closely packed thiol layer causes little or no binding of protein.[20] It appears that when the biotin sites are too closely packed together the streptavidin cannot fully engulf them from solution. Therefore binding does not occur because of steric hindrance and the limited mobility of the densely packed biotin molecules on the metal surface.[21]

The specificity of the interaction was confirmed by two methods. The streptavidin was first exposed to high concentrations of free biotin in order to block all of the biotin binding sites. When this blocked streptavidin was then exposed to the biotinylated mercaptans no measurable change in SPR was observed. In the second method the biotinylated mercaptan layer was replaced with 11-mercaptoundecanol, and the surface exposed to normal streptavidin: no binding was observed. A biotinylated disulfide gave much lower effective thicknesses when bound to gold compared to the thiol. However, its surface gave very effective binding of streptavidin. Again, the correlation is seen between poor packing on the surface and the availability of biotin to bind to the sites on the streptavidin molecule.

From the study of biotin-mercaptans/streptavidin interactions it is clear that thiol self assembly can be succesfully used to form receptive layers. With the assembled thiol layer on the gold sensor surface it is possible to investigate many different immobilization chemistries for receptors by varying the end-group functionality of the thiol. For example, a carboxyl group can bind antibodies through carbodiimide reactions with amine groups on the antibody,[21] thereby forming a covalent bond with the surface. Such assembly techniques are expected to have a key role in improving the reproducibility of the receptor layers on the sensor surface.

16.2.2.4 Reusability of the Sensor/Antibody Surface

An important aspect of any sensing surface is its capability to be used more than once to study immunoreactions. The interaction between the immobilized species and the analyte in solution is usually strong, and this is one of the main reasons why antibody/antigen systems are chosen. For device applications, say, to save time and aid in reproducibility, there is much to be gained from being able to remove the antigen from the immobilized antibody without disturbing the latter. The surface can then be reimmersed in a fresh solution for further study of analyte. Good reproducibility is achieved since the same amount of antibody (hopefully in the same active state) is present for sensing the antigen, and comparison between different concentrations can be readily made. There are, however, different degrees of "regeneration", which can range from a total cleaning of the substrate to the removal of only the last bound antigen layer.

Regeneration of the substrates themselves (i.e., either the glass prism/slide or grating surface) is achieved by removing all the deposited layers, including the coupling metal film. This does not prove successful, however. Apart from the need to fully renew all the layers, the plasmon curves measured from the new metal films are broader in comparison with those freshly formed.[22] This can lead to difficulties in fitting the reflectivity data as well as a reduction in sensitivity.

Removal of the immobilized layer by means of enzymatic digestion has been studied.[6] Adsorbed layers of HSA were removed from the gold by exposure to trypsin solution. The shift in the plasmon resonance is in the opposite direction to that due to HSA adsorption. No data were given to describe the performance of HSA subsequently bound to these surfaces. Without knowing the antibody activity after enzymic treatment it is difficult to assess the viability of this approach.

A more comprehensive study of recycling the sensor surface has been undertaken for immobilized anti-α-feto protein after reaction with α-feto protein in solution.[9] The amount of anti-α-feto protein bound was enhanced by pretreating the metal with glutaraldehyde bound to silane. The anti-α-feto protein was then covalently bound to the glutaraldehyde. After α-feto protein had bound to the immobilized sensing layer of anti-α-feto protein, the surface was exposed to KSCN (3 M) + NaCl (0.5 M) to promote its dissociation over 30 min. Reflectivity measurements indicated that antibodies had been dissociated from the bound antigen, although the removal was incomplete. After each successive binding/dissociation sequence both binding and dissociation were slower. Re-generation was, therefore, not reproducible. Antibody activity was reduced each time the antigen was dissociated.

16.2.2.5 Serum Samples and Nonspecific Binding

One of the hardest challenges for SPR sensing work (and indeed for other transducing methods) lies in detecting the presence of a specific analyte in a real "serum" or solution which has many other molecular species present. Although the antibody-antigen interaction is highly specific, problems due to nonspecific binding of molecules to the receptor surface ultimately limit the detectable range available. In going to real-time sensing as opposed to other assay techniques (for instance, ELISA), detection of the analyte can be made in a direct manner. The various "development" stages necessary for assays generally requiring the labeling of a competitive or sandwich antibody,[23] i.e., enzymic, fluorescent, or radiotracer labeling, are not required for the SPR immunosensor. These indirect methods do, however, suffer less from nonspecific effects since only binding to the reactive sites gives false reading (fluorescence labelling techniques have now been investigated with SPR and improved sensitivity has been achieved, reducing such nonspecific effects.[24] In the case of *direct* measurement of unlabeled protein species with SPR, any binding, specific or nonspecific, to the surface leads to a measurable signal. Nonspecific binding may be reduced with suitable washing steps, but this adds to the measurement time, and moreover the number of necessary wash steps must be predetermined.

Nonspecific antibody-antigen interactions have been studied where the antigen is in a serum.[22,25] Exposure of a goat IgG to a goat serum[22] produced a large shift in the plasmon angle. When the surface was washed, some of the components of the serum that were nonspecifically bound were removed (about 25%). When BSA was exposed to the goat IgG in a similar concentration no plasmon change was recorded. This suggests that it was not the BSA, the most abundant portion of the serum, that had bound nonspecifically. Nonspecific binding can occur through protein-metal or protein-protein interactions. The former can be minimized by ensuring complete coverage of the metal surface with the first IgG layer. The latter may be related to the orientation of the sensing IgG on the surface. In the case studied here, in which the sensing layer was formed by adsorption of IgG directly to gold, there is no inherent orientation of the IgG. Some Fc portions of the antibody are available to the sample solution and uncontrolled binding of protein to these can occur.[22] Improved orientation would no doubt reduce this nonspecific binding by ensuring that the Fc portion of each antibody is adjacent to the metal surface, and hence removed from the receptor/buffer interface.

Nonspecific effects have so far been related to the receptor layer orientation and surface coverage of the metal. However, there are other nonspecific binding effects that need to be assessed, namely those due to the specificity of the antibody/antigen reaction system.

A specific antibody can be raised by injection of the antigen of interest into a host animal. Once antibodies have been raised, and serum obtained from the animal, their specificity to the antigen can be determined by exposure to the original antigen coated onto the SPR sensing surface. The specific antibody may only make up a small portion of the total protein in the serum. As an example, in work by Fontana et al.[25] the sensor surface was exposed to serum obtained from mice which had been immunized with dinitrophenyl conjugated to keyhole limpet hemocyanin (DNP-KLH). KLH was immobilized onto gold surfaces by exposure to different concentrations of the serum (1/10 to 1/10000 dilutions of a stock serum solution of 80 mg/ml). A concentration dependence of the reflectivity was observed, similar to that previously discussed for anti-IgG/IgG interactions. A number of specificity tests were performed to ensure that the reflectivity changes were due to the KLH/anti-KLH reaction.

The stock serum was diluted 140-fold in a 1 mg/ml BSA solution, and this was exposed to one of three different antigens, the KLH, dinitrophenyl bovine serum albumin conjugate (DNP-BSA), or bovine gamma globulin (BGG). For the KLH and DNP layers some of the antibodies were desorbed during rinsing. About 10% of the immobilized KLH was removed, leaving a void where the serum may bind. Such nonspecific binding was reduced when the surface was exposed to a BSA solution prior to exposure to the serum. The BSA blocks "voids" in the receptor layer. Strong response to the serum was observed for the KLH and DNP-BSA coatings whilst a negligible change was observed for the BGG coating. The large changes for DNP-BSA and KLH are expected since the mice were immunized with a DNP-KLH conjugate. The antibodies so raised are specific against both elements of the conjugate. The fact that the largest change was for the DNP-BSA surface may indicate either a higher affinity for binding or a larger concentration of antibodies in the serum. The low response of the BGG-coated surface reflected the absence of BGG antibodies in the serum, since exposure to anti-BGG resulted in a significantly larger response.

It is clear then that antibody receptor binding needs to generate a complete coverage of the metal surface if subsequent protein from direct binding to the underlying metal is to be avoided. The "cross-reactivity" nonspecific binding effects can only be reduced through careful screening of the serum prior to usage.

16.2.2.6 Enhanced Receptor Binding

In the preceding sections methods for immobilizing antibody receptors to the SPR transducing surface have been discussed. It is quite apparent that there are some limitations in these approaches which ultimately reduce the overall sensitivity of the SPR system when detecting immunoreactions.Typically, not all of the receptor sites on the antibodies are available for interaction with analyte. Different pretreatments of the metal surface or chemical modification of the receptor have been investigated in attempts to improve orientation and thereby increase the number of receptor sites available for interaction. It is hoped that such modifications will increase sensitivity due to an increase in the number of reaction sites and a reduction of nonspecific effects, and that regeneration of the surface may also be possible. However, improvements may also be achieved by increasing the overall number density of receptors immobilized onto the surface rather than specifically orienting them; this would increase the signal due to antigen binding, since the larger the number of receptors bound to the metal, the larger the amount of antigen that can subsequently bind to them.

16.2.2.7 Particulate Additives

Latex particles have been utilized to enhance the amount of antibody that can be bound to the surface of the metal by enlarging the surface area available for antibody immobilization. The latex particles are first coated with antibody receptors and surface immobilized. The interaction of the antibodies with their antigens is increased, compared to that of a single layer of receptors, since there are greater numbers of receptors available for interaction.

This method has been used to study the interaction between HSA and anti-HSA, as in work by Schasfoort[26] (see Figure 16.6). HSA was first immobilized directly to the metal surface, by absorption. The immobilized HSA was then exposed to carboxylated microspheres (diameter 100 nm) which bound to the HSA. The surface was then reexposed to HSA, and the amount of immobilized HSA was further increased. When this surface was reacted with anti-HSA the shift in the plasmon angle was about twice that of a single HSA monolayer. Improved sensitivity is thus demonstrated.

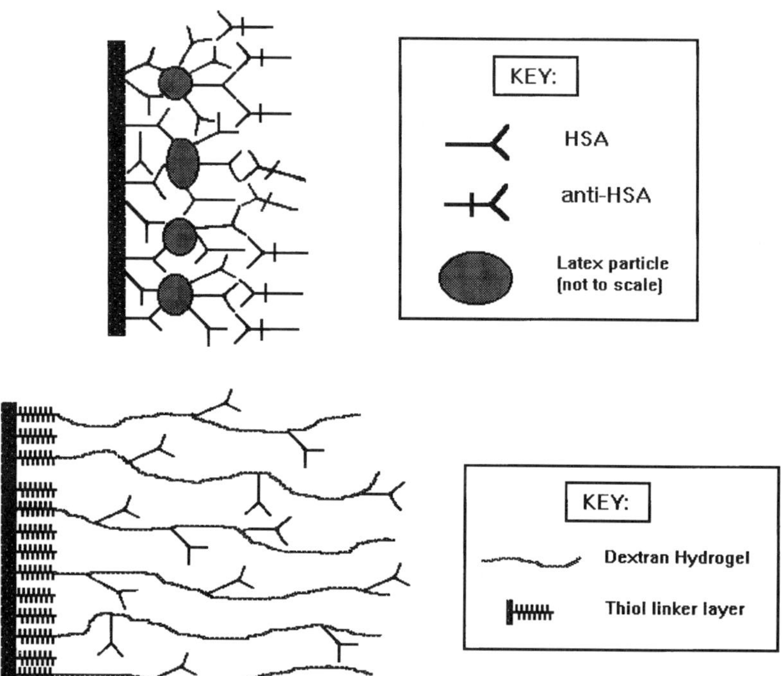

FIGURE 16.6 Increased loading of IgG receptors to the metal surface via the use of either latex particles (above) or a dextran hydrogel layer (below).

Other types of particle can be utilized, e.g., polystyrene, polymethyl methacrylate, or silica. Alternatively, metal sol particles (usually silver or gold) can be immobilized to the surface to form the support particle.[26]

16.2.2.8 Use of Dextran Hydrogels

A novel hydrogel matrix has recently been utilized to increase the number of receptors bound to the sensor surface (see Bergstrom et al.,[27] Löfås and Johnsson,[28] and Liedberg et al.[29]). The hydrogel is constructed from a composite metal protection layer and a carboxymethyl-modified dextran (see Figure 16.6). The metal (in this case, gold) is first pretreated with a hydroxyalkyl thiol layer. This both protects the gold surface from protein absorption and partly functionalizes it for further modification. The hydroxyl groups of the thiol are then converted to epoxide by exposure to a solution of epichlorohydrin. The dextran then binds to the epoxide surface. It is activated towards protein binding via reactions which form reactive *N*-hydroxysuccinimide esters.[28,30] Protein binding to the immobilized and activated dextran depends on the ionic strength, pH, reaction time, and concentration of protein. Once a monoclonal antibody, for instance, has been immobilized, excess esters are deactivated to reduce nonspecific binding which would otherwise occur as a result of subsequent exposure of the surface to the antigen of interest. The binding of antibody and antigen within the gel are monitored by the change in the plasmon angle, such changes having been calibrated to an absolute surface concentration of protein[31] using ^{14}C and ^{35}S radiolabeled proteins.

The change in reflectivity of the plasmon mode is linearly dependent on the surface protein concentration and can be quantitatively correlated to protein loadings, and loadings of up to 50 ng/mm^2 (see Stenberg et al.[31]) are possible. This upper level corresponds to the equivalent of several monolayers of protein,[32] indicating the high capacity of the hydrogel matrix. When a nonactivated hydrogel is exposed to an antibody a shift in the plasmon resonance is also observed. However, all this "bound" protein is easily removed by exposure to a salt solution,[28] indicating that specific binding effects in the system are minimal after deactivation. The reproducibility between measurements using the hydrogel matrix is better than 4% (relative standard deviation[30]).

The exact amount of protein immobilized into the dextran depends on the immunoreaction of interest. It is typically lower than the maximum loading quoted above. The amount bound is optimized for maximum reaction with the antigen and for conservation of the protein, since it is important to avoid wasting possibly rare and expensive receptor material. The thickness of the matrix is typically[32] about 100 nm. The entire gel is within the probing range of the plasmon mode, allowing interactions through the hydrogel to be evaluated. In the case of, for instance, anti-transferrin/transferrin interactions, a monoclonal anti-transferrin antibody was immobilized into the hydrogel to a 10 ng/mm^2 loading capacity. Interactions were monitored as a shift in the plasmon angle as transferrin flowed past the hydrogel surface, binding to the anti-transferrin receptors. The antibody surface was regenerated for further studies using a short pulse of glycine solution (pH 2.5). The bond between antibody and antigen was disrupted, leaving the antibody ready for further interaction. Up to 50 repeat analyses can be performed without loss of response.[28] Transportation of the receptors and analytes to the surface of the hydrogel is important, and this has been achieved with a highly efficient flow injection system containing pneumatically activated microvalves to control the flow of buffer and analyte.[33,34] Solution volumes as low as a few microliters can be used. Therefore only small amounts of antibody are required to generate the receptors in the hydrogel matrix.

The binding events themselves are monitored as optical changes at the interface and recorded continuously with time. A "sensorgram" is thus registered.[34] The change in the reflectivity of the surface is in reflectance units (RU), where 1000 RU correspond to shifts of 0.1°, or a protein loading of about 1 ng/mm^2 into the dextran layer. Reflectance at a certain angle is monitored with time. The signal contains contributions from the sensor surface, the particular captured antibodies and/or antigens of interest, and the buffer. Contributions due to the buffer alone are determined by flowing buffer solution past the surface after protein binding has occurred. The consequent change in RU can then be compared with the original reflectance before protein binding started (i.e., the same buffer each time), allowing protein loadings to be calculated. For more details regarding the kinetic analysis of binding events using the above system the reader is referred to a paper by Karlsson et al.[35]

16.2.2.9 Advances in the Detection of Immunoreactions Using Dextran Hydrogels

The development of the hydrogel matrix for receptor loading, in combination with the liquid handling system to expose the matrix to receptor and analytes, has led to numerous new applications of SPR for immunosensing. A few examples are now discussed.

The subclass of, for instance, different mouse antibodies can readily be determined by first immobilizing a rabbit anti-mouse Fcγ antibody into the hydrogel. The antibodies, which can be in a culture medium, are separately injected to flow past the surface. After each antibody a series of anti-IgG are sequentially injected, anti-IgG_1, IgG_{2a}, IgG_{2b}, or IgG_3, with binding of one of them indicating the subclass of the bound antibody. Once this sequence is completed the surface can be regenerated to leave just the anti-mouse Fcγ antibody. Another antibody subclass can then be identified.[34]

Interactions of both animal and plant viruses have been studied using various monoclonal antibody receptors. The antibodies themselves are specific to different conformational states of the viral protein. The viruses retain their conformational integrity when immobilized on the dextran matrix, allowing their conformation to be evaluated through the subsequent binding of the antibodies. In more conventional solid-phase immunoassays the protein on the virus is usually partly denatured.[36]

The dextran hydrogel coating has also been successfully used for the epitope mapping. of antigens.[37,38] Epitope mapping is the process of defining the unique binding characteristics of individual antibodies to an antigen molecule. One approach involves the simultaneous binding of pairs of antibodies to the antigen. Antibodies which can bind at the same time are directed against separate epitopes, whilst those that interfere with each other may be directed towards common or neighboring epitopes. Epitope mapping studies produce a reactivity pattern matrix showing the ability of antibody pairs to bind simultaneously to the antigen. By way of example, Fägerstam et al.[38] considered the capture of a monoclonal antibody by the use of immobilized rabbit anti-mouse IgG_1 (previously loaded into the dextran). Epitope specificities are determined through the subsequent introduction of the antigen (in these experiments the antibody was raised against recombinant HIV-1 core protein P24) and via the ability of a second monoclonal antibody to bind to the captured antigen. After the first antigen is bound, unreacted sites on the anti-mouse IgG_1 are blocked with a different antibody to reduce false positive readings.

Monoclonals that recognize different epitopes on an antigen are then introduced sequentially. The mapping of their binding efficiencies allows the different epitopes on these antigens to be determined.[38] The labeling necessary for more conventional assays is not needed, and possible interferences are thus avoided. There have been a number of extensions to this work where, for instance, peptide inhibition of the monoclonals has been studied.[38,39] Peptides can be introduced after the antigen has bound to the captured Fcγ antibody in the dextran film. The influence on the binding of the second antibody is subsequently studied. Using the combined use of the epitope map for the secondary antibody binding and protein inhibition indicates site specificity of the peptides.[40]

For high molecular weight species such as proteins, i.e., mol wt 70,000 to 150,000 (IgG and anti-IgG), the direct measurement of the immunoreaction between an antibody and its antigen is straightforward since binding events cause large and easily measurable shifts to the plasmon angle. However, there is a need to measure low molecular weight analytes which cannot, themselves, be monitored directly with the hydrogel arrangement, i.e., hormones, haptens, or drugs. For molecular weights below about 1000 the change in SPR is not sufficient to confidently determine which species are present or their concentrations. To overcome this, indirect methods have to be employed.

Theophylline is an example of a low molecular weight analyte. It is of clinical importance in asthma treatment and has a molecular weight of 180. Its concentration in serum samples over clinically relevant concentration ranges has been evaluated by adding known amounts of a monoclonal anti-theophylline antibody to the sample.[40] The analogue aminotheophylline was first coupled covalently to the sensor surface. Theophylline samples were then mixed in bulk solution with known amounts of anti-theophylline, and left to react before the mixed solution was injected over the aminotheophylline surface. The measured response is inversely related to the concentration of the theophylline, since the higher the theophylline concentration the more it binds to the anti-theophylline prior to exposure to the immobilized aminotheophylline, thus reducing the amount of antibody that is available to bind to the sensor. Comparison of the response with those of known concentrations enables unknown levels to be determined. The useful range of the assay is determined by the affinity of the antibody for theophylline. Different antibodies can be screened to determine which is the most appropriate one for the concentration range of interest (typically in the 1 to 30 μg/ml range).[40]

An alternative approach for enhancing the SPR signal in the monitoring of low molecular weight species is through competition of the small molecule with a larger "conjugate" analyte, i.e., competitive binding. This is accomplished by conjugating (or binding) a larger molecular species to the low weight analyte of interest. The analyte and its conjugated analogue are then mixed together in solution and this solution exposed to a "capture" receptor antibody immobilized in the dextran layer.[41] As pointed out above, the concentration of the analyte of interest is determined from the inverse of the response, i.e., a large shift in the plasmon angle corresponds to greater amounts of analyte-conjugate binding and therefore lower amounts of the analyte. It is also found that the larger the response from conjugate binding, the higher the sensitivity. Therefore, it has been proposed that the conjugate should have a significantly higher molecular weight than the analyte. The conjugate could be then a polystyrene latex,[42] a virus, a microorganism, or a high molecular weight protein. It is also better if the conjugate has a refractive index greater than the surrounding media (glass beads of lithium niobate or colloidal metals), such that larger changes in the plasmon resonance are induced during binding events.[41] These analyte-conjugate systems can be combined with the hydrogel pretreatment to allow more accurate determination of low molecular weight species.

Where the analyte has more than one epitope a sandwiching method can be used to increase signals from low molecular weight material or where low concentrations require study. For instance, β_2-microglobulin is of clinical interest since variations in its concentration reflect changes in the function of the immune system.[43] If anti-β_2-microglobulin is covalently attached to the dextran, β_2-microglobulin in serum can bind to it, producing a plasmon shift. If a polyclonal β_2-microglobulin antibody which binds to the β_2-microglobulin is then injected, this shift is increased, effectively amplifying the signal. This procedure has enabled measurements of β_2-microglobulin in the 10- to 1000-ng/ml range. In these investigations, primary amine groups in the antibody were linked to derivatized carboxyl groups on the sensor surface (carbodiimide chemistry). Other chemistries like thiol-disulfide exchange have also been studied. One of two approaches is used depending on whether the thiol group is on the protein/ligand or on the surface of the matrix.[27,44] Ligands can be immobilized via intrinsic thiol groups, or via groups introduced by derivatization of carboxyl or amine groups where amine coupling may be unsatisfactory, or for ligands or other small proteins where the number of amine groups is limited. Investigations with, for instance, the β_2-microglobulin/anti-β_2-microglobulin system discussed above have found that the concentration dependence of β_2-microglobulin over the 10- to 1000-ng/ml range was the same for both the amine and thiol types of immobilization. The effectiveness of the thiol coupling is thus indicated.

The above section details much of the recent work by the Pharmacia group, and if further information is required the reader is referred to a number of recent review-type papers by the group.[45-48]

16.3 CONCLUSIONS

There are a number of conventional assay methodologies available for the study of interactions between biospecific partners, i.e., between antibodies and antigens. Such methods include ELISA, and fluoro- or radioimmunoassays. They require the labeling of species of interest, either enzymatic, fluorescent, or radioactive, and sufficient time for the reactions to reach equilibrium before analysis can be performed. Also, whilst the sensitivity of ELISA techniques is excellent, there are separation and washing steps involved in the technique, as well as a prolonged incubation period, and training is required if the user is to obtain reliable results.

An SPR immunosensor will generally offer shorter preparation and waiting times and, moreover, can provide dynamic antibody-antigen binding data that can enable a "quick" estimate of analyte concentration, as well as providing a method by which an alarm sensor could be designed (i.e., a biosensor that could be used to constantly monitor the presence of a given impurity within a system, producing a signal *if and when* that impurity is introduced).

The sensitivity of SPR-based sensors depends upon the exact geometry used, since it can be either the wavelength, intensity, or angle of the output that is measured. In the case of angular measurements the sensitivity will generally be around 0.01° for a typical $\theta/2\theta$ rotating table, which corresponds to the detection of a 0.12-nm nonabsorbing dielectric film for which $\varepsilon_r = 2.5$ (a typical value for an organic material), using 632.8-nm-wavelength (HeNe laser) light to excite an SPP (surface plasmon-polariton) on a silver-coated prism. As mentioned previously, differential measurement techniques could improve this angular sensitivity by at least two orders of magnitude, but it is vital to protect the equipment from vibrational and thermal effects if this sensitivity is to be maintained.

The refractive indices of prisms, gratings, and metal overlayers all possess a certain temperature dependence, but this is not generally a consideration when designing an SPR-based sensor: the variation of the critical angle with temperature is less than 2×10^{-6} K^{-1} for BK7 glass (a typical prism material[49]), whilst silver's variation of ε_r with temperature of 8.5×10^{-4} K^{-1} (as given by van Exter and Lagendijk[50]) gives rise to a plasmon angle shift of approximately 1.96×10^{-6} °/K for an SPP (surface plasmon-polariton) excited with an HeNe laser, indicating that thermally induced changes of refractive index are inconsequential under most circumstances. The thermal effects in differential experiments are thought to be due to small-scale expansion and contraction of the apparatus that does not affect less sensitive detection methods.

The stability of the plasmon-supporting surface is purely a function of the chosen metal, as has previously been discussed. Whilst silver produces a sharp reflectivity profile which enhances the sensitivity of an SPR immunosensor, the metal is highly prone to degradation, and is adversely affected by buffer solutions (as discussed by Kooyman et al.[5]). Gold is a far better choice, since whilst its SPR reflectivity profiles are somewhat broader than those of silver, the metal is inert and is unaffected by most buffer solutions, irrespective of pH or temperature (although it should be pointed out that thermally evaporated gold does not always adhere well to glass — the above discussion presumes that the gold has been sputtered). This stability would be invaluable in the design of a disposable biosensor that did not require calibration (on condition that gold films of identical thickness could be produced) and, indeed, the sensing heads within Pharmacia's biosensors[37,38,40,42] have been designed in exactly this manner. As stated previously, whilst it is possible to reuse transducer surfaces by removing bound material from the receptor layer, this leads to a reduction in sensitivity after a given number of experiments, and therefore the use of disposable sensing heads is desirable.

It is believed that the ultimate limiting factor upon an SPR immunosensor's sensitivity lies in the choice of the active biochemical layer, since this is the true interface between the target molecule and the SPP-supporting surface. As has been discussed, binding efficiency can be improved by making more receptor sites available to the target protein molecules, either by improving the orientation of the sites or increasing their number density, and this can be achieved in a variety of ways (e.g., thiolation, particulate additives, the use of dextran hydrogels — see Table 16.2). The previously mentioned Pharmacia biosensor utilizes hydrogels to capture target analytes, achieving sensitivities down to 20 pg/mm^2. Saturation of the sensing surface does occur for concentrations above 35 ng/mm^2, but the system's sensitivity is *proportional* to the bulk concentration at lower values, and is independent of the molecular weight of the analyte. This has allowed an extensive study of many biospecific interactions, and the system can be considered to be representative of the optimum sensitivity available from an SPR-based biosensor at present.

TABLE 16.2
Binding Techniques

Method	Comment
Adsorption to metal	Molecules bound by hydrophobic forces Alignment (and hence availability) of binding sites within the protein layer is poor due to random orientation.
Biotinylation	Biotin binds to the metal, avidin (or streptavidin) to the biotin, and a biotinylated protein binds to the avidin to form the receptor layer High specificity has been demonstrated, but the method is unlikely to improve the alignment of binding sites
Thiolation	Thiol monolayers are chemisorbed onto a gold film, functionalizing the metal according to the choice of end-groups on the thiols[18] Creates efficient and reproducible receptor layers
Particulate additives	Particles (e.g., of latex) are coated with molecules that bind to proteins at a metal surface, increasing the surface area available for subsequent immunoreactions Improves sensitivity[26]
Dextran hydrogels	A dextran hydrogel matrix is attached to a gold film via an epoxide layer[27,29] Molecules bind to activated portions of the dextran and the equivalent of several monolayers can become attached[31] providing a large surface area for subsequent immunoreactions. Sensitive, capable of taking real-time measurements,[35] and resuable[30]

A point worth making is that, whilst the sensitivity of a system is independent of molecular weight, the binding efficiency is of particular importance when the target proteins are small (i.e., below a molecular weight of 10,000) since they will only form a relatively thin overlayer and the signal will be weak. When dealing with such small analytes, further complementary techniques such as sandwiching and competitive binding may also be of use.

Perhaps the biggest problem in the field of immunosensing is that of specificity, since the ideal sensor would be able to detect the presence of a specific analyte within a solution that contained a variety of materials (e.g., blood, milk). SPR immunosensors are particularly sensitive to nonspecific binding since *any* material that collects onto the transducer surface will produce a signal, and hence it is important to ensure that the active receptive layer provides full coverage of the metal's surface. Further, "cross-reactivity" (the blocking of receptor sites by molecules other than those under scrutiny) is a problem that needs to be addressed. Ideally a molecule-specific membrane across the sensing head would filter out foreign material (i.e., molecules other than those of the analyte), but at present the problems of cross-reactivity have only been dealt with directly via screening of the analyte solution: further work is necessary.

Hence it is the sensitivity and stability of the bound antibody layer that is the prime consideration in the fabrication of an SPR immunosensor: the SPR transducer can be designed so as to meet these criteria, but it is the physical attachment of the target proteins to the transducer's surface that places the upper limit on sensitivity. The use of SPR techniques is now recognized as being a direct method for measuring biospecific reactions, with devices now being commercially available from companies such as Pharmacia AB, and the pursuit of the first truly portable SPR-based immunosensor will ensure that this field of research will be further developed by a number of research groups over the coming years.

ACKNOWLEDGMENTS

The authors thank both Professor J. R. Sambles (Exeter University, U.K.) and Dr. N. Furlong (C.S.I.R.O., Melbourne) for many useful discussions during the preparation of this review, and are also grateful for the support of the Defense Research Agency at Malvern who helped support one of the authors (C.R.L.) at the beginning of this work.

REFERENCES

1. Hurn, B. A. L. and Chantler, S. M., Production of reagent antibodies, *Methods Enzymol.*, 70, 104, 1980.
2. Engvall, E. and Perlmann, P., Enzyme linked immuno-sorbent assay (ELISA): quantitative assay of IgG, *Immunochemistry*, 8, 871, 1971.
3. MacRitchie, F., The adsorption of proteins at the solid/liquid interface, *J Colloid Interface Sci*, 38, 484, 1972.
4. Liedberg, B., Nylander, C., and Lundström, I., Surface plasmon resonance for gas detection and biosensing, *Sensors Actuators*, 4, 299, 1983.
5. Kooyman, R. P. H., Kolkman, H., Van Gent, J., and Greve, J., Surface plasmon resonance immunosensors: sensitivity considerations, *Anal. Chim. Acta.*, 213, 35, 1988.
6. Cullen, D. C., Brown, R. G. W., and Lowe, C. R., Detection of immuno-complex formation via surface plasmon resonance on gold-coated diffraction gratings, *Biosensors*, 3, 211, 1987/88.
7. Mayo, C. S. and Hallock, R. B., Immunoassay based on surface plasmon oscillations, *J. Immunol. Methods*, 120, 105, 1989.
8. Daniels, P. B., Deacon, J. K., Eddowes, M. J., and Pedley, D. G., Surface plasmon resonance applied to immunosensing, *Sensors Actuators*, 15, 11, 1988.
9. Sun, X., Shiokawa, S., and Matsui, Y., Experimental studies on biosensing by SPR, *Jpn. J. Appl. Phys.*, 28, 1725, 1989.
10. Cowen, S. and Sambles, J. R., Resolving the apparent ambiguity in determining the relative permittivity of metal film using optical excitation of surface plasmon-polaritons, *Opt. Commun.*, 79, 427, 1990.
11. Tanford, C., *Physical Chemistry of Macromolecules*, 3rd ed., John Wiley & Sons, New York, 1965, 307.
12. Flanagan, M. T. and Pantell, R. H., Surface plasmon resonance and immunosensors, *Electron. Lett.*, 20, 968, 1984.
13. Wilchek, M. and Bayer, E. A., The avidin-biotin complex in immunology, *Immunol. Today*, 5, 39, 1984.
14. Bayer, E. A. and Wilchek, M., The use of the avidin-biotin complex as a tool in molecular biology, *Methods Biochem. Anal.*, 26, 1, 1980.
15. Morgan, H. and Taylor, D. M., A surface plasmon resonance immunosensor based on the streptavidin-biotin complex, *Biosens. Bioelectron.*, 7, 405, 1992.
16. Morgan, H., Taylor, D. M., and D'Silva, C., Surface plasmon resonance studies of chemisorbed biotin-streptavidin multilayers, *Thin Solid Films*, 209, 122, 1992.
17. Folkers, J. P., Laibinis, P. A., and Whitesides, G. M., Self-assembled monolayers of alkanethiols on gold: comparisons of monolayers containing mixtures of short and long-chain constituents with CH_3 and CH_2OH terminal groups, *Langmuir*, 8, 1330, 1992.
18. Prime, K. L. and Whitesides, G. M., Self-assembled organic monolayers: model systems for studying adsorption of proteins at surfaces, *Science*, 252, 1164, 1991.

19. Häussling, L., Ringsdorf, H., Schmitt, F. J., and Knoll, W., Biotin-functionalized self-assembled monolayers on gold: surface plasmon optical studies of specific recognition reactions, *Langmuir*, 7, 1837, 1991.
20. Häussling, L., Michel, B., Ringsdorf, H., and Rohrer, H., Direct observation of streptavidin specifically adsorbed on biotin-functionalized self-assembled monolayers with the scanning tunneling microscope, *Angew. Chem. Int. Ed. Engl.*, 30, 569, 1991.
21. van den Heuvel, D. J., Kooyman, R. P. H., Welling, G. W., Bloemhoff, W., and Greve J., Application of mini-antibodies in surface plasmon resonance sensor, in *Proceedings of the Second World Congress on Biosensors*, Elsevier, London, 1992, 392.
22. Cullen, D. C. and Lowe, C. R., A direct surface plasmon-polariton immunosensor: preliminary investigations of the nonspecific adsorption of serum components to the sensor interface, *Sensors Actuators,* B1, 576, 1990.
23. Miles, L. E. M. and Hales, C. N., Labelled antibodies and immunological assay systems, *Nature*, 219, 186, 1968.
24. Attridge, J. W., Daniels, P. B., Deacon, J. K., Robinson, G. A., and Davidson, G. P., Sensitivity enhancement of optical immunosensors by the use of a surface plasmon resonance fluorimmunoassay, *Biosens. Bioelectron.*, 6, 201, 1991.
25. Fontana, E., Pantell, R. H., and Strober, S., Surface plasmon immunoassay, *Appl. Optics*, 29, 4694, 1990.
26. Schasfoort, R., International Patent Number WO 91/17427, 1991.
27. Bergstrom, J., Löfås, S., and Johnsson, B., International Patent Number WO 90/05303, 1990.
28. Löfås, S. and Johnsson, B., A novel hydrogel matrix on gold surfaces in surface plasmon resonance sensors for fast and efficient covalent immobilisation of ligands, *J. Chem. Soc. Chem. Commun.*, 21, 1526, 1990.
29. Liedberg, B., Lundström, I., and Stenberg, E., Principles of biosensing with an extended coupling matrix surface plasmon resonance, *Sensors Actuators,* B11, 63, 1993.
30. Johnsson, B., Löfås, S., and Lindquist, G., Immobilization of proteins to a carboxymethyldextran-modified gold surface for biospecific interaction analysis in surface plasmon resonance sensors, *Anal. Biochem.*, 198, 268, 1991.
31. Stenberg, E., Persson, B., Roos, H., and Urbaniczky, C., Quantitative determination of surface concentration of protein with surface plasmon resonance using radiolabeled proteins, *J. Colloid Interface Sci.*, 143, 513, 1991.
32. Löfås, S., Malmqvist, M., Rönnberg, I., Stenberg, E., Liedberg, B., and Lundström, I., Bioanalysis with surface plasmon resonance, *Sensors Actuators,* B5, 79, 1991.
33. Sjölander, S. and Urbaniczky, C., Integrated fluid handling system for biomolecular interaction analysis, *Anal. Chem.*, 63, 2338, 1991.
34. Fägerstam, L. G., A non-label technology for real-time biospecific interaction analysis, in *Techniques in Protein Chemistry II* , Academic Press, New York, 1991, p65.
35. Karlsson, R., Michaelsson, A., and Mattsson, L., Kinetic analysis of monoclonal antibody-antigen interactions with a new biosensor based analytical system, *J. Immunol. Methods*, 145, 229, 1991.
36. Dubs, M., Altschuh, D., and Van Regenmortel, M. H. V., Interaction between viruses and monoclonal antibodies studied by surface plasmon resonance, *Immunol. Letts.,* 31, 59, 1991.
37. Malmqvist, M., Karlsson, R., Larsson, A., and Sjödahl, J., International Patent Number WO 90/05306, 1990.
38. Fägerstam, L. G., Frostell, Ä., Karlsson, R., Kullman, M., Larsson, A., Malmqvist, M., and Butt, H., Detection of antigen-antibody interactions by surface plasmon resonance, *J. Mol. Recognition*, 3, 208, 1990.
39. Application note 102, Pharmacia Biosensor AB.
40. Application note 202, Pharmacia Biosensor AB.
41. Drake, R. A. L., Sawyers, C. G., and Robinson, G. A., Australian Patent Number AU-A-10631/88, 1988.
42. Severs, A. H. and Schasfoort, R. B. M., Enhanced surface plasmon resonance inhibition test (ESPRIT) by using latex particles, in *Proceedings of the Second World Congress on Biosensors,* Elsevier, London, 1992, 363.
43. Application note 201, Pharmacia Biosensor AB.

44. Application note 601, Pharmacia Biosensor AB.
45. Jönsson, U. and Malmqvist, M., Real-time biospecific interaction analysis, in *Advances in Biosensors*, JAI Press, London, 1992, 291.
46. Jönsson, U., Fägerstam, L., Ivarsson, B., Johnsson, B., Karlsson, B., Lundh, K., Löfås, S., Persson, B., Roos, H., Rönnberg, I., Sjölander, S., Stenberg, E., Ståhlberg, R., Urbaniczky, C., Östlin, H., and Malmqvist, M., Real-time biospecific interaction analysis using surface plasmon resonance and a sensor chip technology, *BioTechniques*, 11, 620, 1991.
47. Chaiken, I., Rose, S., and Karlsson, R., Analysis of macromolecular interactions using immobilized ligands, *Anal. Biochem.*, 201, 197, 1992.
48. Fägerstam, L. G., Frostell-Karlsson, A., Karlsson, R., Persson, B., and Rönnberg, I., Biospecific interaction analysis using surface plasmon resonance detection applied to kinetic, binding site and concentration analysis, *J. Chromatogr.*, 597, 397, 1992.
49. Anon., *Optical Glass*, technical manual of Schott-Glass Optics division.
50. van Exter, M. and Lagendijk, A., Ultrashort surface-plasmon and phonon dynamics, *Phys. Rev. Lett.*, 60/1, 49, 1988.
51. Matsubara, K., Kawata, S., and Minami, S., Multilayer system for a high-precision surface plasmon resonance sensor, *Opt. Lett.*, 15/1, 75, 1990.

17 Fluorimetric Immunosensors

Monika Wortberg, Marjan Orban, Reinhard Renneberg, and Karl Cammann

CONTENTS

0-8493-8905-4/97/$0.00+$.50
© 1997 by CRC Press, Inc.

17.1 INTRODUCTION

The recent development of a vast number of new immunosensor systems reflects the increasing demand for sensitive and efficient screening tools in the fields of environmental, agricultural, pharmaceutical, food, and clinical chemistry. Based on the highly specific interaction of an antibody with its corresponding antigen, mostly the target analyte, immunosensors offer a high selectivity for a single component or a whole class of compounds, even at trace levels. Thus they can help monitor human exposure to hazardous chemicals in water, food, or the environment.

The basic principles of immunosensors have been adopted from the well-established technique of immunoassays. Their initial development dates back as early as 1959 with the introduction of the radioimmunoassay (RIA) by Yalow and Berson.[1] This achievement broadened the horizon of the enormous field of analytical chemistry in a revolutionary way. However, since immunoassays tend to be labor intensive and are not designed for continuous monitoring, much effort has been directed toward the challenge of developing easy to handle immunosensor devices. On one hand, the development has been supported by the enormous technological advances in microfabrication of various optical and electronic transducers and the availability of cheaper instrumentation, especially laser-based devices. On the other hand, achievements in synthetic chemistry, biotechnology, and bioengineering contributed to the idea of utilizing tailored immunoreagents, such as antibody fragments and recombinant antibodies, and labels with improved performance characteristics.

Modern immunosensors are a smart combination of sophisticated instrumentation and advanced (bio)chemical strategies. Thus, immunosensors now can supplement or in some cases even replace conventional instrumental analytical methods.

This chapter will focus on optical immunosensors based on fluorescence detection. First, some basic considerations concerning an immunosensor setup are presented. After the introduction of basic immunochemical principles, being valid for immunoassays as well as for immunosensors, the advantage of fluorescent labels is described. The following presentation of fluorimetric immunosensors comprises fiberoptical devices in a traditional setup or as planar, miniaturized waveguides as well as the combined techniques of affinity chromatography and flow-injection analysis. Special features of different sensor approaches are demonstrated and further illustrated by selected interesting examples of environmental and clinical analysis.

17.2 THE IDEA OF IMMUNOSENSING

Immunosensors are a special form of biosensors.[2] In general, a biosensor combines the step of selective analyte recognition by means of an immobilized receptor molecule with signal generation near or directly at the surface of a transducer as is depicted in Figure 17.1. The specific recognition process can be described as a key fitting into its keyhole or, considering the molecule's flexibility, as a hand fitting into a glove (induced fit concept). The receptor in an immunosensor is an antibody but can be an antigen as well, as discussed below. For signal

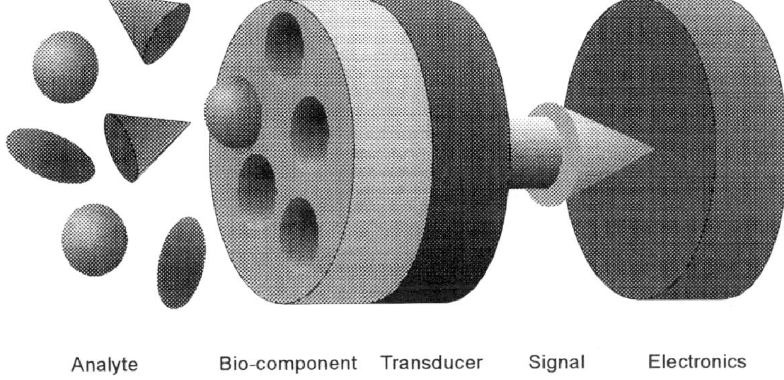

FIGURE 17.1 General principle for a biosensor.

transduction, various optical, electrochemical, mass, or temperature-sensitive devices are available.

Originally, one demand for all biosensors was reversibility, which means that the signal changes with both concentration increase or decrease.[3] In a more general recent definition this requirement no longer exists for immunosensors, since due to the high affinity of antibodies immunosensors are not strictly reversible. A new suggestion of the IUPAC refers to immunosensors as "immunoprobes", which accounts for the inherent reversibility problem. However, some immunoprobes are regenerable or continuously release immunoreagents, respectively and therefore show quasi-reversibility.[4]

Since the binding reaction between an antibody as the receptor and the analyte does not generate any reaction product, some knowledge of signal generation is necessary. The following description mainly focuses on optical sensors though it applies in a general way to all other transducers.

If binding takes place on the transducer surface, the properties of the solid phase are altered. The increase in layer thickness or surface coverage can be measured in terms of change in refractive index, mass increase, or reflectivity properties. A device capable of determining any of these parameters directly associated with the immunoreaction on the surface is referred to as direct immunosensor.

Another immunosensor approach is signal generation by tagging one of the complementary reaction partners (e.g., the antigen) with some label capable of signal generation. A typical label common in immunoassays would be a radioactive marker, an enzyme, an electroactive compound, or a fluorophore. The use of a label yields an indirect immunosensor whose signal is produced by a secondary compound or reaction. In rare cases where the analyte itself has fluorescent properties no label is required, thus yielding a sensor of the direct type although measuring fluorescence.

The working principle of direct immunosensors, namely measuring alterations on the transducer surface, implies also their most important limitation: all direct immunosensors suffer severely from nonspecific binding (NSB), also named nonspecific adsorption, which increases the limit of detection. NSB naturally occurs at a solid-liquid interface, but is especially crucial for immunoreactions where proteins, of course, are involved. The adsorptive effect, usually described as a hydrophobic interaction, is further increased when the analyte matrix is very complex, such as whole blood, urine, or sewage samples. In immunoassays the problem is partly overcome by sample dilution and addition of detergents and other reagents reducing hydrophobic interactions. However, since in direct immunosensors the signal caused by specific binding to the surface cannot be further enhanced over the nonspecific adsorption, the signal-to-noise ratio tends to be smaller compared to a sensor using specific signal enhancement by labeling. General aspects of labeling are discussed in more detail in Section 17.3.

17.3 ANALYTE RECOGNITION BY IMMUNOREACTION

17.3.1 MONOCLONAL AND POLYCLONAL ANTIBODIES

Antibodies, proteins of the class of immunoglobulins, are the most important molecules of the vertebrate immune system. They are produced in B lymphocytes after the organism is exposed to a "foreign" substance, called antigen, and responds with an immunoreaction. If the foreign molecule has a molecular weight lower than 3000 to 5000 Da (mol wt 3000 to 5000), no immunoreaction will take place unless this molecule, the hapten, is attached to a large carrier protein.

Those immunoglobulins being part of a special subgroup named immunoglobulin G (IgG) have an average mass of 150 kDa (mol wt 150,000). The general structure of an antibody of the IgG type is given in Figure 17.2. Antibodies consist of four chains, namely, two identical "heavy" and "light" chains, respectively, consisting of 440 and 220 amino acids, respectively. These chains are linked by disulfide bonds, forming a molecule the size of approximately 10 nm. For convenience of graphic display, antibodies are regarded as Y-shaped molecules. The "arms" of the Y contain the specific antigen binding sites, the paratope, being responsible for the recognition process. The two paratopes of an antibody are usually identical. If the antibody is cleaved enzymatically, fragments containing these binding sites are obtained separately, therefore they are named fragments antigen binding (F_{ab}).[5] The remaining "core" of the antibody molecule can be crystallized and is referred to as F_c, fragment crystallizing. The F_c fragment contains carbohydrate residues which can be used for immobilization. It has no antigen binding properties but plays a biologically important role in an organism. The specificity of one antibody over another is only achieved by slight variations in the amino acid sequence in small parts of the paratope, and are therefore called variable regions. The remaining parts of the four chains are constant over a wide range.

Antibodies generated during an immunoreaction can bind to only one specific area of the antigen molecule, called the epitope. If the antigen is very large, a heterogeneous population of different antibodies is generated during immunization. Each stimulated B cell or clone produces its own characteristic antibodies, but all antibodies expressed by the same B cell are identical. Since the antibodies from different B cells cannot be separated, the resulting "antiserum" is polyclonal in its nature, meaning the antibodies are generated by different clones of cells.

On the other hand, modern biotechnology enables production of so-called monoclonal antibodies by fusing single B cells with tumor cells.[6] If each of these fused, immortal cells is cultivated separately, monoclonal antibodies can be obtained. Besides uniformity, the advantage of monoclonal antibodies is that the same cell line can produce a virtually unlimited number of antibodies, whereas the supply of a polyclonal antiserum is limited to that from one individual immunized animal.

Both types of antibodies, mono- and polyclonal, show different characteristics but are equally useful for immunoassays or immunosensors. To understand the differences, a closer look at the antibody-antigen interaction is necessary.

17.3.2 ANTIBODY-ANTIGEN INTERACTIONS

The binding between an antibody's binding site and an epitope of an antigen can be described as an equilibrium association reaction:

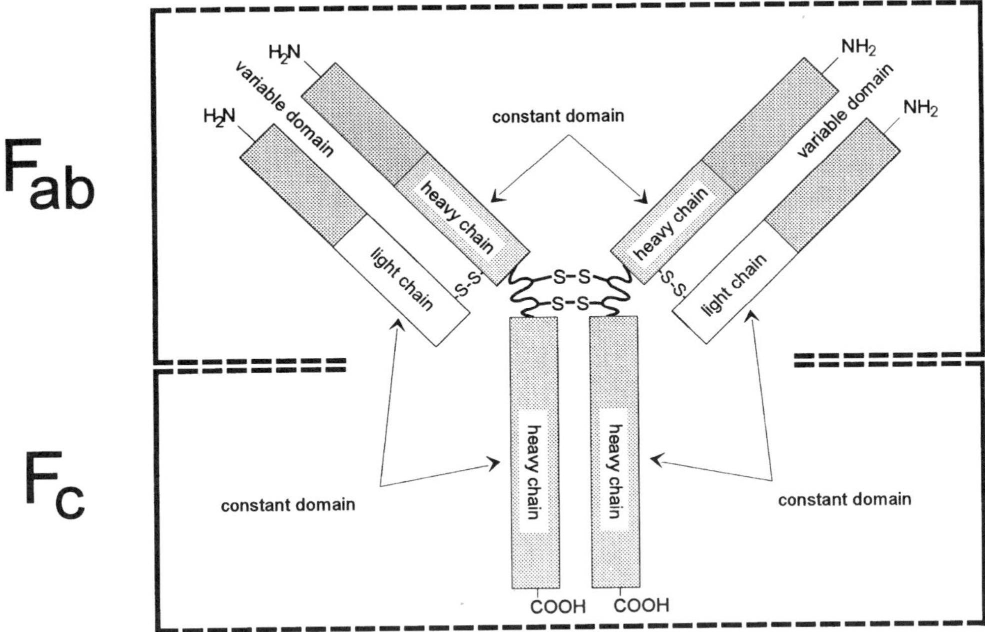

FIGURE 17.2 General structure of an antibody of the IgG type composed of two heavy and two light chains. The domains are formed by intrachain disulfide bonds.

$$Ab + Ag \rightleftharpoons Ab - Ag \qquad \begin{aligned} &Ab: \text{ antibody} \\ &Ag: \text{ antigen} \end{aligned}$$

with

$$K = \frac{[Ab - Ag]}{[Ab][Ag]} \qquad \begin{aligned} &Ab - Ag: \text{ antibody} - \text{antigen complex} \\ &K: \text{ binding constant} \end{aligned}$$

In principle the binding reaction is reversible, but since binding constants K usually range between 10^5 and 10^{12}, the reaction is virtually irreversible. The affinity constant is a measure for the "tightness" of binding between antibody and antigen, with binding forces being of merely noncovalent nature, e.g., hydrogen bonding, van der Waals forces, and electrostatic interactions.[7] These forces can be released, though, by altering the protein structure. This lowering of the binding constant can be achieved by changing the pH, increasing the ionic strength of the solution, or by simply replacing the previously bound antigen by a compound with an even higher affinity constant. These approaches make the antibody-antigen reaction quasi-reversible and enable the reuse of an antibody for subsequent antigen bindings as is common in immunoaffinity chromatography.

Antibodies are not monospecific, although sometimes monoclonal antibodies are believed to be so. In general, an antibody will bind to structurally related compounds, thus yielding group specificity towards a class of compounds rather than to a single compound. This phenomenon referred to as cross-reactivity is a very important feature of immunoassays. The more closely related these compounds are, the higher is the cross-reactivity for both mono- and polyclonal antibodies. Although cross-reactivity may be undesirable in some applications where a single analyte cannot be sufficiently discriminated from interfering compounds, the cross-reactivity can be an advantage for screening a whole class of analytes in the same assay.

Since polyclonal antibodies are heterogeneous, so are their binding constants towards different epitopes of the same antigen. Thus, some binding events are less reversible than others and there is an antibody fraction of the antiserum which does not contribute to specific binding at all. This is not necessarily a disadvantage, but if a uniform affinity toward an antigen is desired, monoclonal antibodies are preferred. For haptens which do not offer a variety of epitopes both mono- and polyclonal antibodies should fulfill the requirement of uniformity.

Since the interaction between an antibody and an antigen involves only the binding sites, it is also possible to use F_{ab} fragments rather than whole antibodies for performing immunoassays.

17.3.3 Basics of Immunoassays

A typical heterogeneous immunoassay involves a specific poly- or monoclonal antibody attached (immobilized) to a solid support which is subsequently reacted with the analyte and a labeled reagent. The antibody usually is simply bound to the solid phase by adsorption. Assays are frequently performed in 96-well microtitration plates made of polystyrene with optimized adsorptive properties. Between consecutive assay steps the wells are rinsed with buffer to wash out excess unbound reagents.

Two basic types of heterogeneous immunoassays can be performed. The first type is called a sandwich assay, because it involves two antibodies directed toward different epitopes of the antigen, forming an antibody sandwich trapping the antigen in the middle. The principle is shown in Figure 17.3a. The first antibody is immobilized; subsequently the analyte molecules are reacted (incubated). To visualize the binding event, a labeled second antibody is introduced. Since the second, labeled antibody is also specific to the antigen, it will only tag analyte molecules previously bound to the first antibody; therefore the signal generated by the label is proportional to the analyte concentration. A typical calibration curve obtained in a sandwich assay is shown in Figure 17.3b. For this noncompetitive approach a high antibody loading on the solid phase is desired to bind even minute amounts of analytes present in the sample solution. The sandwich assay approach is only feasible for large molecules with at least two different epitopes and two different antibodies available. It is therefore not applicable to small analytes (haptens) like pesticides or drugs and thus is not suitable for most environmental applications. The second assay type shown in Figure 17.4a is called a competitive immunoassay, involving competition between analyte and labeled analyte for a limited number of antibody binding sites. This approach is feasible for analyte molecules of any size, but it requires the preparation of a labeled analyte derivative, which sometimes cannot easily be obtained or is too expensive. To circumvent this problem, the antigen can be immobilized instead of the antibody and competes with free analyte antigens in solution for binding sites of the now-labeled antibody, as is shown in Figure 17.4b. In this case, a distribution of the antibody molecules between the solid phase antigens and the analytes in solution takes place according to the respective affinities. Figure 17.4c shows a calibration curve obtained with either approach of the competitive assay type. In contrast to the sandwich approach, the competitive assay has its lowest limit of detection when the number of antibodies (or antigens, respectively) on the solid phase is very low. Also, this assay works faster than the sandwich assay since, ideally, only one incubation and assay step is necessary, thus being more suitable for an immunosensor.

To achieve competition, analyte and labeled compounds may also be incubated sequentially without intermediate washing steps. If in a first step the analyte molecules are preconcentrated on the solid phase antibodies, fewer unoccupied binding sites remain for binding of the labeled compounds, which are only added in a second step.[6] This lowers the limit of

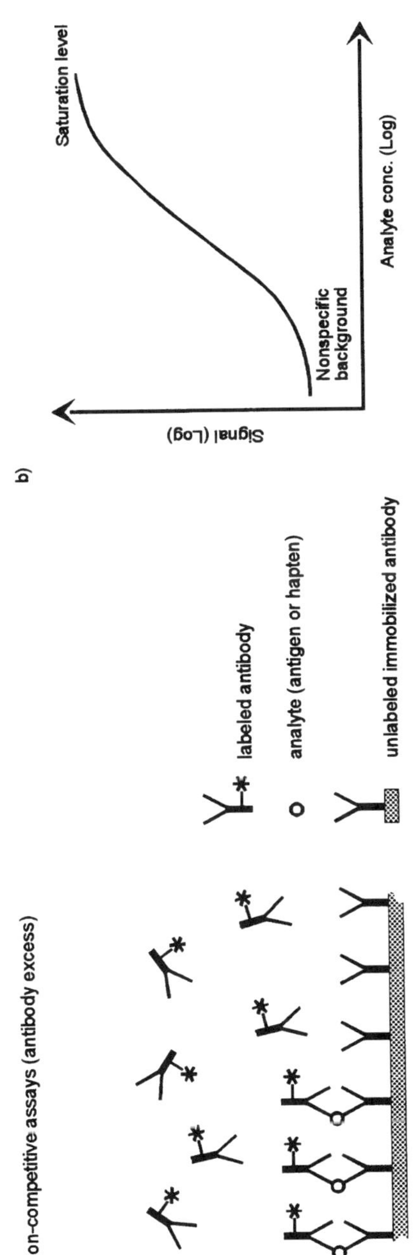

FIGURE 17.3 Schematic drawing of a sandwich immunoassay with typical calibration curve.

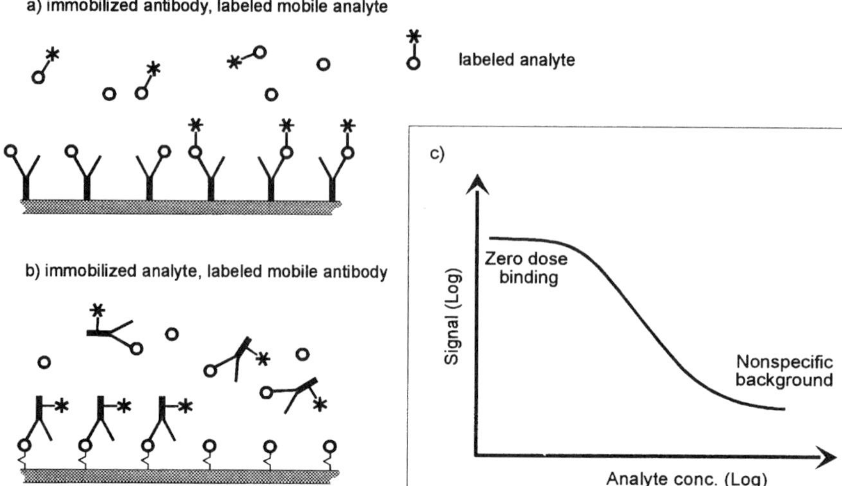

FIGURE 17.4 Competitive immunoassay: (a) competitive binding of analyte and labeled analyte to a limited number of antibody binding sites, (b) immobilized antigen competes with free antigens in solution for binding sites of the labeled antibody, (c) calibration curve obtained with either approach of the competitive assay type.

detection if the assay is performed under nonequilibrium conditions. However, if the reaction is allowed to reach equilibrium, the distribution of labeled molecules and analyte molecules on the solid phase is the same as with simultaneous incubation. Practically, performing nonequilibrium assays means an increased assay speed since there is no need to wait for equilibrium to be achieved.

Another modification of the competitive assay especially useful for immunosensors is the replacement approach (Figure 17.5). Immobilized antibodies are saturated with labeled antigens prior to the assay. When the sample containing the antigen is added, an amount of labeled molecules proportional to the analyte concentration is released from the antibodies. One might determine the concentration of labeled antigens released or bound to the antibodies. The replacement approach, however, is only feasible when the labeled compound shows a sufficiently low affinity to the antibodies to be replaceable at all. As yet, it has been demonstrated for haptens only. This approach is useful for flow-injection systems based on an affinity column preloaded with labeled molecules obtaining a sensor which can repeatedly be used without intermediate regeneration.

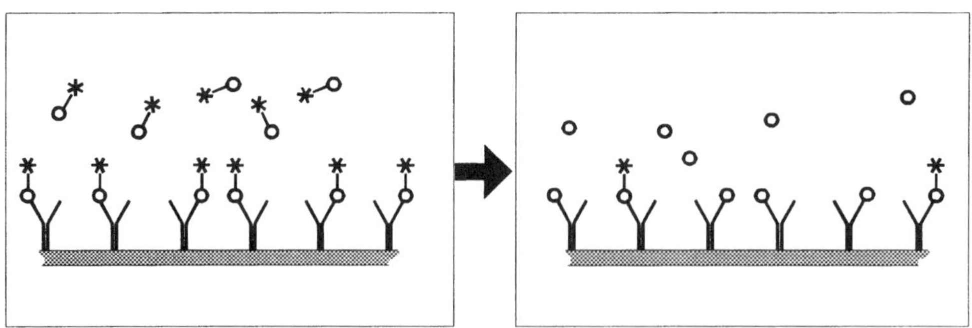

FIGURE 17.5 Modification of the competitive assay — replacement approach. After antibody saturation with labeled antigen, the sample containing the antigen is added. Labeled molecules proportional to the analyte concentrations are released from the antibodies. Calibration curve shows the same characteristics as in Figure 17.4c.

The idea of immobilizing the antigen rather than the antibody is especially applicable to immunosensors. The main reason is the practical stability: if the solid phase is supposed to be reused, for example, in a fiberoptic immunosensor, an immobilized antigen may be less affected by repeated irradiation than the respective antibody might be. In addition the antigen might withstand repeated cleavage of the binding by some regenerating agent much better than the antibody does.

17.3.4 Labels for Immunoassays

The first immunoassays involved radioactive tracers as labels. However, due to the disadvantage of limited shelf life, costly equipment, and the hazards of handling and disposing of radioactive compounds, alternative classes of labels have been employed. The most heavily used labels are enzymes, but also fluorescent markers are common. Immunoassays using luminescence, spin labels, or any class of electroactive markers are less widely applied although useful. Table 17.1 gives an overview of immunoassay techniques, the labels, and their detection principles.[8]

TABLE 17.1
Overview of Immunoassay Techniques

Assay method	Label	Detected	Detector
RIA (radioimmunoassay)	^{125}I, ^{3}H, ^{14}C	Radiation	Scintillation counter
EIA (enzyme immunoassay)	HRP AP β-D-galactosidase	Color change (absorbance)	Photometer
	HRP, AP, galactosidase	Fluorescence	Fluorimeter
	HRP	Luminescence	Luminometer
	HRP, AP, GOD, catalase	Current	Amperometric electrode
FrIA (fluoroimmunoassay)	Fluorescein rhodamines, dansyl chloride, cumarines, phycoerythrin, also liposomes	Fluorescence	Fluorimeter
TR-FrIA (time-resolved FIA)	Lanthanoid cations: Eu^{3+}, Tb^{3+}, Sm^{3+}	Delayed fluorescence	Time-resolved fluorimeter
LIA (luminescence immunoassay)	Acridinium esters Dioxetanes Peroxyoxalates Luminol Luciferase/luciferin Peroxidase	Chemi- and bioluminescence	Luminometer
	Pyrene	Electroluminescence	Electrode luminometer
Electrochemical immunoassays	Metallocenes Metals GOD, catalase	Current	DPP (differential pulse polarograph) DPASV (differential pulse anodic stripping voltammetry)
	Urease Liposomes	Ions (potential change)	Potentiometric electrode

Note: AP: alkaline phosphatase, GOD: glucose oxidase, HRP: horseradish peroxidase.

Most approaches listed in Table 17.1 are based on the principle of heterogeneous assay, thus requiring separation of surface-bound and free labels. Obviously, the different categories overlap, especially enzyme immunoassays which can be combined with photometric, fluorimetric, luminometric, or electrochemical detection principles, depending on the product being generated. Thus, the intention of the present table is to give an overview of the variety of possible assay or sensor designs, but not to delineate a definite classification system.

The signal enhancement associated with enzymes can be mimicked by using liposomes instead. If these liposomes contain a colored or a fluorescent dye or an electroactive marker, the signal can be generated immediately after lysis of the vesicles. This class of assay is referred to as particle immunoassay. It also comprises assays utilizing fluorescence or enzyme-labeled latex beads, which may additionally contain a magnetic core.

In addition to the heterogeneous assay techniques, some homogeneous assays not requiring a solid phase and thus no separation between bound and free molecules will be described. Examples for this category include fluorescence quenching, fluorescence energy transfer, or fluorescence polarization associated with the binding process, which can also be utilized in optical immunosensors. Homogeneous techniques have inherently higher limits of detection due to interferences.[9] Some of these approaches are discussed in more detail in Section 17.4.

17.3.5 Immobilization Strategies

In immunoassays the antibody is usually immobilized to a polystyrene support simply by adsorption.[10] The immobilization is sufficiently stable to perform a single assay, including washing steps with detergents present. The effects of differences between individual assay plates are minimized by assaying unknown samples and standards together on the same plate. Since the immobilized compounds are not intended to be used several times, this technique is satisfactory. In contrast, an immunosensor has to be calibrated and used for sample measurement. Thus, stable immobilization allowing repeated use has to be applied. When repeated use is not desirable, as for example in clinical analysis, the sensor surface has to be exchanged prior to each measurement. Here, it has to be ensured that surface preparations emerging from the same batch show uniform response properties for performing reliable calibration.

A second important issue is the orientation of the immobilized antibody. If the binding sites are attached to the surface, the antibody loses its binding ability. Therefore, directed immobilization is desirable. This has routinely been applied in immunoassays by using two approaches. A "capture" antibody with binding specificity towards the Fc region of the "active" antibody can be preimmobilized. Alternatively, special proteins isolated from bacteria membranes (protein A, protein G) with similar affinity properties can be used. The subsequently bound "analytical" antibody will be spatially orientated and has an improved assay performance compared to a randomly orientated adsorbed antibody. Another technique to immobilize antibodies in an oriented way is to take advantage of the carbohydrate moiety located at the F_c fragment. The carbohydrates can selectively be oxidized via simple standard procedures and subsequently be covalently linked to aminogroups or any nucleophile in general.[7]

Both approaches, random or directed immobilization, can be achieved by adsorption or covalent binding. The terms covalent and adsorptive, however, refer only to the first immobilization step. For example, protein G can be immobilized randomly oriented by adsorption, but still the coupled antibody subsequently will be aligned. If protein G were attached covalently, the resulting immobilization of the antibody would be oriented as well. Methods yielding only random orientation include entrapment (into a gel or a membrane) and cross-linking. In general, covalent binding is preferred over the other approaches because of enhanced stability.

In the case of antigen immobilization, attaching a spacer molecule between the antigen and the surface is advantageous due to increased accessibility. Presenting the antigen to the antibody by means of a six-carbon chain is frequently used to minimize steric hindrance that might reduce antibody-antigen binding.

17.4 FLUORESCENT LABELS FOR IMMUNOSENSORS

17.4.1 Luminescence Phenomena

Luminescence is defined as the emission of electromagnetic radiation in the ultraviolet (UV), visible (VIS), and infrared (IR) spectra from atoms or molecules as a result of the transition of an electronically excited state to a lower energy state, usually the ground state. Luminescent molecules absorb energy, for example, in the form of radiation or through a chemical reaction and subsequently emit energy as photons. In photoluminescence, absorption of light creates an excited state species (the S_1 state) which, after a vibrational relaxation, can return to the S_0 state in various ways including radiative deactivation (fluorescence) or radiationless deactivation. Another path is the delayed return to the ground state via the metastable triplet (unpaired electron) state by either phosphorescence or radiationless relaxation. A popular method to depict the absorption and emission process is the Jablonski diagram shown in Figure 17.6. It is often used to describe the energy levels of a molecule. A typical energy flow for luminescence in the case of Eu(III)-chelates is also shown and will be described later. The small loss of energy in luminescence, which is observed as a difference between excitation and emission energies (frequencies), is determined as the Stokes shift (expressed as a wavelength difference). In fluorescent organic molecules the shift is normally about 30 to 50 nm; in phosphorescence the shift is longer, especially in luminescent lanthanide chelates (even over 200 nm).

Background is present in all fluorimetric determinations and is due, among other things, to light scattering, emissions from the samples' endogenous fluorescence, autofluorescence of cells and tissues, luminescent properties of solid matrixes, cuvettes, test tubes, lenses, etc. In time-resolved fluoroimmunoassays the difference between the fluorescence lifetimes (τ) of the specific signal and the nonspecific background has been used to increase the signal-to-noise ratio and thus the sensitivity. When the τ of the probe is sufficiently longer than the average background decay time, the specific signal can be integrated after the background signal has decayed. The efficient use of the time-resolved (TR) detection requires luminescent probes exhibiting excited state lifetimes longer than the lifetime of the background. Typical fluorophore lifetimes range from 2 to 20 ns, while phosphorescence lifetimes are much longer (1 μs to 10 s). The development of new long-lifetime probes — rare earth metal chelates for which τ ranges from 10 to 1000 μs (more than 4 orders of magnitude longer than the average background duration) — presents interesting possibilities for increasing the sensitivity of the fluoroimmunoassay (FrIA) by reducing the background signal to practically zero.[11-13] Therefore, time-delayed fluorimetry holds great potential for optical time-resolved immunosensing with its scatter and background problems. The principle of time-resolved fluorescence measurement is presented in Figure 17.7.

Exothermic chemical reactions generally release energy in the form of vibrational or rotational excitation. Luminescent reactions result in products that are capable of emitting light instead of generating heat. This phenomenon is called chemiluminescence (CL), if the electronically excited state is reached by a chemical reaction.

Other classifications according to how the excited state is produced include photoexcitation (photoluminescence), electricity (electroluminescence), stress (triboluminescence), and others. In most chemiluminescent reactions, however, the source of energy is the cleavage of an energy-rich bond, such as that of peroxides, hydroperoxides, 1,2-dioxetanes, or dioxytenones. Luminescent labels from biological sources such as luciferin tend to be more expensive and less stable than those of chemical origin such as acridinium esters. The latter can produce luminescence without need for a catalyst. The main advantage of CL methods

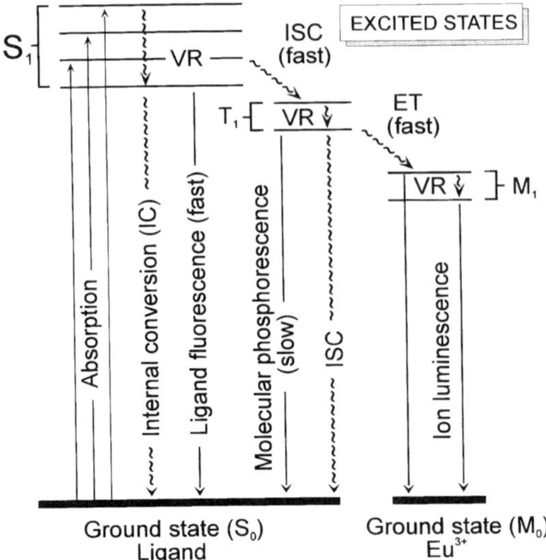

FIGURE 17.6 Jablonski diagram showing the relative energies of ground state (S_0) and first excited singlet (S_1) and triplet states (T_1), and some of their vibrational subniveaus. Rotational energy levels are omitted for clarity. Electronic absorption from S_0 to S_1 is followed by rapid radiationless internal conversion (IC) and vibrational relaxation (VR) to the lowest vibration level of S_1. Competing for deactivation of S_1 are the radiationless internal conversion and singlet-triplet (paired-unpaired spins) intersystem crossing (ISC) as well as fluorescence. Intersystem crossing is followed by vibrational relaxation (VR) in the triplet state (T_1). Both nonradiative ($T_1 \rightarrow S_0$) intersystem crossing and phosphorescence return the molecule from the T_1 to the S_0 state. In the case of an energy flow with a chelate, where the excited metal level (M_1) is under both the T_1 and S_1 levels of the ligand, the chelated metal ion receives excitation energy by a fast energy transfer (ET) from the ligand triplet state. The chelated metal, e.g., Eu, efficiently quenches the ligand fluorescence and produces its typical ion luminescence characterized by d-d* of f-f* transitions.

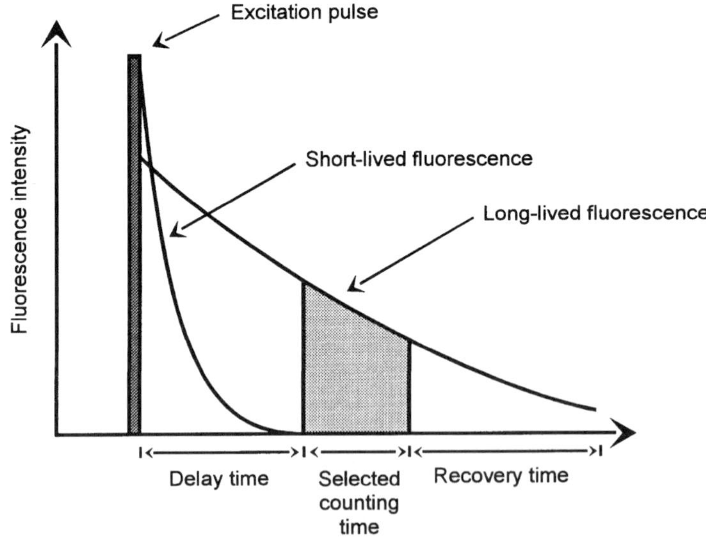

FIGURE 17.7 Schematic diagram of pulse fluorescence shows the fluorescence decay profile of an europium chelate as used in a time-resolved fluoroimmunoassay for discrimination of scattering and short decay-time background from longer decay-time emissions. Background fluorescence disappears after a few nanoseconds, whereas the chelate decays in the millisecond time regime.

is the wide dynamic range. Another point is the fact that there is no need for a monochromator or light source with its power requirements since the chemically sensitive material itself is the emitter. Therefore, detection is accomplished by using simple instrumentation. However, some chemiluminescent labels such as acridinium esters require automated reagent injection inside the luminometer due to the short luminescence lifetime. Since problems caused by background and light source interferences are alleviated, detection limits for CL assays can be as low as the femtomolar or attomolar range (10^{-15} to 10^{-18} M).

17.4.2 Fluorophores and Immunosensing

In optimizing detection sensitivity, the probe must have a high fluorescence intensity, the fluorescence signal must be distinguishable from the background, and the binding of the probe to an antibody or antigen should not adversely affect their properties. In fluoroimmunoassay (FrIA) the fluorescent probe should have fluorescence wavelengths far from the sample background, emission at higher than 600 nm, and preferably a large Stokes shift of more than 50 nm. Commonly, fluorescein and rhodamine derivatives have been used in the past as labels. The maximum sensitivity attainable with such fluorophore labels is about 10^{-9} to 10^{-10} M.[9] The major reason for this limited sensitivity is the high background signal mentioned before. Scattering interference is aggravated by the small Stokes shift of conventional fluorophores, which is usually 25 to 50 nm. Background fluorescence from biological samples usually arises between 350 to 600 nm and overlaps extensively with the emission spectrum of many fluorophores.[14]

Different fluorescent probes have been developed for biological, biochemical, and clinical purposes.[15] Table 17.2 lists the properties of some of the most frequently used probes. Fluorescein as an isothiocyanate, FITC, is the probe most widely used both in immunofluorescence and FrIA.[16] Different rhodamines are widely used for labeling antibodies, particularly for use in immunofluorescence studies. Compared with fluorescein, their fluorescence occurs at longer wavelength but the quantum yield is somewhat lower.[17,18] Comparison of rhodamines with fluorescein for antibody labeling shows certain advantages associated with their use, for example, stability and homogenity.[19-21]

In addition to the conventional organic probes used in FrIA, some new interesting types of labels have been introduced. The only group of long-lifetime photoluminescent labels successfully applied in TR-FrIAs so far are chelates of rare earth metals.[8] Only four lanthanides (Sm (III), Eu (III), Tb (III), and Dy (III)) form highly fluorescent chelates with appropriate organic ligands. In these chelates the strong ion luminescence emission originates from an intrachelate energy transfer, where the organic ligand absorbs the excitation radiation in the UV range and transfers the excited energy through its triplet state to the ion (Figure 17.6). The chelated central ion collects the absorbed energy and produces a strong, narrow-banded line-type emission at long wavelengths, well distinguishable from the interfering background. The exceptionally long luminescence decay time of these chelates allows the efficient use of time-resolved detection.

The red, far-red, and near IR (NIR) spectral regions (600 to 1000 nm) are of special interest, since here only a few classes of chemical compounds exhibit significant absorption or fluorescence.[24] These features of the NIR spectral region make it ideal for using fluorogenic labels, especially since the introduction of appropriate instrumentation, e.g., NIR semiconductor lasers. Porphyrines are one class of compounds with fluorescence in the IR region. Especially in the clinical field of photodynamic therapy (PDT), porphyrines with strong absorption in the far-red at 783 nm and a fluorescence maximum at 990 nm have been investigated by Franck et al.[25] These porphyrines, with a large Stokes shift and the advantage of absorption and emission in a region with little interference, may be potential labels. Polymethine dyes are another group known to have absorption maxima in the near IR.[26] Based on the concentration limit of detection (LOD) and the volume of sample, the mass

TABLE 17.2
Spectral Characteristics of Fluorophores

Fluorophore	λ abs/exc [nm]	λ emis [nm]	Decay time [ns]	Quantum yield [%]	Ref.
Fluorescein	492	520	4.5	0.85	9
Rhodamine B-isothiocyanate	550	585	3.0	0.7	9
Texas red (sulforhodamine sulfonyl chloride)	489	615	—	—	22
Umbelliferones	380	450	—	—	22
Dansyl chloride	340–350	510–560	14	0.03–0.3	8
Lucifer yellow	430	540	3.3	0.2	8
B-phycoerythrin	546, 565	575	3	0.98	8
Porphyrins	400–410	619–633	—	—	22
Chlorophylls	430-453	648-669	2–6	—	8
Carboxymethyl-indocyanines	550–764	566–794	—	0.08–-0.3	23
Eu-(β-NTA)$_3$	340	590, 613	500,000	—	9
Tb-EDTA-sulfosalicyclic acid	300	490, 545	~150,000	—	9
Nd-benzoyltrifluoroacetone	800	900, 1060, 1350	—	—	9

Note: β-NTA: β-naphthoyltrifluoroacetone.

LOD is 59 ag (6×10^{-17} g), or 46,000 molecules of the polymethine dye IR-140. This best absolute LOD has been reached with the liquid jet fluorescence spectrometer system, since this technique resulted in the smallest detection volume (56 nl).[27]

17.4.3 Instrumentation for Luminescence Detection

The principle components of a fluorimeter are a light source, monochromator, sample housing, light detector, signal processor recorder, and data processor. Arc lamps, tungsten lamps, lasers, or laser diodes are often used as light sources; possible detectors are photodiodes (PD) or photomultiplier tubes (PMT), the latter showing higher sensitivity in the VIS and UV region. Fiberoptics are used to bring light from a variety of sources to the sample compartment, and to take light from the sample, e.g., in a conventional cuvette, to the detector. Figure 17.8 presents a schematic diagram of a fiber-based and non-fiber-based fluorimeter.

In the past, fluorescent measurements have been limited from the UV up to the yellow part of the visible spectrum. Various lasers such as the continuous wave (CW) argon ion laser and a pulsed nitrogen-laser-pumped dye laser are used as a light source for fluorimetric detectors. The oscillating wavelengths of the semiconductor lasers used in fluorimetry are limited to discrete lines in the range 630 to 1600 nm (red to NIR), and it is difficult to find suitable organic dyes for covalent labeling. Imasaka et al. have reported the first application of a visible semiconductor laser to fluorescence spectrometry.[26] One of these lasers with a low emission wavelength (670 nm) is the NEC NDL 3200, with an output of 3 mW. However, with the development of tunable solid-state lasers such as Nd:YAG lasers or new tunable dye lasers, fluorescence measurements are now being extended out into the NIR region where there is less possibility for interferences with the emitted light. As mentioned above, fluorogenic dyes that emit light with wavelengths in the range from 700 to 1500 nm are now being investigated for use with the new lasers.

IR fluorescence measurements can be performed using a great variety of instrumentation. For many researchers, the simplest approach will be to use a conventional fluorescence spectrometer with a photodiode for IR. The simplest instrumentation for IR fluorimetry

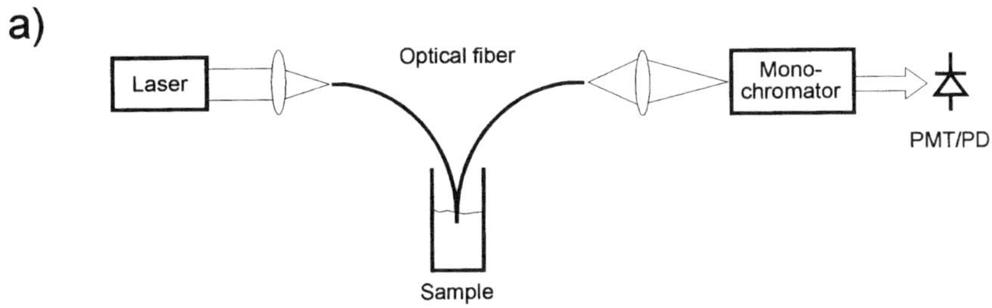

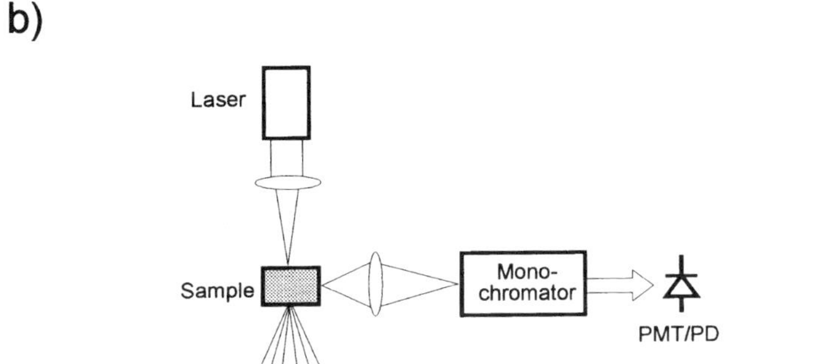

FIGURE 17.8 Schematic diagram for a fluorimeter, (a) fiber-based, (b) non-fiber-based.

utilizes bright light-emitting diodes as sources and photodiodes as detectors. Such systems are capable of determinations at micromolar and nanomolar levels, and lower limits of detection are probably feasible with avalanche photodiodes as detectors.[28]

The difference between a time-resolved fluorimeter and a conventional one is the use of lanthanide chelates as label, pulsed light source, and a gated detector reader. In comparison to the fluorescence lifetime of the chemical system, the excitation light is a flash of very short duration. After each flash the photomultiplier is inactive while any short-lived fluorescence decays. Subsequently the photomultiplier measures the long-lived fluorescence of the rare earth metal chelate for a certain period of time. Depending on the pulse frequency of the lamp, the excitation-emission cycle is repeated many times per second.

The Arcus fluorimeter from Pharmacia LKB is commercially available.[29,30] A xenon flash lamp with a fixed integrated photon emission is used as the pulsed excitation light source. For distinction of the fluorescence wavelength of interest various emission filters can be used. By measuring different lanthanides it is possible to detect at different emission wavelengths. A newer time-resolved fluorimeter, available from CyberFluor Inc., Toronto, Canada is the CyberFluor 615 Immunoanalyzer. The nitrogen laser source has an emission wavelength at 337.1 nm and excellent characteristics. Both instruments measure samples automatically with speeds of one sample per second.

The light emitted by chemiluminogenic compounds or reactions can often be measured with sufficient sensitivity using relatively simple equipment. Due to the fact that no light source is needed, in principle every device capable of measuring light can be used for this purpose. The essential compounds for the measurement and recording of the chemiluminescence are a sample chamber, filter or monochromator, and a light-detecting device, e.g., PMT in a single-photon counting mode. The instrumentation is strongly dependent on the kinetics of the chemiluminescent reaction. Measurement of transient labels such as luminol and acridinium esters, which show very fast kinetics (seconds), requires a number of extra features to perform a homogeneous and reproducible chemiluminescent reaction.[31] A chemiluminescence reader for microtiter plates is available (from Labsystems, Finland) which is also capable of performing injections into the sample position, opening the possibility of measuring transient labels in microtiter plates.[31]

17.5 FLUORESCENCE-BASED OPTICAL IMMUNOSENSORS

17.5.1 CONCEPTS FOR FLUORIMETRIC IMMUNOSENSORS

If the goal of immunosensor development is the construction of a fluorescence-based system, several options are possible. In the unlikely case of a fluorescent target analyte no label has to be introduced and the sensor will be of the direct type. In all other cases the fluorescent label has to be used, yielding an indirect type sensor.

When using fibers, two approaches are possible.[32] To illustrate this, a general picture of the light-guiding process in an optical fiber is shown in Figure 17.9. Light propagates through the fiber inside the core by total internal reflection at the interface between the core (higher refractive index) and cladding (lower refractive index). In the case of the receptor molecules being immobilized on the distal tip, the fiber merely serves as a pipe guiding the light to the tip. When the cladding surrounding the core is partly removed, the total internal reflection necessary for light-guiding occurs at the newly created interface between the core and the surrounding medium. The reflected wave partly penetrates into the adjacent layer and interacts with it.[33] Figure 17.10 shows schematically how the light intensity decreases exponentially in the medium surrounding the fiber core. This phenomenon, referred to as an evanescent wave, gives additional options for the use of a fiber, which is no longer a passive light guide. Fluorescent molecules as close as several hundred nanometers to the surface of the stripped fiber can be excited via the evanescent wave, whereas fluorophores in the bulk solution cannot be excited and therefore are virtually "invisible".

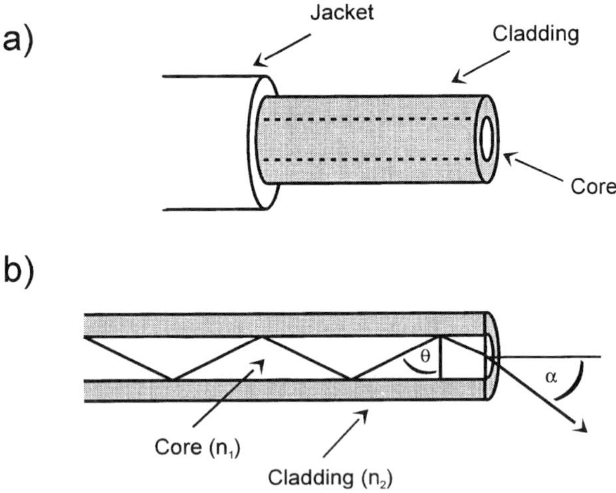

FIGURE 17.9 (a) Schematic of an optical fiber. (b) Path of light in a waveguide: α is the acceptance angle; θ is the critical angle for total internal reflection to occur; n_1 and n_2 are the refractive indices for core and cladding.

Either of the approaches based on fibers yields a dip-stick format device or a sensor which is exposed to the analyte by mechanical pumping in a flow-through cuvette. Alternatively, the fiber can be substituted by a planar chip composed of light-guiding materials of differing refractive indices. If the chip is patterned with "integrated" waveguides an integrated optical device is obtained.

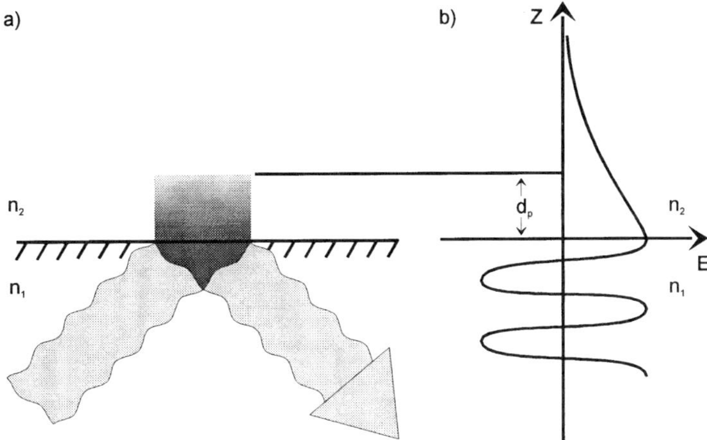

FIGURE 17.10 Generation of the evanescent wave at an interface between two optical media. (a) Light is totally reflected at the interface between an optical dense medium and an optical rare one ($n_1 > n_2$), when the angle of refraction is larger than a critical angle. The evanescent wave is generated at the reflecting surface. (b) Same as (a), but showing the electric field amplitude E on both sides of the reflecting surface (z = distance into the rarer medium, d_p is the characteristic penetration depth of the evanescent wave).

The solid phase (immobilized antibody) may also be remote from any transducer or the fluorescence reading device, thus creating a sensor with the receptor separated from the transducer. This is achieved by the technique of flow-injection immunoanalysis (FIIA) involving an "immunoreactor" as the receptor part in the recognition process and an on-line detector (fluorimeter) placed downstream or directly on-column in the flow setup. This immunosensing system is similar to a liquid chromatography setup with post- or on-column detection.

17.5.2 Fiberoptic-Based Immunosensors

If a fiberoptic immunosensor (FIS) is to be developed, it may either be based on a single or a bifurcated fiber. The two possible setups are shown in Figure 17.11. In case of a single fiber, both the excitation and the fluorescence light are guided in the same fiber. Separation of incident from fluorescence light is achieved, e.g., by a dichroic filter. This approach, however, gives rise to background fluorescence, which is suppressed more efficiently in the bifurcated fiber setup.[34] For both of the two basic fiber types there are several locations for antigen or antibody immobilization: on the fiber tip, on the core of the stripped fiber, or remote from the tip on an external surface near the fiber. Figure 17.12 shows several configurations.[35]

The most common immobilization approaches for fiberoptic immunosensors utilize functionalized silanes which are initially reacted with the glass or quartz fiber surface to activate it for further coupling reactions. Examples for suitable and widely used silanes are aminopropyl-triethoxysilane (ATS), mercaptopropyltriethoxysilane (MTS), or 3-glycidoxypropyltrimethoxysilane (GOPS).[36-38] A new and superior class of silanes are the recently described silanes with aldehyde functional groups.[39]

If photostability of the immobilized compound and the labels being subsequently introduced is a problem, direct illumination should be avoided. For higher surface loading capacity and avoidance of direct light exposure, stripping off the cladding and immobilizing on the fiber core is suitable. However, photodegradation may also occur when evanescent wave excitation is used. The most effective means of preventing photodegradation is to use short excitation intervals rather than permanent illumination.

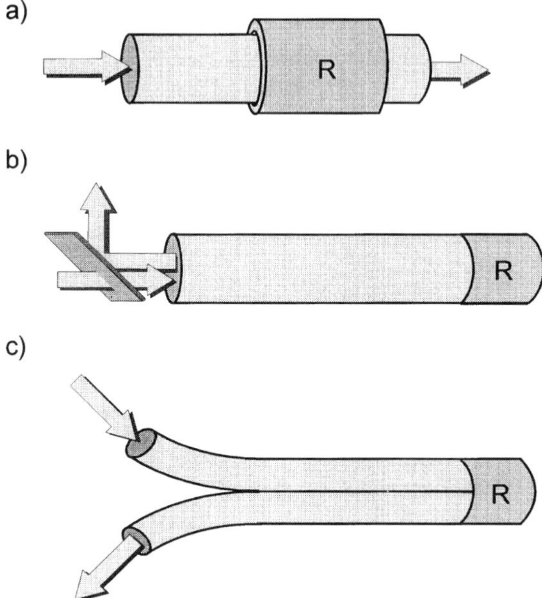

FIGURE 17.11 Possible configurations for a single or bifurcated fiber. R: chemically sensitive reagent. (a) single fiberoptic in which the reagent phase is coated on the outside of the fiber; (b) single fiberoptic in which the same fiber carries light to and from the reagent, a beam splitter separates incident and reflected light; (c) bifurcated fiberoptic sensor.

Photobleaching is also minimized in the unique approach of the continuous release polymer sensor, where fluorescently labeled reagents are embedded in a polymer reservoir which is never directly illuminated.[4]

The advantage of evanescent wave excitation (Figure 17.12e) is that no bulk fluorescence is excited. This yields a wash-free sensor which can inherently discriminate free from bound fluorophores. However, evanescent wave immunosensors are sensitive to NSB as well. Thus, fluorophore-labeled molecules approaching the surface nonspecifically cannot be discriminated from fluorophores held in the proximity of the fiber core due to binding to antibodies.

17.5.3 Planar Waveguide Sensors Based on Total Internal Reflection Fluorescence (TIRF)

Instead of a regular fiber, a planar device can serve as a light guide. To achieve total internal reflection as is required for light propagation, the planar device functions as a fiber core with the surrounding medium serving as the cladding. As for optical fibers, suitable materials are quartz or glass, the simplest version being a microscope glass slide. Usually the use of planar waveguides automatically implies evanescent wave techniques since the advantage of a large surface area applies. Since light propagation is achieved by total internal reflection between the waveguide surface and the surrounding solution, these devices are often referred to as total internal reflection fluorescence (TIRF) sensors. The setup of a TIRF-based sensor is shown in Figure 17.13. To achieve evanescent wave excitation with a planar waveguide, light is coupled into the waveguiding layer, e.g., by a prism mounted onto the planar device. Fluorescence signals are conveniently monitored through the bottom of the glass slide with a PMT, but fluorescence reading at the edge of a waveguide is also feasible.[40-43]

Another possibility is to use the planar glass substrate simply as a support for a light-guiding layer with a higher refractive index. Suitable surface modifications to achieve higher refractive indices on top of the substrate include deposition of metal phosphate glassy films

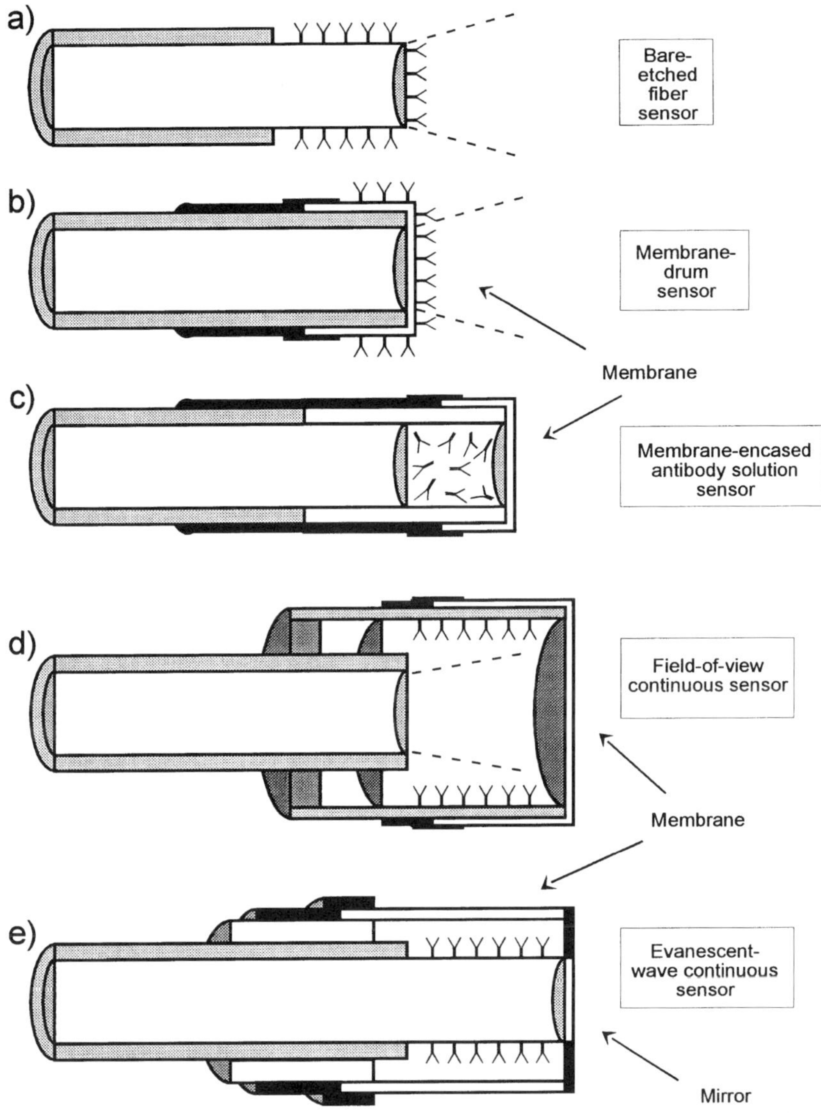

FIGURE 17.12 Several configurations for fiberoptics immunosensor probe.

or ion exchange in the substrate surface.[44-46] With either technique, the waveguide can additionally be patterned.

17.5.4 Flow-Injection Immunosensors

17.5.4.1 General Principle

The technique of affinity chromatography is well established in the field of preparative biochemistry.[47] It involves the specific interaction between an immobilized "ligand" with its complementary substance of interest. The binding on the solid phase enables separation of the desired species from its sample matrix. After all interfering compounds are washed off, the specifically bound molecules are released from the immobilized ligands by applying an eluting solution. Usually, this technique does not require any labeling since the purpose is a simple cleanup. Immunoaffinity chromatography can serve as an analytical rather than a

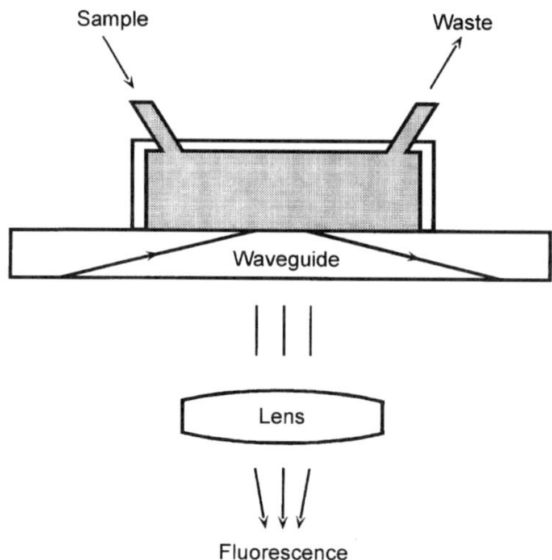

FIGURE 17.13 Construction of a TIRF-based sensor.

cleanup method. In contrast to the large volume (in the milliliter range) of preparative affinity columns, useful volumes of analytical columns are in the 50 to 500 µl range.

By combining such a miniaturized column, the immunoreactor, with flow-injection analysis (FIA), another variation of an immunosensor is obtained. Since the affinity column can be remote from any detector, this method is immunochromatography with on- or postcolumn detection. A very general setup of a reactor-based flow-injection immunoanalysis (FIIA) is shown in Figure 17.14. Establishing an FIA system is especially suitable when a high degree of automation is desired. Usually, FIIAs have a throughput between 1 to 60 samples per hour, depending on the immunochemical assay setup and the affinity constants of the immunoreactants involved.

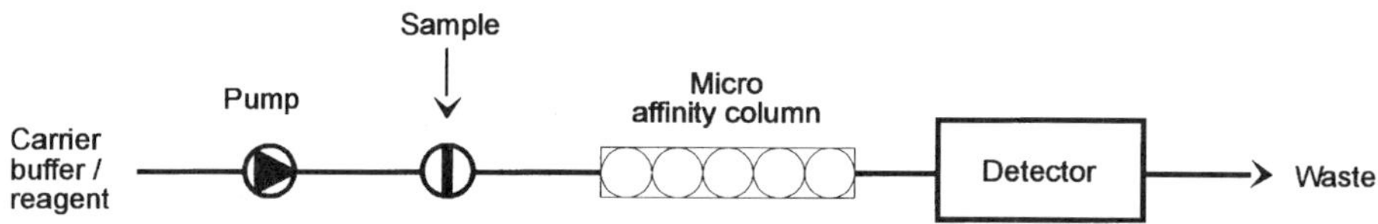

FIGURE 17.14 General setup of a flow-injection immunoanalysis (FIIA) system.

17.5.4.2 Solid Supports for Immunoreactors

In general, any kind of solid support employing immobilized antibodies or antigens/haptens is suitable for an FIIA immunoreactor. According to experiences of conventional chromatography, carrier particles trapped in a column are most common. Usually the particle sizes are in the micrometer to submillimeter range, since conventional FIA pumps, unlike HPLC pumps, do not operate under high pressure. These beads are either porous or nonporous. Examples for useful carrier beads for covalent immobilization are agarose, Sepharose, polyacrylamide, trisacryl, oxirane acrylic beads, or controlled pore glass. A good description of immobilization methods on various materials is given by Dean et al.[47] Latex or polystyrene beads as nonporous particles are less widely used. Due to their smaller surface, their loading capacity is too low for affinity chromatography. For FIIA however, they are suitable since they are available in various sizes and functionalities. Also latex beads with magnetic cores are available which allows the use of a magnet rather than a column to keep the particles localized. Nonfunctionalized beads have adsorptive properties similar to polystyrene ELISA plates, thus immobilzation conditions can easily be adapted to this carrier. Another approach is the membrane-type reactor, utilizing either adsorptive or covalent ligand immobilization on carriers such as (nitro)cellulose or immunodyne membranes.

17.5.4.3 Elution and Detection

Since on-column fluorescence detection is inconvenient due to light scattering by the particles and illumination of only a few layers of beads, postcolumn detection is the approach of choice. For chemiluminescence-based FIIA, however, on-column luminescence detection is more feasible due to the lack of an excitation light source.

For postcolumn fluorescence detection, labeled molecules have to be released from the beads during the assay. Two general approaches are possible. As is shown in Figure 17.5, labeled antigens can be simply displaced from the solid-phase antibody by adding free analyte molecules in a sample. The number of fluorescent molecules that are detected downstream is proportional to the concentration of free antigens in the sample solution. An eluant to remove all bound molecules from the column is not required and the antibody binding sites only need to be saturated with a fresh portion of labels after a measurement. Alternatively, the column volume can be increased to serve as a reservoir to which samples are repeatedly injected without intermediate regeneration.

The second approach is to perform a competitive type assay and to elute all bound species subsequently. This elution is at the same time the regeneration for the next determination. One class of suitable eluants are acidic solutions (0.1 M HCl, propionic acid, glycine-HCl pH 1.5–3.0) or bases (0.1 M NaOH). Lowering the polarity by adding organic solvents (dioxane, ethylene glycol) is another means of disrupting the binding. Very effective is elution with high salt concentrations (4 to 8 M urea or guanidine hydrochloride) to dissociate the antibody-antigen complex. Some anions are strongly disruptive and therefore referred to as chaotropic ions, e.g., Cl^-, I^-, ClO_4^-, SCN^-. All these eluants elute nonspecifically adsorbed molecules as well. Therefore, especially when strong eluants are applied, nonspecific binding during the assay has to be minimized. With porous beads, this is sometimes critical. Also, the nature of the label, the stability of the ligand, or the ruggedness of the solid matrix determine the choice of the eluant. Some fluorophores suffer from quenching in several media, while some eluants denature the immobilized antibodies. In general, a matrix with low NSB and an easy, covalent coupling method is preferred. Elution should be avoided if possible. Controlled pore glass (CPG) as a carrier for immunoreactors seems to be disadvantageous for elution approaches due to the high degree of nonspecific adsorption and the general slight solubility of glass in buffers above pH 7. However, this does not interfere with the use of CPG in biotechnology for enzyme immobilization.

For luminescence-based systems, column regeneration is necessary for further measurements only, but not for detection itself which can be performed on-column. However, for this mode of detection the design of the (now transparent) immunoreactor is more critical, since the use of particles will yield scattering of emitted light. Therefore, membrane-based transparent reactors offer an alternative.

Specific differences in the reactor capacity may require a replacement of particles or the membrane after each measurement. Due to the lower specific surface area, a membrane-based reactor will require immediate or at least frequent replacement. Also, most membrane-type FIIAs cannot operate without enzymatically enhanced fluorescence. The number of fluorophores that can bind to the relatively small surface area of a membrane is insufficient to generate a higher fluorescence signal. The use of columns with a sufficient volume (200 to 500 μl) allows repeated measuring cycles without reloading when a replacement approach is utilized. If beads are to be replaced automatically between subsequent assay cycles, the use of magnetic polystyrene particles is convenient. Since they can be held in place simply by a magnetic field, not even a column is required. Also, the idea of operating several columns in parallel for higher sample throughput is feasible. In many cases, incorporation of a stopped-flow interval into the flow-injection protocol is required. Depending on the actual antibody affinity, replacement or competitive binding cannot be achieved by simply lowering the buffer flow speed.

In general, once suitable carrier beads, fluorophores, eluants, FIIA protocols, detectors, etc. are chosen for a special application, parameters can in principle be adapted to the determination of other analytes. However, individual differences in antibody affinity or label stability may require major changes in the assay conditions. Methods suitable for the determination of large proteins will strongly differ from those for the determination of small haptens. Also, for some clinical analytes a relatively insensitive method yielding a high detection limit may be feasible, whereas the same limit of detection may not be sufficient for an environmental analyte. Therefore the inherent limits of a system have to be evaluated and matched with the goal to be achieved with the special sensor.

17.6 APPLICATIONS OF FLUORIMETRIC IMMUNOSENSORS IN ENVIRONMENTAL AND CLINICAL ANALYSIS

17.6.1 Environmental Monitoring of Water and Soil Pollution

17.6.1.1 Fiberoptic Sensors for Pesticides

Since environmental regulations require monitoring of organic compounds, especially in water at the parts per billion level, methods applied to achieve this goal have to be very sensitive. Methods using fiberoptics combined with fluorescence detection have background fluorescence as an inherent barrier to low limits of detection. As was mentioned earlier, with the evanescent wave technique the signal-to-noise ratio can be increased by eliminating bulk fluorescence. Therefore the method of choice to determine, e.g., pesticides, involves evanescent wave fluorescence excitation.

A class of pesticides being target analytes of interest are triazine herbicides. Triazines have a low mammal toxicity but, in general, the presence of triazine herbicides in water or soil is an indicator for the likelihood of finding other pollutants. Since triazines are one of the most heavily used classes of agrochemicals, monitoring triazines is a means of spotting polluted water resources. Therefore, after developing the appropriate antibodies, many immunosensors for the determination of triazine herbicides have been described.

One approach combining evanescent wave excitation with triazine monitoring was described by Oroszlan et al.[48] Monoclonal anti-triazine antibodies were immobilized on a stripped, silanized quartz fiber and were competitively reacted with atrazine and an FITC-labeled atrazine derivative. The excitation source was a xenon lamp equipped with interference filters; the detector consisted of a photodiode. By replacing fibers after each determination a calibration curve from 0.1 to 10 μg/l could be obtained. The intrabatch variation of the individual fibers in terms of signal reproducibility was shown to be less than 5%. A major advantage of this evanescent wave sensor setup was that even crude, colored soil extracts with significant fluorescence at the wavelength of the label FITC could be analyzed.

Instead of disposing of the fiber after each measurement, Bier et al. presented a regenerable evanescent wave immunosensor for the triazine herbicide terbutryn.[49] A triazine derivative was immobilized on the stripped, silanized fiber. FITC-labeled monoclonal antibodies served as labels in a competitive type assay format involving simultaneous incubation of the triazine sample. After each measurement the binding between the labeled antibodies and the immobilized hapten was disrupted by acidic glycine-HCl buffer alone or additional incubation with proteinase. The detection limit was 0.1 μg/l for terbutryn, and the same fiber could be reused 200 times, thus fulfilling an important requirement for quasi-continuous monitoring.

Wong et al. described a reusable fiberoptic immunosensor for the herbicide imazethapyr, a compound of the imidazolinone class.[50] The polyclonal sheep anti-imazethapyr antibodies were immobilized on the fiber core and used for two assay modes. One assay mode, referred to as the association approach, involved competitive incubation of fluorescein hydrazino methylene imazethapyr (FHMI) and the unlabeled herbicide. The increase of fluorescence was inversely proportional to the concentration of imazethapyr in the sample solution. For the dissociation approach, the antibodies were saturated with FHMI, which was subsequently partially replaced by imazethapyr. Here, an initially high fluorescence signal was decreased during displacement, the decrease being directly proportional to the analyte concentration. With the latter approach an enormously extended dynamic range of 6 orders of magnitude (10^{-3} to 10^{-9} M) was achieved with both buffered imazethapyr solutions and soil extracts. The replacement approach yielded a 100-fold lower limit of detection than the competitive association. Due to the reversibility of binding of both FHMI and the analyte, regeneration of the sensor surface could be achieved by simply applying PBS buffer solution for more than 20 min.

Anis et al. and Rogers et al. demonstrated a fiberoptic evanescent wave sensor for the determination of the insecticide parathion, which is highly toxic to mammals due to metabolic conversion to the oxygen analogue paraoxon.[51,52] The principle was to perform a competitive immunoassay on the surface of a quartz glass fiber using adsorptively immobilized parathion-protein conjugates. The assay consisted of three consecutive incubations performed in a flow cell. In the competitive step a nonmodified polyclonal parathion antibody and parathion were incubated with the fiber. After blocking empty surface sites with casein, a secondary, FITC-labeled antibody was introduced and the fluorescence signal was read. With this approach, a detection limit of 0.3 ppb parathion was achieved. The oxygen analogue only cross-reacted at very high concentrations. A disadvantage of this sensor is the use of two antibodies, which requires additional reagents and a more complex flow-injection protocol.

A preliminary study for the determination of pyrethroid pesticides described by Northrup et al. also used the evanescent wave principle.[53] Pyrethroid derivatives coupled to BSA were immobilized on the fiber core. The binding of fluorescamine-labeled monoclonal anti-pyrethroid antibodies to the fiber-immobilized haptens was studied in a noncompetitive approach.

17.6.1.2 Flow-Injection Immunoanalysis (FIIA) for Triazine Herbicides and Explosives

As was mentioned earlier, a fiberoptic-based immunosensor needs either to be regenerated after each measurement or the fiber has to be replaced. Using a new fiber each time is costly, but regeneration is time-consuming, lowers the sample throughput, and may denature the immobilized compounds. Additionally, with fiberoptic sensors, intrabatch variation of the surface preparation is critical. Therefore, sensors based on affinity columns filled with batch-immobilized particles are an alternative. Many recent publications are based on the replacement approach, mostly taking advantage of the reservoir a column provides.

An affinity-column based FIIA for the determination of triazine herbicides was presented by Wortberg et al.[54] Here, an Eu(III)-chelate conjugated to monoclonal anti-triazine antibodies served as fluorescent label. Oxirane acrylic beads as the solid carrier particles were subsequently reacted with poly-L-lysine and a functionalized triazine derivative. On one hand this preimmobilization of poly-L-lysine provided a large number of amino groups for attachment of the carboxyfunctionalized atrazine derivative. On the other hand the bulky protein blocked smaller pores, which helped to minimize nonspecific binding. Prior to the measurement the haptens were loaded with the Eu(III)-chelate-labeled antibodies. After analyte injection the flow was stopped for 20 min to allow replacement of labeled antibodies. The postcolumn fluorescence detector, especially designed for Eu(III)-chelates, consisted of a pulsed nitrogen laser (337.1 nm excitation wavelength) and a photomultiplier equipped with an interference filter and an integrator connected to the laser trigger. Since the Stokes shift between excitation and fluorescence at 613 nm was extremely large, background interference was greatly reduced.

The linear range of the calibration curve for atrazine was three orders of magnitude with a limit of detection of 1 μg/l and a CV of <10%. Figure 17.15 shows part of a calibration curve. The oxirane acrylic beads were stable for at least 2 weeks at room temperature.

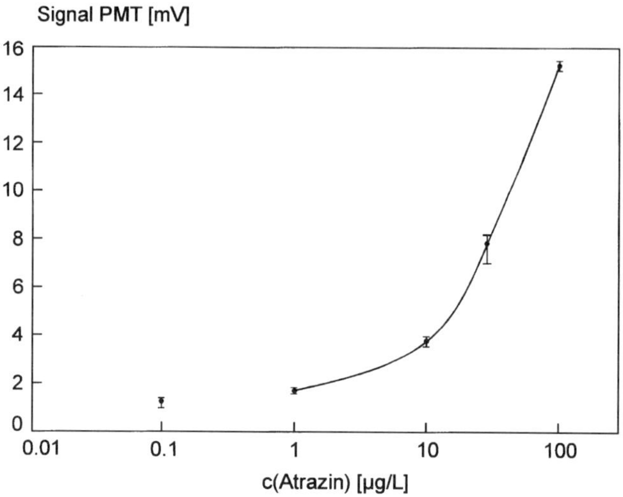

FIGURE 17.15 Part of a calibration curve for atrazin. (From Wortberg, M. et al., *Anal. Chim. Acta*, 289, 177, 1994. With permission.)

Atrazine determination with a membrane-based FIIA was described by Krämer and Schmid.[55] This system was based on enzymatic conversion of the nonfluorescent substrate hydroxypropionic acid (HPPA) to a fluorescent product. Polyclonal anti-atrazine antibodies were immobilized on a Pall immunodyne membrane that was exchanged after each assay. In a nonequilibrium assay mode involving stopped flow, atrazine and atrazine-labeled horseradish peroxidase were reacted subsequently with the membrane-bound antibodies. After HPPA was added, a fluorescence signal was measured. With this approach the cycle time was less than 7 min, yielding a calibration curve with a very low limit of detection and a dynamic concentration range of 0.02 to 0.3 μg/l. However, the coefficient of variation (CV) was observed to be 10 to 40%, significantly higher than the CV of the respective ELISA performed with the same enzyme label.

Monitoring explosives is an important issue in aircraft safety. As an example, an FIIA for the explosive trinitrotoluene (TNT) based on the replacement principle was recently presented by Whelan et al.[56] The method developed was based on previous investigations with 2,4-dinitrophenol as a model hapten by Kusterbeck et al.[57] Monoclonal anti-TNT antibodies were immobilized on tresyl chloride-activated Sepharose® 4B. The antibody binding sites were saturated with a hapten-fluorophore conjugate prior to the assay. The conjugate consisted of FITC-modified cadaverin to which a TNT derivative was coupled. To simulate the presence of explosives in air, TNT vapors were generated on board a sealed airplane and collected into distilled water. The samples were run with GC-ECD in parallel to verify the data given by the immunosensor. With the present FIIA configuration a linear calibration curve with a range of 20 to 1200 μg/l could be obtained. Since the 200 to 500 μl reactor provided a reservoir of labeled molecules, it could be used for 10 to 50 subsequent measurements of TNT-positive samples without reloading. Interestingly, the sensitivity increased when, e.g., ethanol was added to the assay buffer. This was ascribed to the enhanced fluorescence of FITC in this solution compared to purely aqueous buffers.

The same replacement FIIA principle was applied to the determination of the drug of abuse cocaine, using also an FITC-labeled hapten preloaded to a Sepharose column.[58,59] Here the detection limit was 5 μg/l with an assay cycle time of less than 1 min.

17.6.2 Clinical Analysis

17.6.2.1 Planar Optical Devices

One example of a commercial optical immunosensor is the Fluorescent Capillary Fill Device (FCFD) which was first presented by Badley et al.[43] This evanescent wave-based disposable immunosensor incorporates a novel capillary fill design. The system consists of two small glass plates which are separated by a narrow gap of 100 μm. Figure 17.16 shows the principle of the FCFD. The lower plate acts as an optical waveguide and contains on its surface a layer of immobilized antibodies. Due to capillary forces, a fixed volume of a sample is drawn into the space between the plates regardless of the actual sample volume, e.g., a blood droplet. Thus, volume errors are automatically avoided. The immunosensing format involves either a competitive or a sandwich-type assay. For the competitive format, the upper plate contains on its surface a layer of fluorescently labeled analyte molecules trapped in a water-soluble matrix. For the sandwich approach labeled secondary antibodies are embedded in the matrix. On addition of the analyte the labels are released into the sample solution, thereby competing for antibody binding sites with the analye or forming a sandwich complex, respectively. After a fixed incubation period the fluorescence signal generated by fluorophores specifically bound to the lower plate is measured. The optical setup ensures discrimination of bound from free fluorophores.

To overcome the inherent problem of quality control of a single-use device, in a more recent approach the device was patterned into discrete regions.[41] Assuming that lateral diffusion takes much longer than the binding equilibrium between the immunoreactants, two separated reference zones were incorporated in the chip. One zone did not contain fluorophores and therefore monitored matrix fluorescence effects, whereas in the second reference zone nonspecific binding of fluorophores to a "neutral" antibody was observed. The FCFD has been applied to various clinical parameters such as estrone-3-gluconuride, human chorionic gonadotrophin (hCG), and opiates.[41,43,60] The performance of the device was tested in various biological matrices such as whole blood, serum, plasma, saliva, and urine. With the competitive assay format, morphine could be determined with a limit of detection of 300 ng/ml and a precision at the cut-off level with a CV between 10 to 15%.[41] The sandwich assay for hCG yielded a limit of detection of 50 mIU/ml.[60]

The advantage of the system is that all reagents are contained in the chip. Additionally, the automatic filling of the gap avoids volume errors. The FCFD is well suited as a hygienic single-use device for clinical analysis, but continuous monitoring is not possible. Also, calibration with real samples is critical. For highly viscous samples such as whole blood, the time required for filling of the gap and achieving equilibrium conditions takes longer than for other matrices. Additionally, filling volumes may change with changes in sample viscosity.

The use of an indium phosphate waveguide on top of a glass substrate was demonstrated by Sloper et al. for the determination of hCG. In this sensor, the glassy metal film deposited by spin-coating and baked in a low-temperature process served as the light guide, onto which monoclonal anti-hCG antibodies were immobilized.[44] To perform a sandwich-type assay, hCG-spiked horse serum was preequilibrated with QFITC-labeled monoclonal anti-hCG antibodies and then applied to the chip in a single assay step. Equilibrium binding was achieved after 5 min, the actual fluorescence reading was performed after 15 min by monitoring the fluorescence through the bottom of the glass slide. This low-cost disposable device yielded a limit of detection of 300 mIU (0.83 nM), being higher than the limit achieved with the FCFD. However, this sensor proved to be more sensitive than a noncoated glass slide which was used for evanescent wave excitation via multiple internal reflections.[44]

In contrast to the disposable sensors described above, a regenerable planar waveguide chip for the clinical analyte theophylline was presented by Choquette et al.[42] Here, the

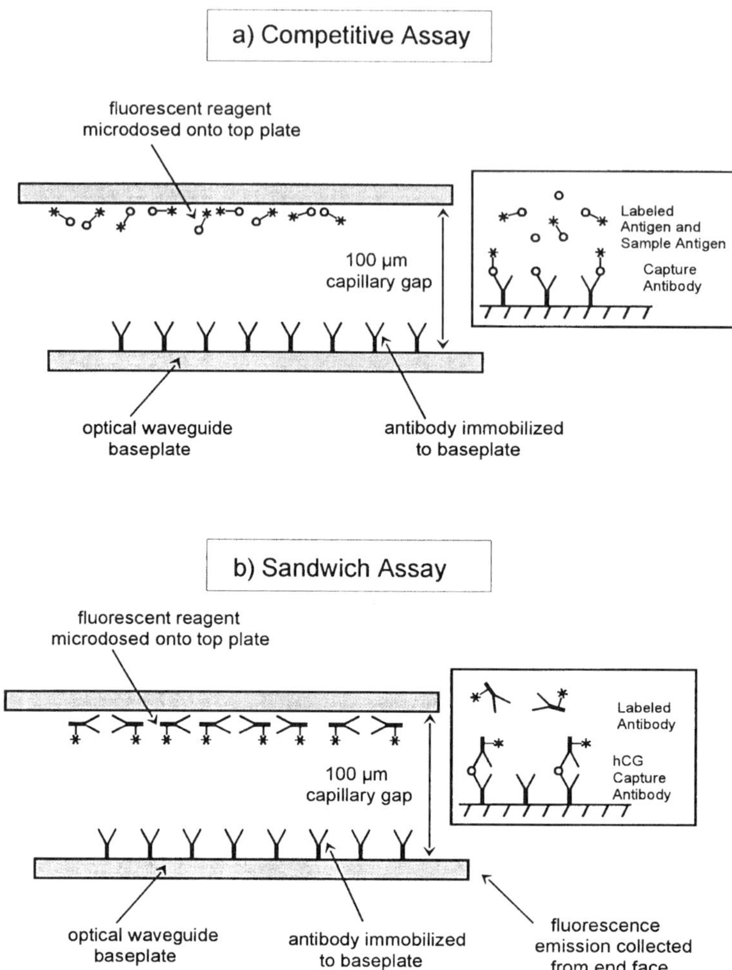

FIGURE 17.16 Schematic diagram of the fluorescence capillary-fill device (FCFD): (a) for competition, and (b) for the sandwich assay, e.g., for human chorionic gonadotropin (hCG).

light-guiding layer was prepared by a silver ion-diffusion process performed on the surface of a glass slide. The chip was integrated into a flow-injection setup with a fiberoptic-based fluorometer for signal reading. A special feature of this sensor was liposome amplification: the fluorescent dye carboxyfluoresceine was entrapped in phospholipid vesicles that were further modified with theophylline derivatives attached to phospholipids.[61] These liposomes were used as tracers in a competitive binding format. Anti-theophylline antibodies were covalently immobilized to the silanized waveguide. After competitive binding the liposomes were disrupted by applying 1-*O*-octyl-β-D-glucopyranoside (OG) to release fluorophores. Since the immobilized antibodies had only moderate affinity to theophylline and to the tracer, regeneration was achieved by rinsing the sensor surface in buffer stream for 20 min. The limit of detection was approximately 5×10^{-9} M theophylline and the sensor response was linear for 1.5 orders of magnitude. After 15 regenerations the sensor signal decreased, which was suggested to be primarily due to physical loss of proteins from the waveguide.

17.6.2.2 Fiberoptic Sensors for Proteins and Drugs

The clinically important human enzyme creatine kinase (CK) was determined fiberoptically using a sandwich-type approach.[40] Monoclonal antibodies were immobilized on fused silica fiber rods of 1 mm diameter. Prior to the determination, creatine kinase was mixed with B-phycoerythrin-labeled antibodies. The second monoclonal antibody was specific to a different antigen determinand than the first one. After 15 min incubation time the fluorescence signal was recorded. The limit of detection was 10^{-12} M or 0.1 ng/ml CK and therefore useful for the clinically relevant range of 2 to 50 ng/ml.

Self-contained fiberoptic systems for the determination of the anticonvulsant drug phenytoin based on homogeneous fluorescence energy transfer were described by Anderson and Miller[62] and by Astles and Miller.[63,64] B-phycoerythrin-labeled phenytoin and Texas red labeled monoclonal antibodies were sealed inside a dialysis tubing mounted on the tip of a single fiber. An Ar^+ laser served as the excitation source. While the labeled phenytoin was bound to the labeled antibodies, the fluorescence of the donor B-phycoerythrin was quenched by the acceptor Texas red. When free analyte molecules diffused into the dialysis tubing, they competed for binding sites. The release of labeled phenytoin from the antibodies generated a fluorescence signal since the energy transfer decreased. Therefore, the sensor response was directly proportional to the analyte concentration. Both whole antibodies and Fab fragments yielded good results. The sensor was applicable for the clinically important range of 1 to 20 μM phenytoin, and in latest investigations the measurement was performed in whole blood and serum.[64]

Another interesting approach was based on reduced fluorescence quenching in the presence of haptens as analytes.[65,66] The principle of this immunosensor was to covalently immobilize antibody fragments on a quartz plate mounted onto the tip of a bifurcated fiber and to subsequently label the fragments with the fluorophore dansyl chloride. The unique property of dansyl is a strong fluorescence quenching in aqueous media. Thus, in the initial sensor state the dansyl fluorescence is quenched and only a low background signal is recorded. However, when antigen molecules bind to the immobilized antibody fragments, the fluorophore dansyl is shielded from its aqueous environment and the fluorescence signal increases. Using human albumin as a model for a large antigen molecule and theophylline, digoxin, and phenytoin as small haptens, the working principle was demonstrated. With the albumin sensor the same fiber could be regenerated up to 50 times before the signal decreased. The limit of detection for albumin was 1.2 μg/ml. The sensor for the haptens had a shorter shelf life. The main achievement of this technique is the realization of a reagent-free sensor. Since no additional compounds are required for analysis this approach is especially useful as a potential *in vivo* application in clinical analysis.

17.6.2.3 Fiberoptic Immunosensors for Carcinogens

Polynuclear aromatic compounds (PNA) such as benzo(a)pyrene (BaP) are byproducts of the incomplete combustion of organic matter. BaP is known to metabolize in humans to the reactive intermediate which forms DNA adducts, thereby gaining its carcinogenic potential.[67] Therefore, monitoring BaP as an indicator of exposure to carcinogens is of interest in the field of cancer research.

Vo-Dinh et al. demonstrated a fiberoptic immunosensor for BaP.[35,68] Since BaP as a polyaromatic hydrocarbon has fluorescent properties, no fluorescent label was needed for this sensor. In the initial version, polyclonal anti-BaP antibodies were covalently immobilized onto the tip of a single fused silica fiber. To excite the BaP fluorescence, an HeCd laser (325 nm) was used. The fiber was simply placed in a 5-μl drop of analyte solution for 10 min. After rinsing the fiber, the fluorescence signal was measured which was directly proportional to the BaP concentration in the sample solution. The absolute detection limit was 10^{-15} mol per droplet or 2×10^{-8} mol/l. The advantages of this sensor setup are its self-confinement and the obviation of additional reagents.

Using the technique of phase-resolved fluorescence detection the authors could distinguish BaP from its DNA adduct BaP-tetrole.[69] For this approach a microcavity was mounted on the fiber tip. The cavity was filled with anti-BaP antibodies prior to each measurement and sealed with a dialysis membrane. The probe was dipped into a BaP or BaP-tetrole solution to allow analyte molecules to diffuse into the cavity. The probe then was removed and immersed into buffer solution, thereby washing off all nonbound BaP or interfering molecules. Thus, only fluorescence of specifically bound and therefore "trapped" BaP molecules inside the cavity was excited with the HeCd laser. The limit of detection with this homogeneous-type immunosensor was 5×10^{-10} M.

17.6.2.4 FIIA Systems for Theophylline, Transferrin, and Insulin

For the determination of the clinical analyte theophylline an approach using fluorescence enhancement by carboxyfluorescein-filled liposomes was presented by Locasio-Brown et al.[61,70] Anti-theophylline antibodies were covalently immobilized to silanized nonporous silica beads trapped in an affinity column. As was described above for the planar waveguide sensor, derivatized liposomes were used as tracers in a competitive binding format.[42] To disrupt the liposomes, 1-*O*-octyl-β-D-glucopyranoside (OG) or KSCN was used. The fluorescence was detected downstream after a total assay time of 15 min. When using the denaturing KSCN solution, the fluorescence signal was quenched dramatically and also a severe decrease in antibody affinity occurred, whereas no quenching was observed with OG. The linear dynamic range of the calibration curve was found to be between 3×10^{-5} to 3×10^{-8} M theophylline. Since this is more sensitive than required for clinical analysis, the serum samples tested had to be diluted 1:400. Using OG as eluant, the same columns were stable for more than 270 consecutive measurements in an interval of 3 months. This excellent lifetime indicates that the relatively limited reusability of the waveguide sensor which was developed in the same group using the same reagents is a function of the immobilization rather than antibody stability.[42]

Palmer et al. demonstrated the determination of transferrin using a controlled porous glass (CPG) reactor with immobilized protein A.[71] Lucifer yellow served as a pH-independent fluorescent label with a larger Stokes shift than FITC. PH independence of the label fluorescence was necessary because the FIIA was based on elution with an acidic buffer. The assay involved binding of a specific sheep antibody to the beads followed by competitive binding of transferrin and labeled transferrin. For downstream detection the column was flushed with citrate buffer pH 2.5 and could be reused up to 60 times since the reactor had a high protein A loading. Although the nonspecific background signal was relatively high, being about 25% B/Bo even when the highest analyte concentrations were applied, the limit of detection was 25 mg/l which is sufficient for the clinically relevant range of this analyte.

Protein G immobilized on agarose was employed in a monitoring system for insulin as described by Khokhar et al.[72] The immunoreactands anti-insulin antibodies, insulin, and rhodamine-labeled insulin, were mixed prior to injection into the FIIA system. After competitive binding and washing off the excess material, an acidic elution buffer also containing the detergent Triton® X was used, similar to the previous examples. For samples containing 50 pg/ml insulin the RSD was only 4%.

17.6.3 Other Applications

17.6.3.1 Bioprocess Monitoring

An FIIA for bioprocess monitoring which did not require labeling at all was presented by Stöcklein et al.[73] The idea was to monitor the expression of monoclonal antibodies in cell culture fluid. Oxirane acrylic beads served as a support for immobilized protein A or anti-mouse IgG. Monoclonal mouse antibodies present in the culture fluid were bound to the affinity column in a noncompetitive way. Subsequently they were eluted with citrate buffer pH 2.5–3 and the natural protein fluorescence at 340 nm was measured. With protein A the calibration curve ranged from 1 to 200 μg/ml antibody, whereas with anti-mouse IgG the curve shifted to 75 to 400 μg/ml IgG. The oxirane beads were reusable up to 1000 times.

In a previous version, bioprocess monitoring was performed using anti-mouse antibodies immobilized on membranes or magnetic beads.[74] Using either a competitive or noncompetitive assay format, peroxidase-labeled anti-mouse antibodies served as labeled species. Fluorescent molecules were generated by substrate conversion of HPPA. The sandwich approach required a 25-min assay time, whereas the competitive assay could be performed in only 10 min.

17.6.3.2 Model Analytes and Miscellaneous Methods

A novel type of a quasi-continuously working fiberoptic immunosensor was described by Barnard and Walt.[4] It was based on the slow release of two fluorophores which were entrapped separately in a polymer matrix attached to the fiber tip. The idea was to monitor the fluorescence energy transfer due to binding between a fluorescein-labeled anti-IgG and a Texas red-labeled IgG. Both immunoreagents constantly diffused into the small reaction chamber and a constant fluorescence signal was generated. When IgG was presented in the sample, less Texas red-labeled IgGs would bind to fluorescein-labeled anti-IgG antibodies, thus changing the fluorescence signal. The signal was measured as the ratio of two emission maxima. Using ethylvinylacetate copolymers as the slow release matrix, the sensor was continuously supplied with fresh reagents for a period of at least 30 days.

The concept was recently adapted to the determination of small molecules. It was demonstrated for atrazine using FITC-labeled anti-atrazine antibodies and rhodamine-labeled atrazine-protein conjugates or atrazine-rhodamine conjugates, respectively.[75]

A fiberoptic sensor based on time-resolved fluorescence of Eu(III)-chelates was described by Petrea et al.[76] The primarily nonfluorescent Eu-chelate was linked to IgG, which served as the model analyte. To measure the fluorescence, the fiber tip was subsequently dipped into the sample solution containing the labeled analytes, rinsed, and immersed into the enhancement solution. In the enhancement solution the Eu(III)-chelate was converted into highly fluorescent Eu-complex which could be excited with an excimer laser at 308 nm. Using the model protein IgG a limit of detection of 0.1 μg/ml was achieved.

A system for the model protein human albumin involving evanescent wave detection was described by Eenink et al.[77] Anti-human albumin antibodies were immobilized on the silanized fiber, which was further blocked with bovine albumin prior to the assay. The fluorophore used for labeling the antigen human albumin was rhodamine B which was excited with a HeNe laser as light source. However, this assay did not involve competitive binding, therefore only the detection limit for the labeled compound was given (10^{-9} M or 0.06 mg/l).

Zhou et al. demonstrated the application of a potassium exchanged, buried planar waveguide as a wash-free evanescent wave fluoroimmunosensor.[15,16] The waveguide was covered and patterned with a photoresist to create separate microwells which were accessible by the evanescent wave.[46] To monitor specific vs. nonspecific binding, anti-rat IgG coupled to FITC as a model analyte was reacted with several species IgG and proteins, each immobilized in a separate well. By partly blackening the bottom of the chip, fluorescence excited in the wells could be monitored separately by scanning with a PMT. The patterned waveguide offers the advantage of internal background correction or even a calibration at the same time a sample is analyzed. However, this device is not reusable.

A simple nonmodified planar quartz waveguide was used for IgG determination by Lu et al.[78] The aim was to develop a reusable instead of a disposable system based on immobilized antibodies, thus several regenerating agents were tested. The eluants diethylamine, glycine-HCl, propionic acid, and ethylene glycol resulted in similar remaining antibody activities. The application of chemo- and bioluminescent markers is mostly demonstrated for IgG as a model analyte. One example is reported by Osipov et al. who used 6 mm polystyrene beads for antibody immobilization and peroxidase-labeled antibodies competing with unlabeled IgG.[79] However, the beads had to be transferred into the detection cell where they were reacted with luminol, iodophenol, and hydrogen peroxide to generate luminescence.

A sandwich assay for IgG using a membrane-type reactor and peroxidase-labeled secondary antibodies was demonstrated by Liu et al.[80] Here the light was directly collected from a transparent flow cell. After acidic regeneration the membranes were reusable for 2 more determinations, yielding a limit of detection of 1 fmol (10^{-15} mol) absolute in an 8-min assay cycle. A method using acridinium esters as labels instead of an enzyme has been developed by Shellum and Güblitz.[81] In a transparent flow cell a two-site (sandwich) immunoassay for mouse IgG was performed. Although the assay protocol required extreme pH change, from initiating chemiluminescence at pH 12.7 to regeneration at pH 1.8, the trisalkyl beads with covalently immobilized anti-mouse IgG were stable for 1 week. Since acridinium ester luminescence has a half life of only 0.9 s, luminescence was initiated in front of the PMT and the emitted light was directly collected from the 20-µl immunoreactor. Depending on the flow rates, the assay cycle lasted from 10 to 18 min, yielding a limit of detection of 500 to 50 atto mol mouse IgG in a 20-µl sample volume.

A fiberoptic system for the protein human albumin based on chemiluminescence detection was reported by Hara et al.[82] Human albumin was determined in competitive and noncompetitive fashion, using anti-human albumin antibodies immobilized on the tip of a fiber. The label, attached to either human albumin or the secondary antibody, was a catalytic metal complex, iron(III)2,9,16,23-tetrakis(chlorocarbonyl)phthalocyanine (TCCP-Fe(III)). This complex accelerates the chemiluminescence reaction between luminol and hydrogen peroxide and therefore replaces an enzyme. Chemiluminescence was immediately monitored with a photon counter. Since regeneration of the fiber surface with acidic solution (pH 2.3) reduced the signal in the following determination, a newly prepared fiber was used for each measurement. With the competitive approach the limit of detection for albumin was 0.1 mg/ml, whereas the sandwich approach was ten times more sensitive.

17.7 SUMMARY

To give a summerized overview of the variety of analytes as well as the variety of possible approaches to fluorimetric immunosensors, Table 17.3 lists the sensors presented in this chapter. Clinical analytes such as drugs, hormones, and proteins and organic environmental pollutants such as pesticides are the compounds of major interest. The most widely used fluorophore is still FITC, although numerous other "more sophisticated" fluorescent dyes are available.

The two dominating technical approaches are (1) evanescent wave-based planar or fiberoptic systems, and (2) affinity column-based flow-through systems with postcolumn fluorescence detection. The reusability of a device as well as self containment are important issues in the development of most fluorimetric immunosensors.

17.8 CONCLUSIONS

The field of immunosensing has been rapidly expanding in the last few years and offers powerful tools for detecting chemicals and studying biological systems. Several areas that will benefit from the development of immunosensors include biomedical applications, environmental monitoring, process control, defense, biotechnology, food quality control, and

TABLE 17.3
Overview of Fluorimetric Immunosensors Reported in This Chapter

Analyte	Principle	Label	LOD	Remarks	Ref.
Albumin	Fiberoptic, direct excitation	Metal-complex + luminol/H_2O_2	0.1 mg/ml	Chemiluminescence-based Disposable	82
Albumin	Fiberoptic, direct excitation	Dansyl chloride	1 μg/ml	50 × reusable	65,66
Atrazine	Fiberoptic, evanescent wave	FITC	0.1 μg/l	Disposable	47
Atrazine	FIIA, membrane reactor	HRP/HPPA	0.02 μg/l	Enzyme enhancement disposable membrane	55
Atrazine	FIIA, affinity column	Eu(III)-chelate	1 μg/l	Stable >2 weeks at room temp.	54
Benzo(a)-pyrene	Fiberoptic, direct excitation	Fluorescent analyte	$5 \cdot 10^{-10}$ M	Homogeneous	69
Cocaine	FIIA, affinity column	FITC	5 μg/l	Regenerable	58,59
Creatine Kinase	Fiberoptic, evanescent wave	Phycoerythrin	0.1 ng/ml (10^{-12}M)	—	40
hCG	Planar waveguide Evanescent wave (FCFD)	FITC	$1.4 \cdot 10^{-10}$M	Disposable	60
hCG	Planar waveguide Evanescent wave	FITC	$8.3 \cdot 10^{-10}$M	Disposable	44
IgG	FIIA, membrane reactor	HRP, luminol/ iodophenol/H_2O_2	10^{-15}M	Enzyme enhancement, 3 × reusable	80
IgG	FIIA, affinity column	Acridinium ester	$2.5 \cdot 10^{-12}$M	Chemiluminescence-based	81
IgG	Fiberoptic, direct excitation	Eu(III)-chelate	0.1 μg/ml	Enhancement required	76
IgG	FIIA, affinity column	Protein fluorescence	1 μg/ml	1000 × reusable	73
IgG	Fiberoptic, direct excitation, energy transfer	FITC + Texas red	Not reported	Polymer release sensor, self-contained >30 days homogeneous	4
Imazethapyr	Fiberoptic, evanescent wave	Fluorescein derivative	10^{-9} M	Dynamic range 6 orders of magnitude, reusable	50
Insulin	FIIA, affinity chromatography	Rhodamine isothiocyanate	0.05 ng/ml	Reusable	72
Parathion	Fiberoptic, evanescent wave	Fluorescein derivative	0.3 μg/l	Sandwich assay	51,52
Phenytoin	Fiberoptic, direct excitation, energy transfer	Phycoerythrin + Texas red	10^{-6} M	Homogeneous, self-contained	62–64
Terbutryn	Fiberoptic, evanescent wave	FITC	0.1 μg/l	200 × reusable	49
Theophylline	Planar waveguide, evanescent wave	Carboxyfluorescein	$5 \cdot 10^{-9}$ M	Liposome enhancement, reusable	42
Theophylline	FIIA, affinity column	Carboxyfluorescein	$3 \cdot 10^{-8}$ M	Liposome enhancement, >270 × reusable	61, 70
TNT	FIIA, affinity column	FITC	20 μg/l	10–50 × reusable	56
Transferrin	FIIA, affinity column	Lucifer yellow	25 mg/l	60 × reusable	71

agriculture. In this context fluorimetric immunosensors have been promoted due to several advantages.

Fluorimetric immunosensors are well suited to the analysis of trace contaminants in environmental samples due to their high sensitivity, especially compared to direct immunosensors. Compared to the immunoassays using an enzyme label, the fluorescence dye is much more stable and guarantees a shelf life of several years. Sensitivity reported for fiberoptic immunosensors is in the 10^{-8} to 10^{-12} M range. These devices require very small sample volumes (40 nl to a few microliters) to detect attomole amounts (10^{-18} M) of toxic chemicals and related biomarkers for monitoring environmental exposure and human health.

An advantage is the elimination of matrix interferences by laser-induced time-resolved spectroscopy. Time-resolved fluoroimmunoassay (TR-FrIA) using lanthanide chelates as labels has already gained wide acceptance in a variety of routine clinical and research applications. Although the ultimate sensitivity of the assays is determined by antibody affinity, increased sensitivity afforded by new labels allows detection in the femtomolar and attomolar (10^{-15} and 10^{-18} M) range. The possibility of carrying out fluorimetric analysis with two or three different time domains could be exploited in multianalyte imaging studies.

The development of new, very near IR (VNIR) fluorophores (780 to 1100 nm), and further advances in solid-state light sources and detectors, will certainly expand the use of VNIR methods instead of the UV-visible fluorophores used at present. Especially, the signal-to-noise-ratio with biological samples will be drastically improved because no biological compound is fluorescent in this region. Together with newly developed "humanized" antibody F_{ab} fragments an optical tumor marker device is possible since this is the "open wavelength window" of biological tissue. Such an "optical tomography" would be able to localize deviations within the tissue as small as 0.1 mm, thus being of great benefit for the health care business. In the near future most conventional lasers or even less sophisticated incoherent light sources will be replaced by semiconductor lasers.

There is no doubt that all steps leading to real-time monitoring of intermolecular interactions are of advantage. The available optical and opto-electronic systems like BIAcore (Pharmacia Biosensor AB, Uppsala, Sweden and Piscataway, NJ), IAsys (Fisons Applied Sensor Technology, Cambridge, U.K.), and BIOS-1 (Artificial Sensing Instruments, Zürich, Switzerland) are more costly than the fluorimetric sensors and mainly designed for research labs. Using the displacement principle, fluorimetric immunosensors also can cope with the problem and reach "near real time" measurements, i.e., they give the result of displacement within minutes.

Finally, fluorimetric immunosensors have proved to be practical — and this is the best argument one can find for a sensor!

ABBREVIATIONS

Ab:	Antibody
Ab-Ag:	Antibody-antigen complex
Ag:	Antigen
α:	Acceptance angle
AP:	Alkaline phosphatase
ATS:	Aminopropyltriethoxysilane
B/B_0:	Binding relative to zero dose
BaP:	Benzo(a)pyrene
β-NTA:	β-Naphthoyltrifluoroacetone
BSA:	Bovine serum albumin
CK:	Creatine kinase
CL:	Chemiluminescence
CPG:	Controlled pore glass
CV:	Coefficient of variation
CW:	Continuous wave

Da:	Dalton, relative molecular weight unit
DNA:	Desoxyribonucleic acid
dp:	Characteristic penetration depth of the evanescent wave
DPASV:	Differential pulse anodic stripping voltammetry
DPP:	Differential pulse polarography
E:	Intensity of electric field
EDTA:	Ethylenediaminetetraacetic acid
EIA:	Enzyme immunoassay
ET:	Energy transfer
F_{ab}:	Fragment antigen binding
F_c:	Fragment crystallizing
FCFD:	Fluorescent capillary fill device
FHMI:	Fluorescein hydrazino methylene imazethapyr
FIA:	Flow-injection analysis
FIIA:	Flow-injection immunoanalysis
FIS:	Fiberoptic immunosensor
FITC:	Fluorescein isothiocyanate
FrIA:	Fluoroimmunoassay
GC-ECD:	Gas chromatography-electron capture detector
GOD:	Glucose oxidase
GOPS:	3-Glycidoxypropyl-trimethoxysilane
hCG:	Human chorionic gonadotrophin
HPLC:	High-performance liquid chromatography
HPPA:	Hydroxypropionic acid
HRP:	Horseradish peroxidase
IC:	Internal conversion
IgG:	Immunoglobulin G
IR:	Infrared
ISC:	Intersystem crossing
IUPAC:	International Union of Pure and Applied Chemistry
K:	Binding constant
KSCN:	Potassium thiocyanate
LIA:	Luminescence immunoassay
LOD:	Limit of detection
M_0:	Ground electronic state, metal ion
M_1:	Excited electronic state, metal ion
MTS:	Mercaptopropyltriethoxysilane
Mol wt:	Molecular weight
n_1:	Refractive index for core
n_2:	Refractive index for cladding
NIR:	Near infrared
NSB:	Nonspecific binding
OG:	1-*O*-octyl-β-D-glucopyranoside
PBS:	Phosphate-buffered saline
PD:	Photodiodes
PDT:	Photodynamic therapy
PMT:	Photomultiplier tube
PNA:	Polynuclear aromatic compounds
ppb:	Parts per billion
θ:	Critical angle
QFITC:	Quinolizino-substituted fluorescein isothiocyanate
R:	Chemically sensitive reagent

RIA: Radioimmunoassay
S_0: Ground electronic state
S_1: Excited electronic state
T: Triplet unpaired electron state
τ: Fluorescence lifetime
TCCP-Fe(III): Iron(III)2,9,16,23-tetrakis(chlorocarbonyl)phthalocyanine
TIRF: Total internal reflection fluorescence
TNT: Trinitrotoluene
TR-FrIA: Time-resolved fluoroimmunoassay
TR: Time-resolved
UV: Ultraviolet
VIS: Visible
VNIR: Very near infrared
VR: Vibrational relaxation
z: Distance into the rarer medium

REFERENCES

1. Yalow, R. S. and Berson, S. A., Immunoassay of endogeneous plasma insulin in man, *Nature*, 184, 1648, 1959.
2. Turner, A. P. F., Karube, I., and Wilson, G. S., *Biosensors. Fundamentals and Applications*, Oxford University Press, New York, 1989.
3. Hulanicki, A., Glab, S., and Ingman, F., IUPAC Discussion Paper, Commission V.I., July 1989.
4. Barnard, S. M. and Walt, D. R., Chemical sensors based on controlled release polymer systems, *Science*, 251, 927, 1991.
5. Stryer, L., *Biochemie,* Spectrum, New York, 1991, chap. 6.
6. Köhler, G. and Milstein, C., Continuous cultures of fused cells secreting antibodies of predefined specificity, *Nature*, 256, 495, 1975.
7. Tijssen, P., Practice and theory of enzyme immunoassay, in: *Laboratory Techniques in Biochemistry and Molecular Biology*, Burdon, R. H. and van Knippenberg, P. H., Eds., Elsevier, New York, 1990.
8. Hemmilä, I., *Application of Fluorescence in Immunoassays*, John Wiley & Sons, New York, 1991.
9. Hemmilä, I., Fluoroimmunoassays and immunofluorometric assays, *Clin. Chem.*, 31, 359, 1985.
10. Hartmeier, W., *Immobilisierte Biokatalysatoren,* Springer, New York, 1986, chap. 2.
11. Soin, E. and Hemmilä, I., Fluoroimmunoassay: present status and key problems, *Clin. Chem.*, 25, 353, 1979.
12. Wieder, I., Background rejection on fluorescence immunoassay, in *Immunofluorescence and Related Staining Techniques,* Knapp, W., Holubar, H., and Wick, G., Eds., Elsevier/North Holland, New York, 1978, 67.
13. Wieder, I. and Hidgson, K. O., German Patent 2,628,158, 1977; U.S. Patent 4,058,732, 1977.
14. Diamandis, E. P., Immunoassay with time-resolved fluorescence spectroscopy: principles and applications, *Clin. Biochem.*, 21, 139, 1988.
15. Kanaoka, Y., Organic fluorescence reagents in the study of enzymes and proteins, *Angew. Chem. Int. Ed. Engl.*, 16, 137, 1977.
16. The, T. H. and Feldkamp, T. R., Conjugation of fluorescein isothiocyanate to antibodies, *Immunology*, 18, 865, 1970.
17. Brandtzaeg, P., Rhodamine conjugates: specific and nonspecific binding properties in immunochemistry, *Ann. N.Y. Acad. Sci.*, 254, 35, 1975.
18. McKinney, R. M. and Spillane, J. T., An approach to quantitation in rhodamine isothiocyanate labeling, *Ann. N.Y. Acad. Sci.*, 254, 55, 1975.
19. Brandtzaeg, P., Conjugates of immunoglobulin G with different fluorochromes. I. Characterisation by anionic-exchange chromatography, *Scand. J. Immunol.*, 2, 273, 1973.

20. Brandtzaeg, P., Conjugates of immunoglobulin G with different fluorochromes. II. Specific and nonspecific binding properties, *Scand. J. Immunol.*, 2, 333, 1973.
21. Chadwick, C. S., McEntegard, M. G., and Nairn, R. C., A trial of new fluorochromes and the development of an alternative to fluorescein, *Immunology*, 1, 315, 1958.
22. Wood, P., Heterogeneous fluoroimmunoassay, *Principles and Practice of Immunoassay*, Price, C. P. and Newman, D. J., Eds., Stockton Press, New York, 1991.
23. Southwick, P. L., Ernst, L. K., Tauriello, E. W., Parker, S. R., Mujumdar, R. B., Mujumdar, S. R., Clever, H. A. and Waggoner, A. S., Cyanine dye labeling reagents — carboxyethylindocyanine succinimidyl esters, *Cytometry*, 11, 1990, 418.
24. Patonay, G. and Antoine, M. D., Near-infrared fluorogenic labels. New approach to an old problem, *Anal. Chem.*, 63, 321A, 1991.
25. Schermann, G., Schmidt, R., Völcker, A., Brauer, H. D., Mertes, H., and Franck, B., Potential photosensitizers for photodynamic therapy. II. Photophysical properties of [26] porphyrin, *Photochem. Photobiol.*, 52, 741, 1990.
26. Imasaka, T., Tsukamoto, A., and Ishibashi, N., Visible semiconductor laser fluorometry, *Anal. Chem.*, 61, 2285, 1989.
27. Johnson, P. A., Barber, T. E., Smith, B. W., and Winefordner, J. D., Ultralow detection limits for an organic-dye determined by fluorescence spectroscopy with laser diode excitation, *Anal. Chem.*, 61, 861, 1989.
28. Miller, J. N., Brown, M. B., Seare, N. J., and Summerfield, S., Analytical applications of very near-IR fluorometry, in *Fluorescence Spectroscopy*, Springer, Berlin, 1993, chap.14.
29. Soini, E., Pulsed light, time resolved fluorometry immunoassay, in *Monoclonal Antibodies and New Trends in Immunoassays*, Bizollon, C. A., Ed., Elsevier Science, Amsterdam, 1984, 197.
30. Soine, E. and Kojola, H., Time-resolved fluorometer for lanthanide chelates — a new generation of nonisotopic immunoassays, *Clin. Chem.*, 29, 1983, 65.
31. Jansen, E. H. J. M., Chemiluminescence detection in immunochemical techniques. Applications to environmental monitoring, in *Fluorescence Spectroscopy*, Wolfbeis, O. S., Ed., Springer, Berlin, 1993, chap. 19.
32. Seitz, W. R., Chemical sensors based on immobilized indicators and fiberoptics, *Crit. Rev. Anal. Chem.*, 19, 135, 1988.
33. Sutherland, R. M. and Dähne, C., IRS devices for optical immunoassays, in *Biosensors. Fundamentals and Applications*, Turner, A. P. F., Karube, I., and Wilson, G. S., Eds., Oxford University Press, New York, 1989, chap. 33.
34. Seitz, W. R., Optical sensor based on immobilized reagents, in *Biosensors. Fundamentals and Applications,* Turner, A. P. F., Karube, I., and Wilson, G. S., Eds., Oxford University Press, New York, 1989, chap. 30
35. Vo-Dinh, T., Alarie, J. P., and Sepaniak, M. J., Laser-based fiberoptic immunosensors, *Proc. SPIE Int. Soc. Opt. Eng.*, 1716, 37, 1992.
36. Weetall, H. H., in *Methods in Enzymology,* Mosbach, K., Ed., Academic Press, New York, 1976, pp. 134-148
37. Mandenius, C. F., Welin, S., Danielsson, B., Lundström, I., and Mosbach, K., The interaction of proteins and cells with affinity ligands covalently coupled to silicon surfaces as monitored by ellipsometry, *Anal. Biochem.*, 137, 106, 1984.
38. Bhatia, S. K., Shriver-Lake, L. C., Prior, K. J., Georger, J. M., Calvert, J. M., Bredenhorst, R., and Ligler, F. S., Use of thiol-terminal silanes and heterobifunctional crosslinkers for immobilization of antibodies on silica surfaces, *Anal. Biochem.*, 178, 408, 1989.
39. Brüning, C., Dissertation: Aldehydfunktionalisierte Silane als neue Immobilisierungsreagenzien — Synthese und Anwendung, Münster, 1993.
40. Walczak, I. M., Lowe, W. F., Cook, T. A., and Slovacek, R. E., The application of evanescent wave sensing to a high-sensitivity fluoroimmunoassay, *Biosens. Bioelectron.*, 7, 39, 1992.
41. Robinson, G. A., Attridge, J. W., Deacon, J. K., and Whiteley, S. C., The fluorescent capillary fill device, *Sensors Actuators,* B11, 235, 1993.
42. Choquette, S. J., Locasio-Brown, L., and Durst, R. A., Planar waveguide immunosensor with fluorescent liposome amplification, *Anal. Chem.*, 64, 55, 1992.

43. Badley, R. A., Drake, R. A. L., Shanks, I. A., Smith, A. M., and Stephenson, P. R., Optical biosensors for immunoassays: the fluorescent capillary fill device, *Philos. Trans. R. Soc. London Ser. B*, 316, 143, 1987.
44. Sloper, A. N., Deacon, J. K., and Flanagan, T. M., A planar indium phosphate monomode waveguide evanescent field immunosensor, *Sensors Actuators*, B1, 589, 1990.
45. Zhou, Y., Laybourn, P. J. R., Magill, J. V., and de la Rue, R. M., An evanescent fluorescence biosensor using ion-exchanged buried waveguides and the enhancement of peak fluorescence, *Biosens. Bioelectron.*, 6, 595, 1991.
46. Zhou, Y., Magill, J. V., de la Rue, R. M., and Laybourn, P. J. R., Evanescent fluorescence performed with a disposable ion-exchanged patterned waveguide, *Sensors Actuators,* B11, 245, 1993.
47. Dean, P. G. D., Johnson, W. S., and Middle, F. A., *Affinity Chromatography,* IRL Press, Washington, D.C., 1991.
48. Oroszlan, P., Duveneck, G. L., Ehrat, M., and Widmer, H. M., Fiber-optic atrazine immunosensor, *Sensors Actuators,* B11, 301, 1993.
49. Bier, F.F., Stöcklein, W., Böcher, M., Bilitewski, U., and Schmid, R. D., Use of a fibre optic immunosensor for the detection of pesticides, *Sensors Actuators,* B7, 509, 1992.
50. Wong, R. B., Anis A. N., and Eldefrawi, M. E., Reusable fiber-optic-based immunosensor for rapid detection of imazethapyr herbicide, *Anal. Chim. Acta*, 279, 141, 1993.
51. Anis, A. N., Wright, J., Rogers, K. R., Thompson, R. G., Valdes, J. J., and Eldefrawi, M. E., A fiber-optic immunosensor for detecting parathion, *Anal. Lett.*, 25(4), 627, 1992.
52. Rogers, K. R., Anis, N. A., Valdes, J. J., and Eldefrawi, M. E., Fiber-optic biosensor based on total internal-reflection principle, ACS Symp. Ser. 511, 165, 1992, in: *Biosensor Design and Application,* Mathewson, P. R. and Finley, J. W., Eds., American Chemical Society, Washington, D.C., 1992.
53. Northrup, M. A., Stanker, L. H., Vanderlaan, M., and Watkins, B. E., Development and characterization of a fiberoptic immuno-biosensor, *NATO ASI Ser. C*, 280, 229, 1989.
54. Wortberg, M., Middendorf, C., Katerkamp, A., Rump, T., Krause, J., and Cammann, K., Flow injection immunosensor for triazine herbicides using Eu(III)-chelate label fluorescence detection, *Anal. Chim. Acta*, 289, 177, 1994.
55. Krämer, P. and Schmid, R. D., Flow injection immunoanalysis (FIIA) — a new immunoassay format for the determination of pesticides in water, *Biosens. Bioelectron.*, 6, 239, 1991.
56. Whelan, J. P., Kusterbeck, A. W., Wemhoff, G. A., Bredenhorst, R., and Ligler, F. S., Continuous-flow immunosensor for detection of explosives, *Anal. Chem.*, 65, 3561, 1993.
57. Kusterbeck, A. W., Wemhoff, G. A., Charles, P. T., Yaeger, D. A., Bredenhorst, R., Vogel, C. W., and Ligler, F. S., A continuous flow immunoassay for rapid and sensitive detection of small molecules, *J. Immunol. Methods*, 135, 191, 1990.
58. Ogert, R. A., Kusterbeck, A. W., Wemhoff, G. A., Burke, R., and Ligler, F. S., Detection of cocaine using the flow immunosensor, *Anal. Lett.*, 25(11), 1999, 1992.
59. Ligler, F. S., Kusterbeck, A. W., Ogert, R. A., and Wemhoff, G. A., Drug detection using the flow immunosensor, ACS Symp. Ser. 511, 73, 1992, in: *Biosensor Design and Application,* Mathewson, P. R. and Finley, J. W., Eds., American Chemical Society, Washington, D.C., 1992.
60. Deacon, J. K., Thomson, A. M., Page, A. L., Stops, J. E., Roberts, P. R., Whiteley, S. C., Attridge, J. W., Love, C. A., Robinson, G. A., and Davidson, G. P., An assay for human chorionic gonadotropin using the capillary fill immunosensor, *Biosens. Bioelectron.*, 6, 193, 1991.
61. Locasio-Brown, L., Plant, A. L., Horváth V., and Durst, R. L., Liposome flow injection immunoassay: implications for sensitivity, dynamic range, and antibody regeneration, *Anal. Chem.*, 62, 2587, 1990.
62. Anderson, F. P. and Miller, W. G., Fiberoptic immunochemical sensor for continuous, reversible measurement of phenytoin, *Clin. Chem.*, 34(7), 1417, 1988.
63. Astles, J. R. and Miller, W. G., Reversible fiber-optic immunosensor measurements, *Sensors Actuators,* B11, 73, 1993.
64. Astles, J. R. and Miller, W. G., Measurement of free phenytoin in blood with a self-contained fiber-optic immunosensor, *Anal. Chem.*, 66, 1675, 1994.
65. Bright, F. V., Betts T. A., and Litwiler, K. S., Regenerable fiber-optic-based immunosensor, *Anal. Chem.*, 62, 1065, 1990.

66. Betts, T. A., Catena, G. C., Huang, J., Litwiler, K. S., Zhang, J., Zagrobleny, J., and Bright F. V., Fiber-optic based immunosensors for haptens, *Anal. Chim. Acta*, 246, 55, 1991.
67. Vollhardt, K. P. C., *Organische Chemie,* VCH Publishers, New York, 1988, chap.25.
68. Vo-Dinh, T., Tromberg, B. J., Griffin, G. D., Ambrose, K. R., Sepaniak, M. J., and Gardenhire, E. M., Antibody-based fiberoptics biosensor for the carcinogen benzo(a)pyrene, *Appl. Spectrosc.*, 41(5), 735, 1987.
69. Vo-Dinh, T., Nolan, T., Cheng, Y. F., Sepaniak, M. J., and Alarie, J. P., Phase-resolved fiber-optics fluoroimmunosensor, *Appl. Spectrosc.*, 44(1), 128, 1990.
70. Locasio-Brown, L., Plant, A. L., Chesler, R., Kroll, M., Rudel, M., and Durst, R. A., Liposome-based flow-injection immunoassay for determining theophylline in serum, *Clin. Chem.*, 39(3), 386, 1993.
71. Palmer, D. A., Xuezhen, R., Fernandez-Hernando, P., and Miller, J. N., A model on-line flow injection fluorescence immunoassay using a protein A immunoreactor and lucifer yellow, *Anal. Lett.*, 26(12), 2543, 1993.
72. Khokhar, M. Y., Miller, J. N., and Seare, N. J., Heterogeneous fluorescence immunoassay using flow-injection analysis with protein G solid phase reactors, *Anal. Chim. Acta*, 290, 154, 1994.
73. Stöcklein, W., Jäger, V., and Schmid, R. D., Monitoring of mouse immunglobulin G by flow-injection analytical affinity chromatography, *Anal. Chim. Acta*, 245, 1, 1991.
74. Stöcklein, W. and Schmid, R. D., Flow-injection immunoanalysis for the on-line monitoring of monoclonal antibodies, *Anal. Chim. Acta*, 234, 83, 1990.
75. Walt, D., Polymer release biosensors, *Third World Congress on Biosensors,* June 1-3, 1994, Elsevier, New York, 1994.
76. Petrea, R. D. and Sepaniak, M. J., Fiber-optic time-resolved fluorimetry for immunoassays, *Talanta*, 35(2), 139, 1988.
77. Eenink, R. G., de Bruijn, H. E., Kooyman, R. P. H., and Greve, J., Fibre-fluorescence immunosensor based on evanescent wave detection, *Anal. Chim. Acta*, 238, 317, 1990.
78. Lu, B., Lu, C., and Wei, Y., A planar waveguide immunosensor based on TIRF principle, *Anal. Lett.*, 25(1), 1, 1992.
79. Osipov, A. P., Arefyev, A. A., Vlasenko, S. B., Bavrilova, E. M., and Yegorov, A. M., Flow-injection enzyme immunoassay for human IgG by using enhanced chemiluminescence reaction for horseradish peroxidase label quantitation, *Anal. Lett.*, 22, 1841, 1989.
80. Liu, H., Yu, J. C., Bindra, D. S., Givens, R. S., and Wilson, G. S., Flow injection solid-phase chemiluminescent immunoassay using a membrane-based reactor, *Anal. Chem.*, 63, 666, 1991.
81. Shellum, C. and Güblitz, G., Flow injection immunoassays with acridinium ester-based chemiluminescence detection, *Anal. Chim. Acta*, 227, 97, 1989.
82. Hara, T., Tsukagoshi, K., Arai, A., and Imashiro, Y., A highly sensititve fiber-optic immunosensor using a metal-complex compound as a chemiluminescent catalyst, *Bull. Chem. Soc. Jpn.*, 62, 2844, 1989.

Part IV

On-Line and *In Vivo* Monitoring and Control

18 Optimized Biosensors in Clinical Applications

Danila Moscone and Marco Mascini

CONTENTS

18.1 INTRODUCTION

One of the major interests in biosensors arises from the possibility of continuous monitoring *in vivo* or *ex vivo* of a specific metabolite or therapeutic drug with electrochemical devices. Situations in which such monitoring would be desired include

- Critical-care units or surgery in life-threatening situations, where rapid assessment of blood concentrations of a drug is required for dosage regulation;
- Premature infant care, where the removal of large volumes of blood is prohibitive;
- Long-term drug maintenance, where implanted probes would allow periodic assessment of drug concentration;
- Therapeutic treatment with extracorporeal circuits, such as the heart-lung bypass machine;
- Hemodialysis;
- The artificial pancreas;

0-8493-8905-4/97/$0.00+$.50
© 1997 by CRC Press, Inc.

- Reactor perfusion to remove toxins, drug overdose, etc.;
- Organ preservation to maintain viability and assess functionality prior to transplantation into a suitable donor.

There is almost an infinite number of situations where the evaluation of the level of a specific metabolite can provide the basis for a decision in real time.[1-6] Biosensors can be interfaced to microcomputers in order to evaluate their performance and provide a facility for control loops. Drift compensation and automatic recalibration can be facilitated by flow cell designs and microprocessor control.

The idea of a detector capable of direct measurement in blood or urine without recourse to a reagent or the need for measurements of sample volume is attractive. Although in some cases the development of such sensors is currently in the formative stages, some are very close to realization, and several scientists claim the priority and the patent for some applications. In this chapter we will analyze some *in vivo* or *ex vivo* applications of electrochemical biosensors published recently where the final goal is approached more closely and where the results justify the general interest in this area.

18.1.1 Enzyme Immobilization

The most critical step in electrochemical biosensor manufacturing is the enzyme immobilization and coupling to the electrochemical device. These two steps are in sequence and should be related and well defined. Because the most valuable part of the biosensor is the electrochemical sensor, it is not advisable to fix the enzyme to the electrode surface permanently unless necessary. This technique, in fact, leads to the need for an electrode surface treatment when the enzyme lifetime is expired and it is generally an impractical solution unless a disposable biosensor can be realized.

In the preferred realization, the immobilization of the enzyme should lead to a high loading confined by a thin membrane physically coupled with the electrochemical surface and secured to it by an O ring or other suitable means. The electrode surface should contact the thin membrane as much as possible, and when the enzyme has lost its activity the membrane should peel off easily from the electrode surface. With this concept in mind, several solutions have been presented; in the following paragraphs we review the most successful realizations for practical applications of *in vivo* analysis.

18.1.2 Problems Concerning the Biocompatibility of the Biosensor

The major drawback of the electrochemical biosensor is that it needs to be in direct contact with the biological fluid and it may be affected by sample constituents. The surface fouling will alter the response by altering the substrate diffusion into the immobilized enzyme layer.

Generally, many devices reported so far often have impressive steady state and dynamic performance characteristics and the nonspecialist can be forgiven for wondering why they are not already in regular clinical use. The explanation is almost entirely that the studies have been conducted in controlled aqueous solution and not in the hostile environment of a biological fluid.

The presence of the enzyme coating increases the electrode dependence on solution variables such as ionic strength, pH, and stirring rate, thus altering the rate of the enzymatic reaction. The stirring rate together with the sample viscosity influences the substrate access to the enzyme layer. The effects of viscosity will be most evident in proteinaceous fluid. In whole blood complications arise from the diffusion barrier of red cells.

Oxidase enzymes are often employed in metabolite sensors (glucose, lactate, and pyruvate). The requirement for oxygen cosubstrate at these devices is a drawback in samples having a low oxygen content, and restrict the linear range of the substrate response.

Conventionally, air equilibration or sample dilution in aerated buffer is used to overcome the problem. It is possible to use diffusion-limiting membranes over the enzyme layer whereby the local concentration of substrate is lowered relative to that of oxygen.

Such diffusion-limiting, low-permeability membranes have the added advantage of being the major control step for mass transfer, and the electrode signal is then independent of sample stirring, viscosity or hematocrit. Furthermore, electrochemically active species in biological fluids (ascorbate, urate) will generate a false signal at amperometric detectors; electrochemical interference may be reduced either by lowering the polarizing voltage of the detector, or by covering it with a protective, permselective membrane. The last-mentioned solution is simpler and up to now more often utilized.

A range of proteins, from albumin to fibrinogen, are adsorbed onto the electrode membrane within seconds of its exposure to blood, regardless of whether a membrane is hydrophilic or hydrophobic. The amounts adsorbed do not generally compromise sensitivity, but the composition of the protein layer conditions subsequent interactions with elements in whole blood; fibrinogen promotes platelet adhesion whereas albumin reduces it. The surface coating of platelets, leukocytes, and eventually of red cells acts as a serious barrier to diffusion, and produces cumulative losses of response in blood. Electrodes made using either external Cuprophan (hydrophilic) or polycarbonate (hydrophobic) membranes are equally susceptible to surface fouling, but the treatment of such membranes with organosilane reagents (e.g., methyltrichlorosilane) can improve hemocompatibility.[7-8] Regardless of the membrane used, the decay in signal experienced in blood is considerably greater than that in aqueous solution, and overshadows altered responses due to enzyme denaturation.

The problems of surface fouling, particularly in whole blood, are common to all enzyme electrodes and make it imperative that greater efforts are made towards the investigation of biocompatible membranes for these devices (see also Chapter 5).

18.1.3 Considerations for Implantable Sensors

While the intravascular compartment is the most obvious choice for *in vivo* monitoring, it is also the most hazardous. Intravascular catheters, regardless of design, pose a finite risk of vascular injury, infection, or thrombosis; the risks increase when the catheter tip bears a complex structure such as an enzyme electrode. The turbulence generated in the vicinity of the probe increases the shear stress on platelets and also the platelet-surface contact times with a high risk of clotting. With extracorporeal electrodes, a good cell design permits laminar flow to occur, helping to reduce fouling.

Enzyme electrodes located either subcutaneously or intraperitoneally offer a much safer monitoring route;[6,9-11] however, metabolite levels at these sites are likely to be quite different from those in blood, making interpretation, especially of dynamic change, quite difficult. Ready access to subcutaneous tissue sites allows easy insertion and replacement of implanted electrodes, but it is possible that in future a simplified vascular access may be gained by a chronic access port or an extracorporeal circulatory loop; this would reduce risks from vascular monitoring.

The possibility of local and systemic side effects must also be considered as these effects are important for chronic implantation; thus, Ag or AgCl reference electrodes can have local toxic effects. The enzyme protein is immunogenic, and masking it behind a membrane is vital. The integrity of such a membrane has to be checked after sterilization procedures, as these can have an adverse effect on the behavior of the probe and need to be assessed in detail.

18.2 THE BEDSIDE ARTIFICIAL PANCREAS

Diabetic patients have a relative or absolute lack of insulin which causes the blood glucose concentration to exceed the normal narrow limits (about 3.5 to 5 mmol/l in the fasting state).

About 20% of diabetics, who mostly contract the disease under the age of about 30 years, have suffered a complete or near complete destruction of the insulin-secreting cells (islets of Langerhans) in the pancreas; this type of diabetes is called insulin-dependent or type I diabetes and these patients need insulin replacement to live. Insulin is usually given by subcutaneous injection but this treatment cannot maintain the normal blood glucose levels. The values sometimes slip too low (hypoglycemia), causing unpleasant symptoms and dangerous impairment of consciousness, or they often are too high, causing serious long-term tissue complications in the eyes, nerves, kidney, and blood vessels. There has, therefore, been intensive research in the last few years to improve diabetic control.[12]

A logical development of these studies is the "closed-loop" feedback control of the insulin rate via an implanted glucose sensor. The scheme of the glucose sensor is summarized below:

$$\text{Glucose} + \text{Oxygen} \xrightarrow{\text{Glucose oxidase}} \text{Gluconic Acid} + \text{Hydrogen Peroxide}$$

$$\text{Hydrogen Peroxide} \xrightarrow{\text{Pt at +650 mV vs. Ag/AgCl}} \text{Oxygen} + 2\text{H}^+$$

Clemens et al.[13,14] were the first to adapt such a sensor for use in a bedside-type artificial pancreas. Similar sensors have been adapted for the same purpose by several groups. Over the last ten years, improvements have been made in the sensor design, the binding of the enzyme to its support, and the functional characteristics of the electrodes.

Recently a new artificial pancreas was developed and it is shown in Figure 18.1; it is called Betalike (Esacontrol SpA, Genoa, Italy) and represents an improvement with respect to the devices available previously. One of the most interesting features is a miniaturized hollow fiber hemofiltering cartridge (filtration surface: 50 cm; membrane cut off: about 35,000 Da) which allows only the hemofiltrate to reach the sensors while the blood cells and proteins are reinfused into the patient. It results in a more stable signal, longer life for the membranes, and avoids loss of blood.

The blood is taken from the patient via a double lumen catheter (6 ml/h) and is diluted (1:9) with a buffer solution (Normosol, pH 7.4, Abbott, Italy) with the addition of 3 units/ml of heparin. The diluted blood is then dialyzed by the miniaturized hemofilter, and the dialysate passed through the glucose sensor. Results of one experiment are reported in Figure 18.2.

This instrument has an insulin feedback delivery system regulated by an algorithm function of the blood glucose concentration.[13,14] It represents a great improvement in the treatment of diabetes, but it still does not completely normalize altered concentrations of intermediary metabolites such as lactate, pyruvate, alanine, and ketone bodies. Information on the concentration of these metabolites is useful in establishing the metabolic pattern in diabetic patients and eventually for deriving a more precise algorithm for the insulin infusion. Biosensors for lactate and pyruvate have been assembled and placed downstream from developed artificial pancreas to monitor changes in lactate and pyruvate concentrations during insulin infusion. Figure 18.3 shows the result of an "extracorporeal" determination of glucose, lactate, and pyruvate in heparinized blood from a normal subject.[15] A good correlation was observed between results obtained by continuous monitoring and by spectrometry.

Another application of the use of electrochemical biosensors for extracorporeal measurements has been performed in sports medicine.[16] Lactate and glucose were measured in the blood of athletes running on a treadmill by using two extracorporeal electrochemical biosensors. It is well demonstrated that a progressive increase in the intensity of physical exercise results in parallel increase in the concentration of lactic acid in the blood. Moreover, at a certain point during a progressive increase in physical exercise, a sharp increase in the blood lactate is observed.[17] This increase of lactate can be related to the anaerobic muscle metabolism and allows for the evaluation of the aerobic as well as the anaerobic threshold, especially in sports such as cycling, cross-country skiing, and marathon running. Experiments were

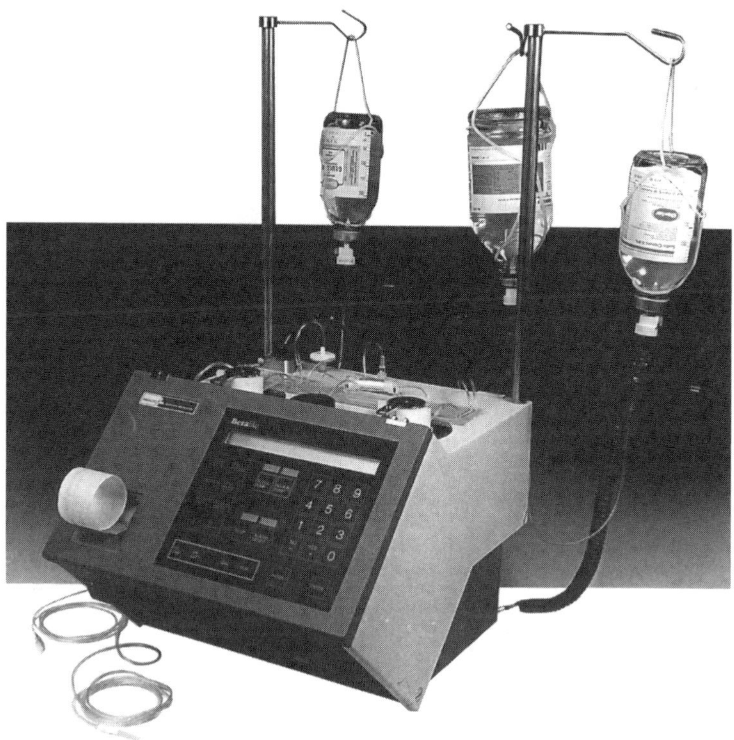

FIGURE 18.1 A general view of the Betalike, the artificial pancreas developed and marketed by Esacontrol (Genoa, Italy).

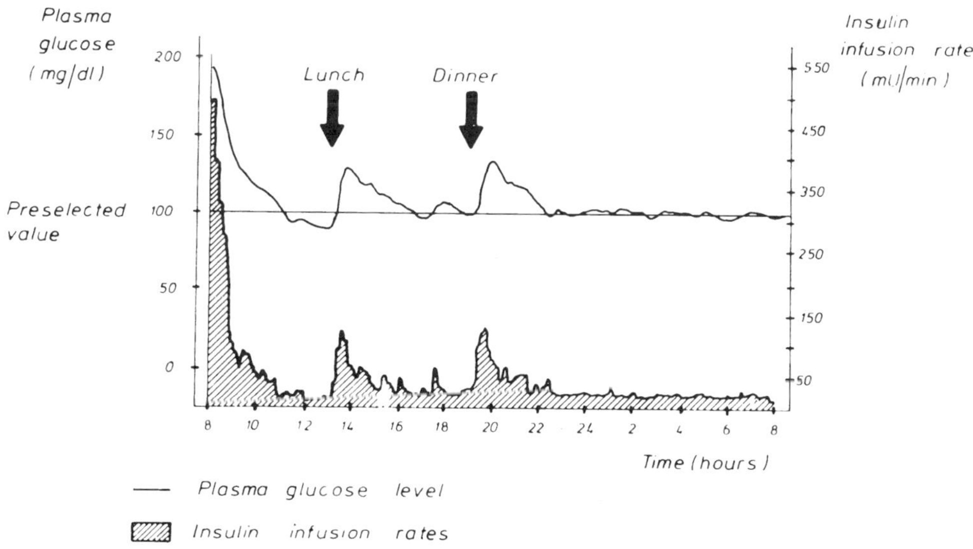

FIGURE 18.2 A typical experiment performed by clamping a "normal" value of glucose.

carried out using the artificial pancreas Betalike. In this case the glucose sensor and a lactate sensor were added in series.

200
mg/dl
GLU
100
STOP
EX
EX
STOP
INF
INF
GLU
MEAL
LACT
4·10^{-3}
mol/l
2
1
st
cal
PYR
2·10^{-4}
mol/l
11 a.m.
12
13
14
15
16
HOURS

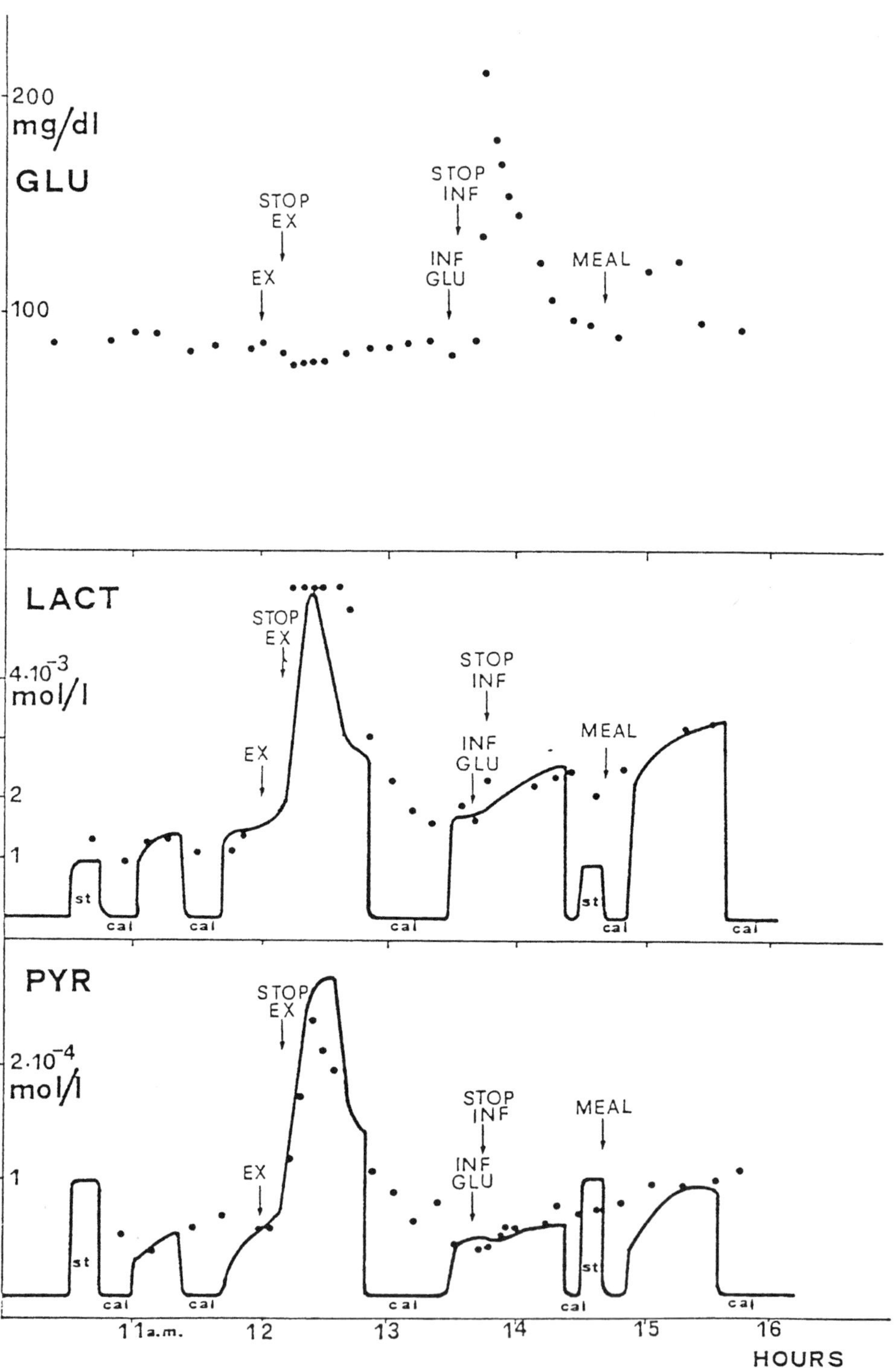

FIGURE 18.3

FIGURE 18.3 Continuous monitoring of glucose, lactate, and pyruvate during an *ex vivo* experiment with the artificial pancreas Betalike. At the time marked st, a standard solution of lactate and pyruvate was passed through the cell to calibrate the sensors. At the time marked cal, the glucose sensor of Betalike was calibrated. The blood flow was disconnected from the sensors during such periods. At the time marked EX, the patient was requested to do a short physical exercise, which was stopped at the time marked STOP EX. At the time INF GLU, a 50 g load of glucose was rapidly infused, which was terminated at STOP INF. MEAL indicates the time at which the patient ate a normal meal. Dots represent lactate and pyruvate analysis in blood taken from the subject every 15 to 20 min, using a spectrophotometric procedure.

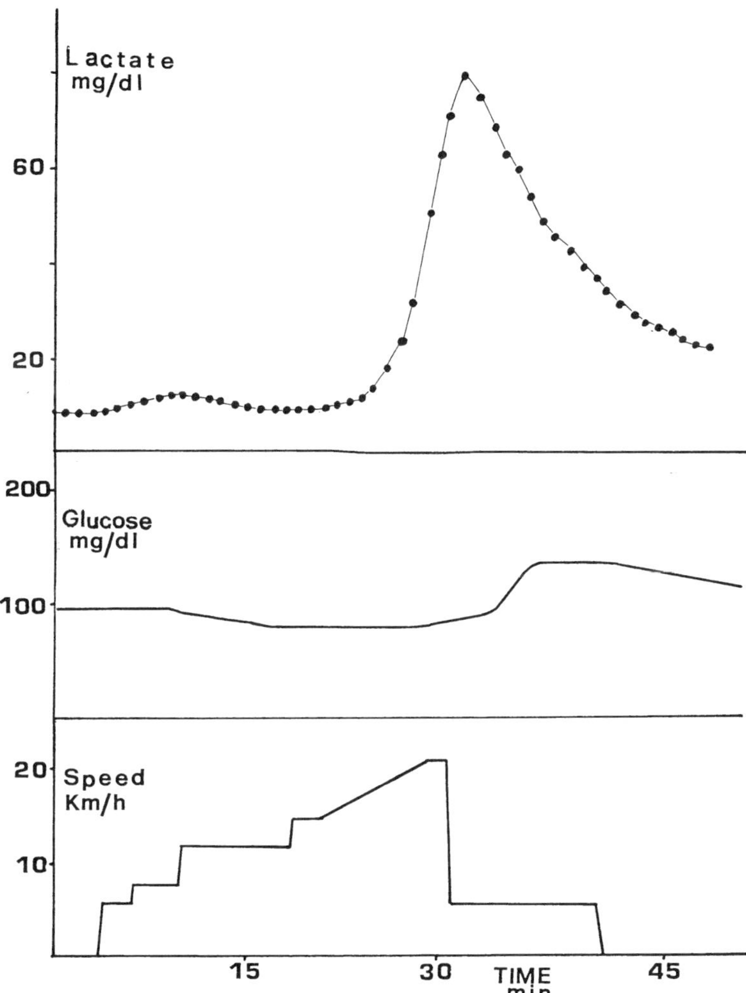

FIGURE 18.4 Continuous monitoring of lactate and glucose in a high-level marathon runner during an anaerobic threshold experiment with lactate and glucose probes and the artificial pancreas Betalike. (See text for explanation and procedure).

Figure 18.4 illustrates continuous monitoring in a high-level marathon runner during an anaerobic threshold experiment with lactate and glucose probes. His speed was varied several times, and at a running speed of 18 km/h the lactate concentration began to rise markedly. The results obtained gave a precise and real-time determined lactate curve during the exercise;

moreover, it was possible to identify the onset of blood lactate accumulation, which according to Mader et al.,[18] is approximately 2 mmol/l (18 mg/dl). The blood lactate interval from this point to a level of 4 mmol/l was well defined and an appreciable variation of the slope between these two points was observed. This transition point is most important for long-distance runners. Beyond this point athletes run under anaerobic conditions; thus it can be considered the maximum speed to be maintained to remain in aerobic metabolism. The glucose concentration showed a constant value throughout this period. During recovery the lactate concentration decreased, but an increase in the glucose concentration was observed. The glucose behavior supports the theory that anaerobic glycolysis in muscle is supplied mainly by glycogen storage rather than blood glucose.

18.3 NEEDLE ELECTRODES FOR *IN VIVO* MEASUREMENT

Shichiri et al. at the University of Osaka reported the most advanced experiments with needle electrodes.[9,10] The needle electrode was the most obvious approach for the procuring a wearable artificial pancreas. However, attaining a reproducible needle electrode is not easy and lack of repeatability is often found. In this section we report the details of the needle electrode preparation along with some experimental results obtained in our laboratory.

To obtain a suitable selectivity, the platinum anode (working electrode) was covered with a cellulose acetate membrane which excluded interfering molecules (uric or ascorbic acid). Thus a first layer of cellulose acetate covers the platinum surface. Then a glucose oxidase immobilized membrane was attached as a second layer; however, to obtain a current linearly related to the glucose concentrations in the clinical range (5 to 20 mmol/l) a third layer was necessary which reduced the glucose diffusion to the enzyme active sites without affecting oxygen availability.

This outer membrane was in the first part of our research a polyurethane layer as is described in several similar experiments in the literature.[19-21] However, poor reproducibility was obtained in our laboratory and a different approach was proposed; a commercially available polycarbonate membrane, treated with organochlorosilanes was fixed on the tip of the needle electrode by fine silk threads. Analytical reproducibility was highly improved and the needles show mechanical ruggedness. Preliminary experiments of *in vivo* measurements in rabbits are reported and reliable results over a short period (4 h) are obtained.

18.3.1 Preparation

Teflon®-coated Pt wire was inserted into an hypodermic needle and the lumen then filled with epoxy glue. The platinum wire was soldered to the central wire of a coaxial cable, whose external wire was moreover soldered to the steel stem of the same needle inside its cone, so that it can act as reference electrode. The needle cone with the coaxial cable inside was then filled with epoxy glue and allowed to harden for 48 h. The tip of the needle was polished by a rotating disk equipped with several grinding papers and alumina powders and, after cleaning with acetone, the needle was dipped into a 4% solution of cellulose acetate and 0.04% of polyvinylacetate in an acetone-cyclohexanone mixture (33.3% cyclohexanone and 66.6% acetone) for 30 s and then dried at room temperature for 24 h. For enzyme coating, the needle electrode was dipped into an enzyme solution with 3% GOD, 6% BSA, and 2% glutaraldehyde for 5 s, and allowed to dry for 2 h. The enzyme solution was prepared just before dipping and it was used for a few minutes only.

After this time, the needle was dipped into a glycine solution, 0.1 M for 30 min, and after drying, dipped for 10 s in polyurethane solutions (several formulations) and allowed to dry for 12 h in different solutions or covered with a polycarbonate membrane.

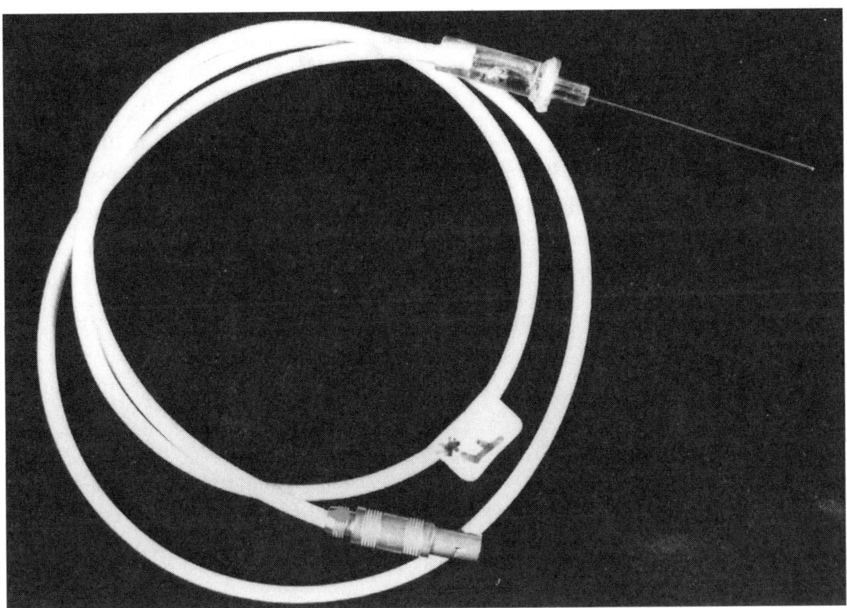

FIGURE 18.5 Picture of the needle electrode.

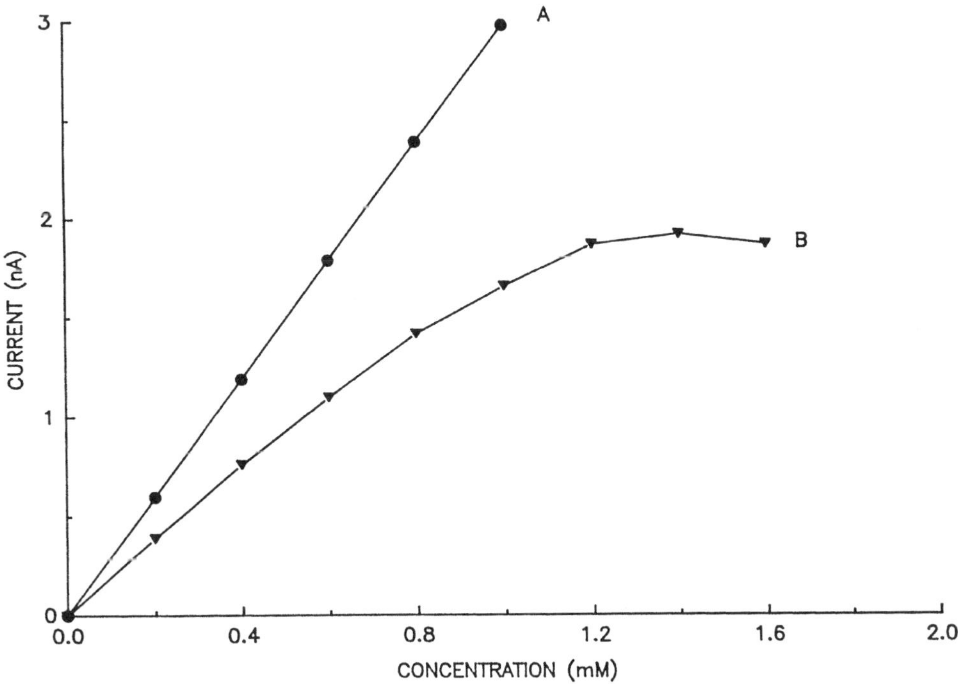

FIGURE 18.6 Calibration curve obtained by a needle electrode: A = needle dip-coated with cellulose acetate: response to hydrogen peroxide. B = needle dip-coated with cellulose acetate and immobilized enzyme: response to glucose. The linearity range was not suitable for "in vivo" glucose measurements. (Normal range 4.4–6.6 mM; pathologic range 1.5–30 mM).

18.3.2 Procedure for Subcutaneous Needle Insertion in Rabbits

A Teflon® intravenous needle catheter with internal needle in stainless steel was inserted subcutaneously in the rabbit back, then holding the Teflon catheter, the steel needle was withdrawn and replaced with the glucose needle sensor so that the sensor tip covered by the enzymatic membrane exceeded the Teflon needle by 1 to 2 mm. The glucose needle sensor was fixed to the Teflon needle by a bayonet lock already present on its cone.

18.3.3 Experimental Data

Figure 18.5 shows an electrode produced by this procedure. Figure 18.6 shows calibration curves obtained with a needle electrode covered by a cellulose acetate membrane and GOD membrane for hydrogen peroxide and glucose. A linear calibration curve can be obtained up to 10^{-3} M without an external polyurethane membrane.

The presence of a polyurethane membrane decreases the diffusion of glucose by about ten times (Figure 18.7), and it seems suitable for a biosensor with extended linearity. However, in the same Figure 18.7 we show the lack of reproducibility of successive calibration curves prepared with the polyurethanes. Generally, only one electrode out of five shows a linear calibration curve with a reproducible result.

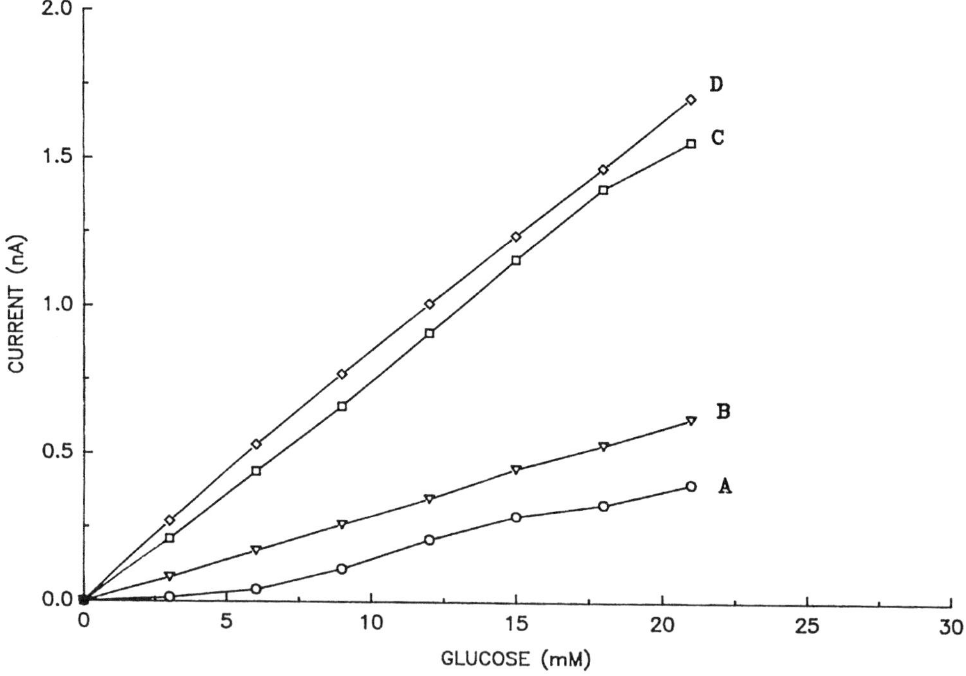

FIGURE 18.7 Successive calibration curves (A,B,C,D) obtained by adding a glucose concentrated solution to a Dulbecco Buffer pH 7.4 of a single glucose biosensor covered by polyurethane. The linearity was substantially extended but the reproducibility was very poor.

Figure 18.8 shows the behavior of polycarbonate coverage. The values refer to successive calibration curves. The behavior seems to be more regular and it shows an adequate response for an *in vivo* measurement. From a practical point of view, it is essential that the membrane tightly adheres to the tip of the needle and that the tip of the needle is finely beveled in order not to scratch the membrane. Optimum results can be obtained after few trials; folds in the membrane should be avoided to obtain prompt responses. Figure 18.9 shows an experiment

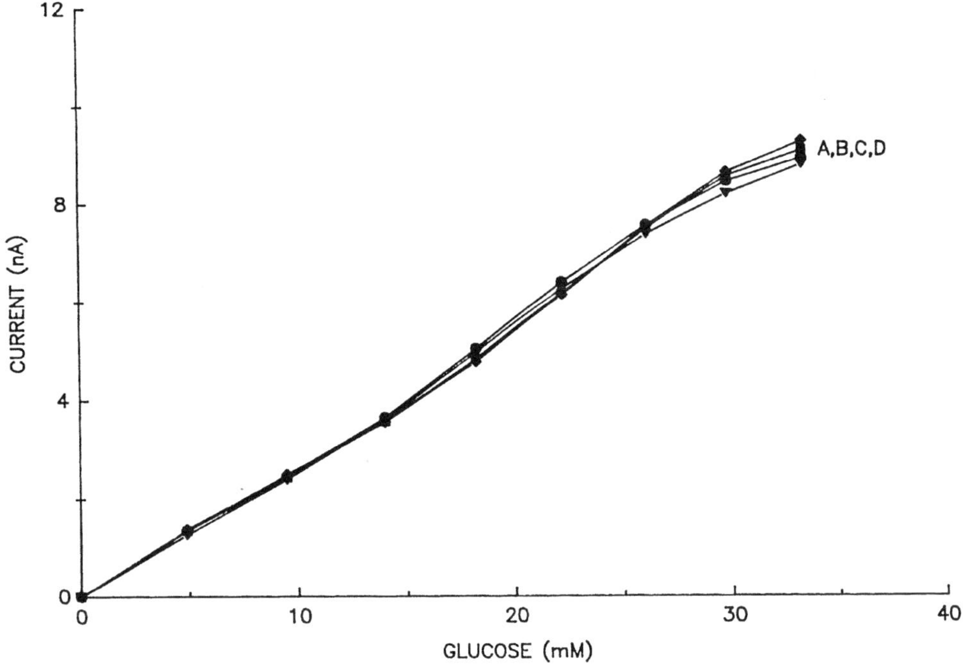

FIGURE 18.8 Successive calibration curves of a glucose needle biosensor covered by silanized polycarbonate membrane. Both linearity and reproducibility are more suitable for "in vivo" measurements.

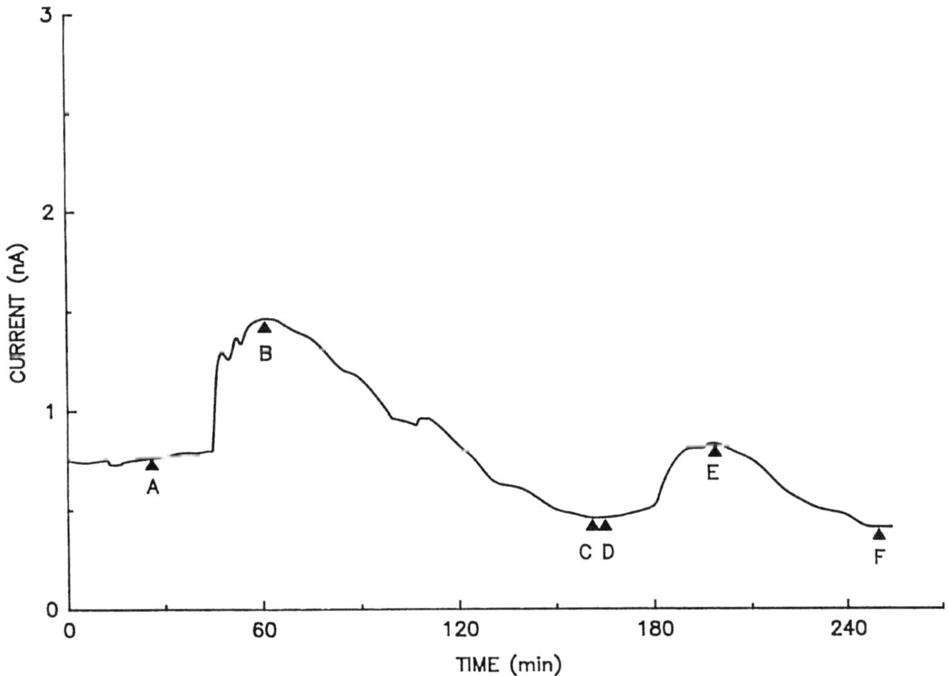

FIGURE 18.9 Nonanesthetized rabbit glucose monitoring. A: oral ingestion of 5 ml glucose solution 4.2 M; B: current intensity maximum (C_{glu} = 12.5 mM); C: base line (C_{glu} = 4.2 mM); D: oral ingestion of 5 ml glucose solution 4.2 M; E: current intensity maximum (C_{glu} = 7.8 mM); F: base line (C_{glu} = 4.2 mM).

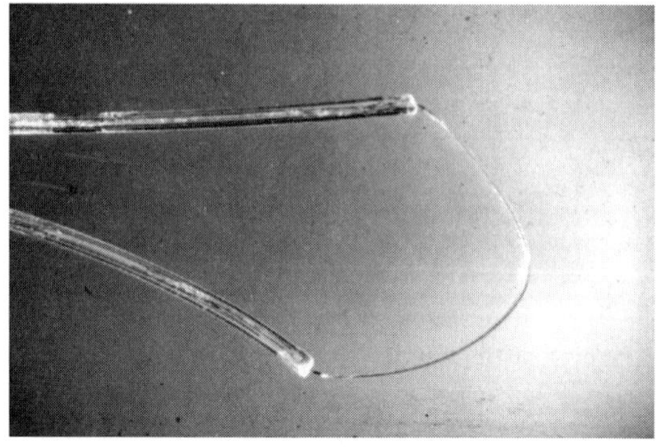

a

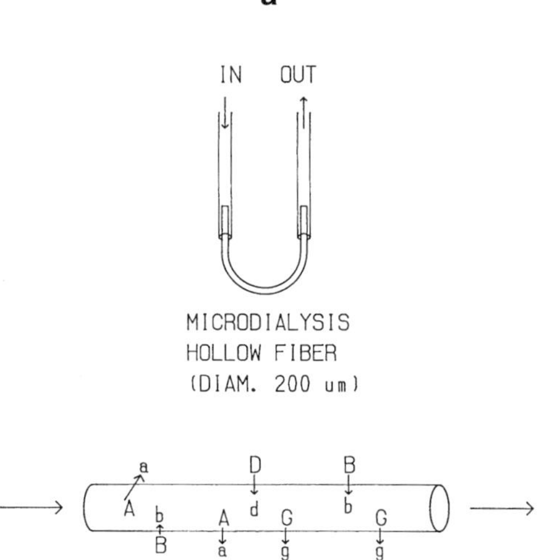

b

FIGURE 18.10 (a) Microdialysis probe for subcutaneous continuous measurement of glucose. (b) Scheme of the operation of the microdialysis probe.

obtained *in vivo* with a fasting rabbit submitted to glucose loads. The experiment lasted 4 h. The initial glucose concentration of the subcutaneous liquid was 7.1 mM.

18.4 MICRODIALYSIS FOR *IN VIVO* MEASUREMENTS

A new technique for sampling in vivo has recently been applied in our laboratory for the purpose of developing an artificial wearable pancreas; it is called microdialysis. This technique is a complementary approach to the implantable biosensors. The idea is to mimic the function of a blood vessel by implanting a "microdialysis probe" into the tissue.[22] The essential component of the probe is a thin dialysis tube perfused with a physiological solution much like the blood perfuses a blood vessel (Figure 18.10). Substances in higher concentration in the extracellular fluid outside the probe diffuse in. Once substances are carried out of the body by the perfusion liquid their concentration can be determined by analytical techniques. Biosensors can easily be coupled to the microdialysis device and can monitor the appropriate metabolite without any preseparation step. A flow cell assembled with a glucose biosensor has been connected in series to microdialysis probes. Analytical evaluation of the probes has been carried out by studying the reproducibility, lifetime, and stability of the probe by varying the type, temperature, flow rate, and the length of the dialysis membrane.[23]

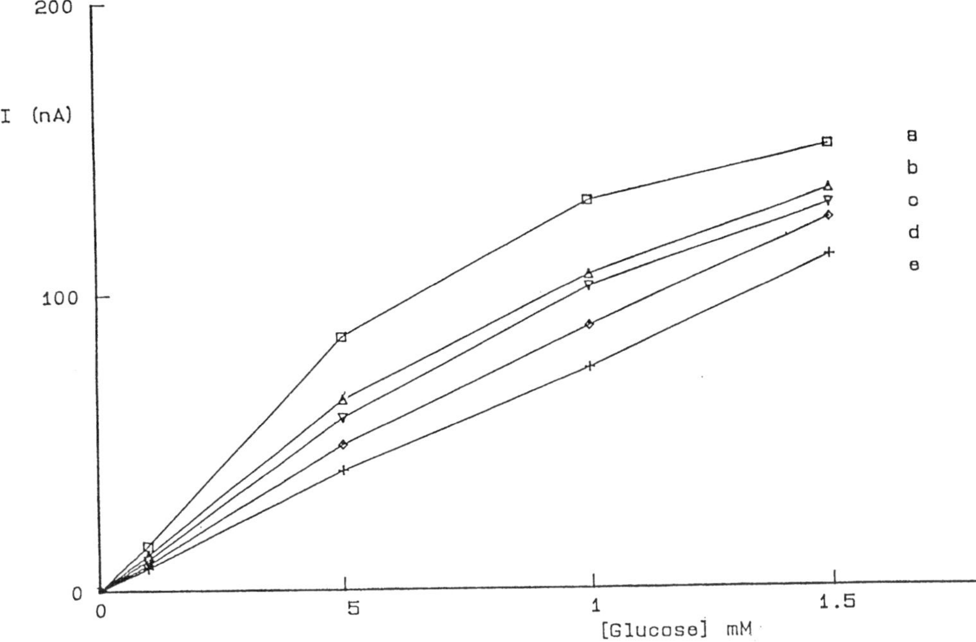

FIGURE 18.11 Calibration curves of glucose biosensor at different flow rates (without the microdialysis probe); a = 10 μl/min, b = 20 μ/min, c = 30 μl/min, d = 40 μl/min, e = 50 μ/min. Room temperature.

18.4.1 Microdialysis *In Vitro*

Typical calibration curves for a glucose flow cell, without the microdialysis probe, at different flow rates are shown in Figure 18.11. Increasing the flow rate causes the linear range of the calibration curve to increase and the current values to decrease. This is a common experience with glucose biosensors with hydrogen peroxide detection in a flow cell. The logical explanation is that hydrogen peroxide reaching the electrode surface decreases by increasing the flow rate. This is due partly to a lower conversion of glucose and partly to a lower fraction of hydrogen peroxide reaching the electrode surface.

The nonlinearity of the calibration curve at a concentration higher than about 1 mmol/l is mainly due to depletion of molecular oxygen, a cofactor in the glucose oxidase reaction. In Figure 18.12, the above calibration curves are shown (for a diagram of the apparatus, see Figure 18.15). The upper limit of concentration attained in this case (20 mmol/l) is much higher and is due to the limited diffusion of glucose through the microdialysis probe and reaching the glucose biosensor. In addition to this effect we observed a flow rate influence as in Figure 18.11, but in this case the diffusion rate through the microdialysis probe also affects the results.

In Figure 18.13 the length of the microdialysis probe (hollow fiber) was varied and the linearity range and the current values were greatly affected by this parameter. To obtain a linear calibration curve up to 20 mmol/l (the high value for glucose in blood for diabetes) we chose a hollow fiber 1 cm long and a flow rate of 30 μl/min. This flow is feasible for a wearable instrument, since it corresponds to less than 50 ml/day which can be stored easily.

In Figure 18.14 the dynamic curves are reported for the hollow fiber. The system, microdialysis and biosensor, shows fast response and recovery; only a few seconds are necessary to reach a stable current value corresponding to a defined concentration. The reproducibility of the current response is very high, it was evaluated in several experiments

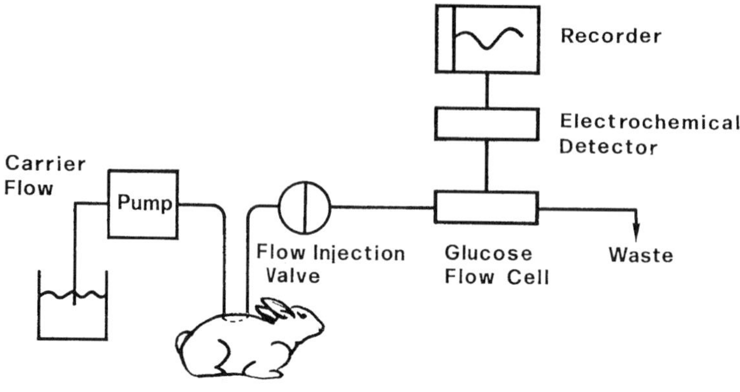

FIGURE 18.12a Diagram of the microdialysis system. The valve enables the user to inject (FIA) a standard solution of glucose to control the variation of the sensitivity of the glucose cell. The microdialysis probe (the hollow fiber) for the "in vitro" experiments was only immersed in a beaker with a standard solution with a suitable glucose concentration.

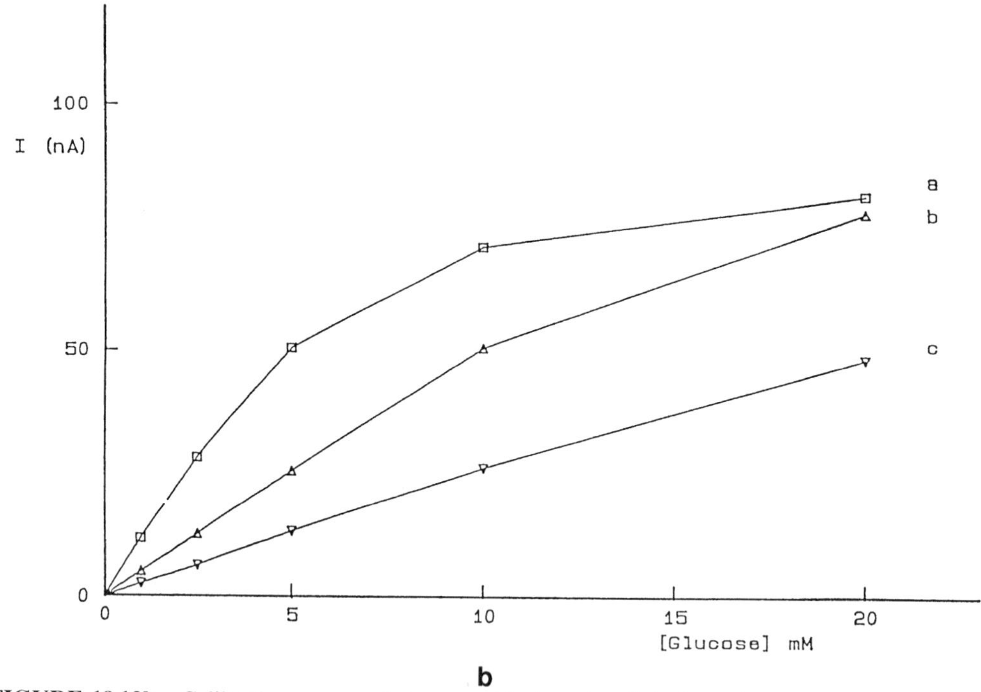

FIGURE 18.12b Calibration curves of glucose with the microdialysis probe at different flow rates. Hollow fiber, length = 20 mm, T = 37°C; a = 10 μl/min, b = 30 μl/min, c = 50 μl/min.

as less than 5% over 10 consecutive assays. Delay time was greatly reduced by using a narrow-bore tubing (Teflon® tube 0.3 mm) between the microdialysis probe and the glucose biosensor (volume under 50 μl).

The influence of temperature on the dialysis probe was evaluated. At 37°C the current is about 30% higher and the linearity range is slightly reduced; this reflects the variation of the diffusion coefficient of the glucose through the microdialysis probe. The stability of the signal with a hollow fiber during a 10-h period was followed *in vitro*. Fluctuations smaller than 15% were generally obtained due to random variations in the experimental parameters. The

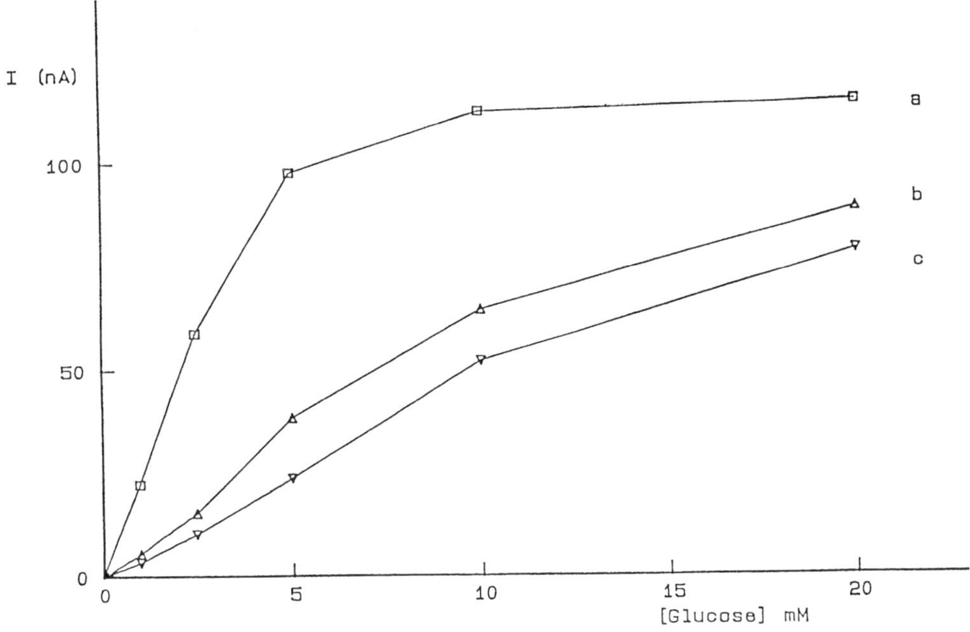

FIGURE 18.13 Calibration curves of glucose with different lengths of membrane microdialysis probes. Flow rate = 30 μl/min, T = 37°C, a = 40 mm, b = 20 mm, c = 10 mm.

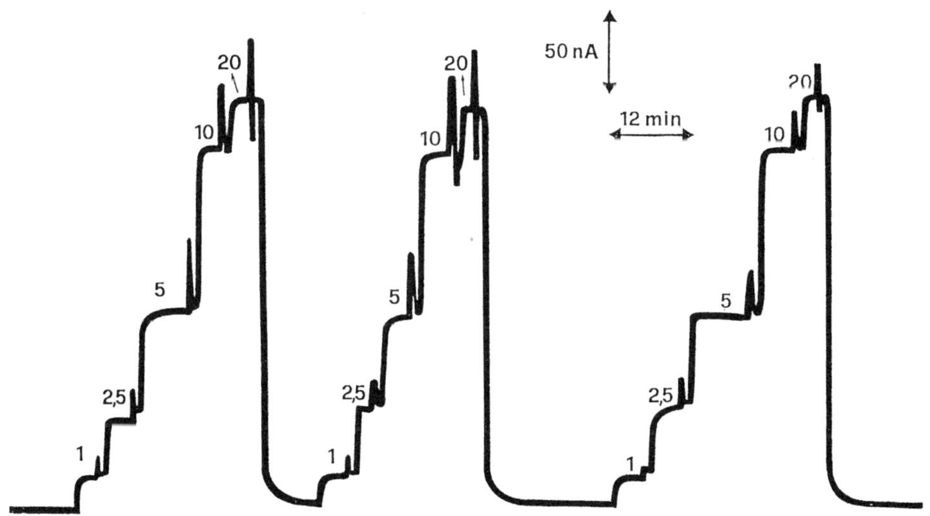

FIGURE 18.14 Response time of the hollow fiber used as a microdialysis probe. Flow rate = 30 μl/min, room temperature, membrane length = 20 mm.

glucose biosensor is known to be stable during such an interval of time, so it is not the primary source of fluctuation.

18.4.2 Procedures and Results *In Vivo*

Fast response and recovery, and a simple apparatus and procedures have allowed the proposed method to be directly applied in *in vivo* experiments. The fiber can be sterilized; it is rugged and easily handled; the material is reported to be highly biocompatible.[24]

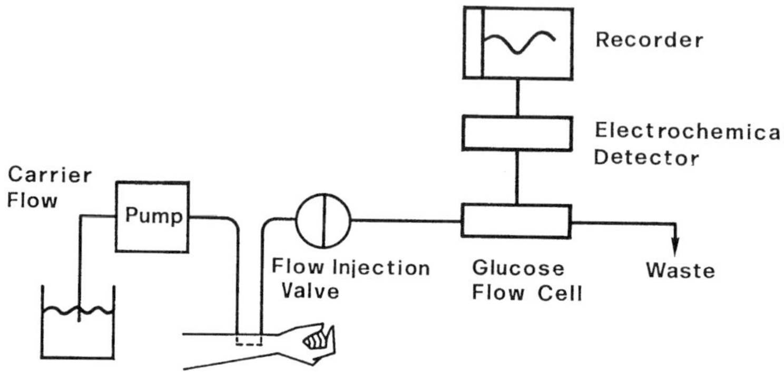

FIGURE 18.15 Diagram of the flow system for the microdialysis experiments.

To place the microdialysis hollow fiber subcutaneously, a sterilized needle was inserted transcutaneously for about 1 cm and the needle tip was pulled out. Then the sterilized fiber was inserted from the needle tip and the needle was taken out, leaving the hollow fiber under the skin. The fiber was connected to nylon tubes and fixed with cyanoacrylic glue. For checking variations in sensitivity during the experiments, a flow injection system was used. An injection valve with a 20-μl sample loop was introduced in the flow system just after the microdialysis probe (Figure 18.15). A glucose standard buffered solution filled the loop of the injection valve and flowed through the glucose biosensor to obtain a current profile similar to a peak. Figure 18.16 shows preliminary results obtained monitoring glucose by sampling with a hollow fiber inserted subcutaneously in a rabbit (Figure 18.16a) and in a human volunteer (Figure 18.16b) during a glucose load experiment. The stability of the signal before the glucose load shows how the removal of glucose by the probe does not disturb the physiological process. After a glucose load the current increases and then decreases following a normal behavior. The variation of sensitivity was checked regularly by the flow injection apparatus described.

A sharp decrease of the sensitivity is evident after about 2-h in both experiments (Figures 18.16a and b). This effect was not previously detected.[25] If the microdialysis probe was disconnected and buffer as carrier was pumped through the cell, the glucose biosensor recovered the initial sensitivity within 15 to 30 min. We attribute this observation to an unknown substance produced in the physiological liquid, probably in response to the fiber introduction. We believe it is released as a consequence of an inflammatory reaction and is able to diffuse through the hollow fiber and interferes with the enzyme or the electrode reaction. This sensitivity variation can explain why attempts to measure glucose *in vivo* by directly inserting needle glucose biosensors in blood or subcutaneously fail more or less rapidly, and it may explain the variation in sensitivity (slope of the response curve current vs. glucose concentration) reported in the literature.[26-28a] It is the first time that this phenomenon was followed during an "*in vivo*" experiment. The problem of tissue reaction was reported recently in a few cases[28a] to explain the high failure of subcutaneous glucose monitoring.

We succeeded in overcoming the problem by changing the flow cell with the glucose biosensor. Replacing the thin-layer-type flow cell with a wall jet-type cell, the results improved drastically. The two cells are depicted in Figure 18.17. We think that the jet of the flow

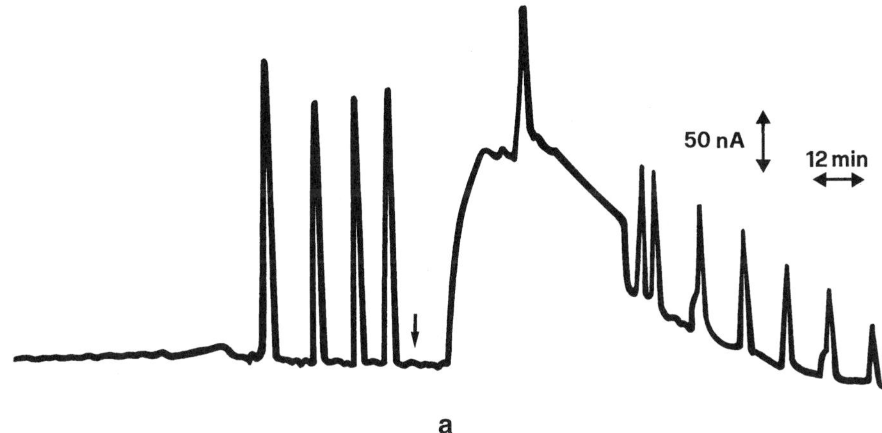

FIGURE 18.16a *In vivo* experiments during a glucose loading. Hollow fiber as microdialysis probe; flow rate = 30 μl/min, membrane length = 10 mm, rabbit weight 2.5 kg, fasting, unanesthetized (intravenous glucose loading = 3.5 g (glucose).

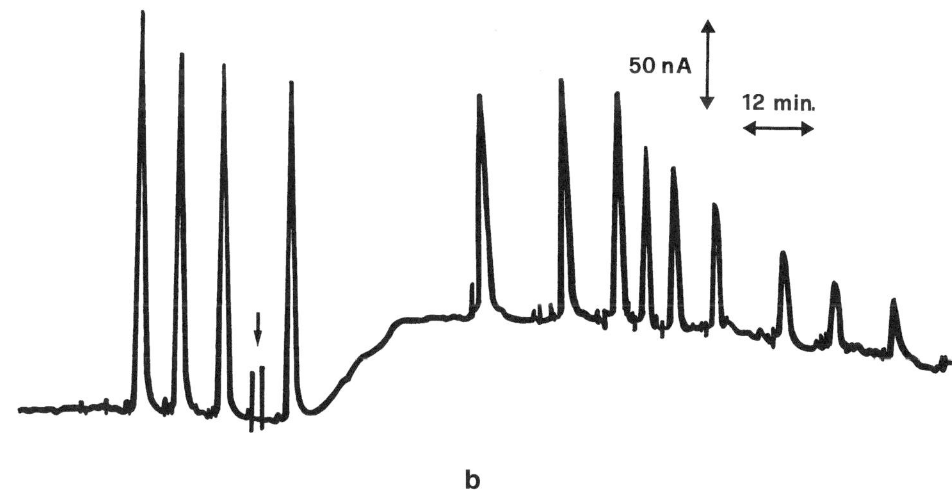

FIGURE 18.16b *In vivo* experiment on a human volunteer (oral loading = 70 g). The arrow shows the glucose administration.; the peaks show the monitoring of sensitivity variation; and the glucose standard solution was 1 mM.

obtained by the nozzle in front of the glucose biosensor cleans the surface of the electrode, eliminating the proteinaceous deposit (sometimes visible) formed in the thin-layer cell in "*in vivo*" operation. Figure 18.18 shows the experiment with a rabbit (3 kg) where a glucose load of 2 g (30 ml of glucose solution 7%) was infused in the ear vein during about 8 min. After about 2 to 3 minutes from the start of the infusion procedure we could notice a variation of current measured by the cell. Such an increase due to the subcutaneous glucose reached a maximum value after 15 min, then the current decreased, reaching the basal value after about 1 h. During this time the sensitivity of the biosensor was checked and we could notice only a slight decrease, less than 5% after the 3 h of monitoring. During the experiment, blood aliquots were taken from the ear of the rabbit and analyzed in the clinical laboratory for glucose.

The constant value of current before the glucose load was proportional to the concentration measured in the corresponding blood sample, and assuming a linear relation of

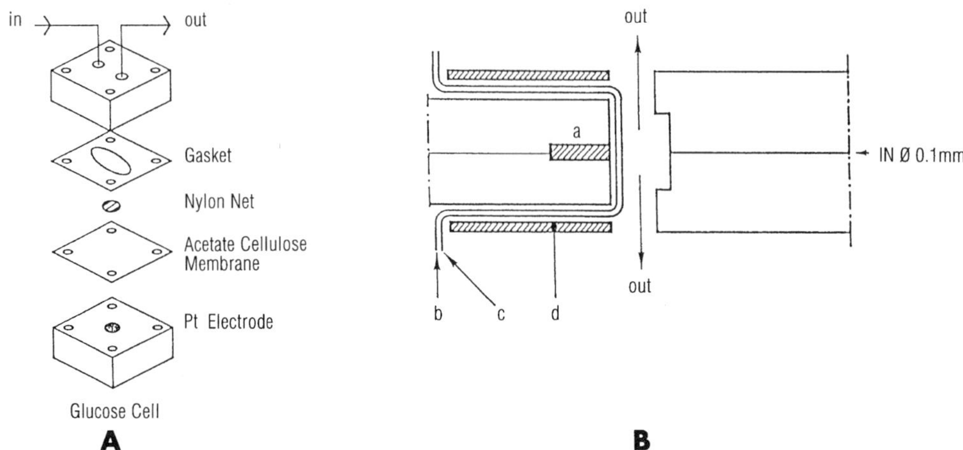

FIGURE 18.17 Thin layer(A) and wall jet (B) flow cells. In (B): a = platinum electrode, b = cellulose acetate membrane, c = glucose oxidase immobilized on nylon net, and d = plastic ring.

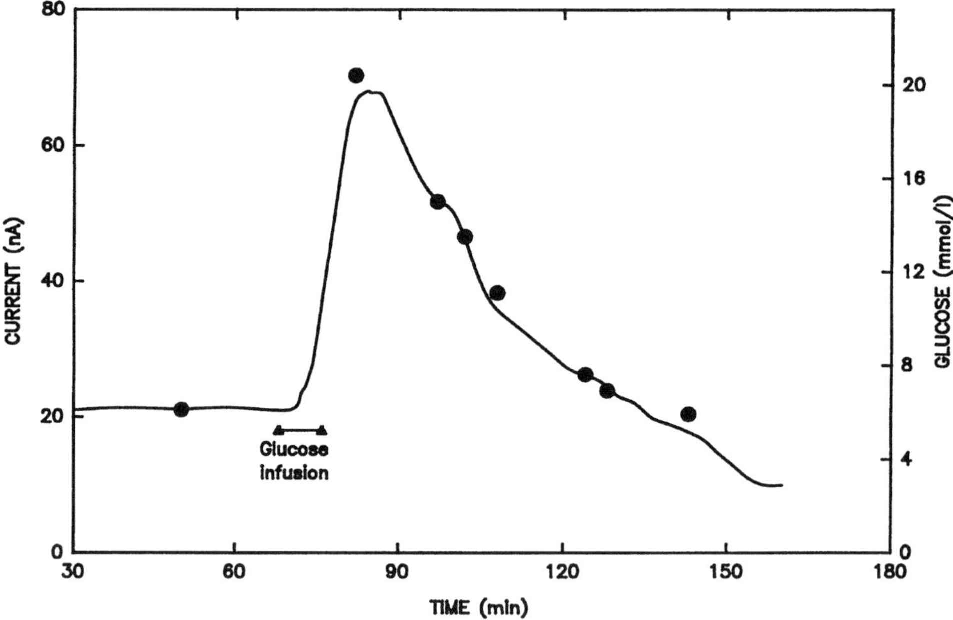

FIGURE 18.18 *In vivo* glucose load with a 3-kg rabbit. The glucose load was accomplished by infusing a glucose concentrated solution in the ear vein during 8 min. The hollow fiber has MWCO of 9.000 and was inserted subcutaneously. By adjusting the stable value before the load with the clinical value, we could plot the right ordinate (current proportional to concentration) according to the one-point calibration. The values plotted are the clinical values of blood taken out during the experiment (correlation coefficient r = 0.993).

biosensor output (current) to concentration in the range of interest (one-point calibration), we could obtain the continuous monitoring of glucose concentration during the experiment (right side of the plot). In the plot of Figure 18.18 we also inserted the values of the control procedure.

It can be seen how this system follows with high accuracy the concentration value of blood in rabbits with a simple one-point calibration. The response time of the overall system is 2 to 3 min and the stability of the sensitivity of the biosensor is perfectly acceptable.

18.4.3 Human Volunteers

In Figure 18.19 we report 15 experiments on human volunteers submitted to a glucose oral load; we follow them by continuously monitoring the subcutaneous glucose value and by normal clinical methods by taking blood samples every 30 min. The glucose value of the blood was measured by clinical standard procedures. In four cases (numbers 5,6,8,13) the microdialysis probe had to be replaced during the course of the experiment, due to accidental breakage or malfunctioning of the probe.

To correlate the continuous monitoring of the current output with the glucose value we assumed that the current value before the load corresponded to the glucose value of the first blood sample (one-point calibration). Experiments reported as numbers 2,14,15 did not perfectly correlate (Figure 18.20), but the correlation increases (Figure 18.20 right side) if we assume a delay between the blood glucose value and subcutaneous values of 30 min.

In our experiments the microdialysis probe was located in the forearm or in the arm, but other sampling sites could be more suitable for a better correlation with the glucose values in blood. This has been considered in a similar experiment[29] where up to 18 min of delay was calculated between the blood glucose and subcutaneous glucose values. Three other experiments (1,11,12) show a low correlation; the trend of glucose in blood seems at glance dissimilar or opposite to the trend of the subcutaneous values.

Experiments 3,4,7,8,9,10 seem to correlate much better and give hope for real portable subcutaneous glucose monitoring. One of the effects of the position of the microdialysis probe was the involuntary muscle contraction near the sampling point. Often, this contraction (generally when the blood sample was taken for clinical analysis) leads to a sudden variation of the continuous monitoring due in our opinion to a collapse of the subcutaneous fiber.

By exploiting this microdialysis technique a new instrument has been realized and the presentation is reported in Figure 18.21. The functions are completely microprocessor controlled. The blood glucose values, updated every minute, are shown on an LCD and can be radiotransmitted. The data arc stored in an internal memory and are transmitted at the end of a 24-h period. A buzzer and several display messages warn about hypoglycemias, malfunctions, and wrong data input.

18.5 UREA SOLID STATE BIOSENSORS FOR CONTINUOUS CONTROL OF DIALYSIS

The problem of monitoring the course of the dialysis treatment in order to allow a personalized treatment (length and frequency) is still a challenge even if several suitable approaches have been published recently.[30-35] During the dialysis treatment the concentration of urea in blood decreases from 50 mM to below 10 mM. Nowadays, no on-line monitoring of the dialysis performance is available and of course the treatment is rarely interrupted at the optimum point.

Recently we succeeded in assembling[36] a solid state potentiometric sensor (nonactin-based with immobilized urease) which is very practical and easy to change for every dialysis treatment, together with an FIA apparatus for continuous monitoring of ultrafiltrate of blood. The FIA procedure was found necessary for controlling the shift occurring at the potentiometric urea sensor continuously, and probably due to a continuous extraction of the ionophore (nonactin) by the ultrafiltrate of lipophilic character. We specifically refer to the dialysis treatment where the ultrafiltration of blood accomplished in a suitable filter precedes the true dialysis process carried out by a second filter where the dialysis liquid reequilibrates the blood (MULTIMAT SYSTEM from Bellco, Italy).

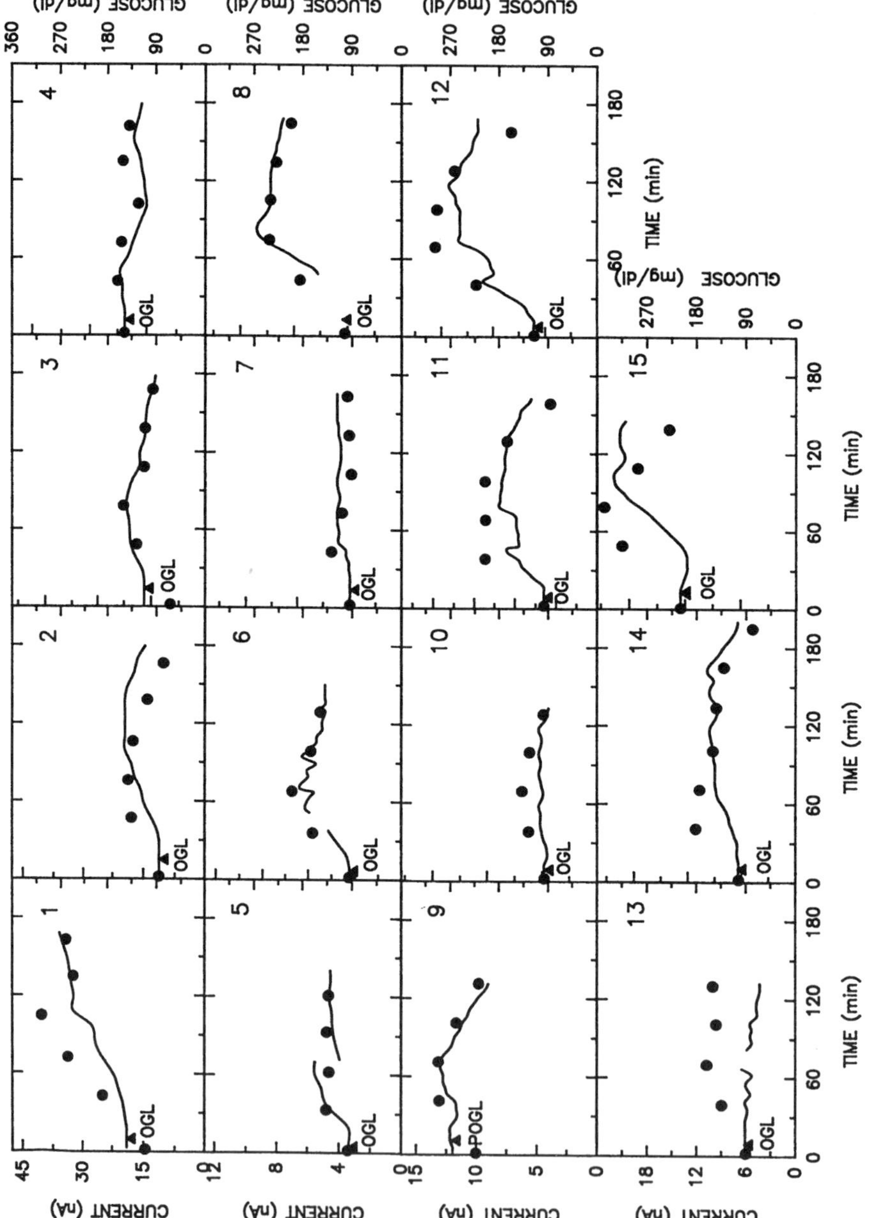

FIGURE 18.19 Glucose oral load of 15 volunteers. The glucose load was accomplished by drinking 75 g of glucose at the time indicated by the arrowhead. The values obtained by clinical analysis are reported as dots.

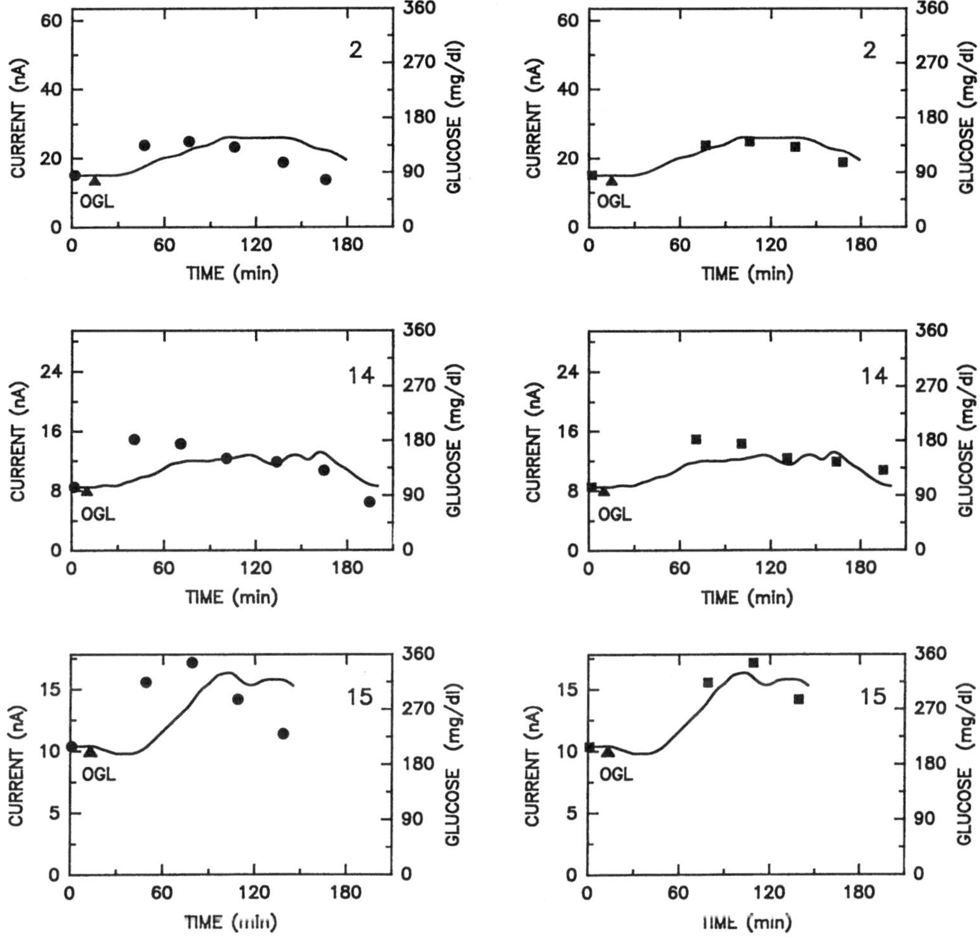

FIGURE 18.20 The subcutaneous experiments in numbers 2, 14 and 15 have been shown delayed 30 min with respect to their glucose value in blood. Better agreement was later obtained.

The ultrafiltrate of blood obtained in the first filter consists of a proteinaceous pale yellow liquid which contains all low molecular weight compounds and is wasted in the dialysis treatment. This liquid was considered the most suitable for the continuous monitoring of urea because the urea concentration in this liquid corresponds perfectly to the blood concentration.

18.5.1 The Sensor

The sensor was obtained by immobilizing over a graphite electrode a layer of PVC-nonactin solution in tetrahydrofuran, and over it a layer of urease immobilized by bovine serum albumin and glutaraldehyde.[37] The sensor has been used or placed in a flow cell (preliminary experiments) or in a wall jet cell provided with a sampling valve in an FIA procedure. The valve was actuated automatically with a pneumatic actuator and an electronic timer to obtain a peak every 4 min. A diagram of the instrumentation is presented in Figure 18.22.

18.5.2 Experimental Results

Different solid state sensors show a Nernstian behavior in the range of 1 to 100 mM; they have E_0 values differing up to ±200 mV for unpredictable reasons and this value can shift from day to day. However the potential slope value is very stable during a period of several

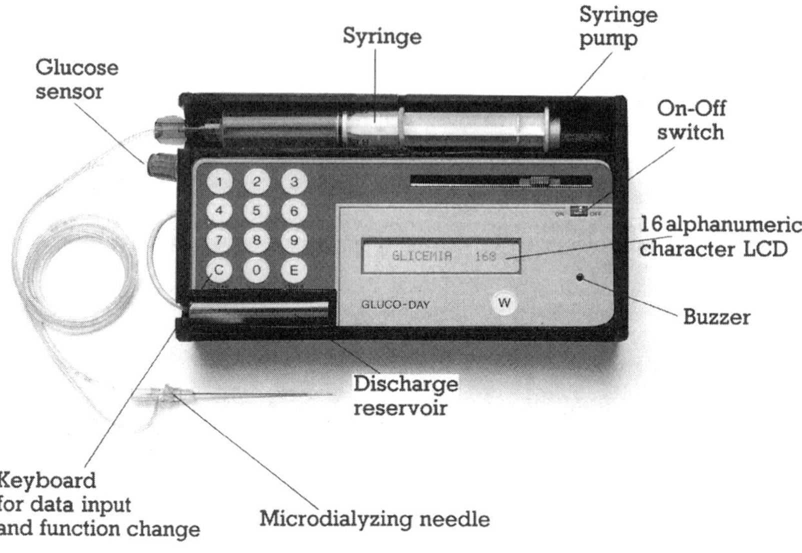

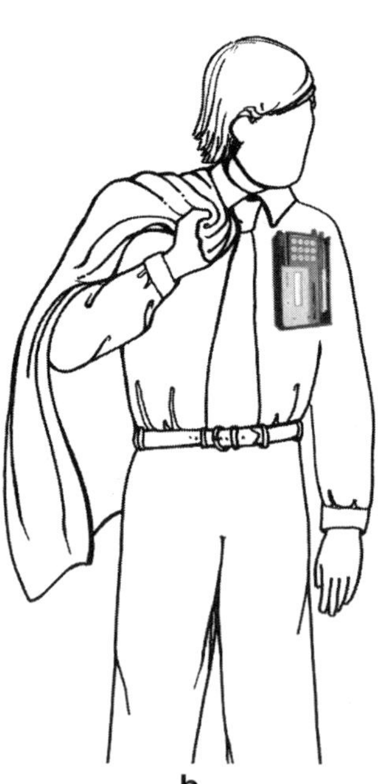

FIGURE 18.21 The Gluco-Day instrument for diabetes monitoring: (a) photograph and specifications, (b) diagram of patient carrying the instrument.

hours and permits an easy determination in flow systems. In contrast, Figure 18.23 depicts the shift observed in an experiment where ultrafiltrate at constant urea concentration (obtained from heparinized bovine blood and adjusted to 40% v/v for the hematocrit value) flowed in

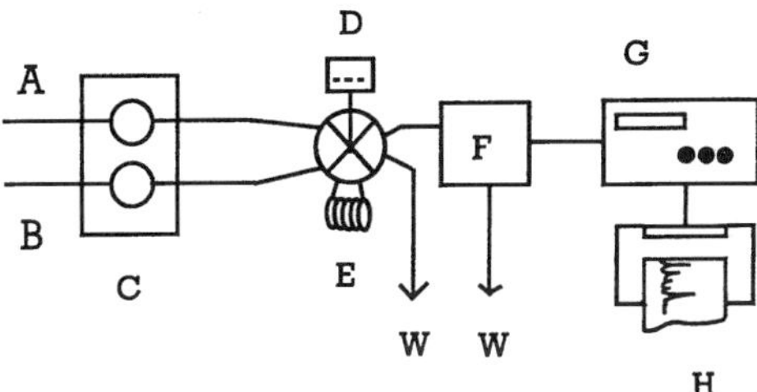

FIGURE 18.22 Scheme of FIA measurement. A: buffer phosphate as carrier; B: ultrafiltrate; C: peristaltic pump; D: timer; E: sampling valve, 50 µl; F: wall-jet cell; G: potentiometer; H: recorder; W: waste. The sampling valve was operated through a pneumatic actuator controlled through a solenoid valve and a Crouzet timer.

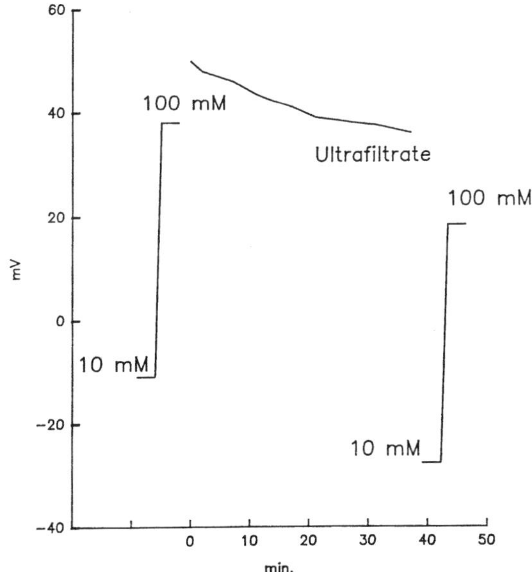

FIGURE 18.23 Experiment with the ultrafiltrate. Two standard solutions, 10 and 100 mM, were prepared and flowed at the beginning and at the end of a 40-min experiment where the ultrafiltrate (urea content 200 mM) flowed.

a continuous mode. We can see how the signal shifted during the 40 min of continuous monitoring and that the signal obtained with two standard solutions (10 and 100 nM) of urea was shifted in the same period by about 25 mV.

Figure 18.24 reports how several calibration curves obtained in continuous flow in another experiment during a 5-h period demonstrate a continuous shift, while the slope was maintained almost constant. After assembling an FIA procedure (50 µl sampling valve) we obtained the results reported in Figure 18.25 with standard solutions prepared in buffer phosphate and in ultrafiltrate for a long period (5 h), while we consecutively sent into the sampling probe standard solutions of urea, ultrafiltrate, and ultrafiltrate with urea added in suitable concentration (10, 30, and 100 mmol/l), simulating a real dialysis process.

The baseline obtained in the last experiment is very stable and the sensitivity of the probe is not impaired by contact with the ultrafiltrate and the long period of the experiment. Therefore we can conclude that this sensor preparation and this analytical procedure are very suitable for the continuous monitoring of urea in such application.

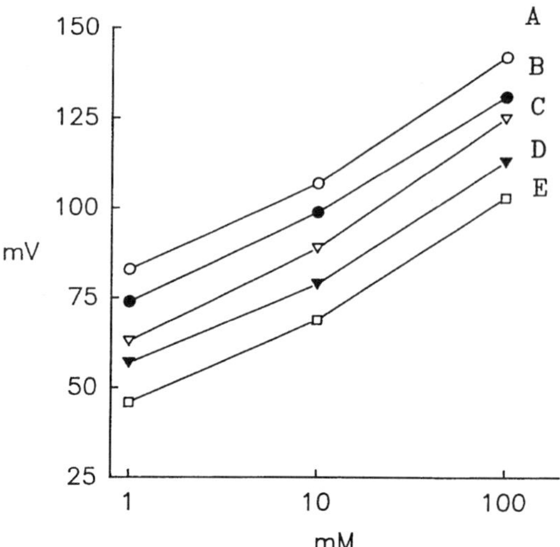

FIGURE 18.24 Successive calibration curves obtained with continuous flow of ultrafiltrate during a 5-h period. Each calibration curve was recorded every hour.

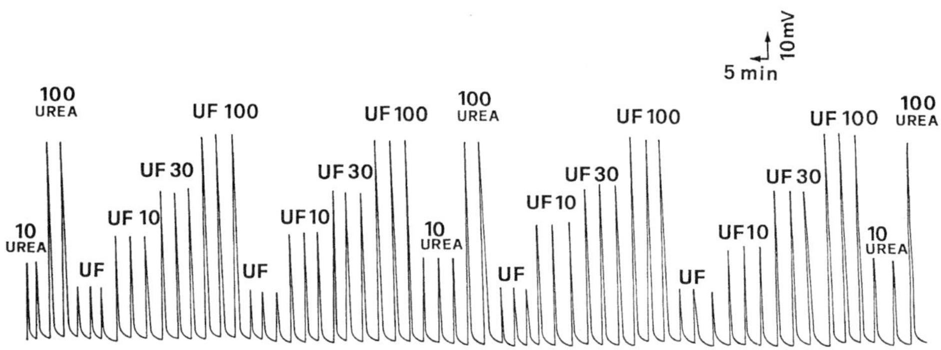

FIGURE 18.25 Continuous recording over a 5-h period of calibration curves of standard solutions and ultrafiltrate spiked with standard urea content.

In Figure 18.25 we can observe how in the low range of urea concentration the peaks obtained in ultrafiltrate are higher than the same urea concentrations in buffer. This result was expected and it is due to the well-known interference of potassium ions at the nonactin-based ammonium sensors. However, the low range of urea is the least important part of the calibration curve for clinical purposes.

The drift observed in the continuous flow experiment (Figure 18.23) can be ascribed to the lipophilic nature of the ultrafiltrate which probably extracts the constituents of the PVC membrane (ionophore or softener). This was reported with other ISE (ion-selective electrodes) with neutral carriers when in contact with blood or proteinaceous fluids.[38] However, the FIA procedure eliminates the problem for at least up to 5 h. It is logical that the small period of contact between the ultrafiltrate and the sensor membrane allows generation of a very reproducible signal, but does not alter the composition and the structure of the membrane. We think that this approach solves the problem of continuous monitoring of urea during dialysis treatment with a cheap, disposable, and easily fabricated sensor, which can be even printed for mass production and distribution (screen printing, etc.) and can be considered a real disposable sensor.

ACKNOWLEDGMENTS

This work has been supported by the C.N.R. Target Project on Biotechnology and Bioinstrumentation, which is gratefully acknowledged.

REFERENCES

1. Guilbault, G. G. and Mascini, M., *Uses of Immobilized Biological Compounds,* NATO ASI Series E, Vol. 252, 1993.
2. Scheller, F. and Schmid, R. D., Eds., *Biosensors, Fundamentals, Technologies and Applications,* VCH Publishers, New York, 1992.
3. Heineman, W. R., Higgins, I. J., Potter, W. G., Turner, A. P. F., and Wingard, L. B., Jr., Eds., *Biosensors, An International Journal,* Elsevier, New York, 1985.
4. Cheung, P. W., Fleming, D. G., Neuman, M. R., and Ko, W. H., Eds., *Theory, Design and Biomedical Application of Solid State Chemical Sensors,* CRC Press, Boca Raton, Fl, 1978.
5. Turner, A. P. F., Ed., Chemical sensors for *in vivo* monitoring, *Advances in Biosensors,* JAI Press, Oxford, 1993.
6. Alcock, S. J., and Turner, A. P. F., Eds., *In Vivo Chemical Sensors: Recent Developments,* Cranfield Press, Cranfield, U.K., 1993.
7. Vadgama, P., *Advanced Models for the Therapy of Insulin Dependent Diabetes,* Brunetti, P. and Waldhouse, W. K., Eds., Raven Press, New York, 1987, 235.
8. Mullen, W. H., Keedy, F. H., Churchouse, S. J., and Vadgama, P., *Anal. Chim. Acta,* 183, 59, 1986.
9. Shichiri, M., Yamasaki, Y., Saito, Y., Hoshiyama, S., and Kamada, T., *Advanced Models for the Therapy of Insulin Dependent Diabetes,* Brunetti, P. and Waldhouse, W. K., Eds., Raven Press, New York, 1987, 261.
10. Shichiri, M., Kawamori, R., and Yamasaki, Y., *Biosensors, Fundamentals and Applications,* Turner, A. P. F., Karube, I., and Wilson, G. S., Eds., Oxford Science Publishers, Oxford, 1987, 261.
11. Shichiri, M, Yamasaki, Y., Kawamori, R., Ueda, N., and Sekiya, M., Biosensors, International Workshop 1987; Gesellschaft für Biotechnologische Forschung, Braunschweig, Stockeim, Germany, 95, June 23-26, 1987.
12. Brunetti, P., and Waldhouse, W. K., Eds., *Advanced Models for the Therapy of Insulin Dependent Diabetes,* Raven Press, New York, 1987.
13. Clemens, A. H., Chang, P. H., and Myers, R. W., *Horm. Metab. Res. Suppl.,* 7, 23, 1977.
14. Clemens, A. H., Chang, P. H., and Myers, R. W., *J. Annu. Diabetol. Hotel,* 269, 1976.
15. Mascini, M., Mazzei, F., Moscone, D., Calabrese, G., and Massi-Benedetti, M., *Clin. Chem.,* 24, 1366, 1978.
16. Palleschi, G., Mascini, M., Bernardi, L., Zeppilli, P., *Med. Biol. Eng. Comput.,* 28, B25, 1990.
17. Karlsson, J. and Jacobs, I., *Int. Sports Med.,* 3, 190, 1982.
18. Mader, A., Leisen, H., Heck, H., Philippi, H., Rost, R., Schurch, P., and Hollman, W., *Sportarzt Sportmed.,* 4, 80, 1976.
19. Shichiri, M, Kawamori, R., Yamasaki, Y., and Ueda, N., *Medical Applications of the Glucose Sensor in Chemical Sensor Technology,* Vol. 1, Seiyama, T., Ed., Kodansha, Tokyo, 1988, p. 209.
20. Churchouse, S. J., Battersby, C. M., Mullen, V. H., and Vadgama, P. M., *Biosensors,* 2, 325, 1986.
21. Velho, G., Reach, G., and Thevenot, D. R., *Biosensors, Fundamentals and Applications,* Turner, A. P. F., Karube, I., and Wilson, G., Eds., Oxford Science, Oxford, 1987, p. 390.
22. Kissinger, P. K., *J. Chromatogr.,* 488, 31, 1989.
23. Moscone, D., Pasini, M., and Mascini, M., *Talanta,* 39(8), 1039, 1992.
24. **Anon.,** Information obtained from Hospal Industrie, Mizandala, Italy, 1990.

25. Huang, T. and Kissinger, P., *Curr. Separations,* 9(1/2), 9, 1989.
26. Sternberg, R., Barrau, M. B., Gangiotti, L., Thevenot, D., Bindra, D., Wilson, G., Velho, G., Froguel, P., and Reach, G., *Biosensors,* 4, 27, 1988.
27. Pickup, J., Shaw, G., and Claremont, D., *Diabetologia,* 32, 213, 1989.
28a. Rebrin, K., Fisher, U., Woedtke, T. , Abel, P., and Brunstein, E., *Diabetologia,* 32, 57320, 1989.
28b. Moscone, D. and Mascini, M., *Ann. Biol. Clin.,* 50, 323, 1992.
29. Meyerhoff, C., Bischof, F., Sternberg, F., Zier, H., and Pfeiffer, E. F., *Diabetologia,* 35, 1087, 1992.
30. Martorell, D., Martínez-Fábregas, E., Bartroli, J., Alegret, S., and Tran-Minh, C., *Sensors Actuators,* B15-16, 448, 1993.
31. Alegret, S., Bartroli, J., Jiménez, C., Martínez-Fábregas, E., Martorell, D., and Valdés-Pérez-gasga, F., *Sensors Actuators,* B15-16, 453, 1993.
32. Thavarungkun, P., Hakanson, H., Holst, O., and Mattiasson, B., *Biosens. Bioelectron.,* 6, 101, 1991.
33. Sansen, W., Jacobs, P., Claes, A., and Lamprechts, M., 2nd Workshop of Biomedical Engineering Action of the European Community on Chemical Sensors for In Vivo Monitoring, 12-15 November 1989, Florence, Italy.
34. Karube, I., Tamiya, E., Dicks, J. M., amd Gatoh, M., *Anal. Chim. Acta,* 185, 195, 1986.
35. Palleschi, G., Mascini, M., Martínez-Fábregas, E., Alegret, S., *Anal. Lett.,* 21(7), 1115, 1988.
36. Zamponi, S., Lo Cicero, B., Mascini, M., Della Ciana, L., and Sacco, S., *Talanta,* submitted.
37. Mascini, M. and Guilbault, G. G., *Anal. Chem.,* 49, 795, 1977.
38. Mascini, M. and Marrazza, G., *Anal. Chim. Acta,* 231, 125, 1990.

19 Biosensors for Process Monitoring

Ursula Bilitewski and Ingrid Rohm

CONTENTS

0-8493-8905-4/97/$0.00+$.50
© 1997 by CRC Press, Inc.

19.1 INTRODUCTION

In recent years the number of analytical systems developed for process monitoring, mainly bioprocess monitoring, has increased continuously. Research in this field is driven by an increasing demand for analytical information about processes for several reasons:

1. Monitoring physical, chemical, and biological parameters of a process allows judgment of the state of the cultivation. This can help to optimise cultivation conditions, duration of the cultivation, time of product harvesting, etc., which leads to a reduction of time required to establish a process and of costs related to nonoptimised cultivation conditions.
2. Improved process and product documentation is required as soon as products of high economic value are produced, or where the health and safety of consumers are implicated, e.g., for pharmaceutical purposes using recombinant microbial strains, or if production occurs according to the guidelines of Good Manufacturing Practices.
3. During development and establishment of production processes analytical information is required for understanding mechanisms in the process, which in turn allows modification and control of cultivation conditions to achieve high reproducibility in the performance of the process and by this in product quality.[1]

Process analysis is accomplished in two basically different ways: the classical method is off-line determination of parameters, which involves manual sampling during the process and analysis of the samples in the lab. This leads to a certain time delay of data, especially if the samples collected during cultivation are analysed altogether only at the end of the cultivation, and additionally requires a high amount of manual work. Thus, this method is the method of choice only for slow or well-established and intensively characterised processes requiring no frequent sampling and in situations where just a final documentation of the process is required. However, the majority of bioprocesses are microbial batch processes or continuous feed batch cultivations where control of various parameters is essential. Therefore, instrumentation for on-line monitoring of processes is being developed. This can be achieved by systems suitable for *in situ* monitoring directly in the fermenter or by application of sampling modules allowing automated and sterile removal of samples from the process in combination with automated analytical devices.[2] In Figure 19.1 various possibilities for the positioning of on-line devices are shown. Automated on-line analysis minimises on one hand the requirement for manual work and on the other hand the time delay of data, thus allowing effective monitoring even of fast processes and also control of process conditions.

A bioprocess is characterised by its physical, chemical, and biological state. That means that analytical information is required about physical parameters, e.g., temperature, pressure, and stirring speed, and about chemical parameters, e.g., pH, pO_2, composition of the gas phase, concentrations of substrates, metabolic products or other constituents of the media and the desired product, and about the biological state, i.e., biomass, total cell count, cell viability, etc. To date, only physical data such as temperature and pressure, some chemical parameters such as pH, pO_2, composition of the exhaust gas, and further properties such as the capacitance,[3] fluorescence,[4-6] turbidity,[7] and relative density[8] of the medium as indicators of biomass concentration and viability (see below) can routinely be monitored by commercially available *in situ* sensing devices.

Due to the complexity of media containing a large number of components, analytical devices of high specificity are required to obtain detailed information about concentrations of single compounds. Various chromatographic procedures such as LC[9] or GC[10], or mass spectrometry,[11,12] applied to process monitoring achieve the specificity by separation of

1. In situ sensor

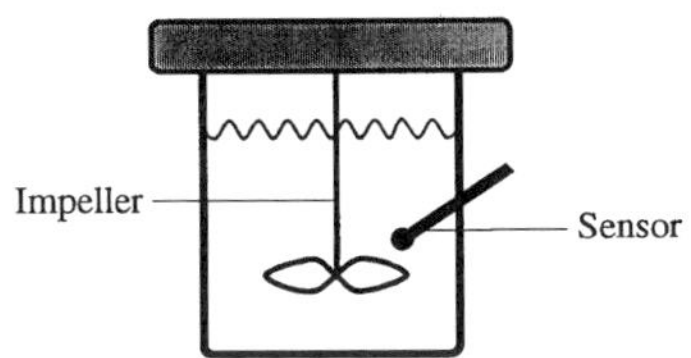

2. In situ sampling

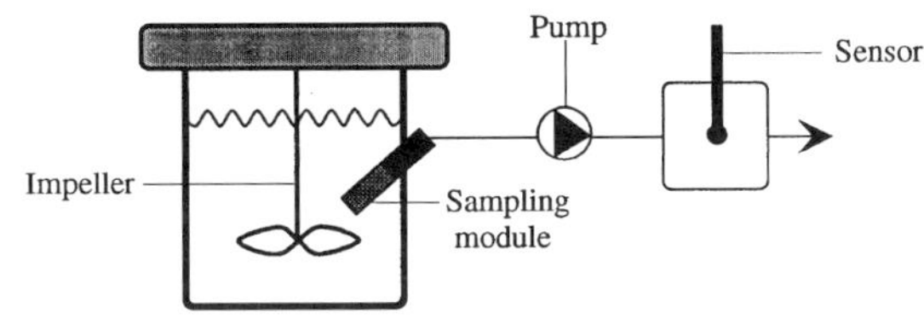

3. Bypass sampling

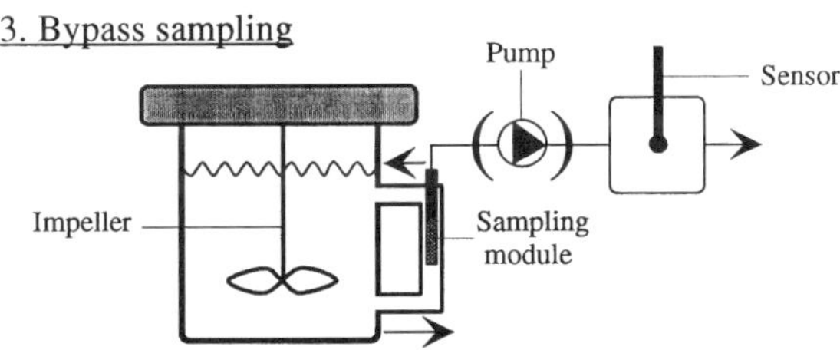

FIGURE 19.1 Various locations for on-line sampling and monitoring devices in a bioreactor.

medium components allowing simultaneous determination of several compounds if required. Additionally, biochemical analytical procedures are used utilising the specificity mainly of enzymatic[13-16] and immunochemical,[17] but also of microbial[18] reactions, allowing the design of simplified, automated devices with high measurement frequencies. However, all these devices cannot be sterilised and demand a suitable interface to the process, guaranteeing the sterility of the cultivation. In the case of biosensing devices this can be achieved by *in situ* sensors[16] or, generally, by a combination of automated devices with suitable sampling modules. Biochemical determination of medium components is automated in most cases by using flow injection analysis (FIA) and using immobilised enzymes or antibodies as recognition elements for the analyte.[14,19]

Additional to this chemical information, biological information about the process, i.e., biomass, total cell count, cell viability, and productivity is required.[20] This is obtained by off-line methods, such as determination of the dry cell weight or cell counting using a microscope. As these methods are time consuming, alternative or supplementary methods were developed allowing on-line or even *in situ* determination of parameters which are directly or indirectly related to biomass or cell viability. Schügerl et al.[7] demonstrated, for example, that *in situ* turbidity determination of media generally correlated well with biomass, whereas fluorescence sensing of NADH showed good correlation to off-line determinations of biomass only as long as the cell state did not change, indicating that this signal is not only dependent on the cell number but also on the metabolic processes in the cells. Similar observations were reported by Ding et al.,[21] who used an on-line FIA system with electrochemical determination of reduced mediators which were reduced by *E. coli*. Here, a good correlation of the electrochemical data to the oxygen uptake rate (OUR) was found, thus indicating again not only cell number but also cell viability.

Within this whole area of analytical methods required for effective process monitoring this review will focus on requirements, possibilities, and limitations of methods and devices used for on-line determination of components in fermentation media with biochemical analytical systems. Already, numerous books and reviews dealing with the development of biosensors[22-30] and their applicability to bioprocess monitoring exist;[13-19,31] we want to mention only briefly the general principles and then concentrate on new developments and systems applied to on-line monitoring of processes.

Analytical systems based on biochemical principles can be divided roughly into three categories:

1. Biosensors designed as *in situ* sensors with the biological component (enzyme, microorganism, antibody) being immobilised in close proximity to the transducer (see Section 19.2).
2. Flow injection analysis (FIA) systems and related flow-through devices with the biological component (enzyme, antibody) being immobilised either on the transducer or on any other kind of solid support which can be used in an enzyme or antibody column (see Section 19.4).
3. Systems for the on-line determination of the biological component, e.g., for the determination of enzyme activities[32-36] or of biomass.[7,20,21] As these systems do not contain an immobilised biochemical receptor they are not considered in this review.

19.2 Sensors For *In Situ* Measurements

Insertion of sensors into a fermenter allows determination of compounds in real time, thus providing information necessary for effective process control. Additionally, *in situ* sensors are less sensitive to external disturbances than external instruments, as they are integrated in the reaction vessel. Thus, generally the development of *in situ* sensors is highly desirable. However, to date *in situ* sensors for some parameters can only be used routinely. The reason is that by insertion into the fermenter the probe must withstand sterilisation of the reaction vessel. Concentrations of substrates, metabolic products, or intracellular components are often determined by biochemical methods using the specificity of enzymatic or immunochemical reactions (see also Section 19.4). As enzymes and antibodies cannot be sterilised without loss of activity, special probes were designed allowing *in situ* determination of glucose[37-39] and penicillin.[40,41]

The sensors consisted of two parts (see Figure 19.2): an outer housing made of stainless steel with one end closed by a membrane permeable to the analyte and at the same time acting as sterile barrier, and an inner sensor component containing the immobilised enzymes.[38] The outer housing could be inserted into the fermenter during sterilisation, and the inner sensor part was inserted after sterilisation with the membrane guaranteeing the sterility of the process. By an internal buffer flow, the analyte diffusing through the membrane to the immobilised enzyme was removed from the probe and by adjusting the flow rate the linear range of the sensor could be adapted to practical requirements. Additionally, *in situ* calibration of the sensor was possible by injection of a standard solution into the internal buffer. Detailed descriptions of these systems are given in the corresponding literature[37-41] and were reviewed by Bradley et al.[16]

Though the applicability of these sensors to bioprocess monitoring was shown and continuous monitoring of glucose would be highly desirable, the widespread use of these sensors is restricted by some practical problems. As for all *in situ* devices, the position of the sensor within the reaction vessel must be optimised to obtain representative information from the process and achieve sufficient movement of liquid at the sensor head to minimise

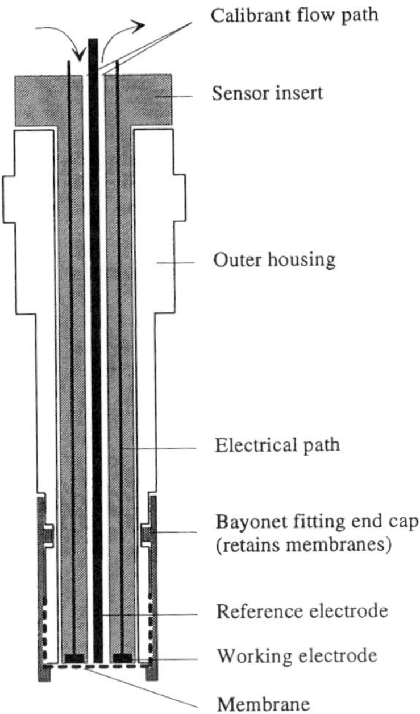

FIGURE 19.2 Simplified scheme of an *in situ* biosensor probe.

effects of fouling and clogging by attached cells which would change transport characteristics of the membrane thus influencing the sensor response. Additionally, if transportation through the membrane was changed by other parameters, e.g., changes of pressure in the reaction vessel or within the sensor, this also affected the sensor signals.[31]

19.3 SAMPLING SYSTEMS

19.3.1 General Remarks

As described in Section 19.2, biochemical analysis by *in situ* sensors is restricted to some selected examples. The best established principle to achieve continuous information from the process is the application of FIA devices (Section 19.4) together with suitable sampling modules. In these cases the value of the analytical information is not only dependent on the performance of the analytical device but also on the quality of the sampling procedure.

In an ideal situation a representative sample is taken from the process, analysed in an accurate and reproducible manner before any changes of the sample occur, and analysis of the process is achieved in real time.[42] Additionally, the sampling device should be applicable to different kinds of processes, and the analysis of extra- and intracellular compounds should be possible. These requirements cannot be met to date by a single module, and R&D efforts are underway to approximate this situation as closely as possible.

As pointed out in Figure 19.1, on-line instrumentation can be coupled to a process in different positions, leading to development of different suitable sampling devices. They have to fulfill at least two requirements:[16] the sample must be removed from the medium and transported through the analytical device (e.g., FIA manifold) to the detector, and the sterile integrity of the process must be maintained. For most analytical purposes the application of cell-free samples to the sensing device is preferred to prevent metabolic processes within the sample and, by this, changes in composition during transportation, and to prevent contamination of the analytical device with cells which would require additional cleaning steps.

Therefore, most of the sampling devices used for on-line monitoring of processes contain a barrier for whole cells, e.g., a suitable membrane through which the target molecules have to be transported. An exception is the sampling module described by Ding et al.,[21] who removed samples containing whole cells (*E. coli*) from fermentation broth and ensured the sterility of the process by a chemical barrier consisting of valves and a tubing between the bioreactor and the measurement device which was filled with a disinfectant when no sampling was executed. It is also described that specific inhibitors had to be added to samples after removal from the cultivation to inhibit extracellular enzymes which decompose sample ingredients.[43] Separation of cells was done after sampling by a dialysis chamber placed in front of the immobilised enzyme.

Depending on their position within the reaction vessel, systems being inserted directly into the medium have to be distinguished from those being placed in a bypass with circulation of the sample. With the sampling module placed in the bypass it is possible to change the membrane within the module during cultivation, but circulation of the sample may affect the performance of the cultivation due to substrate depletion, anaerobic conditions, or shear forces.[44] *In situ* placed modules have the advantage that a true picture of the conditions in the bioreactor is obtained, but the membrane cannot be changed during the process. Different approaches and resulting systems, mainly applied to microbial cultivations, were recently reviewed by Mattiasson and Hakanson[42] and by Bradley et al.[16] Sampling during animal cell cultivations was simplified due to the presence of a perfusion line, to which analytical instruments were connected through a chemical barrier,[45] and due to longtime constants of the processes allowing low sampling rates and time delays of data of several minutes.

19.3.2 *In Situ* Sampling Devices

Most of the *in situ* sampling devices are used in combination with the determination of low molecular weight compounds in cell-free medium, allowing removal of cells by (micro)dialysis or filtration. Removal generally occurs directly in the fermenter as the modules contain a suitable membrane. However, it is also possible to remove samples containing whole cells by adding an inhibitor and separating the cells in a dialysis chamber integrated in the analytical instrument.[43]

Dialysis or filtration membranes are incorporated into the fermenter with a receiving carrier buffer being circulated on the permeate side of the membrane and transporting the sample to the detector of the FIA device.[31,44,46,47] This buffer can be added from outside the fermenter, as no contamination of the process occurs as long as the membrane is intact. The *in situ* device used most frequently in combination with FIA is known as the ABC probe and consists of a membrane-supporting unit which contains on the permeate side 16 grooves in which the sample is collected and unified to a continuous sample stream. Suitable tubular membranes are made of polypropylene, polycarbonate, or ceramics.[39] Flow rates of 1 ml/min were achieved allowing easy combination with FIA instrumentation. When using a microdialysis module for sampling,[46] flow rates of only 2 to 10 μl/min can be encountered, leading to longer response times, reduced sampling frequencies, and the requirement for microelectrodes.[42]

Since dialysis systems have no pressure gradient which forces material through a membrane, the tendency to build up a cell layer on the membrane from the fermenter side is reduced compared to filtration modules. However, even on dialysis modules cells may attach and grow and form a film, acting as a biologically active filter, thus changing sample composition during the sampling process and clogging the membrane. Therefore, a dialysis module was developed in which a tangential flow across the membrane was created either by a built-in impeller or by directing the existing turbulent flow inside the fermenter over the membrane surface.[47]

19.3.3 Bypass Sampling Modules

If the sampling module is placed outside the fermenter, fermentation broth has to be pumped out of the fermenter to the sampling module and, after filtration, back to the fermenter. This circulation increases the risk of infection of the cultivation. Additionally, the morphology of the microorganisms may be affected due to shear forces present during pumping, and cultivation conditions in the bypass may differ from those in the fermenter due to ineffective mixing, substrate depletion, or anaerobic conditions. On the other hand, the performance of externally placed sampling modules can be controlled more easily, membranes can be changed during cultivation, and there are less restrictions with the design and size of the module than for *in situ* modules. Thus, several types of modules were developed and are commercially available. They differ mainly in the principle used to avoid build up of cells and thus clogging of the filtration membrane.

Buttler et al.[48,49] used a tangential flow filtration assembly (Waters FAM filtration unit) to divide the bioreactor solution into a particle-enriched retentate and a particle-free filtrate. In this module the solution is driven in a path parallel to the filter. This movement of liquid keeps the surface of the filter clean and prevents sedimentation of cells. The rate of filtration is dependent on the pressure drop across the membrane and therefore on the rate of the feed pump. The filtrate flow rate was not controlled by a filtrate pump, which would generate an additional pressure drop and could lead to air bubbles in the filtrate, but by a restrictor situated inside the assembly, reducing the filtrate rate by generating a backpressure. Controlling the restrictor allowed discontinuous sampling[49] which is essential for monitoring small-scale fermentations. Different types of membranes were tested with the pore size influencing both the purity of the filtrate and the filtrate rate.

The same principle of tangential or cross-flow of the fermentation broth is used in the A-SEP™ module,[50] where the following criteria were additionally considered during development: (1) use of standard-sized filter discs, (2) use of a rapid linear recycle rate, (3) minimisation of the filtrate dead volume, and (4) no damage to shear-sensitive organisms. The filtrate rate was controlled to 0.15 or 0.3 ml/min by a filtrate pump. In the Biopem module[51] movement of liquid across the membrane surface is achieved by a magnetic stirrer placed above the membrane. During cultivation of *Penicillium chrysogenum* a decrease in the permeate flow rate from 1.8 to 0.4 ml/min was observed,[44] due to a buildup of material on the membrane. It was concluded that the Biopem can successfully be applied to bacteria and yeast fermentations, but is very poor for sampling during cultivations of filamentous fungi. Another drawback is the response time of 2 min with a circulation flow of 30 l/min, which may lead to anaerobic conditions in the circulation loop.

A hollow-fibre UF module was used by van de Merbel et al.[9] in combination with a liquid chromatography system. This module was chosen due to its high membrane area-to-volume ratio necessary for a high filtrate rate. However, dead times of 5 to 12 min, depending on the viscosity of the medium, were reported. Additionally, a decreasing filtration rate was observed during cultivation.

These descriptions of some sampling modules show that the proper choice of the sampling device strongly influences the applicability of automated analytical systems to on-line process monitoring.

19.4 FLOW INJECTION ANALYSIS SYSTEMS

19.4.1 Principles of FIA

19.4.1.1 Fundamentals

Flow injection analysis (FIA) was introduced in 1975 by Ruzicka and Hansen[52] as a method of automated liquid handling. An exact volume of the sample is injected into a continuous, nonsegmented carrier stream. When the sample zone moves through the tubes of the system in a laminar flow fashion (Figure 19.3), the original square-wave concentration profile disperses through complex diffusion and convection processes. This dispersion can be monitored by injecting a coloured dye into a colourless carrier stream and monitoring the resulting peak by a photometer equipped with a suitable flow-through cuvette. Increasing dispersion is indicated by a reduced peak height and an increased peak width. Using a very simple, single-line manifold comprising a pump for the carrier stream, an injection valve, another pump for filling the injection valve with the sample, and a detector (Figure 19.4), the dispersion can be manipulated by the injected sample volume, the tube length, and pumping rate. Increasing the sample volume leads to a less effective mixing of the sample with the carrier, i.e., to a reduced dispersion, whereas the degree of dispersion increases with the length of the tube through which the sample has travelled. In order to obtain maximum sampling frequencies it is necessary to prevent peak spreading, i.e., limit the dispersion, as otherwise the sample would mix with the next oncoming sample zone. On the other hand, an excessively low dispersed sample zone is not sufficiently mixed with the carrier stream, which may contain reagents, and thus the chemical reaction cannot take place.

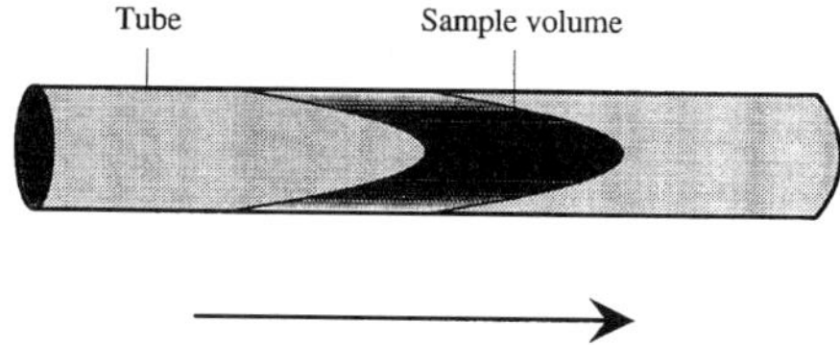

FIGURE 19.3 Laminar flow of a sample within an FIA tube.

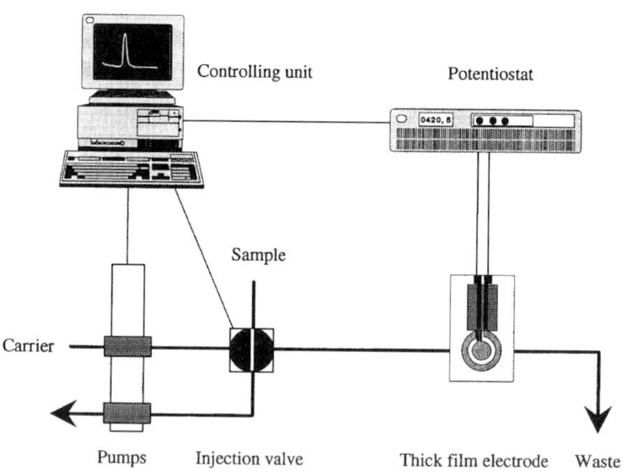

FIGURE 19.4 Schematic view of a simple flow injection analysis device.

The dispersion D is defined as the ratio of the original analyte concentration c_0 to the concentration of the analyte in that element of fluid which corresponds to the maximum of the peak c_{max}:

$$D = c_0/c_{max} \tag{19.1}$$

It is determined by comparing the signals H_0, obtained when the sample is not diluted, i.e., used as the carrier, and H_{max}, obtained when the sample is injected into the carrier, provided that the signals H are linearly related to the concentrations of the analyte. The value of D characterises an FIA manifold because it quantifies the dilution of the sample through the carrier solution and facilitates the comparison of different FIA manifolds. Reproducible results can only be obtained if the dispersion in the device is controlled, i.e., not all parameters of the manifold such as sample volume or pumping rate must be accurately known, but they must be constant and reproducible. If this is achieved, chemical reactions do not have to reach equilibrium and thus the sampling frequency can be increased and sample consumption be decreased. Typical parameters in FIA devices are sample volumes of 20 to 300 μl, flow rates of 0.5 to 3.5 ml/min, dispersions larger than 2, and measuring frequencies of up to several hundred samples per hour.

FIA has found wide application in analytical chemistry because nearly all detection principles can be used if suitable flow-through cells exist (see Section 19.4.1.5). Thus, physical parameters such as absorbance at a given wavelength or conductivity, and chemical parameters such as pH and concentrations of other ions or of oxygen, can be determined by using suitable flow-through detectors. The typical form of the signal is a peak, representing the concentration gradient between carrier and sample (Figure 19.3), with the peak height generally being proportional to the concentration of the analyte. The basic FIA-manifold, a single-line manifold, can be adapted to a variety of analytical methods by the development of additional components and special procedures[53-61] (see below). Commonly used components are mixing chambers, confluence points, small columns containing immobilised reagents[62] or catalysts, gas diffusion[63] or pervaporation[64] units, dialysis chambers, 2/3-way valves, and additional injection valves (Figure 19.5). All these modifications of the manifold again influence the dispersion of the sample, but they lead to a large variability of FIA and its applicability to different kinds of analysis.

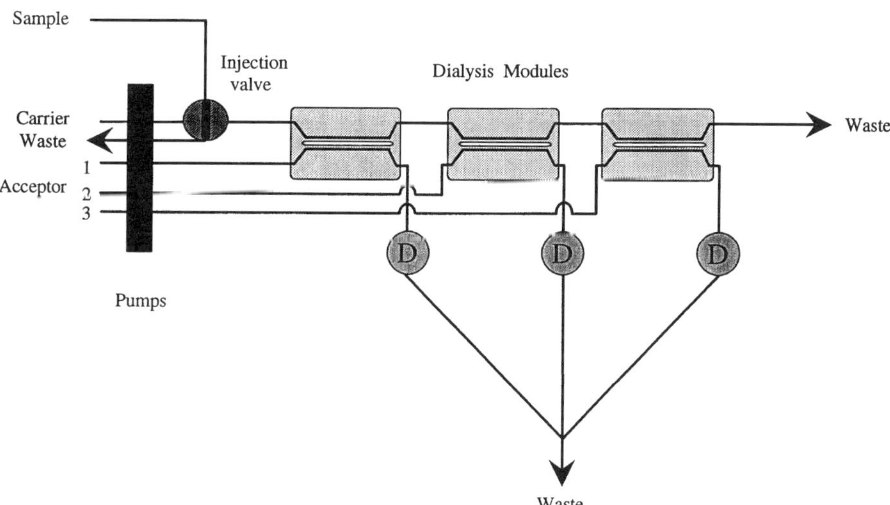

FIGURE 19.5 Three-channel FIA system with dialysis modules for the dilution and separation of analytes.

19.4.1.2 FIA Procedures

Using enzymes or antibodies in FIA improves the specificity and selectivity of analytical procedures. However, the kinetics of the biochemical reaction have to be taken into account. This implies that (1) special FIA modes have to be applied in order to prolong the contact time of the analyte solution and the biochemical reagent, and (2) FIA configurations have to be adapted to the limited linear range of the biological reaction and the detection units.

Condition (1) is fulfilled by the concept of "stopped flow", which is of paramount importance especially in the case of enzyme activity determination. Advantage is taken of the fact that the dispersion of the sample zone does not change significantly even if its residence time is increased by stopping the carrier stream. The stopped-flow technique[53,54] was used for the measurement of enzymatic reaction rates (kinetic stopped-flow) as well as for the measurement of analytes (nonkinetic stopped-flow). Condition (2) is accomplished by gradient techniques such as "electronic dilution" and zone sampling.[64,65] By coupling two manifolds in line (Figure 19.6), the analyte concentration reaching the detector can be controlled by zone sampling over a dilution range of 10^4 and more.

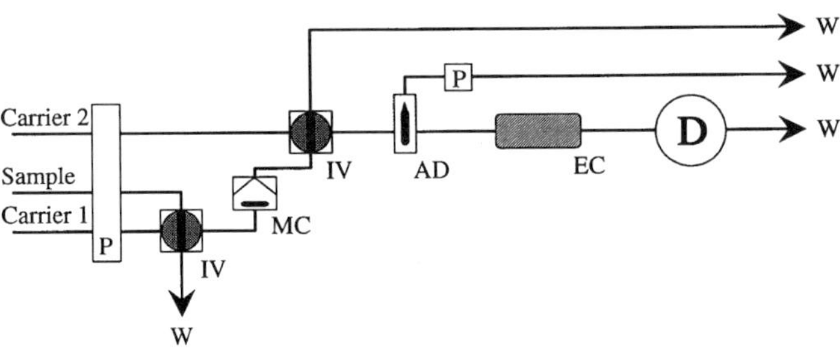

FIGURE 19.6 Flow injection analysis system based on zone sampling: P, peristaltic pump; IV, injection valve; MC, mixing chamber; AD, air damper; EC, enzyme column; D, detector; W, waste.

19.4.1.3 Reactor Design

As already mentioned above, FIA devices can comprise reaction coils or columns containing immobilised reagents or catalysts. This leads to a further extension of methods which can be used in flow injection analysis, for example, the performance of biochemical reactions by immobilising enzymes or antibodies on suitable carriers which can be placed in flow-through reactors.

Though it is not necessary that (bio)chemical reactions performed in FIA reach equilibrium, a close to 100% conversion of the analyte, e.g., by a reaction catalysed by an enzyme, is preferred because such devices are less sensitive to conditions affecting the enzyme activity than those where only incomplete conversion is achieved.[66] The rate of conversion in the reactor depends on the rate of the (bio)chemical reaction as well as on the rate of the mass transfer. The chemical rate depends on the kinetics and on the amount of the enzyme. With surface-bound enzymes, the amount of enzyme will depend on the total surface area and on the number or molecules per unit surface.

Two different types of reactors are described here. A packed-bed reactor generally is a small column which is filled with a pressure-resistant support material such as controlled pore glass. The amount of enzyme in this reactor is dependent on the length (typically 1 to 10 cm) and diameter (typically 1.5 to 3 mm) of the column, and on the surface area of the support to which the enzyme is bound. The highest enzyme loading is obtained using a support with pores of the smallest possible pore diameter compared to the size of the enzyme.

In an open tubular reactor the enzyme is immobilised in a thin layer on the walls, with the surface area being several orders of magnitude less than in a packed-bed reactor of the same volume. Additionally, mass transfer of the analyte to the enzyme is more important in the tubular reactor, but dispersion is less. Thus, signals obtained with systems comprising packed-bed reactors are often higher and less sensitive to changes of experimental conditions than those obtained with systems comprising tubular reactors.

19.4.1.4 Immobilisation Methods

Enzymes and antibodies can be immobilised by various methods based on either physical or chemical binding. As FIA devices are developed for the analysis of a large number of samples, high stability and reliability of these devices are required. Thus, most of the immobilisation methods used in FIA are based on covalent binding of the enzymes or antibodies to a carrier, requiring suitable functional groups on the protein and on the carrier. Functional groups of the protein are provided by the amino acids, the most important one being the amino group provided by lysin residues. In some cases, proteins can be modified without loss of activity resulting in additional groups suitable for covalent binding, for example the carbohydrate residue of glucose oxidase can be removed by oxidation with $NaIO_4$ resulting in active aldehyde groups.[67]

Suitable carriers for immobilised enzymes or antibodies are in some cases the transducer surfaces onto which an enzyme or antibody layer is formed,[68-71] or membrane materials which are preactivated such as nylon,[72,73] or finely divided materials such as glass (controlled pore glass = cpg),[74-76] ion exchangers,[70] or polymers[45,77] which are chemically modified resulting in suitable functional groups on the surface.

No immobilisation method can be given which is superior to others, because the influence of the immobilisation on the enzyme depends on the structure, hydrophobicity, pH sensitivity, etc. of the enzyme, and therefore the immobilisation method has to be optimised for each enzyme.

19.4.1.5 Detection Principles

19.4.1.5.1 Enzymatic detection principles

Mainly, three different types of enzymes are used for analytical purposes: oxidases, dehydrogenases, and hydrolases. They catalyse different types of chemical reactions allowing the combination of a given detection principle or detector with different enzymes of the same class, and thus the determination of different analytes using the same detector and changing only the enzyme.

Oxidases generally catalyse the oxidation of a compound by oxygen:

$$\text{substrate} + O_2 \rightarrow \text{product} + H_2O_2 \qquad (19.2)$$

This offers the possibility to determine the concentration of the substrate via the consumption of O_2 or the production of H_2O_2.

O_2 can be determined by Clark-type oxygen electrodes, as was done in the first biosensor published by Clark.[78] They consist of a Pt cathode at which O_2 is reduced to H_2O, and an Ag/AgCl anode. The whole electrode system is covered with a gas-permeable membrane. Alternatively, O_2 can be determined optically, because it quenches the fluorescence of several dyes.[79] Thus, decacyclen as indicator was immobilised in a silicon membrane on top of an optical fibre, and integrated in a flow-through chamber.[61] With increasing O_2 concentration the intensity of the fluorescence decreased, thus allowing determination of substrates of oxidases.

The amount of H_2O_2 produced by an enzymatic reaction is routinely determined via its oxidation at Pt electrodes. Several flow-through cells are commercially available comprising a working electrode made as a Pt wire or Pt disc, an Ag/AgCl reference electrode, and a counter electrode again made from Pt as a wire, disc, tube, or foil. They are designed either as electrochemical detectors which can be used for any kind of electrochemical detection or as enzyme electrodes integrated in enzyme analysers for glucose, lactate, etc. To date the applicability of technologies suitable for mass production of electrodes, such as thin[80] and thick-film technologies,[81] is being intensively investigated. Electrodes made by these technologies can be integrated into suitable flow-through cells and can either be used just as electrochemical detectors[83] or as enzyme electrodes if the enzyme is immobilised on the surface of the working electrode.[84] The electrochemical determination of H_2O_2 is affected by other components of the sample which are also oxidised at the working electrode. Thus, efforts were made to minimise these interferences by the reduction of the applied potential using working electrodes made of metallised carbon.[85] Less widespread than the electrochemical methods are optical methods for the determination of H_2O_2. They are based on the reaction of H_2O_2 with suitable dyes or luminol catalysed by peroxidase, which is required as a second enzyme. This allows photometric,[34,63] fluorimetric,[86] and luminometric[87] determination of substrates of oxidases.

Dehydrogenases catalyse the oxidation or reduction of compounds by cofactors such as NAD(P)H or NAD(P), respectively:

$$\text{substrate} + \text{NAD(P)}^+ \rightarrow \text{product} + \text{NAD(P)H}^+ \quad (19.3)$$

Generally, determination of substrate concentration is done via the determination of the concentration of NAD(P)H. This can be done either electrochemically, i.e., oxidation of NAD(P)H at carbon electrodes[88] which are modified by chemical modifiers, facilitating the oxidation of NAD(P)H,[89-91] or optically via the absorbance[92] or fluorescence[93,94] of NAD(P)H. As detectors, conventional electrochemical flow-through cells and photometers or fluorimeters equipped with a flow-through cell are used.

Hydrolases catalyse the hydrolysis of compounds. Therefore, generally no common compounds or compounds which can easily be oxidised or reduced are involved. However, often NH_3, CO_2 or H^+ or OH^- are formed which can be determined by potentiomentric gas or ion-selective electrodes or ion-selective field effect transistors (ISFET).[95] In other cases, the first enzyme has to be combined with a second one, e.g., an oxidase or dehydrogenase, generating an easily detectable reaction product.

All detection principles described so far are related to a special class of enzymes, as common substrates or products are detected. However, these combinations are not limited to these general principles; for example, glucose oxidation is also related to a pH shift and can therefore be determined by a pH electrode. A variety of enzymatic reactions are combined with the production of heat, independent of the class of enzyme[96,97] which can be measured by thermistors placed in close proximity to the immobilised enzyme. Though this principle can be adapted to all kinds of enzymatic reactions it has not found widespread application, probably due to the complexity of the required device.

19.4.1.5.2 Detection principles in antibody-based systems

In bioprocess monitoring, immunological reactions are mainly used for the determination of high molecular weight proteins such as antibodies or enzymes, and only some systems are described which were applied to on-line process monitoring. Immunological assays can be divided into two major groups: (1) direct assays, requiring no additional reagents; (2) indirect assays, requiring tracers, such as conjugates of the antibodies or analytes with enzymes, fluorescent dyes, radioactive elements, etc.

The major characteristic of an immunological reaction is the formation of the antigen-antibody complex without catalysis of a chemical reaction and without regeneration of the antibody. Thus, immunological reactions can only be used for analytical purposes if the formation of the complex can be determined and, at least in on-line bioprocess monitoring, if regeneration is possible.

The latter requirement is met by using special regeneration buffers of extremely acidic[45] (pH 1–2) or alkaline[17] (pH 10–11) pHs. For the determination of the antigen-antibody complex several formats were developed using, e.g., direct or indirect assays. Direct assays are based on optical (refractive index,[69] turbidimetry[98]) or electrical (capacitance[68]) methods.

The most common indirect assays are based on enzyme conjugates with the antigen (competitive assays) or with the antibody (sandwich assays), requiring the additional supply with these tracers and the enzyme substrates. Thus the resulting FIA manifold is much more complicated. The antibodies can be immobilised on a membrane[72] or on polymeric[45] or glassy beads, the reactors being separated from the detection unit. Generally, the different steps (supply of the sample, the tracer, the enzyme substrates) are separated by washing steps. To date, indirect assays are more sensitive than direct ones, and they are less sensitive to matrix effects.

19.4.2 Examples of FIA Systems Used for On-Line Bioprocess Monitoring

There are hundreds of publications dealing with biosensor systems which are in principle applicable to bioprocess monitoring. In comparison there is a significant lack of literature dealing with real applications of these systems, which is caused by several reasons: (1) the degree of automation of the system may not be sufficient for on-line monitoring, (2) due to the limited concentration range of the systems samples may require manual dilution, (3) a suitable sampling device may not be available, and (4) the specific detection of analyte caused by a biochemical enzyme or antibody reaction and the signal conversion by the transducer could interfere with different medium components.

19.4.2.1 Carbohydrates

19.4.2.1.1 Glucose

Due to the following reasons, β-D-glucose, a hexose, is the most often detected component of bioprocess media by biosensors (see Table 19.1):

1. The first biosensor described in the literature was a glucose sensor, and glucose developed into a model analyte for new developments concerning enzyme sensors.
2. In a plurality of microbial fermentations as well as in animal cell cultures glucose is an important carbon source guaranteeing the energy supply of cell metabolism.
3. A variety of enzymes used for the specific detection of glucose are commercially available and due to the large demand for homogeneous or heterogeneous (ELISA) assay systems these biocatalysts can be obtained in a relatively purified and stabilised form.

The often used glucose oxidase (GOD) from *Aspergillus niger* (EC 1.1.3.4) is an oxidoreductase — a flavo enzyme containing two FAD molecules as cofactors which are strongly associated within the two enzyme subunits, but not covalently bound. These cofactors mediate the electron transfer from glucose to oxygen.[99]

$$\beta\text{-D-glucose} + O_2 \rightarrow \text{D-glucono-}\delta\text{-lactone} + H_2O_2 \qquad (19.4)$$

The determination of glucose is mainly done via quantification of the cosubstrate oxygen or the coproduct hydrogen peroxide by electrochemical or optical detection principles (Table 19.1; Section 19.4.1.5). Sensor systems based on this principle do not require substances except of the analyte glucose and the natural occurring oxygen.

However, the main problems are unspecific reactions, which can be reduced by special configurations of the flow systems. Christensen et al.[44] demonstrated the successful elimination of a penicillin interference during chemiluminescence detection of H_2O_2. Hydrogen peroxide oxidises the sulfur in the penicillin V molecule to a sulfoxide leading to a significant decrease of the signal. The problem could be solved by favouring the chemiluminescence

TABLE 19.1
FIA Systems for Glucose Monitoring

Analyte	Enzyme	Enzyme carrier	Detection	Linear range	Stability	Sampling	Bioprocess	Ref.
Glucose	GDH (*Bacillus megaterium*)	Graphite electrode	Amperom. NADH by BPT mediator		At least 3 days in continuous use	Filtration		91
Glucose	GOD (*Aspergillus niger*)	VA-epoxy biosynth in column or FET	Oxygen electrode or FET				*E. coli*	7
Glucose	GOD	Enzyme membrane	Amperom. H_2O_2 YSI-Analyser				Cellobiase reactor	104
Glucose	GOD	CPG enzyme column	Chemilumin. H_2O_2	0.01–50 mmol l^{-1}	4 Weeks in continuous use	Sterile filtration	BHK cells, animal cell culture	76
Glucose	GOD	Oxirane acrylic resin in column	Thermistor		60 h on line	Hollow fibre micro-filtration module	*Cephalosporium acremonium*	105
Glucose	GOD	Graphite electrode	Amperom. DMF	0–20 g l^{-1}	3 Days fermentation	*In situ* electrode	*Saccharomyces cerevisiae*	38
Glucose	GOD	Enzyme membrane	Amperom. H_2O_2 YSI-Analyser	0.05–41 g l^{-1}	19 h in continuous use	Off line	*Saccharomyces cerevisiae*	101
Glucose	GOD	Graphite electrode	Amperom. TTF	0.02–10 mmol l^{-1}	After 2000 measurements 50 %	Degassing chamber within a bypass	Acidophilic methylotrophic bacterium MB 53	102
Glucose	GOD	CPG column	Chemilumin. H_2O_2	0.005–0.7 g l^{-1}		BIOPEM ABC cross flow filtr.	*Penicillium chrysogenum*	44
Glucose	GOD	Ion-selective electrode	pH shift by ion-sel. electrode	0–30 g l^{-1}		ABC	*E. coli, Saccharomyces cerevisiae, Cephalosporium acremonium*	106

reaction relative to the penicillin oxidation by modifying the setup and increasing the amounts of chemicals used for chemiluminescence. Thus, up to a penicillin concentration of 18,000 U ml^{-1} no interference was detectable.

Another popular method to reduce interferences is the utilisation of membranes to exclude interfering substances from penetration into the flow system by filtration,[38] by dialysis,[100] or from the detector itself[101] by coverage with a membrane. Reduction of the applied potential can also be used to minimise interferences in amperometric glucose measurements. In this case oxygen as electron acceptors is replaced by mediators such as dimethylferrocene[38] or tetrathiafulvalene[102] which are reduced by the enzyme and are reoxidised at the electrode. A disadvantage of the mediated sensors is the limited long-term stability due to a washing out of the adsorbed mediators.[103]

Other glucose-converting enzymes are used for bioprocess monitoring, especially glucose dehydrogenase (GDH, EC 1.1.1.47). This enzyme also catalyses the conversion of β-D-glucose to D-glucono-δ-lactone.

$$\beta\text{-D-glucose} + NAD^+ \rightarrow \text{D-glucono-}\delta\text{-lactone} + NADH + H^+ \quad (19.5)$$

The cofactor NAD^+ is only weakly associated with the enzyme and is easily removed in aqueous solutions, which leads to the necessity of a continuous supplement of NAD^+. Therefore, the costs of an assay system are relatively high, but, on the other hand, the detection of the reduced cofactor offers some interesting advantages. The amperometric detection of NADH by a mediator-modified electrode allows the detection at a relatively low working potential[91] and, additionally, NADH is a fluorescent and can be directly optically detected.[100] Both properties allow reliable detections combined with low interferences.

19.4.2.1.2 Galactose

D-galactose can be oxidised by galactose oxidase (EC 1.1.3.9) yielding hydrogen peroxide as a coproduct.

$$\text{D-galactose} + O_2 \rightarrow \text{D-galactohexodialose} + H_2O_2 \quad (19.6)$$

The mechanism of this reaction is complex and the details are not understood completely. The enzyme is liable to deactivation, but it can be reactivated by oxidants, e.g., hexacyanoferrate(III). Galactose oxidase is not highly specific for galactose, since the enzyme catalyses the oxidation of several compounds carrying D-galactopyranosyl residues, e.g., lactose, raffinose, and glycerol. This indicates the necessity of a safe exclusion or reliable differentiation of such compounds if this enzyme is used for galactose monitoring. By injection of samples with equal concentrations of lactose and galactose, Nielsen et al.[87] found that the lactose accounted for approximately 5% of the response of the used chemiluminescent biosensor. If the galactose concentration was negligible it was possible to use the galactose analyser for measuring the lactose concentration.

19.4.2.1.3 Fructose

Fructose is of greater importance in the food industry than it is for bioprocess monitoring. It can be determined by biosensors containing the enzyme fructose dehydrogenase. The enzyme catalyses the oxidation of fructose to 5-keto-D-fructose, leading to a reduction of the covalent bound cofactor PQQ to $PQQH_2$.[107] Reoxidation of $PQQH_2$ is achieved by mediators such as hexacyanoferrate(III). The mediators can be reoxidised at an electrode generating a current depending on the fructose concentration.[108]

Up to now, no available fructose oxidase has been isolated; that is the reason for the utilisation of an assay format containing hexokinase, phosphoglucose isomerase, and glucose-6-phosphate dehydrogenase.[109]

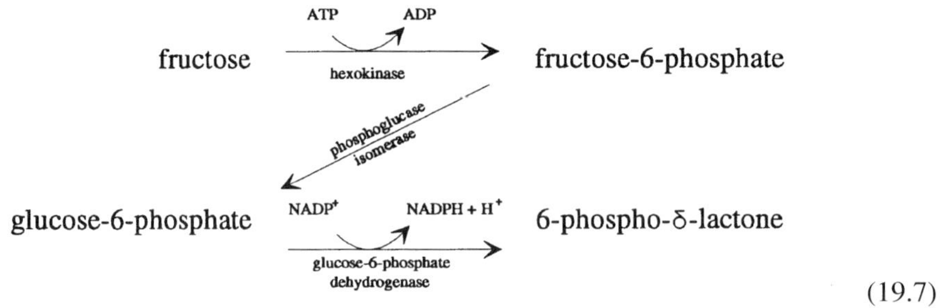

(19.7)

An interesting type of fructose-converting enzyme is the recently described biocatalyst glucose-fructose oxidoreductase,[110] which contains a confined NADPH cofactor molecule in the protein complex allowing a simplified layout of the analytical device.

glucose → gluconolactone

NADP+ NADPH + H+

sorbitol ← fructose (19.8)

The enzyme produced by *Zymomonas mobilis* oxidises glucose to gluconolactone and reduces fructose to sorbitol via a ping-pong mechanism. The protein consists of four 40,000 Da subunits. During the reduction of fructose to sorbitol, the NADPH is oxidised to $NADP^+$ and is reduced to NADPH by the oxidation of glucose to gluconolactone. Thordsen et al.[110] used this enzyme, confined by an ultrafiltration membrane within a measuring chamber, to determine fructose by measuring the fluorescence of NADPH (excited at 360 nm, measured at 450 nm) during the fermentation of *Pseudomonas pseudoflava* cultures.

19.4.2.1.4 Lactose

The disaccharide lactose is present in milk and dairy products but can also be a relevant substance within some fermentation processes. A suitable enzyme for lactose detection is β-galactosidase, hydrolysing lactose into the two monosaccharides β-D-galactose and β-D-glucose.

$$\text{lactose} + H_2O \rightarrow \beta\text{-D-galactose} + \beta\text{-D-glucose} \quad (19.9)$$

The combination with GOD reaction allows lactose determination on the basis of glucose sensors. Glucose present as an additional compound in fermentation processes obviously interferes with the lactose determination and it causes several times higher signals in conventional bioprocesses due to the relatively high specific GOD activity compared with the specific activity of β-galactosidase. A possibility to overcome this problem is to differentiate between the glucose signal generated by GOD and the lactose signal, using individual chemiluminescent detection channels for both compounds.[87]

19.4.2.1.5 Sucrose

The best known enzyme applied to sucrose determination is invertase. It catalyses the hydrolysis of the disaccharide sucrose into the monosaccharides α-glucose and fructose. Mandenius et al.[111] described the utilisation of the enzyme within a CPG reactor in combination with a thermistor during *Saccharomyces cerevisiae* fermentations. The thermistor measured the heat generated by the analyte conversion of invertase. To distinguish between the specific enzymatic reaction and nonspecific signals generated by medium compounds, the establishment of a second enzyme-free thermistor channel was useful, as described by Hundeck et al.[112] for cultivations of *Bacillus licheniformes* and *Spodoptera frugiperda*.

19.4.2.1.6 Oligosaccharides

A biosensor for the sum of oligosaccharides present in a sample can be developed based on a sequence of different immobilised enzymes. First, enzymatic hydrolysis of poly- and oligoglucans such as starch, maltodextrins, and saccharides, is catalysed by the relatively unspecific enzyme amyloglucosidase (EC 3.2.1.3). Hereby, α-D- and β-D-glucose molecules are generated. α-D-glucose is converted to β-D-glucose by mutarotase. The last enzymatic step is the conversion of β-D-glucose by GOD or GDH (Section 19.4.2.1.1). The latter enzyme was used by Marko-Varga[113] during *Penicillium* and *Fusarium oxysporum* fermentations. The NADH was detected amperometrically by a phenoxacine-modified graphite electrode with a potential of 50 mV (vs. SCE). Hundeck et al.[112] described the bioconversion of saccharides by signals which represented the concentrations of present sugars assimilable by immobilised *Saccharomyces cerevisiae* cells. Measurements were done by a thermistor probe monitoring the generated heat. An overview on all systems mentioned here is given in Table 19.2.

19.4.2.2 Alcohols

Alcohols, mainly ethanol and methanol, are important products or byproducts, for example, during the cultivation of yeast. Besides the development of nonenzymatic methods, e.g., near-infrared spectroscopy,[114] semiconductor sensors,[115,116] gas chromatography, or NMR,[117] enzyme-based flow-through devices were developed. To allow simultaneous determination of several alcohols an enzyme electrode was used as detector in column liquid chromatography,[118] which is planned to be applied to bioprocess monitoring. This system utilised the nonspecificity of the enzyme alcohol oxidase, which was immobilised together with peroxidase in a carbon paste electrode. Alcohol oxidase (EC 1.1.3.13) catalyses the oxidation of short-chain primary alcohols[63] by oxygen to the corresponding aldehyde,

$$\text{alcohol} + O_2 \rightarrow \text{aldehyde} + H_2O_2 \tag{19.10}$$

allowing determination of alcohol concentration via hydrogen peroxide. The main enzyme substrate is methanol, but other primary alcohols are also oxidised with the affinity decreasing with increasing chain length of the alcohol. In an FIA system applied to monitoring of a yeast fermentation,[63] electrochemical and spectrophotometric determination of hydrogen peroxide were compared. The photometric test required peroxidase as a second enzyme and ABTS as electron donator and showed a shorter linear range than the electrochemical test. Specificity of the system was improved and modulated by the integration of a diffusion module containing a gas-permeable membrane allowing only diffusion of volatile compounds. Material and thickness of this membrane modified the specificity of the whole system.[63]

A comparable principle was described by Ogbomo et al.[64] who used a pervaporation module to improve specificity. The main characteristic of this module was an air gap between analyte and membrane thus avoiding any direct contact of the sample with the membrane, and minimising problems of membrane fouling. Some problems were reported when the sample contained significant amounts of carbon dioxide, as this led to changes by the evaporation of the ethanol. Nevertheless, the system was successfully applied to a cultivation of baker's yeast. The system was used in combination with alcohol oxidase (electrochemical determination of hydrogen peroxide) and with alcohol dehydrogenase (fluorimetric determination of NADH) (for the generalized equation, see Section 19.4.1.5.1, Equation 19.3).

19.4.2.3 Acids

19.4.2.3.1 Lactic acid

Due to its cell toxicity, lactic acid, a final product of carbohydrate metabolism, is next to glucose the most important analyte which has to be monitored and controlled during

TABLE 19.2
FIA Systems for Carbohydrate Determination

Analyte	Enzyme	Enzyme carrier	Detection	Linear range	Stability	Sampling	Bioprocess	Ref.
Glucose Galactose Lactose	GOD GalOD ß-Galactosidase	CPG column, nylon tubing	Chemilumin. H_2O_2	Gluc. 0.001–2 g l^{-1} Galac. 0.003–3 g l^{-1} Lact. 0.025–5 g l^{-1}		Chem. barrier + sample cooling	*Streptococcus cremoris*	87
Oligosaccharides Glucose	Amyloglucosidase Mutarotase GDH	CPG column	Amperom. NADH, phenoxazine-modified electrode		4 Days	Off line samples	Malt beer, *Penicillium, Fusarium oxysporum*	113
Fructose	Glucose-fructose-oxidoreductase	Membrane separation in flow-through cell	Fluorescence NADPH		After 50 h long-term measurement 22 % residue	Off line samples	*Pseudomonas pseudoflava*	110
Sucrose	Invertase	CPG column	Themistor	2–100 mmol l^{-1}	6 Months	Degassing chamber within a bypass	*Saccharomyces cerevisiae*	111
Glucose Maltose Sucrose Assimilable sugars	GOD + Catalase α-Glucosidase Invertase *S. cerevisiae* cells	VA-Epoxy Biosynth in column Cells in Ca-alginate	Thermistor			Filtration	*Bacillus licheniformes Spodoptera frugiperda*	112

bioprocesses to achieve optimal product yield. This is done by a variety of different enzymes mainly in animal cell cultivations.

1. Lactate oxidase (LOD) from *Pediococcus* spec. This enzyme catalyses the oxidation of lactate to pyruvate by O_2:

$$\text{L-lactate} + O_2 \rightarrow \text{pyruvate} + H_2O_2 \tag{19.11}$$

In contrast to glucose oxidase only one description of a mediated lactate sensor based on LOD is available, indicating only slow charge transfer rates from LOD to artificial acceptors.[119]

2. Lactate oxidase from *Mycobacterium smegmatis* (EC 1.13.12.4.). This enzyme is a lactate-2-monooxygenase which oxidises and decarboxylises L-lactate to acetic acid and carbon dioxide in the presence of oxygen:

$$\text{L-lactate} + O_2 \rightarrow \text{acetic acid} + CO_2 + H_2O \tag{19.12}$$

A biosensor based on this oxidase designed by Weaver and Vadgama consisted of an oxygen-electrode which measured the O_2 consumption during catalysis.[120]

3. Lactate dehydrogenase (LDH) from muscle tissue (EC 1.1.1.27):

$$\text{L-lactate} + NAD^+ \rightarrow \text{pyruvate} + NADH + H^+ \tag{19.13}$$

Descriptions of biosensors containing this enzyme deal with electrochemical detection principles, whereby the cofactor NAD^+ was confined before an enzyme electrode by membranes.[88]

4. Lactate dehydrogenase type cytochrome b_2 from aerobic yeasts (EC 1.1.2.3.). This enzyme catalyses the oxidation of lactate to pyruvate in the presence of a hydrogen acceptor, e.g., hexacyanoferrate(III). The reduced mediator can be reoxidised electrochemically, thus allowing the development of mediated amperometric lactate sensors.[121]

$$\text{L-lactate} + 2\ Fe(CN)_6^{-3} \rightarrow \text{pyruvate} + 2\ Fe(CN)_6^{-4} + 2\ H^+ \tag{19.14}$$

To date, particularly LOD and LDH are used in biosensor systems (Table 19.3) due to the stability and the constant quality of these enzymes. Dremel et al. examined lactate concentrations by optical measurement of oxygen consumption (Section 19.4.1.5.1). LOD was either immobilised on CPG and placed in an enzyme column[61] or directly on top of the membrane containing the O_2-sensitive dye.[65] The sensor was stable for over 2 days of continuous measurements. A chemiluminometric system for lactate determination was established by Nielsen et al.[122]

Though the same sensor principles could be used for lactate determination as for glucose determination, only a few electrochemical lactate sensors were applied to bioprocess monitoring,[123,124] with only a few examples of on-line application.[124] One of the reasons may be that optical systems are less affected by electrical noise and have advantages, therefore, when sensor systems are to be used in close proximity to the complex instrumentation required in bioprocess technology. Another reason is probably that lactate is mainly monitored during animal cell cultivations, which are run as continuous cultivations with the need for high stability of the sensors, which has only been achieved by a few sensor systems containing enzyme columns (see also Table 19.7) in FIA systems based on optical determination.

TABLE 19.3
FIA Systems for Organic Acid Determination

Analyte	Enzyme	Enzyme carrier	Detection	Linear range	Stability	Sampling	Bioprocess	Ref.
Lactate	LOD	Carbon black at optrode	Fluorescence of oxygen	0.02–20 mmol l^{-1}	2 Days		Kefir cultures	65
Lactate	LOD	Column	Chemilumin. H_2O_2	0.1–2 g l^{-1}	Few days, fouling of the membrane	Chem. barrier and filtration within the flow system	Lactic acid bacteria	123
Lactate	LDH	CPG column	Fluorescence NADH	0.1–20 mmol l^{-1}	70% after 120 h	Cross flow microfiltration module	Animal cell culture	100
Lactate	LOD	Enzyme membrane covered with polycarbonate membrane	Amperom. H_2O_2			Harvesting tube of a hollow fibre reactor	Animal cell culture	125
Acetic acid	Acetate kinase Pyruvate kinase LDH	CPG column	Photometric NADH	10–60 mmol l^{-1}	60% After 6 days	Harvesting tube of a hollow fibre reactor	Acetic acid production	126

19.4.2.3.2 Acetic acid

Acetic acid was determined during several bioprocesses,[50] but only a few examples of enzymatic assays are known, probably due to the complexity of the required enzymatic sequence:

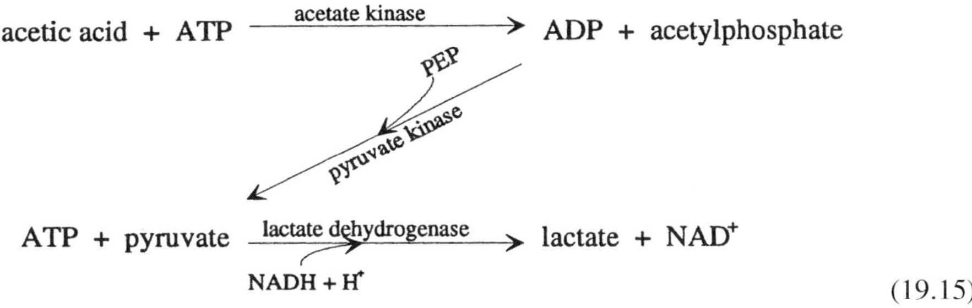

(19.15)

Becker et al.[125] integrated the enzymes in an FIA system by immobilisation on CPG and using enzyme columns. The required substances ATP (adenosine triphosphate), PEP (phosphoenol pyruvate), and NADH were mixed and injected in the carrier, thus increasing the complexity of the device. The detector was a flow-through photometer for monitoring NADH consumption. During 6 days of continuous measurements the signals decreased to 60%.

19.4.2.3.3 Amino acids

Various FIA systems were described suitable for the determination of amino acids in fermentation broth, with the most important analyte being glutamine in mammalian and insect cell culture media. They were based on various biological elements and detection principles (see Table 19.4).

Due to the complexity of the composition of the samples all systems had to deal with nonspecific reactions either of the biological element or of the detector. This problem was solved by the following different approaches.

Tosa et al.[126] described a microbial sensor for aspartic acid determination based on a potentiometric CO_2 electrode. They observed a good selectivity of *P. dacunhau* for aspartic acid but had to remove endogenous CO_2 from the samples by aeration after lowering the pH.

Glutamine is often determined by coimmobilisation of glutaminase and glutamate oxidase:

$$\begin{aligned} &\text{glutamine} + H_2O \xrightarrow{\text{glutaminase}} \text{glutamate} + NH_3 \\ &\text{glutamate} + O_2 \xrightarrow[\text{oxidase}]{\text{glutamate}} \alpha - \text{ketoglutarate} + H_2O_2 \end{aligned} \tag{19.16}$$

In this case endogenous glutamate interfered with specific glutamine determination. Thus, removal of glutamate by preceding anion exchange columns was suggested.[127,128] Alternatively, a differential measurement of only glutamate and the sum of glutamate and glutamine may be used.[129] Matuszewski et al.[75] tried to avoid the problem by using glutaminase alone in combination with an NH_4^+ ion-selective electrode. However, they had to use a split-stream single-detector arrangement to measure endogenous NH_4^+.

All systems were only applied off-line to samples taken from mammalian or insect cell cultivations and diluted 10- to 100-fold. In all cases a sufficient correlation to HPLC data was found.

On-line determination of amino acids is only described by Dremel et al.,[130] who monitored an *E. coli* K12 HB 101-cultivation over a period of approximately 35 h. This strain required proline and leucine as essential amino acids, which were added during cultivation as casein.

TABLE 19.4
FIA System for Amino Acid Determination

Analyte	Biolog. comp.	Immob. matrix	Detect. princip.	Linear range	Stability	Application	Ref.
Aspartic acid	*P. dacunhae*	Carrageenan membrane	CO_2-electr.	0.2–5 mM	70 Days or 140 assays	Off-line data	126
Glutamine	Glutaminase + glutamate oxidase	Aminopropyl glass	Amperom. H_2O_2	0.01–1 mM	500 Assays	Off-line mammalian + insect cell culture	127
Glutamine	Glutaminase + glutamate oxidase	Gelatine membrane	pO_2	0.2–2 mM	300 Assays	Off-line media	131
Glutamine	Glutaminase + glutamate oxidase	Aminopropyl glass	Chemiluminescence	1–100 μM	500 Assays	Cell culture supernatants	128
Glutamine	Glutaminase	Controlled pore glass	NH_4^+-ion selective electrode	0.5–4.5 mM	—	Off-line samples	130
Glutamine	Glutaminase - glutamate oxidase	Nylon membrane	H_2O_2		300 Assays (60% activity)	Off-line	129
Lysine	Lysine decarboxylase	Glass tubes	Photometric pH-det.	2 mM	500 Assays	Recovery in ferm broth	132
Total amino acids	Amino acid oxidase	CPG	O_2-optode	15 g/l Leucine		*E. coli* K 12 HB 101	130

The analytical system was based on immobilised amino acid oxidase from *Crotalus adamanteus* and an oxygen optode. Due to the broad substrate specificity of the enzyme, only the sum of all amino acids could be determined. However, no correlation to HPLC data was given.

19.4.2.4 Antibiotics

Antibiotics, mainly penicillin, but also cephalosporin, are monitored as products of biotechnological processes. Determination can be done by using the photometric properties of cephalosporin[133] or by enzyme assays. Even the photometric determination of cephalosporin was combined with hydrolysis of cephalosporin by cephalosporinase immobilised on Eupergit-C™ to improve selectivity of the device.

In penicillin fermentations the fermentation broth contains mainly penicillin G, but also penicillin F, N, V, O, X, and so on,[134] which are all hydrolysed by penicillinase, also called β-lactamase:

$$\text{penicillin} + H_2O \rightarrow \text{penicilloate}^- + H^+ \quad (19.17)$$

Thus, most of the biosensor systems designed for penicillin determination in fermentation broth are based on this enzymatic reaction in combination with either pH measurements or with determinations of the penicilloic acid (Table 19.5). Penicilloic acid can be determined by utilising its reducing properties, e.g., the classical photometric assay is based on the reduction of iodine to iodide monitored by the decolorisation of a starch-iodine solution.[66,135]

Besides penicillinase other enzymes are known to hydrolyse penicillin, mainly penicillin G, e.g., penicillin G amidase, which is used for the industrial production of 6-aminopenicillanic acid (6-APA), an important precursor for semisynthetic penicillins,[136] and penicillin acylase[134] hydrolysing only penicillin G.

All enzymatic reactions lead to a decrease of pH and can thus be monitored by pH-electrodes, pH FETs, or pH optodes (Table 19.5). Therefore, the common problem of all these sensor systems is the dependence of the sensor signals on the pH and buffer capacity of the sample.[134,136–139] It is solved by either diluting the sample to a sufficient degree to minimise these matrix effects or by measuring additionally the pH of the sample by a reference sensor and calculating the penicillin concentration on the basis of the known pH dependence of the penicillin sensor.[139]

Sensor systems based on other detection principles do not have to deal with this problem, but the systems are more complicated[66,140] and require additional reagents, such as iodine-starch[66] or mercury(II) chloride and molybdoarsenic acid.[135]

19.4.2.5 Proteins

Products of bioprocesses of high economic value are often proteins or peptides, e.g., enzymes, monoclonal antibodies, hormones, interferon. They are determined either by suitable biochemical or biological activity tests or, if available, by immunoassays. The corresponding processes are run as continuous processes requiring no frequent sampling but high stability of the analytical devices.

Several FIA systems based on different types of immunological detection were applied mainly to on-line monitoring of IgG in cultivations of hybridoma cell lines. But the same principles were applied also to pullulanase, antithrombin III, and recombinant tissue-type plasminogen activator monitoring.[141] The groups of Scheper and Schügger[17,98,141] established a turbidimetric immunoassay based on monitoring turbidity of immunocomplexes at 340 nm. The detection range of micrograms per millilitre was suitable for process monitoring, with the advantage of a short assay time of 1 to 5 min. The major disadvantages of this system

TABLE 19.5
FIA Systems for Penicillin Determination

Analyte	Enzyme	Detection principle	Immobilisation	Linear range	Application	Remarks	Ref.
Penicillin	Penicillinase	H^+-FET	Cross-linking with glutaraldehyde	0.5–25 mM	Off-line	5 Months storage, more than 1000 assays	134
Penicillin G	Penicillin acylase	H^+-FET	Cross-linking with glutaraldehyde	5 mM		More selective for penicillin G	134
Penicillin G	Penicillin-G-amidase	H^+-FET	Glutaraldehyde binding to the gate	0.3–30 mM	Planned	90 s Response time Up to 100 days storage (85% remaining activity)	136
Penicillin V	Penicillinase	pH-electr.	Cross-linking with glutarald.	100 mM	Off-line		137
Penicillin V	Penicillinase	pH-electr.	Cross-linking with glutaraldehyde	40 mM	Off-line	200 Samples/h Stable for 12 days at room temp.	138
Penicillin G	Penicillinase	Thermistor	Controlled pore glass, nylon tubing	100 mM 10 mM	Off-line		140
Penicillin V	Penicillinase	Photometric (molybdenum blue) Photometric (iodine-starch) pH-electr.	Controlled pore glass, nylon tubing	10–100 mg/l 2.5–150 mg/l 100–800 mg/l	Off- and on-line *P. chrysogenum*	Iodine-det. preferred, 60 samples/h, reference channel	135
Penicillin V	Penicillinase	pH-electr. Photometric(iodine-starch)	Nylon tube (1 m)	0.5–30 g/l 0.1–30g/l	On-line *P. chrysogenum*	200 h Cultivation 3 Samples/h	66
Penicillin G	Penicillin-G-amidase	pH-optode (FITC-fluorescence)	PVA-membrane cross-linked with glutaraldehyde		Off-line *P. chrysogenum*	Reference pH-optode	139

were its complexity due to the need for a reference channel[141] and its high cost, as the immunocomplexes had to stay in suspension and were discarded after each assay.

Mainly, the latter aspect is avoided if the binding protein of the analyte is immobilised. This was done by Stöcklein et al.[72] who immobilised protein A or anti-mouse IgG antibodies onto oxirane beads and determined bound antibodies of the sample by their fluorescence (ex: 280 nm; em: 360 nm) after elution with acidic buffer. Six assays per hour were run, and a protein A column could be used for more than 1000 assays.

Further simplification of the system was achieved when immunosensors were used as detectors.[69] Monitoring physical properties of the transducers, i.e., capacitance[68] and refractive index,[69] allowed direct observation of the binding of the analyte, thus reducing the FIA system to a pump for the carrier solution and the injection valve. Assay times were 17 min[45] and approximately 25 min,[68] including washing and regeneration steps. The main problems of these systems were their limited stability (e.g., 50% loss of signals after 50 cycles[69]) and unspecific binding to the sensor surface.

The first drawback was reduced by using sufficient amounts of active immobilised antibodies placed in an antibody column,[142] and the second is less important if indirect assay formats, i.e., labelled compounds, are used.[17,45,72,141] Generally, the principle of an ELISA was used, either as a sandwich[45,72] assay or as a competitive assay.[17,72,141] Only the system based on the sandwich test, with the first antibody bound to oxiran beads and the second labelled with β-galactosidase, was applied to on-line monitoring of mouse IgG.[45] A decrease of the signals of 50% was observed during cultivation time of 8 days due to aging of reagents and loss of activity of the immobilised antibodies.

A summary of characteristic features of these systems is given in Table 19.6.

TABLE 19.6
FIA Systems for Protein Determination

Assay format	Detection principle	Immobilisation matrix	Assay time	Stability	Ref.
Direct homogeneous	Turbidity	—	1–5 min	—	17
Direct heterogeneous	Fluorescence	Oxiran beads	6 Assays/h	After 1000 assays decrease by 22 %	142
Direct	Capacitance	Ta-oxide-capacitor	22 min	After 8 d cultivation decrease by 21%	45
Direct	Refractive index	Ta-oxide grating coupler	29.5 min	After 50 cycles decrease by 50%	69
Indirect, heterogeneous	Fluorescence	Oxiran-acrylic beads	14 min.	After 8 d decrease by 50%	45

19.4.2.6 Multichannel Devices

Effective optimisation of bioprocesses and maintenance of optimal conditions requires knowledge about the concentrations of all important compounds such as nutrients, vitamins, inhibitors, metabolites, or products. Therefore, systems suitable for simultaneous determination of analytes were developed and applied mainly to monitoring of animal cell cultivations. Animal cells usually require complex cultivation media of rather high costs and, additionally, products of these cultivations are of high economic value. This even allows the application of expensive analytical instrumentation, if this guarantees constant product quality and yield. The most important analytes are glucose, lactate, and glutamine, which are most often combined in multichannel devices due to their physiological relevance in the cells (Table 19.7). Beyond glucose, the primary carbon

TABLE 19.7
FIA Systems for Multichannel Analysis

Analyte	Enzyme	Enzyme carrier	Detection	Linear range	Stability	Sampling	Bioprocess	Ref.
Glucose Lactate Glutamine Glutamate	GDH LDH Glutamic pyruvic-transaminase Glutaminase GlutamatDH	CPG column	Fluorescence NADH	0.1–50 mmol l^{-1} 0.1–20 mmol l^{-1} 0.1–5 mmol l^{-1} 0.1–5 mmol l^{-1}	After 120 h between 55% and 72% depending on the individual enzyme	Cross flow micro-filtration module	Animal cell culture	100
Glucose Lactate	GOD LOD	CPG column	Fluorescence of an indicator quenched by oxygen	0–30 mmol l^{-1} 0–30 mmol l^{-1}	4 Weeks	Sterile filtration	Animal cell culture	61
Glucose Maltose Sucrose Assimilable sugars	GOD + Catalase α-Glucosidase Invertase *Saccharomyces cerevisiae* cells	VA-epoxy biosynth in column Cells in Ca-alginate	Thermistor			Filtration	*Bacillus licheniformes* *Spodoptera frugiperda*	112
Glucose Lactate	GDH LDH	CPG column	Photometric. NADH	Up to 3 g l^{-1} Up to 3 g l^{-1}		Sterile filter connected to the harvest stream of a perfusion fermenter	Mammalian cell culture	92
Ammonia Glutamine	Glutaminase	Enzyme column	Potentiometric detection of ammonium ions by ionsel. electrode			Off line	Animal cell culture (pMFG/Crip cells)	143
Glucose Lactate	GOD LOD	Enzyme column	Chemilumin. H_2O_2	0.01–2 g l^{-1} 0.1–2 g l^{-1}	Few days, fouling of the membrane	Chemical barrier + filtration within FIA	Lactc acid bacteria	122
Glucose Lactate Glutamine	GOD LOD Glutaminase Glutamate oxidase	Membranes	Amperom. H_2O_2	30 mmol 20 mmol 15 mmol		Sterile filtration	Mammalian cell culture	144

source of higher cells, glutamine is the most abundant constituent of tissue culture media. In low-serum or serum-free media, mammalian cells utilise both glucose and glutamine as energy sources and produce lactate and ammonia.[143] Accumulated amounts of lactate and ammonia can modify cell behaviour leading to a significant reduction in cell multiplication rates.

With the complexity of media the amount of interfering compounds could increase, which has to be taken into consideration during the development of analytical devices. Spohn et al.[100] separated the low molecular weight analytes (glucose, lactate, glutamine, glutamate) and the higher molecular weight medium compounds by dialysis modules within the flow system to prevent fouling processes and unspecific reactions. During application the system could be simplified, because the glutamate concentrations were negligible in contrast to the glutamine concentrations which had to be determined continuously. Another interesting property of dialysis modules utilised in FIA systems is automated sample dilution,[63] allowing the on-line determination of even higher analyte concentrations.

In general, the complexity of analytical devices increases with the number of analytes, at the same time reducing the reliability of the device. Thus, instruments should be simplified as much as possible. Figure 19.5 shows schematically the concept of a multichannel flow-injection system — in this example suitable for the determination of three different analytes, using just a single injection valve. The sample is transported by the carrier through three dialysis modules placed in series. A small amount of sample constituents diffuses into acceptor streams, leading to dilution of the analytes.

19.5 DISCUSSION

In modern biotechnology there is a need for intensive information about parameters and conditions in the fermenter at any time during cultivation. As a consequence, a variety of concepts of analytical instruments suitable for on-line monitoring were developed. They range from expensive instrumental methods, such as nuclear magnetic resonance[117] and mass spectrometry,[12,145] to chromatographic procedures with more or less elaborate derivatisation procedures or with biosensors as detectors,[118] to flow injection analysis systems comprising several biochemical receptors and thus allowing simultaneous determination of several compounds (see Section 19.4.2.6) to simple devices suitable for the determination of just a single compound (see Sections 19.4.2.1 to 19.4.2.5). Generally, information about more than one parameter is required, at least in the establishment of a process, thus the application of systems allowing simultaneous determination of several compounds is favoured. However, these devices are either rather expensive or show a degree of complexity which increases with the number of analytes which can be determined. Additionally, most of the systems require recalibration in regular terms, integrated sample pretreatment such as dilution to varying degrees, regeneration procedures, and data processing.[146] These features increase the complexity further and generate the need for sophisticated software to control only the analytical instrument, which has to communicate with the software required to control the process. Thus, reliable data can often only be obtained if the instruments are used by well-trained specialists. Consequently, these devices are used only in research laboratories and not routinely during biotechnological production processes.

Nevertheless, the number of applications of even complex systems to on-line bioprocess monitoring is increasing, at least during optimisation of processes, and even some examples are known where information about concentrations of medium components obtained with suitable (bio)chemical sensors was used to control the process.[50,147-149] As increased volumetric productivity and increased product concentrations, which are required to reduce production costs and to increase product yield by maintaining quality of metabolic products, can be achieved by application of advanced control techniques, there is now considerable interest in many bioindustries in monitoring and controlling strategies.[150] Fortunately, sampling modules and several FIA devices for important analytes (glucose, lactate, ethanol) are commercially available even as multichannel systems. Thus, it can be expected that their application to even routine production processes will increase.

REFERENCES

1. Locher, G., Hahnemann, U., Sonnleitner, B., and Fiechter, A., Automatic bioprocess control. 4. A prototype batch of *Saccharomyces cerevisiae, J. Biotechnol.*, 29, 57, 1993.
2. Scheper, T.-H. and Lammers, F., Fermentation monitoring and process control, *Curr. Opin. Biotechnol.*, 5, 187, 1994.
3. Fehrenbach, R., Comberbach, M., and Pêtre, J. O., On-line biomass monitoring by capacitance measurement, *J. Biotechnol.*, 23, 303, 1992.
4. Peck, M. W. and Chynoweth, D. P., On-line monitoring of the methanogenic fermentation by measurement of culture fluorescence, *Biotechnol. Lett.*,12, 17, 1990.
5. Müller, W., Wehnert, G., and Scheper, T., Fluorescence monitoring of immobilized microorganisms in cultures, *Anal. Chim. Acta*, 213, 47, 1988.
6. Scheper, T., Lorenz, T., Schmidt, W., and Schügerl, K., On-line measurement of culture fluorescence for process monitoring and control of biotechnological processes, *Ann. N. Y. Acad. Sci.*, 15, 431, 1987.
7. Schügerl, K., Brandes, L., Wu, X., Bode, J., Ree, J. I., Brandt, J., and Hitzmann, B., Monitoring and control of recombinant protein production, *Anal. Chim. Acta*, 279, 3, 1993.
8. Kilburn, D. G., Fitzpatrick, P., Blake-Coleman, B. C., Clarke, D. J., and Griffiths, J. B., On-line monitoring of cell mass in mammalian cell cultures by acoustic densitometry, *Biotechnol. Bioeng.*, 33, 1379, 1989.
9. Van de Merbel, N. C., Lingeman, H., Brinkman, U. A. T., Kolhorn, A., and De Rijke, L. C., Automated monitoring of biotechnological processes using on-line ultrafiltration and column liquid chromatography, *Anal. Chim. Acta*, 279, 39, 1993.
10. Filippini, C., Sonnleitner, B., and Fiechter, A., On-line monitoring of fast bioprocesses with flow injection analysis and gas chromatography, *GBF Monogr.*, 17, 531, 1992.
11. Hayward, M. J., Kotiaho, T., Lister, A. K., Cooks, R. G., Austin, G. D., Narayan, R., and Tsao, G. T., On-line monitoring of bioreactions of *Bacillus polymyxa* and *Klebsiella oxytoca* by membrane introduction tandem mass spectrometry with flow injection analysis sampling, *Anal. Chem.*, 62, 1798, 1990.
12. Heinzle, E., Present and potential applications of mass spectrometry for bioprocess research and control, *J. Biotechnol.*, 25, 81, 1992.
13. Brooks, S. L., Higgins, I. J., Newman, J. D., and Turner, A. P. F., Biosensors for process control, *Enzyme Microbiol. Technol.*, 13, 946, 1991.
14. Schügerl, K., Which requirements do flow injection analyser/biosensor systems have to meet for controlling the bioprocess?, *J. Biotechnol.*, 31, 241, 1993.
15. Scheper, T., Biosensors for process monitoring, *J. Ind. Microbiol.*, 9, 163, 1992.
16. Bradley, J., Stöcklein, W., and Schmid, R. D., Biochemistry based analysis systems for bioprocess monitoring and control, *Process Control Quality*, 1, 157, 1991.
17. Degelau, A., Freitag, R., Linz, F., Middendorf, C., Scheper, T., Bley, T., Müller, S., Stoll, P., and Reardon, K. F., Immuno- and flow cytometric analytical methods for biotechnological research and process monitoring, *J. Biotechnol.*, 25, 115, 1992.
18. Karube, I., Tamiya, E., Sode, K., Yokoyama, K., Kitagawa, Y., Suzuki, H., and Asano, Y., Application of microbiological sensors in fermentation processes, *Anal. Chim. Acta*, 213, 69, 1988.
19. Locher, G., Sonnleitner, B., and Fiechter, A., On-line measurement in biotechnology: techniques, *J. Biotechnol.*, 25, 23, 1992.
20. Sonnleitner, B., Locher, G., and Fiechter, A., Biomass determination, *J. Biotechnol.*, 25, 5, 1992.
21. Ding, T., Bilitewski, U., Schmid, R. D., Korz, D. J., and Sanders, E. A., Control of microbial activity by flow injection analysis during high cell density cultivation of *Escherichia coli*, *J. Biotechnol.*, 27, 143, 1993.
22. Cammann, K., Lemke, U., Rohen, A., Sander, J., Wilken, H., and Winter, B., Chemo- und Biosensoren - Grundlagen und Anwendungen, *Angew. Chem.*, 103, 519, 1991.

23. Schmidt, H.-L., Schuhmann, W., Scheller, F. W., and Schubert, F., Specific features of biosensors, in *Sensors — A Comprehensive Survey,* Vol. 3, Göpel, W., Hesse, J., and Zemel, J. N., Eds., VCH Publishers, Weinheim, 1992, 717.
24. Griffiths, D. and Hall, G., Biosensors — what real progress is being made?, *TIBTECH*, 11, 122, 1993.
25. Bardeletti, G., Séchaud, F., and Coulet, P., Amperometric enzyme electrodes for substrate and enzyme activity determinations, *Bioprocess Technol.*, 15, 7, 1991.
26. Vadgama, P. and Crump, P. W., Biosensors: recent trends. A review, *Analyst*, 117, 1657, 1992.
27. Scheller, F. W. and Schubert, F., *Biosensors*, Elsevier, Amsterdam, 1992.
28. Cass, A. E. G., Ed., *Biosensors A Practical Approach*, Oirl Press, Oxford, 1990.
29. Hall, E. A. H., Biosensors, in: *The Biotechnology Series,* Open University Press, Milton Keynes, 1990.
30. Turner, A. P. F., Karube, I., and Wilson, G. S., Eds., *Biosensors Fundamentals and Applications*, Oxford University Press, Oxford, 1987.
31. Scheper, T. and Reardon, K. F., Sensors in Biotechnology, in *Sensors — A Comprehensive Survey,* Vol. 3, Göpel, W., Hesse, J., and Zemel, J. N., Eds., VCH Publishers, Weinheim, 1992, 1023.
32. Kracke-Helm, H.-A., Brandes, L., Hitzmann, B., Rinas, U., and Schügerl, K., On-line determination of intracellular β-galactosidase activity in recombinant *Escherichia coli* using flow injection analysis (FIA), *J. Biotechnol.*, 20, 95, 1991.
33. Steube, K. and Spohn, U., On-line monitoring of intracellular enzyme activities with flow injection analysis, *Anal. Chim. Acta*, 287, 235, 1994.
34. Künnecke, W., Kalisz, H. M., and Schmid, R. D., Flow injection zymography — a novel procedure for the on-line detection of enzyme activity, *Anal. Lett.*, 2, 1471, 1989.
35. Silfwerbrand-Lindh, C., Nord, L., Häggerström, L., and Ingman, F., FIA for down-stream processing — determination of β-galactosidase in viscous extraction media, *Bioprocess Eng.*, 7, 47, 1991.
36. Flygare, L., Larsson, P.-O., and Danielsson, B., Control of affinity purification procedure using a thermal biosensor, *Biotechnol. Bioeng.*, 36, 723, 1990.
37. Cleland, N. and Enfors, S. O., Monitoring glucose consumption in an *Escherichia coli* cultivation with an enzyme electrode, *Anal. Chim. Acta*, 163, 281, 1984.
38. Bradley, J. and Schmid, R. D., Optimisation of a biosensor for *in situ* fermentation monitoring of glucose concentration, *Biosens. Bioelectron.*, 6, 669, 1991.
39. Rishpon, J., Shabtai, Y., Rosen, I., Zibenberg, Y., Tor, R., and Freeman, A., *In situ* glucose monitoring in fermentation broth by "sandwiched" glucose oxidase electrode (SGE), *Biotechnol. Bioeng.*, 35, 103, 1990.
40. Enfors, S. O. and Nilsson, H., Design and characterisation of an enzyme electrode for measurement of penicillin in fermentation broth, *Enzyme Microbiol. Technol.*, 1, 260, 1979.
41. Hewetson, J. W., Jong, T. H., and Gray, P. P., Use of an immobilised penicillinase electrode in the monitoring of the penicillin fermentation, *Biotechnol. Bioeng. Symp.*, 9, 125, 1979.
42. Mattiasson, B. and Hakanson, H., Sampling and sample handling — crucial steps in process monitoring and control, *TIBTECH*, 11, 136, 1993.
43. Hakanson, H., Nilsson, M., and Mattiasson, B., General sampling system for sterile monitoring of biological processes, *Anal. Chim. Acta*, 249, 61, 1991.
44. Christensen, L. H., Nielsen, J., and Villadsen, J., Monitoring of substrates and products during fed-batch penicillin fermentations on complex media, *Anal. Chim. Acta*, 249, 123, 1991.
45. Gebbert, A., Alvarez-Icaza, M., Peters, H., Jäger, V., Bilitewski, U., and Schmid, R. D., On-line monitoring of monoclonal antibody production with regenerable flow-injection immuno systems, *J. Biotechnol.*, 32, 213, 1994.
46. Buttler, T., Gorton, L., Jarskog, H., Marko-Varga, G., Hahn-Hägerdal, B., Meinander, N., and Olsson, L., Monitoring of ethanol during fermentation of a lignocellulose hydrolysate by on-line microdialysis sampling, column liquid chromatography, and an alcohol biosensor, *Biotechnol. Bioeng.*, 44, 322, 1994.
47. Mandenius, C. F., Danielsson, B., and Mattiasson, B., Evaluation of a dialysis probe for continuous sampling in fermentors and in complex media, *Anal. Chim. Acta*, 163, 135, 1984.

48. Buttler, T., Gorton, L., and Marko-Varga, G., Characterization of a sampling unit based on tangential flow filtration for on-line bioprocess monitoring, *Anal. Chim. Acta*, 279, 27, 1993.
49. Buttler, T. A., Johansson, K. A. J., Gorton, L. G. O., and Marko Varga, G. A., On-line fermentation process monitoring of carbohydrates and ethanol using tangential flow filtration and column liquid chromatography, *Anal. Chem.*, 65, 2628, 1993.
50. Forman, L. W., Thomas, B. D., and Jacobson, F. S., On-line monitoring and control of fermentation processes by flow-injection analysis, *Anal. Chim. Acta*, 249, 101, 1991.
51. Kroner, K. H., Stach, W., and Kuhlmann, W., Kontinuierliche Probenahmeverfahren für die Bioprozeßanalytik, *Chemie-Ing. Technol.*, 15, 72, 1986.
52. Ruzicka, J. and Hansen, E. H., Flow injection analysis. I. A new concept of fast continuous flow analysis, *Anal. Chim. Acta*, 106, 207, 1975.
53. Olsen, S., Ruzicka, J., and Hansen, E. H., Gradient techniques in flow injection analysis. Stopped flow measurements of the activity of lactate dehydrogenase with electronic dilution, *Anal. Chim. Acta*, 136, 101, 1982.
54. Ruzicka, J. and Hansen, E. H., Stopped flow and merging zones — a new approach to enzymatic assay by flow injection analysis, *Anal. Chim. Acta*, 106, 207, 1979.
55. Ruzicka, J. and Hansen, E. H., Flow injection analysis, in *Chemical Analysis*, Vol. 62, 2nd ed., Wiley Intersciences, New York, 1988.
56. Valcarcel, M. and Luque de Castro, M. D., *Flow Injection Analysis, Principles and Applications*, Ellis Horwood Ser. Anal. Chem. John Wiley & Sons, New York, 1987.
57. Fang, Z., *Flow Injection Separation and Preconcentration*, VCH Publishers, Weinheim, 1993.
58. Schmid, R. D., Ed., Flow injection analysis (FIA) based on enzymes or antibodies, *GBF Monographs*, Vol. 14, VCH Publishers, Weinheim, 1991.
59. Schmid, R. D. and Künnecke, W., Flow injection analysis based on enzymes or antibodies — applications in the life sciences, *J. Biotechnol.*, 14, 3, 1990.
60. Kindervater, R., Künnecke, W., and Schmid, R. D., Exchangeable immobilized enzyme reactor for enzyme inhibition tests in flow-injection analysis using a magnetic device. Determination of pesticides in drinking water, *Anal. Chim. Acta*, 234, 113, 1990.
61. Dremel, B. A. A., Li, S. Y., and Schmid, R. D., On-line determination of glucose and lactate concentrations in animal cell culture based on fibre optic detection of oxygen in flow-injection analysis, *Biosens. Bioelectron.*, 7, 133, 1992.
62. Johansson, G., Ögren, L., and Olsson, B., Enzyme reactors in unsegmented flow injection analysis, *Anal. Chim. Acta*, 145, 71, 1983.
63. Künnecke, W. and Schmid, R. D., Development of a gas diffusion FIA system for on-line monitoring of ethanol, *J. Biotechnol.*, 14, 127, 1990.
64. Ogbomo. I., Steffl, A., Schuhmann, W., Prinzing, U., and Schmidt, H.-L., On-line determination of ethanol in bioprocesses based on sample extraction by continuous pervaporation, *J. Biotechnol.*, 31, 317, 1993.
65. Dremel, B. A. A., Yang, W., and Schmid, R. D., On-line determination of lactic acid during kefir fermentation based on a fibre optic lactic acid biosensor and flow-injection analysis, *Anal. Chim. Acta*, 234, 107, 1990.
66. Carlsen, M., Johansen, C., Wei Min, R., Nielsen, J., Meier, H., and Lantreibecq, F., On-line monitoring of penicillin V during penicillin fermentations: a comparison of two different methods based on flow injection analysis, *Anal. Chim. Acta*, 279, 51, 1993.
67. Bradley, J., Kidd, A. J., Anderson, P. A., Dear, A. M., Ashby, R. E., and Turner, A. P. F., Rapid determination of the glucose content of molasses using a biosensor, *Analyst* , 114, 375, 1989.
68. Gebbert, A., Alvarez-Icaza, M., Stöcklein, W., and Schmid, R. D., Real-time monitoring of immunochemical interactions with a tantalum capacitance flow-through cell, *Anal. Chem.*, 64, 997, 1992.
69. Polzius, R., Bier, F. F., Bilitewski, U., Jäger, V., and Schmid, R. D., On-line monitoring of monoclonal antibodies in animal cell culture using a grating coupler, *Biotechnol. Bioeng.*, 42, 1287, 1993.
70. Scheper, T., Brandes, W., Maschke, H., Plötz, F., and Müller, C., Two FIA-based biosensor systems studied for bioprocess monitoring, *J. Biotechnol.*, 31, 345, 1993.
71. Romette, J. L. and Cooney, C. L., L-glutamine enzyme electrode for on-line mammalian cell culture process control, *Anal. Lett.*, 20, 1069, 1987.

72. Stöcklein, W. and Schmid, R. D., Flow-injection immunoanalysis for the on-line monitoring of monoclonal antibodies, *Anal. Chim. Acta*, 234, 83, 1990.
73. Cattaneo, M. V., Luong, J. H. T., and Mercille, S., Monitoring glutamine in mammalian cell cultures using an amperometric biosensor, *Biosens. Bioelectron.*, 7, 329, 1992.
74. Male, K. B., Luong, J. H. T., Tom, R., and Mercille, S., Novel FIA amperometric bisensor system for the determination of glutamine in cell culture systems, *Enzyme Microbiol. Technol.*, 15, 27, 1993.
75. Matuszewski, W., Rosario, S. A., and Meyerhoff, M. E., Operation of ion-selective electrode detectors in the sub-Nernstian/linear response range: application to flow injection/enzymatic determination of L-glutamine in bioreactor media, *Anal. Chem.*, 63, 1906, 1991.
76. Huang, Y. L., Li, S. Y., Dremel, B. A. A., Bilitewski, U., and Schmid, R. D., On-line determination of glucose concentration throughout animal cell cultures based on chemiluminescent detection of hydrogen peroxide coupled with flow-injection analysis, *J. Biotechnol.*, 18, 161, 1991.
77. Dullau, T., Reinhardt, B., and Schügerl, K., High reliability and stability of enzyme cartridges in flow injection analysis, *Anal. Chim. Acta*, 225, 253, 1989.
78. Clark, L. C. and Lyons, C., Electrode systems for continuous monitoring in cardiovascular surgery, *Ann. N.Y. Acad. Sci.*, 102, 29, 1962.
79. Wolfbeis, O. S. and Carlini, F. M., Long-wave fluorescent indicators for the determination of oxygen partial pressures, *Anal. Chim. Acta*, 160, 301, 1984.
80. Moser, I., Schalkhammer, T., Mann-Buxbaum, E., Hawa, E., Rakohl, M., Urban, G., and Pittner, F., Advanced immobilization and protein techniques on thin film biosensors, *Sensors Actuators*, B7, 356, 1992.
81. Prudenziati, M., Ed., Thick film sensors, in: *Handbook of Sensors and Actuators,* Vol. 1, Elsevier, Amsterdam, 1994.
82. Wollenberger, U., Paeschke, M., and Hintsche, R., Interdigitated array microelectrodes for the determination of enzyme activities, *Analyst*, 119, 1245, 1994.
83. Günther, A. and Bilitewski, U., Characterisation of inhibitors of acetylcholinesterases by an automated amperometric flow-injection system, *Anal. Chim. Acta*, 300, 117, 1995.
84. Schmidt, A., Rohm, I., Rüger, P., Weise, W., and Bilitewski, U., Application of screen printed electrodes in biochemical analysis, *Fresenius J. Anal. Chem.*, 349, 607, 1992.
85. White, S. F., Turner, A. P. F., Schmid, R. D., Bilitewski, U., and Bradley, J., Investigations of platinized and rhodinized carbon electrodes for use in glucose sensors, *Electroanalysis*, 6, 625, 1994.
86. Krämer, P. M. and Schmid, R. D., Automated quasi-continuous immunoanalysis of pesticides with a flow injection system, *Pestic. Sci.*, 32, 451, 1991.
87. Nielsen, J., Nikolajsen, K., Benthin, S., and Villadsen, J., Application of flow-injection analysis in the on-line monitoring of sugars, lactic acid, protein and biomass during lactic acid fermentations, *Anal. Chim. Acta*, 237, 165, 1990.
88. Blaedel, W. J. and Engstrom, R. C., Reagentless enzyme electrodes for ethanol lactate and malate, *Anal. Chem.*, 52, 1691, 1980.
89. Kulys, J. J., Bilitewski, U., and Schmid, R. D., Reagentless biosensors for substrates of dehydrogenases, *Anal. Lett.*, 24, 181, 1991.
90. Dominguez, E., Lan, H. L., Okamoto, Y., Hale, P. D., Skotheim, T. A., and Gorton, L., A carbon paste electrode chemically modified with phenothiazine polymer derivative for electrocatalytic oxidation of NADH. Preliminary study, *Biosens. Bioelectron.*, 8, 167, 1993.
91. Appelqvist, R. and Hansen, E. H., Determination of glucose in fermentation processes by means of an on-line coupled flow-injection system using enzyme sensors based on chemically modified electrodes, *Anal. Chim. Acta,* 235, 265, 1990.
92. Becker, T., Schuhmann, W., Betken, R., Schmidt, H.-L., Leible, M., and Albrecht, A., An automatic dehydrogenase-based flow-injection system. Application for the continuous determination of glucose and lactate in mammalian cell-cultures, *J. Chem Tech. Biotechnol.*, 58, 183, 1993.
93. Chemnitius, G. C. and Schmid, R. D., L-Malate determination in wines and fruit juices by flow injection analysis. Adaptation of a coupled dehydrogenase/transferase system, *Anal. Lett.*, 22, 2897, 1989.

94. Scheper, T. and Bückmann, A. F., A fibre optic biosensor based on fluorometric detection using confined macromolecular nicotinamide adenine dinucleotide derivatives, *Biosens. Bioelectron.*, 5, 125, 1990.
95. Shul'ga, A. A., Strikha, V. I., Soldatkin, A. P., El'skaya, A. V., Maupas, H., Martelet, C., and Clechet, P., Removing the influence of buffer concentration on the response of enzyme field effect transistors by using additional membranes, *Anal. Chim Acta*, 278, 233, 1993.
96. Jespersen, N. D., Thermistor probes, *Bioprocess Technol.*, 6, 193, 1990.
97. Danielsson, B., Enzyme thermistor devices, *Bioprocess Technol.*, 15, 83, 1991.
98. Freitag, R., Fenge, C., Scheper, T., Schügerl, K., Spreinat, A., Antranikian, G., and Fraune, E., Immunological on-line detection of specific proteins during fermentation processes, *Anal. Chim. Acta*, 249, 113, 1991.
99. Hecht, H. J., Kalisz, H. M., Hendle, J., Schmid, R. D., and Schomburg, D., Crystal structure of glucose oxidase from *Aspergillus niger* refined at 2*3 Å resolution, *J. Mol. Biol.*, 229, 153, 1993.
100. Spohn, U., van der Pol, J., Eberhardt, R., Joksch, B., and Wandrey, C., An automated system for multichannel flow-injection analysis, *Anal. Chim. Acta*, 292, 281, 1994.
101. Lelong, P., Cellard, H., Pardo, D., and Cavalie, J. M., Automation of glucose measurement in fermentor broths, *Appl. Microbiol. Biotechnol.*, 36, 173, 1991.
102. Gründig, B., Strehlitz, B., Kotte, H., and Ethner, K., Development of a process-FIA system using mediator-modified enzyme electrodes, *J. Biotechnol.*, 31, 277, 1993.
103. Schuhmann, W., Wohlschläger, H., Lammert, R., Schmidt, H.-L., Löffler, U., Wiemhöfer, H.-D., and Göpel, W., Leaching of dimethylferrocene, a redox mediator in amperometric enzyme electrodes, *Sensors Actuators,* B1, 571, 1990.
104. Leung, K. K., Petersen, J. N., and Lee, J. M., A system for the on-line determination of glucose concentration, *Bioprocess Eng.*, 7, 19, 1991.
105. Wehnert, G., Sauerbrei, A., Bayer, T., Scheper, T., Schügerl, K., and Herold, T., Application of an enzyme thermistor for the determination of glucose in complex fermentation media, *Anal. Chim. Acta,* 200, 73, 1987.
106. Brand, U., Brandes, L., Koch, V., Kullik, T., Reinhardt, B., Rüther, F., Scheper, T., Schügerl, K., Wang, S., Wu, X., Ferretti. R., Prasad, S., and Wilhelm, D., Monitoring and control of biotechnological production processes by Bio-FET-FIA-sensors, *Appl. Microbiol. Biotechnol.*, 36, 167, 1991.
107. Yamada, Y., Aida, K., and Uemera, T., A new enzyme, D-fructose dehydrogenase, *Agric. Biol. Chem.*, 30, 95, 1966.
108. Ikeda, T., Matsushita, I., and Senda, M., Amperometric fructose sensor based on direct bioelectrocatalysis, *Biosens. Bioelectron.,* 6, 299, 1991.
109. Bergmeyer, H. U., Bernt, E., Schmidt, F., and Stork, H., in *Methods of Enzymatic Analysis*, 2nd ed., Bergmeyer, H. U., Ed., Academic Press, New York, 1974.
110. Thordsen, O., Lee, S. J., Degelau, A., Scheper, T., Loos, H., Rehr, B., and Sahm, H., A model system for a fluorometric biosensor using permeabilized *Zymomonas mobilis* or enzymes with protein confined dinucleotides, *Biotechnol. Bioeng.*, 42, 387, 1993.
111. Mandenius, C. F., Danielsson, B., and Mattiasson, B., Process control of an ethanol fermentation with an enzyme thermistor as a sucrose sensor, *Biotechnol. Lett.*, 3(11), 629, 1981.
112. Hundeck, H.-G., Hübner, U., Lübbert, A., Scheper, T., Schmidt, J., Weiß, M., and Schubert, F., Development and applications of a four-channel enzyme thermistor system for process control, *GBF Monogr.*, 17, 321, 1992.
113. Marko-Varga, G. A., Determination of mono- and oligosaccharides in fermentation broths by liquid chromatographic separation and amperometric detection using immobilized enzyme reactors and a chemically modified electrode, *Anal. Chem.*, 61, 831, 1989.
114. Cavinato, A. G., Mayes, D. M., Ge, Z., and Callis, J. B., Nonivasive method for monitoring ethanol in fermentation processes using fibre-optic near-infrared spectroscopy, *Anal. Chem.*, 62, 1977, 1990.
115. Austin, G. D., Sankhe, S. K., and Tsao, G. T., Monitoring and control of methanol concentration during polysaccharide fermentation using an on-line methanol sensor, *Bioprocess Eng.*, 7, 241, 1992.

116. Dumoulin, E. D., Mazette, S. L., Cogat, P. O., and Guerain, J. T., Determination of ethanol in complex liquid media for continuous processing control, *J. Agric. Food Chem.*, 37, 680, 1989.
117. Tellier, C., Guillou-Charpin, M., Grenier, P., and Le Botlan, D., Monitoring alcoholic fermentation by low-resolution pulsed nuclear magnetic resonance, *J. Agric. Food Chem.*, 37, 988, 1989.
118. Johansson, K., Jönsson-Pettersson, G., Gorton, L., Marko-Varga, G., and Csöregi, E., A reagentless amperometric biosensor for alcohol detection in column liqiud chromatography based on co-immobilized peroxidase and alcohol oxidase in carbon paste, *J. Biotechnol.*, 31, 301, 1993.
119. Palleschi, G. and Turner, A. P. F., Amperometric tetrathiafulvalene-mediated lactate electrode using lactate oxidase adsorbed on carbon foil, *Anal. Chim. Acta*, 234, 459, 1990.
120. Weaver, M. R. and Vadgama, P. M., An O_2-based enzyme electrode for whole blood lactate measurements under continuous flow conditions, *Clin. Chim. Acta*, 155, 295, 1986.
121. Dubinin, A. G., Li, F., Li, Y., and Yu, J., A solid state immobilized enzyme polymer membrane microelectrode for measuring lactate-ion concentration, *Bioelectrochem. Bioenerg.*, 25, 131, 1991.
122. Nielsen, J., Nikolajsen, K., and Villadsen, J., FIA for on-line monitoring of important lactic acid fermentation variables, *Biotechnol. Bioeng.*, 33, 1127, 1989.
123. Bilitewski, U., Drewes, W., Neermann, J., Schrader, J., Surkow, R., Schmid, R. D., and Bradley, J., Comparison of different biosensor systems suitable for bioprocess monitoring, *J. Biotechnol.*, 31, 257, 1993.
124. Yoda, K., Tsuchida, T., and Takasugi, H., Application of enzyme electrodes for monitoring of mammalian cell cultures, *Ann. N.Y. Acad. Sci.*, 613, 410, 1990.
125. Becker, T., Kittsteiner-Eberle, R., Luck, T., and Schmidt, H.-L., On-line determination of acetic acid in a continuous production of *Acetobacter aceticus*, *J. Biotechnol.*, 31, 267, 1993.
126. Tosa, T., Senuma, M., Nakagawa, Y., and Morimoto, T., Industrial application of microbial sensors for process control, *Ann. N.Y. Acad. Sci.*, 672, 184, 1992.
127. Male, K. B., Luong, J. H. T., Tom, R., and Mercille, S., Novel FIA amperometric biosensor system, for the determination of glutamine in cell culture systems, *Enzyme Microbiol. Technol.*, 15, 26, 1993.
128. Cattaneo, M. V. and Luong, J. H. T., Monitoring glutamine in animal cell cultures using a chemiluminescence fibre optic biosensor, *Biotechnol. Bioeng.*, 41, 659, 1993.
129. Cattaneo, M. V., Luong, J. H. T., and Mercille, S., Monitoring glutamine in mammalian cell cultures using an amperometric biosensor, *Biosens. Bioelectron.*, 7, 329, 1992.
130. Dremel, B. A. A., Huang, Y., and Schmid, R. D., Improvement of an *E. coli* fermentation by on-line monitoring of glucose and total amino acids using a fibre optic FIA-system, GBF *Monogr.*, 17, 221, 1992.
131. Romette, J. L. and Cooney, C. L., L-Glutamine enzyme electrode for on-line mammalian cell culture process control, *Anal. Lett.*, 20(7), 1096, 1987.
132. Tanaka, A., Hagi, N., Itho, N., and Fukui, S., Application of immobilized lysine decarboxylase tubes for automated analysis of L-lysine, *J. Ferment. Technol.*, 58, 391, 1980.
133. Bayer, T., Herold, T., Hiddessen, R., and Schügerl, K., On-line monitoring of media components during the production of cephalosporin c, *Anal. Chim. Acta*, 190, 213, 1986.
134. Zhong, L.-C. and Li, G.-X., Biosensor based on ISFET for penicillin determination, *Sensors Actuators*, B13-14, 570, 1993.
135. Carlsen, M., Christensen, L. H., and Nielsen, J., Flow-injection analysis for the measurement of penicillin v in fermentation media, *Anal. Chim. Acta*, 274, 117, 1993.
136. Brand, U., Scheper, T., and Schügerl, K., Penicillin G sensor based on penicillin amidase coupled to a field effect transistor, *Anal. Chim. Acta*, 226, 87, 1989.
137. Meier, H., Lantreibecq, F., and Tran-Minh, C., Application of flow injection analysis (FIA) using fast responding enzyme glass electrodes to detect penicillin in fermentation broth and urea in human serum, *J. Autom. Chem.*, 14, 137, 1992.
138. Meier, H. and Tran-Minh, C., Determination of penicillin V in standard solution and in fermentation broth by flow-injection analysis using fast responding enzyme glass electrodes in different detection cells, *Anal. Chim. Acta*, 264, 13, 1992.
139. Scheper, T., Brandes, W., Maschke, H., Plötz, F., and Müller, C., Two FIA-based biosensor systems studied for bioprocess monitoring, *J. Biotechnol.*, 31, 345, 1993.

140. Mattiasson, B., Danielsson, B., Winquist, F., Nilsson, H., and Mosbach, K., Enzyme thermistor analysis of penicillin in standard solutions and in fermentation broth, *Appl. Environ. Microbiol.*, 41, 903, 1981.
141. Middendorf, C., Schulze, B., Freitag, R., Scheper, Th., Howaldt, M., and Hoffmann, H., On-line immunoanalysis for bioprocess control, *J. Biotechnol.*, 31, 395, 1993.
142. Stöcklein, W., Jäger, V., and Schmid, R. D., Monitoring mouse immunoglobulin G by flow-injection analytical affinity chromatography, *Anal. Chim. Acta*, 245, 1, 1991.
143. Palsson, B. O., Shen, B. Q., Meyerhoff, M. E., and Trojanowicz, M., Simultaneous determination of ammonia nitrogen and L-glutamine in bioreactor media using flow injection, *Analyst*, 118, 1361, 1993.
144. Renneberg, R., Trott-Kriegeskorte, G., Lietz, M., Jäger, V., Pawlowa, M., Kaiser, G., Wollenberger, U., Schubert, F., Wagner, R., Schmid, R. D., and Scheller, F., Enzyme-sensor-FIA-system for on-line monitoring of glucose, lactate and glutamine in animal cell cultures, *J. Biotechnol.*, 21, 173, 1991.
145. Goodacre, R. and Kell, D. B., Rapid and quantitative analysis of bioprocesses using pyrolysis mass spectrometry and neural networks. Application to indole production, *Anal. Chim. Acta*, 279, 17, 1993.
146. Filippini, C., Sonnleitner, B., and Fiechter, A., "Intelligent" analytical subsystems for on-line control and monitoring of bioprocesses, *Anal. Chim. Acta*, 265, 63, 1992.
147. Vigié, P., Dahhou, B., Queinnee, I., Lakrori, M., Chéruy, A., and Pourciel, J. B., Control of substrate concentration in a continuous bioprocess, *Bioprocess Eng.*, 6, 259, 1991.
148. Oishi, K., Tominaga, M., Kawato, A., Abe, Y., Imayasu, S., and Nanba, A., Development of on-line sensoring and computer aided control systems for sake brewing, *J. Biotechnol.*, 24, 53, 1992.
149. Schügerl, K., Brandes, L., Dullau, T., Holzhauer-Rieger, K., Hotop, S., Hübner, U., Wu, X., and Zhou, W., Fermentation monitoring and control by on-line flow injection and liquid chromatography, *Anal. Chim. Acta*, 249, 87, 1991.
150. Shimizu, K., An overview on the control systems design of bioreactors, in *Advances in Biochemical Engineering/Biotechnology*, Vol. 50, Fiechter, A., Ed., Springer-Verlag, Berlin, 1993.

20 Fuzzy Logic in the Evaluation of Sensor Data

Peter G. Berrie

CONTENTS

20.1 INTRODUCTION

The current interest in fuzzy logic can be traced back to the appearance on the market in 1990 of a number of Japanese consumer articles which boasted fuzzy control as a means to simplify and improve operation. Although earlier industrial applications had been reported, it was the commercial exploitation of fuzzy set theory which set off the subsequent boom. The stimulus it created has resulted in a greater awareness in industry of the benefits to be reaped from a discipline which, if known at all, has too often been seen as purely academic.

The first paper on fuzzy set theory was published by Zadeh[1] in 1965. In this and subsequent publications, he examined the problems of uncertainty as mirrored in human reasoning, and sought to provide a mathematical algorithm on which this could be modelled. According to Zadeh,[2] fuzzy analogues can be found for all »crisp« mathematical terms, producing a new set of tools able to more closely model human thinking. Since 1965, many thousands of papers have been published on fuzzy sets and systems, establishing a sound

0-8493-8905-4/97/$0.00+$.50
© 1997 by CRC Press, Inc.

theoretical foundation for the subject. Today fuzzy set theory has applications in the following fields:

- Data banks and expert systems, e.g., for medical or business purposes
- Decision support systems for business and production management
- Pattern recognition, e.g., for computer-aided evaluation of aerial photographs
- Classification for fault recognition, e.g., in materials testing
- Data analysis in sensor or multisensor applications
- Fuzzy control

In this chapter we shall be concerned primarily with fuzzy set theory, data analysis, and fuzzy control. The chapter assumes no previous knowledge of fuzzy logic and has been deliberately kept as descriptive as possible. The fuzzy applications quoted are in the main concerned with physical and chemical measurands; however, since the problems faced by biosensor designers and users are essentially the same, no matter what their discipline, it is thought that there are sufficient parallels between the two to make them interesting. Readers seeking more detailed information on fuzzy set theory and applications are directed to books such as that by Zimmermann[3] as well as the references at the end of the chapter. These are by no means comprehensive and have a European bias, but should provide the springboard to more intensive research.

20.2 FUZZY SET THEORY

In order to understand the ideas behind fuzzy set theory and fuzzy logic, it is useful to compare the way in which humans and computers (or more precisely their designers and programmers) go about solving problems. Real systems are usually extremely complex. When a computer programmer sets out to model such a system he first analyses its constituent parts and the way in which they interact. He then proceeds to describe them in terms of equations and operations which can be programmed on his computer. It might be assumed that the more detailed a model is, the more accurate are its predictions. In practice, however, this is not always true. The more detailed a model, the more complex it becomes. As the complexity increases, so does the uncertainty in the interactions of its components. The number of input parameters also increases and values for these are often difficult to determine accurately by experiment or to estimate reliably. The choice of input parameters can be a problem even with the simplest models. Despite the computing power at its disposal, therefore, very often the model fails.

Humans, on the other hand, are able to master complex situations despite a short-term memory which allows us to handle only five to seven concepts at a time. In personal communication, for example, we do this by using verbal models which are understandable and significant to us, but which are seldom mathematically precise. The uncertainties which are associated with the contents of words and sentences pose us no problems. Only when such linguistic wisdom is to be reproduced on a computer do difficulties arise.

The discrepancy between intuitive human behaviour and the numerical precision required by computers to imitate the same actions can be seen in practically every human activity. Take the case of the baseball player in the outfield running to catch a ball as shown in Figure 20.1. The pitcher throws, the batter makes contact, and the ball flies into the air. The fielder watches all these actions, and intuitively sets off in the direction in which the ball is carrying and catches the ball. In doing so he uses no mathematical model. Rather, he pictures in his mind's eye where the ball will fall and moves off in the right direction, correcting his movements as he runs, and homes in on the ball. A computer, on the other hand, must be fed with the minutest physical data of both players and equipment for even the simplest model of the sequence.

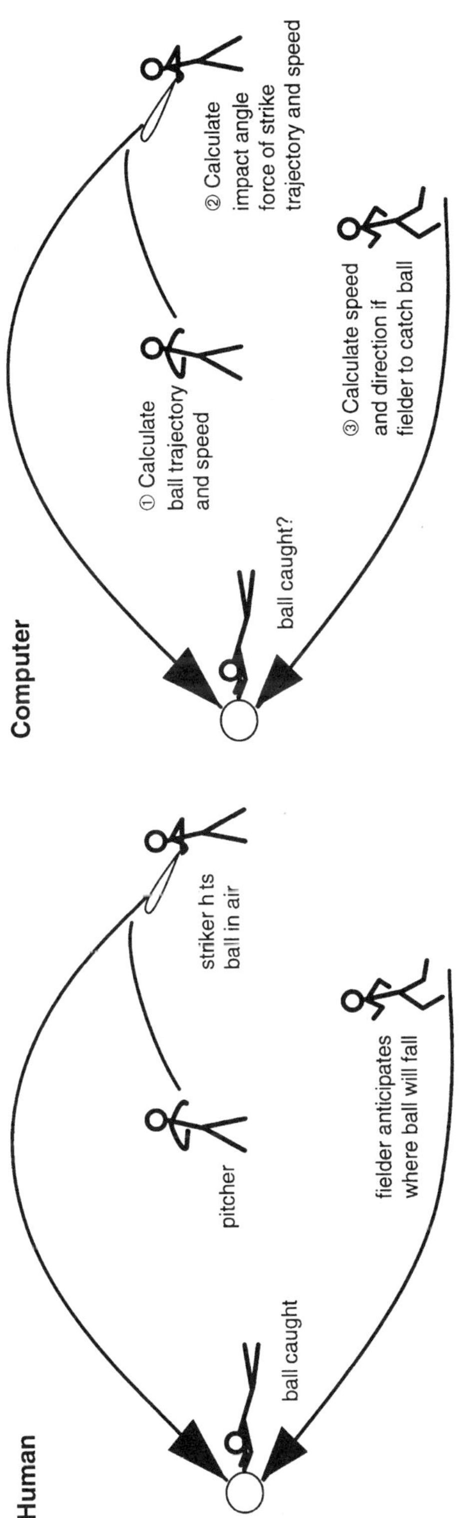

FIGURE 20.1 Comparison of human and computer ball-catching strategies.

Another example of imprecise yet effective human communication can be seen in cooperative human activities. When two people solve a problem together they automatically express their commands in terms such as *a little to the left, more to the right, up a bit, down some more, a lot hotter, a lot colder, turn it a bit,* etc. Both partners find nothing unusual in this type of communication and the job gets done. Of course it is also possible that one partner gives his commands in the following form: *5.3 cm to the left, 12" to the right, 2.8 cm upwards, 4" down; 34 ℃, 50 ℉, 5° 30′ clockwise.* Although the final result might be the same, it is obvious that this type of communication, which is fine for controlling technical processes, is not appropriate to human psychology.

Many of the expressions humans use are dependent upon the context and on inflection, many are simply unquantifiable. The expression *"you are driving too fast"* covers a whole range of speeds: over 5 mph in a play street, 15 mph in a residential area, 30 mph in a built-up zone, 40 mph on an urban thoroughfare, and 70 mph on a motorway — plus, of course, the various national differences which are met across the world. And what of such abstract concepts as *ugly, plain, good-looking, beautiful?* Here, there is not even a numerical basis on which to work — one person's idea of good-looking is radically different from that of another. Simply transferring such expressions to the computer, therefore, will not provide an adequate model of human wisdom because the information must be interpreted within its context before it takes on any meaning. Thus, human reasoning can be used only when its contents are defined. It was with the objective of making human knowledge and reasoning quantifiable, and thus acceptable to the computer, that fuzzy set theory was developed.

The principles of fuzzy logic will now be introduced in Sections 20.2.1 to 20.2.7, before the applications in the evaluation of sensor data are discussed in the remainder of the chapter.

20.2.1 Fuzzy Sets

The theory of fuzzy sets can be looked upon as a generalisation of both classical set theory and binary logic. The membership of a fuzzy set is no longer a question of yes or no (1 or 0) but rather each element x is linked to a degree of membership $\mu(x)$, a so-called membership function. Put formally, if X is a classical crisp set of objects, then the fuzzy set A is defined by

$$A: = \{(x, \mu_{A'}(x)); x \in X\}$$

where $\mu_{A'}(x) \rightarrow \Re$ is a real-valued function. Thus A is the fuzzy set containing the elements x with the degrees of membership of A, $\mu_A(x)$. (The elements x also form the crisp set X, but here the degree of membership is 1 (= 100%) for each element x). The objects in the fuzzy set are termed its supports, the number of objects its cardinality. If the values of the membership function are restricted to the interval between 0 and 1, e.g., by dividing by the maximum value or supremum, then one speaks of a normalised fuzzy set.

Figure 20.2 shows the crisp set "temperature 25 ± 5°C" together with the fuzzy set "temperature about 25°C". For example, a temperature of 25°C is part of both sets with a degree of membership of 100% (i.e., $\mu = 1$), a temperature of 18°C is not part of the crisp set, but is an element of the fuzzy set with the degree of membership 10% ($\mu = 0.1$). The representation of the fuzzy set is not restricted to the Gaussian function shown here: discrete values, triangles, and trapeziums are often preferred because they are simpler to handle on the computer and require less computing time. Further information on computing with fuzzy sets can be taken from the literature, e.g., from Tilli.[4]

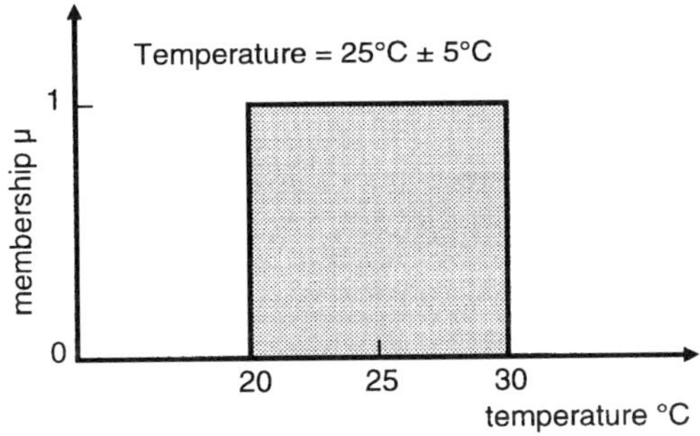

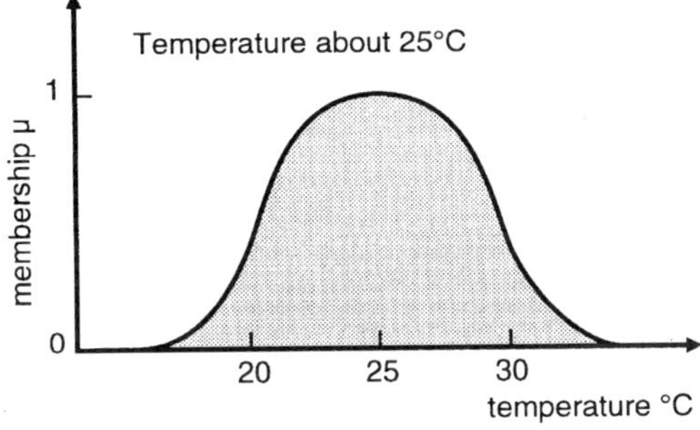

FIGURE 20.2 Comparison of crisp and fuzzy temperature sets.

Like their crisp counterparts, fuzzy sets can be subject to a number of logical and algebraic operations. Table 20.1 lists the basic operators and laws together with their formal mathematical definitions. The elementary operators originally suggested by Zadeh were

- The minimum operator for the intersection of two fuzzy sets C = A∩B
- The maximum operator for the union of two fuzzy sets C = A∪B as well as
- The complement C of a fuzzy set A.

The intersection can be interpreted as a logical "AND" (objects of set C have to satisfy conditions for sets A and B), the union as a logical "OR" and the complement as a logical "NOT". The shaded areas in Figures 20.3, 20.4, and 20.5 show the effects of these operators on two fuzzy sets "hot" and "cold".

TABLE 20.1
Logical Operators, Algebraic Operators and Modifiers

Operator	Definition	Function
Intersection, A∩B	$\mu_C(x) = \min\{(\mu_A(x), \mu_B(x)\}, x \in X$	logical "AND" for fuzzy sets (t_3)
Union, A∪B	$\mu_C(x) = \max\{(\mu_A(x), \mu_B(x)\}, x \in X$	logical "OR" for fuzzy sets (s_3)
Complement C	$\mu_C(x) = 1 - \mu_A(x), x \in X$	logical "NOT" for fuzzy sets
Concentration	$\mathrm{con}(\mu(x)) = \{\mu(x)\}^2$	"very" in approximate reasoning
Dilation	$\mathrm{dil}(\mu_A(x)) = \{\mu_A(x)\}^{1/2}$	"more or less" in approx. reasoning
Contrast intensifier	$\mathrm{int}(\mu_A(x)) = 2\{\mu_A(x)\}^2$ if $\mu_A(x) < 0.5$ else $1 - 2\{1 - \mu_A(x)\}^2$	
Commutative law	$\mathrm{op}(\mu_A, \mu_B) = \mathrm{op}(\mu_B, \mu_A)$	
Associative law	$\mathrm{op}(\mu_A, \mu_B, \mu_C) = \mathrm{op}(\mathrm{op}(\mu_A, \mu_B), \mu_C)$	

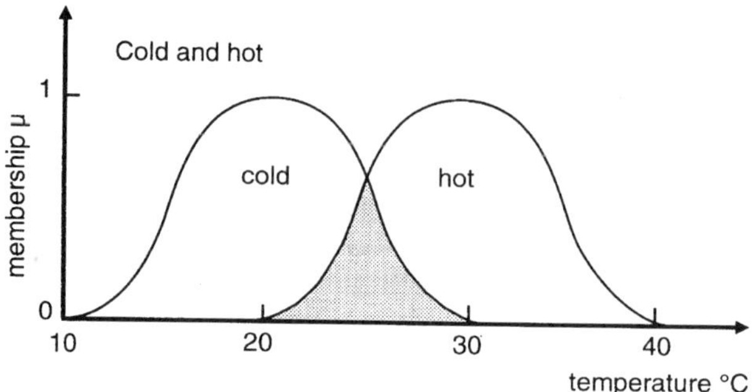

FIGURE 20.3 Fuzzy set "hot and cold".

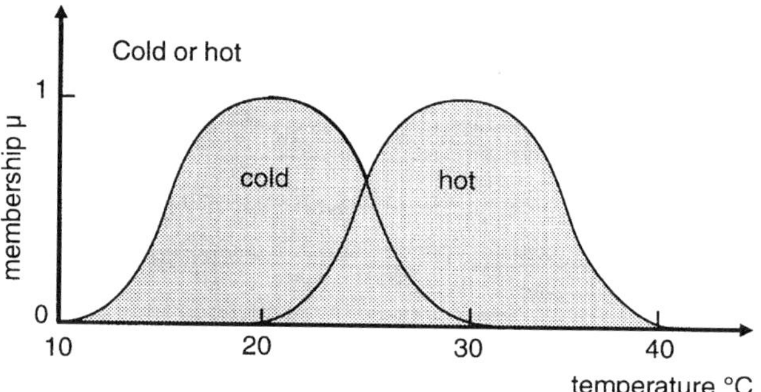

FIGURE 20.4 Fuzzy set "hot or cold".

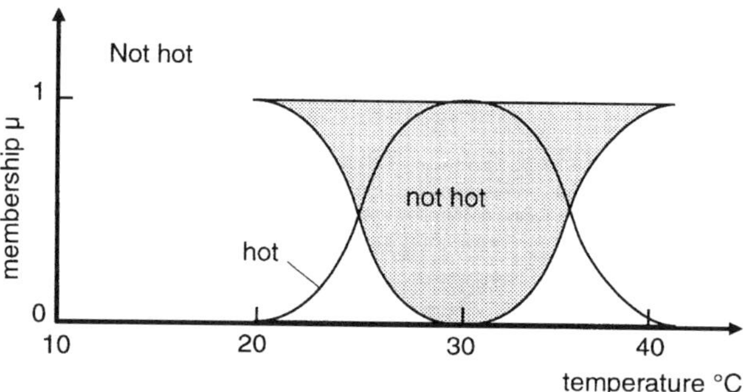

FIGURE 20.5 Fuzzy set "not hot".

Two important properties of the minimum and maximum operators are that they are both cumulative and associative. This means that the result of an operation on more than two values is dependent neither upon the order in which they are taken nor on the arrangement of the arguments. As regards effect, the minimum operator is seen to be relatively pessimistic, taking always the smallest value of the membership function $\mu(x)$, i.e., a small value of μ_A is not compensated by a large value of μ_B. Similarly, the maximum operator is relatively optimistic.

20.2.2 Fuzzy Operators

The minimum operator is a member of a class of operators called the triangular norms or t-norms[5] which can be used to model the "AND" operator. The maximum operator is a member of the cotriangular norm operators or s-norms which model the "OR" operator. Both classes are cumulative, associative, and monotonic. When the value of the membership function is restricted to zero or one, all the operators behave as the classical "AND" or "OR" of binary logic (see Table 20.2). When this restriction is removed each behaves differently, varying from the minimum and maximum operator at one extreme of the class to the drastic product and sum at the other. The choice of operator depends on the application and is generally influenced by its adaptability, numerical efficiency, degree of compensation, and its suitability as a model for a real system.

TABLE 20.2
t-norms and s-norms

Operator	Definition
Drastic product t_w	$t_w(\mu_A(x), \mu_B(x)) = \min(\mu_A(x), \mu_B(x))$ if $\max(\mu_A(x), \mu_B(x)) = 1$ else $= 0$
Drastic sum s_w	$s_w(\mu_A(x), \mu_B(x)) = \max(\mu_A(x), \mu_B(x))$ if $\min(\mu_A(x), \mu_B(x)) = 0$ else $= 1$
Bounded difference t_1	$t_1(\mu_A(x), \mu_B(x)) = \max(0, \mu(x) + \mu_B(x) - 1)$
Bounded sum s_1	$s_1(\mu_A(x), \mu_B(x)) = \min(1, \mu_A(x) + \mu_B(x))$
Einstein product $t_{1.5}$	$t_{1.5}(\mu_A(x), \mu_B(x)) = (\mu_A(x) \cdot \mu_B(x))/(2 - [\mu_A(x) + \mu_B(x) - \mu_A(x) \cdot \mu_B(x)])$
Einstein sum $s_{1.5}$	$s_{1.5}(\mu_A(x), \mu_B(x)) = (\mu_A(x) + \mu_B(x))/(1 + (\mu_A(x) \cdot \mu_B(x))$
Algebraic product t_2	$t_2(\mu_A(x), \mu_B(x)) = \mu_A(x) \cdot \mu_B(x)$
Algebraic sum s_2	$s_2(\mu_A(x), \mu_B(x)) = \mu_A(x) + \mu_B(x) - \mu_A(x) \cdot \mu_B(x)$
Hamacher product $t_{2.5}$	$t_{2.5}(\mu_A(x), \mu_B(x)) = (\mu_A(x) \cdot \mu_B(x))/(\mu_A(x) + \mu_B(x) - \mu_A(x) \cdot \mu_B(x))$
Hamacher sum $t_{2.5}$	$t_{2.5}(\mu_A(x), \mu_B(x)) = (\mu_A(x) + \mu_B(x) - 2\mu_A(x) \cdot \mu_B(x)/(1 - \mu_A(x) \cdot \mu_B(x))$
Relationship t-/s-norms	$t(\mu_A(x), \mu_B(x)) = 1 - s(1 - \mu_A(x), 1 - \mu_B(x))$

In addition to these "pure" AND and OR operators, there exist a number of adjustable operators (see Table 20.3). The "Fuzzy AND" and "Fuzzy OR" operators proposed by Werners[6] combine the minimum or maximum operators with the arithmetic mean, ranging between the two extremes. More general still are the "compensatory and" — commonly known as the "Gamma-operator" — proposed by Zimmermann and Zysno[7] and the MIN-MAX operator, for which there are several forms. These operators are often encountered in decision support systems and support programs for developing fuzzy controllers, since it is generally assumed that the linguistic "AND" used by humans is not as unambiguous as the logical "AND" used in classical set theory and thus requires a greater degree of compensation.

TABLE 20.3
Fuzzy Operators

Operator	Definition
Fuzzy "AND"	$\mu(\mu_A(x), \mu_B(x)) = \gamma \min(\mu_A(x), \mu_B(x)) + {}^1/_2(1 - \gamma)(\mu_A(x) + \mu_B(x))\ \gamma \in [0,1]$
Fuzzy "OR"	$\mu(\mu_A(x), \mu_B(x)) = \gamma \max(\mu_A(x), \mu_B(x)) + {}^1/_2(1 - \gamma)(\mu_A(x) + \mu_B(x))\ \gamma \in [0,1]$
Compensatory "AND"	$\mu_{comp}(x) = (\Pi\ \mu_i(x))^{(1-\gamma)}\ (1 - \Pi(1 - \mu_i(x)))^{\gamma}\ i = 1 \ldots m,\ \gamma \in [0,1]$
Min-Max operator	$\mu(\mu_A(x), \mu_B(x)) = \gamma \min(\mu_A(x), \mu_B(x)) + (1 - \gamma) \max(\mu_A(x), \mu_B(x))\ \gamma \in [0,1]$

20.2.3 Modifiers

In addition to the operators used for aggregating two fuzzy sets, there also exists a series of operators which modify a set. These modifiers are

- The normalisation operator — in this case all the membership values are divided by the maximum value to produce a normalised set
- The concentration operator — in this case the set becomes crisper
- The dilation operator — in this case the set becomes fuzzier
- The contrast intensifier — here the flanks of the fuzzy set become crisper

The mathematical definitions of these operators are also to be found in Table 20.1. The concentration operator is often associated with the linguistic qualifier or hedge "very" in respect of the truth value of the set on which it operates, the dilation operator with "more or less". Figure 20.6 shows the effect of both operators on the fuzzy set "hot". Note that in our case the concentration operator does not produce the fuzzy set "very hot", rather the set "hot" is more sharply defined. Where the membership function is of S-form or a ramp, however, the concentration does produce a shift towards hotter (or colder) values and may be used in this manner.[2]

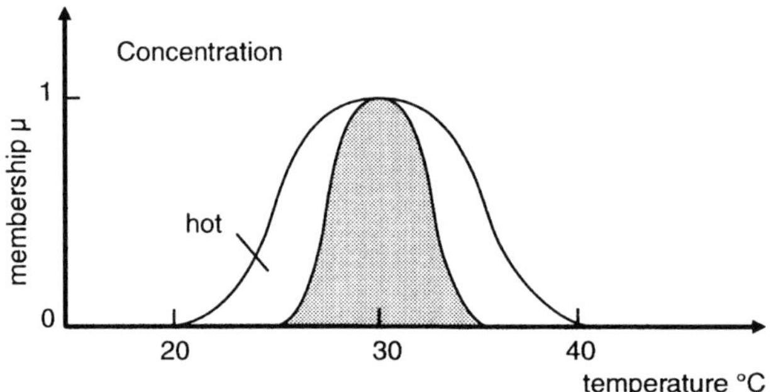

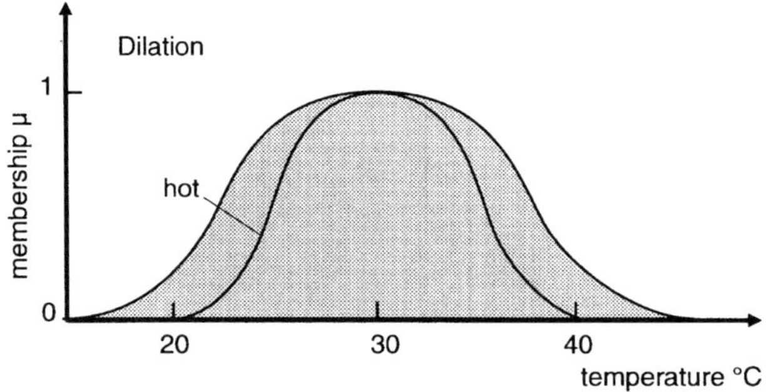

FIGURE 20.6 Effect of concentration and dilation on fuzzy set "hot".

The set may also be modified by taking a so-called α-cut to produce the α-level set: in this case only the supports with a degree of membership greater than or equal to α are used in any set operations. A so-called strong α-cut uses only those supports with degree of membership greater than α.

20.2.4 Fuzzy Numbers

In 1973, Zadeh published a paper in which crisp mathematical concepts were extended to fuzzy mathematical concepts.[2] The extension principle, as it is known, lays down the theoretical basis for the addition, subtraction, multiplication, and division of fuzzy numbers and intervals as well as for the formation of transcendental functions. A fuzzy number is defined as having several values, but only one of these with the membership value 1.0; a fuzzy interval can have several. In addition, the membership function must be convex, i.e., rises monotonically to and falls monotonically from the supremum.

For computational purposes it is usual to define the membership values of fuzzy numbers as continuous functions. This is primarily to save computing time, but also because some operations on discretely defined fuzzy numbers, e.g., multiplication, lead to sets with more than one support having the value 1 or which are not convex, i.e., the result is not a fuzzy number. It should also be noted that the addition of a fuzzy set A′ with –A′ does not result in crisp 0, and the division of A′ by A′ does not result in crisp 1. For this reason fuzzy equations are very difficult to solve because the variables do not cancel as usual. Readers wanting to know more about fuzzy numbers are referred to the literature;[2-4,8] the formal mathematical definitions are given in Table 20.4. To illustrate the use of the extension principle, the two fuzzy sets below will be added together:

$$A_1 = \{(4, 0.4), (5, 1.0), (6, 0.5)\}$$

$$A_2 = \{(2, 0.3), (3, 0.8), (4, 1.0), (5, 0.4)\}$$

The first number in the brackets is the support, the second its degree of membership, i.e., the number 4 is contained in the fuzzy set A_1 to a degree of membership 0.4. The first step is to calculate the Cartesian product $A_1 \times A_2$ and the membership functions for each pair of values, whereby the minimum operator is used (see Table 20.5).

TABLE 20.4
Fuzzy Number Functions and Operators

Operator/Function	Definition
Cartesian product	$\mu_{cart}(x_1, \ldots, x_n) = \min(\mu_{A1}(x_1), \ldots, \mu_{An}(x_n))$
Fuzzy cartesian product	$\mu_B(y) = \sup \mu_C(x_1, \ldots, x_n)$ if $f^{-1} \neq 0$ otherwise = 0, whereby $y = f(x_1, \ldots, x_n)$,

TABLE 20.5
Cartesian Product of $A_1 \times A_2$

X1	X2			
	2	3	4	5
4	0.3	0.4	0.4	0.4
5	0.3	0.8	1.0	0.4
6	0,3	0.5	0.5	0.4

The fuzzy Cartesian product is now calculated by performing the desired transformation on each support pair, then taking the largest membership function (supremum) where two or more results are identical. Taking addition for the function f, i.e., $y := f(x_1, x_2) = x_1 + x_2$, the following membership values are obtained from Table 20.5 for the addition of the fuzzy sets A_1 and A_2:

$$\mu_B(y = 6) = \mu_B(4 + 2) = \sup(0.3) = 0.3$$

$$\mu_B(y = 7) = \mu_B(4 + 3 \text{ or } 5 + 2) = \sup(0.4, 0.3) = 0.4$$

$$\mu_B(y = 8) = \mu_B(4 + 4 \text{ or } 5 + 3 \text{ or } 6 + 2) = \sup\,(0.4, 0.8, 0.3) = 0.8$$

$$\mu_B(y = 9) = \mu_B(4 + 5 \text{ or } 5 + 4 \text{ or } 6 + 3) = \sup\,(0.4, 1.0, 0.5) = 1.0$$

$$\mu_B(y = 10) = \mu_B(5 + 5 \text{ or } 6 + 4) = \sup\,(0.4, 0.5) = 0.5$$

$$\mu_B(y = 11) = \mu_B(6 + 5) = \sup\,(0.4) = 0.4$$

The result of our fuzzy addition, also shown in Figure 20.7, is thus

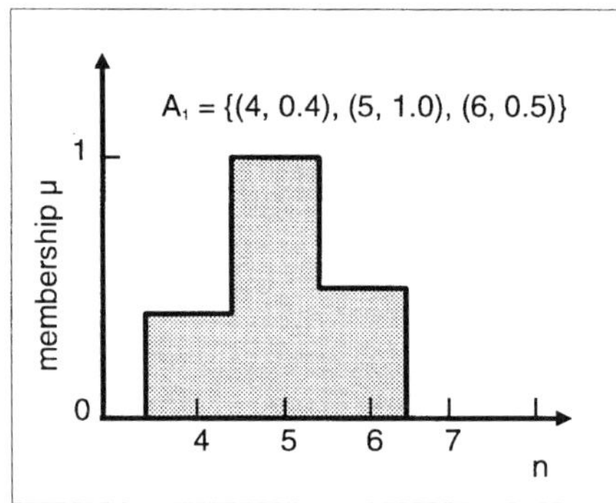

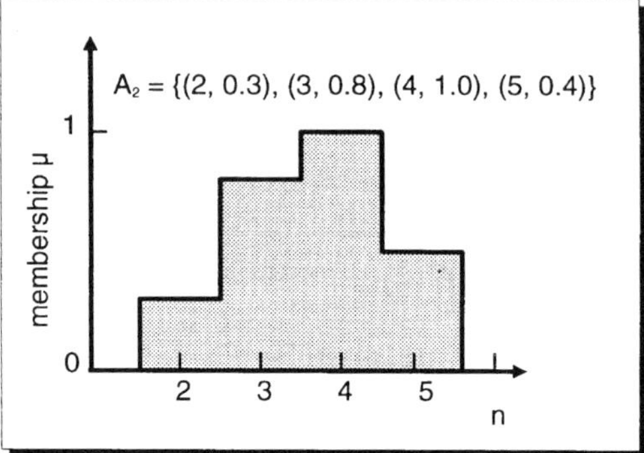

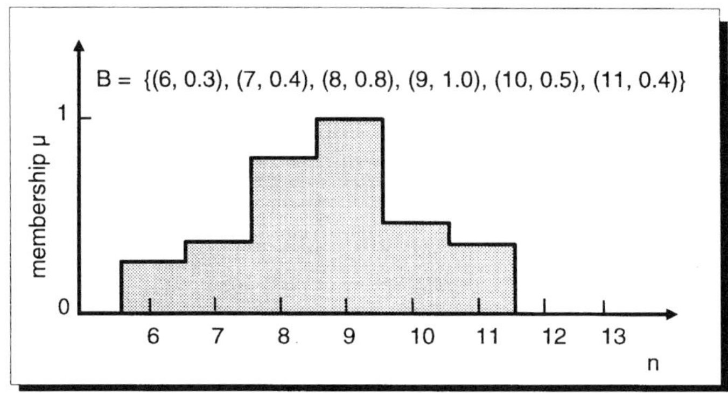

FIGURE 20.7 Addition of two fuzzy numbers.

$$B = A_1 + A_2 = \{(6, 0.3), (7, 0.4), (8, 0.8), (9, 1.0), (10, 0.5), (11, 0.4)\}$$

20.2.5 Fuzzy Relations

Fuzzy relations are concerned with the interdependencies of two fuzzy sets. Examples might be *Y is greater than X, X is equal to Y, Y is close to X*. The relationship between two fuzzy sets might be expressed in terms of a function, such as the following for *X is much smaller than Y*:

$$\mu_R(x,y) = \begin{cases} 1 \text{ if } 10x < y; \\ (y-x)/0.9y \text{ if } 0.1y \le x \le y, \\ 0 \text{ if } x > y \end{cases}$$

or if X and Y are discrete sets, fuzzy relations can be defined by means of matrices. Table 20.6 shows an example for the fuzzy sets *Temperature T1* and *Temperature T2* for the relation *Temperature T1 is close to Temperature T2*.

TABLE 20.6
Fuzzy Relation: Temperature T1 is Close to Temperature T2

T1	T2				
	20	22	24	26	28
20	1.0	0.9	0.6	0.3	0.1
25	0.5	0.7	1.0	1.0	0.7
30	0.0	0.1	0.3	0.6	0.9

We might also define a second fuzzy relation for temperatures T1 which are about 3° lower than T2, as shown in Table 20.7.

TABLE 20.7
Fuzzy Relation: Temperature T1 About 3° Lower Than Temperature T2

TI	T2				
	20	22	24	26	28
20	0.2	0.9	0.9	0.5	0.2
25	0.0	0.0	0.1	0.5	1.0
30	0.0	0.0	0.0	0.0	0.0

Since fuzzy relations are fuzzy sets in product space, they can be subject to set and algebraic operations. Thus the union operator is obtained by taking the maximum and the intersection by taking the minimum membership function of the connected relations, with the usual interpretation. Table 20.8 shows the result for the union of our two relations, which can be interpreted as *T1 close to or about 3° lower than T2,* and Table 20.9 the intersection, which can be interpreted as *T1 close to and about 3° lower than T2* .

TABLE 20.8
Fuzzy Relation: Temperature T1 Is Close to or About 3° Lower Than Temperature T2

T1	T2				
	20	22	24	26	28
20	1.0	0.9	0.9	0.5	0.2
25	0.5	0.7	1.0	1.0	1.0
30	0.0	0.1	0.3	0.6	0.9

Fuzzy relations are an important aspect of fuzzy set theory and provide the theoretical basis for the realisation of fuzzy controllers and expert systems. They can also be used in

TABLE 20.9
Fuzzy Relation: Temperature T1 Is Close to and About 3° Lower Than Temperature T2

T1	T2				
	20	22	24	26	28
20	0.2	0.9	0.6	0.3	0.1
25	0.0	0.0	0.1	0.5	0.7
30	0.0	0.0	0.0	0.0	0.0

the **evaluation of sensor data**. Table 20.10 lists the definition of a fuzzy relation R as well as the union and intersection of two fuzzy relations P and R.

TABLE 20.10
Fuzzy Relations

Operator	Definition
Relationship	$R = \{((x,y), \mu_R(x,y)) \mid (x, y) \in X \times Y$
Union	$\mu_{R \cup P}(x, y) = \max(\mu_R(x, y), \mu_P(x, y) \mid (x, y) \in X \times Y$
Intersection	$\mu_{R \cap P}(x, y) = \min(\mu_R(x, y), \mu_P(x, y) \mid (x, y) \in X \times Y$

20.2.6 Linguistic Variables

A linguistic variable is a variable where value is expressed in terms of sentences and words rather than numbers.[2] For the linguistic variable "temperature" used in our examples, such values might be icy, cold, cool, tepid, warm, very warm, hot, very hot, red hot, white hot. These values are obviously not as precise as numerical values: the value "warm" is not as precise as 25°C, 25°C ± 5°C, or even "about 25°C", and its interpretation depends very much upon the context in which it is used. Similarly, the values "tepid, warm, hot" are not sharply defined as is the case for the temperatures 24°C, 25°C, 26°C, but overlap to a greater or lesser degree.

Figure 20.8 shows the relationship between the linguistic and numerical variables "temperature" for the case of outdoor temperature in a temperate zone. The totality of possible values of a linguistic variable — in this case: icy, cold, cool, warm, hot — constitute its term-set. The numerical variable –20…40°C constitutes its base variable. The degree to which each numerical value of the base variable belongs to the linguistic values of the term set is called its compatibility. Looking at Figure 20.8, it is easy to see how the linguistic values can be represented as the fuzzy sets shown in Figure 20.9, the compatibilities being equivalent to the membership functions. It is also simple to imagine a so-called composite linguistic variable "temperate climate" at a higher level, with the linguistic variables "temperature", "rainfall", "humidity", 'hours of sunshine", etc. forming its constituent parts.

Central to the concept of a linguistic variable is some knowledge, either already known or empirically gathered, which can be used to define the fuzzy sets for the linguistic values in terms of the base variable. For the case in point, most people in a temperate zone would agree that above 30°C it is hot, and below 0°C it is icy. Similarly, a consensus can be reached on the meaning of the other linguistic values, and where the transition from one term to another begins and where it ends.

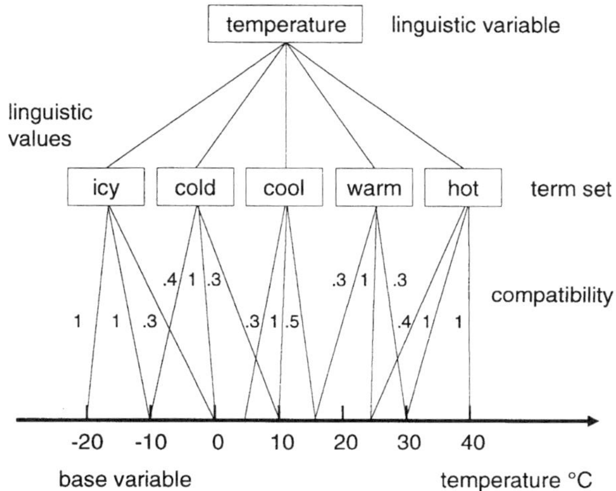

FIGURE 20.8 Linguistic variable "temperature in temperate zone".

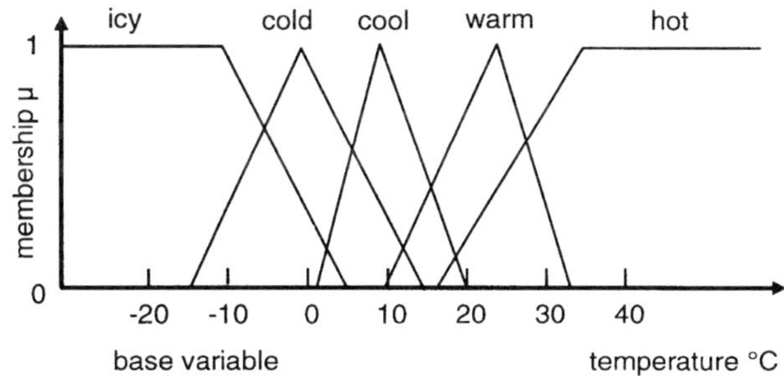

FIGURE 20.9 Fuzzy sets for temperature in temperate zone.

The assignment of numerical values and memberships to linguistic values turns out to be one of the most important steps when fuzzy concepts are applied to engineering problems. In order to do this successfully, a sound knowledge of the process being modelled and of the effects of altering operating parameters is required. In contrast to mathematical modelling, however, the knowledge base can be built up by a combination of questions and answers, expert opinion, and intuition, i.e., it is not restricted to quantifiable statements. Through his personal experience, therefore, the unskilled man on the job can contribute just as much as the mathematician with his theoretical knowledge.

20.2.7 Fuzzy Logic

With the linguistic variable at our disposal, we are now able to interpret human statements in such a way that they can be allocated numerical values and be processed by the computer. Fuzzy logic takes this process a step further by emulating human reasoning.[2,9,10] It has already been pointed out that fuzzy set theory can be seen as a generalisation of binary logic, allowing states between true and false. Take the following example:

Premise:	A is true
Implication:	If A is true, then B is true
Conclusion:	B is true

In binary logic, the premise and the implication can take on the values of true or false only, the rule must be precisely defined and deterministic, and the observed value of A must be identical to the value of A stipulated in the premise, otherwise the conclusion is false.

Premise:	T = 31°C
Implication	If T >30°C, then I eat ice cream
Conclusion	I eat ice cream

If T = 29.9°C, however, no conclusions can be made.

In *fuzzy logic*, the terms A and B are replaced by linguistic variables, but remain precise and deterministic. The degree of truth can also vary, as expressed by terms such as "untrue, sometimes untrue, half true, true". For example:

Premise:	A is true
Implication:	If A is true, then B is sometimes true
Conclusion:	B is sometimes true

Premise:	It is hot
Implication:	If it is hot, then I sometimes eat an ice cream
Conclusion:	I sometimes eat an ice cream

Again there is no conclusion for other values such as warm or cold, but the degree of membership of an observed temperature, say 28°C to the fuzzy set "hot" influences the conclusion to be drawn from the premise. An example of this type of fuzzy logic is given in Section 20.4.

In so-called *approximate reasoning*, the terms A and B may also contain fuzzy statements such as "usually, more or less, now and again" or the identity of B may be slightly relaxed. For example:

Premise:	A is more or less true
Implication:	If A is true, then B is sometimes true
Conclusion:	B is now and again true

Premise:	It is more or less hot
Implication:	When it is hot, I sometimes eat ice cream
Conclusion:	I now and again eat ice cream

In this case, the fuzzy statement "more or less hot" might be obtained by dilating the fuzzy set "hot" as indicated in Section 20.2.3, "Modifiers". In the least constrained form of fuzzy logic, *plausible reasoning*, the identity between the components of the rules is dispensed with and replaced by similarity

Premise:	A′ is true
Implication:	If A is true, then B is true
Conclusion:	B′ is true

At one extreme A and A′ or B and B′ might be identical, and at the other extreme, opposite in meaning.

Premise:	It is not hot
Implication:	If it is hot, then I eat ice cream
Conclusion:	I do not eat ice cream

The above example makes clear that plausible reasoning may lead to partially wrong conclusions. For this reason, it is possible to weight the rules according to their truth values. If the degree of truth in premise A is expressed as υA and that of the rule as $\upsilon(A \rightarrow B)$, then the relation between the two can be calculated by means of an implication operator. Table 20.11 lists a number of operators which are based on the MIN-MAX method of calculation.

TABLE 20.11
Implication (Truth) Operators

Operator	Definition
Zadeh	$\max(1 - \upsilon(A), \min(\upsilon(A), \upsilon(B))$
Lukasiewicz	$\min(1, 1 - \upsilon(A) + \upsilon(B))$
Mamdani	$\min(\upsilon(A), \upsilon(B))$
Kleene-Dienes	$\max(1 - \upsilon(A), \upsilon(B))$
Yager	$(\upsilon(A))^{\upsilon(B)}$

20.2.8 Fuzzy Applications

It can be seen from this brief introduction, that fuzzy set theory provides a surprisingly solid basis for making human reasoning and experience accessible to a computer. As far as its application to practical engineering problems is concerned, two distinct directions may be discerned:

Fuzzy algorithms — In this case existing crisp models or methods are *fuzzified* in order to create more realistic algorithms. This assumes that the original models are in some way or other not totally able to describe all the situations encountered in practice. The fuzzification enables them to react more flexibly.

Knowledge based applications — These form the majority of the applications described in the literature and use fuzzy sets and approximate reasoning to model human knowledge on the computer. Implicit in these applications are the steps: **knowledge acquisition** — e.g., from people, books, or experiment; **documentation** — usually in the form of rules; **knowledge processing**; and **translation**. The latter encompasses the conversion of numerical information into linguistic information on the input side — fuzzification, and the conversion of the membership functions into numbers — and defuzzification, or linguistic expression — so-called linguistic approximation — on the output side.

As far as **sensors** are concerned, applications are more practically subdivided into expert systems, fuzzy data analysis, and fuzzy control. For further information on expert systems which, other than as an aid to fuzzy control are beyond the scope of this book, the reader is referred to the literature,[11-14] where a number of applications relevant to biochemistry, medicine, and the environment are to be found.

20.3 FUZZY DATA ANALYSIS

Instrumentation and control is an area of activity which is characterised by its striving for precision and accuracy. More often than not, sensors are purchased on the grounds of their performance data, and manufacturers vie with each other to offer higher precision, better linearity, less temperature dependence on long-term drift, etc. than their competitors. It seems paradoxical, therefore, that a theory which has the recognition of uncertainty as its central concept should have any application at all within this field. In fact there are many areas of uncertainty in sensor systems and it is generally agreed that fuzzy set theory offers possibilities in the following:

- The internal processing of sensor signals, for example, the evaluation of relatively noisy signals
- Automatic fault diagnosis
- The use of indirect measured values to measure process variables
- The automation of measurement and evaluation procedures based on expert knowledge
- The fusion of sensor information in a multisensor environment
- The presentation of "crisp" measured values in a manner more readily understandable to the unskilled operator.

20.3.1 Internal Processing of Sensor Signals

Sensors can be categorised into three general groups according to the signal they deliver:

- Those that give a direct representation of the process value, e.g., as for pressure with a manometer
- Those that provide an indirect measurement by using a property which is dependent upon the variable to be measured, e.g., the resistance of a thermocouple, and
- Those which require a more sophisticated interpretation, e.g., spectral measurements as found in chemical analysis or time of flight in ultrasonic level measurement. (Interpretation is also complex for sensor arrays used in odour analysis — see Part V, "Towards the Electronic Nose" of this book — or in the analysis of biosensor equilibrium traces, e.g., during conditioning.)

Uncertainty can be introduced into all three categories by the presence of interference, be it as the result of imprecise readings, drift, cross-sensitivities, or noise. Of the three, the interpretation of spectra has probably the most to gain by using fuzzy methods and there are already a number of publications on this subject. Since the principles used in spectral analysis are also suited, for example, to fault detection and analysis — an area which will become increasingly important for the sensors of the future — all three areas can benefit from a fuzzy approach. Chemical analysis applications are discussed in Section 20.3.4 of this chapter.

20.3.2 Fuzzy Thresholds

A simple example of the use of fuzzy methods in signal processing is the fuzzy threshold. This may be implemented at either the sensor or control level. Adaptive thresholds are used to detect failures or eliminate noise. An event is usually detected by comparing the predicted and measured performance of the sensor. To this end it is necessary to

- Model the normal operation
- Find any differences (symptoms) between normal and predicted operation
- Decide whether the difference is significant

Figure 20.10 shows a block diagram of the detection system. The comparison of the measured and predicted performance leads to the building of a residual. The residual evaluation, e.g., done by thresholds, identifies the symptoms, which are then analysed to find the associated fault. Ideally the residual is zero when there are no faults, and not zero when a fault is present. The system must be modelled exactly and the decision is strictly yes/no. In practice, the residuals are often greater than zero even when no fault is present. This may be due to:

- Noisy measurements
- Unknown disturbances (e.g., temperature dependence), or
- Uncertainties in the models

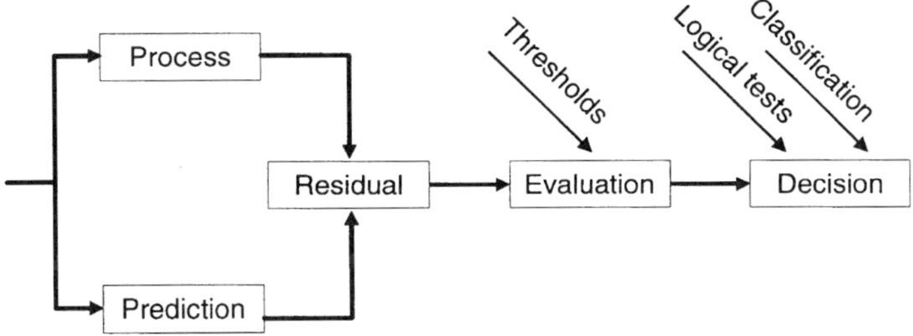

FIGURE 20.10 Model-based fault detection.

How can these facts be taken into account? One answer to these problems, demonstrated by Sauter et al.[15] and Schneider,[16] is to update the threshold according to the operating conditions. To a basic threshold is added a fuzzy factor which is dependent upon the difference between the current and original state of the system. The size of the fuzzy factor is determined by a set of fuzzy rules which describe the possible relations between the state variables. The larger the difference between the residual and threshold, the larger the likelihood that a fault has been detected. Figure 20.11 shows an example based on this method.

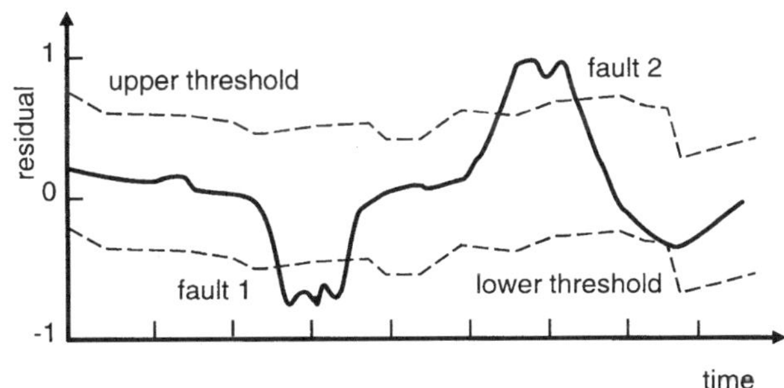

FIGURE 20.11 Use of fuzzy thresholds to detect sensor faults.

A similar method can be used to separate the noise component from an ultrasonic signal (see Figure 20.12). In this case, there is no predictive model and the events are the acoustic peaks which characterise the measured value, i.e., the elements in the spectrum which are to be identified and classified. The threshold used is conceived such that it models the actions of an expert who, in seeing the whole, readily identifies the peaks as projecting above the general background noise level. To this end, the threshold decreases monotonically, is weighted towards shorter distances where any interference is stronger, and adapts itself to the general noise level of the signal.[17]

20.3.3 Fuzzy Classification

Having positively identified the events of interest within a signal, the next step is to classify them. Here again, fuzzy methods offer interesting possibilities. A prerequisite for correct classification is a good knowledge of the system. This is either already existent in the form of expert knowledge or operator's experience, or can be accumulated by the system by a training phase — it is in this respect that fuzzy logic is often associated with neural networks (see also Section 20.3.5, and Section 20.4). The knowledge is usually expressed as rules which are then used to classify the events.

For the example of the ultrasonic level sensor, which is used to measure the level of solids and liquids in tanks and silos, it is known that the level echo is usually the largest

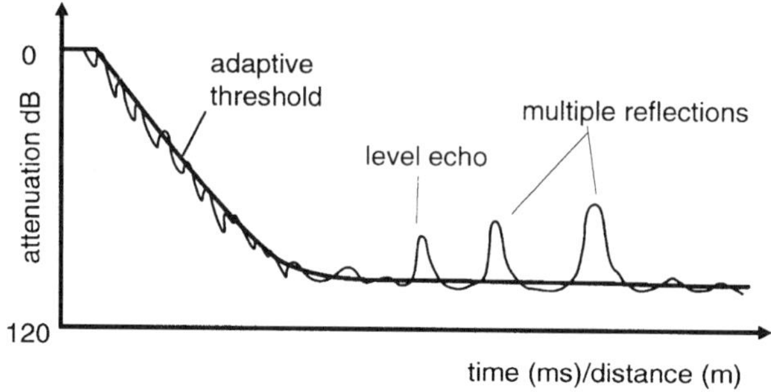

FIGURE 20.12 Adaptive threshold for ultrasonic level sensor.

echo. This statement must be qualified by the knowledge that when liquids in closed tanks or fine-grained solids in silos are measured under steady conditions, multiple echoes can be present in the echo profile which are larger than the level echo, i.e., there is a built-in uncertainty in the system under specific operating conditions. Multiple echoes can be readily identified by the human observer because they appear at regular intervals behind the level echo (see Figure 20.12). If conditions are unsteady within the vessel due to filling, vapour, dust, or turbulence, the multiple echoes quickly decay, only to reappear again when the disturbance has passed.

The fuzzy algorithm chosen (see Figure 20.13) classifies the echoes above the threshold as large or small, according to their amplitude. Of the large echoes, that with the largest amplitude is temporarily assumed to be the level echo. A cut is then made in the normalised fuzzy set, the size of which is dependent upon the amplitude of the temporary level echo. A search is now made for echoes with membership functions which still lie above the cut, i.e., those which can be considered "possible level echoes", the foremost being taken as the true level echo. Critical to the algorithm is the correct choice of cut, which was selected with the help of experienced service technicians.

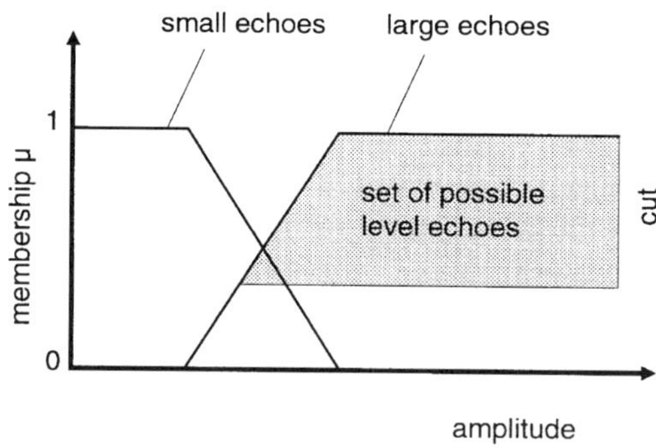

FIGURE 20.13 Fuzzy classification of possible level echoes.

A second ultrasonic sensing application is reported by Poloni,[18] in which a robot has to map a room. Taking the first echo as always being of interest, the fuzzy algorithm is used to assign belief values to the signal received. To this end, fuzzy sets are assigned representing the emptiness and fullness of the space being investigated. The membership functions are also selected such that the belief in the signal decreases at the edge of the field of sight. As the robot moves into the space it has to map, signals from adjacent positions are aggregated using the AND operator, producing a complete map of the room.

It is not always the case that an event can be identified on the basis of a single characteristic — more often than not several features are required. In the ultrasonic distance-sensing application described by Kroemer et al.,[19] a robot detects objects in its path. These may be either real or virtual, depending upon whether the echoes arrive at the sensor unhindered or by way of a multiple reflection. In general there is no reinforcement of the multiple echoes, so that they are always smaller than the true echoes. On the other hand, there is a general decrease in intensity as the distance from the sensor increases. In order to identify the real objects, the shape of each detected echo is analysed according to several characteristic dimensions (see Figure 20.14a), and the type of echo is determined by a set of fuzzy rules.

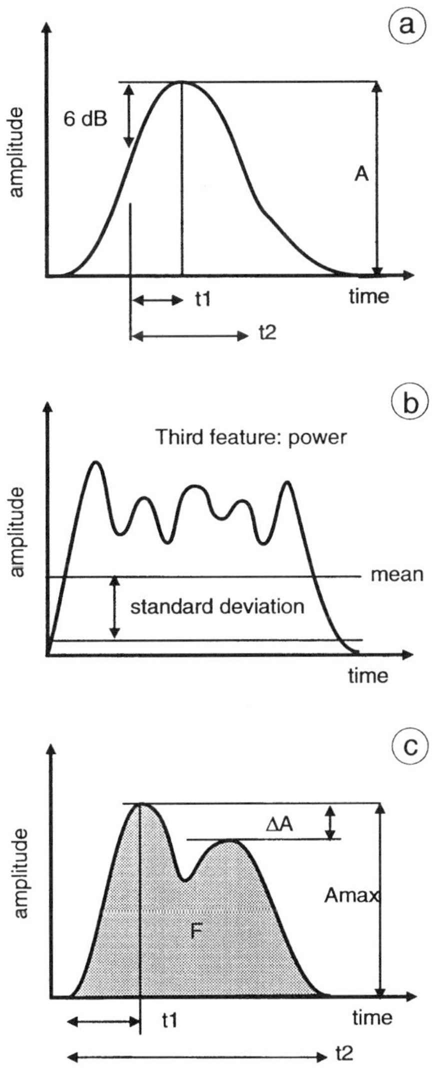

FIGURE 20.14 Simple signal classifiers.[18-20]

A similar approach is adopted in two simple sorting applications. In the first, beer crates are sorted according to their labels by a signal generated as they pass by a photosensor.[20] The lettering is detected as the variation in time of the degree of blackness of the full logo. Two classes, "own crates" and "other crates", are built according to the characteristic features of the signal: mean value, standard deviation, and power (Figure 20.14b). The system was trained by measuring several crates of the same type in various conditions of dirtiness. The sorting was then made on the basis of fuzzy IF and THEN rules.

The second application, described by Zühlke and Lauzi,[21] is the sorting of metal objects on the basis of characteristic electrical signals which are generated as they pass through an inductive coil. Figure 20.14c shows a typical signal. The features used for sorting were the amplitude and time of the signal maximum, the difference between local and absolute maximum, the area and duration of the signal, and the rise time to the first maximum. Fuzzy sets of, e.g., "large" and "small" area were built up on the basis of experimental observations, and the classification made on the basis of a rule set for each object. The model tested was designed for the identification of cutlery; the classes being knife, fork, tablespoon, and teaspoon. The orientation of the object was also detected. The success rate of detection was 95% on a trained system.

Other applications or feasibility studies which use similar techniques are the testing of ceramic tiles on the basis of their acoustic spectrum,[22] the classification of plating defects in roller bearings by optical sensor,[23] and the determination of tool wear from the force-time diagrams.[24] In the latter case, the system outputs the classification as a fuzzy statement such as "the tool is heavily worn" which is easily understood by the machine operator.

Two other classification applications might also be mentioned at this point. In the one, the behaviour with time of the current and voltage supply curves generated by a welding robot could be used to check the composition of the gas shielding, dirty workpiece surfaces, wear in the electrical contacts, incorrect feeding and ill-adjusted electrical parameters.[25] In the other, a quality control system for refrigerators was set up on the basis of the information received from an array of 6 temperature sensors placed at strategic points on the cooling circuit; 11 typical features were extracted from the 6 temperature vs. time curves which were then used to form 7 quality classes for good and bad products.[26] These applications use fuzzy classification and pattern recognition methods in multidimensional space. They are interesting because they point the way towards a possible early-warning system for more sophisticated sensors such as flowmeters or for sensor arrays in process control systems, whereby several parameters are monitored and features indicating fault conditions are searched for and extracted. The basis of a successful system is, as always, expert knowledge.

20.3.4 Chemical Analysis

With the exception of the last two examples, the applications just described are characterised by the fact that the signal provided by the sensor carries information on one measurand only, the fuzzy analysis providing a reliable means of extracting and interpreting it. There exist, however, a number of fuzzy applications where either the data provided by the sensor contain information from several variables or the information from several sensors is used to provide a measurement of a single variable. Bandemer and Otto[27] have examined several potential uses of fuzzy set theory in analytical chemistry: data handling for calibration of analytical methods, classification of chromatographic and spectral patterns, component identification, and multicomponent analysis, as well as the design of an expert system for selection of analytical methods.

The standard method of modelling a system with two dependent variables is to calibrate with known standards and perform a least-squares fit on the results. Very often there is a degree of uncertainty in both dependent and independent variables which might lead to poor estimates in the behaviour of the system, in particular when the sample size is small. By using a fuzzy approach, the observational error can be modelled by an elliptical membership function, i.e., the measured value is surrounded by an oval within which the membership function decreases from 1 to 0 (see Figure 20.15). The resulting fuzzy prediction for an unknown value reflects not only the error in observation, but its membership function also provides a valuation of the result.[28]

Gas chromatography is another analytical tool in which peaks must be evaluated with respect to position and size. Here, classical pattern recognition methods can be applied only when the signals can be separated in a reproducible manner. This is usually accomplished by selecting particular bands of the spectrum and scanning for the appearance or nonappearance of the peak. In practice, however, the natural variability of the sample composition causes peaks to be missing, and changes in concentration cause the peak width to vary. In addition, there is an uncertainty in the retention time for a particular compound. When position and height of the peak vary, classical methods cannot be used.

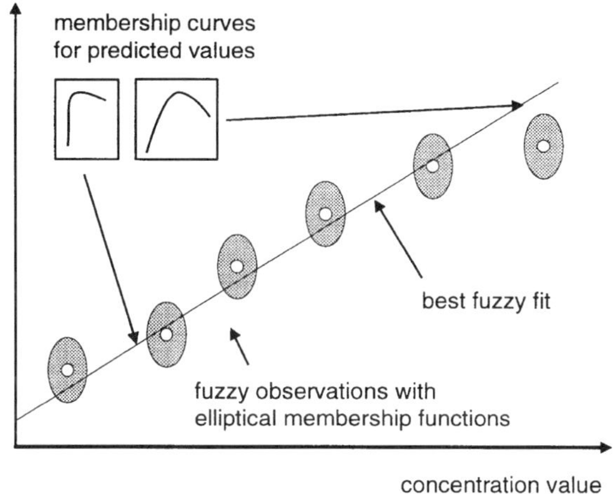

FIGURE 20.15 Calibration signal vs. concentration value based on fuzzy observations.[27]

Fuzzy pattern recognition allows a more robust method of classification. Crisp training patterns, obtained by overlaying the retention times of the available training samples, are fuzzified by imposing a bell-shaped or triangular membership function to each peak (see Figure 20.16) and stored in a library as a reference pattern. The retention times in the unknown sample are read in as crisp spectra with membership = 1 at the actual retention time and zero elsewhere. The classification is performed in a fuzzy associative memory by intersecting the unknown pattern with the fuzzy reference pattern. Absolute correspondence in a peak position results in a membership value of 1; complete disagreement in a value of 0. The resulting membership functions (or sympathy values) are summed across the spectrum and compared with the reference sample to give a grade of containment, which is 1 for absolute correspondence.

The ability to discriminate is improved further if the signal response is included in the classification scheme. This is done by reducing the peaks to a dot pattern and assigning each an elliptical membership function, as in Figure 20.15, which describes its possible membership in terms of the absorbence (y) and retention time (x) to a crisp peak appearing at the same position in the spectrum. This method has been successfully applied to the quality control of pain-relieving tablets, whereby the method of analysis was ultraviolet spectroscopy.[29]

Pattern recognition and component identification in unknown samples are of course closely related, and the first application of fuzzy set theory was proposed by Blaffert[30] who, with a similar method to the above, used it to identify chemical species in infrared spectra. (Pattern analysis techniques in odour analysis are discussed in Chapter 27 by Gardner and Hines.) Where the spectra can be strongly modified due to solvent effects, however, e.g., in

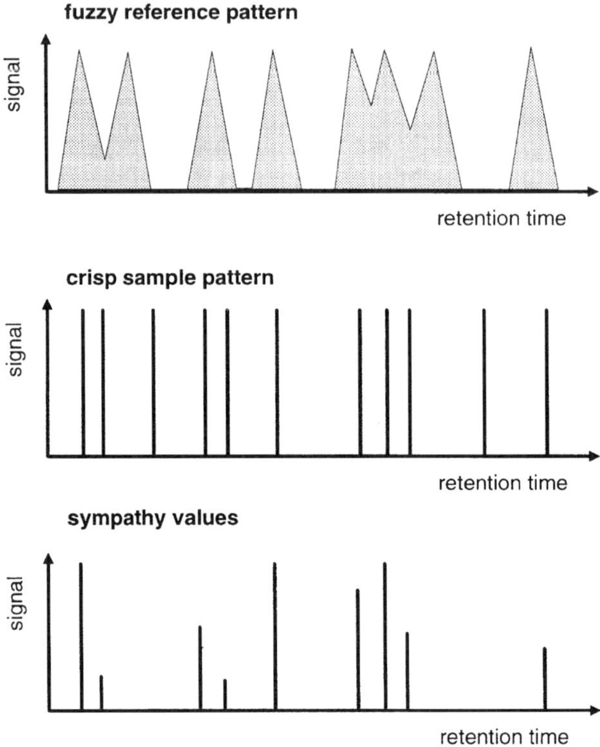

FIGURE 20.16 Spectral classification using fuzzy associative memory.[28]

the visible/ultraviolet range, a more sophisticated method is required.[31] In order to compare blurred experimental with blurred reference spectra, the fuzzified data are subtracted from each other and the quality of coincidence obtained by manipulating the membership functions of the resulting residuals. When compared to standard methods, fuzzy component identification exhibits greater tolerance of solvent effects and better discrimination of spectrally similar but chemically different species than the standard Euclidean distance measure.

The component identification algorithm can also be extended to mixture analysis. In this case, the sample spectrum at every band position is considered to be composed of the concentration-weighted spectrum according to Beer's law. From the resulting membership functions, the difference between the reference and sample spectrum is calculated and the coincidence of the spectra derived. The optimum combination of component concentrations is then obtained by minimising the coincidence function.

20.3.5 Cross-Sensitivities and Sensor Fusion

Chemical and biological sensors are notorious for the fact that very few are specific to a particular species; more often than not there is cross-sensitivity to other components such as pH and temperature as well as to the concentration of a related compound or ion. Thus it is often the case that several sensors are used in an array to extract information on the composition and concentration of a particular analyte. The cross-sensitivities are corrected by multivariate calibration and evaluation by multiple linear regression or major component regression. Since the interfering species have also to be determined, their simultaneous analysis is also possible. Where the sensor dependencies are linear, this method gives reliable results; for nonlinear dependencies, however, precise determination using mechanistic methods is practically impossible.

One possible solution to these problems is to proceed as in the case of mixture analysis as mentioned above. Another alternative is fuzzy logic, usually used in combination with a training technique (see Figure 20.17), and a simple example using sensors sensitive to different wavelengths in the optical spectrum for sorting cans by colour has been described by von Altrock.[32] The sensor data from each sensor in the array are first fuzzified, i.e., the numerical value is translated into a linguistic variable as described previously. The results of this step are analysed by a fuzzy rule base which describes the various relationships between all possible sensor array outputs. The possible outcomes of the fuzzy analysis are then combined and defuzzified to produce the crisp measured values. In fact, this is exactly the same principle as is used by the fuzzy controller described in the next section.

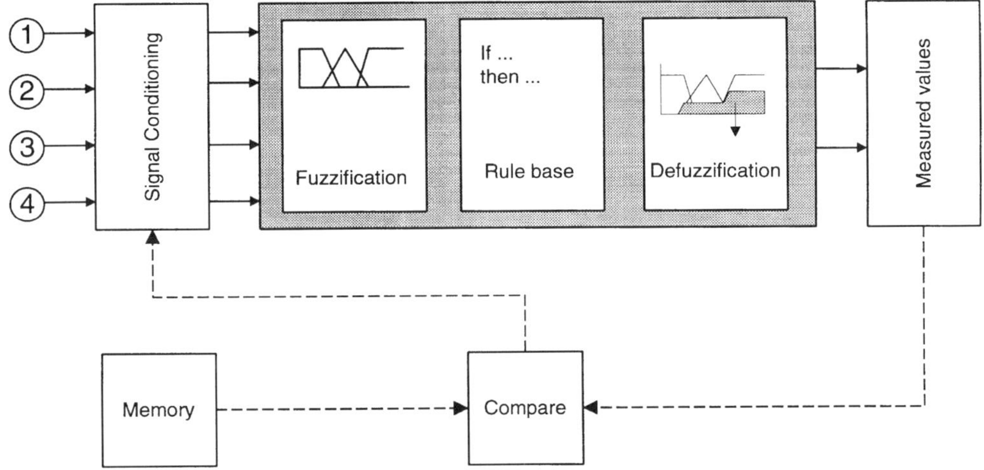

FIGURE 20.17 Sensor fusion with fuzzy evaluation.

For example, it might be that Sensor 1 of a sensor array measures species A well, B not so well, and C not at all. Sensor 2 measures B well, A not so well, and C a little. Sensor 3, on the other hand, measures A and C equally well, but B not at all, etc. If the output of each sensor is now expressed as a linguistic variable, e.g., high, medium, and low, and the possible significance of the signals is expressed as a fuzzy rule, then it is possible to extract information on the presence or not of the components and their concentrations. Specimen rules might be as follows:

If Signal 1 is low and Signal 2 is medium, then the amount of B is medium.
If Signal 1 is low and Signal 3 is high, then the amount of C is high.

The result of such an analysis depends, of course, on the expertise at hand when the rules are formulated and the fuzzy sets representing the linguistic variables are dimensioned. The system can be improved, however, by comparing the sensor signal combinations with those obtained from standard solutions, then using a fuzzy associative memory to train it by altering the rule base and linguistic variables. It is in this context that fuzzy logic is often associated with neural networks: an example has been described by Otto[33] in the analysis of Na^+, K^+, Ca^{2+}, and Mg^{2+} ions in blood and urine samples. Another example is the measurement of methane and butane concentrations in air by microcalorimetric sensors.[34] (Details on neural networks are presented in Chapter 27).

A good example of the combination of various fuzzy techniques with classical methods is the interpretation of laser-induced fluorescent spectra for the automatic analysis of oil-polluted water as described by Schödel[35] and shown schematically in Figure 20.18. In this case, samples of polluted water were subjected to a short laser pulse and the intensity distribution in the spectral band 350 to 600 nm of the resulting fluorescence was observed as a function of time. This is known to be dependent upon the age, composition, and concentration of the oil in the sample. From the information provided by the sensor system, the intensities and relaxation times of the signal were calculated for specific wavelengths. The questions to be answered by the fuzzy algorithm, which was designed to mirror the procedure adopted by the geologists who provided the expert knowledge for the system, were

- Does the distribution under consideration point to any oil at all being present in the sample
- What are the possible correct solutions from the results available at each wavelength
- Does information from other wavelengths have to be taken into consideration

In the first step, the local fusion of data for a particular wavelength, the intensities and spectra are analysed to provide concentration and oil sort predictions. Measurement uncertainty is accounted for by fuzzy look-up tables. These fuzzy associative memories consider both tolerance bands, implemented as fuzzy numbers, and additive properties, which give information on the oil sorts present. Deviations from the nominal spectra stored in the memory result in decreasing activation of the solution. In the global data fusion step which follows, the intersection of all possible outcomes of the local data fusion are calculated and ranked. The final result is output as a list of oil sorts and their concentrations.

20.4 FUZZY CONTROL

As far as the present fuzzy boom is concerned, by far the most attention is being paid towards fuzzy control. In the past two years a number of papers have appeared describing how fuzzy algorithms have been successfully employed to solve a number of control problems which are not conducive to standard linear methods. The impression might be gained that all this is new, but in fact we are now experiencing the third wave of applications, the origins of which can be traced back to the mid-1970s.

The success of the method lies in the fact that fuzzy control seeks to build human experience into its control models. The knowledge gained by the experienced plant operator is taken and interpreted as a number of linguistic rules which describe the control strategies. The words are defined as fuzzy sets and their interactions are fuzzy rules. As Kickert and Mamdani explain,[36] the advantages of this method, based on rule of thumb, experience, and intuition, lie in the fact that it does not require a rigorous mathematical model of the process.

Complex industrial processes are difficult to control. They are characterised by non-linear, time-dependent behaviour, often accompanied by process measurement of poor quality. (Similar considerations apply to the monitoring of patients during surgery or in environmental monitoring.) Automatic control is limited to those parts of the process which can be adequately measured and controlled, usually flow, pressure, and level tasks. Overall objectives such as the quality and quantity of the product produced has in the past been left to the human operator. Even with modern process controllers, adequate control has proven elusive because the processes are often so complex that the modelling is only approximate and requires a large amount of computing time. Difficulties arise particularly where the process operates over a wide range of conditions and suffers from stochastic disturbances.[37]

The theoretical origins of fuzzy control lie in Zadeh's paper "Outline of a New Approach to the Analysis of Complex Systems and Decision Processes".[38] The first application was reported by Mamdani and Assilian[39] in 1975, who used it to control a laboratory steam engine. Subsequent developments showed fuzzy control to be effective and a promising future was foreseen, the first industrial application being reported in 1977.[40,41] The initial impetus petered out at the end of the 1970s, however, possibly due to a lack of suitable hardware and software

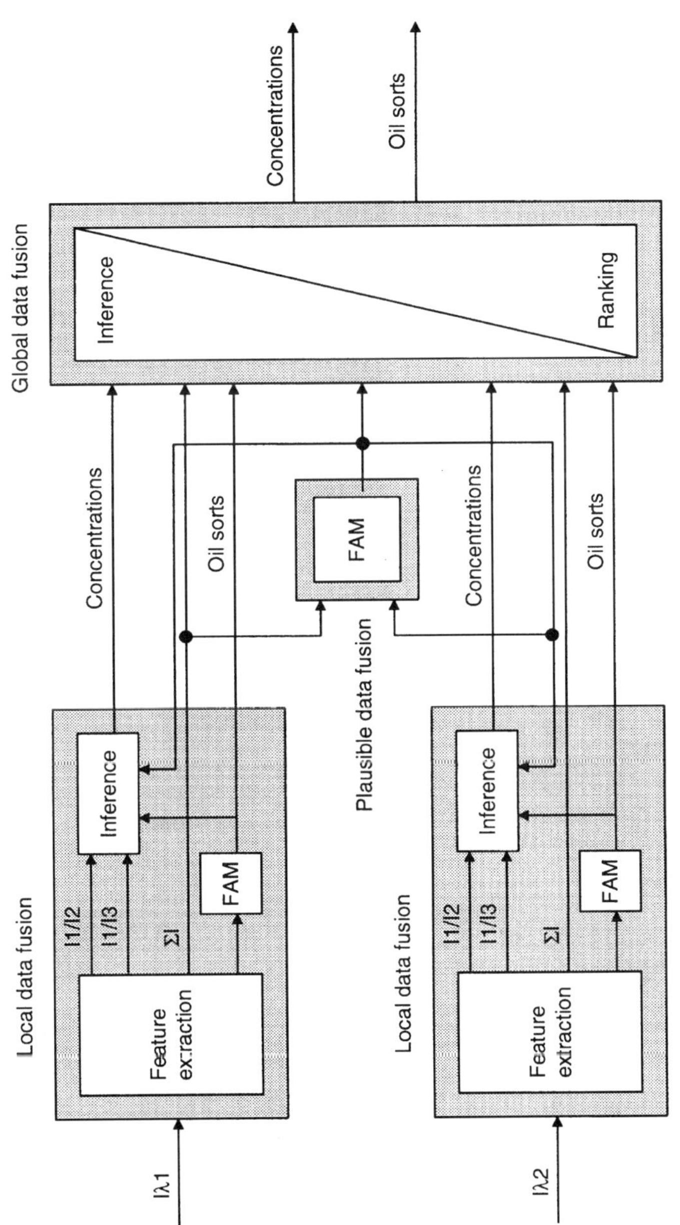

FIGURE 20.18 Fuzzy system for the detection of oil contamination. (From Schödel, H.[24] With permission.)

for more complex problems with many input variables.[42] The second wave of interest, this time in Japan, started in the mid-1980s and included such developments as the use of fuzzy logic for automatic train control in the Sendai public transport system.[43] It was this and the publicity given to the fuzzy video camera which touched off interest in Europe again, and started the third fuzzy control wave. This time around, its practitioners are supported by better hardware and a number of sophisticated fuzzy tools which aid in the modelling and development of fuzzy controllers.

Although there are several ways in which fuzzy control can be used, the control model might be fully or only partly fuzzy, the basic design still follows the rules laid down in the 1970s. Figure 20.19 shows a schematic diagram of the essentials. Five steps must be considered:

- *Input and control variables* — The first step is to determine which process variables are to be observed and the resulting control actions.
- *Conditional interface* — The second step is to fuzzify the observations by expressing them as appropriate fuzzy sets.
- *Rule base* — The rule base contains the control logic. The rules that are to be applied and the conditions under which they act are obtained by questioning process operators, using expert knowledge, or simply by analysing the process to obtain a rough model.
- *Computational unit* — At this point it must be determined which algorithms are to be used to perform the fuzzy computations. As a rule these will lead to fuzzy outputs.
- *Transformation* — The final step is to determine the rules according to which fuzzy control statements can be transformed into crisp control actions.

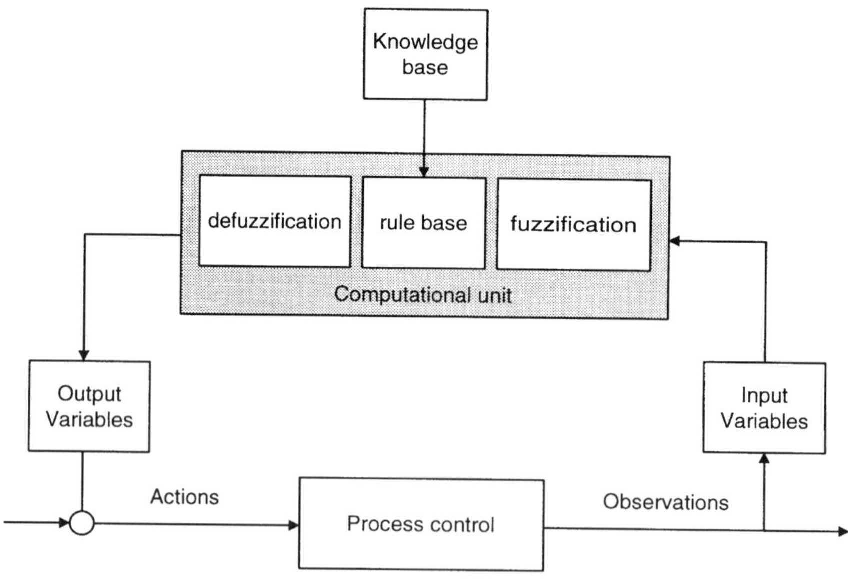

FIGURE 20.19 A simple fuzzy logic control system.

The ideas which have developed from these premises are best explained on the basis of a simple example. Figure 20.20 shows an imaginary reactor with an inflow valve V1, an outflow valve V2, and a level measurement system which delivers the measured value L. The two valves can be controlled across their entire opening range. The task is to keep the level at about 50% by observing the amount by which the level deviates from the setpoint value as well as the amount leaving the vessel (position of valve 2) and controlling the amount of fluid entering the reactor (position of valve 1).

The fuzzy sets for the variables are also shown in Figure 20.20. For simplicity only three sets have been designated to each base variable and the valve position sets are identical. In practice, it is usual for up to nine sets to be defined, whereby most applications use five or seven. The level L is represented by the sets too low, normal, or too high; valve 1 and 2 by the terms closed, half open, and open.

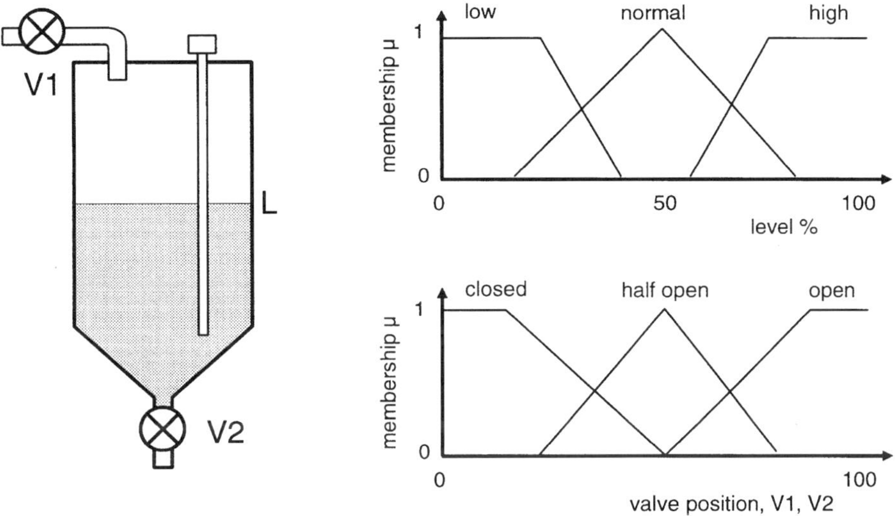

FIGURE 20.20 Level control problem with associated fuzzy sets.

Having defined the fuzzy sets, the next step is to formulate the rule base. In our example these might be

1. IF the level is normal AND valve 2 is open, THEN open valve 1
2. IF the level is high AND valve 2 is half-open, THEN close valve 1 etc.

The rule base might include other direct actions or OR statements such as

3. IF the level is low THEN open valve 1
4. IF the level is low OR valve 2 is open THEN half-open valve 1

Figure 20.21 shows what happens when, e.g., a level measurement of 70% (membership of "normal" 0.4 and of "high" 0.7) and a valve 2 position of 60% (membership of "half-open" 0.6 and of "open" 0.4) are used as input variables. Those rules where the level fuzzy sets "normal" and "high" appear alone, or in combination with valve 1 fuzzy sets "half-open" and "open" are activated and combined according to the logical operator they possess to form the inference. For this step two methods are possible:

- *The MIN-method* — The membership function of the rule results from the limitation of the membership function of the THEN part to the momentary truth value of the IF part.
- *The PROD-method* — The membership function of the rule results from the multiplication of the membership functions of the THEN part with the momentary truth value of the IF part.

Rule 1: IF the level is normal AND valve 2 is open, THEN open valve 1

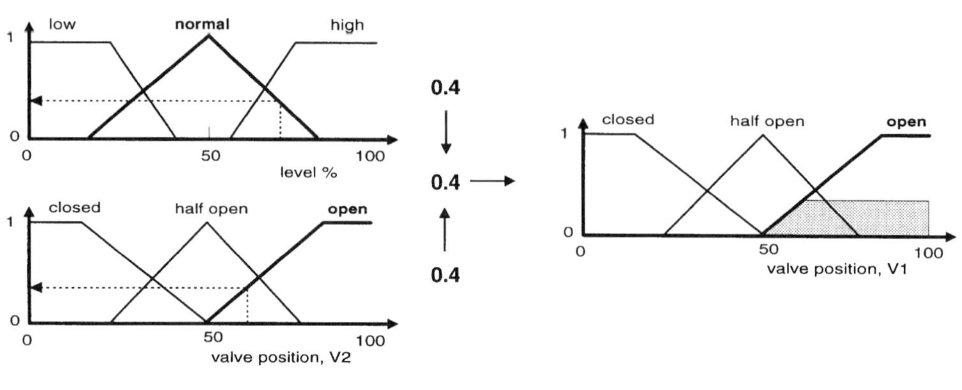

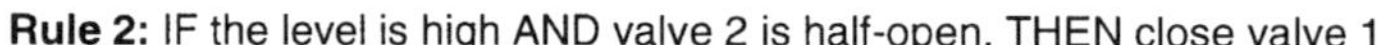
Rule 2: IF the level is high AND valve 2 is half-open, THEN close valve 1

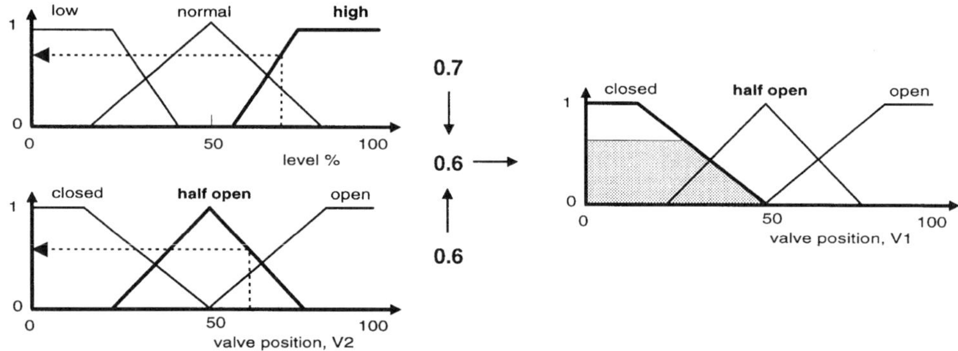

Rule 4: IF the level is low OR valve 2 is open THEN half-open valve 1

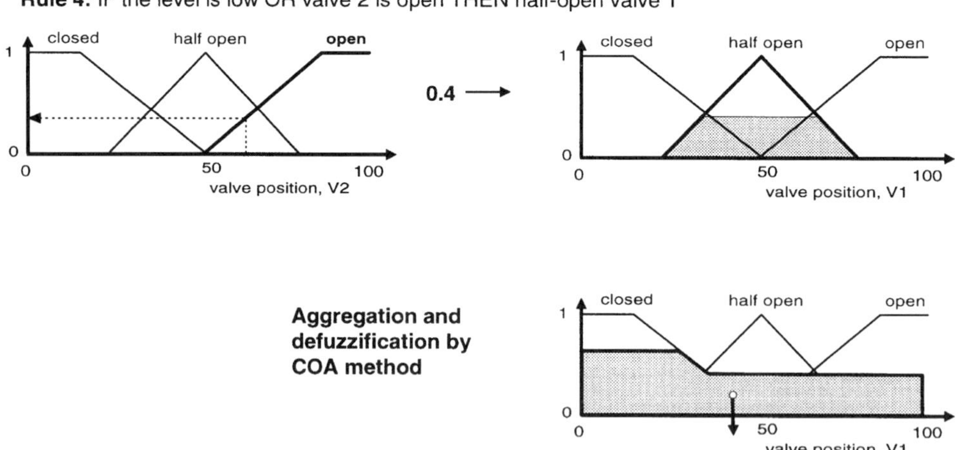

FIGURE 20.21 Fuzzification, inference, and defuzzification steps for the example shown in Figure 20.20. Rule 3 is not activated because the level is not "low".

Having computed the membership values for each rule, all activated rules are now aggregated by using the MAX operator to form a MAX-MIN or MAX-PROD inference. In our worked example the MAX-MIN method was used; for comparison, Figure 20.22 shows the result of a MAX-PROD inference of the same parameters.

The final step is the transformation of the fuzzy inference into a crisp control output variable for the position of valve 1 (in our example approximately 40%). This so-called

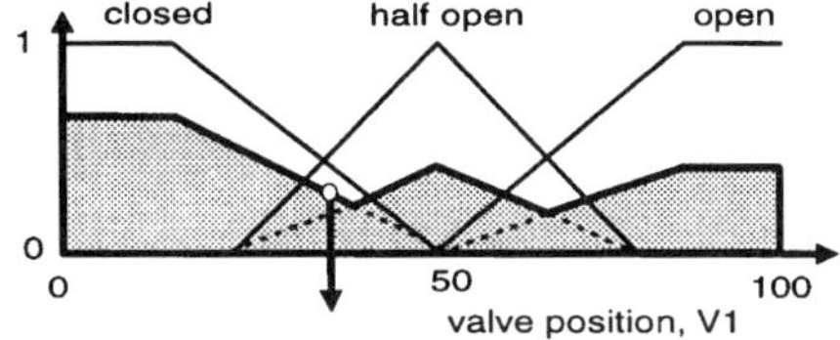

FIGURE 20.22 Result of MAX-PROD inference for the example shown in Figure 20.21.

defuzzification step may also be performed in different ways. The most common is the COA method, in which the centre of gravity of the membership function of the inference is calculated and its position on the abscissa is used as control variable. Also used, mainly because it is quicker to calculate, is the COM or centre of maximum method, in which the positions of the weighted maxima of all activated fuzzy sets on the abscissa are averaged to form the crisp control variable.

There is general agreement that the methods used for inference and defuzzification are less critical to the performance of the controller than the definition of the linguistic variables and rules. It is often the case that the first rough design for a fuzzy control works surprisingly well, but that the fine tuning proves to be more difficult. For this reason, there has been an increasing interest in expert systems and self-learning controllers where the fuzzy sets are modified through neural networks: an example for food engineering is described by Eerikäinen et al.[44] Two applications in bioprocessing are described by von Numers et al.[45] and Kishimoto et al.[46]: in the former the control knowledge is implemented in the form of a fuzzy expert system which selects an appropriate control strategy on the basis of the output variable. Three wastewater treatment applications are also included in the references.[47-49] This is by no means a comprehensive list and the interested reader is referred to the technical press or to recent conference proceedings, where such applications are being reported with increasing frequency.

20.5 FUZZY DEVELOPMENT TOOLS

It is beyond the scope of this book to go into detail about the relative merits of the fuzzy tools which are currently on the market. Regular reviews[50.52] are to be found in the technical press, which list the currently available software and hardware. These may be divided into five categories:

- PC programs which support the writing of fuzzy control programs. Most use a Windows-type interface and allow fuzzy rules and membership functions to be entered directly. The inference and defuzzification can be performed according to a number of methods and the results graphically displayed. The most modern systems allow programming in C and downloading to a chip.
- PC programs for building fuzzy data banks and assisting in decision-making processes. These tools are often offered as part of a package which includes customisation to specific tasks.
- PC programs for fuzzy data analysis. Here the choice is restricted, but those on the market offer, for example, data acquisition interfaces, fast Fourier transformations, fuzzy operations, fuzzy functions, etc. As the interest in fuzzy set theory increases, it is to be expected that more programs of this type will follow.
- Fuzzy chips. There are already several fuzzy chips from the U.S., Japan, and Europe on the market. These contain the standard membership functions, operators, and aggregation strategies which are required for fuzzy control tasks, but differ in the type and number implemented. It is often the case that a fuzzy algorithm for a

sensor is either too slow or too large for a conventional chip, so that these devices offer the developer much more scope.

- Programmable logic controllers with fuzzy modules. Following their introduction by Japan, Europe and the U.S. have been quick to bring out their own fuzzy PLCs. Most allow the user complete freedom of programming, definition of rule base, etc. and some can be programmed directly from a PC fuzzy tool. A few, however, use fuzzy control to smooth the output variable and the user decides only whether the fuzzy filter is to be switched on or not.

20.6 CONCLUSION

It was stated at the beginning of this chapter that interest in fuzzy logic has never been so great. The question arises, of course, Will this interest be maintained when the current publicity subsides or will fuzzy logic be quietly put aside as another technology which did not make the grade? There are several arguments which suggest that fuzzy logic will survive.

- Fuzzy logic mirrors human thinking and makes it easier for human experience to be integrated into decision-making or control algorithms.
- Fuzzy tolerates uncertainties in input data and is capable of producing crisp output data from noisy or incomplete data.
- Fuzzy complements classical control methods by offering better solutions where mathematical modelling reaches its limits.
- Fuzzy algorithms can be developed and implemented more quickly than is the case for classical control methods.
- Fuzzy controls just as well as traditional control circuits, in particular cases even better, e.g., where processes are nonlinear.

Up to now, applications involving the internal processing of signals within a sensor are comparatively rare; however, a start has been made and more can be expected in future. More progress has been made in the fuzzy classification of sensor signals, sensor fusion, and expert measuring systems. Sensors are of course an integral part of fuzzy control systems, and in this connection it is often said that simpler, less accurate sensors are sufficient. This statement must be qualified: just as with standard applications, the accuracy requirements on the sensors are determined by the task for which they are used. In all cases, however, the sensor chosen must be capable of withstanding the process conditions which it encounters in practice. With this in mind, it is confidently expected that fuzzy evaluation methods will establish themselves as reliable alternatives to conventional sensor signal processing.

REFERENCES

1. Zadeh, L., Fuzzy Sets, *Inf. Control,* 8, 338, 1965.
2. Zadeh, L., The Concept of a Linguistic Variable and Its Application to Approximate Reasoning, *Inf. Sci.*, 8, 199 and 301, 1975.
3. Zimmermann, H.-J., *Fuzzy Set Theory and Its Applications*, Kluwer Academic, Boston, 1991.
4. Tilli, T., *Fuzzy Logic, Grundlagen, Anwendungen, Hard- und Software,* Francis Verlag, München, 1991; *Building Intelligent Systems with Fuzzy Logic and Neural Networks,* John Wiley & Sons, New York, 1996.
5. Dubois, D. and Prade, H., A Review of Fuzzy Set Aggregation Connectives, *Inf. Sci.*, 36, 85, 1985.
6. Werners, B., Aggregation Models in Mathematical Programming, in *Mathematical Models for Decision Support*, Mitra, G., Ed., Springer-Verlag, Berlin, 1988, 295.

7. Zimmermann, H.-J. and Zysno, P., Latent Connectives in Human Decision Making, *Fuzzy Sets Systems,* 4, 37, 1980.
8. Dubois, D. and Prade, H., Fuzzy Real Algebra, *Fuzzy Sets Systems, 2,* 327, 1979.
9. Dubois, D. and Prade, H., Fuzzy Sets and Approximate Reasoning, *Fuzzy Sets Systems,* 40, 143, 1991.
10. Mizumoto, M. and Zimmermann, H.-J., Comparison of Fuzzy Reasoning Methods, *Fuzzy Sets Systems,* 8, 253, 1982.
11. Jackson, F., *An Introduction to Expert Systems*, Addison-Wesley, Reading, MA, 1989.
12. Kurbel, K., *Entwicklung und Einsatz von Expertensystemen*, Springer-Verlag, Berlin, 1989.
13. Harmon P., Maus R., and Morrisey W., *Expert Systems, Tools and Applications*, John Wiley & Sons, New York, 1988
14. Watermann, D., *A Guide to Expert Systems*, Addison-Wesley, Reading MA, 1986.
15. Sauter, D., Dubois, G., Levrat, E. and Brémont, J., Fault Diagnosis in Systems using Fuzzy Logic, in Proc. Eufit '93, Aachen, 1993, 2, 781.
16. Schneider, H., Implementation of a Fuzzy Concept for Supervision and Fault Detection of Robots, in Proc. Eufit '93, Aachen, 1993, 2, 775.
17. Berrie, P., Fuzzy Logic Elements in Ultrasonic Level Measurements, in Proc. Eufit '93, Aachen, 1993, 1, 181.
18. Poloni, P., A Fuzzy-Based Architecture for Sensor Integration and Fusion, in Proc. Eufit '93, Aachen, 1993, 1, 188.
19. Kroemer, N., Vossiek, M., Eccardt, P.-C., and Mágori, V., Ultrasonic Distance Sensors with Fuzzy Evaluation, in Proc. Sensor 93 in Nürnburg, Paper A6.2
20. Schoder, D. and Geiger, H., The Secret of Neuro-Fuzzy, *Elektronik plus,* 2, 123, 1993 (German).
21. Zühlke, D. and Lauzi, M., Inductive Pattern Recognition Using Fuzzy Logic, in Proc. Eufit '93, Aachen, 1993, 1, 478.
22. Weber, R., Quality Assurance through Acoustic Analysis, Proc. 2. Anwender Symp. Fuzzy Technol., Aachen 1993, 15 (German).
23. Priber, Oberflächenprüfung mittels Beugungslichtsensor und unscharfer Klassifikation, 1991, 7th Conf. "Meßinformationssysteme, TU Chemnitz, 1991.
24. Schödel, H., Automatische Test- und Prüfsysteme mit Fuzzy Logik, in *Fuzzy Logik in der Industriellen Automatisierung*, Bonfig, K., Ed., Expert-Verlag, Renningen, 1992, 27.
25. Bocklisch, S., Burmeister, B., and Paulinus, D., Anwendung eines Klassifikations konzeptes für die Automatisierung in der Schweißtechnik, Part 1: *ZIS Mitt.* 1987 (10), 1005: Part 2, *ZIS Mitt.* 1988 (2), 127.
26. Lorenz, O. and Bocklisch S., Diagnosegestützte Zuverlässigkeitsabschätzungen von Haushaltskühlschränken mittels der unscharfen Klassifikation. VI. Symp. "Zuverlässigkeit", TU Magdeburg, 1990
27. Bandemer, H. and Otto, M., Fuzzy Theory in Analytical Chemistry, *Mikrochim. Acta,* II, 93, 1986.
28. Otto, M. and Bandemer, H., *Chemom. Int. Lab. Syst.*, 1, 71, 1986.
29. Otto, M. and Bandemer, H., *Anal. Chim. Acta*, 184, 21, 1986.
30. Blaffert, T., *Anal. Chim. Acta*, 161, 135, 1984.
31. Otto, M. and Bandemer, H., *Anal. Chim. Acta,* 191, 193, 1986.
32. von Altrock, C., Praktische Umsetzung von Fuzzy-Technologien in der Meßtechnik, *Messung Prüfen,* 6, 486, 1991.
33. Otto, M., Fuzzy Methods and Neural Networks for Analytical Chemistry, Proc. 2. Anwender Symp. Fuzzy Technol., Aachen, 1993, 68 (German).
34. Sommer, V., Tobias, P., and Kohl, D., Methane and Butane Concentrations in a Mixture with Air Determined by Microcalorimetric Sensors and Neural Networks, *Sensors Actuators,* B12, 147, 1993.
35. Schödel, H., Fuzzy Logic and Laser Induced Fluorescent Spectrography for the Detection of Oil Contaminants, *Mikroelektronik*, 1, 26, 1992; see also Reference 24.
36. Kickert, W. and Mamdani, E., Analysis of a Fuzzy Logic Controller, *Fuzzy Sets Systems,* 1, 29, 1978.

37. King, P. and Mamdani, E., The Application of Fuzzy Control Systems to Industrial Processes, in *Fuzzy Automata and Decision Processes*, Gupta, M., Saridis, G., and Gaines, B., Eds., Elsevier/North Holland, Amsterdam, 1977, 321.
38. Zadeh, L., Outline of a New Approach to the Analysis of Complex Systems and Decision Processes, *IEE Trans. Sys. Man Cybern.*, SMC-3 (1), 28, 1973.
39. Mamdani, E. and Assilian, S., An Experiment in Linguistic Synthesis with a Fuzzy Logic Controller, *Int. J. Man.-Mach. Studies*, 7, 1, 1975.
40. Østergaard, J.-J., Fuzzy Control of a Heat Exchanger Process, in *Fuzzy Automata and Decision Processes*, Gupta, M., Saridis, G., and Gaines, B., Eds., Elsevier, North Holland, New York, 1977, 285.
41. Østergaard, J.-J., Fuzzy Control of Rotary Cement Kilns, A Retrospective Summary, in Proc. Eufit '93, Aachen, 1993, 1, 552.
42. Tong, R., A Retrospective View of Fuzzy Control Systems, *Fuzzy Sets Systems,* 14, 199, 1984.
43. Miyamoto, S., Yasunobu, S., and Ihara, H., Predictive Fuzzy Control and Its Application to Automatic Train Operation Systems, in *Analysis of Fuzzy Information,* Vol. II, Bezdec, J., Ed., CRC Press, Boca Raton, FL, 1987.
44. Eerikäinen, T., Zhu, Y.-H., and Linko, P., An Expert System with Fuzzy Variables and Neural Network Estimation, in Proc. Eufit '93, Aachen, 1993, 1, 202.
45. von Numers, C., Nakajima, M., Yada, H., Linko, P., and Endo, I., On-Line Fuzzy Reasoning System for Bioprocesses Control, in Proc. Eufit '93, Aachen, 1993, 1, 270.
46. Kishimoto, M., Kitta, Y., Takeuchi, S., Nakajima, M., and Yoshida, T., Computer Control of Glutamic Acid Production Based on Fuzzy Clusterization of Culture Phase, *J. Ferm. Bioeng.*, 72, 110, 1991.
47. Hou, R. and Lauer, L., A Fuzzy Feedback Controller and Its Application to the Sewage Treatment Process, in Proc. Eufit '93, Aachen, 1993, 1, 275.
48. Maron, C. and Burgert, K., Adaptive pH Value Control in a Neutralization Plant with Fuzzy Logic, in Proc. Eufit '93, Aachen, 1993, 1, 279.
49. Müller-Nehler, U. and Lorenz, O., Anwendung von Fuzzy-Control in der Klärwerkstechnik, Proc. 2. Anwender Symp. Fuzzy Technol., Aachen, 1993, 151.
50. Editorial, *Elektronik plus*, Special Issue on Fuzzy Logic, Market Survey on Fuzzy Products, 1993, 128.
51. Bartos, F., Fuzzy Logic is Clearly Here to Stay, *Control Eng.*, 7, 45, 1992.
52. Bartos, F., Fuzzy Logic Widens Its Appeal to Industrial Controls, *Control Eng.*, 6, 64, 1993.

Part V

Towards the Electronic Nose

21 Mammalian Semiochemistry: Chemical Signalling Between Mammals

Eric Albone

CONTENTS

21.1 CONTEXT, USE, AND APPLICATION

The world is full of chemical information and mammals have adapted to make use of it. Chemical communication was probably the earliest means of communication which life evolved. Through its own natural chemistry, a mammal broadcasts evidence of all aspects of itself: its species, sex, reproductive state, health, group and individual identity, and its relatedness to other individuals. Natural chemicals can signal alarm or mark territory; they can attract others of the same species, or they can attract predators. Besides that, through its natural chemistry a mammal can directly influence the physiological state of another animal, possibly at levels which do not elicit a behavioural response.

The study of mammalian semiochemistry is not only a fascinating science in its own right; it has considerable practical importance. This is a new area of study and although some applications have already been realised, many more remain to be explored.

0-8493-8905-4/97/$0.00+$.50
© 1997 by CRC Press, Inc.

Medicine and Veterinary Medicine

- Scents influence mood (Section 21.3) — possible applications in medical therapy and in modifying behaviour, as well as in quite other areas such as in marketing products.
- Natural chemicals can have major physiological effects on other individuals (Section 21.5) — implications for the control of reproduction remain largely unexplored.
- Body odours can warn of certain diseased states (Section 21.7) — possible applications in medical diagnosis.

Personal Products Industry

- Incorporation of natural pheromones/semiochemicals into a new generation of perfumes (Section 21.3).
- New deodorant research (Section 21.8).
- New products for personal protection against human or animal molestation.

Forensic Science

- Odour identity has a genetically determined component (Section 21.7) — possible forensic applications.

Agriculture and Forestry

- Wider applications to animal breeding programmes suggested by identification and marketing of pig pheromone product; also potential applications of primer pheromones (Sections 21.5 and 21.8).
- Wider applications to pest control and plant protection (Section 21.9).

Environmental Protection

- Possible applications to plant protection with reduced need for pesticides or culling.

Food Industry

- Human sensitivities to and perception of different scent compounds vary considerably between different compounds, between different individuals, and in relation to context, both chemical (concentration and the presence of other substances) and nonchemical (Sections 21.5, 21.7, and 21.8) — implications for food flavour assessment.
- Limitations of chemical analysis; even modern GC-MS cannot always compete with the animal nose in sensitivity; also less volatile compounds tend to be neglected; need to interpret GC-MS spectra of odours with caution (section 21.6) — value in attempting to emulate the mammalian sense of smell with electronic nose approaches.
- Accessory olfactory sense for less volatile substances may also function in humans (Section 21.3) — potential consideration for food flavour assessment?

Semiochemistry, derived from the Greek word for sign or signal, concerns the chemistry of those substances, semiochemicals, by means of which organism interacts with organism in the shared environment. Studies in chemical ecology have shown just how profound and widespread chemically mediated interactions between organisms are although, certainly in the case of mammals, remarkably little is yet known of the underlying chemistry.

Early work on the chemistry of animal scents was directed by the concerns of perfumers and natural product chemists and was undertaken with little attention to their biological and ecological significance. Notable were studies in the 1920s by Ruzicka[1a] on the macrocyclic ketones muscone (Formula A) and civetone (Formula B) from the scent glands of the musk deer and the civet, respectively, and by Lederer[1b] in the 1940s on castor from the scent glands of the beaver.

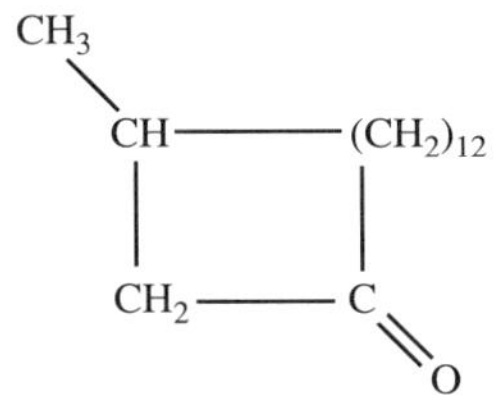

CH_3 — CH — $(CH_2)_{12}$ — $C(=O)$ — CH_2 — (ring)

(Formula A)

$CH{=}CH$, $(CH_2)_7$, $(CH_2)_7$, $C{=}O$ (ring)

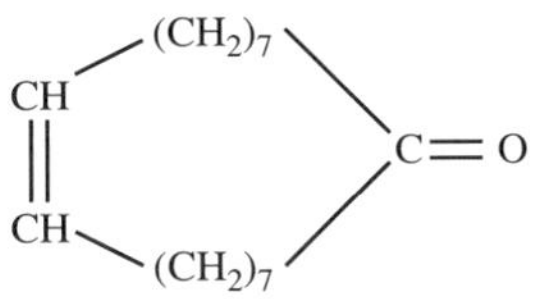

(Formula B)

Today mammalian semiochemistry is a highly interdisciplinary subject. Within the domain of chemistry it draws on techniques and insights derived from such diverse fields as flavour and perfume chemistry, insect pheromone research, and environmental chemistry; in a human context there is also a wealth of relevant information particularly with regard to skin chemistry and urine chemistry. However, this is chemistry set within the context of the biological and ecological sciences such that the divisions become invisible.

This brief review does not and cannot attempt to be exhaustive. Rather it seeks to place earlier detailed accounts of mammalian chemical communication in current context. For amplification of many of the ideas discussed here, and for a wide range of examples, the reader is referred in particular to Albone[1c] and to three further books on the subject.[2-4] The interested reader should also consult the proceedings of the triennial International "Chemical Signals in Vertebrates" Symposia, the last of which was held in Tübingen in 1994.

21.2 COMPLEX SEMIOCHEMICAL SOURCES

Mammals produce a complex array of scents and other semiochemically significant substances through the skin (in humans in the products of eccrine, apocrine, and sebaceous glands, on occasion modified by skin bacteria, and from materials adhering to desquamated [i.e., scaled off] epithelial tissue), from the lungs and the mouth in breath, from the kidneys and the various accessory sex glands, in urine, and in faeces. These substances contain chemical information about the individual animal, its species, sex, reproductive state, health, as well as its individual and group identity.

Mammals also possess a multitude of specific adaptations to generate chemical signals. Specialized scent glands, usually under hormonal control, abound, and the natural bacteria living on or in the animal can also play a significant role. Studies on the anal sacs of carnivores, where secretions from the sac walls are broken down by the remarkably restricted microflora of the sacs, led to speculation about a possible fermentation hypothesis of chemical recognition.[5] This has parallels with some of the ideas currently under discussion concerning microbially generated, genetically controlled individual scents in rodents, discussed later. How far are the recognizable profiles of volatiles a reflection of subtle differences in a stable microflora operating on similar substrates, or a similar microflora acting on different substrates?

To add to the complexity, scents frequently are mixed, whether in a particular scent gland complex which may contain secretory tissues of different types or by the animals actively mixing the scents themselves, spreading them over their own body surface, or depositing them on other conspecifics (animals of the same species) or on objects in their environment.

Thus the androgen-dependent "aversive pheromone" in male mouse urine, which deters investigation and inhibits aggression in other males entering a urine-marked area, derives from contact between the bladder urine and the product of the coagulating gland, and from neither material singly or when placed in close proximity. Similarly, the socially important signal which derives from the secretion of the Harderian gland which is located behind the eye of the Mongolian gerbil, *Meriones unguiculatus,* and is secreted via the nostrils when the animal is excited, requires for its production the contact with saliva which it receives during grooming behaviour.

The red deer stag Cer*vus elaphus* at rut sprays urine over its belly hair where urine compounds and their degradation products are displayed to other animals, while the black-tailed deer O*docoileus hemionus hemionus* displays socially important chemical signals by means of the hairs of its tarsal organ. This is an enlarged area of sebaceous and apocrine skin glands and an associated conspicuous hair tuft located on the inside of its hocks. Its scent however does not derive from the gland complex itself, which merely provides a lipid coating to the hairs, but from urine, which the deer "solvent-extracts" into the lipid by urinating over these hair tufts while rubbing its legs together. The tarsal signals can then be displayed to conspecifics by opening up the hair tuft for inspection as required. In this context, a urine-derived gamma lactone appears to elicit particular interest.

Such specialised scent hairs, or osmetrichia, which are adapted to hold and present scent materials, occur in a number of species, the most notable being the honeycombed hairs on the lateral scent gland of the crested rat *Lophiomys imhausi.*

21.3 THE CHEMICAL SENSES

Olfaction[6] and the vomeronasal sense (accessory olfactory system for less volatile substances, described later in this section) are principally involved in mammalian chemical communication. Gustation (taste) and the trigeminal sense (described below) are much less so. This is a simplification, and detailed analysis can identify five mammalian "olfactory" chemical sense organs including the septal organ, and that associated with the nervus terminalis.[7]

Scents affect mood and emotion at a deep level. Many people also find scents to be remarkably effective in bringing back long-forgotten associated memories. There is speculation, too, that certain scents can assist learning, and there is even a patent for a substance which when impregnated in paper is said to induce people to pay their bills! However this may be, the scent receptors of the olfactory epithelium feed information via the olfactory bulb not only to the neocortex, the part of the brain which allows awareness and recognition of the smells encountered, but also to the much more ancient nonconscious limbic system which controls emotion and sexual behaviour.

The study of olfaction has recently been considerably stimulated by the identification of odorant binding proteins[8] and the identification of a new family of genes which code for putative olfactory receptors.[9,10] Unexpectedly, genes belonging to this family are expressed also in the testis in humans and in dogs, and olfactory receptors have been demonstrated on the surface of mature dog sperm cells where they are presumed to act as receptors for substances involved in sperm maturation, migration, and/or fertilization.[11]

However, along with the higher primates, humankind appeared until recently to lack yet another chemical window on the world that is possessed by most mammals — that of the vomeronasal organ or VNO. The VNO is commonly located above the roof of the mouth, opening into the oral cavity through small ducts. It possesses its own separate nerve pathways to the brain and seems to be sensitive to less volatile substances that are often taken up in solution by licking. It could well be of particular importance in the reception of sex pheromones.[12-14]

It is now believed that a structure within our own nostrils may be a functional human VNO and the opportunity has not escaped notice to use this organ to probe the human skin for potential human pheromones which could be incorporated into a new generation of perfumes.[15]

Trigeminal sensations are sometimes confused with olfactory ones. The chemosensitive endings of the trigeminal nerve are distributed over much of the body surface, including the mucous membranes of the nose and mouth where they respond to aggressive substances (e.g. ammonia) with a stinging sensation.

21.4 BIOLOGICAL CONSEQUENCES

Mammalian chemical signals may act as sex attractants, as alarm substances, as recognition signatures for individuals, for groups, and for species, as trail substances and to mark territory, to signal reproductive state, and to indicate reproductive condition. They can also regulate in profound ways the physiological state of a receiving animal.

Quite often an animal may be involved in making comparisons between scents. This has been discussed by Gosling[16] in terms of "scent matching" where territorial scent marks are matched by an intruder with the scent of the territory owner, and Natynczuk and Macdonald[17] describe scent referencing in their notion of a "self-calibrating rat" by which a male rat judges the reproductive state of a female by comparing the scent of the female's haunch (which as the authors posit on the basis of histological data fluctuates with circulating sex hormones and thus provides the indicator scent), with that of another region of the body which is judged not to do so and can thus act as a built-in reference scent source.

A particular secretion may contain a number of different messages, or as we shall see later, a particular chemical signal may be read in different ways in different situations. A good example of the former is the case of the golden hamster, *Mesocricetus auratus*. This species is unusually dependent on chemical signals in its reproduction. Hamsters live largely solitary lives, so shortly before oestrus the female deposits a complex vaginal scent in her environment. This contains a potent male attractant. Chemical analysis using gas chromatography and mass spectrometry combined with a bioassay showed that a large part of the potency of this complex mixture resided in one minor volatile constituent, dimethyl disulphide, Formula C, which the male senses by olfaction and to which he will respond at subpicogram ($<10^{-12}$ g) levels.[18]

$$CH_3—S—S—CH_3 \qquad \text{(Formula C)}$$

However, on encountering the female the male hamster requires a further signal to trigger mating. This is also a component of the vaginal secretion, but an involatile component sampled by direct contact and sensed by the VNO. It is appropriate that this signal should be involatile, for the response can only occur when male and female are together. This "mounting pheromone" is associated with a small, very specific protein, aphrodisin, present in the vaginal secretion, and related in amino acid sequence to known lipocalycin odorant binding proteins. Related substances also occur in the major urinary proteins of mice and rats, and are also associated with chemical signalling systems in these species.[19]

21.5 PHEROMONES AND SEMIOCHEMICALS

The term "pheromone" arose originally in insect studies where it is used to designate substances produced by one insect which elicit a reproducible response in another member of the same species. Mammal responses, and especially our own, are far more complex, are less "automatic", and depend on many other factors, so that there is concern that the term "pheromone" may not be widely applicable to mammals at all, and that the more general term, semiochemical, or chemosignal, which does not have this emphasis on a reproducible response, should be used.

There remains one category, that of the Primer Pheromone, about which we can feel more confident in using the term.[20] Here the substance immediately elicits not a behavioural response, but a physiological change in the recipient. Primer pheromones in mammals have been most closely studied in rodents and particularly in mice. Thus mouse urine mediates a diverse range of chemical signals including the following primer pheromone effects:

1. Triggering synchronous oestrus cycling in grouped female mice (in which the oestrus cycle has become long and irregular) following exposure to the odour of male mouse urine (Whitten effect).[21]
2. Puberty acceleration in immature females caused by male urine constituents, the effect being greatest when a dominant male is used.[22,23] The active substance appears to be heat labile and associated with a peptide fraction,[24] although this could merely be a carrier for it is very difficult to remove the residual odour from the material; also enzymic hydrolysis of the active peptide fraction did not remove activity, although since not all protein was removed in the process this is not conclusive.[25]
3. Puberty acceleration in immature females by urines taken from singly caged oestrous female mice and from pregnant and lactating females, while grouped female mice kept in isolation from males produce urines which retard puberty in immature females.[26,27]
4. Pregnancy block in a recently mated female may be induced by the scent of a strange male (Bruce effect).[28,29]

In *Homo sapiens*, the menstrual (ovarian cycle) synchrony observed in groups of women living together could be a manifestation of another primer pheromone effect,[30-32] although some studies have failed to find synchrony and there is debate concerning the analysis of data.[33] Evidence in support of this is provided by studies in which axillary secretions from donor females applied to subjects tended to shift timing of the monthly cycle towards that of the donor[34] and an anecdotal account that high levels of certain scents can have an effect on the menstrual cycle. Social and environmental factors could also be important.

21.6 CHEMICAL ANALYSIS STRATEGIES

An understanding of the chemical language of communication in mammals is still very much in its infancy. The chemical senses present an immense challenge to our technology, and rival the best chemical instrumentation available both in their sensitivity and in their discrimination. In addition, the complexity of the mammal's own chemical ambience is vast, and this becomes increasingly more apparent with each technological advance in chemical instrumentation. Were it not for the advent and increasing sophistication of computerised gas chromatographic-mass spectrometric methods over the past three decades, which themselves combine high resolution with high sensitivity, chemical progress in this field would not be possible, but even here the sensitivity may not match that of the nose.

Most attention has been given to the complex profiles of volatile components associated with semiochemical materials, using headspace trapping techniques based on those developed by Zlatkis[35] and by Apps.[36] However, it is increasingly realised that this overlooks semiochemically important less volatile and involatile components.

It is easy to forget that any chemical analysis only examines that part of the chemical ambience of the animal defined by the limits of sensitivity of the method employed and the properties of the substances examined (e.g., volatility, compound class) and can never produce a complete chemical description. Even the relative proportions of those components reported in a gas chromatographic description depend on the precise details of the analytical procedures used. For a good example of this, see Jennings and Filsoof.[37]

There are two complementary strategies[1] which may be employed in the search for chemical messages in the complex chemical mixtures produced by mammals.

21.6.1 Response-Guided Strategy

The powerful response-guided strategy widely used by chemists in many contexts depends on developing a robust bioassay procedure, whether behavioural or physiological, and subjecting the material under examination to a series of increasingly refined fractionations guided by the bioassay, so that eventually a pure active material is obtained and its chemical identity determined.

In many areas of mammalian chemical communication, such a response-guided strategy is not appropriate. For some types of chemical communication, it may be very difficult if not impossible to devise precise, reproducible bioassays which can be used under controlled conditions. The chemical signal may convey information which the animal assesses and responds to in a range of different ways (or perhaps not overtly at all) in the context of a whole range of other sensory inputs and of its own past experience.

In addition, fractionating a biological substrate frequently leads to substantial or total loss of activity. Even in those cases where behaviourally active components have been identified in a biological substrate, they usually do not exhibit the full activity of the total secretion or excretion.

21.6.2 Chemical Image Strategy

The alternative chemical image strategy lies at the other extreme. This is based on the view that the animal is not responding to particular active components hidden in a meaningless mixture of chemicals, but rather that meaning is vested in a particular pattern of what are individually inactive, perhaps very common, natural chemicals. It is this chemical pattern or "chemical image" which contains meaning rather than the substances themselves.

There have been many attempts to analyze biological materials by gas chromatography to search for patterns of occurrence of a range of different components which could, for example, specify an individual or group signature. A major difficulty of interpretation is that the differences in sensitivity of the gas chromatographic detector to different compounds does not correspond to those of the nose. Major components on the gas chromatogram may have little olfactory impact, while trace components may dominate. To take an example,[38] the complex gas chromatogram of components in the steam volatiles of California bell peppers (which themselves account for a mere 10 ppm of whole pepper) contain identified compounds the odour threshold of which vary a millionfold, so that one trace component, 2-methoxy-3-isobutylpyrazine (Formula D), which appears insignificant on the gas chromatogram, dominates the odour profile.

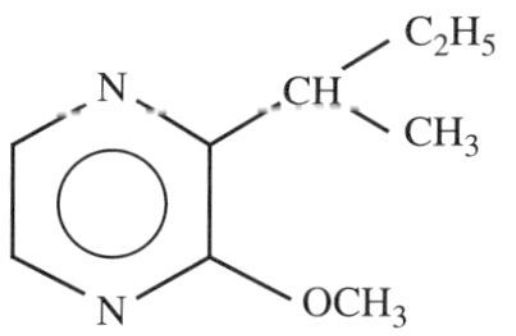

N, CH, C_2H_5, CH_3, N, OCH_3

(Formula D)

Even so, comparisons of gas chromatograms can be used with caution. Thus Belcher et al.[39] studied the scent marks from the circumgenital sebaceous and apocrine gland fields present in the tamarin, *Saguinus fuscicollis*, and showed that the chemist can interpret the resulting GC profiles to deduce *inter alia* the species, subspecies, and gender of the marking animal. The substances responsible for these profiles, which remained stable over a considerable period of time, were the butyl esters of a series of C16 to C24 alcohols. Whether these compounds are used by the tamarins themselves in communication is far from clear.

Although not widely used in animal studies, the procedure by which the effluent from the gas chromatograph is split and part of it assessed for odour descriptors by a trained sniffer and the gas chromatogram annotated accordingly does have merit, even if the observations could be criticised as being subjective.

On occasions, for all their limitations animals have also been used to assess the compounds emerging from the gas chromatograph in the preliminary search for substances of interest. An example[40] is the use of rabbits to assess the components of the headspace volatiles associated with rabbit anal gland material. The rabbit anal glands increase greatly in size with the coming of maturity and are particularly large in dominant animals of either sex. The glands produce a secretion which coats rabbit faecal pellets, and in this way establishes certain sites which act as a kind of olfactory notice board, not only for the resident group but also for intruders. In an effort to select components of semiochemical significance in the complex chromatograms of rabbit anal gland headspace volatiles, CSIRO scientists in Australia constrained a rabbit to sample the headspace volatiles as they emerged from the gas chromatogram while continuously monitoring its heart rate radiotelemetrically. Components of interest which instantaneously depressed the heart rate more than 3% were then selected for future semiochemical study. They consisted of some 13 different C8 to C12 saturated and unsaturated aldehydes. Heart rate monitors have more recently been used to examine the volatiles associated with faecal pellets in wild house mice.[41]

Linking the chemical image and the response guided approaches, profiles may be scanned for components the occurrence of which corresponds with particular biological parameters (e.g., hormone status) which could then be assessed biologically in more detail. However, a negative bioassay result does not necessarily imply lack of significance. On many occasions, activity is manifest only when components are presented in combination with each other or in appropriate contexts.

21.7 RODENT SEMIOCHEMICALS

Chemical communication systems have been studied in more detail in rodents than in any other group of animals. Most work has of course been carried out on laboratory mice and rats, although there is increasing concern with wild species in their natural environments.

Mouse semiochemicals have been found to carry a very wide range of information. Thus there is evidence that female mice can discriminate between the odours of urines of males which are parasitized by a natural enteric parasite and those which are not, finding the odours of the parasitized males more stressful,[42] reminiscent of the ways in which human body or urine odour can give warning of certain disease states.

While some very interesting studies have been undertaken on the chemistry of some of the accessory sex glands which contribute components to urine, for example, the alkyl acetates and other compounds present in the preputial glands, two areas are particularly of note.

21.7.1 Volatile Rodent Urine Pheromones

A great deal of impressive chemical work has been conducted by Novotny's research group[43] on the semiochemistry of the urine of the house mouse *Mus musculus*, and a number of primer pheromone effects have been probed. Here, mouse urine volatiles are trapped on Tenax adsorbents and subjected to analysis based on capillary gas chromatographic procedures. Although biological activity could well be associated with mixtures of simple compounds, it is postulated that unusual volatile compounds, where they occur, could well have special communicatory significance.

The complexity of the profiles obtained was addressed by seeking components which vary with biological parameters, and particularly with endocrine status. Thus, male mouse semiochemicals are frequently under the control of testosterone,[44] which, in turn, is influenced by signals produced in the urine of other conspecifics of either sex.

Following studies using castration and hormone treatment, two testosterone-dependent trace volatile constituents of male mouse urine were identified, synthesised, and found to be semiochemically active in eliciting a fighting response from other male mice. These compounds, unique to mouse urine, were identified as (R,R)-3,4-dehydro-exo-brevicomin (Formula E) and 2-*sec*-butyl-4,5-dihydrothiazole (Formula F).[45] The stereochemistry of the latter was not determined as the compound very readily epimerizes, and a racemic mixture was used in bioassay trials.

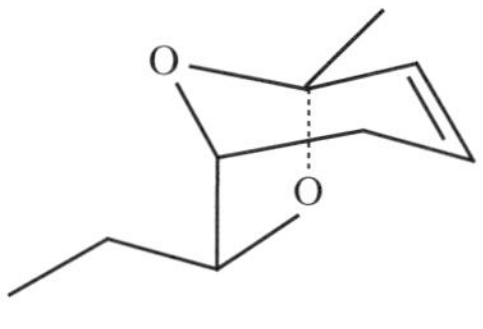

O O

(Formula E)

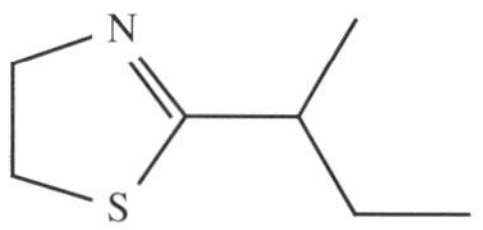

N S

(Formula F)

The remarkable complexity of the biological activity of these substances is evident not only in that they are only active when presented together, but also that they require castrate mouse urine (itself inactive) as a necessary substrate if activity is to be manifested. In addition, they elicit different responses from different animals:

1. For dominant male mice, the mixture in castrate urine elicits a fighting response, which castrate urine alone does not.
2. Female mice are as attracted to castrate urine containing these two substances as they are to intact male mouse urine.
3. Grouped female mice show the Whitten effect (synchronous oestrus cycling, see above) when exposed to the mixture in castrate urine.

A further examination of urine volatile profiles from dominant male mice, from subordinate males, from immature males, from castrates, and from castrates treated with androgen, revealed that overall volatile content of the urine was greatest in dominant males, was greatly reduced in castrates, and was restored on treatment with androgen. These effects were particularly apparent for the brevicomin and the thiazole discussed, but also for 2-isopropyl-4,5-dihydrothiazole, for *p*-toluidine, as well as for α farnesene (Formula G) and for β-farnesene (Formula H) components of the headspace volatiles.

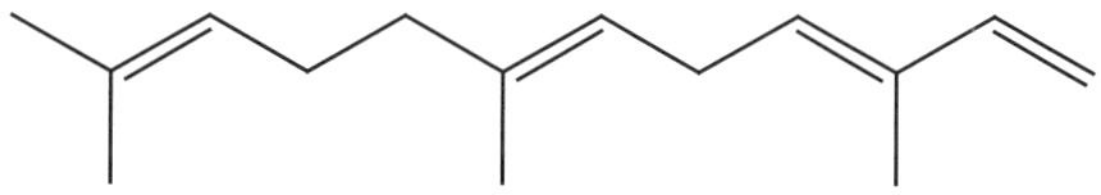

(Formula G)

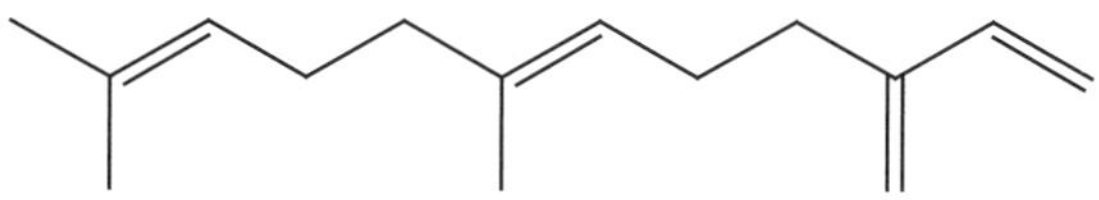

(Formula H)

The farnesenes were particularly in evidence in dominant male mouse urine and are of preputial origin, being present in preputial lipid, but absent from bladder urine (in contrast with the situation with brevicomin and the thiazoles). Behavioural tests show these substances discourage investigation by other mice.[46]

Female mouse urine produced by animals living under crowded conditions contains substances which decrease female mating by delaying puberty. As the adrenal glands respond to stress induced by crowding, urines from intact and adrenalectomized female mice were compared and consistent differences noted. Volatiles which were consistently reduced following adrenalectomy included the ketones heptan-2-one (Formula I), *trans*-hept-5-en-2-one (Formula J), *trans*-hept-4-en-2-one (Formula K), the acetate esters pentyl acetate (Formula L), *cis*-pent-2-en-1-yl acetate (Formula M), and 2,5-dimethylpyrazine (Formula N),[47] while the pyrazine was present at high concentration in the urines of female mice maintained under crowded conditions. The acetate esters and the pyrazine have a substantial puberty delaying effect in males and females.[48]

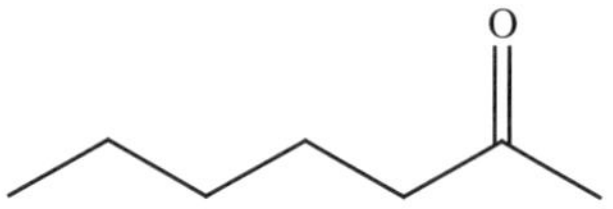

O

(Formula I)

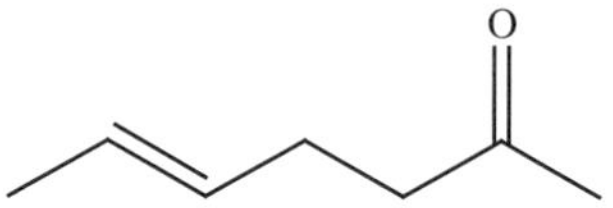

O

(Formula J)

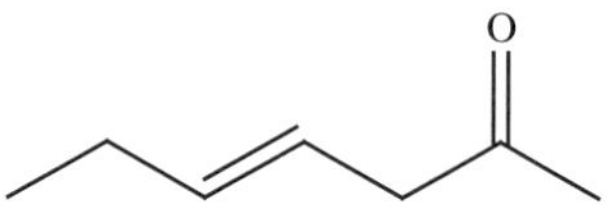

O

(Formula K)

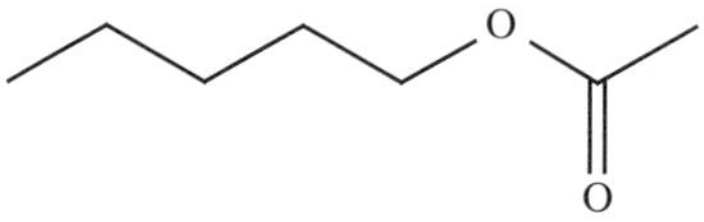

O

O

(Formula L)

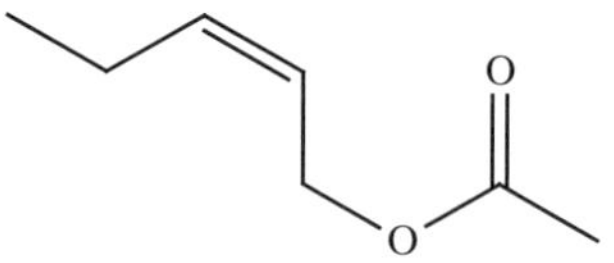

O

O

(Formula M)

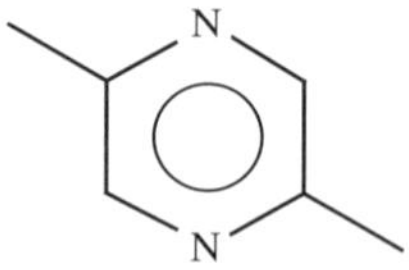

N

N

(Formula N)

Sexual maturation is accelerated in juvenile females by exposure to male urine, and also by female urine whether from oestrous, pregnant, or lactating females.[49] The components responsible for these effects have been identified.[50] In contrast, in another species of rodent, the California mouse *Peromyscus californicus*, a monogamous rather than a polygamous species, reproduction in females is suppressed by female urinary semiochemicals.[51] Sexual maturation is delayed by contact with the mother or with other females. Maternal urinary signals are also involved in maintaining the father's paternal care of the young. A typical gas chromatogram revealed around 40 volatile components in comparison with more than 100 in house-mouse urine, and although many of these are common to the two species, compounds such as brevicomin, thiazole, and the farnesenes present in house-mouse urine are absent from this species. Instead, levels of the pyrazines, 2,5-dimethylpyrazine (Formula N), 2-ethyl-5-methylpyrazine (Formula O), 2,3,5-trimethylpyrazine (Formula P), and 2-ethyldimethylpyrazine are remarkably high (36% of all volatiles in both sexes) and are likely to be involved in reproductive suppression. There are no male-specific or female-specific compounds, but rather the sexes differ in the relative amounts of the substances.

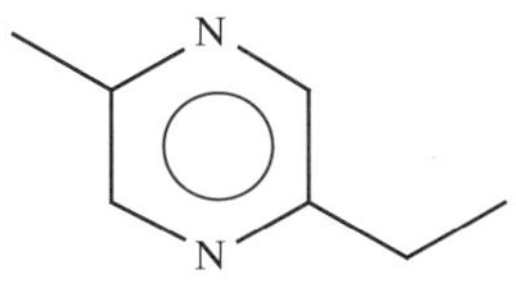

N
N

(Formula O)

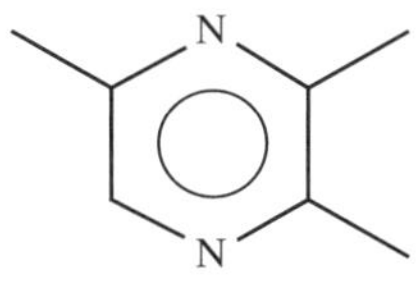

N
N

(Formula P)

21.7.2 Individual Recognition

Remarkable progress has been made in defining the genetic origins of individual rodent scents. Genetically determined individual identifying odours (odourtypes) in laboratory rats and mice have been linked principally to genetic differences in the major histocompatibility complex (MHC), with other genes (including some on the X and Y chromosomes) playing a lesser role. The MHC genes are of central importance in the immune response and code for antigens with which the body recognizes and rejects foreign tissue. It is interesting that this immunological identity also results in odour identity.[52]

These findings and their subsequent development arose from chance observations in the mid 1970s in the Memorial Sloan-Kettering Cancer Center congenic breeding rooms that male and female mice of different MHC types tended to pay greater attention to each other and to nest together. These differences were then linked with odourtypes and mating preferences, the female preferring a male of different MHC. Subsequent experiments by fostering mice on other parents showed that this was an acquired response, the preference being for the scent of a male of different MHC odourtype from that of the family in which the young mouse was reared. It is reasonable to suppose that under natural conditions such a bias would serve to guard against inbreeding.

The major histocompatibility complex (MHC) imparts to each mouse an individual urinary odour, perception of which affects mate selection and embryonic implantation. There is even evidence that paternal genetic MHC substances may be expressed *in utero* and sensed even before birth, with implications for familial identification and communication.[53]

A similar situation is documented for laboratory rats. However, in surprising contrast to the situation in mice, in rats commensal bacteria are essential to the production of these odours — animals raised in germ-free conditions not displaying such odours. This is reflected in differences in the headspace volatiles associated with their urines.[54] In the rat, there appears to be a complex interplay between gut microflora, MHC gene type, diet, and urine odour. The gut microflora in a particular animal are stable over time and show significant individual differences.

Although MHC-related odours have been studied only in rodents, there is speculation that a similar phenomenon might occur in humans, and some progress has been made in a preliminary study using trained rats to discriminate between human urines and linking this with the donor's HLA class I type.[55]

An interesting example of another rodent scent controlled by the gut microflora is provided by the maternal pheromone in the rat. This is a faecal chemical attractant operating between the mother and the preweanling young 16 to 27 days postpartum, a period when they can leave the nest but remain dependent on their mothers.[56,57]

21.8 PHEROMONAL STEROIDS IN PIG AND MAN

Odour signals have considerable significance in humans[58,59] and particularly in mother/child bonding because mothers and children are uniquely sensitive to each others scents, as evidenced by a young child's ability to discriminate its mother's odour.[60]

However, in quite a different context much interest in human chemical communication has focused on the odorous steroids, 5α-androst-16-en-3-one (Formula Q) and 3α-hydroxy-5α-androst-16-ene (Formula R).[59,61]

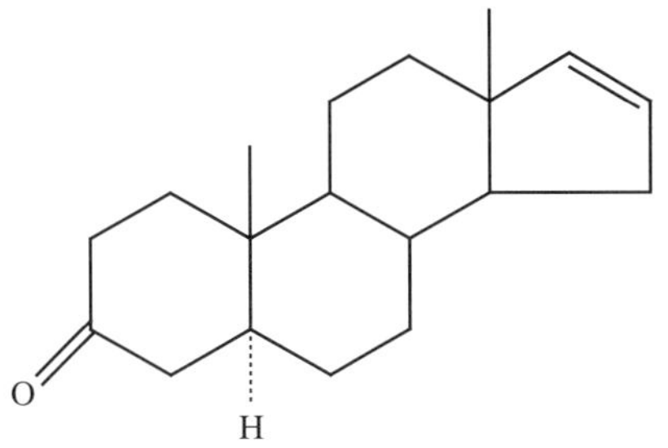

O H

(Formula Q)

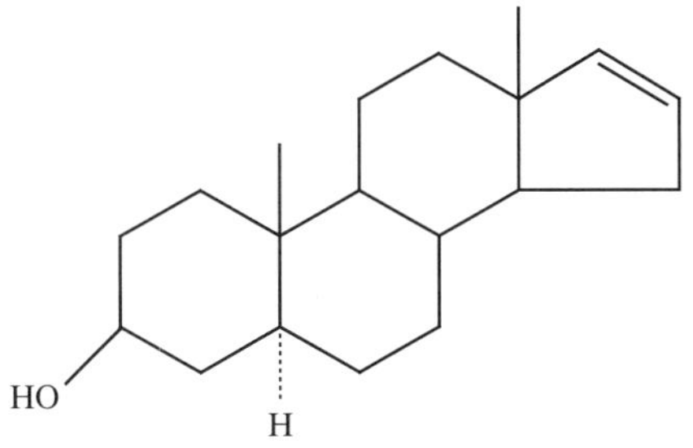

HO H

(Formula R)

Some people have difficulty in smelling certain scent categories (specific anosmia). In 1986 in the largest smell survey ever conducted (in association with the National Geographic Magazine), 1.5 million people worldwide sampled six scents using scratch and sniff sheets and answered a questionnaire: 1.2% of all respondents could not detect any of the scents (the number increasing with age), while only half the respondents could detect all six. Women were overall better scent detectors than men. What is intriguing is that the two substances which people had most difficulty in detecting were musks, one a synthetic musk, galaxolide, and one a substance which some consider to be a possible human pheromone, androstenone (Formula Q). This has been investigated more recently in greater depth by Baydar et al (1993).[62]

Androstenone is a remarkable substance. It is a steroid, related to the sex hormones, but having little hormonal activity yet is produced by a biochemical pathway which leads nowhere else. Its function was at first a mystery. The situation was resolved in a most remarkable fashion. Male pigs are not widely used for meat unless they are neutered, but castrated animals produce a lot of fat. Intact males would be much better for lean meat production, but boar meat has about it a certain flavour (boar taint) which some like but which many find repulsive. In an effort to come to terms with this, pig fat was extracted and the odorous component identified. It was androstenone. Subsequently this finding was linked to the occurrence of the steroid with the alcohol related (Formula R) in the peculiar viscous submaxillary saliva which the male pig drools when it is sexually aroused, and to which the sow responds. It turned out that both the ketone and the alcohol are involved in pig reproductive behaviour, and form an essential male signal to the female. The compounds are produced in the testes and are transferred around the body to the saliva and to the fat. The ketone is now marketed in an aerosol spray for use by pig breeders to assess the state of the sow in artificial insemination programmes. This was the first marketed mammal pheromone.[1]

Having found this unusual steroid to be an active chemical signal in one species, there was great interest in its possible use by other species, and it was discovered at very low levels in human axillary sweat, particularly in male sweat. The supposition is that it could be a human pheromone.[63] Many people are anosmic to the substance. Of those who can detect it, there is a remarkable diversity of response: some report finding it attractive, others quite repulsive. However, as a pheromone acting via the VNO (see Section 21.3 above) it could be effective at a level below that of conscious detection.

The human axillary coryneform bacteria have an important role in producing perceptible levels of 16-androstenes from the odourless secretions produced by the axillary apocrine glands.[64] Microorganisms also produce odorous volatile C6 to C11 fatty acids, of which the unusual (*E*)-3-methyl-2-hexenoic acid (Formula S) is the most abundant.[65,66]

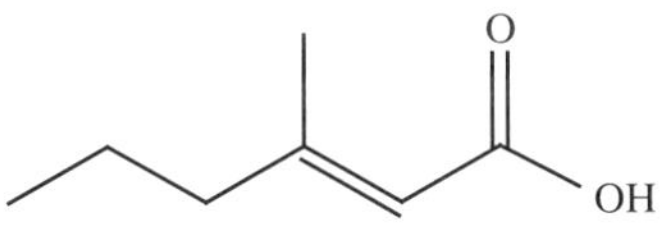

O

OH

(Formula S)

21.9 PREDATOR ODOURS: AN APPLICATION IN PEST CONTROL

A great deal of interest surrounds the development of safe, effective mammal repellents, particularly to limit the damage caused by herbivore species. Deer browse damage to young trees constitutes a major forestry problem and in some places, faeces, particularly predator faeces, have been used to much effect. Deer appear to be particularly repelled by the scent of putrefying animal tissue, that is attractive to many predators such as the fox and coyote,[67] and putrefied fish and egg products have been found to be effective deer repellents, albeit at very short range. Indeed, a putrefied egg product has been marketed commercially for this purpose by a U.S. company.

Lion faeces are known to be very effective as a deer repellent also, even in areas where the lion is not indigenous, and zoo keepers know it to be much in demand by gardeners who want to keep deer out of their gardens. Recently, one company developed an artificial lion dung scent and patented its use for this purpose. Lion dung scent was analyzed gas chromatographically and was found to consist of a complex mixture of common natural substances. A synthetic mixture of many common components was reconstructed and, after some modifications in their proportions by an odour panel, a scent which mimicked lion dung to the human nose was formulated and patented. This material is reported to be effective as a deer repellent in trials, and the company is now examining its use as a rabbit repellent also.[68-70]

This is very much in accord with earlier experiments in North America on the use of predator odours, specifically the sulphur compounds from mustelid anal sacs,[71,72] predator faecal materials,[73] and predator urines[74] to reduce herbivore browse damage. It appears that high levels of sulphur compounds in predator excreta (urines) associated with a meat diet are responsible for some of the repellency.[75]

REFERENCES

1a. Ruzicka, L., Zur Kenntnis der Kohlenstoffringes. I. Über die Konstitation des Zibetons, *Helv. Chim. Acta,* 9, 230, 1926.

1b. Lederer, E., Chemistry and biochemistry of the scent glands of the beaver, *Castor fiber, Nature,* 157, 231, 1946.

1c. Albone, E. S., *Mammalian Semiochemistry; The Investigation of Chemical Signals Between Mammals,* Wiley-Interscience, Chichester, 1984.

2. Brown, R. E. and Macdonald, D. W., Eds., *Social Odours in Mammals,* Vol. 1 & 2, Clarendon Press, Oxford, 1985.
3. Stoddart, D. M., *The Scented Ape; The Biology and Culture of Human Odour*, Cambridge University Press, Cambridge, 1990.
4. Van Toller, S. and Dodd, G. H., Eds., *Fragrance, the Psychology and Biology of Perfume*, Elsevier, London, 1992.
5. Albone, E. S., Gosden, P. E., Ware, G. C., Macdonald, D. W., and Hough, N. G., Bacterial action and chemical signalling in the red fox (*Vulpes vulpes*) and other mammals, in *Flavor Chemistry of Animal Foods,* Am. Chem. Soc. Symp. Ser. 67, Bullard, R. W., Ed., American Chemical Society, Washington, D.C., 1978, 78.
6. Farbman, A. I., *Cell Biology of Olfaction*, Cambridge University Press, Cambridge, 1992.
7. Quay, W. B., Olfaction in central neural and neuroendocrine systems: integrative review of olfactory representations and interrelations, in *Chemical Signals in Vertebrates,* Vol. 3, Müller-Schwarze, D. and Silverstein, R. M., Eds., Plenum Press, New York, 1983, 105.
8. Pelosi, P., Odorant-binding proteins, *Crit. Rev. Biochem. Molec. Biol.*, 29, 199, 1994.
9. Buck, L. B., The olfactory multigene family, *Curr. Opinion Neurobiol.*, 2, 282, 1992.
10. Buck, L. B., Receptor diversity and spatial patterning in the mammalian olfactory system, in *The Molecular Basis of Smell and Taste Transduction,* Ciba Found. Symp. 179, Wiley Interscience, Chichester, 51, 1993.
11. Vanderhaeghen, P., Schurmans, S., Vassart, G., and Parmentier, M., Olfactory receptors are displayed on dog mature sperm cells, *J. Cell Biol.*, 123, 1441, 1993.
12. Wysocki, C. J., Beauchamp, G. K., Reidinger, R. R., and Wellington, J. L., Access of large and non-volatile molecules to the vomeronasal organ of mammals during social and feeding behaviors, *J. Chem. Ecol.*, 11, 1147, 1985.
13. Meredith, M. and Fernandez-Fewell, G., Vomeronasal system, LHRH, and sex behaviour, *Psychoneuroendocrinology*, 19, 657, 1994.
14. Berliner, D. L., Michael, R. P., and Pasqualini, Proceedings of the International Symposium on Recent advances in Mammalian Pheromone Research, in *J. Steroid Biochem. Molec. Biol.*, 39, 4B, 1991.
15. Monti-Bloch, L., Jennings-White, C., Dolberg, D. S., and Berliner, D. L., The human vomeronasal system, *Psychoneuroendocrinology*, 19, 673, 1994.
16. Gosling, L. M., Scent marking by resource holders; alternative mechanisms for advertising the costs of competition, in *Chemical Signals in Vertebrates,* Vol. 5, Macdonald, D. W., Müller-Schwarze, D., and Natynczuk, S. E., Eds., Oxford University Press, Oxford, 1990, 315.
17. Natynczuk, S. E. and Macdonald, D. W., Scent, sex and the self-calibrating rat, *J. Chem. Ecol.*, 20, 1843, 1994.
18. O'Connell, R. J., Singer, A. G., Pfaffmann, C., and Agosta, W. C., Pheromones of hamster vaginal discharge. Attraction to femtogram amounts of dimethyl disulfide and to mixtures of volatile components. *J. Chem. Ecol.*, 5, 575, 1979.
19. Singer, A. G. and Macrides, F., Lipocalycins associated with mammalian pheromones, in *Chemical Signals in Vertebrates,* Vol. 6, Doty, R. L. and Müller-Schwarze, D., Eds., Plenum Press, New York, 1992, 119.
20. McClintock, M. K., Synchronizing ovarian and birth cycles, in *Chemical Signals in Vertebrates,* Vol. 3, Müller-Schwarze, D. and Silverstein, R. M., Eds., Plenum Press, New York, 1983, 159.
21. Whitten, W. K., Bronson, F. H., and Greenstein, J. A., Estrus-inducing pheromone of male mice: transport by movement of air, *Science*, 161, 584, 1968.
22. Vandenbergh, J. G., Acceleration and inhibition of puberty in female mice by pheromones, *J. Reprod. Fertil. Suppl.,* 19, 411, 1973.

23. Drickamer, L. C., Puberty-influencing chemosignals in house mice: ecological and evolutionary considerations, in *Chemical Signals in Vertebrates,* Vol. 4, Duvall, D., Müller-Schwarze, D., and Silverstein, R. M., Eds., Plenum Press, New York, 1986, 441.
24. Vandenbergh, J. G., Finlayson, J. S., Dobrogosz, W. J., Dills, S. S., and Kost, T. A., Chromatographic separation of puberty accelerating pheromone from male mouse urine, *Biol. Reprod.*, 15, 260, 1976.
25. Novotny, M., Jorgenson, J. W., Carmack, M., Wilson, S. R., Boyse, E. A., Yamazaki, K., Wilson, M., Beamer, W., and Whitten, W. K., Chemical studies of the primer mouse pheromones, in *Chemical Signals; Vertebrates and Aquatic Invertebrates*, Müller-Schwarze, D. and Silverstein, R. M., Eds., Plenum Press, New York, 1980, 377.
26. Drickamer, L. C., Delay of sexual maturation in female house mice by exposure to grouped females or urine from grouped females, *J. Reprod. Fertil.*, 51, 77, 1977.
27. Drickamer, L. C. and Hoover, J. E., Effects of urine from pregnant and lactating female house mice on sexual maturation of juvenile females, *Dev. Psychobiol.,* 12, 545, 1979.
28. Bruce, H. M., An exteroceptive block to pregnancy in the mouse, *Nature*, 184, 105, 1959.
29. Hoppe, P. C., Genetic and endocrine studies on the pregnancy-blocking pheromone in mice, *J. Reprod. Fertil.,* 45, 109, 1975.
30. Graham, C. A., Menstrual synchrony, an update and review, *Hum. Nature*, 2, 293, 1991.
31. Weller, L. and Weller, A., Human menstrual synchrony — a critical assessment, *Neurosci. Biobehav. Rev.*, 17, 427, 1993.
32. Weller, A. and Weller, L., The impact of social interaction factors on menstrual synchrony in the workplace, *Psychoneuroendocrinology*, 20, 21, 1995.
33. Wilson, H. C., A critical review of menstrual synchrony research, *Psychoneuroendocrinology*, 17, 565, 1992.
34. Preti, G., Cutler, W. B., Garcia, C. R., Huggins, G. R., and Lawley, H. J., Human axillary secretions influence women's menstrual cycles; the role of donor extract of females, *Horm. Behav.*, 20, 474, 1986.
35. Zlatkis, A. and Shanfield, H., Concentration techniques for volatile samples, in *Practical Mass Spectrometry*, Middleditch, B. S., Ed., Plenum Press, New York, 1979, 151.
36. Apps, P., Dynamic solvent effect sampling for quantitative analysis of mammalian semiochemicals, in *Chemical Signals in Vertebrates,* Vol. 5, Macdonald, D. W., Müller-Schwarze, D., and Natynczuk, S. E., Eds., Oxford University Press, Oxford, 1990, 23.
37. Jennings, W. G. and Filsoof, M., Comparison of sample preparation techniques for gas chromatographic analysis, *J. Agric. Food Chem.,* 25, 440, 1977.
38. Buttery, R. G., Seifert, R. M., Guadagni, D. G., and Ling, L. C., Characterization of some volatile constituents of bell peppers, *J. Agric. Food Chem.*, 17, 1322, 1969.
39. Belcher, A. M., Smith, A. B., Jurs, P. C., Lavine, B., and Epple, G., Analysis of chemical signals in a primate species *(Saguinus fuscicollis)*: use of behavioral, chemical and pattern recognition methods, *J. Chem. Ecol.*, 12, 513, 1986.
40. Goodrich, B. S., Hesterman, E. R., Murray, K. E., Mykytowycz, R., Stanley, G., and Sugowdz, G., Identification of behaviourally significant volatile compounds in the anal gland of the rabbit, *Oryctolagus cuniculus, J. Chem. Ecol.*, 4, 581, 1978.
41. Goodrich, B. S., Gambale, S., Pennycuik, P. R., and Redhead, T. D., Volatiles from the faeces of wild male house mice: chemistry and effects on behavior and heart rate, *J. Chem. Ecol.*, 16, 2091, 1990.
42. Kavaliers, M. and Colwell, D. D., Aversive responses of female mice to the odors of parasitized males; neuromodulatory mechanisms and implications for mate choice, *Ethology*, 95, 202, 1993.
43. Novotny, M., Jemiolo, B., and Harvey, S., Chemistry of rodent pheromones: molecular insights into chemical signalling in mammals, in *Chemical Signals in Vertebrates,* Vol. 5, Macdonald, D. W., Müller-Schwarze, D., and Natynczuk, S. E., Eds., Oxford University Press, Oxford, 1990, 1.
44. Schwende, F. J., Wiesler, D., Jorgenson, J. W., Carmack, M., and Novotny, M., Urinary volatile constituents of the house mouse, *Mus musculus*, and their endocrine dependency, *J. Chem. Ecol.*, 12, 277, 1986.

45. Novotny, M., Schwende, F., Wiesler, D., Jorgenson, J. W., and Carmack, M., Identification of a testosterone-dependent unique volatile constituent in male mouse urine: 7-*exo*-ethyl-5-methyl-6,8-dioxaloicyclo[3.2.1]-3-octane, *Experientia*, 40, 217, 1984.
46. Novotny, M., Harvey, S., and Jemiolo, B., Chemistry of male dominance in the house mouse, *Mus musculus, Experientia*, 46, 109, 1990.
47. Novotny, M., Jemiolo, B., Harvey, S., Wiesler, D., and Marchlewska-Koj, A., Adrenal-mediated endogenous metabolites inhibit puberty in female mice, *Science*, 231, 722, 1986.
48. Jemiolo, B. and Novotny, M., Inhibition of sexual maturation in juvenile female and male mice by a chemosignal of female origin, *Physiol. Behav.*, 55, 519, 1994.
49. Drickamer, L. C., Urinary chemosignals from mice (*Mus musculus*); acceleration and delay of puberty in related and unrelated young females, *J. Comp. Psychol.,* 89, 414, 1984.
50. Jemiolo, B., Harvey, S., and Novotny, M., Puberty-affecting synthetic analogs of urinary chemosignals in the house mouse, *Mus musculus, Physiol. Behav.*, 46, 293, 1989.
51. Jemiolo, B., Gubernick, D. J., Yoder, M. C., and Novotny, M., Chemical characterization of urinary volatile compounds of *Peromyscus californicus*, a monogamous biparental rodent, *J. Chem. Ecol.,* 20, 2489, 1994.
52. Yamazaki, K., Beauchamp, G. K., Imai, Y., Bard, J., Thomas, L., and Boyse, E. A., MHC control of odortypes in the mouse, in *Chemical Signals in Vertebrates,* Vol. 6, Doty, R. L. and Müller-Schwarze, D., Eds., Plenum Press, New York, 1992, 189.
53. Beauchamp, G. K., Yamazaki, K., Curran, M., Bard, J., and Boyse, E. A., Fetal H-2 odortypes are evident in the urine of pregnant female mice, *Immunogenetics*, 39, 109, 1994.
54. Brown, R. E. and Schellinck, H. M., Interactions among the MHC, diet and bacteria in the production of social odors in rodents, in *Chemical Signals in Vertebrates,* Vol. 6, Doty, R. L. and Müller-Schwarze, D., Eds., Plenum Press, New York, 1992, 175.
55. Ferstl, R., Eggert, F., Westphal, E., Zavazava, N., and Muller-Ruchholtz, W., MHC-related odors in humans, in *Chemical Signals in Vertebrates,* Vol. 6, Doty, R. L. and Müller-Schwarze, D., Eds., Plenum Press, New York, 1992, 205.
56. Leon, M., Development of olfactory attraction by young Norway rats, in *Chemical Signals; Vertebrates and Aquatic Invertebrates*, Müller-Schwarze, D. and Silverstein, R. M., Eds., Plenum Press, New York, 1980, 193.
57. Moltz, H. and Lee, T. M., The maternal pheromone of the rat; identity and functional significance, *Physiol. Behav.,* 26, 301, 1981.
58. Schleidt, M., The semiotic relevance of human olfaction: a biological approach, in *Fragrance, the Psychology and Biology of Perfume*, Van Toller, S. and Dodd, G. H., Eds., Elsevier Applied Science, London, 1992, 37.
59. Labows, J. N. and Preti, G., Human semiochemicals, in *Fragrance, the Psychology and Biology of Perfume*, Van Toller, S. and Dodd, G. H., Eds., Elsevier Applied Science, London, 1992, 69.
60. Porter, R. H., Balogh, R. D., and Makin, J. W., Olfactory influences on mother-infant interactions, in *Advances in Infancy Research*, Vol. 5, Rovee-Collier, C. and Lipsitt, L. P., Eds., Ablex, Norwood, NJ, 1988, 39.
61. Gower, D. B., Quantitation of odorous 16-androstene steroids in vertebrates, in *Chemical Signals in Vertebrates,* Vol. 5, Macdonald, D. W., Müller-Schwarze, D., and Natynczuk, S. E., Eds., Oxford University Press, Oxford, 1990, 34.
62. Baydar, A., Petrzilka, M., and Scott, M.-P., Olfactory thresholds for androstenone and galaxolide: sensitivity, insensitivity and specific anosmia, *Chem. Senses,* 18, 661, 1993.
63. Grammer, K., 5-Alpha-androst-16-en-3-alpha-one — a male pheromone? — a brief report, *Ethology Sociobiol.*, 14, 201, 1993.
64. Gower, D. B., Holland, K. T., Mallet, A. I., Rennie, P. J., and Watkins, W. J., Comparison of 16-androstene steroid concentrations in sterile apocrine sweat and axillary secretions — interconversions of 16-androstenes by the axillary microflora — a mechanism for axillary odour production in man, *J. Steroid Biochem. Mol. Biol.*, 48, 409, 1994.
65. Zeng, X.-N., Leyden, J. J., Brand, J. G., Spielman, A. I., McGinley, K. J., and Preti, G., An investigation of human apocrine gland secretion for axillary odor precursors, *J. Chem. Ecol.*, 18, 1039, 1992.
66. Zeng, X.-N., Leyden, J. J., Lawley, H. J., Sawano, K., Nohara, I., and Preti, G., Analysis of characteristic odors from human male axillae, *J. Chem. Ecol.*, 17, 1469, 1991.

67. Bullard, R. W., Wild canid associations with fermentation products, *I&EC Prod. Res. Dev.*, 21, 646, 1982.
68. Abbott, D. H., Baines, D. A., Faulkes, C. G., Jennens, D. C., Ning, P. C. Y. K., and Tomlinson, A. J., A natural deer repellent: chemistry and behaviour, in *Chemical Signals in Vertebrates,* Vol. 5, Macdonald, D. W., Müller-Schwarze, D., and Natynczuk, S. E., Eds., Oxford University Press, Oxford, 1990, 599.
69. Baines, D. A., Faulkes, C. G., Tomlinson, A. J., and Ning, P. C. Y. K., European Patent Application 0,280,443, 1988.
70. Boag, B. and Mlotkiewicz, J. A., Effect of odor derived from lion faeces on behavior of wild rabbits, *J. Chem. Ecol.*, 20, 631, 1994.
71. Sullivan, T. P. and Crump, D. R., Influence of mustelid scent-gland compounds on suppression of feeding by snowshoe hares, J. *Chem. Ecol.*, 10, 1809, 1984.
72. Zimmerling, L. M. and Sullivan, T. P., Influence of mustelid semiochemicals on population dynamics of the deer mouse *(Peromyscus maniculatus), J. Chem. Ecol.*, 20, 667, 1994.
73. Weldon, P. J., Graham, D. P., and Mears, L. P., Carnivore fecal chemicals suppress feeding by alpine goats *(Capra hircus), J. Chem. Ecol.,* 19, 2947, 1993.
74. Swihart, R. K., Pignatello, J. J., and Mattina, M. J. I., Aversive responses of white-tailed deer, *Odocoileus virginianus*, to predator urines, *J. Chem. Ecol.*, 17, 767, 1991.
75. Nolte, D. L., Mason, J. R., Epple, G., Aronov, E., and Campbell, D. L., Why are predator urines aversive to prey?, *J. Chem. Ecol.*, 20, 1505, 1994.

22 Sense Of Smell: Signal Recognition And Transduction In Olfactory Receptor Neurons

Heinz Breer

CONTENTS

22.1 INTRODUCTION

Artificial olfactory devices are expected in the future to replace or complement human sensory tests in many fields of food, drink, cosmetic, and environmental control. Mimicking the biological mechanisms of olfaction is considered a promising approach for constructing artificial odor-sensing systems. Our sense of smell is able to recognize and discriminate extraneous volatile compounds of diverse molecular structure with high sensitivity and accuracy. Certain odorants are detected at concentrations as low as a few parts per trillion and thousands of distinct odors, even stereoisomeric compounds, are discriminated. The recognition of odorants and the primary events of olfactory signal transduction occur in the cilia of olfactory receptor neurons; the cilia, extruding from the dendritic knob, are considered as scaffolding for the chemosensory membrane, providing a large expansion of the surface area.

0-8493-8905-4/97/$0.00+$.50
© 1997 by CRC Press, Inc.

Upon interaction between odorous ligands and specific receptor proteins a multistep reaction cascade is initiated which amplifies the olfactory signal and ultimately leads to the electrical response of the sensory neurons, thus converting the strength, duration, and quality of odorant stimuli into distinct patterns of neuronal signals (Figure 22.1). The information of an odorous stimulus encoded as a pattern of neuronal activity is conveyed to and processed in the olfactory bulb and in higher brain centers.[1,2]

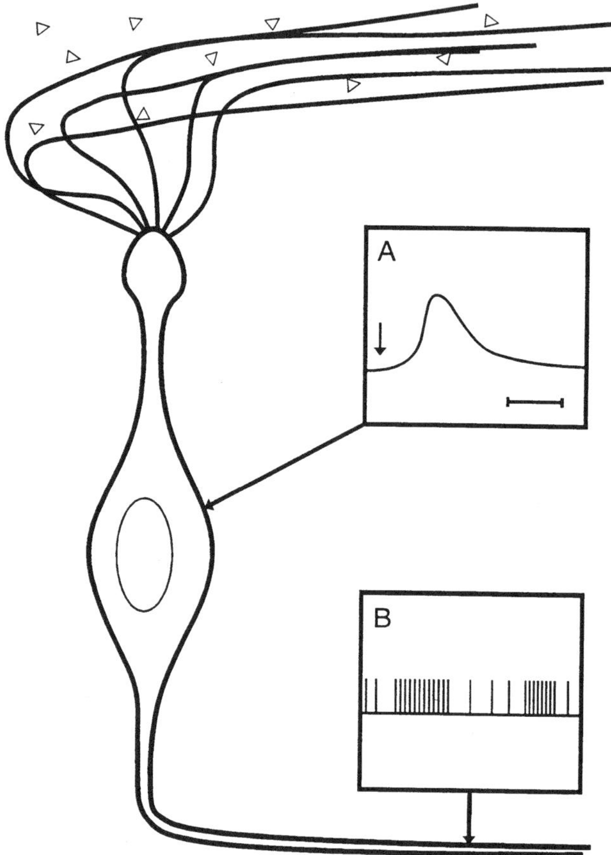

FIGURE 22.1 Chemo-electrical signal transduction in olfactory neurons. Olfactory neurons recognize small, volatile molecules by means of specific receptor proteins located in the ciliary membrane. In a multistep reaction the olfactory signal is converted into a generator potential and ultimately into a frequence of action potentials. Thus, the quality, strength, and duration of odor stimuli are translated into distinct patterns of neuronal activity.

To elucidate the complex molecular machinery mediating the chemo-electrical transduction process in olfactory receptor neurons, the main principles common to transduction operations of most sensory modalities include detection and discrimination, amplification and encoding of the signal, as well as termination and adaptation of the transduction process and these are currently under extensive investigation.

22.2 PERIRECEPTOR EVENTS

The process of olfaction in air-breathing vertebrates begins when volatile odorous molecules are inhaled; the inspired air contains low concentrations of hydrophobic odorants that must traverse an aqueous medium, the mucus layer covering the nasal epithelium, before contacting the chemosensory membrane of olfactory neurons. Processes that influence the entry, exit, or residence time of odorant molecules in the receptor vicinity have been termed perireceptor events.[3] These auxiliary processes include translocation of hydrophobic odorants to their receptor sites as well as inactivation of chemostimulants by enzyme-catalyzed degradation or biotransformation.[4]

22.2.1 Odorant Binding Proteins

The discovery that the nasal mucus contains abundant small, water-soluble proteins which are homologous to carrier proteins for hydrophobic ligands in other body fluids (lipocalins) and which bind odorants, has led to the concept that these odorant binding proteins (OBPs) accommodate hydrophobic molecules in solution and shuttle the odorant towards the chemosensory cilia (Figure 22.2).[5] In addition, it is conceivable that OBPs may play a dual role, as binders of chemostimulants and as initiators of the signal transduction process.[4] Alternatively, it is also a possibility that OBPs may act as scavengers by binding and thereby inactivating odorant molecules. Despite the general agreement that OBPs are important components in the olfactory signaling process, their exact functional role is still elusive. The recent observation that multiple OBPs are expressed in rats supports the notion that binding proteins may be involved in discriminating groups of hydrophobic, volatile molecules.[6]

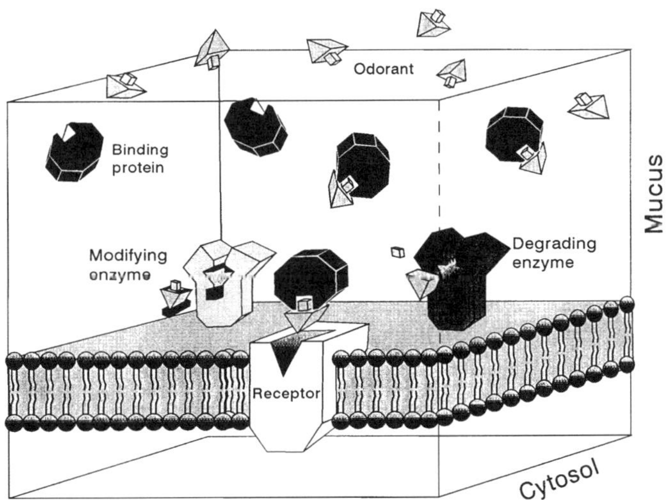

FIGURE 22.2 Perireceptor events. Odorant molecules are thought to be transferred to the receptor sites by means of soluble binding proteins located in the mucus layer. The hydrophobic ligands are inactivated by degrading and/or biotransformation enzymes.

Multiple isoforms of odorant binding proteins have also been discovered in the sensillum lymph of insect antennae.[7,8] In fact, it has been suggested that the acquisition of OBPs may represent one of the molecular adaptions that animals evolved to cope with the terrestrial life style. Interestingly, OBPs from vertebrates and insects display virtually no significant homology in their primary structure; this observation favours the view that vertebrates and insects evolved binding proteins for odorants independently; i.e., OBPs in both phyla represent an evolutionary convergence.

22.2.2 Biotransformation Enzymes

In order to maintain sensitivity for reiterated stimuli of external odors, it is essential that animals can distinguish between what has just been smelled from what is about to be smelled; residual odorant molecules solubilized in the mucus and lipid membrane must rapidly be eliminated in order to recognize new incoming odorant molecules (odorant clearance). Inactivation of odorants displaying a broad spectrum of chemical configurations may be accomplished by the concerted action of biotransformation or detoxification enzymes, which modify and neutralize hydrophobic compounds.[9] In fact, olfactory-specific isoforms of cytochrome P450 monooxygenase (phase I enzyme: introducing chemical changes such as hydroxylation) and UDP glucuronosyl transferase (phase II enzyme: catalyzing conjugation of the phase I-activated compounds with glucuronic acid) have been identified recently.[10] Furthermore, it has been demonstrated that glucuronation of odorants indeed diminishes their ability to stimulate adenylate cyclase in olfactory cilia (Figure 22.2).[10]

22.3 ODORANT RECEPTORS

22.3.1 Recognition and Discrimination of Odorous Ligands

After traversing the mucus layer, odorants reach the chemosensory ciliary membrane of olfactory neurons and elicit an electrical response in a subset of these cells. The reactive neurons are apparently most sensitive for a given odorant. The olfactory system responds to a vast number and variety of volatile compounds;[1] most of them are foreign molecules which are evolutionarily "unknown" to the organism until they are encountered for the first time. Nevertheless, they are readily detected and discriminated. The inherent molecular problems in recognizing and discriminating myriads of foreign compounds appear to be analogous to those of the immune system. Two alternative principles that may underlie the discrimination of odorous molecules have been discussed. By analogy with color vision, specificity of odor detection may be based on only a few receptor types each reacting with a wide range of odorants; alternatively, by analogy with the immune system and the large antibody repertoire there might be thousands of distinct receptors, each specialized for one or a small number of odorants. In the latter case, much of the discrimination between odors may occur in the periphery and thus alleviate input processing in the brain. Unraveling the nature as well as the diversity and specificity of receptors for odorants has long been considered as crucial for understanding the fundamental mechanisms of olfaction.

22.3.2 Molecular Cloning of Genes Encoding Odorant Receptors

The notion that G-protein-coupled transduction cascades play a central role in olfactory transduction has led to the concept that receptors for odorants might be members of the G-protein-linked receptor superfamily.[2] Employing conventional biochemical approaches has led to the discovery of interesting proteins; however, none of them met the criteria of odorant receptors. A breakthrough was achieved when Buck and Axel[11] discovered a novel gene family encoding polypeptides with seven hydrophobic domains that were considered as candidate odorant receptors. The new receptors display all hallmarks of the G-protein-coupled receptor superfamily, but also have some unique motifs. Most notably they appear to be minimal in structure with very short cytoplasmic and extracellular loops; in addition, there is a striking structural diversity in the third, fourth, and fifth transmembrane domains which are supposed to form the hydrophobic core of these proteins; these regions are thought to form the ligand binding site of the receptors (Figure 22.3). In their pioneering study, Buck and Axel found that expression of the receptors appears to be restricted to olfactory epithelium and genomic analyses revealed a surprisingly large number of genes encoding these receptors;

this novel multigene family seems to comprise several hundreds or even thousands of homologous genes.

Meanwhile, numerous members of this new receptor family have been identified in various species including rat,[11-13] mice,[14,15] fish,[16] and also in human.[9,17,18] Their large number, and the fact that these newly discovered genes are only expressed in the olfactory epithelium, were considered as a hint that they may encode the long-sought odorant receptors. This view was strongly substantiated by *in situ* hybridization experiments demonstrating that these receptor proteins are indeed expressed in the actual olfactory receptor neurons.[13,15,16,19]

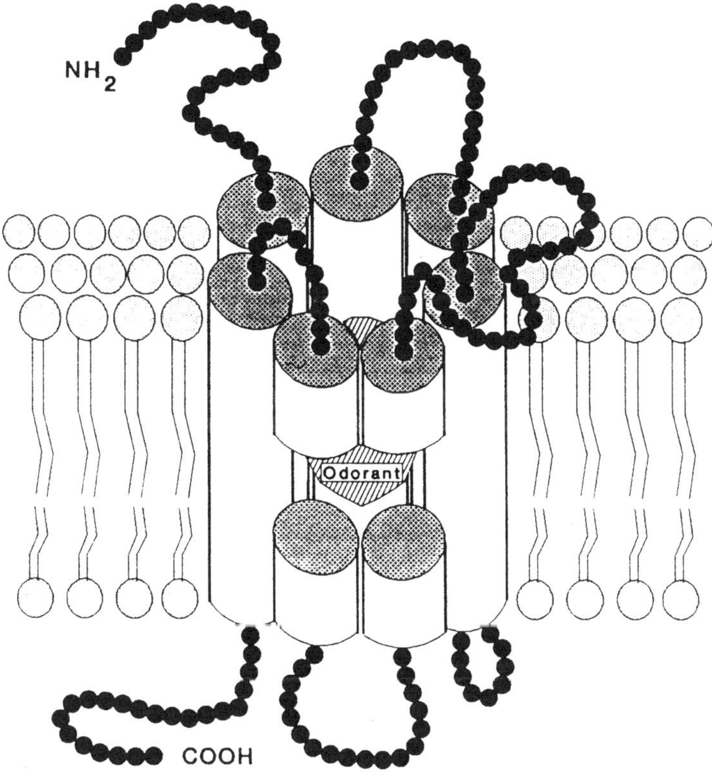

FIGURE 22.3 Model structure of odorant receptors. Odorant receptors identified by molecular cloning approaches are members of the G-protein-coupled receptor superfamily. The polypeptide contains seven hydrophobic domains which are thought to span the membrane and form the binding site for the odorous ligands.

22.3.3 Heterologous Expression of Odorant Receptors

The rigorous proof that the genes indeed encode the receptors for odorous molecules can only be provided by functional expression of receptor-encoding complementary DNA in surrogate cells demonstrating that the polypeptide products can mediate odorant activation of G-protein pathways. The baculovirus-Sf9 cell system was chosen for a heterologous expression of odorant receptor genes. Upon extensive screening to find suitable odorous ligands, it could be demonstrated that receptor proteins expressed in Sf9 cells interact and in turn are activated by certain odorants and functionally couple to the second-messenger cascade of host cells.[13] The graded response to several out of a set of odors indicates that this receptor has a relatively broad but selective ligand specificity. This observation is in line with previous suggestions that olfactory neurons may express only one receptor type, but nonetheless respond to different odorants.[2] Functional expression of odorant receptors may eventually allow successful reconstitution of the complete olfactory signaling cascade in surrogate cells; thus it could provide novel approaches to exploring the functional role of each molecular element in signal recognition and transduction. A functional characterization of an array of receptors will reveal if individual receptors are broadly or narrowly tuned for certain odors, and which type of G-proteins/second-messenger pathways they activate.

Questions concerning the genomic organization of the large family of genes encoding the odorant receptors and the factors that may regulate the expression of defined subsets of these genes in individual olfactory neurons are of great interest and under intensive investigation.[9,20,21]

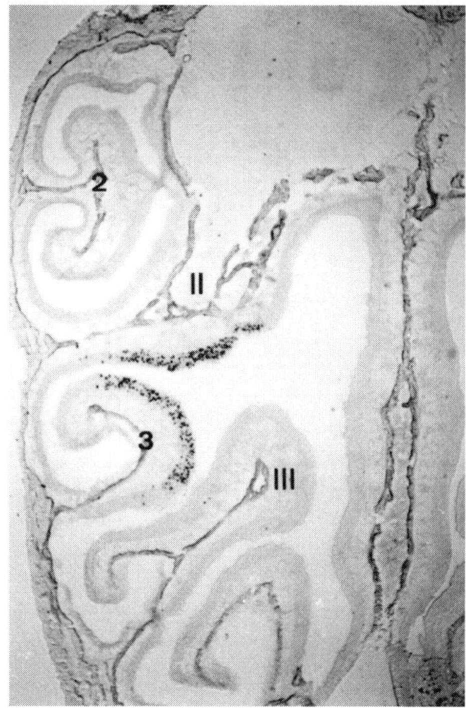

FIGURE 22.4 Zonal expression patterns of receptor types. Olfactory neurons expressing distinct receptor subtypes are spatially segregated in defined zones of the olfactory epithelium. Whether the resulting topographic patterns of chemosensory cells have functional implications for odor coding or are due to developmental processes is unclear.

22.3.4 Spatial Patterns of Receptor Expression in the Olfactory Epithelium

Perception of odorants encountered by an organism requires the identification of that subset of receptor neurons which responds to a given odorant. The position of individual cells in the nasal neuroepithelium and/or their projection patterns to the olfactory bulb may be used to identify the responsive neurons.[22-24] The identification of the odorant receptor genes has provided molecular probes which allow us to explore if olfactory neurons expressing a specific receptor type are spatially segregated in the olfactory epithelium. Recent studies on different species employing a limited number of receptor probes led to quite divergent results. In catfish olfactory epithelium no discernible pattern of receptor expression was observed.[25] In mice, the distribution of odorant receptor mRNA suggests that the nasal cavity is divided into several expression zones, but with a random distribution of positive cells within a given zone.[15] In rat, very similar expression zones were observed (Figure 22.4);[19,26,26a] in addition, for one particular receptor type a spatial segregation of reactive cells in a very restricted region was found.[27] Whether these differences are due to species variations or represent some of many principles underlying the topographic organization of the chemosensory epithelium is now under investigation.

22.4 CHEMO-ELECTRICAL SIGNAL TRANSDUCTION

22.4.1 Second-Messenger Signaling

The primary events of odor detection occur in the olfactory cilia extending from the dendritic knob of receptor neurons. Procedures for isolating olfactory cilia have greatly facilitated molecular studies of olfaction, as much as retinal rods have contributed to the investigation of phototransduction. Olfactory cilia preparations possess high levels of adenylate cyclase which is stimulated by certain odorants in a GTP-dependent (GTP: guanosine triphosphate) manner.[28,29] These observations have led to the concept that cAMP (cyclic adenosine monophosphate; of major metabolic importance through its multiple effects as intracellular messenger controlling enzymes and ion channels) may play a key role in olfactory signal transduction. This view was further consolidated by the discovery of a cyclic nucleotide-gated ion channel in the membrane of olfactory cilia.[30] Furthermore, employing molecular cloning approaches has led to the identification of olfactory-specific isoforms of elements forming the cAMP cascade: a specific G-protein "G_{olf}",[31] an olfactory adenylate cyclase designated "adenylate cyclase III",[32] and an olfactory cyclic nucleotide-gated channel.[33-35] The reason why olfactory neurons express specific rather than conventional isoforms of these proteins is still unclear. It has been suggested that these subtypes may contribute to a high signal-to-noise ratio for signal amplification.[32]

22.4.2 Kinetics of Second-Messenger Responses

Although most of the molecular elements essential for the cAMP cascade were identified and enzyme activity measurements implicated that cAMP may be involved in the transduction process, it was a matter of debate whether stimulation of cyclase activity really resulted in a significant buildup of second-messenger levels and whether the kinetics would be fast enough to elicit the electrical response of olfactory receptor neurons which occurs in the subsecond time range. These problems were approached by using a rapid quench technique to monitor the odorant-induced formation of cAMP in isolated cilia preparations in the subsecond time course. Application of odorants, such as isomenthon or citralva, elicited a rapid elevation of cAMP levels; a peak concentration, severalfold higher than the basal level, was reached after 50 ms. Thereafter, the concentration returned to prestimulated levels within a few hundred milliseconds (Figure 22.5).[36] This "pulse" of cAMP precedes the electrical response and thus could mediate the chemo-electrical transduction in receptor cells.

22.4.3 Dual Pathways of Olfactory Transduction

A survey of numerous odorous compounds indicated that all odorants that have previously been shown to activate adenylate cyclase[29] induced a rapid cAMP response; odorants that failed to elicit cyclic nucleotide accumulation produced another second-messenger response; those odorants induced an increase in inositol-1,4,5-trisphosphate (IP_3), instead.[37] The odorant-induced IP_3 signals displayed similar rapid kinetics; the transient "pulse" of IP_3 also precedes a typical electrical response. Although IP_3-gated ion channels have been discovered in the plasma membrane of olfactory neurons from various species.[38,39] Understanding exactly how the intracellular IP_3 signal is propagated and converted into an electrical response of the cell requires further investigation. Assaying a whole range of odorants on isolated cilia indicated that odorants may be categorized into one of two classes, each class activating a

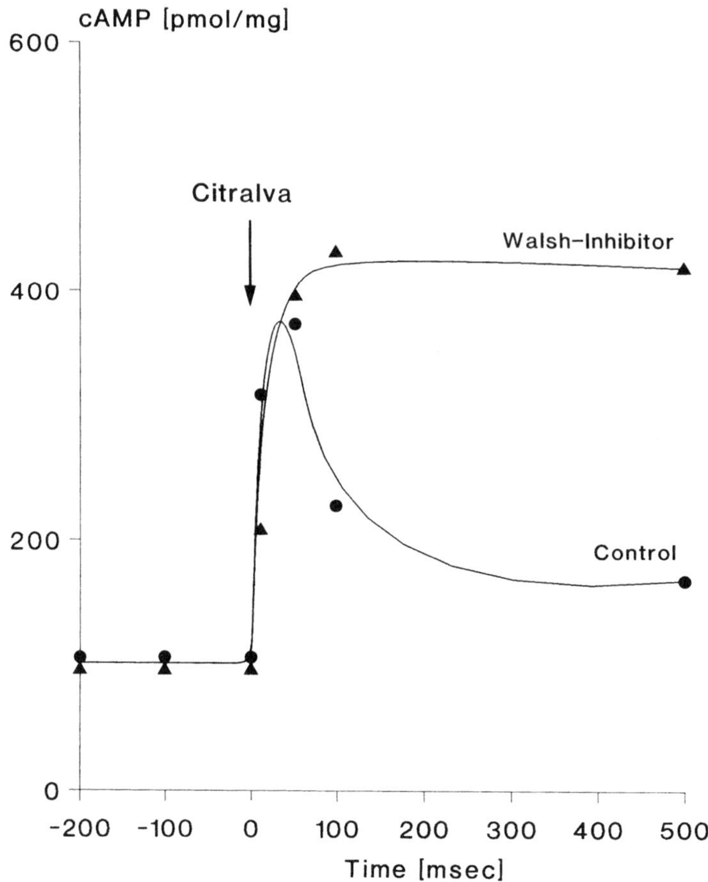

FIGURE 22.5 Kinetics of odorant-induced second-messenger responses. Stimulation of isolated olfactory cilia with low odor doses elicits a rapid and transient elevation of second-messenger concentration, e.g., cAMP. The signaling cascade is turned off by second-messenger controlled protein kinase in a negative feedback reaction.

different transduction pathway;[40] however, a recent study indicates that in cultured receptor cells a given odorant may activate both pathways.[41]

The notion that two alternative pathways for the chemo-electrical transduction of olfactory stimuli exist opens the way for new concepts towards an understanding of olfactory sensory processing. Coexistence of both pathways within the same receptor cell raises the possibility of an efficient interaction between the two systems, thus providing the potential for considerable positive and negative "cross talk" which would affect the generation of electric responses (Figure 22.6). The existence of two alternative transduction cascades would be of particular relevance if they could be related to the observed alternative excitatory or inhibitory response of olfactory neurons to odor stimulation.[42] Such a correlation has recently been clearly demonstrated in elegant studies on olfactory cells from lobster, where the cAMP system mediates hyperpolarization and inhibitory responses, whereas the IP_3 pathway leads to depolarization and excitatory responses.[39] There is some preliminary evidence suggesting that in vertebrates the functional role of the two second-messengers may be reverse: cAMP evokes an inward current and as a result excites the cell, whereas IP_3 evokes an outward current and thereby inhibits the spontaneous activity of the cell.[43] In any case, a convergent integration of different odor stimuli may already begin at the level of primary reactions in the olfactory receptor cells.

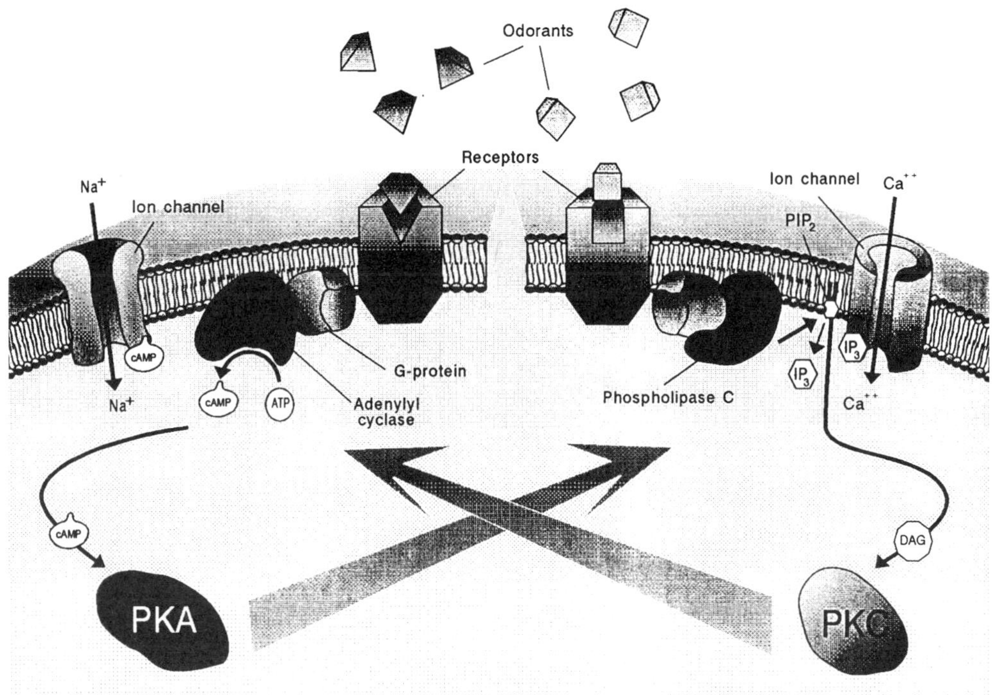

FIGURE 22.6 Dual pathways of olfactory signal transduction. The process of chemo-electrical signal transduction in olfactory neurons is mediated by second-messenger cascades. Interaction of odorous molecules with specific receptor proteins elicits the generation of cAMP or IP_3 signals. Cross-talk between the two pathways may provide a first step for convergent integration of olfactory information.

22.4.4 Termination of Olfactory Signaling (Desensitization)

An essential prerequisite for the precise reaction of chemosensory neurons to iterative stimulation is the characteristic phasic response of the cells. The basis for this characteristic feature is a rapid termination of the odor-induced primary reaction, i.e., the second-messenger cascade initiated by an odorant-activated receptor is rapidly turned off. This is reflected in the kinetics of odorant-induced rapid and transient second-messenger response. The "turning off" reaction cannot be attributed to odorant inactivation or to activation of catabolic enzymes[44] but rather resembles the waning of second-messenger responses to cell-surface receptor activation in other cells (desensitization). This feature, common to many forms of transmembrane signaling, has been attributed to phosphorylation of liganded receptor proteins.[45] Recent studies employing specific kinase inhibitors have indicated that, in the olfactory system, termination of the odorant-induced primary reaction involves a kinase which is stimulated by the second messengers generated in the active cascade. Switching off the cAMP-generating cascade involves protein kinase A (PKA); the pathway producing IP_3 and DAG (diacylglycerol) is controlled by protein kinase C (PKC) (Figure 22.5).[46]

In an extensive study it has previously been shown that specific ciliary polypeptides are rapidly and transiently phosphorylated upon odorant stimulation. Autoradiographic analysis suggested that the polypeptides which were labeled during odorant stimulation may in fact be the receptors for odorants.[47] This notion was recently confirmed by using receptor-specific antipeptide antibodies which allowed immunoprecipitation of the phosphorylated proteins.[48] Thus, the emerging picture suggests that the rapid "turn off" reaction for the olfactory transduction cascade is in line with desensitization in other signaling systems.

22.5 CONCLUSION

Recent studies have led to a more refined understanding of olfactory neurons and the mechanisms involved in odor detection. The collaborative efforts of electrophysiologists and biochemists have elucidated that olfactory receptor neurons accomplish their task of odorant recognition and chemo-electrical signal transduction by recruiting molecular elements common to many other transmembrane signaling systems. Second messengers provide the critical link between the initial odor recognition and the elicitation of generator currents in olfactory receptor cells. Upon interaction of odorous molecules with specific receptors in the chemosensory membrane of olfactory neurons, key enzymes of second-messenger pathways are activated via specific G-proteins, leading to a rapid and transient signal of either cAMP or IP_3. These second-messenger "pulses" are thought to increase the membrane permeability by activation of specific ion channels. Whether multiple signaling pathways are operating in individual receptor neurons is still elusive; however, the diversity of signaling mechanisms allows complex cross-talk reactions which may contribute to the processing of olfactory stimuli in receptor cells. Termination of odor-induced responses is apparently brought about by uncoupling the reaction cascades via kinases catalyzing the phosphorylation of activated odorant receptors. The phosphorylated/dephosphorylated status of odorant receptors controlled by kinase/phosphatase systems may be involved in fine-tuning the sensitivity of olfactory receptor cells. The availability of DNA clones encoding specific elements of the chemosensory transduction apparatus now allows expression of the specialized proteins in surrogate cells; this is considered as a first step towards a functional reconstitution of the complete olfactory cascade. This new information is considered as advantageous in designing artificial olfactory devices which may allow efficient and reliable monitoring of important volatile compounds.

ACKNOWLEDGMENT

The work of this laboratory was supported by the Deutsche Forschungsgemeinschaft.

REFERENCES

1. Getchell, T. V., Functional properties of vertebrate olfactory receptor neurons, *Physiol. Rev.*, 66, 772, 1986.
2. Lancet, D., Vertebrate olfactory reception, *Annu. Rev.* 9, 329, 1986.
3. Getchell, T. V., Margolis, F. L., and Getchell, M. L., Perireceptor and receptor events in vertebrate olfaction, *Prog. Neurobiol.*, 23, 317, 1984.
4. Carr, W. E. S., Gleeson, R. A., and Trapido-Rosenthal, H. G., The role of perireceptor events in chemosensory processes, *Trends Neurosci.*, 13, 212, 1990.
5. Pevsner, J. and Snyder, S. H., Odorant binding protein: odorant transport function in the nasal epithelium, *Chem. Senses*, 15, 217, 1990.
6. Dear, T. N., Boehm, T., Keverne, E. B., and Rabbitts, T. H., Novel genes for potential ligand binding proteins in subregions of the olfactory mucosa, *EMBO J.*, 10, 2813, 1991.
7. Krieger, J., Raming, K., and Breer, H., Cloning of genomic and complementary DNA encoding insect pheromone binding proteins: evidence for microdiversity, *Biochim. Biophys. Acta*, 1088, 277, 1991.
8. Vogt, R. G., Prestwich, G. D., and Lermer, M. R., Odorant-binding-protein subfamilies associate with distinct classes of olfactory receptor neurons in insects, *J. Neurobiol.*, 22, 74, 1991.
9. Lancet, D., Gross-Isseroff, R., Margalit, T., Seidemann, E., and Ben-Arie, N., Olfaction: from signal transduction and termination to human genome mapping, *Chem. Senses*, 18, 217, 1993.
10. Lazard, D., Zupko, K., Poria, Y., Nef, P., Lazarovits, J., Horn, S., Khen, M., and Lancet, D., Odorant signal termination by olfactory UDP-glucuronosyl transferase, *Nature*, 349, 790, 1991.

11. Buck, L. and Axel, R., A novel multigene family may encode odorant receptors: a molecular basis for odor recognition, *Cell,* 65, 175, 1991.
12. Levy, N. S., Bakalyar, H. A., and Reed, R. R., Signal transduction in olfactory neurons, *J. Steroid Biochem. Mol. Biol.*, 39, 633, 1991.
13. Raming, K., Krieger, J., Strotmann, J., Boekhoff, I., Kubick, S., Baumstark, C., and Breer, H., Cloning and expression of odorant receptors, *Nature*, 361, 353, 1993.
14. Nef, P., Hermans-Borgmeyer, I., Artieres-Pin, H., Beasley, L., Dionne, V. E., and Heinemann, S. F., Spatial pattern of receptor expression in the olfactory epithelium, *Proc. Natl. Acad. Sci. U.S.A.*, 89, 8948, 1992.
15. Ressler, K. J., Sullivan, S. L., and Buck, L. B., Azonal organization of odorant receptor gene expression in the olfactory epithelium, *Cell*, 73, 597, 1993.
16. Ngai, J., Dowling, M. M., Buck, L., Axel, R., and Chess, A., The family of genes encoding odorant receptors in the channel catfish, *Cell*, 72, 657, 1993.
17. Reed, R. R., Mechanisms of sensitivity and specificity in olfaction, *Cold Spring Harbor Symp. Quant. Bio.*, 57, 501, 1992.
18. Schurmans, S., Muscatelli, F., Miot, F., Mattei, M. G., Vassart, G., and Parmentier, M., The OLFR1 gene encoding the HGMPO7E putative olfactory receptor maps to the 17p13-p12 region of the human genome and revals an Mspl restriction fragment length polymorphism, *Cytogenet. Cell Genet.*, 63, 200,1993.
19. Vassar, R., Ngai, J., and Axel, R., Spatial segregation of odorant receptor expression in the olfactory epithelium, *Cell*, 73, 597, 1993.
20. Margolis, F. L., Regulation of olfactory neuron gene expression, *Cytotechnology*, 11, 17, 1993.
21. Wang, M. M. and Reed, R. R., Coordinate regulation of olfactory neuronal gene expression, *Chem. Senses*, 18, 199, 1993.
22. Mackay-Sim, A., Shaman, P., and Moulton, D. G., Topographic coding of olfactory quality: odorant specific patterns of epithelial responsivity in the salamander, *J. Neurophysiol.* 48, 584, 1982.
23. Kauer, J. S., Contributions of topography and parallel processing to odor coding in the vertebrate olfactory pathway, *Trends Neurosci.*, 14, 79, 1991.
24. Shepherd, G. M., Computational structure of the olfactory system, in *Olfaction: A Model System for Computational Neuroscience*, Davis, J. L. and Eichbaum, H., Eds., MIT Press, Cambridge, 1991, 3.
25. Ngai, J., Chess, A., Dowling, M. M., Necles, N., Macgno, E. R., and Axel, R., Coding of olfactory information: topography of odorant expression in the catfish olfactory ephithelium, *Cell*, 72, 667, 1993.
26. Strotmann, J., Wanner, I., Helfrich, T., Beck, A., Meinken, C., Kubick, S., and Breer, H., Olfactory neuron expressing distinct odorant receptors subtypes are spatially segregated in the nasal neuroepithelium, *Cell Tissue Res.* 276, 429, 1994.
26a. Strotmann, J., Wanner, I., Helfrich, T., Beck, A., and Breer, H., Rostro-caudal patterning of receptor-expressing olfactory neurones in the rat nasal cavity. *Cell Tissue Res.*, 278, 11, 1994.
27. Strotmann, J., Wanner, I., Krieger, J., Raming, K., and Breer, H., Expression of odorant receptors in spatially restricted subsets of chemosensory neurons, *NeuroReport*, 3, 1053, 1992.
28. Pace, U., Hanski, E., Salomon, Y., and Lancet, D., Odorant-sensitive adenylate cyclase may mediate olfactory reception, *Nature*, 325, 442, 1986.
29. Sklar, P. D., Anholt, R. H., and Snyder, S. H., The odorant-sensitive adenylate cyclase of olfactory receptor cells: different stimulation by distinct classes of odorants, *J. Biol.Chem.*, 261, 15538, 1986.
30. Nakamura, T. and Gold, G. H., A cyclic-nucleotide gated conductance in olfactory receptor cilia, *Nature*, 325, 442, 1987.
31. Jones, D. T. and Reed, R. R., G_{olf}: an olfactory neuron specific G-protein involved in odorant signal transduction, *Science*, 244, 790, 1989.
32. Bakalyar, H. A. and Reed, R. R., Identification of a specialized adenylate cyclase that may mediate odorant detection, *Science*, 250, 1403, 1990.
33. Dhallan, R. S., Yau, K. W., Schrader, K. A., and Reed, R. R., Primary structure and functional expression of a cylic nucleotide-activated channel from olfactory neurons, *Nature*, 347, 184, 1990.

34. Ludwig, J., Margalit, T., Eismann, E., Lancet, D., and Kaupp, U. B., Primary structure of cAMP-gated channel from bovine olfactory epithelium, *FEBS Lett.*, 270, 24, 1990.
35. Goulding, E. H., Ngai, J., Kramer, R. H., Colicos, S., Axel, R., Siegelbaum, S. A., and Chess, A., Molecular cloning and single-channel properties of the cyclic nucleotide-gated channel from catfish olfactory neurons, *Neuron*, 8, 45, 1992.
36. Breer, H., Boekhoff, I., and Tareilus, E., Rapid kinetics of second messenger formation in olfactory transduction, *Nature*, 345, 65, 1990.
37. Boekhoff, I., Tareilus, E., Strotmann, J., and Breer, H., Rapid activation of alternative second messenger pathways in olfactory cilia from rats by different odorants, *EMBO J.*, 9, 2453, 1990.
38. Restrepo, D., Miyamoto, T., Bryant, B. P., and Teeter, J. H., Odor stimuli trigger influx of calcium into olfactory neurons of the channel catfish, *Science*, 249, 1166, 1990.
39. Fadool, D. A. and Ache, B. W., Plasma membrane inositol 1,4,5-trisphosphate-activated channels mediate signal transduction in lobster olfactory neurons, *Neuron*, 9, 907, 1992.
40. Breer, H. and Boekhoff, I., Odorants of the same odor class activate different second messenger pathways, *Chem. Senses*, 16, 19, 1991.
41. Ronnet, G. V., Cho, H., Hester, L. D., Wood, S. F., and Snyder, S. H., Odorants differentially enhance phosphoinosite turnover and adenylyl cyclase in olfactory receptor neuronal cultures, *J. Neurosci.*, 13, 1751, 1993.
42. Dionne, V. E., Chemosensory responses in isolated olfactory receptor neurons from *Necturus maculosus, J. Gen. Physiol.*, 99, 415, 1992.
43. Morales, B., Ugarte, G., Labarca, P., and Bacigalupo, J., Inhibitory K^+-current activated by odorants in toad olfactory neurons, *Proc. R. Soc. London Ser. B,* 257, 235, 1994.
44. Borisy, F. F., Ronnett, G. V., Cunningham, A. M., Juilfs, D., Beavo, J., and Snyder, S. H., Calcium/calmodulin-activated phosphodiesterase expressed in olfactory receptor neurons, *J. Neurosci.*, 12, 915, 1992.
45. Lefkowitz, R. J., Hausdorff, W. P., and Caron, M. G., Role of phosphorylation in desensitization of the β-adrenoreceptor, *Trends Pharmacol. Sci.*, 11, 190, 1990.
46. Boekhoff, I. and Breer, H., Termination of second messenger signaling in olfaction, *Proc. Natl. Acad. Sci. U.S.A.*, 89, 471, 1992.
47. Boekhoff, I., Schleicher, S., Strotmann, J., and Breer, H., Odor-induced phosphorylation of olfactory cilia proteins, *Proc. Natl. Acad. Sci. U.S.A.*, 89, 471, 1992
48. Krieger, J., Schleicher, S., Raming, K., Strotmann, J., Wanner, I., Boekhoff, I., de Geus, P., and Breer, H., Probing odorant receptors with sequence-specific antibodies, *Eur. J. Biochem.*, 219, 829, 1994.

23 Semiconductor and Calorimetric Sensor Devices and Arrays

Dieter Kohl

CONTENTS

0-8493-8905-4/97/$0.00+$.50
© 1997 by CRC Press, Inc.

23.1 INTRODUCTION

Metal oxides (MeO_x) semiconductor devices are already widely used as inexpensive and robust sensors for combustible and other hazardous gases and vapors in safety and automotive applications.[1] The material most frequently used in safety applications is SnO_2, but ZnO, In_2O_3, WO_3, Fe_2O_3 and Ga_2O_3 are also employed. These sensors rely on changes of conductance induced by adsorption of gases and by subsequent surface reactions. Typical operation temperatures are between 100 and 600°C, (Figure 23.1). Semiconducting oxygen probes operating at higher temperatures in the exhaust systems of cars (lambda probes) are made from TiO_2, Ga_2O_3, or titanates, and rely on bulk conductivity effects. No complex devices need to be constructed to apply these materials for gas sensing; a straightforward resistor configuration is sufficient in many cases. A heater needs to be incorporated, however, as the MeO_x semiconductor has to be kept at an elevated temperature to exhibit a reversible response to gases.

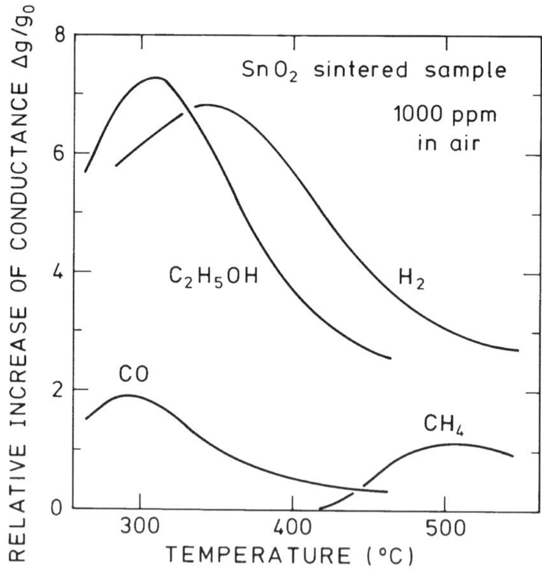

FIGURE 23.1 Sintered layer, thickness 0.05 mm, 0.05 wt% Sb. Relative increase of conductance by reducing gases as a function of temperature. (From Heiland, G. and Kohl, D., *Sensors Actuators*, 8, 227, 1985. With permission.)

In its simplest form, delivered in quantities of some million pieces per year, the MeO_x gas sensor consists of a sintered tin oxide pellet on a tubular heated ceramic former which also carries electrode tracks. The conductance of the MeO_x semiconductor changes in the presence of reducing or oxidizing gases. Some species detectible by oxidic sensors are listed in Table 23.1.

TABLE 23.1
Overview on Analyte Gases and Volatiles

Analyte	Device	Ref.
H_2	SnO_2 350°C thick film	2
H_2	SnO_2 400°C thick film	3
H_2	SnO_2 400°C Sol-Gel	4
H_2	SnO_2(SiO_2 on top) 600°C Sol-Gel	4
H_2	SnO_2 320°C thick film	5
H_2	SnO_2/Pt 150°C thick film	5
H_2	SnO_2/Pd 150°C thick film	5
H_2	SnO_2/Ag 80°C thick film	5
CH_4	SnO_2 500°C thick film	2
CH_4	SnO_2 600°C Sol-Gel	4
CH_4	SnO_2(SiO_2 on top) 400°C Sol-Gel	4
CH_4	SnO_2/Pt 300°C thick film	5
CH_4	SnO_2/Pd 380°C thick film	5
C_3H_8	SnO_2 380°C thick film	5
C_3H_8	SnO_2/Pt 280°C thick film	5
C_3H_8	SnO_2/Pd 260°C thick film	5
C_3H_8	SnO_2/Ag 360°C thick film	5
C_2H_5OH	SnO_2 300°C thick film	2
CH_3COOH	SnO_2 500°C sintered	2
CO	SnO_2 310°C CVD	9
CO	SnO_2 350°C thick film	5
CO	SnO_2/Pt <50°C thick film	5
CO_2	CuO/$BaTiO_3$ 450°C sintered	7
NO, NO_2	La_2CuO_4 400°C sintered	8
NO, NO_2	WO_3 300°C sintered	9
NH_3	In_2O_3/MgO/Ir 450°C thick film	3
$(CH_3)_3N$	TiO_2/In 400°C thick film	3
$(CH_3)_3N$ (TMA)	ZnO/Al 400°C sputtered	10
$(CH_3)_2HN$ (DMA)	ZnO/Al 450°C sputtered	10

The sensitivity and the specificity (ability to respond to a certain species in a gas mixture) of the device can be controlled to some extent by selecting the temperature at which the metal oxide is held. Even so, the specificity of the basic device remains, in general, broad, and the sensitivity does not reach that of more complex gas sensors such as the CHEMFET (see Chapter 6).

It was these broad, overlapping specificity characteristics of metal oxide sensors at differing temperatures that inspired devices mimicking some features of the animal nose. These odor meters (as they are known in their commercial form) consist of an array of two to ten metal oxide sensors held at temperatures selected to provide the desired overlapping response characteristics. Pattern recognition techniques are used in the interpretation of the multiple sensor signal.

Beyond the safety and automotive applications, applications in the food industry have been studied, for example, the monitoring of headspace alcohol concentrations in the brewing process. The reproducibility achieved with MeO_x devices manufactured with the simplest production procedures were, however, not satisfactory for applications demanding high accuracy.

The initial low-tech, cheap-and-cheerful image of the MeO_x devices has changed, however, through more sophisticated preparation procedures based on a better understanding of the device characteristics. These methods provide for enhanced reproducibility, sensitivity, and specificity, thereby opening up a wider range of applications.

Thin-film deposition techniques have improved the reproducibility and response time of MeO_x gas sensors, and the inclusion of catalyst additions such as palladium and controlled heat processing regimes were found to enhance the specificity and the sensitivity of the devices. Current research aims to characterize the function of such additions to the semiconductor material so as to tailor the device properties more closely.

Calorimetric devices are standard for the accurate measurement of explosives up to the lower explosion limit (LEL), usually 2 to 5%. Such precise measurements are of interest in plants; stopping a production process too early because of a small leakage causes a loss of money avoidable by precise monitoring. To guarantee safety, the sum of all concentrations of explosive gases and vapors has to be determined. An active catalyst for total oxidation kept at a sufficiently high temperature can perform the task.

Microcalorimetric sensors are often denoted as pellistors, because they consist typically of a ball (diameter 1 to 2 mm) of highly dispersed catalyst. The quiescent air covering the surface of the ball limits the gas access to the interior as a diffusion barrier. Thus all gas molecules traversing the diffusion barrier are burnt in the interior and contribute to the signal. A platinum coil embedded in the catalyst (Pt, Pd, or Rh, or mixtures) serves to heat the pellistor and also to monitor its temperature. Usually, an electrical circuit measures the resistance of the coil (proportional to its temperature) and adapts the electrical power to keep the temperature constant. The decrease of electrical power in the presence of reducing gases is proportional to the sum of concentrations of combustibles. The stable sensitivity is due to a physical effect, the proportionality of concentration outside the ball to the flux into its interior. Typically the catalyst activity has to decrease by a factor of ten to be noticeable as a decrease in sensitivity. In home and leisure applications oxide sensors are preferred because they are cheaper by a factor of five. However, the sensitivity of oxides decreases with decreasing catalytic activity. The corresponding lack of stability is taken into account by the use of an initially rather low-lying alarm level. For home appliances such a choice is tolerable, because there is no economic reason to delay the repair of small leaks. Special microcalorimetric sensors without a diffusion barrier, e.g., planar thick films, serve as elements in multisensors. An example is given in Section 23.5.2.

23.2 EXPERIMENTAL METHODS

23.2.1 Characterization Techniques

Only a fraction of the spectroscopic methods successfully applied to the investigation of metal surfaces is transferable to semiconductor surfaces, because the achievable adsorbate coverages are lower by some orders of magnitude (10^{-3} to 10^{-5} of a monolayer). With respect to sensor properties SnO_2 is the most frequently investigated oxide, whereas most of the basic studies of electrical and catalytic properties are devoted to zinc oxide. SnO_2 has gained much confidence on the strength of graphs covering more than 10 years, showing that commercial Figaro devices have been operating for a full decade detecting hydrocarbons in air. Investigations of gas response reproducibility for other materials covering more than a month are not published in the literature. There is a high interest towards such stability data accompanied by spectroscopic control of the sample state; however, the usual short-term funding is not in favor of stimulating such research. This situation also has surely helped to concentrate fundamental research efforts on exploiting the SnO_2 potential.

Infrared spectroscopy is a powerful tool to investigate the presence and stability of intermediate surface products. Its application is limited though to polycrystalline samples with a large effective area including internal surfaces. Results from electron spectroscopic investigations of the SnO_2 surface are reviewed in Reference 1. Some results of central importance are discussed in Section 23.3. It should be remarked that the spectroscopic observation of intermediates can be misleading if more than one reaction path is active. The observed surface species may not belong to the channel active in catalysis. Also, the predominant catalytic reaction may be different from the reaction responsible for a conductance change. In this study, thermal desorption spectroscopy was used as the primary technique of characterizing the interaction of gases with the semiconductor surface. It is sensitive enough to identify the reaction products leaving the surface and allows one to establish reaction schemes. Reaction schemes are a precondition to enhance or weaken a reaction path in order to adapt to a desired specificity. An example is given in Section 23.4.1.2.

23.2.2 Sample Preparation

Various sample preparations are possible. In practical use are sintered layers and sputtered or evaporated films. Because of the polycrystalline structure an interpretation of the observed conductance changes is often difficult.[11] By studying the surface of single crystals under well-defined conditions one might try to achieve a better separation of parameters influencing the properties of gas sensors.[12]

In our group the following preparations were employed: SnO_2 crystals were grown from the vapor phase. They exhibit mainly (101) and (110) surfaces of the rutile structure containing equal numbers of Sn and O atoms. Thin films were prepared by vapor deposition of metallic tin on amorphous quartz substrates with oxidation at 830 K for 90 min.[13] Scanning electron microscope pictures show that the tin layers consist of interconnected spheres. The diameter of the tin spheres increases with the film thickness. In a layer with a mean thickness of 25 nm, measured by a mechanical stylus (alphastep), large balls with a diameter of about 200 nm are interconnected by smaller ones. In 280-nm films the large balls have diameters of 2000 nm. All these spheres ideally show smooth surfaces under the microscope. Subsequent oxidation roughens the surface of the spheres. Sintered specimens were prepared by drying and sintering (1170 K, 1 h) a 0.5-mm-thick layer of water/SnO_2 paste on an alumina platelet. In some experiments sputtered SnO_2 films of 100-nm thickness on a porous alumina substrate bearing interdigital conductance electrodes (length-to-width ratio: 267) were used for comparison.[14]

After deposition of eight monolayers of Pd on the SnO_2 films and annealing in UHV, it was shown by XPS that the oxide surface is partially exposed between clusters of Pd. Complete oxidation of palladium to palladium oxide was obtained by annealing for 2 h at 900 K in flowing dry air, as confirmed by XPS. For comparison, not only the films with palladium oxide clusters were heat-treated in air, but also the uncovered samples and those with palladium clusters were treated before the palladium deposition. A summary is given in Table 23.2.

23.2.3 Identification of Reaction Products

A sensitive mass spectrometer (Extranuclear) was used in thermal desorption spectroscopy (TDS). A sample is exposed to a certain gas dose at room temperature and, after pumpdown, heated at a rate of about 1 to 50 K/s. The desorbing products are monitored by the mass spectrometer in ultrahigh vacuum (UHV). Corrections are made for the dissociation within the mass spectrometer by ionization. Usually, all reaction products are offered to the sample in separate TDS runs, too. By a comparison some products are found desorbing immediately after reaction, others are stored in a chemisorbed state before desorption. Products desorbing together are characteristic of a common preceding surface reaction step. The reaction order of the slowest reaction step is also accessible: the peak temperature of the desorption maximum depends on the heating rate for second-order processes. It does not vary in first-order processes. In a thermal desorption experiment the coverage may already be low

TABLE 23.2
MeO_x Gas Sensing Devices Tested Here

SnO_2 Single Crystals Grown by Chemical Vapor Deposition
Growth temperature 1550°C (101) and (110) faces exposed
Dimensions: a few mm, evaporated gold contacts (4 probes)
Characteristics: low reaction rates because of low specific reaction area

Heated Resistor SnO_2 Evaporated Thin Film
Substrate: amorphous quartz
Vapor deposition of metallic tin
Oxidation at 830 K for 90 min

Heated Resistor SnO_2 Thick Film
Substrate: polycrystalline alumina platelet
Paste consisting of water and SnO_2 powder, 0.5 mm thick
Drying and sintering for 1 h at 1170 K

Heated Resistor SnO_2/Pd Sputtered Film
Substrate: porous alumina platelet
Sputtered film, 100 nm thickness[14]
On-top deposition of 8 ml palladium
Pd oxidation for 2 h at 900 K in air

before a temperature high enough for the reaction is attained. This limitation is absent in reactive scattering experiments, where coverage and temperature can be chosen closer to the conditions of practical use: in reactive scattering experiments a gas beam is directed to the surface continuously or in a pulsed mode. The desorbing molecules are monitored by the mass spectrometer. Degradation of catalytic properties is discernible. In some cases the reaction product distribution hints at the type of poisoning by a nondesorbing species. Such products can be desorbed by a heat pulse or by offering a reactive gas. So the effect of surface reactions changing the density of surface donors or acceptors is observed. Table 23.3 gives a compilation of some methods applied for the analysis of sensor surfaces.

TABLE 23.3
Methods of Characterizing the Interaction of the Heated MeO_x Surface With Gases and Volatiles

Method	Properties analyzed	Applicability
Infrared spectroscopy	Binding states of adsorbates	Polycrystalline samples only
Electron loss spectroscopy	Binding states of adsorbates	Single crystals
Photoemission (XPS)	Binding states of adsorbates	Single crystals and polycryst. samples
Auger spectroscopy	Presence of adsorbates	Single crystals and polycryst. samples
Thermal desorption spectroscopy	Reaction products leaving the surface	Single crystals and polycryst. samples

23.3 FUNCTIONS OF LATTICE AND ADSORBED OXYGEN

23.3.1 CONDUCTANCE RESPONSE TO BEAMS OF CO AND O_2 MOLECULES

In the mass spectrometer apparatus described above it is possible to measure the conductance of the sample simultaneously. The apparatus is equipped with two nozzles to vary the flux of the reducing gas and the flux of oxygen independently. In Figure 23.2 (upper trace: a) CO and O_2 are offered sequentially. Only lattice oxygen is available for reaction. In Figure 23.2 (lower trace: b) CO and O_2 molecules impinge simultaneously onto the surface. Under the conditions of (b) adsorbed oxygen ions can also be consumed in the reaction. The conductance slope is less steep. One reason may be that oxygen ions adsorbed near oxygen vacancies "compensate" the donors formed by the oxygen vacancies. A part of the vacancies may also be refilled. The conductance decay immediately after CO flux switch-off at 350°C does not necessarily indicate a desorption of CO acting as surface donor. It can also be assumed that within the grains of the sputtered layer oxygen diffuses to the grain boundary.

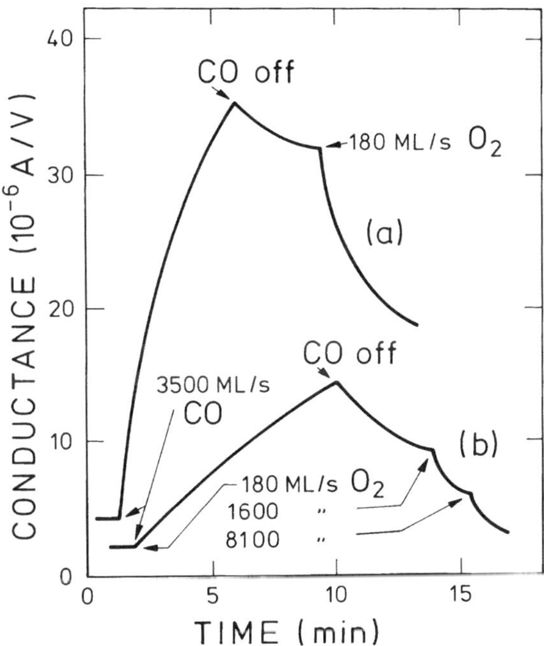

FIGURE 23.2 Conductance of a sputtered SnO_2 film at 350°C exposed to fluxes of CO and O_2 molecules from two nozzles. Before each run an oxygen pretreatment was applied to remove contaminants from the film and to establish a stoichiometric surface: 30 min at 870 K followed by 15 min at 670 K in 0.33 Pa of O_2, 5 min at 640 K during pumpdown to 10^{-7} Pa.

23.3.2 Reactivities of Surface Oxygen Species

Different types of surface oxygen differ in reactivity: the "nucleophilic" O^{-2} ions bound within the lattice at the surface react with activated hydrogen or dehydrogenate hydrides and hydrocarbons.[15] Activation means excitation of a bond and, as a possible consequence, ionization, dissociation or formation of radicals. For example, methane can be activated on the SnO_2 surface and form a CH_3 radical. H_2 molecules are not activated on smooth SnO_2 surfaces of single crystals.[16] The same holds for WO_3 and V_2O_5.[17] However, on the rough surface of sintered SnO_2 specimen activation and reaction to H_2O occur at 470 K.[18] This may be due to exposed oxygen atoms. Hydrogen is strongly and nearly irreversibly adsorbed on surface lattice oxygen of SnO_2 as is typical for semiconducting oxides.[17] On heating, only a small fraction of H_2 can be recovered; predominant is the formation of water.[2,18,20]

23.3.3 Reactivity of n- and p-Type Oxides

When pure n-type oxides (with a nonoxidizable metal ion) are exactly stoichiometric, they cannot chemisorb oxygen. However, when they are oxygen deficient they can chemisorb just as much as is needed to restore their stoichiometry or, more generally, until their charge averaged over the depth of the depletion layer is balanced.[17] Therefore, it is specific for n-type oxides that the concentration of surface oxygen ions remains some orders of magnitude lower than the concentration of lattice oxygen in the uppermost surface layer. In contrast, on p-type semiconductors a full monolayer of oxygen ions typically adsorbs, because the metal ions of the lattice can be oxidized into a higher oxidation state, e.g., from Ni^{2+} into Ni^{3+} in NiO.[17] With respect to oxidation reactions the adsorbed (O_{2ads}) and (O_{ads}) species and also exposed oxygen atoms at steps are classified as "electrophilic" reactants which preferentially attack the C=C double bond of adsorbates abstracting electrons.[15] Therefore, p-type semiconductors are good catalysts for total oxidation resulting in CO_2 and H_2O only.[17] Reaction products of n-type semiconductors include partially oxidized molecules, e.g., acetaldehyde after exposure to ethanol.

23.3.4 Oxygen Vacancies

Exposure to hydrogen and to hydrogen-containing gases at elevated temperatures produces surface oxygen vacancies. They are well known as donors, for example, on TiO_2 (110) faces.[21] Munnix and Schmeits[21] showed by band structure calculations that surface oxygen vacancies on SnO_2 (110) faces do not act as donors. A study[22] comparing the ultraviolet photoemission (UPS) spectra of TiO_2 (110) and SnO_2 (110) demonstrated that oxygen vacancies created by argon ion bombardment produce new surface states in the upper part of the bulk band gap of TiO_2 but not of SnO_2. After the bombardment on the reduced surface tin is present as Sn(II).[23] Conductivity measurements[24] indicate that these surface defects on SnO_2 do not act as donor states in contrast to TiO_2 surfaces. After exposure of a stoichiometric SnO_2 (101) face or a sputtered SnO_2 film to methane in UHV, considerable amounts of water desorb at temperatures near 350 K leaving surface oxygen vacancies, but the conductivity does not increase below 550 K.[16] So the theoretical prediction that surface oxygen vacancies do not act as surface donors on SnO_2 is supported by UPS and by conductance measurements after reducing argon bombardment and also by conductance measurements after exposure to methane.

Annealing of an argon-bombarded SnO_2 (110) face in UHV increases the conductance until a plateau is reached at 550 K.[24] Surface oxygen vacancies may diffuse towards the bulk, where they are able to act as donors as explained above. Oxygen vacancies left after water formation at 670 to 770 K increase the conductance. Again, a migration towards bulk sites can "activate" the vacancies as donors. Since recent cluster calculations by Lannto[25] have shown that the vacancies have to cross only two lattice planes, the temperature of 550 K seems to be sufficient for an "activation".

23.3.5 Methane Decay in the Absence and Presence of O_2

The role of lattice oxygen and ionosorbed oxygen in a reaction is demonstrated in detail by a reactive scattering experiment.[26] First the decomposition of methane in the absence of gaseous oxygen on a sputtered SnO_2 film was investigated. Then a two-nozzle arrangement was used to look for reaction products during simultaneous incident fluxes of methane and oxygen atoms. In the latter case, deeper oxidation (higher oxygen consumption per consumed methane molecule) of methane to only CO, CO_2, and H_2 is observed. If no oxygen is offered, the reaction products C_2H_4, C_2H_5OH, CH_3COOH, H_2CCO, and H_2CO also show up.

23.3.6 Selective and Total Oxidation of Ethanol

In the following, a comparison of ethanol decay reactions on an SnO_2 single crystal and on a sintered sample demonstrates the transition from selective oxidation to total oxidation.

23.3.6.1 Selective Oxidation on Single-Crystal Tin Oxide

23.3.6.1.1 Exposure of single crystals to gaseous ethanol

After exposure of a (110) face to ethanol the desorption spectrum in Figure 23.3 (c) and (d) shows the decomposition products acetaldehyde, ethylene, and water as well as the desorption of ethanol.[27] The ethanol molecule may be weakly bound to the surface, e.g., via the oxygen atom of its OH group, (Figure 23.4a):

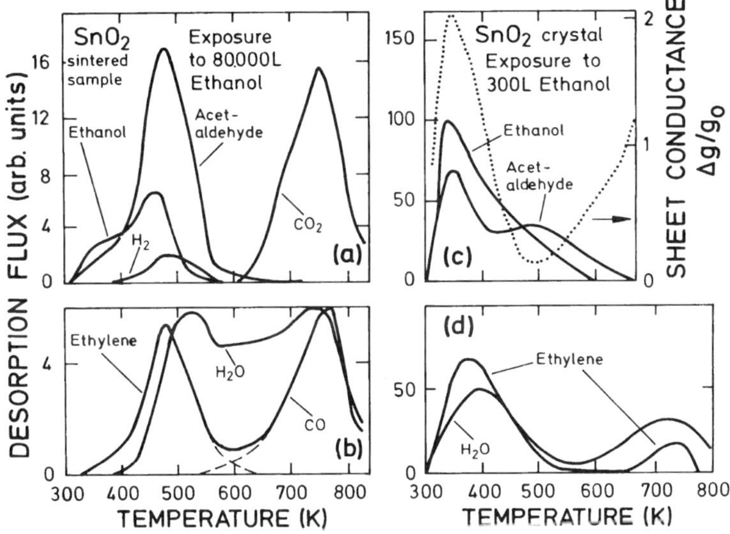

FIGURE 23.3 Thermal desorption spectra (continuous curves) and sheet conductance (dotted curve). Before each run the oxygen pretreatment was applied to remove contaminants from the as-grown surface and to establish a stoichiometric surface: 30 min at 870 K and 15 min at 670 K in 0.25 Pa of O_2, finally 5 min at 670 K during pumpdown. Heating rate 9 K/s in the TDS runs: (a) and (b) sintered sample, (c) and (d) single crystal.

$$CH_3CH_2OH_{gas} \rightarrow CH_3CH_2OH_{ads} \tag{23.1}$$

The TDS maximum at 360 K is near the maximum of acetic acid at 350 K, where the same type of binding is possible. The extended high-temperature tail of the ethanol desorption arises from a reversible dissociation to an ethoxy group (Figure 23.4b) and adsorbed hydrogen (dehydrogenation):

$$CH_3CH_2OH_{ads} \leftrightarrow CH_3CH_2O_{ads} + H_{ads} \tag{23.2}$$

The hydrogen from Reaction 23.2 can react to water and desorb with a maximum at 400 K (Figure 23.3d). For sintered specimens the reversible dissociation has been verified by experiments with deuterated ethanol. The desorption of ethylene and water from single crystals near 400 K and between 660 K and 750 K (Figure 23.3d) can be formally regarded as a dehydration of ethanol:

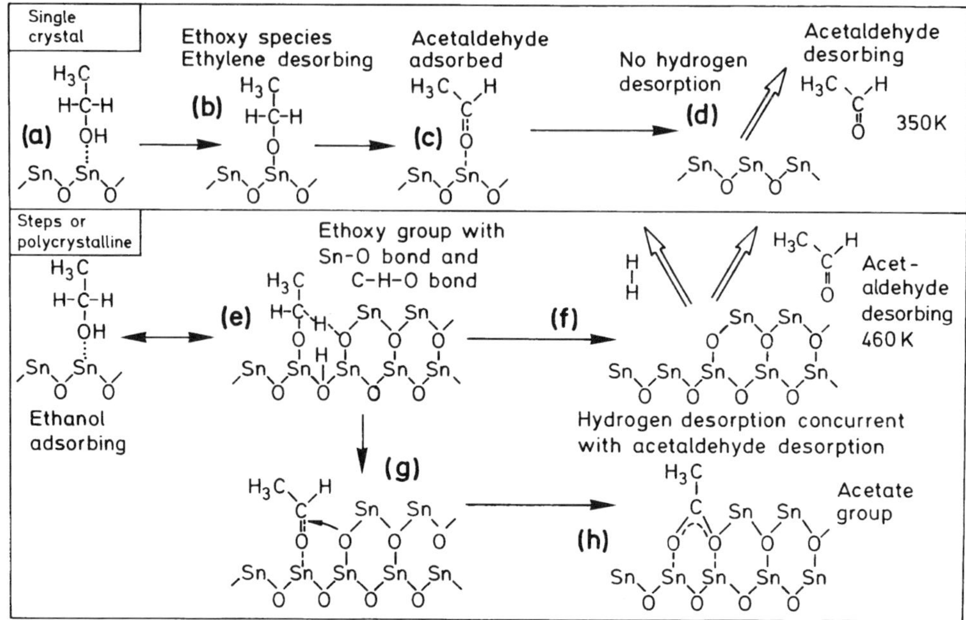

FIGURE 23.4 Surface intermediates after exposure to ethanol. SnO_2 (110) face: (a) molecular adsorption, (b) after dissociation to an ethoxy group and hydrogen (dehydrogenation), (c) after a second dehydrogenation, (d) desorption of acetaldehyde. Polycrystalline or stepped SnO_2 sample: (e) ethoxy group with an additional hydrogen bond, (f) desorption of hydrogen and acetaldehyde, (g) double bond of adsorbed acetaldehyde attacked by electrophilic oxygen, (h) acetate group at a step.

$$CH_3CH_2OH_{gas} \rightarrow C_2H_{4\ gas} + H_2O_{gas} \tag{23.3}$$

The reverse reaction is well known from the industrial ethanol production over Cu/ZnO catalysts. Since ethylene adsorbed on polycrystalline SnO_2 is known to form ethoxy groups,[28] ethylene may be evolved by a decomposition of the ethoxy group of Equation 23.2:

$$CH_3CH_2O_{ads} + H_{ads} \rightarrow H_2O_{gas} + C_2H_{4\ gas} \tag{23.4}$$

No lattice oxygen is required. The desorption spectrum also contains acetaldehyde, CH_3CHO, a dehydrogenation product of the ethoxy group:

$$CH_3CH_2O_{ads} \rightarrow H_{ads} + CH_3CHO_{gas} \tag{23.5}$$

Carbon monoxide and dioxide are absent in desorption for the single-crystal SnO_2, (compare Figure 23.3c and 23.3d). Heating of a (110) face exposed to ethanol leads to a conductance maximum (dotted curve in Figure 23.3c) nearly coinciding with the ethanol desorption maximum.[27]

Molecular ethanol bound via its oxygen lone pair orbital (filled with two electrons) to a surface tin atom can act as a surface donor. The right flank of the conductance maximum contains contributions from hydrogen donors of the dissociated molecule. At high temperatures, above 550 K, vacancies left after condensation of hydroxyl groups and water desorption can act as subsurface donors. The absolute and the relative conductance increase of SnO_2 (110) faces kept at 600 K in air with admixtures of 85 to 950 ppm ethanol reveal a nearly linear response to the ethanol concentration.[29]

23.3.6.2 Total Oxidation on Polycrystalline Tin Oxide

In sintered specimens the main desorption maxima of ethanol, acetaldehyde, and ethylene in Figure 23.3a and 23.3b are found between 460 and 480 K. Smaller fluxes of these gases appear as shoulders in the range between 350 and 380 K, indicating that a minor fraction of the adsorbed ethanol adsorbs and reacts in the same way as on the (110) face. At edge sites on the polycrystalline surface (Figure 23.4e) ethoxy groups can be more tightly bound by an additional hydrogen bond of the methylene hydrogen to an exposed lattice oxygen. The observed shift of the TDS maxima corresponds to about 8 kcal/M, typical for hydrogen bridge bonding. Only on the polycrystalline sample a desorption maximum of hydrogen appears at 480 K. In contrast to the finding on the (110) face, CO and CO_2 also desorb from the polycrystalline samples above 600 K (Figure 23.3a and 23.3b). The C–C bond can be broken by the following mechanism: the acetaldehyde formed in Equation 23.5 contains a double bond (Figure 23.4g). An exposed electrophilic oxygen can attack the double bond and form a carboxylate group (acetate) (Figure 23.4h):

$$CH_3CHO_{ads} + O_{exposed} \rightarrow CH_3COO_{ads} + V_o \tag{23.6}$$

It has been shown that formaldehyde and adsorbed oxygen ions on copper react in a similar process to a formate group.[30] Various ketones adsorbing with their carbonyl group on polycrystalline SnO_2 are attacked by OH groups at the double bond and also form carboxylate groups, e.g., acetone reacts on hydroxylated SnO_2 to form an acetate.[31]

Acetate can decompose to CO and CO_2.[13,16] The second maximum of water desorption appears nearly at the same temperature (750 K) as on the (110) face. Again, the vacancies left after water desorption can act as donors.

23.4 ADMIXTURES OF METALS TO TIN OXIDE

23.4.1 Ion Exchange

23.4.1.1 Homogeneous Phase and Separated Phases

Tin dioxide is known to have pronounced and useful cation exchange properties, which means that the surface tin atoms can be easily replaced by atoms of other metals.[32] For example, palladium can be evenly distributed by ion exchange from $Pd(NH_3)_4(OH)_2$. If the ion exchange capacity of SnO_2 is not exceeded, a homogeneous material results. An effective CO oxidation catalyst, routinely in use to reoxidize CO in sealed CO_2 lasers, is obtained by replacing about 55% of tin ions with copper ions in the SnO_2 surface lattice.[32,33] A consequence of exchanging a foreign metal with surface tin is that pore growth and sintering are significantly retarded during heat treatment. Quantitative data for a range of metal ions are given in Reference 23. A mixture of SnO_2 with a second oxide by impregnation or by mechanical mixing can also form two well-separated phases if the calcination temperature is high enough (450°C in the case of Cu) or if the ion exchange capacity is exceeded.[32] When the phase of a second oxide with different catalytic activity is in intimate contact with SnO_2, radicals can migrate between the crystallites.[34]

Morrison emphasizes an electron exchange between separated oxide phases.[35] He prepared a semiconductor heterojunction by impregnating n-type TiO_2 with n-type V_2O_5. Vanadium pentoxide was present in a submonolayer coverage on the titanium dioxide. Since the vanadium oxide has a very low conduction band energy, it acts as an acceptor on titanium oxide and decreases the conductance. V_2O_5 is a specifically active oxidation catalyst for xylene. The sensing element, operated at 400°C, was by a factor of 1000 more sensitive to xylene than to CO. However, it may need more elaborate work to separate electronic mechanisms from migration effects.

23.4.1.2 Effect of Electronegativity of Surface Metal Atoms

The foreign metal atoms on cation exchanged SnO_2 serve also as adsorption sites with an ionic bond strength depending on the electronegativity of the foreign metal atoms. The electronegativity is a relative measure of how strongly an atom attracts electrons. If the adsorption step or the subsequent dissociation rules the kinetics of the surface reaction and the conductance change, the sensor sensitivity correlates with the electronegativity. As an application of this consideration an odor sensor for hydrogen disulfide has been developed.[36] Hydrogen bridge bonding is ruled out for H_2S adsorption because the atomic number of sulfur (16) is too high. H_2S is of weak acidity. Therefore, the following mechanism for increasing the conductance seems probable: the strong ionic binding of the sulfur (electronegativity 2.44) to the oxide metal atom weakens the sulfur-hydrogen bond ($E_{S\text{-}H}$ = 81 kcal/mol for the gaseous molecule) and facilitates dissociation to an S^{2-} or an SH^- ion and two or one H^+ ions. The hydrogen donors cause a conductance maximum already at 370 K.[37]

An admixture of foreign metal to SnO_2 with a larger electronegativity difference to sulfur, for example Zn (1.66) or Ag (1.42), enhances the conductance increase by a factor of five for 10 ppm H_2S in air. Zn and Ag are weak electron acceptors and weak Lewis acids. Smaller electronegativity differences occur if P (2.06) or Sb (1.82) are added. These atoms are stronger Lewis acids with a weakened ionic bond to sulfur, causing less H_2S dissociation. The addition of P or Sb decreases the sensitivity by a factor of five.[36]

More complicated reactions with intermediates on Pd sites of cation exchanged polycrystalline SnO_2 samples were investigated by infrared spectroscopy after exposure to ethane,[28] ethylene,[28] propylene,[38] formic acid,[39] water,[40] CO_2,[41] and ammonia.[40] In a comparative IR study of CO, NO, and CO/NO, admixtures of Cr, Mn, Fe, Co, Ni, and Cu oxides to SnO_2 were used.[42] In such cases the electronegativity cannot be taken as a reasonable parameter to predict the influence on sensitivity.

23.5 CLUSTERS OF CATALYTICALLY ACTIVE METALS

23.5.1 Metal Clusters on Semiconducting Oxides

23.5.1.1 Spillover Effect

The decomposition of hydrogen and hydrocarbon molecules on catalytically active metals is used in calorimetric-type sensors and in semiconductor-type sensors with metal-cluster deposits. On calorimetric-type sensors, besides high diffusion and reaction rates, total oxidation to CO_2 and H_2O is favorable. However, the sensitivity of semiconductor sensors is enhanced by partial oxidation of the gases on the active metal deposit and subsequent spillover of hydrogen to the semiconductor substrate. The activity of a catalyst depends on its oxidation state. Palladium oxide is known to affect total oxidation supplying oxygen to the adsorbed species and thus preventing spillover of hydrogen. The d orbitals of metallic Pd transfer electronic charge into antibonding levels of the adsorbate, facilitating dissociation or dehydrogenation with subsequent spillover.

23.5.1.2 Formation of the Pd/SnO_2 Interface

In Figure 23.5 the Auger signal of palladium on an SnO_2 (110) face is given as a function of the deposited coverage.[43] The deposition of a small amount of Pd at 300 K and a subsequent Auger measurement are repeatedly applied. A layer-by-layer growth mechanism is observed in its ideal form with straight lines changing slope after completion of the first and second

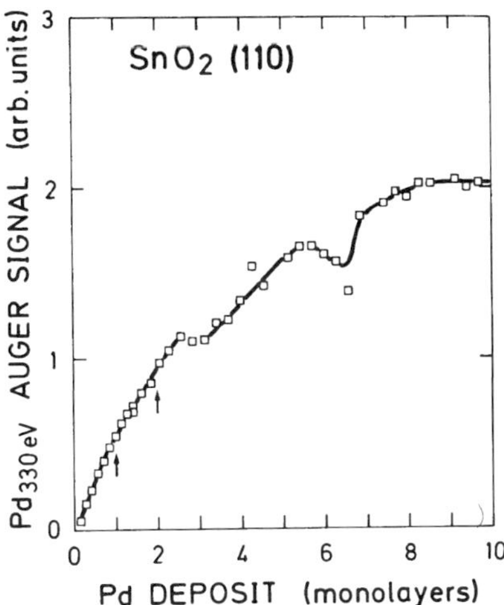

FIGURE 23.5 SnO_2 crystal. Auger signal during deposition of Pd in UHV. The amount of Pd deposited is measured by a quartz microbalance.

layer. The minima at about the 3.5 and 6.5 monolayers may be caused by instabilities of the layers, resulting in cluster formation.

The sequential states of the SnO_2 surface during Pd deposition are sketched in Figure 23.6. During deposition the energetic position and shape of the Sn Auger peak changes from the oxidic type to the metallic type. Lattice oxygen atoms in the surface of SnO_2 are known to be easily available for the oxidation of adsorbates. An infrared investigation[28] revealed that below 450 K SnO_2 is able to oxidize ethylene to acetate. This low-temperature oxidation does not occur with the oxides of Zn, Ni, Cr, and Al. Thus it seems probable that Pd reduces the substrate during deposition. A part of the palladium forms PdO. Surface tin atoms lose their oxygen neighbors and show a metallic-like Auger line. This redox reaction is reversible. During annealing in UHV at temperatures between 600 and 750 K the tin peak converts back to its oxidic form. Oxygen from the PdO or from the substrate bulk migrates back into the vacancies at the substrate surface. XPS investigations[44] showed that thin PdO layers on Pd in UHV are completely reduced to Pd at 750 K. A precondition for this strong metal support interaction is the reducibility of the substrate.[45] Strong metal support interaction was also verified for the systems Pt/TiO_2 and Pt/Nb_2O_5.

23.5.1.3 Influence of the Pd Oxidation State on Gas Sensitivity

Figures 23.7 and 23.8 show the absolute increase of conductance during admixture of hydrogen and methane to dry air, respectively, for sputtered SnO_2 films and (110) faces. The increase is reversible at the indicated temperatures. The conductance of the uncovered surface saturates above 300 ppm H_2. Both Pd and PdO linearize the response, but with Pd the absolute and the relative signal are larger by a factor of 40 at 1000 ppm. Since hydrogen molecules have a sticking coefficient of 1 and dissociate completely at 230°C on Pd films,[46] a strong spillover effect is the probable reason for the marked sensitivity increase.

On admixture of methane the conductance of all three types of films saturates at 200 ppm. The conductance increase is only weakly influenced by Pd or PdO. Since Pd and PdO are effective catalysts in calorimetric sensors for methane,[47] a total oxidation with subsequent desorption of CO_2 and H_2O may not leave any products for spillover. The saturation may be caused by the slow desorption of acetate species at 400°C. At an operating temperature of 450°C the saturation is less pronounced. In the above example the oxidation state of Pd was

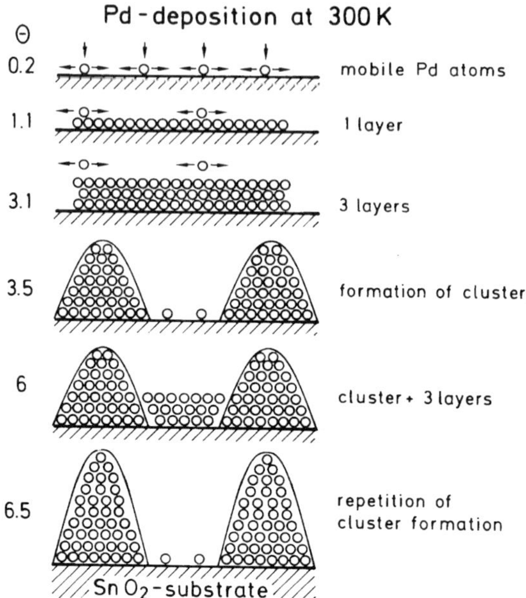

FIGURE 23.6 Model for the subsequent states of cluster formation at room temperature during deposition of palladium.

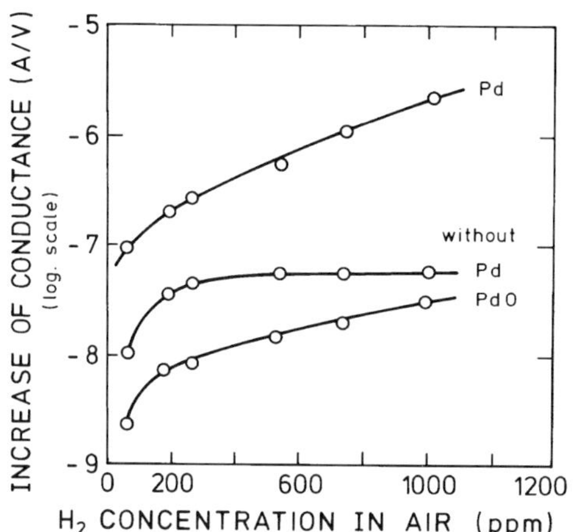

FIGURE 23.7 SnO_2 sputtered films. Increase of conductance as a function of hydrogen concentration in air. Compared are the results of films with palladium clusters, without palladium, and with oxidized palladium clusters. Measurements on a single crystal are also shown.

shown to have a strong influence upon the hydrogen sensitivity of the sensing element. It could be changed by an oxidation or reduction treatment.

23.5.1.4 Au/Fe_2O_3 — An Example of an Electronic Interaction

This example illustrates that even a catalytically ineffective metal, Au, can be provided with "Pt"-like catalytic properties by a charge transfer to its oxide substrate. Kobayashi et al.[48] prepared various α-Fe_2O_3 samples and one SnO_2 sample with small Au clusters by annealing after coprecipitation with an Au salt, or photodeposition, or impregnation, and also without Au clusters. In the presence of Au clusters the sensitivity maxima of CO, H_2, and ethanol

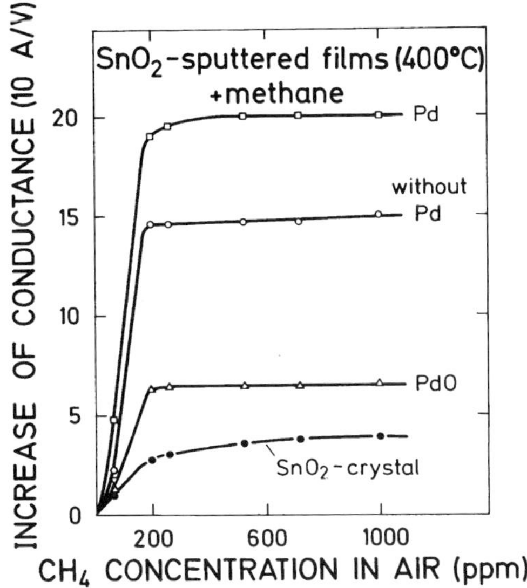

FIGURE 23.8 Same as in Figure 23.7, but increase of conductance as a function of methane concentration in air.

are shifted to lower temperatures, especially, a sensitive detection of CO well below 100°C is possible. On admixture of 100 ppm CO the sensor conductance at 40°C rises within 40 s to 90% of the steady-state value. Return to zero needs about the same time. The enhanced sensitivity is connected with a corresponding catalytic activity increase at low temperature. Bond and Sermon[49] argue that ultrafine Au particles supported on oxides become electron deficient by donating electrons to the support. The catalytic properties of these particles then resemble those of Pt, which is the element to the left of Au in the periodic table. TEM micrographs show that the (111) faces of the Au crystallites in the coprecipitated sample are in close contact with the (110) planes of the α-Fe_2O_3 particles.[48] In the detection of CO this type of "artificial Pt" is more favorable than Pt itself, because the adsorption energies of CO amount to 40 and 120 kJ/mol, respectively.[48] The CO molecule can be activated on the Au cluster and spills over to the oxide, where it reacts with oxygen. However, on Pt the activated CO may be bound too tightly to reach the oxide. Without activation the CO adsorption is the slowest step in the oxidation over α-Fe_2O_3.[50]

23.5.2 Metal Clusters on Insulating Oxides

23.5.2.1 Reactions of Oxygen with Pd/Al_2O_3

The uptake of oxygen from air by noble metal clusters plays an important role in the response of sensor elements. Pd clusters on gamma-alumina have been studied by means of XPS, XRD, and TDS.[51] Figure 23.9 shows XPS results of reduction-oxidation treatments on Pd clusters supported by gamma alumina (Alpha-Ventron: 10 wt% Pd). From the reduced state (a) to the oxidized state (e), the binding energy is shifted by 1.7 eV. The information depth of XPS amounts to about ten atomic layers. From the linewidth of the XRD peaks an average cluster diameter of 13.5 nm was estimated. In the reduced state only the Pd[111] beam was observed, confirming that complete reduction had taken place. In the oxidized state lines of the PdO lattice dominated besides a weak signal of Pd[111]. After annealing in dry air at 770 K bulk oxidation occurs; only a small fraction of the palladium remains metallic.

TDS results of oxygen desorption are shown in Figure 23.10. After annealing in dry air at 300 K, curve (a), a small maximum appears at about 350 K and another maximum, larger

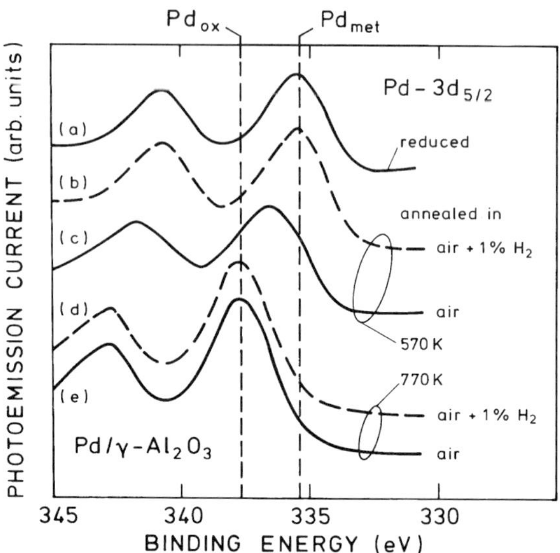

FIGURE 23.9 Reduction-oxidation studies by XPS. Binding energy after 15 min annealing; (a): in ultrahigh vacuum at 1020 K; (b) to (e): in dry air with and without 1% H_2.

by a factor of ten, at about 750 K. By raising the annealing temperature to 770 K, the low-temperature maximum nearly vanishes and the high-temperature maximum is shifted to about 970 K, growing by about two orders of magnitude. A simple model of hemispherical clusters allows some estimations to be made. For the diameter of 13.5 nm about 3,600 surface and 44,000 bulk palladium atoms are calculated, corresponding to 8% surface sites. Palladium is known to form a surface oxide incorporating half a monolayer of oxygen. In dry air at room temperature only the surface is oxidized; at 780 K the bulk oxidation saturates as Figure 23.11 shows. Also, the XRD results after annealing in dry air at 770 K indicate that there is a nearly complete bulk oxidation to PdO. The integral of curve (c) in Figure 23.10 corresponds to the total number of Pd atoms, and the integral of curve (a) to 0.5 ml of oxygen.

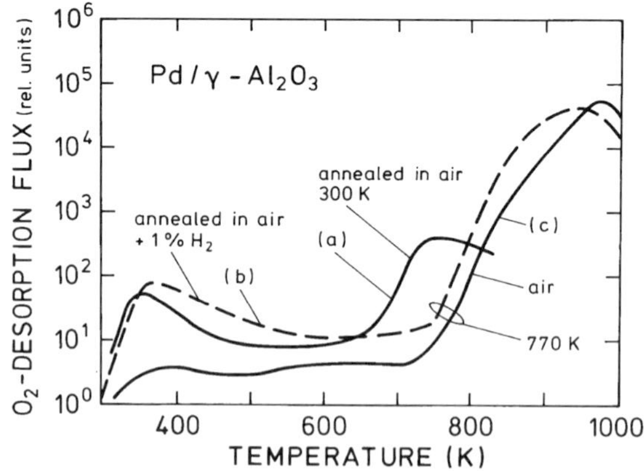

FIGURE 23.10 Flux of desorbing oxygen as a function of increasing temperature after reduction in ultrahigh vacuum at 1020 K. The oxygen was supplied by annealing for 15 min in dry air at 300 K or 770 K. The influence of annealing in dry air with an addition of 1% H_2 at 770 K is also shown. Heating rate: 10 K/s.

Cullis and Willat studied the uptake of oxygen by palladium clusters on gamma-alumina during pulses of 10^5 Pa (1 bar) oxygen as a function of temperature.[52,53] The uptake at high

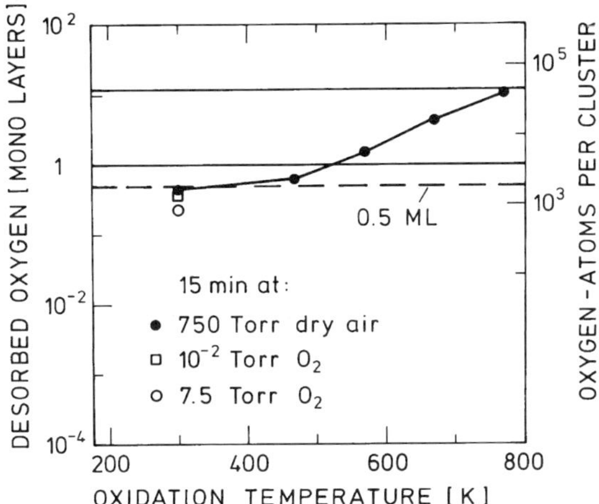

FIGURE 23.11 Desorbed oxygen (log scale) from palladium clusters with a diameter of 13.5 nm on gamma-alumina after various oxygen pretreatments.

temperatures also exceeds by far the number of surface sites. It does not occur at temperatures above 900 K. This fact can be explained by thermodynamics. At 10^5 Pa oxygen pressure the metallic phase is more stable than the oxidic phase above 900 K. During the TDS measurements of Figure 23.10, the oxygen pressure amounts to about 10^{-8} Pa (10^{-10} torr) corresponding to a decomposition of the oxide at 520 K. Therefore the bulk oxygen appears in TDS.

The kinetic limitations of TDS were demonstrated by a simple experiment. After oxidation at 370 K heating was started at a rate of 10 K/s. At 670 K the temperature was kept constant for 2 min. Subsequent heating at the initial rate resulted in a high-temperature peak that was a factor of 200 lower than after heating at a constant rate. As a time-limiting process not only desorption, but also bulk diffusion have to be considered.

23.5.2.2 Response of Microcalorimetric Sensors to H_2 and CH_4

For a simulation of operational conditions, studies with a reducing gas were performed: 1% H_2 was added to dry air during annealing at 770 K. This small amount was sufficient to prevent oxidation at 570 K, as observed by XPS (compare Figure 23.9, curves (b) and (c)). In contrast, at 770 K no influence of the hydrogen addition was visible (curves (d) and (e)). In TDS (Figure 23.10, curves (b) and (c)) the addition of hydrogen considerably increases the maximum near 400 K and shifts the high-temperature peak towards lower temperatures. The increase near 400 K can be attributed to a more metallic state of the surface by superficial reduction, causing an enhanced chemisorption of oxygen. A similar maximum appears after the reducing pretreatment and exposure to oxygen at 300 K (curve (a)). On palladium oxide the adsorption of oxygen is lower (curve (c)).

If a microcalorimetric sensor element does not operate within the mass transport limitation,[54] the sensitivity depends more directly on the catalytic activity. Apparently this holds for silicon microstructured elements.[55] The problem arising for the detection of H_2 is demonstrated by the data given in Figure 23.12. A microreactor was used to check that the production of water corresponds to the generation of reaction heat. The curves of Figure 23.12 show the increase of water desorption after admission of H_2 on the same Alpha-Ventron catalyst (10% Pd on alumina) in the reduced and in the oxidized state. The activity of the oxidized palladium at 100°C is very low initially, and approaches the activity of the metallic catalyst only after about half an hour. This behavior can be dangerous if Pd pellistors are used for warning against hydrogen.

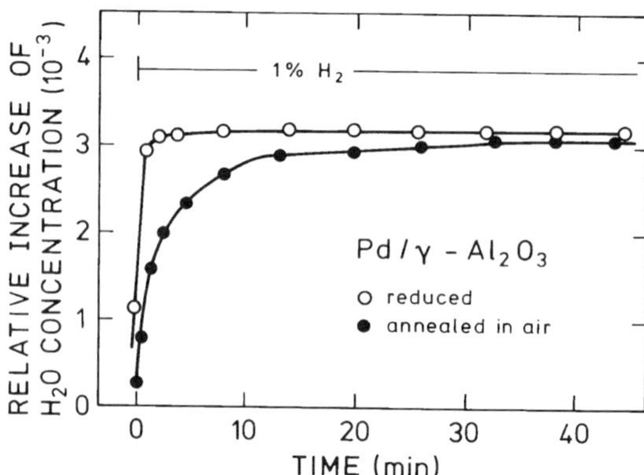

FIGURE 23.12 Relative increase of water concentration in dry air at 370 K as a function of time after admission of 1% H_2 to a microreactor. The reduction was performed at 970 K in 7.6×10^{-4} Pa argon and the oxidation at 770 K in dry air.

Finally, it should be mentioned that the sensitivity of a Pd pellistor to methane is related to the formation/reduction of bulk oxide. Therefore a palladium pellistor for methane has to be operated at higher temperatures, e.g., at 600°C.[53]

23.5.2.3 Cross-Sensitivities of Microcalorimetric Sensors

It is regarded as an advantage of a pellistor that the signal is proportional to the sum of the concentrations of all combustible gases weighted by the respective combustion enthalpies δH of the gas components. Combustion enthalpies at 600°C for methane and butane amount to 800 and 2660 kJ/mol, respectively. Figure 23.13 shows a more complicated behavior for a mixture of methane and butane on the surface of a non-mass-transport-limited platinum pellistor (4 mg of Alpha-Ventron catalyst No. 89100: 10 wt% Pt on gamma-alumina, cluster diameter 13 nm).[56] In Figure 23.13a a linear response to methane is observed to the left of the broken line. However, even in the regime of linear response, the sensitivity to methane depends on the butane concentration: 1.8% butane increases the sensitivity to methane by about 30%. For the higher methane concentrations on the right side of the broken line, the signals increase steeply with concentration till saturation is reached. The onset of the steep increase shifts to lower methane concentrations as the butane concentration is increased. The observed behavior of the sensitivity for methane and butane can be understood qualitatively if three different ranges of concentrations are regarded separately.

For low concentrations of combustibles an excess of oxygen chemisorbed on the surface is probably present. Hicks et al.[57] found that the combustion rate for methane on Pd catalysts under excess oxygen is more than an order of magnitude lower in comparison to the rate under stoichiometric conditions. Under substoichiometric conditions adsorbed oxygen may block sites needed for adsorption and/or reaction of methane and butane. This assumption seems reasonable, since the activation energies for methane combustion are 36 kcal/mol,[57] and for oxygen desorption, 34 kcal/mol.[58,59] In an analogous manner, on Pt pellistor elements the steep increase of combustion rate shown in Figure 23.13a could be due to reaching stoichiometric conditions, where oxygen site blocking is less impeding. At much higher combustible concentrations the signal is limited because of a lack of available oxygen. The reactivity of Pt pellistors to methane is known to be low in comparison to that of higher alkanes.[60] During methane detection a simultaneously present concentration of butane can consume chemisorbed oxygen and increase the density of adsorption and reaction sites for methane combustion. This explains why the methane sensitivity is increased in the presence of butane. In Figure 23.13b the results shown in Figure 23.13a are replotted as a function of

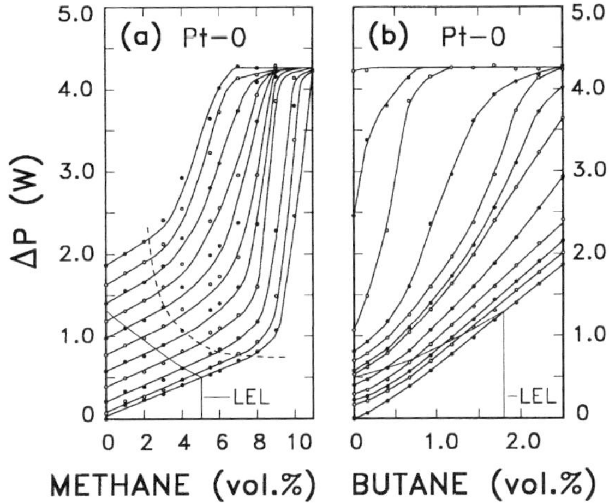

FIGURE 23.13 Microcalorimetric sensor (Pt cluster, 13 nm diameter) operated at 600°C. The loss of power consumption is given for pulses with different methane and butane concentrations. The lower explosion limit values (LEL) for methane, butane, and their mixtures are indicated: (a) the lowest-lying curve belongs to a methane/air mixture. The curves above are taken for pulses with 0.16, 0.40, 0.67, 0.93, 1.18, 1.44, 1.69, 1.95, 2.22, and 2.50 vol% butane added. (b) The lowest-lying curve belongs to a butane/air mixture. The curves above are taken for pulses with 1, 2, 3, 4, 5.5, 6, 7, 8, 9, 10, and 11 vol% methane added.

butane concentrations. Apparently there is no linear response for small butane concentrations. As long as the methane concentrations remain small (below 5%), the signal is proportional to $(c_b)^{1.3}$. A simple description of the sensor response below the lower explosion limit (LEL) in Figure 23.13 is given by (least-squares fit):

$$\delta P = 0.102c_m + 0.606(c_b)^{1.3} + 0.014c_m(c_b)^{1.3} \quad (23.7)$$

where δP is the decrease of power consumption during the exposure to combustibles and c_m, c_b are the concentrations for methane and butane in vol%. The last term in the equation describes the interaction of both gases.

23.6 POISONING AND MODIFICATION OF SENSOR SURFACES

23.6.1 POISONING BY SULFUR COMPOUNDS

Catalytically active surfaces can be deactivated by

1. Tightly bonding species, e.g., sulfur from H_2S or SO_x,
2. Compounds forming protective layers, e. g., hexamethyldisiloxane (HMDS) being oxidized to SiO_x on the active surface of the sensor elements,
3. Carbon-containing compounds.

Sulfur is known as a poison or inhibitor for metal catalysts,[17] oxide catalysts,[17] and calorimetric sensors[61] consisting of supported metal clusters. On metals, sulfur chemisorbs via its occupied lone pair orbital to an unoccupied orbital of the metal. The strongly adsorbed sulfur blocks reactive sites irreversibly. On oxides another process takes place. Sulfur can be substituted for lattice oxygen atoms.[17,62] An H_2S sensor using the sulfidation of WO_3 at 200°C is commercially available; at 300°C the oxide is completely converted to WS_2.[63] WO_3 has a reversible characteristic and is not poisoned. However, the extent of oxygen replacement by sulfur on SnO_2 is connected with an irreversible degradation and seems to depend on the morphology of the surface. It is reported that prolonged exposure to H_2S of a sputtered SnO_2 film at 200°C resulted in slow response.[64] In certain surroundings the life span of sensors is mainly determined by such poisoning effects (Figure 23.14). Porous protective layers binding selectively to tightly binding gas components have to be applied in such cases.

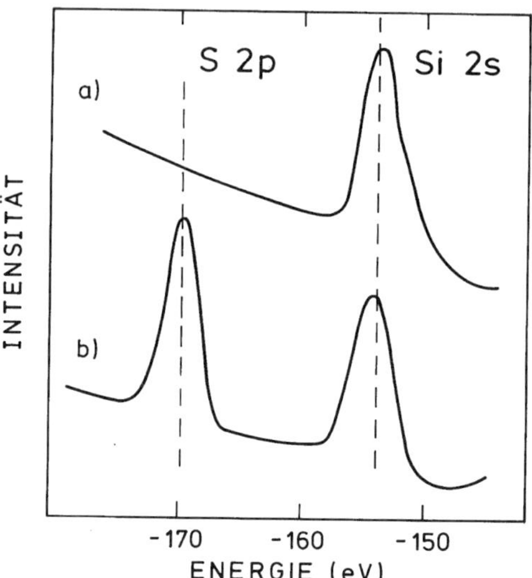

FIGURE 23.14 XPS spectra of an SnO_2 sensor surface before and after 4 months of operation at 300°C for the detection of smoldering fires in a coal power plant (0.5% sulfur in the coal).

23.6.2 Poisoning and Tailoring by Silicon Compounds

Volatile silicon compounds are constituents of materials used for cable insulations. Pellistors intended for the protection of explosion in cable channels or housings must be frequently checked to notice a loss of sensitivity. In a less critical environment a calculated prepoisoning as a constituent of the sensor preparation can modify the specificity of a sensor element. Figure 23.15 shows the XPS spectrum of the pellistor with the characteristics shown in Figure 23.13 before and after an HMDS treatment.[56] The experimental results can be described by a superposition of four peaks positioned at 100.8, 101.8, 102.9, and 104.0 eV. The individual peaks are designated by integers corresponding to the number of Si–O bonds.[65] In the picture of a random bond model[65] a stoichiometry of $SiO_{1.4}$ is obtained. The peak shape was not altered by operation at 600°C for 300 h.

23.6.3 Gas Sensor Arrays

23.6.3.1 Pellistor Array Evaluated by a Neural Network

The general behavior of the characteristics found for the untreated pellistors is also found for HMDS-treated samples, (Figure 23.16). The response below the LEL level can be described by

$$\delta P = 0.018c_m + 0.521(c_b)^{1.3} + 0.010c_m(c_b)^{1.3} \tag{23.8}$$

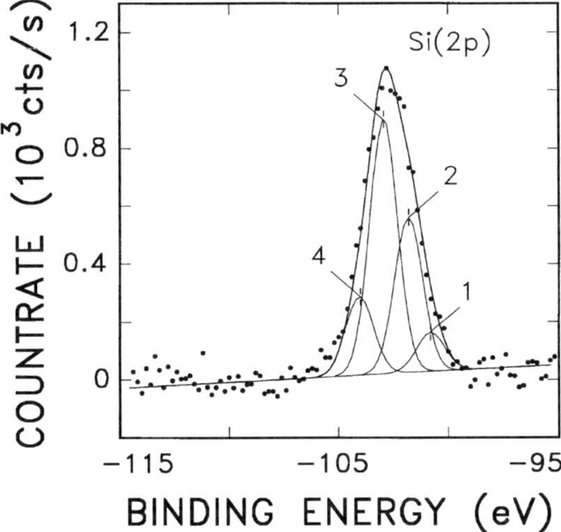

FIGURE 23.15 Photoemission spectrum (XPS) near the 2p peak of Si. The difference before and after a hexamethyldisiloxane treatment is shown.

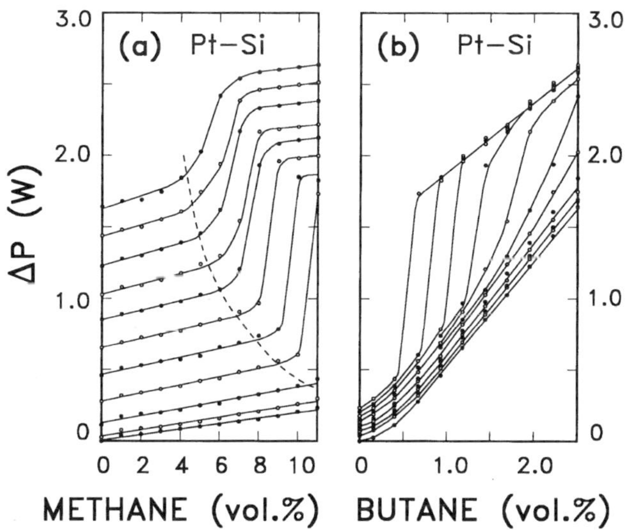

FIGURE 23.16 Pellistor with a hexamethyldisiloxane (HMDS) treatment as described in the text. The gas pulses are applied as described in the caption of Figure 23.13. Only one methane concentration value differs: 5.0 instead of 5.5 vol% methane. For clarity, the curves for 2 and 4 vol% methane are only plotted in the region limited by butane concentrations of 1.18 and 2.5 vol%.

The sensitivities to methane and butane are reduced to about 18 and 86%, respectively, by the HMDS treatment. The interaction between methane and butane remains strong. The description by the response equations of the untreated and the HMDS-treated pellistors allows the methane and butane contents below the LEL limits to be determined with an accuracy of 0.5 vol% for methane and 0.1 vol% for butane. It should be emphasized that in this numeric description the reaction order and an interaction effect is considered in a simple way only. A more accurate modeling of the characteristics for low concentrations and also for concentrations above the LEL levels was achieved by the neural network shown in Figure 23.17.

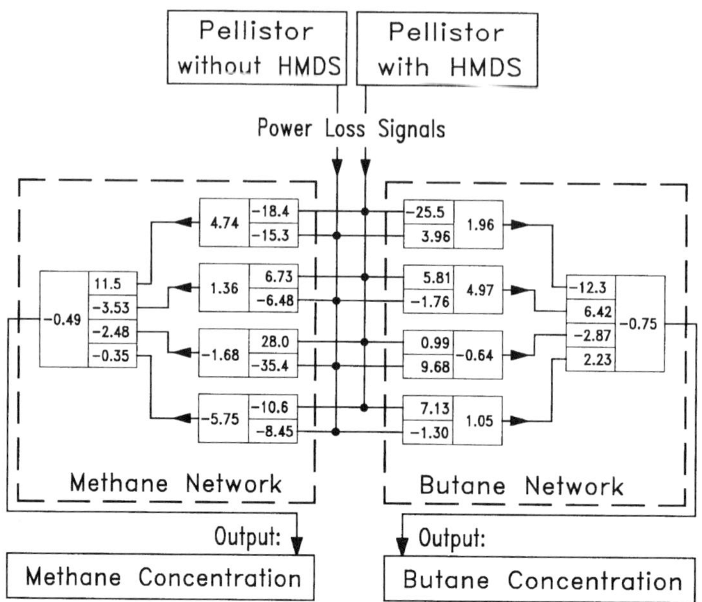

FIGURE 23.17 Neural network for the evaluation of the pellistors with the characteristics shown in Figures 23.13 and 23.16.

The procedure and the results are described in detail by Sommer et al.[66] Neural networks are also discussed in Chapter 27 of this book.

23.6.3.2 Oxide Sensor Array Evaluated by Polynomial Regression

Gas sensor arrays can be evaluated by a polynomial regression, too. Figure 23.18 shows the use of three commercial Figaro sensors for the quantitative determination of benzene (0 to 20 ppm) in mixture with 2-butanone (0 to 240 ppm).[67] A regression software (Abductive Networks, AIM, Abtech Corporation, Virginia, U.S.) known for its applicability to gas sensor arrays[68,69] has been used. AIM synthesizes a feed-forward network using a supervised learning algorithm. The underlying theoretical background can be found in Reference 70. The AIM network consists of nodes acting as functional elements. Different types of nodes are implemented in the algorithm. Normalizers (N in Figure 23.18) transform the original inputs into a common input region with a mean of 0 and a variance of 1. Unitizers reverse the normalization to get the output values. Single, double, and triple elements consist of third-order polynomials having one, two, or three input variables, respectively, and cross-terms between their inputs. These terms are able to consider the interaction of gases on the catalytically active surface of the sensor. The structure of an AIM network is not defined before the learning process as opposed to ANN. Finding the best network structure is part of AIM's learning algorithm. AIM first tests rather simple network structures, proceeding to more complex networks until the results are sufficiently precise. "Sufficiently" means a compromise between model complexity and accuracy concerning the training set. The criterion to classify the network structures, the so-called predicted squared error (PSE),[71] contains a complexity penalty multiplier which is used to choose between network structures with fewer coefficients or with higher precision. The structure shown in Figure 23.18 needed a learning time of a few minutes on an IBM-compatible desktop (386/40 MHz). The accuracy is marked below the scales for the case that the concentration of the other gas in the mixture has any value between zero and the full range. That means a concentration of 10 ppm benzene (can cause cancer) can be detected with an accuracy of +/–1.5 ppm, if butanone in any concentration between 0 and 240 ppm is simultaneously present.

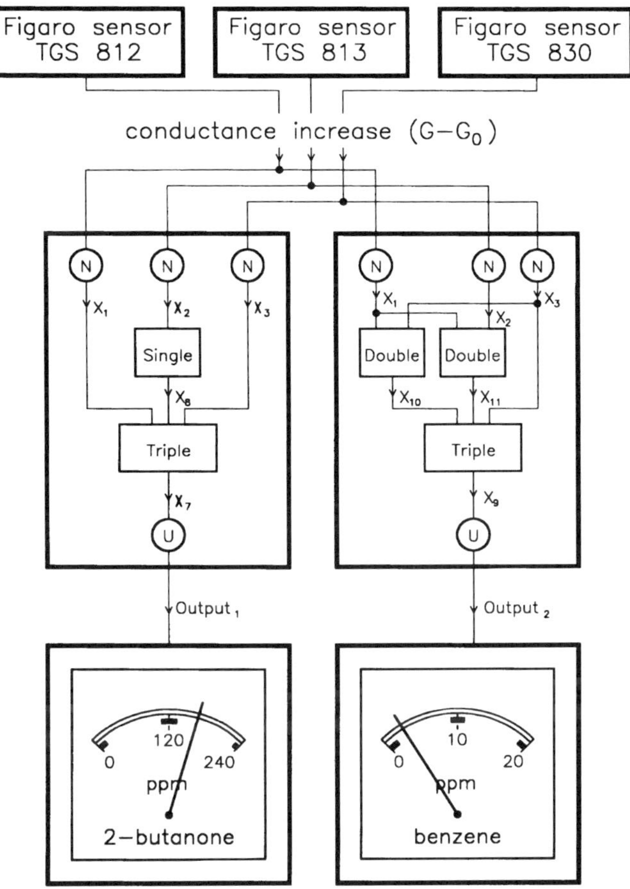

FIGURE 23.18 Array of three oxide sensors evaluated by a polynomial regression.[67] Details are given in the text.

23.6.4 Poisoning by Carbon Deposits

The third type of poisoning, carbon deposition, is a well-known problem in catalyst chemistry. During operation, catalytic sensors can even double their volume by carbon deposition if an efficient catalyst is used.[47] The essential step in carbon deposition on oxides is the attack of a double bond by electrophilic oxygen.[30] During decomposition of acetic acid an intermediate with a double bond is formed, which desorbs from single crystals. On thin films it is cracked and a carbon deposit results. A description of the individual steps is given below.

Exposure of a single crystal to gaseous acetic acid: acetic acid can adsorb on SnO_2 (101) faces as a molecule or dissociatively as acetate.

$$CH_3COOH_{gas} \leftrightarrow CH_3COO_{ads} + H_{ads} \tag{23.9}$$

The decomposition becomes apparent in second-order desorption (TDS maximum at 430 K) and is further proved by a low-temperature desorption of water. A considerable part of the mobile H atoms react with lattice oxygen and form water. The further decomposition of the surface acetate starts with the reaction:

$$CH_3COO_{ads} + 2\ H_{ads} \rightarrow CH_{4\ gas} + HCOO_{ads} \tag{23.10}$$

The TDS spectra of mass 28 (CO or C_2H_4) and of mass 44 (CO_2) look very similar to each other after acetic acid and methane exposure, but are clearly distinct after CO exposure.[16] Therefore, it seems reasonable that the decay reactions of methane via a formate intermediate are also applicable for the acetate decay (Equation 23.10). The increase of electrical conductance at a sample temperature of 473 K may arise from adsorbed hydrogen acting as donor.[72] Above about 650 K acetate can fill a vacancy with one of its oxygen atoms:

$$CH_3COOH_{gas} + V_o \leftrightarrow H_{ads} + CH_3CO - \text{“}O_{lat}\text{”} \quad (23.11)$$

Filling of a vacancy is also possible by oxygen and CO_2, as was shown in an XPS/UPS study on (0,0,0,-1)ZnO.[73] The singly "rooted" acetate with its higher binding energy causes a reincrease of the acetic acid desorption during continuous exposure at high temperatures. A fraction of the rooted acetate species forms keten, observed in desorption, thereby leaving one oxygen atom to fill the vacancy:

$$CH_3CO - \text{“}O_{lat}\text{”} \rightarrow H_2C = C = O_{gas} + H_{ads} + \text{“}O_{lat}\text{”} \quad (23.12)$$

The formate from Reaction 23.10 contains two oxygen atoms of the initial adsorbate. It decomposes into CO and CO_2.[13] The singly rooted acetate from Equation 23.11 can undergo an analogous reaction, delivering a formate including one lattice oxygen atom:

$$CH_3CO - \text{“}O_{lat}\text{”} \rightarrow CH_{2\ ads} + HCO - \text{“}O_{lat}\text{”} \quad (23.13)$$

During continuous exposure to acetic acid in a reactive scattering experiment the CO_2 and the CO desorption fluxes decay. The conductance increases irreversibly. The common reason may be a depletion of lattice oxygen by high-temperature water formation only partly compensated for by Reaction 23.11. In this reaction path, no carbon deposit occurs on the single crystal.

Thin evaporated films: acetic acid increases the surface conductivity at 573 K presumably by the effect of hydrogen donors. At 623 K and 673 K the conductance responds with a transient minimum to acetic acid addition to the ambient air. The minimum possibly reflects the filling of oxygen vacancies by acetate species, thus canceling subsurface donors. Later, in the decomposition process of the singly rooted acetate, the formate extracts oxygen out of the surface producing new donors. Therefore the conductance increases again.

SnO_2 thin-film devices, exposed to acetic acid in air, show after some time an oscillatory conductance behavior. Stable behavior can only be restored by transient heating in air to 870 K. In a reactive scattering experiment with the film kept at 585 K (below the TDS maxima of the formate products) only water desorbs as decomposition product (compare Figure 23.19a). According to a sum equation, elementary carbon must be deposited:

$$CH_3COOH_{gas} \rightarrow 2\ H_2O + 2\ C_{deposited} \quad (23.14)$$

A keten desorption according to Equation 23.12 is missing on thin films. On the rough surface of thin evaporated films keten can react at its carbon-carbon double bond with exposed oxygen atoms at steps. A similar reaction is discussed for the decay of acetaldehyde. This type of electrophilic attack by oxygen, also observed on oxidized copper and silver surfaces, is known to result in carbon deposition on the surface.[30] In the presence of air at sufficiently high temperature it is possible to remove deposited carbon by the formation of CO or CO_2.[30] The curves in Figure 23.19b and Figure 23.19c, recorded at a substrate temperature of 673 and 725 K, also show CO and CO_2 as products of an acetate/formate decay.

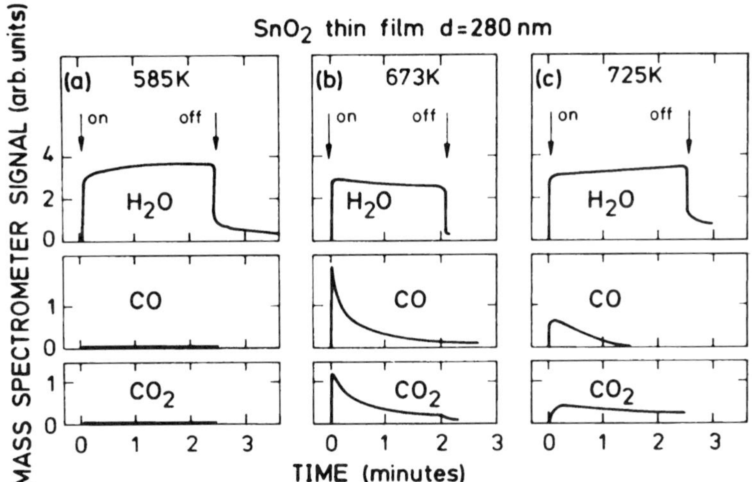

FIGURE 23.19 Fluxes of reactively scattered products from an evaporated film at three different temperatures during exposure to acetic acid. The signals of the decomposition products are corrected for cracking contributions from the acetic acid.

23.7 FUTURE WORK

The results from studies on surface reactions can be used as guidelines to optimize preparation of sensor elements. For example, the parallel routes of dehydrogenation and dehydration of ethanol on SnO_2 described in Section 23.3.6 initiated the exchange of surface tin ions by metal ions of higher electronegativity difference to oxygen (compare Section 23.4). Thereby dehydrogenation is faciliated with the results of a higher ethanol sensitivity. By an exchange of surface tin atoms with metal atoms of lower electronegativity difference to oxygen the dehydration reaction is strengthened and a sensor for other gases (e.g., for CO) with low cross-sensitivity to ethanol is the result. Both types of sensors are now commercially available.

Present investigations in our group are directed towards studies of reactions on sensor surfaces with a chopped molecular beam to eludicate kinetic processes. It is desirable to complement the results of reaction studies by morphological data as available by atomic force or LEED microscopy.

ACKNOWLEDGMENT

The work was supported by the German Bundesminister für Forschung und Technologie (BMFT).

ABBREVIATIONS AND TERMS

UHV: ultra high vacuum (below 10^{-8} Pa)
TDS: thermal desorption spectroscopy using a sensitive mass spectrometer
XPS: X-ray photoemission spectroscopy using X-ray core level excitations
UPS: ultraviolet-light photoemission spectroscopy valence band spectroscopy
XRD: X-ray diffraction analysis for morphology studies
LEED: low-energy electron diffraction
HMDS: hexamethyl disiloxane decomposes to SiO_x on hot surfaces
Auger spectroscopy using an electrons source for core level excitation

REFERENCES

1. Seiyama, T., Ed., *Chemical Sensor Technology,* Vol. I–IV, Kodansha Ltd., Tokyo, in cooperation with Elsevier, Amsterdam, 1988–1992.
2. Heiland, G. and Kohl, D., Problems and possibilities of oxidic and organic semiconductor gas sensors, *Sensors Actuators,* 8, 227, 1985.
3. Egashira, M., Shimizu, Y., and Takao, Y., Configurational design of semiconductor thick film sensors for odor sensing, *Proceedings of the Symposium on Chemical Sensors II*, M. Butler, A. Ricco, and N. Yamazoe, Eds., SENSOR GROUP Proc., Vol. 93-7, Electrochemical Society Inc., Pennington, NJ, 1993, 510.
4. Feng, C.-D., Shimizu, Y., and Egashira, M., Gas-sensing properties of layer-built SnO_2 sensors fabricated by Sol-Gel processing, *Proceedings of the Symposium on Chemical Sensors II*, M. Butler, A. Ricco, and N. Yamazoe, Eds., SENSOR GROUP Proc., Vol. 93-7, Electrochemical Society Inc., Pennington, NJ, 1993, 538.
5. Yamazoe, N. and Miura, N., Some basic aspects of semiconductor gas sensors, in *Chemical Sensor Technology* Vol. IV, T. Seiyana, Ed., Elsevier Science, Amsterdam, 1992, 19.
6. Narducci, D., Cinquegrani, L., D'Acci, E., and Pizzini, S., A study of the surface sensitivity of tin oxide sensors to carbon monoxide and dioxide, *Proceedings of the Symposium on Chemical Sensors II*, M. Butler, A. Ricco, and N. Yamazoe, Eds., SENSOR GROUP Proc., Vol. 93-7, Electrochemical Society Inc., Pennington, NJ, 1993, 482.
7. Ishihara, T., Nishi, Y., Kometani, K., Mizuhara, Y., and Takita, Y., Sensing mechanisms of capacitive type CO_2 sensor, CuO-$BaTiO_3$, *Proceedings of the Symposium on Chemical Sensors II*, M. Butler, A. Ricco, and N. Yamazoe, Eds., SENSOR GROUP Proc., Vol. 93-7, Electrochemical Society Inc., Pennington, NJ, 1993, 474.
8. Morita, T., Miyayama, M., Motegi, J., and Yanagida, H., NO_x gas sensing properties of La_2CuO_4 ceramics, *Proceedings of the Symposium on Chemical Sensors II*, M. Butler, A. Ricco, and N. Yamazoe, Eds., SENSOR GROUP Proc., Vol. 93-7, Electrochemical Society Inc., Pennington, NJ, 1993, 450.
9. Tamaki, J., Zhang, Z., Fujimori, K., Akiyama, M., Harada, T., Miura, N., and Yamazoe, N., Grain size effects on tungsten oxide-based nitrogen oxides sensor, *Proceedings of the Symposium on Chemical Sensors II*, M. Butler, A. Ricco, and N. Yamazoe, Eds., SENSOR GROUP Proc., Vol. 93-7, Electrochemical Society Inc., Pennington, NJ, 1993, 456.
10. Nanto, H., Kawai, T., and Tsubakino, S., ZnO thin film chemical sensor for trimethyl- and dimethylamine gases, *Proceedings of the Symposium on Chemical Sensors II*, M. Butler, A. Ricco, and N. Yamazoe, Eds., SENSOR GROUP Proc., Vol. 93-7, Electrochemical Society Inc., Pennington, NJ, 1993, 522.
11. Matsuurka, Y., Takahata, K., and Ihokura, K., Mechanism of gas sensitivity change with time of SnO_2 gas sensors, *Sensors Actuators,* 14, 223, 1988.
12. Heiland, G. and Kohl, D., Studies on single crystals in relation to the principles of semiconducting metal oxide gas sensors, *Proc. International Meeting on Chemical Sensors*, T. Seiyama, K. Fueki, J. Shiokawa, and S. Suzuki, Eds., Elsevier, Kodansha, 1983, 125.
13. Kohl, D., Thoren, W., Schnakenberg, U., Schüll, G., and Heiland, G., Decomposition of gaseous acetic acid on SnO_2, *J. Chem. Soc. Faraday Trans.,* 87, 2647, 1991.
14. Sputtered films were kindly supplied by Dräger AG, Lübeck, Germany.
15. Haber, J., Catalysis and surface chemistry of oxides, in *Proc. 8th International Congress on Catalysis*, Vol. 1, Verlag Chemie, Weinheim, 1984, 85.
16. Heiland, G. and Kohl, D., Physical and chemical aspects of oxidic semiconductor gas sensors, *Chemical Sensor Technology,* Vol. I, Elsevier Science, Amsterdam, 1988, 15.
17. Bond, G. C., *Heterogeneous Catalysis: Principles and Applications,* Oxford Chemistry Series, Clarendon Press, Oxford, 1987.
18. Yamazoe, N., Fuchigami, J., Kishikawa, M., and Seiyama, T., Interactions of tin oxide surface with O_2, H_2O and H_2, *Surface Sci.,* 86, 335, 1979.
19. Heiland, G. and Kohl, D., Problems and possibilities of oxidic and organic semiconductor gas sensors, *Sensors Actuators,* 8, 227, 1985.
20. Nakamura, Y., Yasunaga, S., Yamazoe, N., and Seiyama, T., Stabilization of SnO_2 gas sensor sensitivity, Proc. of the 2nd Int. Meet. Chemical Sensors, Bordeaux, 1986, 163.

21. Munnix, S. and Schmeits, M., Electronic structure of oxygen vacancies on TiO2 (110) and SnO_2 (110) surfaces, *J. Vac. Sci. Technol.,* A5, 910, 1987.
22. Egdell, R. G., Eriksen, S., and Flavell, W. R., Oxygen deficient SnO_2 (110) and TiO_2 (110). A comparative study by photoemission, *Solid State Commun.,* 60, 835, 1986.
23. Egdell, R. G., Eriksen, S., and Flavell, W. R., A spectroscopic study of electron and ion beam reduction of SnO_2 (110), *Surface Sci.,* 192, 265, 1987.
24. de Fresart, E., Darville, J., and Gilles, J. M., Influence of the surface reconstruction on the work function and surface conductance of (110)SnO_2, *Appl. Surface Sci.,* 11/12, 637, 1982.
25. Lannto, G., private communication, 1992.
26. Kohl, D., Oxidic semiconductor gas sensors, in *Gas Sensors, Principles, Operation and Developments,* G. Sberveglieri, Ed., Kluwer Academic, 1992, 43.
27. Jacobs, H., Mokwa, W., Kohl, D., and Heiland, G., Characterization of structure and reactivity of ZnO and SnO_2 supported Pd catalysts, *Vacuum,* 33, 869, 1983.
28. Harrison, P. G. and Maunders, B., Tin oxide surfaces. Part 14. Infrared study of the adsorption of ethane and ethene on tin(IV) oxide, tin(IV) oxide-silica and tin(IV) oxide-palladium oxide, *J. Chem. Soc. Faraday Trans. I,* 81, 1311, 1985.
29. Böttger, U., Diploma thesis, Aachen, FRG, 1988.
30. Bowker, B. and Madix, R. J., The adsorption and oxidation of acetic acid and acetaldehyde on Cu (110), *Appl. Surface Sci.,* 8, 299, 1981.
31. Harrison, P. G. and Maunders, B. M., Tin oxide surfaces. Part 11. Infrared study of the chemisorption of ketones on tin(IV) oxide, *J. Chem. Soc. Farad. Trans.,* 80, 1329, 1984.
32. Warwick, M. E., The oxidation of CO by O_2, N_2O and NO over tin oxide catalysts, Proc. Properties Uses Inorg. Tin Chemicals, Bruxelles, Belgium, 1986.
33. Harrison, P. G. and Thornton, E. W., Tin oxide surfaces. Part 9. Infrared study of the adsorption of CO, NO and CO+NO mixtures on tin(IV) oxide gels containing ion-exchanged Cr(III), Mn(II), Fe(III), Co(II), Ni(II) and Cu(II), *J. Chem. Soc., Faraday Trans. I,* 74, 2703, 1978.
34. Ruiz, P. and Delmon, B., Selective oxidation of hydrocarbons, Proc. Properties Uses Inorg. Tin Chemicals, Bruxelles, Belgium, 1986, 1.
35. Morrison, S. R., Semiconductor gas sensors, *Sensors Actuators,* 2, 329, 1982.
36. Takahata, K., Tin oxide sensors — development and applications, highly sensitive SnO_2 gas sensor for volatile sulfides, in *Chemical Sensor Technology,* Vol. I, T. Seiyama, Ed., Elsevier Science, Amsterdam, 1988, 39.
37. Pijolat, C., Etude des Proprietes Physico-chimiques et des Proprietes Electriques du Dioxide d'Etain en Fonction de l'Atmosphere Gazeuse Environnante. Application a la Detection Selective des Gaz, Thesis, Grenoble, 1986.
38. Harrison, P. G. and Maunders, B. M., Tin oxide surfaces. Part 15. Infrared study of the adsorption of propene on tin(IV) oxide, tin(IV) oxide-silica and tin(IV) oxide-palladium oxide, *J. Chem. Soc. Farad. Trans.,* 81, 1329, 1985.
39. Harrison, P. G. and Maunders, B., Tin oxide surfaces. Part 16. Infrared study of the adsorption of formic acid, acrylic acid and acrolein on tin(IV) oxide, tin(IV) oxide-silica and tin(IV) oxide-palladium oxide, *J. Chem. Soc. Faraday Trans. I,* 81, 1345, 1985.
40. Harrison, P. G. and Maunders, B. M., Tin oxide surfaces. Part 12. A comparison of the nature of tin(IV) oxide, tin(IV) oxide-silica and tin(IV) oxide-palladium oxide. Surface hydroxyl groups and ammonia adsorption, *J. Chem. Soc. Farad. Trans.,* 80, 1341, 1984.
41. Harrison, P. G. and Maunders, B. M., Tin oxide surfaces. Part 13. A comparison of the nature of tin(IV) oxide, tin(IV) oxide-palladium oxide and tin(IV) oxide-silica. An infrared study of the adsorption of carbon dioxide, *J. Chem. Soc. Farad. Trans.,* 80, 1357, 1984.
42. Schierbaum, K. D., Elektrische und spektroskopische Untersuchungen an Dünnschicht-SnO_2-Gassensoren, Doctoral Thesis, Tübingen, FRG, 1987.
43. Huck, R., Böttger, U., Kohl, D., and Heiland, G., Spillover effects in the detection of H_2 and CH_4 by sputtered SnO_2 films with Pd and PdO deposits, *Sensors Actuators,* 17, 355, 1989.
44. Peukert, M., XPS study on surface and bulk palladium oxide, its thermal stability and a comparison with other noble metal oxides, *J. Phys. Chem.,* 89, 2481, 1985.
45. Narayanan, S., Strong metal support interaction, *J. Sci. Ind. Res.,* 44, 580, 1985.

46. Dannetun, H., Lundström, I., and Petersson, L.-G., Reactions between hydrocarbons and an oxygen covered palladium surface, *Surface Sci.*, 193, 109, 1988.
47. Gentry, S. J. and Walsh, P. T., The influence of high methane concentrations on the stability on catalytic flammable-gas sensing elements, *Sensors Actuators*, 5, 229, 1984.
48. Kobayashi, T., Haruta, M., Sano, H., and Nakane, M., A selective CO sensor using Ti-doped alpha-F_2O_3 with coprecipitated ultrafine particles of gold, *Sensors Actuators*, 13, 339, 1988.
49. Bond, G. C. and Sermon, P. A., Gold catalysts for olefin hydrogenation. Transmutation of catalytic properties, *Gold Bull.*, 6, 102, 1973.
50. Kim, K. H., Han, H. S., and Choi, J. S., Kinetics and mechanisms of the oxidation of carbon monoxide on α-Fe_2O_3, *J. Phys. Chem.*, 83, 1286, 1979.
51. Hoogers, G., Huck, R., Kohl, D., and Heiland, G., The uptake of oxygen by noble metal clusters on gas sensors, *Sensors Actuators*, B9, 123, 1992.
52. Cullis, C. F. and Willat, B. M., Oxidation of methane over supported precious metal metal catalysts, *J. Catal.*, 83, 267, 1983.
53. Kohl, D., The role of noble metals in the chemistry of solid-state gas sensors, *Sensors Actuators*, B1, 158, 1990.
54. Moseley, P. T. and Tofield, B. C., Eds., *Solid State Gas Sensors*, Adam Hilger, Bristol, 1987.
55. Gall, M., The Si planar pellistor: a low-power pellistor sensor in Si thin-film technology, *Sensors Actuators*, B4, 533, 1991.
56. Sommer, V., Rongen, R., Tobias, P., and Kohl, D., Detection of methane/butane mixtures in air by a set of two microcalorimetric sensors, *Sensors Actuators*, B6, 262, 1992.
57. Hicks, R. F., Qi, H., Young, M. L., and Lee, R. G., Structure sensitivity of methane oxidation over platinum and palladium, *J. Catal.*, 122, 280, 1990.
58. Alnot, M., Cassuto, A., Fusy, J., and Pentenero, A., Comparative adsorption of O_2 and N_2O on platinum recrystallized ribbons, *Jpn. J. Appl. Phys.*, Suppl. 2, 79, 1974.
59. Ehrhardt, J. J., Colin, L., Accorsi, A., Kazmierczak, M., and Zdanevitch, I., Catalytic oxidation of methane on platinum thin films, *Sensors Actuators*, B7, 656, 1992.
60. Anderson, R. B., Stein, K. C., Feenan, J. J., and Hofer, L. J. E., Catalytic oxidation of methane, *Ind. Eng. Chem.*, 53, 809, 1961.
61. Gentry, S. J. and Walsh, P. T., The theory of poisoning of catalytic flammable gas-sensing elements, in *Solid State Gas Sensors*, P. T. Moseley and B. C. Tofield, Eds., Adam Hilger, Bristol, 1987, 32.
62. Stoneham, A. N., Oxide surfaces: the basic processes of sensor behaviour, in *Solid State Gas Sensors*, P. T. Moseley and B. C. Tofield, Eds., Adam Hilger, Bristol, 1987, 159.
63. Morrison, S. R., Semiconductor gas sensors, *Sensors Actuators*, 2, 329, 1982.
64. Lagois, J., private communication.
65. Finster, J., Schulze, D., and Meisel, A., Characterization of amorphous SiO_x layers with ESCA, *Surface Sci.*, 162, 671, 1985.
66. Sommer, V., Tobias, P., and Kohl, D., Methane and butane concentrations in a mixture with air determined by microcalorimetric sensors and neural networks, *Sensors Actuators*, B12, 147, 1993.
66a. Sommer, V., Tobias, P., Kohl, D., Sundgren, H., and Lundström, I., Neural networks and abductive networks for chemical sensor signals: a case comparison, *Sensors Actuators*, B28, 217, 1995.
67. Bläser, G., Diploma thesis, Gießen, 1994.
68. Sundgren, H., Vollmer, H., and Lundström, I., Chemical sensor arrays and abductive networks, *Sensors Actuators*, B9, 127-131, 1992.
69. Sundgren, H., Winquist, F., Lukkari, I., and Lundström, I., Artificial neural networks and gas sensor arrays: quantification of individual components in a gas mixture, *Meas. Sci. Technol.*, 2, 464-469, 1991.
70. Farlow, S. J., Ed., *Self Organizing Methods in Modeling: GMDH Type Algorithms*, Marcel Dekker, New York, 1984.
71. Barron, A. R., Predicted squared error: a criterion for automatic model selection, *Proceedings of the Symposium on Chemical Sensors II*, M. Butler, A. Ricco, and N. Yamazoe, Eds., SENSOR GROUP Proc., Vol. 93-7, Electrochemical Society Inc., Pennington, NJ, 1993, 87-113.

72. Thoren, W., Kohl, D., and Heiland, G., Kinetic studies on the decomposition of CH_3COOH and CH_3COOD on SnO_2 single crystals, *Surface Sci.,* 162, 402, 1985.
73. Au, C. T., Hirsch, W., and Hirschwald, W., Adsorption of carbon monoxide and carbon dioxide on annealed and defect zinc oxide (0,0,0,-1) surfaces studied by photoelectron spectroscopy (XPS and UPS), *Surface Sci.,* 197, 391, 1988.

24 Arrays of Broad Specificity Films for Sensing Volatile Chemicals

Krishna C. Persaud and Paul J. Travers

CONTENTS

24.1 INTRODUCTION

The natural function of the human sense of smell is to assess the quality of food or of the immediate environment. It is easy for us to distinguish between the fragrance of a perfume and the putrid odour of rotting meat, and our reactions towards these odours vary accordingly. However, it is not so easy to describe or explain this difference in perception. It is difficult to describe an odour except by comparing it with a more familiar one. There is no scale for measuring the intensity of odours as there is for sound (decibels) or light measurements

0-8493-8905-4/97/$0.00+$.50
© 1997 by CRC Press, Inc.

(lumens). A coherent theory to explain how the nose and brain detect, identify, and recognise an odour is still to be developed. However the biochemical mechanisms involved in odorant perception are now being investigated by a number of laboratories around the world and rapid progress is being made. This section outlines some of the current understanding of the nature of odours, the biological mechanisms involved, odour measurements, and the importance of particular odour classes in food and drink.

24.1.1 ODORANTS

The expertly trained human nose can detect differences between about 10,000 odorous stimuli. The human observer has a large descriptive vocabulary for different olfactory experiences. Odorants which can interact with the olfactory epithelium range from very small molecules such as ammonia (mol wt 17) (pungent), hydrogen sulphide (mol wt 34) (putrid), to larger molecules such as hexadecanolide (musk) (mol wt 254). The structures of the chemicals that give odour sensation are very diverse, and a few of these are illustrated in Figure 24.1. There appears to be no structural requirement for a molecule to be an odorant provided that it is sufficiently volatile to reach the olfactory epithelium, but some common molecules met in everyday life such as saturated hydrocarbons may have little perceptible odour. Molecules of molecular weight greater than about 300 are odourless.

The size and shape of an odorant molecule, together with the distribution of polar groups, determine the odour description. However the exact structural requirements specifying a particular odour type are still ill-defined. Examination of some enantiomeric odorants show that both enantiomers have relatively minor odour differences, indicating a rather "loose" stereospecific requirement at the level of the olfactory receptors. On the other hand, the (+) and (-) isomers of carvone smell like oil of spearmint and caraway, respectively. The presence of polar groups in certain odorant series can be correlated with a distinctive odour type, e.g., the lower fatty acids have a sweaty odour, the lower amines have a fishy odour, and the lower thiols have a putrid odour. With such small molecules, the polar groups will play an important part in any interaction with the olfactory receptors. With large molecules also containing polar groups, the influence of these polar groups on the odour description will be much less.

The most important parameters of an odorant molecule that determine the olfactory response are adsorption and desorption energies of the molecule from an air/lipoprotein interface, the partition coefficients between water and lipoprotein, the electron donor/acceptor interactions which depend on the polarisability of the molecule, and the molecular size and shape.

24.1.2 THE OLFACTORY SYSTEM

The olfactory system of vertebrates may be divided into three main parts shown in Figure 24.2. These are

1. the olfactory epithelium that presents an exposed odour-sensitive surface to the external environment;
2. the olfactory bulb which is important in the processing of signals from the olfactory epithelium;
3. the cerebral hemispheres, where the inputs from the olfactory bulb are combined with inputs from the other senses and with feedback systems within the brain. At this level, the message which is generated at the level of the olfactory epithelium by an odour, is recognised as such, and appropriate behavioural action is initiated if necessary.

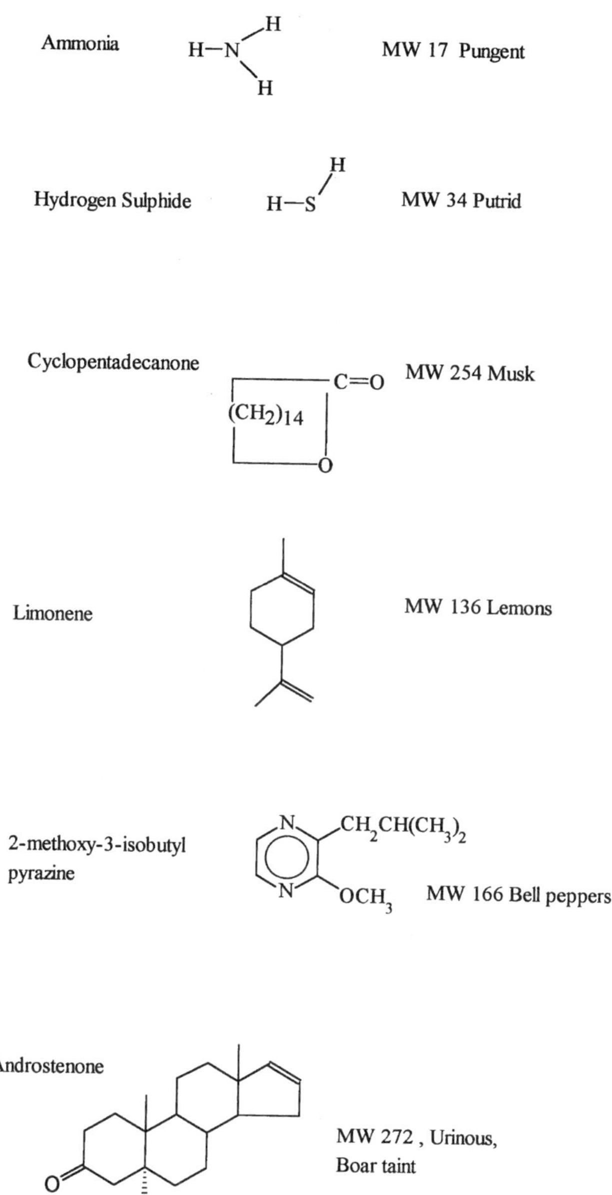

FIGURE 24.1 Chemical structures of a range of odorant molecules showing the range of molecular sizes, shapes, and polar groups that may be involved in defining the odour that is perceived.

24.1.3 Biochemical and Peripheral Events

Much research effort has been focused on the nature of the olfactory receptor proteins, the mechanisms of olfactory transduction, and perireceptor events involved in the overall process of odour sensing (secretion, odorant clearance, detoxification).[1,2] Where the transduction mechanisms are concerned, it is now thought that the binding of an odorant molecule to a receptor protein on the ciliary membranes of receptor cells initiates a sequence of biochemical interactions which culminate in the opening of a sodium ion channel. However the olfactory receptor proteins still have not been isolated and characterised, although recent progress has been made in identification of the genes coding for a large number of olfactory receptor

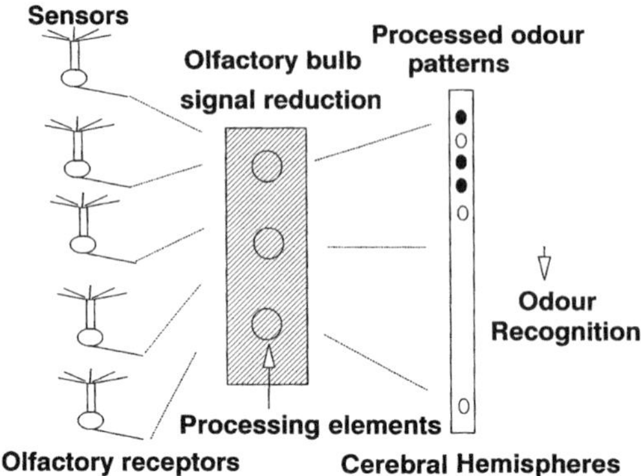

FIGURE 24.2 The olfactory system. The olfactory mucosa contains large numbers of specialised protein receptors that transduce chemical signals. The specificity characteristics are broad, but several families of receptors exist. The signals are integrated and processed in the olfactory bulb, where patterns of output may provide descriptions of odours that are being sensed. The higher processing centers in the brain are involved in interpretation of these patterns to produce odour recognition.

proteins.[3] It has been established that the molecules of the odorant must enter into contact with the receptor cells in order to excite them. Only a few molecules are necessary to excite the receptors and some substances inhibit the activity of the sensory cells. In vertebrates, the inflow of signals from the receptor cells undergoes nervous integration in the olfactory bulb and inhibition of neuronal activity is an important process in the integration. Olfaction plays an important role in many kinds of behaviour such as feeding, mating, and reproduction, and this correlates to the close structural function between the olfactory pathways and the rest of the brain, particularly those parts related to affective and endocrine functions like the pituitary. The ultrastructure of the olfactory system is well characterised; however, the biochemical events involved in olfactory transduction and the nature of the signal processing pathways still need much investigation.

The chemical stimulus alters the properties of a specialised area of the receptor cell membrane, such that the ionic permeability changes and a change in conductance occurs. The change in conductance, together with the electrochemical gradient across the membrane, causes an inward current (receptor or transduction current). The summated change in current across the olfactory mucosa shows an approximately logarithmic relationship to the concentration of the stimulus.

The receptor current produces a change in membrane potential (receptor potential). The receptor potential spreads to an area of membrane that has a regenerative current-voltage relation. This is the spike-initiating region located on the axon hillock of the olfactory neuron. The electrotonic spread of the receptor potential is called the generator potential.

The neural spikes generated in response to an odour stimulus are transmitted to the olfactory bulb via the synapses of the olfactory nerve. In the olfactory bulb much data reduction and processing of information is carried out, resulting in characteristic patterns of activity of output neurons that may be interpreted by the higher centres as descriptors of the odour being sensed.

24.1.4 Olfactory Measurements

Human perception of odour is descriptive. Scales of human perception are subjective, yet carefully designed questions can produce surprisingly precise answers. In the context of evaluating a particular odorous compound, or a mixture, typical questions to which a psychophysical scale can be assigned are the following:

1. How potent is the odour?
2. Are there different notes identifiable?
3. How pleasant or unpleasant is the odour?

These are the usual unconscious assessments that one makes in everyday life for food, drink, perfumes, and other odours of the immediate environment.

24.1.5 Measures of Sensitivity and Discrimination

In general, there are two main concepts used in the measurement of odour: detectability and intensity. Olfactory psychophysics specifies sensitivity and discrimination in terms of either the absolute or differential threshold. A method commonly used in the food and beverage industry is the triangular test. The human subject is presented with six sets of three flasks for each stimulus concentration or stimulus class, depending on what is being measured. The stimulus to be measured is presented in a carefully balanced arrangement or randomised arrangement of all groups of stimuli of the types XXY and YYX (Figure 24.3). There are six possible arrangements of the flasks and one chance in nine that the human subject will select the correct combination by random choice. Usually the task faced by the subject is to pick out the sample that is different from the others in the set of three, after being told that two of the samples in each set are the same. The method may be used with both quantitative and qualitative differences. If one of the samples is a blank then the procedure determines the absolute threshold. If the differences between the samples are known in advance and are quantifiable, then the triangular test determines the differential threshold. Many variations of this method exist, such as the method of Paired Comparisons between samples, or defining one set of samples as a standard to be compared to others as in the Duo-Trio test (Figure 24.3).

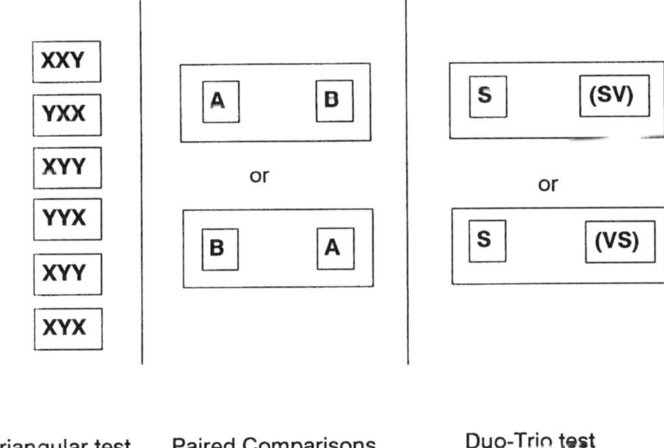

FIGURE 24.3 Psychophysical tests. *The triangular test*: the human subject is asked to pick out the odd sample from the group of three of the odorant sequence type XXY, and other variants of this arrangement totalling six groups of three samples. *Paired comparisons*: the human subject is asked to compare two samples designated A and B with one another. *The Duo-Trio test*: a standard sample S is provided and this is followed by a pair of samples, one of which is the same as the standard. Denoting this as S and V, the subject is asked which of the second pair is the same as the standard S.

Also, several statistical methods have been used to evaluate the results of such tests. These psychophysical evaluations are surprisingly accurate providing a large population is tested. Amoore has used these techniques to show the existence of specific anosmia to several classes of odorants, and to quantify the extent of these anosmia in the human population.[4] The number of these genetic defects of smell discovered have indicated that there are at least 30 different families of odour receptors. Since the existence of an olfactory defect may not preclude the detection of a particular odour class, even though that perception may be different or require much higher concentrations before detection can occur, there is evidence that a given odour may interact with different receptor sites to different extents. This indicates that individual olfactory receptors are not tuned to individual odorants, but that they have a rather broad specificity.

Olfactometric methods are also common, especially in the area of malodour assessment.[5] Detectability is measured by the number of times an odour sample must be diluted with an equal volume of odour-free air until the odour can just be detected in half of the instances. This is referred to as dilution to odour threshold. The number of dilutions can be expressed as odour units per cubic metre, where the odour unit is defined as a cubic metre of air at its odour threshold. Intensity is a measure of the strength of the perceived odour stimulus. The power law formulated by Stevens[6] for many psychophysical events such as taste, loudness, or brightness may approximate to a certain extent to human odour perception as well, and may be expressed as

$$I = k\,C^{p}$$

where I is the perceived intensity, C is the odour concentration, and k and p are constants. Because the human nose surpasses many analytical instruments in sensitivity, many industries that produce foods, beverages, perfumes, or flavourings, rely on human panel judgment as to the quality of the raw materials used and of the final product.

24.1.6 Requirements and Applications of Odour-Sensing Devices With Emphasis on the Food Industry

Before going on to describe artificial odour sensing devices, it is useful to reflect on why such devices are needed and how they may be used. The chemical species to be sensed are diverse and the complexity of measurement becomes greater when it is considered that the headspace of foods, beverages, or the odours of the normal human environment may contain many hundreds of compounds, all interacting with the chemical senses to allow perception of an infinite number of odour nuances. Evaluation of the organoleptic qualities of cooked foods and the identification of contaminants or off-odours are major preoccupations of many food product manufacturers and involves panels of humans trained in distinguishing subtle variations in odours.

24.1.6.1 The Odour of Cooked Foods

Possibly the most important contributor to the odour and flavour of cooked foods is the Maillard reaction (nonenzymic browning).[7] This sequence of carbonyl-amino reactions occurs widely during the heating or prolonged storage of foodstuffs and is a major source of browning and flavour production. The reaction is named after the French chemist Louis Maillard, who first described the formation of brown pigments when heating a solution of glucose and glycine. It now comprises the reactions of aldehydes, ketones, and reducing sugars with amines, amino acids, peptides, and proteins. In foodstuffs, the reactions normally occur between reducing sugars and amino acids or proteins. In food proteins most primary amino groups are represented by the ε-amino group of lysine, and to a small extent the α-amino groups of N-terminal amino acids. In addition, most foods contain a certain proportion of free amino acids.

The most important consequence of the Maillard reactions is flavour and aroma production. However, protein-sugar interactions may severely reduce the nutritional value of foods and some of the products may be toxic. The flavours and aromas from Maillard reactions are generated by heat processes such as baking, roasting, frying, concentration, and dehydration. These include the food aromas described as toasted, baked, nutty and roasted; the corn-like aroma of heated grains, the desirable and undesirable burnt and bitterish tastes of roasted malt, roasted nuts, coffee and cocoa, the burnt and bitter flavours of overheated or long-stored dehydrated foods.

The first step involves the condensation between the carbonyl group of a reducing sugar and the free amino group of an amino acid or protein. The condensation product rapidly loses a molecule of water and is converted into a Schiff's base. This undergoes cyclisation to the corresponding N-substituted glycosylamine which is converted to the 1-amino-1-deoxy-2-ketose by the Amadori rearrangement, a step which involves the transition from an aldose to a ketose derivative. These early reactions do not cause browning or give flavour. However, the 1-amino-1-deoxy-2-ketoses are important nonvolatile flavour precursors.

There are three main pathways in the advanced Maillard reaction, all of them leading to the production of brown pigments or melanoidins, and two of these pathways begin with the Amadori compound. In the first pathway, the 1-amino-1-deoxy-2-ketose enolises C-3 irreversibly and eliminates the amine from C-1 to form a methyl dicarbonyl intermediate, which further reacts with fission products such as C-methyl aldehydes, keto aldehydes, dicarbonyls, and reductones. The reaction products include such flavour and aroma products as acetaldehyde, pyruvaldehyde, diacetal, and acetic acid (Figure 24.4a).

In the second pathway, 3-deoxyhexosones are formed from the enol form of the Amadori compounds by the elimination of the hydroxy group at C-3. Dehydration then occurs yielding flavour compounds such as 2-furaldehydes. The reactions which follow the formation of these intermediates are complex and little understood. They result finally in the production of dark-brown nitrogen-containing pigments, and are believed to involve aldol condensations, aldehyde-amino polymerisation, and the formation of the heterocyclic nitrogen compounds such as pyrazines, pyrroles, and pyridines, which appear to be largely responsible for the roasted, bready, and nutty flavours of heated foods (Figure 24.4b). Many of these compounds have extremely low olfactory thresholds in humans.

The third pathway is the Strecker degradation which involves the oxidative degradation of free amino acids by the α-dicarbonyls and other conjugated dicarbonyl compounds produced by the breakdown of the Amadori compound in pathways one and two. In the Strecker degradation, amino acids are degraded to the corresponding aldehydes of one atom less, with the loss of carbon dioxide. For the reaction to proceed satisfactorily, the amino group must be in the alpha position and the carbonyl compound must contain a –CO–CO– or a –CO–(CH=CH)–CO– grouping. The transamination could be an important reaction in the incorporation of nitrogen into melanoidins. Most of the carbon dioxide released during Maillard reactions is derived from the carboxyl groups of amino acids during Strecker degradation. The Strecker aldehydes appear to be important auxiliary flavour compounds, but they can also condense with themselves, with furfurals, or with other dehydration products to form melanoidins.

The typical aromas of the Maillard reaction products appear to be due mainly to the N-heterocyclic compounds (Figure 24.4b). However, the fragrant caramel aroma fraction seems to consist mainly of oxygen heterocyclics, with rather specific, related molecular structures. They are mainly cyclic enolones that have planar or nearly planar, O-cyclic or alicyclic structures. The structure common to all compounds is the CH –CO–C=C(OH)–C=O grouping (e.g., maltol) or the CH –CO–C=C–OH (e.g., isomaltol). Other compounds of this type include the dehydrofuranones, dehydropyrone, aminoreductones, and cyclopentenolones.

The smell of burnt food is characteristic, and many Maillard reaction products can contribute to the pungent, burnt aroma. The structures generally involved are α,β-unsaturated

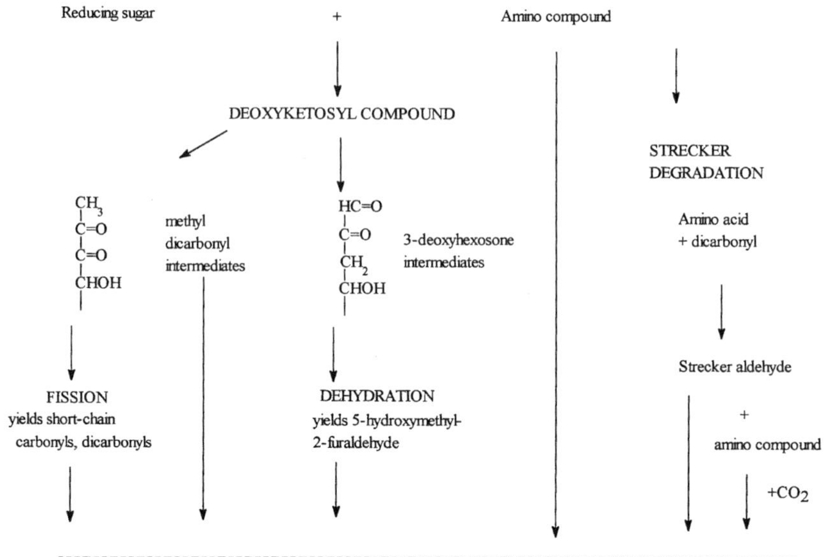

a

green,vegetable

nutty, roasted

green

green,nutty

nutty, roasted

green

roasted,nutty,green

green, nutty

green

cocoa, nutty

nutty, roasted

sweet, nutty

nutty, roasted, meaty

nutty, roasted

O OH CH3

Thiazoles

Pyrazines

Pyridines

Maltol

burnt

b

FIGURE 24.4 The Maillard Reaction and its odorous products. (a) A simplified scheme of the Maillard reactions. Reducing sugars and amino compounds combine together to produce a large variety of odorous compounds. (b) A selection of some odorous products of the Maillard reaction.

aldehydes or the corresponding acids. The groups involved are –CO–CO– as in glyoxal, pyruvaldehyde, and diacetal and the –C=C–CHO grouping such as in acrolein. These reactive Maillard intermediates are more volatile than the N-heterocyclic or caramel flavours and they register burnt aromas at extremely low concentrations.

As part of the odour of cooked food, aldehydic and ketonic aromas may contribute to the flavour of food without being characteristic of them. These aromas are given by monocarbonyls with the general structure R–CHO and R–CO–CH. A detailed account of the Maillard reactions is given by Morton and Macleod.[8]

24.1.6.2 The Odour of Spices

Spices are very commonly used to enhance the flavour and odour of foods. Take ginger for example. This is a prepared rhizome from *Zingiber officinale*. It has been used as a spice and a medicine from early times by the Chinese and Indians. The spice reached Europe in the ninth century. It gives a pungent, pleasant flavour to many foods and beverages. The spice contains 1 to 3% of a volatile oil. The main constituent is a sesquiterpene, and two terpenes d-camphene and β-phellandrene. Also present is borneol, a sesquiterpene alcohol called zingiberol, and linalol. The aldehydes present are citral, decylic aldehyde, and nonylic aldehyde. In addition there is cineole, methyl-heptenone, and acetic and caprylic esters.

Another commonly used flavouring agent is garlic. Garlic is the bulb of *Allium sativum*, a member of the lily family. The most important flavouring products of the Allium genus include onions, shallots, leeks, and chives. These form a well-defined group of flavours called alliaceous. These flavours can be highly appreciated in some contexts, but not in others where they may be repellent. The predominant constituent of garlic is a volatile oil. The main components of the oil are diallyl disulphide (60%), allyl propyl disulphide (6%), diallyl trisulphide (20%), and other higher sulphides.

Coriander seed, the dried ripe fruit of *Coriandrum sativum* is one of the earliest spices used by humans. It is mentioned in the Sanskrit literature and was one of the drugs used by Hippocrates. About 1% of the fruit is a volatile oil. The major constituent of the oil is the terpene alcohol linalol (60%). Associated with d-linalol are various terpenes, including d-α-pinene, dl-α-pinene, β-pinene, dipentene, α-terpinene, g-terpinene, p-cymene, geraniol, l-borneol, C10-aldehyde, and acetic esters of the alcohols present.

These examples give only a tiny proportion of the volatile chemicals used to enhance the aroma of foods, and in the kitchen one may find vanilla, cardamoms, fennel, cumin, celery, and many other spices.

24.1.6.3 Off Odours

Many compounds may give an unpleasant or off-odour to foods and beverages. These may be due to decomposition, or to contamination, or to naturally occurring biochemical reactions. Some of these may be part of the normal odour characteristics of a particular food or beverage, but once the particular component increases above a certain level, the odour note becomes unpleasant to human perception. Such compounds may include mercaptans, amines, and fatty acids. Other compounds such as chloroanisoles, chlorophenols, and geosmin may give musty or medicinal character to the product.

24.1.7 Criteria for the Design of Artificial Odour-Sensing Devices

The sections above give some idea of the complexity of the chemical species that are sensed by the human nose when evaluating odour quality and intensity. Furthermore, it must be realised that under normal circumstances, the olfactory system is evaluating a complex mixture of these substances, where small differences in the relative proportion of one component to others can make the difference between an odour being classed as unpleasant or pleasant. The human nose accomplishes this evaluation by processing information from large numbers of chemical sensors, each of which may have relatively broad specificity to a number of chemical species, but responding mainly to particular families of chemicals.

An electronic system reproducing the characteristics of the human nose could make use of an array of sensors, each designed to match the odour specificity of the single types of olfactory receptors. This would be very difficult to accomplish, as we do not have enough information on the physicochemical characteristics of the olfactory receptors. It would be a major challenge for organic chemists to design artificial sensors with the desired characteristics. Fortunately, it is not necessary to reproduce the human olfactory code in an artificial system as long as we provide the artificial sensing system with enough information for translating the patterns produced by different stimuli into odour descriptions, using the terms that humans use.

In analogy to the biological system, the design of an artificial odour-sensing system would require volatile chemical sensors of broad overlapping specificity that are able to recognize stereochemical parameters of the odorants to a greater extent than functional groups. In order for the information from the artificial sensing system to be applied practically, information is required from the biological system, in terms of odour/structure relationships, to provide the basis for translation criteria between the patterns produced by the sensor arrays and odour descriptions. More thought has to be given to the system as a whole and not just to the chemical sensing elements. The use of multi-element sensor systems for discrimination between odours was reported for the first time by Dodd and Persaud,[9] who showed that discrimination of complex odours could be achieved by three tin oxide Taguchi sensors with broad, but overlapping specificity of response. Since then, many groups have developed sensor arrays based on several technologies that may in the future create complex sensory systems that mimic a large number of odour-sensing characteristics of the human nose.

24.2 SENSING TECHNOLOGIES BASED ON ARRAYS

There are many phenomena which have been exploited as potential gas detectors and a number have been incorporated into sensing arrays in an attempt to achieve better discrimination.

24.2.1 Tin Oxide Detectors

Many researchers have chosen the commercially available Taguchi Gas Sensors (TGS) (Figaro Inc., Japan) as the core sensing element in their investigation of array based odour detectors. These devices consist of an electrically heated ceramic pellet onto which a thin porous film of SnO_2 doped with various precious metals has been deposited. The doped SnO_2 behaves as an n-type semiconductor and the chemisorption of oxygen at the surface results in the removal of electrons from the conduction band. Gases interact with the surface-adsorbed oxygen and thereby affect the conductivity of the SnO_2 film. The devices are run at elevated temperatures (typically 300 to 400°C) to achieve rapid response/recovery times and to avoid interference from water. This results in relatively high power consumption. The response characteristics can be tailored by varying the operating temperature and the doping agent. A more detailed description of the reactions that can take place at the SnO_2 surface is given by Kohl[10] (see Chapter 23 in this handbook). Sensors have been developed for the detection (down to the parts per million level) of a range of target molecules including H_2, CO, NH_3, H_2S, NO_x, SO_x, ethanol, and hydrocarbons.

Gardner and co-workers[11-17] (see also Chapter 27 in this book) have carried out extensive work with these devices, constructing arrays with up to 12 different sensors. Generally, the commercial sensors have been used without modification, but in a recent paper[17] a standard device was catalytically modified with Pd, Au, and Rh. Typically the fractional conductance change was used as the output signal for pattern generation. This could be normalised to the largest change in the array, or the average change across the array, to reduce the concentration dependence of the patterns. Investigation of pattern recognition has been carried out with alcohols,[11-14,16] alcoholic beverages,[11] roasted coffee,[14] and tobacco smoke.[11] A variety of pattern recognition techniques has been utilised including partial least-squares analysis, discriminant function analysis, principal component analysis, cluster analysis, and neural networks.

Nakamoto et al.[18] used an array of three similar TGS sensors operating at different temperatures to differentiate between acetone, ammonia, and hexane. In subsequent experiments[19] three different TGS sensors were used, together with an analogue back-propagation neural network circuit for pattern recognition. After training, the system could discriminate between n-hexane (166 ppm), acetone (166 ppm), and ammonia (3320 ppm) with an output error of less than 5%. The same array was also successfully trained to differentiate between benzene, gasoline, and 2-methyl-1-butene.

The response of an array of 8 TGS sensors to 30 different substances was investigated by Abe et al.[20] Individual sensor responses $r = \log10(R_{air}/R_{gas})$ were normalised by dividing by the total change for the whole array to reduce the concentration dependence of the patterns. Cluster analysis of the patterns produced classes corresponding to ethereal, ethereal-minty, ethereal-pungent, and pungent substances. In subsequent work[21] the measurements were extended to 47 different volatiles and the number of sensors in the array was reduced to 7. Normalisation was carried out relative to one of the sensors to produce a six-component vector for pattern recognition. Classification using a potential function method produced ethereal, pungent, and minty categories. A five-sensor element array[22] has been used to characterise acetone, acetic acid, and ethanol at four different concentrations (10 to 100 ppm) under various environmental conditions.

Modified TGS sensors have also been studied by Schierbaum et al.[23,24] Standard devices were immersed in solutions of transition metal salts and subsequently sintered at various temperatures to modify their behaviour. Arrays of up to six sensors have been studied with changes in both conductivity (G_{gas}/G_{air}) and the work function providing pattern information. The target gases selected were CO (10 to 800 ppm), CH_4 (10 to 15,000 ppm), H_2 (10 to 15,000 ppm), and water (0 to 50% relative humidity). Multicomponent analysis was used to extract partial pressures from gas mixtures.

Walmsley et al.[25] used an array of four TGS sensors to generate patterns for ethanol, ether, hexane, petrol, chloroform, and benzene. Principal component analysis, cluster analysis, and star symbol plots were used to visualise the multivariate data. Discrimination of the aromas from a range of beers, wines, and spirits has been achieved with an array of six TGS sensors.[26] A headspace concentrator was used to pretreat the aroma volatiles and remove ethanol from the samples. Resistance changes were measured relative to a set of reference sensors; responses were normalised by dividing by the total change across the array, and the resulting six component patterns were analysed using a variety of pattern recognition techniques. TGS sensors have been used in conjunction with electrochemical gas sensors by Utsumi et al.[27] Quantitative analysis was carried out on gasoline vapours in the presence of interfering odorants such as toluene, n-butyl acetate, and triethylamine. Olafsson et al.[28] have used arrays of between two and six TGS sensors to evaluate fish freshness. Initially, the response to a number of pure odorants (propanone, butanol, and trimethylamine), present in the headspace of fish, was investigated. Subsequent measurements were then made to investigate the aging of fish samples, both stored in ice and at room temperature, and the results were compared to readings from a pellistor-based commercial odour meter (by Sensidyne, U.S.) and from a fish freshness meter using dielectric measurements.

As an alternative to the commercially available TGS sensors, several research groups have recently investigated the possibility of fabricating thin-film SnO_2 arrays using planar microelectronic technology. Potentially, these could have a number of advantages including a reduction in size and lower power consumption. Gardner et al.[29] have sputtered thin tin oxide films onto silicon substrates with a thermally grown SiO_2 layer (1 μm) for electrical insulation. Metal interdigitated electrodes and a heater/thermometer were fabricated on top of the SnO_2 layer by a combination of vacuum sublimation, electrodeposition, and subsequent photolithography. The response of a typical sensor to ether was presented. Power loss through the ceramic package on which the devices were mounted proved to be a major problem.

Walmsley et al.[30] used an array of three thin-film sensors produced in-house by chemical vapour deposition. The sensor characteristics were varied either by doping with ZnO or by varying the thickness of the tin oxide layer. Response curves for ethyl acetate, acetone, ethanol, pentane, and mixtures of the above were generated and the maximum resistance change was taken as a descriptor for the analyte. Characteristic response patterns were produced for each solvent. A variety of chemometric techniques was used to identify and quantify the components in solvent mixtures.

Thin-film sensors (50 nm) have been sputtered onto alumina substrates and then catalytically doped with an overlayer of either silver or palladium (2 nm).[31] A four-sensor array (two devices of each type) shows high sensitivity to H_2S (measurable response for <5 ppb) and has been used to monitor environmental pollution in a city atmosphere. Faglia et al.[32] have also investigated thin SnO_2 films sputtered onto alumina and then doped with an ultrathin metal layer (palladium or platinum). A nine-sensor array was constructed from SnO_2, SnO_2-Pd, and SnO_2-Pt devices operating at three different temperatures. Conductance changes were used for a quantitative analysis of NO_2, H_2S, and mixtures of both (0 to 9 ppm).

Finally, screen printing has been used to fabricate thick-film sensors of tin oxide. Sensors can be doped by mixing different materials into the basic SnO_2 paste used in the printing process. A four-sensor array was produced in this way consisting of an undoped device and sensors doped with ZnO, MoO, and CdS.[33] Measurements were made on a number of solvent volatiles and the pattern data were analysed by transformed cluster analysis. Dutronc et al[34] used two screen-printed SnO2 sensors doped with palladium or platinum to differentiate between ethanol and methane.

24.2.2 Quartz Resonator and SAW Devices

Quartz resonator odour sensors consist of a piezoelectric quartz crystal oscillator coated with a sensing membrane. The adsorption of odorant molecules onto the membrane results in a decrease in the resonant frequency due to the increased mass. This frequency shift can be used as the sensor output and the device response can be varied by using different membrane materials. (On specifically sorbent films see Chapter 25 in this book.)

Nakamoto and co-workers[35-39] carried out extensive work with quartz resonator arrays containing up to eight different sensors. A wide range of membrane materials was screened including celluloses, gas chromatographic stationary phase materials, and lipids (both natural and synthetic). Frequency changes were normalised relative to either the largest change in the array or the length of the pattern vector. To emphasise differences within a particular set of analytes the response pattern for one sample is subtracted from the others. The arrays have been tested on alcoholic drinks[35,36] and perfume/flavour odorants.[38,39] Principal component analysis has been used to visualise the differences in the multivariate data and identification was achieved using neural network pattern recognition. (On data analysis see Chapter 20 and Chapter 27 in this book.)

Quartz resonator devices coated with plasma polymer films (e.g., polyethylene, polytetrafluoroethylene) deposited by rf sputtering have been studied by Nakamura and co-workers.[41,42] An array of six oscillators was used with both the maximum change in frequency and the time constant of the response contributing pattern information. The pattern data from a range of solvent vapours have been analysed by principal component analysis and using a self-organising map neural network.[42]

Surface acoustic wave (SAW) devices consist of interdigitated electrodes fabricated onto a piezoelectric substrate (e.g., quartz) onto which a thin film coating of a selective material is deposited. An applied radio frequency voltage produces a Rayleigh surface acoustic wave (i.e., a surface oscillation). Adsorption of odours onto the coating increases its mass and elastic modules and thereby perturbs the wave leading to a shift in frequency. To compensate for pressure and temperature effects the sample sensor is usually connected to a reference SAW device and the frequency difference is detected. As with quartz resonator devices, the selectivity is determined by the coating material. SAW devices, however, can be operated at higher frequencies which results in improved sensitivity.[43] (See also Chapter 9 in this book.)

Rose-Pehrsson et al.[44] constructed an array of ten SAW sensors, each coated with a different polymer. Responses were normalised by dividing by the resonant frequency of the coated substrate in the absence of the vapour. This improves the reproducibility in the response of sensors coated with the same polymer. Patterns were generated for a range of solvent vapours at different concentrations. For pattern recognition the concentration dependence was reduced by dividing each response by the largest change in the array. Principal component analysis and clustering methods show that individual vapours could be easily distinguished. The same raw data was later analysed by Zellers et al[45] using principal component regression analysis. In this instance concentration normalisation was not carried out in order that information on vapour concentration should be retained during classification. In a subsequent study by Grate et al.[46] an array of four polymer-coated sensors was used to detect trace amounts of toxic organophosphorus and organosulphur vapours (nerve gases or nerve gas analogues), both individually and in the presence of interfering organic solvents (present at much higher concentrations). An automated sampling system was used which included thermally desorbed preconcentrator tubes and allowed agent vapours to be detected at very low concentrations (minimum 0.01 mg m^{-3}).

Reichart et al.[47] have also investigated the response of polymer-coated SAW sensors. Vapours from octane, methanol, water, and fuel (concentration range 16 to 3600 ppm) were investigated using an array of four devices. Partial least-squares analysis when applied to the sensor responses from analyte mixtures was able to determine the methanol concentration.

24.2.3 Other Technologies

Before considering gas detectors based on conducting polymers some of the other technologies which have been used in sensor arrays will be reviewed.

Stetter et al.[48] used an array consisting of four amperometric sensors (fabricated in-house) operating with different working electrodes and working electrode potentials. The performance of one sensor was optimised for CO detection. This array was used in conjunction with a catalytic microreactor (a heated platinum filament) designed to oxidise organic vapours into detectable decomposition products. In a later paper[49] the CO-optimised sensor was used together with a commercial CO detector (which exhibited significant cross-sensitivity to other chemicals) to analyse mixtures of CO, formaldehyde, benzene, and perchloroethylene.

MOSFETs (see Chapter 6) have been configured as gas detectors (CHEMFET), the vapour producing a shift in the conductance-voltage characteristic. Muller and Lange[50] investigated an array of four MOSFET sensors whose behaviour was modified with coatings of zeolite of various pore sizes. The initial rate of change of capacitance on exposure to the gas was used as the signal for each sensor. Patterns were generated for a range of solvent volatiles, ammonia, and hydrogen. Palladium and platinum gate MOSFETs operating at three different temperatures were used by Sundgren et al.[51] to estimate hydrogen concentration in the presence of ammonia, ethene, and ethanol. In later work[52] a third MOSFET with an iridium gate was introduced and the devices were operated at six different temperatures.

Si-planar-pellistor sensors detect combustible gases by measuring the heats of reaction as they are oxidised at a heated catalyser surface. Gall[53] has produced arrays of such sensors whose behaviour can be modified by adjusting the operating temperature or changing the catalyser. The power needed to maintain a constant temperature at a particular sensor is reduced when gases are burning and this reduction is converted to an output voltage. Patterns generated for trichloroethylene, pentane, methane, CO, ethanol, and methanol by an eight-sensor array could be resolved by cluster analysis.

An array of five metal-substituted phthalocyanines, each acting as a simple chemiresistor, has been produced by Cranny and Atkinson[54] The organic semiconductors were vacuum sublimed onto interdigitated electrodes with each sensor having a separate platinum heater. Optimisation of film thickness and operating temperature for each device maximised the dissimilarity in response to the two target gases, NO_2 and H_2S. The logarithmic resistance change was chosen as the output signal and five-component patterns were generated for various concentrations of NO_2 (20 to 500 ppb) and H_2S (0.2 to 5.0 ppm). In addition the system was tested with various mixtures of the two analytes.

24.2.4 Conducting Polymers

The unique electrical properties of organic conducting polymers, derived from aromatic and hetero-aromatic materials, have led to a large amount of research and application of these materials in different areas, and since 1979 when Diaz et al.[55] first prepared polypyrrole as a free-standing film, many thousands of publications have appeared. Persaud and Pelosi presented an application of conducting polymers for odour sensing at the European Chemoreception Organisation Conference in 1984, and a detailed publication appeared in 1985.[56]

Conducting polymer gas sensors based on measuring resistance changes in thin film structures have been studied by a number of researchers.[57-62] The response to electron-deficient (e.g., NO_2) and electron-rich (e.g., NH_3) species[57-59] can be accounted for in terms of a chemical reaction at the surface which directly generates or removes charge carriers within the semiconducting film. Bartlett and co-workers[60,61] have studied the response of polypyrrole films grown electrochemically across a narrow electrode gap. The response and recovery to organic vapours such as methanol is more rapid than for NO_2 or NH_3 but the sensitivity tends to be reduced. Possible mechanisms by which the gases may affect the behaviour of a conducting polymer chemiresistor are discussed by Bartlett and Gardner.[62]

Josowicz and co-workers[63-66] have developed gas-sensing devices based on measuring changes in the electron work function of an electrochemically deposited polypyrrole layer. Both FET (field effect transistor, see Chapter 6) and Kelvin probe configurations (measuring the contact potential between the film and a suspended gold electrode) have been used to measure the shifts in the work function caused by the adsorption of a range of organic volatiles. The response of the polypyrrole film (i.e., the magnitude and the sign of the work function shift) is determined by the electrochemical deposition conditions and, in particular, the electrolyte/solvent system used. Measurements have also been made of the change in the optical absorption spectra on exposure to organic vapours. This data together with the work function shifts, suggest a small but reversible charge transfer (either donor or acceptor) when a gas is adsorbed at the polymer surface.

A third type of gas sensor using polypyrrole films deposited as an overlayer onto quartz resonator devices has been investigated by Slater and co-workers.[67-69] In addition to monitoring the mass loading effect of adsorbed volatiles a simultaneous measurement of conductivity changes was made on a separate device. A number of volatiles has been studied including NH_3, methanol, cyclohexane, acetone, and H_2S.

Conducting polymer chemiresistor arrays have been developed by Slater et al.[70] in which a single polymer (polypyrrole or a derivative thereof) is used, but the distance between electrodes is varied from sensor to sensor. The relative change in conductance (G_{gas}/G_{air}) was used as the output signal and the four component patterns were subjected to principal component analysis. An array coated with poly(N-methylpyrrole) was able to resolve patterns from methanol, ethanol, and propanol. A range of alcoholic beverages could be discriminated using an array coated with a polymer bilayer.

Following on from their work with polypyrrole, Bartlett and Ling-Chung[71] incorporated several other conducting polymers such as poly(N-methylpyrrole), poly(5-carboxyindole), and polyaniline into chemiresistor structures by electrochemical deposition across narrow electrode gaps. These materials were screened against a range of solvent vapours (methanol, ethanol, toluene, acetone and ether) to assess their suitability for incorporation into sensing arrays. In subsequent work[72] arrays of up to 12 conducting polymer sensors predominantly polypyrrole with different counterions but including polyaniline and poly(3-methylthiophene) were investigated. The fractional change in resistance was measured for each sensor and then normalised by dividing by the vector length. The instrument was used to monitor the head-space above a variety of beers. Cluster analysis of the patterns generated by a six-element array for beers of different strengths (strong lager, normal-strength lager, and a low-alcohol ale) could easily classify the various samples. A 12-element array was able to differentiate between lagers of the same strength and to detect artificial tainting of a particular beer.

Shurmer et al.[73] investigated the possibility of constructing arrays of polypyrrole sensors whose characteristics were modified by coating with Langmuir-Blodgett films of various thicknesses. The arachidic acid/cadmium arachidate layers deposited can be skeletonised with organic solvents to produce holes which may function as a molecular sieve.

Persaud et al.[74,75] have continued to develop conducting polymers as odour-sensing devices, and many materials have been synthesised and characterised for odour transduction. The reasons for choosing conducting polymers as odour sensor elements are as follows:

1. The sensors show rapid adsorption and desorption kinetics at room temperature.
2. The sensor elements feature low power consumption (in the order of microwatts) as no heater element is required.
3. The structure of the polymer can be closely correlated to specificity towards particular classes of chemical compounds.
4. The sensors are resilient to poisoning by compounds that would normally inactivate inorganic semiconductor-type sensors, such as sulphur-containing compounds.

An instrument called "OdourMapper", based on conducting polymer sensors was commercialised from instrumentation developed by Persaud's group. This has now been developed into an analytica instrument, "AromaScan"™ that is being used by a wide variety of industries.

24.3 RECOGNITION OF ODOURS USING MULTIELEMENT SENSOR ARRAYS

It must be recognised that the human nose is a very fallible chemosensory system and is full of contrasts. On the one hand, there is exquisite sensitivity to some chemicals, while on the other hand there is very low sensitivity to other classes such as hydrocarbons. Also, the estimation of odour intensity is on a very poor and compressed scale. A trained human nose is able to discriminate subtle differences in the odour notes between almost identical mixtures of chemicals, yet the perception of odour quality is changeable and dependent on the concentration of the mixture of chemicals being assessed. The human nose can also be abused and yet contains so much redundancy that the discriminatory powers may be decreased only marginally. There are many reasons favouring the development of electronic noses. The human nose is fallible, subject to infection and poisoning, affected by the mental state of the subject, and changes in sensitivity with age.

In many areas of industry, panels of human noses continually assess the quality of raw materials, their processing, and the quality of the final product. This makes the use of artificial odour-sensing devices attractive, except that it must not be forgotten that human judgment is subjective in nature and each individual has preferences and dislikes that are dependent on the past experiences of the individual, or reflect the views of the society. Human judgment is also very context dependent, e.g., the odour of butyric or isovaleric acid is highly prized in the odour of many cheeses; however, when confronted with the same odour in the context of sweaty socks, the general human reaction is one of revulsion. A considerable amount of psychophysics is required to understand human sensory perception.

When confronted with an artificial odour-sensing device, the first reaction of a human user is to expect it to perform better than the human nose. In the design of artificial odour-sensing devices, much attention needs to be paid to the analysis of the requirements of the human user, and in what areas the instrument is likely to be used. Like any instrument, an odour-sensing device will perform well in a particular defined context where a specific question is being asked of the apparatus. For such an instrument to be useful to a wide variety of users, it needs to be flexible enough to adapt to changing requirements of odour discrimination and intensity estimation. The chemosensory systems of humans and vertebrates consist of arrays of chemical transducers, where each type of sensing element has chemical specificities that are broad, but distinct from each other. The signals from this system are processed to produce descriptors of the odour of individual chemicals, or mixtures of chemicals, as well as the intensity of the odour. It thus makes sense to design artificial chemical sensing arrays on this basis, where the application of neural network odour classifier software for such systems may be a less rigid approach than use of statistically based classifiers. (See also Chapter 20 and Chapter 27.) Conducting polymer sensor arrays can produce unique patterns in response to individual volatile chemicals, and these patterns show only slow change with time (Figure 24.5), allowing reliable pattern recognition over a long period of time. The longevity of such sensors may be several years, depending on usage.

Neural network research has been developing in at least two separate directions. In one direction, small systems are being applied as discrete adaptive pattern classifiers. These may not be any better than traditional statistically based classifiers, but they are often easier to use and train, giving them large practical advantages. In another direction, scientists are deliberately attempting to understand psychology and physiology with ideas adapted from artificial neural networks. Generally, only fairly small systems have been attempted, because of limitations in electronic hardware and software. Where artificial odour-sensing devices are concerned, if the goal is limited to simply discriminating odour A from odours B and C, then a simple classifier is adequate. If the goal is not only to carry out discrimination, but to associate the odour with the human perception of the odours, then a more sophisticated classifier is required. Thus, in this case, the directions of movement in neural network research need to reconverge. The section below outlines the directions that we have been exploring in neural net applications to multielement odour-sensing devices.

24.3.1 Artificial Neural Networks

The principles of artificial neural networks are described in a variety of texts[76,77] (including Chapter 27 here), and are not described in any detail here. We have applied algorithms mainly based on supervised learning strategies, where the problem is to discriminate between sets of previously defined odour classes.

An important aspect of an artificial chemosensory system is signal processing. It is almost impossible to guarantee a nonoverlapping orthogonal response of the sensor array when multiple odours have to be compared against each other. Responses to different odours will be correlated to a large extent and statistical classification methods may not be applicable.

We initially applied a correlative template matching pattern recognition approach to classify odours. This algorithm works with a majority of linearly discriminable pattern classes. However, several disadvantages became apparent with use. It required a search through a

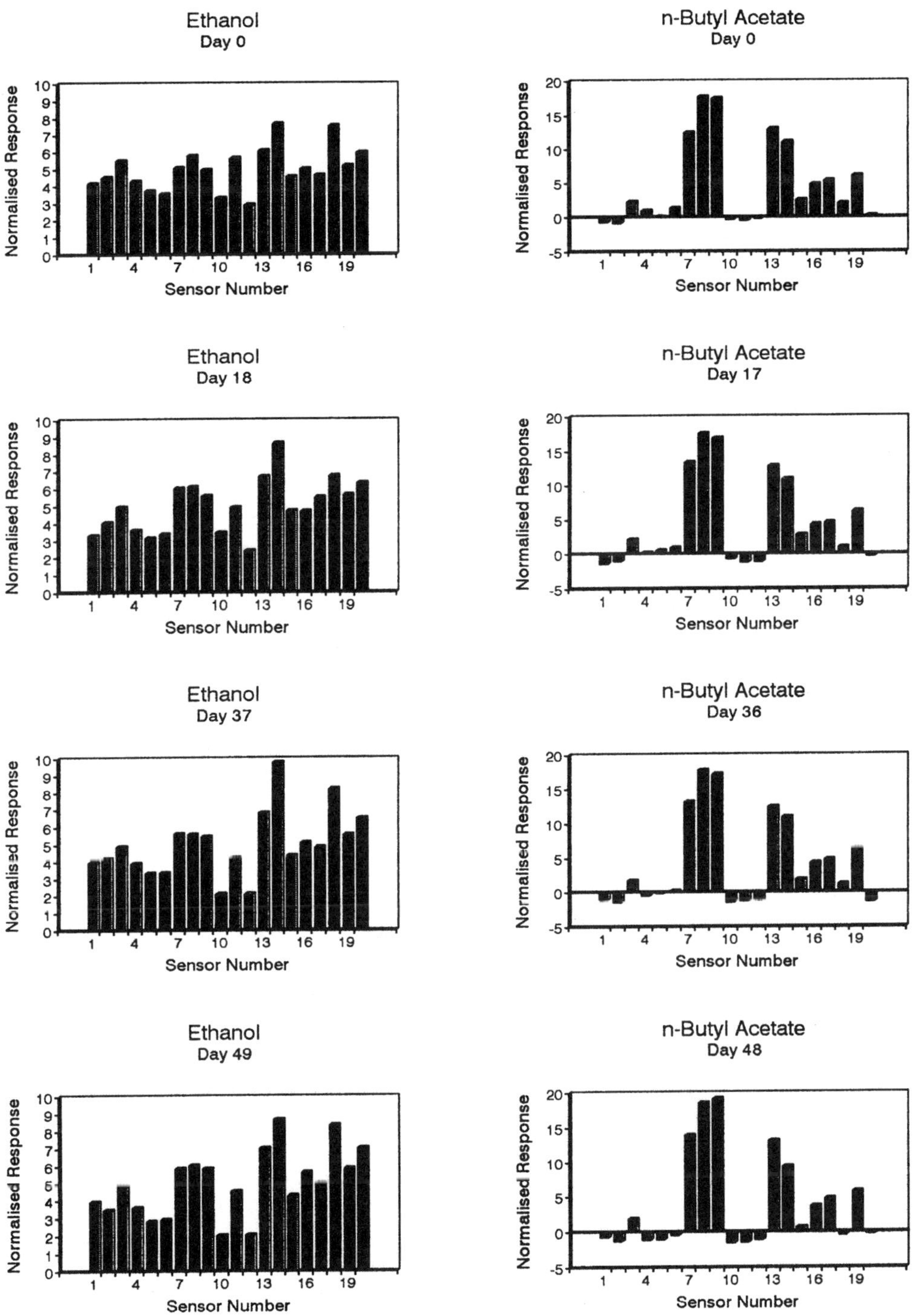

FIGURE 24.5 Variation with time of the normalised response patterns produced by a 20-polymer array on exposure to ethanol (2200 ppm) and n-butyl acetate (990 ppm). The diagram shows the relative responses of individual sensors in the array producing characteristic patterns that can be used to identify a particular chemical or odour. Good stability of patterns is seen over a long period of time.

large database in order to classify incoming odour patterns, thus making real-time recognition difficult. There was also some difficulty in coping with drift of the sensors that may be caused by temperature or humidity variations or by aging. Cases of discrimination caused by nonlinear sensor responses in the presence of mixtures of volatile chemicals could be resolved only with difficulty using this approach, and also high noise immunity of the system could not be achieved.

A computationally simple algorithm was needed that would fulfil several criteria discussed below. In order to cope with nonlinearly separable patterns, there had to be some nonlinear transformation of the input data. The ability to deal with partially redundant and intercorrelated input patterns was necessary. Also, the knowledge acquired during training of the system had to be stored in a compact, easily accessible form that would eliminate the need to access the training database during the recognition process. The strategy chosen had to be able to learn to recognise features when the input data was noisy, both during training and recognition. Also desirable was that the system should perform to an acceptable degree even if there was partial damage or saturation of the sensor array due to a high concentration of odour or amplifier saturation. Saturation of the sensors or of the amplifiers is an especially difficult problem to detect and to deal with since no information is delivered to the classification system and the corresponding feature becomes excluded from influencing the output of the system.

The following algorithms were investigated to determine if they would fulfil the above criteria. These consisted of

1. Two-layer Artificial Neural Networks (ANN) using linear and thresholding activation functions;
2. Multilayer ANN using the continuous sigmoid activation function;
3. Multilayer perceptron (MLP) architecture;
4. Error back-propagation (BP) learning paradigm. Network structures with one layer of hidden units with three hidden neurons, were investigated.

Training of the classifier was conducted in three steps described below.

1. There was an iterative presentation of the training data set to the system until convergence level was reached. After each presentation (training epoch) the errors were computed, and the weights and biases were correspondingly modified. If the error rate could be decreased below the specified level then the steps (2) and (3) were carried out. If this proved impossible then training stopped after a user-specified number of training epochs, and it was the responsibility of the user to deal with this nonconvergence situation.
2. There is a test of the resulting classifier on the same training data set. During the test, no weights or biases are modified. For a long training data set and an inappropriately selected input pattern sequence, it is possible that an error self-cancellation effect may occur. So, the most recent modification of weights may decrease the error for the current input pattern, but could destroy effects of training on the previously presented input patterns. In this case, the total output error reported at the end of the presentation sequence may drop below the requested threshold level, but the classifier still remains not fully trained and training should be continued. In order to eliminate such a situation, the training data set has to be presented once again to the system without changing any weights. If the reported output error conforms to the training convergence criterion then the testing step follows. Otherwise, the training in the processing step (1) has to be continued.
3. There was a full test of the resulting classifier on a data set not used for training, in order to determine how reliably the system performed in the recognition mode. During testing, no weights or biases in the network were modified.

Each of the input training datasets was processed by the algorithms summarised above, attempting to achieve convergence. From the performance of the algorithms it is found that the iteration cycle is shortest for the linear and thresholding two-layer networks, and approximately one order of magnitude longer for the BP networks. We observed that the relatively simple modified two-layer architecture with linear or thresholding activation functions leads to the best results. It has the shortest training times and also guarantees training convergence, reducing the training error rate to zero. It has also been proved, with the data tested, that it delivers the lowest recognition error rate of the algorithms used.

The results indicate that it is unnecessary to employ back-propagation-related algorithms at all. The BP algorithm also fails for another reason. It normally requires very "clean" (noise-free) training data for it to be trained in a reasonable time. After being trained, it is relatively noise-robust, although it is much weaker than the 2-layer thresholding networks.

24.4 APPLICATION OF CONDUCTING POLYMER ARRAYS TO ODOUR SENSING

The system developed at UMIST by Persaud and co-workers has been used to investigate the response of a 20-sensor array to the homologous series of n-alcohols (methanol to 1-pentanol).[78] Some of the data presented in that paper are discussed here. The array, consisting of ten different conducting polymers deposited in pairs, was placed in a sealed glass vessel fitted with an electrically driven PTFE stirrer. Alcohols were injected either as neat liquids or in solution in pentane for the lower concentrations. Typically, three to five injections were made within a particular experiment to give several points on the concentration-response profile. After the final injection the flask was opened to ambient in order to monitor the recovery of the sensors.

The results of four such experiments are shown in Figure 24.6 for a single sensor made of a heterocyclic conducting polymer (No.2) exposed to methanol (3 × 1600 ppm), ethanol (3 × 1100 ppm), 1-propanol (3 × 870 ppm), and 1-butanol (3 × 200 ppm). The response and recovery times of all the polymers tend to increase along the series of alcohols, although it should be noted that part of the delay in the response is a result of the injected sample taking a finite time to evaporate.

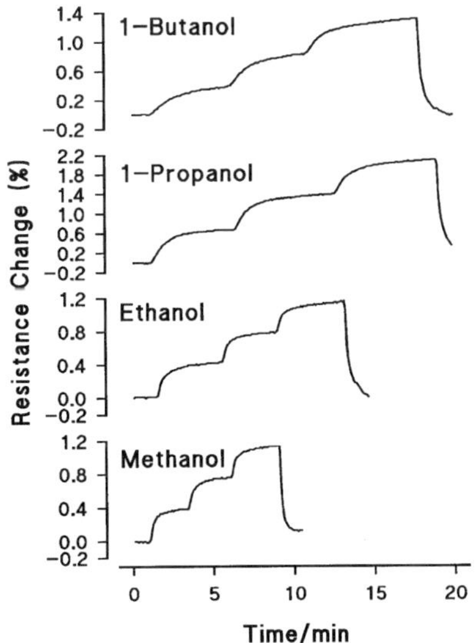

FIGURE 24.6 Response of a sensor of polymer **2** on exposure to methanol (3 × 1600 ppm), ethanol (3 × 1100 ppm), 1-propanol (3 × 870 ppm), and 1-butanol (3 × 200 ppm).

The concentration-response profiles are approximately linear in the concentration regions studied (e.g., Figure 24.7). The gradient of each fitted line in Figure 24.7 is a measure of the respective sensor's sensitivity to methanol (i.e., the percentage in device resistance as a function of volatile concentration in the ambient gas, expressed in parts per million). To compare the response of the ten polymers to the five alcohols, the slopes of each sensor pair have been averaged and plotted as a bar chart in Figure 24.8. The reason for the dramatic increase in sensitivity on moving to the higher alcohols (a factor of almost 30 when comparing the response of polymer 6 to methanol and 1-pentanol) is as yet unclear. One would expect the enthalpies of adsorption to increase with molecular mass as a result of stronger van der Waals interactions with the polymer surface. Evidence for this comes from the observed decrease in recovery rate along the homologous series (Figure 24.6). The rate of adsorption at the surface will depend on the collision frequency and the sticking probability.[79] As molecules are adsorbed at the surface the sticking probability drops due to unfavourable interactions with molecules already bound, until the rates of adsorption and desorption are equal and an equilibrium surface concentration is established. By increasing the adsorption energy the rate of desorption is reduced and equilibrium is reached at a higher surface concentration. In addition, it should be noted that the time taken to establish equilibrium is also increased. It is possible that this may partially account for the observed behaviour.

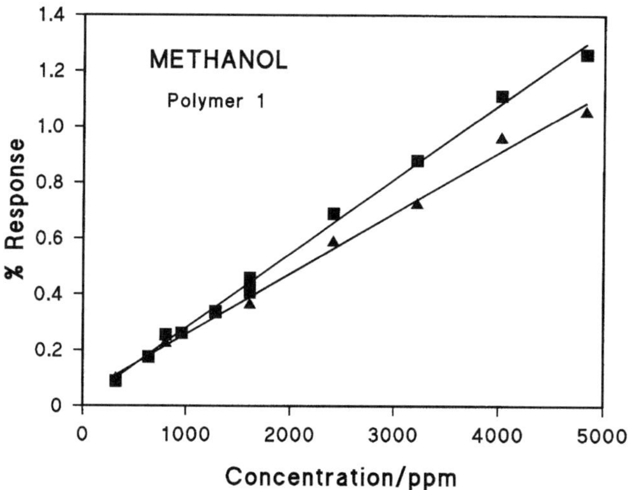

FIGURE 24.7 Methanol concentration-response profiles for the pair of polymer 1 sensors. Lines of linear least-squares fit have been plotted through both data sets.

The response patterns of the 20-sensor array to each alcohol are shown in Figure 24.9. These patterns have been normalised so that the resistance change on each sensor is expressed as a percentage of the total change for the whole array. At low concentrations, where it is reasonable to assume that the concentration-response profiles are linear with zero intercept, patterns normalised in this way become concentration independent. Such patterns can be used to train a neural network to recognise a particular sample irrespective of vapour concentration. Nonlinear mapping is a technique through which a high-dimensional multivariate set of data can be reduced to two or so dimensions in order to observe possible correlations, and is described by Sammon[80] An analysis of the normalised patterns generated for each of the alcohols at four different concentrations is displayed in Figure 24.10. Within each cluster it is possible to pick out subclusters corresponding to patterns for a particular concentration, indicating that the normalisation process is not completely successful.

Half of the patterns represented in Figure 24.10 (two concentrations for each alcohol) were used to train a two-layer artificial neural network. This was then tested with the

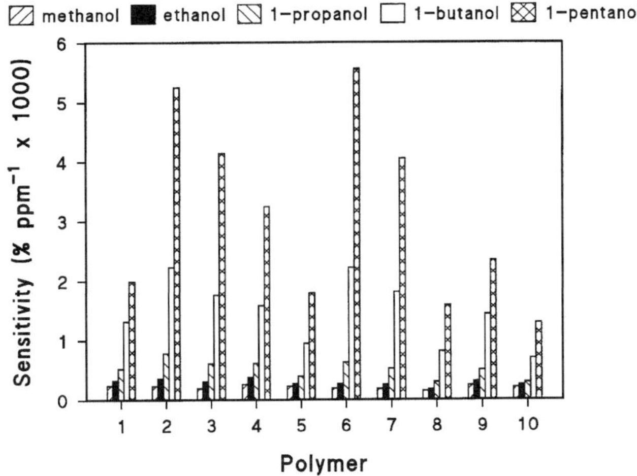

FIGURE 24.8 Bar chart illustrating the average sensitivity of each polymer pair to the five alcohols studied.

remaining patterns and the results are shown in Table 24.1. The only patterns incorrectly assigned were from 1-pentanol which was predominantly identified as 1-butanol. As was illustrated by Figure 24.10, the patterns for 1-butanol and 1-pentanol lie relatively close together in multidimensional space. The overall success rate of the trained neural network was 83%.

An array of 20-sensing elements with 5 different conducting polymers deposited in groups of 4, was tested with a number of flavour/fragrance compounds. Citral (3,7-dimethyl-2,6-octadien-1-al, boiling point = 229°C) is an acyclic terpene aldehyde with a strong lemon odour. A mixture of the cis and trans isomers was used in these experiments. Citronellol (3,7-dimethyl-6-octen-1-ol, boiling point = 222°C) is an acyclic terpene alcohol with a sweet rose-like odour. Cineole (1,8-epoxy-*p*-menthane, boiling point = 176 to 177°C) is a cyclic ether with a characteristic fresh odour and is the main constituent of eucalyptus oil. Isoamyl acetate (boiling point = 142°C) is a saturated aliphatic ester with a strong fruity odour and is the main component of banana aroma.

In this initial investigation the sensor was exposed to the saturated vapour produced by each of the liquids. The response and recovery times, particularly for the less volatile citral and citronellol, are relatively long and vary considerably from polymer to polymer. Rather than wait for an equilibrium to be established, a protocol was adopted in which the patterns generated in the 2 to 4-min period after the initial presentation of the vapour were taken as representative of that sample. Typical patterns for the four odours are presented in Figure 24.11. Cluster analysis using the Sammon method has been carried out with the patterns generated for each odorant during four separate data acquisitions (Figure 24.12).

Two sets of data from each odorant were used to train a neural network and testing was carried out with the remaining patterns. The results are summarised in Table 24.2. The neural network had a 95% success rate in recognising the presented patterns.

Different samples of English cheddar cheese (mild, medium, and mature) were tested with an array with the same polymer configuration as that used for the alcohols. Samples were placed in sealed gas bottles and left for 30 min for the volatiles to reach equilibrium in the headspace. The sensor array was clamped in a polytetrafluoroethylene (PTFE) gas cell (approximate volume 5 ml) which was connected to a small air pump. During sampling, air was pulled from the cheese headspace across the sensor array at a rate of 100 ml/min and patterns were generated at 5-s intervals. Once an equilibrium response had been reached,

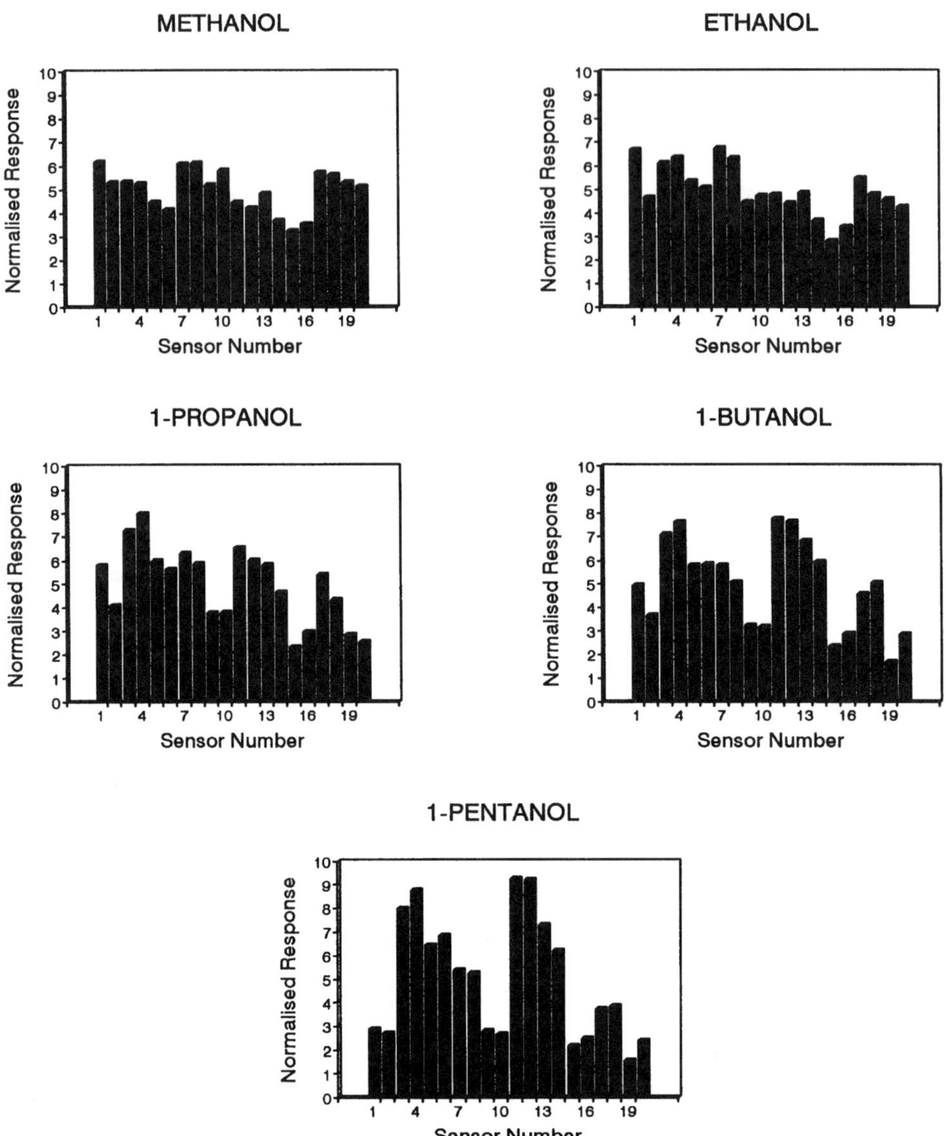

FIGURE 24.9 Normalised response patterns for the first five members of the homologous series of n-alcohols.

sampling was continued for 30 to 40 s, producing 6 to 8 patterns per experiment. Typical response patterns, averaged across the sampling window, are shown in Figure 24.13.

The results of a cluster analysis on three sets of data collected for each cheese are shown in Figure 24.14. It should be noted that the scale of this plot is reduced compared to Figures 24.10 and 24.12, which is a result of the relatively small differences within the data analysed. The patterns arising from separate experiments with the same cheese sample are clearly differentiated. In the sampling procedure for cheese, close control of the equilibration temperature was crucial. The recognition rate achieved with a neural network was 80% for cheese.

Figure 24.15 shows a cluster analysis of results obtained from biscuits containing fats that are sometimes rancid. The data were collected over a period of 3 months. Good discrimination between control samples and rancid population was achieved.

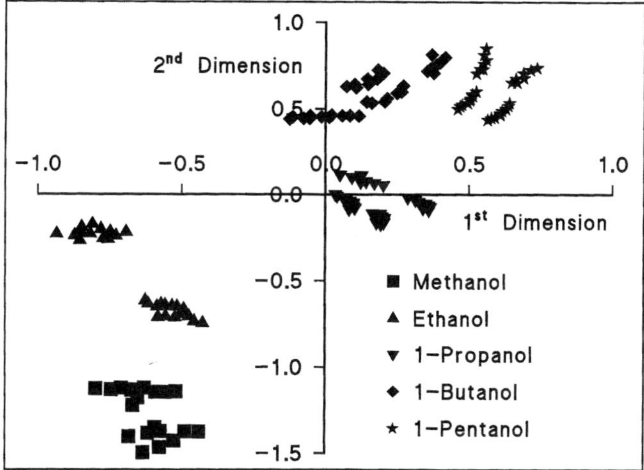

FIGURE 24.10 Nonlinear mapping of the patterns generated for each alcohol at four different concentrations.

TABLE 24.1
Response From Trained Neural Networks

Alcohol (No. of patterns tested)	Methanol	Ethanol	Propanol	Butanol	Pentanol
Methanol (10)	10	0	0	0	0
Ethanol (14)	0	14	0	0	0
Propanol (17)	0	0	17	0	0
Butanol (14)	0	0	0	14	0
Pentanol (14)	0	0	0	12	2

24.5 CONCLUSION

This chapter demonstrates that array-based sensors may be used to discriminate both single chemicals (Figure 24.9) as well as complex mixtures of chemicals (Figures 24.14 and 24.15). The sensing technology utilised may be diverse and tailored to the application. Providing the responses are reproducible, and the sensors have good stability, the choice of technology is governed by the need to have sensor elements that have discrete spectra of responses to individual chemical families. In terms of technologies currently available, conducting polymers have some characteristics that allow their responses to be correlated to human perception of odour. This is because they respond preferentially to polar chemical species and these are the chemicals that have predominantly low odour thresholds in humans. They also work at ambient temperatures, giving rapidly reversible responses to most odours. While metal oxide sensors have good long-term stability, they need to operate at higher temperatures and this means that chemical species adsorbed may be oxidized or "cracked" to produce other species that may then change the odour headspace that is being sampled.

The information from an array of sensors may be utilised in several ways to give quantitative and qualitative information on odours. Since traditional human evaluation of odour is very subjective, this new type of instrumentation should open a new frontier of objective odour measurements.

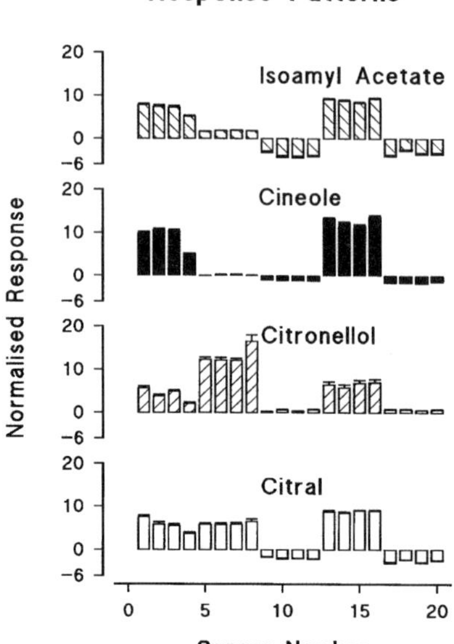

FIGURE 24.11 Typical normalised response patterns for citral, citronellol, cineole, and isoamyl acetate.

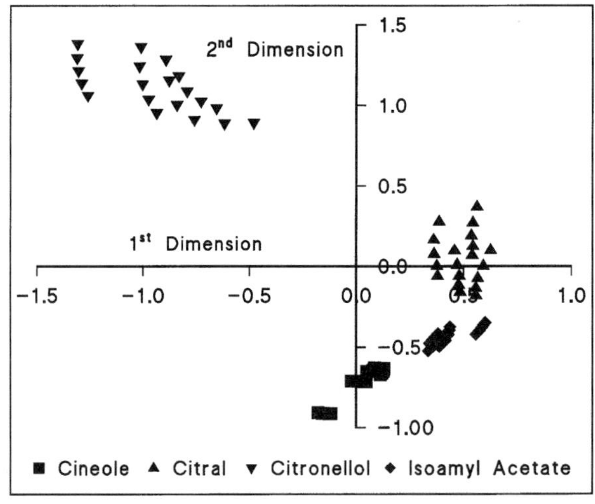

FIGURE 24.12 Nonlinear mapping of the patterns generated for citral, citronellol, cineole, and isoamyl acetate. The database used for each volatile contains patterns from four data acquisitions.

ACKNOWLEDGMENTS

This work was supported by Cogent Ltd., the Science and Engineering Research Council, and the European Space Agency. Mr. A. Qutob carried out the electronic design of the sensing system, Dr. A. M. Pisanelli carried out a study of cheese odour discrimination, and Mr. J. S. Payne a study of rancidity in food products.

TABLE 24.2
Response From Trained Neural Networks

Odorant (No. of patterns tested)	Citral	Citronellol	Cineole	Isoamyl acetate
Citral (10)	10	0	0	0
Citronellol (10)	0	10	0	0
Cineole (10)	0	0	10	0
Isoamyl acetate (10)	2	0	0	8

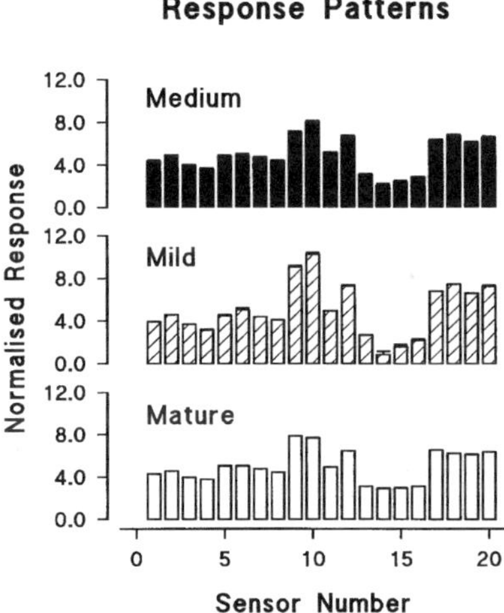

FIGURE 24.13 Typical normalised response patterns for mild, medium, and mature cheddar cheeses.

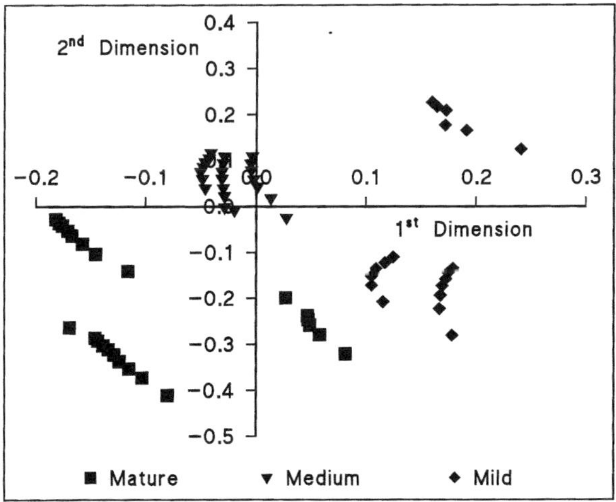

FIGURE 24.14 Nonlinear mapping of the response patterns generated for mild, medium, and mature cheddar cheeses using data from three separate experiments with each cheese sample.

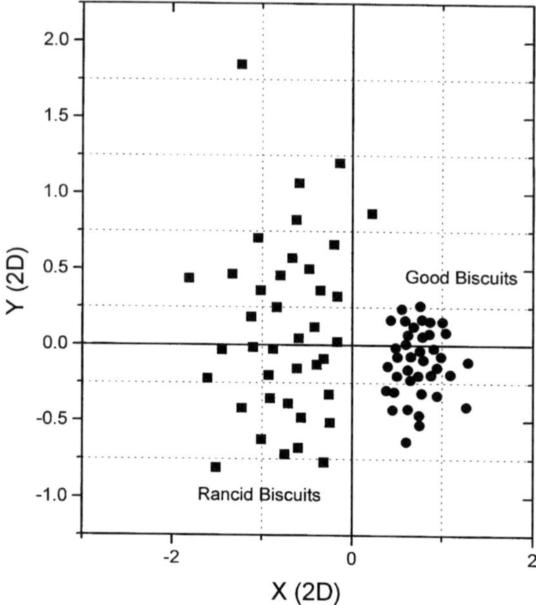

FIGURE 24.15 Differentiation between rancid and nonrancid biscuits. The Sammon map shows that two populations of products can be discriminated.

REFERENCES

1. Schild, D., Ed., *Chemosensory Information Processing,* NATO ASI Series, Springer-Verlag, Berlin, 1990.
2. Getchell, T. V., Functional properties of vertebrate olfactory receptor neurons, *Physiol. Rev.*, 66, 772, 1986.
3. Buck, L. and Axel, R., A novel multigene family may encode odorant receptors: a molecular basis for odor recognition, *Cell*, 65, 175, 1991.
4. Amoore, J. E., *Molecular Basis of Odor*, Charles C Thomas, Springfield, IL, 1970.
5. Hangartner, M., Hartung, J., Paduch, M., Pain, B. F., and Voorburg, J. H., Improved recommendations on olfactometric measurements. *Environ. Technol. Lett.*, 10, 231, 1989.
6. Stevens, S. S., Ed., *Handbook of Experimental Psychology.* John Wiley & Sons, New York, 1951.
7. Maillard, L. C., Action des acides amines sur les sucres: formation des melanoidines par voie methodique, *C. R. Natl. Acad. Paris,* 154, 66, 1912.
8. Morton, I. D. and Macleod, A. J., Eds., *Developments in Food Science,* 3A. Food Flavours (Part A. Introduction), Elsevier, Amsterdam, 1982.
9. Persaud, K. C. and Dodd, G. H., Analysis of discrimination mechanisms in the mammalian olfactory system using a model nose, *Nature*, 299, 352, 1982.
10. Kohl, D., Fundamentals and recent developments of homogenous semiconducting sensors, in *Sensors and Sensory Systems for an Electronic Nose,* NATO ASI Series E: Applied Sciences, Vol. 212, Gardner, J. W. and Bartlett, P. N., Eds., Kluwer Academic, Dordrecht, 1992, chap. 5.
11. Shurmer, H. V., Gardner, J. W., and Chan, H. T., The application of discrimination techniques to alcohols and tobaccos using tin-oxide sensors, *Sensors Actuators*, 18, 361, 1989.
12. Shurmer, H. V., Gardner, J. W., and Corcoran, P., Intelligent vapour discrimination using a composite 12-element sensor array, *Sensors Actuators,* B1, 256, 1990.
13. Gardner, J. W., Hines, E. L., and Wilkinson, M., Application of artificial neural networks to an electronic olfactory system, *Meas. Sci. Technol.*, 1, 446, 1990.

14. Gardner, J. W., Shurmer, H. V., and Tan, T. T., Application of an electronic nose to the discrimination of coffees, *Sensors Actuators,* B6, 71, 1990.
15. Gardner, J. W., Hines, E. L., and Tang, H. C., Detection of vapours and odours from a multisensor array using pattern-recognition techniques. 2. Artificial neural networks, *Sensors Actuators,* B9, 9, 1992.
16. Shurmer, H. V., Corcoran, P., and James, M. K., Sensitivity enhancement for gas sensing and electronic nose applications, *Sensors Actuators,* B15-16, 256, 1993.
17. Moore, S. W., Gardner, J. W., Hines, E. L., Gopel, W., and Weimar, U., A modified multilayer perceptron model for gas mixture analysis, *Sensors Actuators,* B15-16, 344, 1993.
18. Nakamoto, T., Fukuda, T., and Moriizumi T, Gas identification system using plural sensors with characteristics of plasticity, *Sensors Actuators,* B3, 1, 1991.
19. Nakamoto, T., Takagi, H., Utsumi, S., and Moriizumi T, Gas/odour identification by semiconductor gas-sensor array and an analog artificial neural-network circuit, *Sensors Actuators,* B8, 181, 1992.
20. Abe, H., Yoshimura, T., Kanaya, S., Takahashi, Y., Miyashita, Y., and Sasaki, S., Automated odour sensing system based on plural semiconductor gas sensors and computerised pattern recognition techniques, *Anal. Chim. Acta*, 194, 1, 1987.
21. Abe, H., Kanaya, S., Takahashi, Y., and Sasaki, S., Extended studies of the automated odour-sensing system based on plural semiconductor gas sensors and computerised pattern recognition techniques, *Anal. Chim. Acta*, 215, 155, 1988.
22. Abe, H., Kanaya, S., Takahashi, Y., and Sasaki, S., Combined semiconductor gas sensor system for detection of specific substances in particular environments, *Anal. Chim. Acta*, 219, 213, 1989.
23. Weimar, U., Schierbaum, K. D., and Gopel, W., Pattern recognition methods for gas mixture analysis. Application to sensor arrays based upon SnO_2, *Sensors Actuators,* B1, 93, 1990.
24. Schierbaum K. D., Weimar, U., Gopel, W., and Kowalskowski, R., Multicomponent gas analysis. An analytical approach applied to modified SnO_2 sensors, *Sensors Actuators,* B2, 71, 1990.
25. Walmsley, A. D., Haswell, S. J., and Metcalfe, E., Methodology for the selection of suitable sensors for incorporation into a gas sensor array, *Anal. Chim. Acta*, 242, 31, 1991.
26. Aishima T., Discrimination of liquor aromas by pattern recognition analysis of responses from a gas sensor array, *Anal. Chim. Acta*, 243, 293, 1991.
27. Utsumi, S., Yamashita, N., Nakamoto, T., Moriizumi, T., and Sonoda, Y., Active gas sensing system using automatically controlled gas blender and numerical optimisation technique. Presented at 7th Int. Conf. Solid-State Sensors and Actuators (Transducers 1993), Yokohama, June 7 to 10, 1993.
28. Olafsson, R., Martinsdottir, E., Olafsdottir, G., Sigfusson, S. I., and Gardner, J. W., Monitoring of fish freshness using tin oxide sensors, in *Sensors and Sensory Systems for an Electronic Nose,* NATO ASI Series E: Applied Sciences, Vol. 212, Gardner, J. W. and Bartlett, P. N., Eds., Kluwer Academic, Dordrecht, 1992, chap. 16.
29. Gardner, J. W., Shurmer, H. V., and Corcoran, P., Integrated tin oxide odour sensors, *Sensors Actuators,* B4, 117, 1991.
30. Walmsley, A. D., Haswell, S. J., and Metcalfe, E., Evaluation of chemometric techniques for the identification and quantification of solvent mixtures using a thin-film metal oxide sensor array, *Anal. Chim. Acta*, 250, 257, 1991.
31. Mizsei, J. and Lantto, V., Air pollution monitoring with a semiconductor gas sensor array system, *Sensors Actuators,* B6, 223, 1992.
32. Faglia, G., Sberveglieri, G., Nelli, P., Di Natale, C., Davide, F., and D'Amico, A., H_2S and SO_2 quantitative measurement by SnO_2 based sensor array, presented at 7th Int. Conf. Solid-State Sensors and Actuators (Transducers 1993), Yokohama, June 7 to 10, 1993.
33. Nayak, M. S., Dwivedi, R., and Srivastava, S. K., Transformed cluster analysis: an approach to the identification of gases/odours using an integrated gas-sensor array, *Sensors Actuators,* B12, 103, 1993.
34. Dutronc, P., Lucat, C., Menil, F., Loesch, M., Horrillo, M. C., Sayago, I., Gutierrez, J., and de Agapito, J. A., A potentially selective methane sensor based on the differential conductivity responses of Pd- and Pt-doped tin oxide thick layers, *Sensors Actuators,* B15-16, 384, 1993.

35. Ema, K, Yokoyama, M., Nakamoto, T., and Moriizumi, T. Odour-sensing system using a quartz-resonator sensor array and neural network pattern recognition, *Sensors Actuators*, 18, 291, 1989.
36. Nakamoto, T., Fukunishi, K., and Moriizumi, T., Identification capability of odour sensor using quartz-resonator array and neural-network pattern recognition, *Sensors Actuators,* B1, 473, 1990.
37. Nakamoto, T., Fukuda, A., Moriizumi, T., and Asakura, Y., Improvement of identification capability in an odour-sensing system, *Sensors Actuators,* B3, 221, 1991.
38. Moriizumi, T., Nakamoto, T., and Sakuraba, Y., Pattern recognition in electronic noses by artificial neural network models, in *Sensors and Sensory Systems for an Electronic Nose,* NATO ASI Series E: Applied Sciences, Vol. 212, Gardner, J. W. and Bartlett, P. N., Eds., Kluwer Academic, Dordrecht, 1992, chap. 14.
39. Nakamoto, T., Fukuda, A., and Moriizumi, T., Perfume and flavour identification by odour-sensing system using quartz-resonator sensor array and neural-network pattern recognition, *Sensors Actuators,* B10, 85, 1993.
40. Ide, J., Nakamoto, T. and Moriizumi, T., Development of odour-sensing system using an auto-sampling stage, *Sensors Actuators,* B13-14, 351, 1993.
41. Nakamura, M., Sugimoto, I., Kuwano, H., and Lemos, R., Chemical sensing by analysing dynamics of plasma-polymer-film coated sensors, presented at 7th Int. Conf. Solid-State Sensors and Actuators (Transducers 1993), Yokohama, June 7 to 10, 1993.
42. Lemos, R. A., Nakamura, M., Sugimoto, I., and Kuwano, H., A self-organizing map for chemical vapour classification, presented at 7th Int. Conf. Solid-State Sensors and Actuators (Transducers 1993), Yokohama, June 7 to 10, 1993.
43. Wohltjen, H., Mechanism of operation and design considerations for surface acoustic wave device vapour sensors, *Sensors Actuators*, 5, 307, 1984.
44. Rose-Pehrsson, S. L., Grate, J. W., Ballantine, D. S., Jr., and Jurs, P. C., Detection of hazardous vapours including mixtures using pattern recognition analysis of responses from surface acoustic wave devices, *Anal. Chem.*, 60, 2801, 1988.
45. Zellers, E. T., Pan, T-S., Patrash, S. J., Han, M., and Batterman, S. A., Extended disjoint principle components regression analysis of SAW vapour sensor-array responses, *Sensors Actuators,* B12, 123, 1993.
46. Grate, J. W., Rose-Pehrsson, S. L., Venezky, D. L., Klutsky, M., and Wohltjen, H., Smart sensor system for trace organophosphorus and organosulphur vapour detection employing a temperature-controlled array of surface acoustic wave sensors, automated sample preconcentration and pattern recognition, *Anal. Chem.*, 65, 1868, 1993.
47. Reichert, J., Coerdt, W., and Ache, H. J., Development of a surface acoustic wave sensor array for the detection of methanol in fuel vapours, *Sensors Actuators,* B13-14, 293, 1993.
48. Stetter, J. R., Findlay, M. W., Maclay, G. J., Zhang, J., Vaihinger, S., and Gopel, W., Sensor array and catalytic filament for chemical analysis of vapours and mixtures, *Sensors Actuators,* B1, 43, 1990.
49. Vaihinger, S., Gopel, W., and Stetter, J. R., Detection of halogenated and other hydrocarbons in air. Response functions of catalyst/electrochemical sensor systems, *Sensors Actuators,* B4, 337, 1991.
50. Muller, R. and Lange, E., Multidimensional sensor for gas analysis, *Sensors Actuators*, 9, 39, 1986.
51. Sundgren, H., Lundstrom, I., Winquist, F., Lukkari, I., Carlsson, R., and Wold, S., Evaluation of a multiple gas mixture with a simple MOSFET gas sensor array and pattern recognition, *Sensors Actuators,* B2, 115, 1990.
52. Lundstrom, I., Hedborg, E., Spetz, A., Sundgren, H., and Winquist, F., Electronic noses based on field effect structures, in *Sensors and Sensory Systems for an Electronic Nose,* NATO ASI Series E: Applied Sciences,Vol. 212, Gardner, J. W. and Bartlett, P. N., Eds., Kluwer Academic, Dordrecht, 1992, chap. 18.
53. Gall, M., The Si-planar-pellistor array, a detection unit for combustible gases, *Sensors Actuators,* B15-16, 260, 1993.

54. Cranny, A. W. J. and Atkinson, J. K., The use of pattern recognition techniques applied to signals generated by a multi-element gas sensor array as a means of compensating for poor individual element response, in *Sensors and Sensory Systems for an Electronic Nose,* NATO ASI Series E: Applied Sciences, Vol. 212, Gardner, J. W. and Bartlett, P. N., Eds., Kluwer Academic, Dordrecht, 1992, chap. 13.
55. Diaz, A. F., Kanazawa, K. K., and Gardini, G. P., Electropolymerisation of pyrrole. *J. Chem. Soc. Chem. Commun.,* 14, 635, 1979.
56. Persaud K. C. and Pelosi, P., An approach to an artificial nose, *Trans. Am. Soc. Artif. Organs,* 31, 29, 1985.
57. Miasik, J. J., Hooper, A., and Tofield, B. C., Conducting polymer gas sensors, *J. Chem. Soc. Faraday Trans.* 1, 82, 1117, 1986.
58. Hanawa, T., Kuwabata, S., and Yoneyama, H., Gas sensitivity of polpyrrole films to NO_2, *J. Chem. Soc. Faraday Trans.* 1, 84, 1587, 1988.
59. Jiakun, W. and Hirata, M., Research into normal temperature gas-sensitive characteristics of polyaniline material, *Sensors Actuators,* B12, 11, 1993.
60. Bartlett, P. N., Archer, P. B. M., and Ling-Chung, S. K., Conducting polymer gas sensors. Fabrication and characterisation, *Sensors Actuators*, 19, 125, 1989.
61. Bartlett, P. N. and Ling-Chung, S. K., Conducting polymer gas sensors. II. Response of polypyrrole to methanol vapour, *Sensors Actuators*, 19, 141, 1989.
62. Bartlett, P. N. and Gardner, J. W., Odour sensors for an electronic nose, in *Sensors and Sensory Systems for an Electronic Nose,* NATO ASI Series E: Applied Sciences, Vol. 212, Gardner, J. W. and Bartlett, P. N., Eds., Kluwer Academic, Dordrecht, 1992, chap. 4.
63. Josowicz, M. and Janata, J., Suspended gate field effect transistor modified with polypyrrole as alcohol sensor, *Anal. Chem.*, 58, 514, 1986.
64. Josowicz, M., Janata, J., Ashley, K., and Pons, S., Electrochemical and ultraviolet-visible spectroelectrochemical investigation of selectivity of potentiometric gas sensors based on polypyrrole, *Anal. Chem.*, 59, 253, 1987.
65. Blackwood, D. and Josowicz, M., Work function and spectroscopic studies of interactions between conducting polymers and organic vapours, *J. Phys. Chem.*, 95, 493, 1991.
66. Topart, P. and Josowicz, M., Characterisation of the interaction between poly(pyrrole) films and methanol vapour, *J. Phys. Chem.*, 96, 7824, 1992.
67. Slater, J. M. and Watt, E. J., Examination of ammonia-poly(pyrrole) interactions by piezoelectric and conductivity measurements, *Analyst*, 116, 1125, 1991.
68. Slater, J. M. and Watt, E. J., Piezoelectric and conductivity measurements of poly(pyrrole) gas interactions, *Anal. Proc.*, 29, 53, 1992.
69. Slater, J. M., Watt, E. J., Freeman, N. J., May, I. P., and Weir, D. J., Gas and vapour detection with poly(pyrrole) gas sensors, *Analyst*, 117, 1265, 1992.
70. Slater, J. M., Paynter, J., and Watt, E. J., Multi-layer conducting polymer gas sensor arrays for olfactory sensing, *Analyst*, 118, 379, 1993.
71. Bartlett, P. N. and Ling-Chung, S. K., Conducting polymer gas sensors. III. Results for four different polymers and five different vapours, *Sensors Actuators*, 20, 287, 1989.
72. Pearce, T. C., Gardner, J. W., Friel, S., Bartlett, P. N., and Blair, N., Electronic nose for monitoring the flavour of beers, *Analyst*, 118, 371, 1993.
73. Shurmer, H. V., Corcoran, P., and Gardner, J. W., Integrated arrays of gas sensors using conducting polymers with molecular sieves, *Sensors Actuators,* B4, 29, 1991.
74. Pelosi, P. and Persaud, K.C., Gas sensors: towards an artificial nose. In: *Sensors and Sensory Systems for Advanced Robots,* Dario P., Ed., NATO ASI Series F: Computer and Systems Science, Springer-Verlag, Berlin, 1988, 361.
75. Persaud, K. C., Bartlett, J., and Payne, P. Design strategies for gas and odour sensors. In: *Robots and Biological Systems*, Dario P., Sandini, G., and Aebisher, P., Eds., NATO ASI Series, Springer-Verlag, Berlin, 579, 1992.
76. Rumelhart, D. E., Hinton, G. E., and Williams, R. J. Learning internal representations by error propagation. In: *Parallel Distributed Processing: Explorations in the Microstructures of Cognition.* Vol. 1, Rumelhart, D. E. and McClelland, J. L., Eds., MIT Press, Cambridge, MA, 1986, 318.

77. Pao, Y.-H., *Adaptive Pattern Recognition and Neural Networks*. Addison-Wesley, Reading, MA, 1989.
78. Hatfield, J. V., Hicks, P. J., James-Roxby, P., Neaves, P., Persaud, K. C., and Travers, P. J., Towards an integrated electronic nose using conducting polymer sensors, paper presented at Eurosensors VII, Budapest, Sept. 1993.
79. Atkins, P. W., *Physical Chemistry*, 3rd ed., Oxford University Press, Oxford, 1986, chap. 28.
80. Sammon, J. W., A nonlinear mapping for data structure analysis, *IEEE Trans. Computers*, C-18, 401, 1969.

25 Sorbent Polymer Materials for Chemical Sensors and Arrays

Jay W. Grate, Michael H. Abraham, and R. Andrew McGill

CONTENTS

25.1 INTRODUCTION

Although chemical microsensors for gas phase analysis can take many forms, a typical configuration consists of an electronic, acoustic, or optical device with an applied chemically selective layer. This layer interacts with the analyte(s) of interest in such a way that its physical properties change. The device measures those physical changes and produces a signal related to the analyte concentration. Polymer-coated acoustic wave vapor sensors epitomize this definition of a microsensor.[1,2] Many optical microsensors also fit this definition, as do some chemiresistor and field effect transistor sensors.

The sensitivities and selectivities of these types of sensors depend on two processes, sorption and transduction. Sorption of the analyte from the gas phase by the applied chemical layer collects and concentrates analyte molecules at the sensor's surface, either in or on the selective layer. If the sorbed molecules reside on the surface of the selective layer, then

0-8493-8905-4/97/$0.00+$.50
© 1997 by CRC Press, Inc.

adsorption has occurred. If the sorbed molecules dissolve into the layer, then absorption has occurred. Sorption processes are involved in the response mechanisms of all gas phase chemical sensors fitting the general description above. Therefore, the science of sorption is relevant to the development of a variety of chemical sensors.[3]

Transduction is the generation of an analytical signal in response to the presence of the sorbed molecules at the sensor's surface. This process involves the sensitivity of the device to physical changes in the sorbent material on its surface. Consequently, an understanding of transduction mechanisms requires combinations of devices and materials to be considered individually, as well as an understanding of how the material properties are altered by the sorbed molecules. A comprehensive treatment of transduction mechanisms is beyond the scope of this chapter.

However, it is useful to illustrate how sorption principles can be used in the development of sensors and sensor systems. We will use polymer-coated surface acoustic wave (SAW) sensors as examples in this chapter.[1,2] (This is the type of sensor with which the authors have the greatest direct experience.) These sensors respond to the increase in mass and decrease in elastic modulus of the polymer layer when it absorbs vapors.[4] Arrays of acoustic wave vapor sensors used in conjunction with pattern recognition or neural network data processing techniques can form the basis for smart sensor systems or "electronic noses".[5-10] (See also Chapters 9 and 27 in this book.)

Several issues arise in the development of a sensor or sensor array for a particular application. How can the sensor be made sensitive to the analyte(s) of interest? How selective will it be? Which interactions have the most influence on these characteristics? Will the sensor's response be reversible? What will be the response time? Is there a rational basis for choosing a material for use as the selective layer? How can a material be designed to maximize particularly desirable properties? Can estimates for a sensor response be predicted prior to actually making and testing a sensor? How does one best select a set of sensors, or a set of sensor materials, for use in a sensor array? In this chapter we will describe models for the absorption of organic vapors that can help to address these issues in sensor development. (This approach was first proposed in Reference 11, and described in detail in Reference 3.) It is assumed throughout this chapter that reversible sensors are of primary interest.

25.2 PARTITION COEFFICIENT AND SENSOR RESPONSES

Figure 25.1 illustrates the sorption of vapor molecules from the gas phase into a sorbent thin film on a solid substrate, such as a sensor device surface. The partition coefficient, K, is a thermodynamic parameter that measures the equilibrium distribution of vapor between the gas phase and the sorbent phase, as defined according to Equation 25.1.

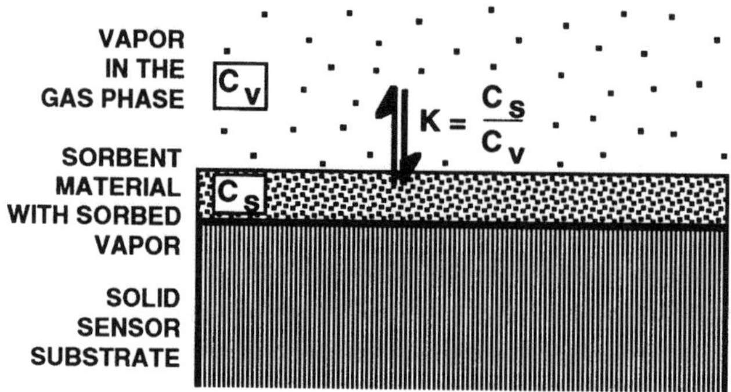

FIGURE 25.1 Illustration of the absorption of a vapor from the gas phase into a sorbent material on a solid substrate, such as a sensor device.

$$K = C_s/C_v \tag{25.1}$$

The concentrations of vapor in each phase are given by C_s and C_v, where C_s is the concentration in the sorbent phase (the polymer in the case of a polymer-coated sensor) and C_v is the concentration in the gas or vapor phase. The larger the partition coefficient, the greater the strength of absorption. The partition coefficient is related to the standard Gibb's free energy of solution of a gaseous solute, ΔG_s^o, by

$$\Delta G_s^o = -RT \ln K \tag{25.2}$$

where the standard states are unit concentration in the gas phase and unit concentration in the sorbent phase.

The response, Q, of a gas phase chemical sensor can be related to the parameters in Equation 25.1 according to the following functions.

$$Q = f(C_v) \tag{25.3}$$

$$Q = f(C_s) \tag{25.4}$$

$$Q = f(KC_v) \tag{25.5}$$

The empirically observed response is the signal obtained from the sensor upon exposure to a particular gas phase vapor concentration (Equation 25.3). However, the sensor does not directly detect the vapor molecules in the gas phase. Rather, the mechanism of sensor response is dependent on the concentration of vapor collected in the sorbent film (Equation 25.4). Therefore, combining Equations 25.1 and 25.4 yields Equation 25.5, which shows the dependence of the response on the partition coefficient. This very general relationship illustrates the key role of sorption and the partition coefficient in the response of a gas phase chemical sensor utilizing an absorbent thin film. The influence of the sorption process is given by KC_v, while the transduction process is represented by the function operating on KC_v.

25.3 ABSORPTION AND SOLUBILITY INTERACTIONS

The process of absorption can be considered in terms of a solubility model with endoergic (endo-energetic) and exoergic steps. In this model, the vapor molecules dissolving into a sorbent material are the solutes, while the sorbent material is the solvent. The creation of a cavity in the solvent involves the disruption of solvent/solvent interactions, and is endoergic. When this cavity is filled with a solute, attractive interactions are formed between the solute and solvent. These interactions are exoergic, favoring sorption, and, by definition, are solubility interactions. The properties of a molecule that contribute to forming these interactions are referred to as its solubility properties.

The solubility interactions relevant to the sorption of organic vapors by nonionic organic materials (or inorganic materials with organic substituents, such as polysiloxanes or polyphosphazenes) include hydrogen-bonding interactions, dipole/dipole interactions, dipole/induced-dipole interactions, and induced-dipole/induced-dipole interactions. The last three types of interactions are also known as orientation, induction, and dispersion interactions, respectively, and are often grouped together as van der Waals interactions. (However, some authors use van der Waals interactions to refer primarily to dispersion interactions.) Dispersion interactions are also called London forces.

Hydrogen-bonding interactions are well known and recognized to be important in many chemical and biochemical processes. They involve the directional interaction between a hydrogen-bond acidic site and a hydrogen-bond basic site. Typical hydrogen-bond acids have hydroxyl groups whose hydrogen atom serves as the acid. A multitude of hydrogen-bond bases exist, typically with a lone pair on an oxygen or nitrogen atom serving as the base. It should be emphasized that hydrogen-bond acidity and basicity are to be distinguished from proton-transfer acidity and basicity. The proton-transfer acidity of an acid, for example, is strongly dependent on the stability of its conjugate base, a factor that is not relevant to hydrogen-bonding interactions. Correlations between hydrogen-bond and proton transfer acidities and basicities can sometimes be made within chemical families, but no general relationship exists.[12,13]

Dipole-dipole interactions are electrostatic interactions involving the attraction between the positively and negatively charged regions of dipolar species. These interactions are strongest for certain orientations of the dipoles. The interaction of a dipole with an uncharged nondipolar polarizable species can shift the position of the electron cloud and induce a dipole, giving rise to a dipole/induced-dipole interaction. The strength of this interaction depends on the polarizability of the nondipolar species and the strength of the perturbing dipole.

Dispersion interactions arise even in molecules without significant permanent dipoles because of momentary dipoles formed when mobile electrons around a nucleus are not evenly distributed. These momentary dipoles induce dipoles in neighboring polarizable species resulting in an attractive force. (Thus, these could be called instantaneous-dipole/induced-dipole interactions.) Although this attraction falls off rapidly with distance, and an individual attractive event may be weak, the net dispersive attraction increases rapidly with increasing molecular volume and the number of polarizable electrons.

The relative importance of each individual type of interaction described above depends on the particular species interacting. Hydrogen-bonding is usually significant and sometimes dominant when hydrogen-bond acids and bases interact. Dipole/induced-dipole interactions are generally weak, but dipole-dipole interactions can be dominant between strongly dipolar species. Dispersion interactions are the principal interactions between nonpolar species, and are generally a significant contributor to the sorption of all vapors by organic polymers.

25.4 SOLVATION PARAMETERS

Solvation parameters have been developed to provide a measure of the abilities of the solute molecules to participate in the interactions discussed above. Thus, these parameters measure the solubility properties of monomeric solutes. They are to be distinguished from other scales of solubility parameters that measure the solubility properties of solvents. A listing of selected representative solvation parameters is given in Table 25.1. A more comprehensive listing can be found in a review by one of the authors.[14]

Hydrogen-bonding properties are described by the α_2^H and β_2^H parameters, which measure solute hydrogen-bond acidity and basicity, respectively. These parameters were derived from measurements of 1:1 complexation between hydrogen-bond acids and bases in tetrachloromethane, and thus are free-energy related.[14-16] To derive the α_2^H scale for hydrogen-bond acidity, the equilibrium constants between a series of acids against a reference base were measured and compared with additional series of acids against additional reference bases. A total of 45 reference bases were considered, providing 45 series of equilibrium values as a basis for the α_2^H scale. Similarly, the complexation of 34 series of bases against 34 reference acids was used to develop the β_2^H scale for hydrogen-bond basicity. These scales refer to 1:1 complexation. For complexation involving a solute surrounded by solvent, "effective" or "summation" α_2^H and β_2^H scales, sometimes denoted as $\Sigma\alpha_2^H$ and $\Sigma\beta_2^H$, were developed based on the original 1:1 complexation α_2^H and β_2^H scales. In general, the 1:1 complexation parameters are successful in describing hydrogen-bonding when the solute is surrounded by solvent, so in most cases the values in the scales of effective α_2^H and β_2^H parameters are the same as or very similar to the 1:1 complexation α_2^H and β_2^H parameters. In this chapter, the α_2^H and

TABLE 25.1
Solvation Parameters for Various Organic Vapors[a,b]

Solute	Polarizability R_2	Dipolarity/ polarizability π_2^H	Acidity α_2^H	Basicity β_2^H	Dispersion/ Cavity $\log L^{16}$
n-Hexane	0.000	0.00	0.00	0.00	2.668
n-Heptane	0.000	0.00	0.00	0.00	3.173
n-Octane	0.000	0.00	0.00	0.00	3.677
2,2,4-Trimethylpentane	0.000	0.00	0.00	0.00	3.106
Cyclohexane	0.305	0.10	0.00	0.00	2.964
Buta-1,3-diene	0.320	0.23	0.00	0.10	1.543
Cyclohexene	0.395	0.20	0.00	0.10	3.021
Dichloromethane	0.387	0.57	0.10	0.05	2.019
Trichloromethane	0.425	0.49	0.15	0.02	2.480
Tetrachloromethane	0.458	0.38	0.00	0.00	2.823
1,2-Dichloroethane	0.416	0.64	0.10	0.11	2.573
Tetrachloroethene	0.639	0.44	0.00	0.00	3.584
Dibromomethane	0.714	0.67	0.10	0.10	2.886
Diiodomethane	1.453	0.69	0.05	0.23	3.857
Diethyl ether	0.041	0.25	0.00	0.45	2.015
Ethylene oxide	0.250	0.59	0.00	0.35	1.371
Formaldehyde	0.220	0.70	0.00	0.33	0.730
Acetaldehyde	0.208	0.67	0.00	0.45	1.230
Propanone	0.179	0.70	0.04	0.49	1.696
Butanone	0.166	0.70	0.00	0.51	2.287
Ethyl acetate	0.106	0.62	0.00	0.45	2.314
Acetonitrile	0.237	0.90	0.07	0.32	1.739
Diethylamine	0.154	0.30	0.08	0.69	2.395
Triethylamine	0.101	0.15	0.00	0.79	3.040
Nitromethane	0.313	0.95	0.06	0.31	1.892
N,N-Dimethylformamide	0.367	1.31	0.00	0.74	3.173
N,N-Dimethylacetamide	0.363	1.33	0.00	0.78	3.717
Acetic acid	0.265	0.65	0.61	0.44	1.750
Water	0.000	0.45	0.82	0.35	0.260
Methanol	0.278	0.44	0.43	0.47	0.970
Ethanol	0.246	0.42	0.37	0.48	1.485
Propan-2-ol	0.212	0.36	0.33	0.56	1.764
2,2,2-Trifluoroethanol	0.015	0.60	0.57	0.03	1.224
Hexafluoropropan-1-ol	-0.240	0.55	0.77	0.10	1.392
Triethyl phosphate	0.000	1.00	0.00	1.06	4.750
Benzene	0.610	0.52	0.00	0.14	2.786
Toluene	0.601	0.52	0.00	0.14	3.325
Styrene	0.849	0.65	0.00	0.16	3.856
1,3-Dichlorobenzene	0.847	0.73	0.00	0.02	4.410
Phenol	0.805	0.89	0.60	0.30	3.766
3-Fluorophenol	0.667	0.98	0.68	0.17	3.842
Aniline	0.955	0.96	0.26	0.41	3.934
Pyridine	0.631	0.84	0.00	0.52	3.022

[a] These are for the solute surrounded by excess of solvent. Therefore, the α_2^H and β_2^H parameters, for example, are really "effective" or "summation" $\Sigma\alpha_2^H$ and $\Sigma\beta_2^H$ parameters, but we retain the simpler nomenclature here.

[b] A more extensive listing of solvation parameters can be found in Reference 14.

β_2^H parameters are always those referring to the solute surrounded by solvent (i.e., "effective" or "summation" values, but denoted by the simpler notation α_2^H and β_2^H, rather than $\Sigma\alpha_2^H$ and $\Sigma\beta_2^H$).

Dipolarity and polarizability are described by the R_2 and π_2^H parameters. The π_2^H parameter measures the ability of a molecule to stabilize a neighboring charge or dipole.[17] It is derived from measurements of the partition coefficients of solutes on polar gas-liquid chromatography (GLC) stationary phases, and is free-energy related. For nonprotonic, aliphatic solutes with a single dominant dipole, π_2^H values are proportional to molecular dipole moments. However, polarizability can also contribute to positive values of this parameter. The R_2 parameter is an excess molar refraction parameter that provides a quantitative indication of polarizable n and p electrons.[18] It is calculated by taking the difference in molar refraction between the solute and an alkane of the same characteristic volume.

The parameter denoted by log L^{16} is the experimentally measured gas-liquid partition coefficient of the solute on hexadecane at 25°C, and is therefore free-energy related.[19] (L is the symbol for the Ostwald solubility coefficient, which is defined identically to the partition coefficient as in Equation 25.1.) Hexadecane is a completely nonpolar sorbent, precluding the possibility of any dipole-dipole or hydrogen-bonding interactions with solute vapors. Log L^{16} is therefore a combined measure of exoergic dispersion interactions (leading to an increase in log L^{16}) and the endoergic cost of forming a cavity (leading to a decrease in log L^{16}).

These various parameters, or descriptors, provide a detailed description of the solubility properties of solutes, and are useful in linear solvation energy relationships (LSERs).

25.5 LINEAR SOLVATION ENERGY RELATIONSHIPS

Linear solvation energy relationships aid in understanding how particular interactions contribute to the overall sorption process, and provide models for the predictions of partition coefficients that have not been measured.[3,14,16,18,20-24] In addition, the coefficients in these relationships provide a measure of the solubility properties of the sorbent material. For the sorption of an organic vapor into a sorbent material, the LSER takes the form

$$\log K = c + r\, R_2 + s\, \pi_2^H + a\, \alpha_2^H + b\, \beta_2^H + l \log L^{16} \tag{25.6}$$

The measure of sorption, log K, is modeled as a linear combination of terms related to particular solubility interactions. R_2, π_2^H, α_2^H, β_2^H, and log L^{16} are the solvation parameters described above that characterize the solubility properties of the vapor. The coefficients s, r, a, b, and l characterize the complementary properties of the sorbent material. (The constant c arises from the regression method used to derive the equation.) The terms r R_2, s π_2^H, a α_2^H, b β_2^H, and l log L^{16} measure the contributions of particular interactions to the overall sorption process, where s π_2^H is a polarity term, r R_2 is a polarizability term, a α_2^H is a hydrogen-bonding term in which the vapor is the hydrogen-bond acid, b β_2^H is a hydrogen-bonding term in which the vapor is the hydrogen-bond base, and l log L^{16} is a combined dispersion interaction and cavity term.

The data required to determine an LSER for a sorbent material are the partition coefficients of about 30 vapors at a single temperature. In this approach, the solvent is held constant as solute properties are varied. The set of solute vapors measured must adequately represent all the solubility properties of interest. It must include simple hydrocarbons, polarizable molecules, dipolar molecules, hydrogen-bond bases, and hydrogen-bond acids. The resulting experimental data encode information about the properties of the sorbent phase that interact with the properties of the test vapors. This information is extracted by regressing the measured partition coefficients against the solvation parameters of the solute vapors by the method of multiple linear regression, and thus generating the LSER. In most laboratories, the required partition coefficients are most easily obtained from GLC retention times. Gas-liquid chromatography is a well-established and precise method of making these measurements.[25] It is also possible to derive LSER relationships from the sensor responses, provided that the sensor responses are directly proportional to the amount of vapor absorbed.[26]

The solubility properties of the sorbent material are then indicated by the LSER coefficients as follows. The r-coefficient measures the ability of the sorbent material to interact with solute n and π electrons, and is an indication of polarizability. The r-coefficient is generally slightly positive, but it can be negative if the material contains fluorine atoms. The s-coefficient measures the sorbent phase dipolarity/polarizability. The a-coefficient, being complementary to the solute hydrogen-bond acidity, measures the sorbent phase hydrogen-bond basicity. Similarly, the b-coefficient, being complementary to the solute hydrogen-bond basicity, measures the sorbent phase hydrogen-bond acidity. The l-coefficient is a combined measure of dispersion interactions that tend to increase l, and cavity effects that tend to decrease l.

Table 25.2 lists the LSER coefficients and constants for 14 polymers, all determined at 298 K.[27] The chemical structures of these polymers are shown in Figure 25.2. These polymers were selected for study in an effort to represent a diverse set of properties and structures, and because many of these polymers have been utilized as sorbent layers on SAW vapor sensors.[7,28-30] Although similar relationships are available for over a hundred other sorbent materials through the analysis of GLC data in the literature, the partition coefficients were determined at elevated temperatures, and are therefore not as useful in connection with chemical sensors to be operated near room temperature.[18,22,31,32] Moreover, sorption decreases exponentially with increasing temperature, so a sensor whose response is related primarily to the amount of vapor sorbed will become much less sensitive as its operating temperature is raised.

TABLE 25.2
LSER Results for Fourteen Polymers

Solvent:	Polarizability	Dipolarity/ polarizability	Basicity	Acidity	Dispersion/ cavity	
Polymer[a]	r	s	a	b	l	Constant
P4V	–1.538	2.493	1.507	5.877	0.904	–1.329
SXFA	–0.417	0.602	0.698	4.250	0.718	–0.084
FPOL	–0.672	1.446	1.494	4.086	0.810	–1.207
ZDOL	–0.750	0.606	1.441	3.668	0.709	–0.486
PEI	0.495	1.516	7.018	0.000	0.770	–1.580
SXPYR	–0.189	2.425	6.780	0.000	1.016	–1.938
PEM	–1.032	2.754	4.226	0.000	0.865	–1.653
SXCN	0.000	2.283	3.032	0.516	0.773	–1.630
PVPR	0.674	0.828	2.246	1.026	0.718	–0.571
PVTD	–0.016	0.736	2.436	0.224	0.919	–0.591
PECH	0.096	1.628	1.450	0.707	0.831	–0.749
OV202	–0.480	1.298	0.441	0.705	0.807	–0.391
PIB	–0.077	0.366	0.180	0.000	1.016	–0.766
SXPHB	0.177	1.287	0.556	0.440	0.885	–0.846

[a] The structures of these polymers are found in Figure 25.2.

From Abraham, M. et al., *J. Chem. Soc. Perkin Trans.*, 2, 369-378, 1995; *CHEMTECH*, 24(9), 27-37, 1994; *Analytical Chem.*, 67, 2162-2169, 1995. With permission.

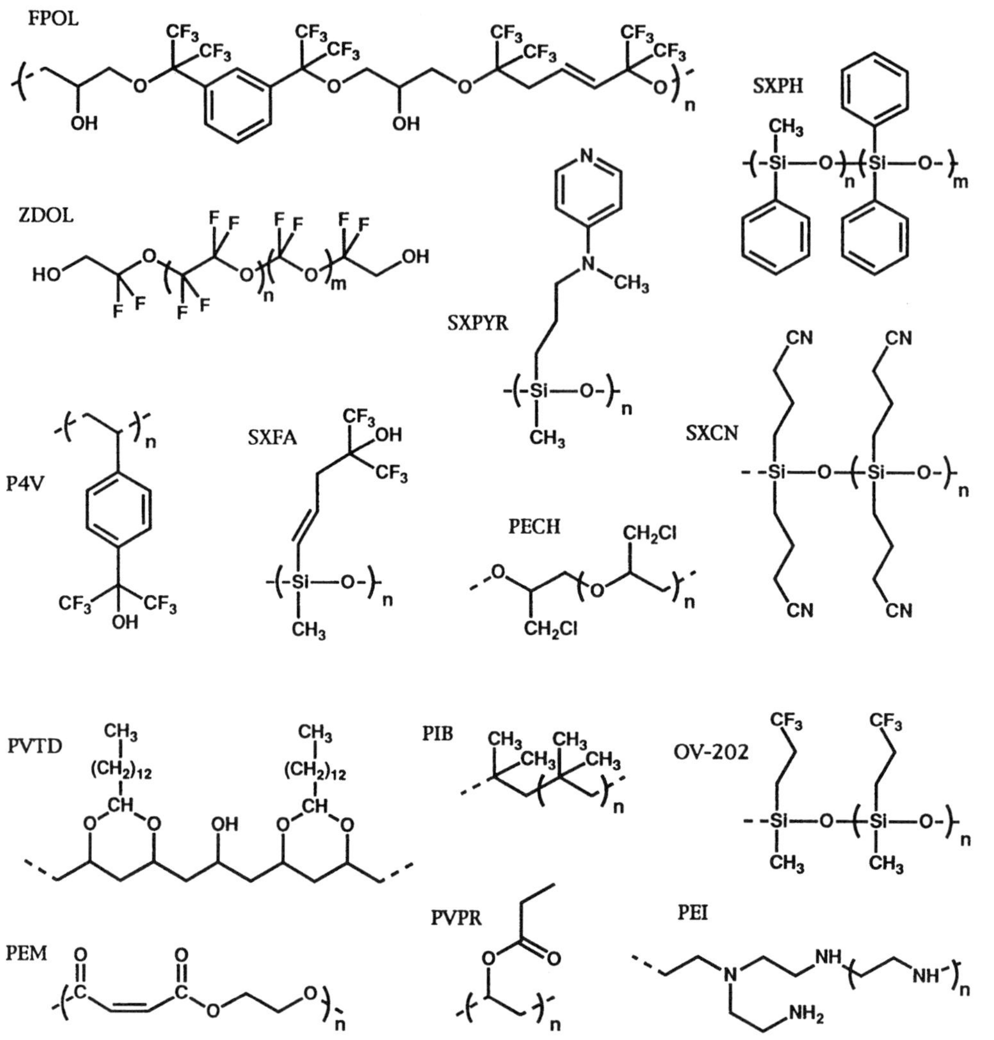

FIGURE 25.2 Structural units of the sorbent polymers and oligomers characterized by the LSER method. In some cases, more than one repeat unit has been shown to illustrate structural characteristics or the chemical environment that a sorbed vapor would experience. The polymers are fluoropolyol (FPOL), Fomblin-ZDOL (ZDOL), a 75%-phenyl-25%-methylpolysiloxane (SXPH), an alkylaminopyridyl-substituted polysiloxane (SXPYR), poly(4-vinylhexafluorocumyl alcohol) (P4V), a hexafluoroisopropanol-substituted polysiloxane (SXFA), poly(epichlorohydrin) (PECH), polybis(cyanopropyl)siloxane (SXCN), poly(vinyl tetradecanal) (PVTD), poly(isobutylene) (PIB), poly(trifluoropropyl)methylsiloxane (OV-202), poly(ethylene maleate) (PEM), poly(vinyl propionate) (PVPR), and poly(ethylenimine) (PEI). (Reprinted with permission from Abraham, M. et al, *J. Chem. Soc. Perkin Trans.*, 2, 369-378, 1995.)

25.6 APPLICATION OF SOLUBILITY MODELS TO ISSUES IN SENSOR DEVELOPMENT

The strength with which a vapor is sorbed by a particular material depends on the solubility interactions between the vapor and the material. These interactions depend on the respective solubility properties of the interacting species, which in turn depend on their chemical structures. The design and selection of sorbent materials for use on sensors therefore relies on understanding the relationships between structures, properties, and interactions.

25.6.1 Vapor Properties

While a general understanding of molecular properties can be gained from typical organic chemistry texts, a more detailed understanding requires a method of comparing the properties of one molecule against another. The solvation parameters described above provide scales of individual solubility properties, and do so for hundreds of molecules.[14] The properties of vapors to be detected as analytes can be determined simply by looking up their solvation parameters. These properties must be known before a material can be chosen or designed that will interact strongly and selectively with the analyte molecule.

Tables of solvation parameters can also be examined to see how particular structural features of the monomeric solutes give rise to particular solubility properties. Thus, the following observations can be made about typical organic functional groups in monomeric solutes.[3] (Some of these same functional groups will appear in the polymers to be discussed below.)

Aliphatic alcohols are moderate hydrogen-bond acids and hydrogen-bond bases, whereas phenols are more strongly hydrogen-bond acidic, and fluoroalcohols and fluorophenols are particularly strong hydrogen-bond acids. Fluorosubstitution also reduces the basicity of alcohols.

Ethers, ketones, esters, and nitriles are weak to moderate bases, while amines, amides, sulfoxides, N-oxides, and phosphoryl-containing species are strong bases. Most bases are also dipolar, with simple aliphatic amines having the least dipolarity, ethers being weakly dipolar, and esters and ketones having moderate dipolarity. All the strongest bases except amines have strong dipolarity. Nitriles are strongly dipolar species with only moderate basicity.

Dipolarity is most commonly associated with basic molecules, but weak to moderate dipolarity is also associated with uneven distributions of electron-withdrawing halogen atoms in a molecule. These provide modest dipolarity without significant basicity, as in 1,1,1-Trifluoroethane, for example. (1,1,1-Trifluoroethane is more dipolar than ethyl acetate, but less so than acetone.) The presence of pi-electrons and lone pairs often results in significant polarizability, as in aromatic molecules like benzene and toluene, or chlorinated and brominated molecules. Highly fluorinated molecules, on the other hand, are among the least polarizable.

25.6.2 Sorbent Material Properties

Scales of individual solubility properties for large numbers of polymers (or other sorbent materials), similar to the solvation parameters for solutes, are unfortunately not available. However, as we have described above, the LSER approach provides a method for determining polymer solubility properties in detail. Table 25.2 provides 14 examples of polymers so characterized at 298 K. With this many examples, it is also possible to begin elucidating relationships between polymer structure and properties.

Several strongly hydrogen-bond acidic polymers are represented, as indicated by their large b-coefficients. These include FPOL, P4V, SXFA, and ZDOL, with b-coefficients of 4.086, 5.877, 4.25, and 3.668, respectively. The hydrogen-bond acidic character of these phases is due to the presence of fluoroalcohol substituents. The fluoro-substitution increases the acidity of the hydroxyl group while simultaneously decreasing its basicity. The polymer P4V is one of a series of fluoroalcohol-containing polymers examined by Snow et al. as selective layers on SAW devices.[33] Fluoroalcohol-substituted polystyrenes similar to P4V were first suggested for sensor applications by Barlow et al.[34,35] FPOL is an oligomeric material that has proven to be useful in chemical sensor studies for the detection of basic compounds such as phosphonates.[7,11,28,29,33,36] The SXFA polymer incorporates the hexafluoroisopropanol group into a siloxane polymer. ZDOL is a commercially available liquid.

The four strongly hydrogen-bond acidic polymers in Table 25.2 are all based on fluoroalcohols. It is also possible to obtain strongly hydrogen-bond acidic sorbents based on phenols. A series of nonvolatile phenolic liquids have been examined at 298 K, and the fluoro-substituted phenol was the most acidic of these.[23]

The polymer PVTD in Table 25.2 and Figure 25.2 also contains hydroxyl groups in its structure and therefore might be expected to be a hydrogen-bond acid. Simple aliphatic alcohols are in general only moderate hydrogen-bond acids, so this polymer is expected to be less acidic than the fluoroalcohol-substituted polymers described above. However, the b-coefficient of 0.224 for PVTD is very small. Since this polymer also contains basic sites (a = 2.436), it is expected to be internally hydrogen-bonded and this can be confirmed in its FTIR spectrum.[27] Self-association reduces the availability of the hydroxyl groups for interactions with vapors that might be sorbed, and therefore reduces the effective hydrogen-bond acidity of the material. Comparing the properties of PVTD with those of the more acidic phases discussed above illustrates the importance of fluoro-substitution for obtaining acidic properties from the hydroxyl groups of alcohols.

Several of the polymers in Table 25.2 are basic, including two that are particularly strong in this property, PEI and SXPYR. These polymers have a-coefficients of 7.02 and 6.78, respectively. In PEI, the basicity is due to the alkylamine functionalities. Alkylamines (see Table 25.1) are in general strong bases with little dipolarity. In this regard the moderate s-coefficient of 1.516 of PEI is somewhat larger than expected. This result is most likely a consequence of quaternized ammonium groups that are usually present in commercial samples of PEI, which could give rise to charge-dipole interactions. PEI has been used in chemical sensor studies.[29,37] The basicity of SXPYR is due to the pendant alkylaminopyridyl groups, which are expected to be quite basic.[38] The large s-coefficient of 2.425 for SXPYR indicates strong dipolarity/polarizability, a result that is consistent with the large dipolarity of the 4-dimethylaminopyridine (dipole moment: 4.33 D).[39]

The next most basic polymers are PEM and SXCN, with a-coefficients of 4.23 and 3.03, respectively. These polymers are also strongly dipolar, with s-coefficients of 2.75 and 2.28. The properties of the SXCN polymer arise from the appended nitrile groups, which are strongly dipolar and moderately basic. PEM contains a pair of ester groups conjugated with the carbon-carbon double bond in the maleate portion of the repeat unit. This structure apparently gives rise to the strong basicity and dipolarity. Simple organic esters are generally of only moderate dipolarity and moderate basicity. The moderate s- and a-coefficients for PVPR (0.828 and 2.246, respectively) are consistent with these expectations.

As is evident from the consideration of basicity above, dipolarity and basicity generally occur simultaneously. Indeed, strong dipoles are invariably also moderately to strongly basic. The least basic polymer with strong dipolarity is SXCN, whose s-coefficient of 2.28 confirms that it is very dipolar, while its a-coefficient of 3.032 is less than half those of the more strongly basic phases PEI and SXPYR. The most dipolar phase in Table 25.2 is found in PEM, which is slightly more basic than SXCN. The polymer OV202 exhibits moderate dipolarity (s-coefficient of 1.298) without appreciable basicity. The dipolarity of this polymer is expected from the polarizing effect of the trifluoromethyl groups on the pendant trifluoropropyl substituents. An additional polymer with a significant s-coefficient (1.628) is PECH. Dipolarity in this material must arise from the polarizing effects of the electron-withdrawing Cl and O atoms. The ether linkages also give rise to weak basicity, a = 1.45. PECH has been used in a number of chemical sensor studies.[4,28,29]

Nonpolar phases that interact primarily by dispersion interactions are represented by SXPH and PIB. PIB is a simple aliphatic hydrocarbon polymer that can interact mainly by dispersion interactions. It has one of the largest l-coefficients in the data set. In nonpolar phases such as PIB, the cost of forming a cavity is expected to be less than in more polar phases where solvent/solvent interactions are stronger. In practice, PIB-coated SAW vapor sensors are more selective for hydrocarbons than are other SAW devices with more polar polymer coatings.[29] The SXPH polymer contains phenyl groups that could render the material more polarizable than a simple aliphatic hydrocarbon polymer such as PIB.[24] It does have more positive r- and s-coefficients than PIB, but the effect is not large. The synthesis or identification of a more polarizable nonpolar phase may require further study.

We have noted a number of instances where the LSER coefficients indicated a property that was not expected based on the notional polymer structure, only to find by infrared spectroscopy that the material actually contained additional functionalities. The SXPH samples exhibited weak hydrogen-bond acidity as indicated by the b-coefficient, although there are no acidic sites in the repeat unit structure shown in Figure 25.2. However, the infrared spectra of these samples demonstrated that hydroxyl groups were present.[24] Similarly, it was surprising that the PVPR sample, whose structure has no acidic groups in its repeat unit, had weak hydrogen-bond acidity (b = 1.026). However, the presence of acidic groups in the sample was confirmed by the observation of hydroxyl groups at 3600 cm^{-1} in the infrared spectrum.[27] The OV202 also exhibited unexpected weak hydrogen-bond acidity (b = 0.705).[27] In this case, the infrared spectrum indicated that hydroxyl groups were not detectable, but it is possible that the weak acidity arises from CH groups activated by adjacent trifluoromethyl groups. We suggest that candidate polymers for use as sensor materials should be examined by infrared spectroscopy or other methods as a matter of course.

25.6.3 Interactions Governing Sorption

Although a sorption process often involves multiple interactions all occurring simultaneously, the LSER method allows these various interactions to be distinguished and their relative importances examined. This is accomplished by calculating the values of the interaction terms $r\ R_2$, $s\ \pi_2^H$, $a\ \alpha_2^H$, $b\ \beta_2^H$, and $l\ \log L^{16}$ for individual polymer/vapor pairs. This approach is illustrated in Table 25.3 with results from five polymers and four vapors, showing all possible combinations. The vapors selected are ethanol, a hydrogen-bond acid that is also moderately basic; triethylamine, a basic nondipolar vapor; dimethylformamide, a strongly basic very dipolar vapor; and hexane, a nonpolar vapor. The polymers selected are SXFA, a strongly hydrogen-bond acidic polymer; PEI, a strongly hydrogen-bond basic polymer; SXCN, a strongly dipolar basic polymer; OV202, a moderately dipolar nonbasic polymer; and PIB, an nonpolar polymer.

Particularly strong specific interactions are seen when the properties of the vapor and polymer are complementary. Strong hydrogen-bonding interactions occur between the hydrogen-bond acidic polymer SXFA and the basic vapors (triethylamine, dimethylformamide, and ethanol), and also between the hydrogen-bond basic polymer PEI and the only hydrogen-bond acidic vapor, ethanol. Dipolar interactions are particularly strong between the very dipolar polymer SXCN and the most dipolar vapor, dimethylformamide. OV202 also has significant dipolar interactions with this vapor. The only significant interactions between PIB and any of the vapors are dispersion interactions. Dispersion interaction make a significant contribution to sorption in all the polymer/vapors pairs shown, although the strength varies significantly.

The last column of Table 25.3 shows the partition coefficients calculated for all the polymer/vapor pairs, with measured values in parenthesis. Partition coefficients vary over five orders of magnitude, from log K calculated to be 0.43 for SXCN/hexane to 5.97 for SXFA/dimethylformamide.

25.6.4 Strategies for Sensitivity and Selectivity

It is generally the case that organic vapors will be absorbed by organic materials. Indeed, any vapor derived from an organic compound that is liquid at room temperature will be absorbed to some degree by all of the polymers in Table 25.2 (as well as numerous other

TABLE 25.3
Calculated Interaction Terms[a] for Four Vapors Sorbed by Each of Five Polymers

Vapor	Polarizability $r\ R_2$	Dipolarity/ polarizability $s\ \pi_2^H$	Hydrogen-bonding $a\ \alpha_2^H$	Hydrogen bonding $b\ \beta_2^H$	Dispersion/ cavity $l\ \log L^{16}$	Partition coefficient[b] $\log K$
SXFA						
n-Hexane	—	—	—	—	1.92	1.83 (1.74)
Triethylamine	–0.04	0.09	—	3.36	2.18	5.50
Dimethylformamide	–0.15	0.79	—	3.15	2.28	5.97
Ethanol	–0.10	0.25	0.26	2.04	1.07	3.43 (3.54)
PEI						
n-Hexane	—	—	—	—	2.05	0.47
Triethylamine	0.05	0.23	—	—	2.34	1.04
Dimethylformamide	0.18	1.99	—	—	2.44	3.03
Ethanol	0.12	0.64	2.60	—	1.14	2.92 (3.26)
SXCN						
Hexane	—	—	—	—	2.06	0.43 (0.23)
Triethylamine	—	0.34	—	0.41	2.35	1.47
Dimethylformamide	—	2.99	—	0.38	2.45	4.20
Ethanol	—	0.96	1.12	0.25	1.15	1.85 (1.94)
OV202						
n-Hexane	—	—	—	—	2.15	1.76 (1.73)
Triethylamine	–0.05	0.19	—	0.56	2.45	2.77 (2.76)
Dimethylformamide	–0.18	1.70	—	0.52	2.56	4.22
Ethanol	–0.12	0.55	0.16	0.34	1.20	1.74 (1.72)
PIB						
n-Hexane	—	—	—	—	2.71	1.94 (1.87)
Triethylamine	–0.01	0.05	—	—	3.09	2.37
Dimethylformamide	–0.03	0.48	—	—	3.22	2.91
Ethanol	–0.02	0.15	0.07	—	1.51	0.94

[a] Dashes indicate terms calculated to be zero.

[b] These are calculated values, each derived from the sum of the interaction terms plus the constant. Values in parenthesis are measured values.

organic materials). Sorption occurs because there will, at the very least, be dispersion interactions that occur between the vapor and the polymer. Therefore, application of a sorbent polymer to an acoustic wave device will easily yield a vapor sensor. However, the usefulness of such a sensor will depend on whether it is adequately sensitive for the application at hand, and whether it is sufficiently selective.

To maximize the sensitivity of a sensor to a given vapor, a material should be chosen (or designed) whose properties are complementary to those of the vapor, with the aim of maximizing all possible interactions. This will maximize the partition coefficient, and hence, the sensor response. As an example, sorption of a dipolar, basic vapor will be best promoted by a polymer that is both dipolar and hydrogen-bond acidic. P4V and FPOL are examples of polymers with these properties, and both have been shown to be effective in sorbing dipolar, basic phosphonates.[7,28,29,33,36] (This approach involving maximizing all possible interactions is subject to the caveat that self-association in the sorbent material must be avoided. A polymer that is both a strong acid and a strong base, for example, will be self-associated and thus will have less tendency to interact with other species such as the vapors to be sorbed. PVTD is an example of this phenomenon.)

Obtaining the best selectivity possible, however, requires a different strategy. In this case, one should attempt to maximize a single property that will interact favorably with the vapor of interest, and minimize all others. This will limit the types of vapors with which the material will interact. Thus, for example, the SXFA polymer, which is less dipolar than the FPOL and P4V polymers, would be expected to be a more selective sorbent for simple bases. SXFA would have less tendency to interact with potentially interfering dipolar vapors.

Finally, sensors may be used in sensor arrays in combination with pattern recognition or neural network techniques (see Chapter 27), in which case an entire array of materials must be selected to obtain sensitivity and selectivity. Factors governing the selection of materials for arrays is discussed later in this chapter.

25.6.5 Sorbent Material Design

Given strategies for sensitivity and selectivity expressed in terms of interactions and properties, the task remains to design materials with chemical structures that afford the desired properties. In addition to chemical properties to promote particular interactions, the material must have suitable physical properties to promote sorption and to facilitate application of the material as an adherent thin film to the sensor device's surface.

Polymers are well suited for meeting all these requirements. Polymers can easily be applied as thin films by a variety of techniques, including spin-casting, airbrushing, and in some cases by the Langmuir-Blodgett technique. Adhesion is generally good provided that the device surface is thoroughly cleaned prior to film application.

Sorption is both rapid and reversible in polymers whose static glass-to-rubber transition temperatures are below the sensor's operating temperature. Although glassy polymers are able to sorb vapors, diffusion is more rapid through rubbery polymers because of greater free volume and the thermal motion of polymer chain segments. This property facilitates vapor transport to sites for selective interactions, and leads to sensors with rapid response times and simple response kinetics. So long as the interactions between the vapor and polymer are all solubility interactions (i.e., no chemical reactions with bond-making or bond-breaking occur), the polymer-coated sensors will be reversible. All the polymers (and oligomers) in Table 25.2 have static glass-to-rubber transition temperatures below room temperature except P4V.

Therefore, the objective in polymer design is to include structural features that promote particular interactions in an overall structure that gives the polymer favorable physical properties. For selectivity, one would attempt to create a structure that maximizes a particular interaction, while minimizing all others. This is a challenge within the constraints of real materials, which usually have multiple possible interactions. All sorbent polymers will be capable of dispersion interactions to some degree. This property can be increased or decreased by the degree of polarizability. A highly fluorinated polymer, for example, would be less polarizable than one based on aliphatic hydrocarbon chains or aromatic groups. Hydrogen-bond acidity can be incorporated into a polymer while minimizing other properties (other than dispersion) through incorporation of fluoroalcohol substituents, as in SXFA. In this case the siloxane backbone of the polymer afforded the desirable physical property of glass-to-rubber transition temperature below room temperature. Selective hydrogen-bond basicity can, in principle, be incorporated into a polymer by alkylamino-functionality, as in PEI, although quaternary ammonium groups must be avoided. Dipolarity is more difficult to incorporate into a polymer without simultaneously incorporating other properties as well, because most strongly dipolar functional groups are also basic. Therefore a trade-off must be made, choosing very high dipolarity and accepting some basicity, as in SXCN, or minimizing basicity at the cost of lower dipolarity, as in OV202. It is not particularly challenging to find materials that can interact only by dispersion interaction, PIB and SXPH for example, but some care must be taken to be sure the chain ends of the polymers do not have polar functional groups. (As mentioned earlier, examination by infrared spectroscopy and other methods is a useful precautionary measure.)

25.6.6 Sensor Array Design

The purpose of a sensor array is to collect sufficient chemical information through the use of multiple sensors to distinguish responses from the analyte(s) of interest from responses due to potentially interfering vapors. This is especially important if the sensors being used are only semiselective. With a single sensor, there is no way to tell if the observed response is due to a low concentration of a vapor to which the sensor is very sensitive, or if it is actually due to a high concentration of a vapor to which the sensor has modest sensitivity. The same situation exists, for example, in a spectrophotometric determination if absorption is measured at only one wavelength. These single-point measurements are referred to as zero-order. Using an array of sensors, or determining spectral absorption at multiple wavelengths, represents a first-order system. In this case, different chemical species can be distinguished by the pattern or spectrum of responses recorded, using statistical pattern recognition methods or neural network analysis[6-10,28,29,40-42] (see Chapter 27 in this book).

Accordingly, the design principle to be used in selecting sensors or sensor materials for a sensor array is to maximize the relevant chemical information obtained. For this discussion, it will be assumed that a vapor or class of vapors must be detected in an environment where other vapors with diverse properties may be present, as in a field environment. In addition, this discussion pertains primarily to sensors whose selectivity is based on sorption, such as polymer-coated acoustic wave sensors. The objective, then, is to include in the array a set of sensors where each is selective for different classes of vapors. Therefore, each sensor should emphasize a different solubility interaction or combination of solubility interactions. Ideally, these sensors would produce completely orthogonal responses, although this is not rigorously achievable using real materials. (Dispersion interactions will occur in all sorbent materials.) Nevertheless, it is possible to maximize particular solubility interactions in a given material while minimizing others.

The importance of including sensing materials with diverse properties can be seen by considering how statistical pattern recognition is done. If there are n sensors, then the set of responses collected in response to one vapor exposure is plotted in n-dimensional space, called feature space. Each axis defining this space is the response of one sensor in the array, and the single exposure then plots as a single point in n-dimensional feature space. If several test exposures are made, say five, then the results will plot as five different points. If the five test vapors had similar properties, they will plot near each other in feature space. If they are different, and the sensor array is capable of sensing these differences, they will plot out in different regions of feature space, and they will be distinguishable. Thus it is apparent how a sensor array with the most diverse set of coatings will best spread a diverse set of vapors out in feature space, and facilitate discrimination. It is worth noting as well that a sensor material that can interact strongly by a particular interaction with a given vapor will produce a sensor signal that plots farther out on the axis representing that sensor's response than a similarly coated sensor whose sorbent material is less effective at promoting that particular interaction. Therefore, in addition to including materials with diverse properties in an array, each property should be maximized in order to best spread the sensor responses out in feature space.

Based on the solubility approach set out above, a sensor array with diverse properties might include a hydrogen-bond acidic material with minimal basicity and modest dipolarity, a hydrogen-bond basic material with no acidity and minimal dipolarity, a dipolar material minimizing basicity and having no acidity and a nonpolar polarizable material. This type of array would prove the full range of solubility properties discussed above, and when used in combination with pattern recognition methods, provide very good selectivity. The array might also include one or more materials that have combinations of properties in order to maximize sensitivity to particular vapors of interest. The five polymers considered in Table 25.3 could form the basis for a sensor array where each sensor's selectivity is distinct from those of the others. The differing patterns of sorption for each of the four vapours in Table 25.3 on these five polymers are shown in Figure 25.3.

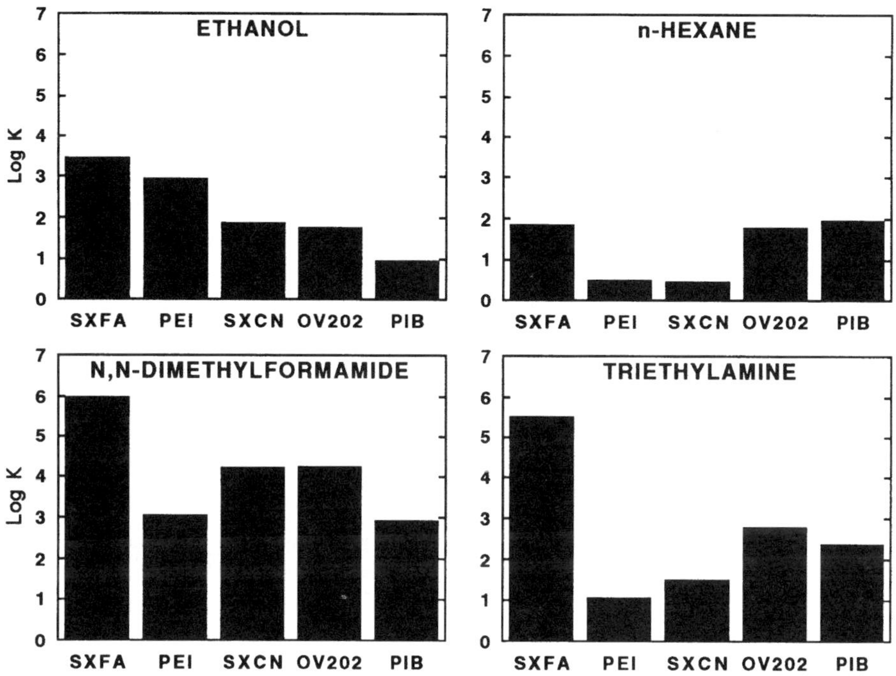

FIGURE 25.3 Log K values for each of four different vapors on the five polymers in Table 25.3.

The combination of a sensor array with data processing techniques such as statistical pattern recognition or neural networks is somctimes referred to as a smart sensor system. Since such a system may be able to "sniff out" and recognize more than one type of vapor, they have also been referred to as electronic noses.[5-10] A number of types of applications for such systems can be envisioned. In some cases, it may only be necessary to detect and identify a single vapor or class of vapors that is of particular interest because of acute toxicity, for example.[7] In this case, all other vapors in the background must either not be detected by the sensors, or if detected, their signals must be distinguished and then ignored. Alternatively, given the wealth of chemical information provided by an array, a single system may be capable of detecting and identifying multiple known species. Yet another use would be to train such a system to recognize a particular odor or condition, even if the vapors giving rise to that condition are not known. Detecting and distinguishing fires based on different origins (i.e., types of materials burning) could be such an application, as could be the detection and recognition of foul odors from a fermentation system.

25.6.7 Elucidation of Transduction Mechanisms

The typical method of evaluating a sensor is to measure its response to a calibrated vapor stream, as indicated by Equation 25.3. However, as discussed in Section 25.2, the observed response actually depends on two processes, sorption and transduction. Therefore, empirical sensor responses alone are insufficient for the investigation of the transduction mechanisms. It is also necessary to know the concentration of vapor absorbed by the film on the sensor under the experimental conditions. One method for obtaining vapor concentrations in the sorbent layer is to know the concentration of the test vapor in the gas phase, and its partition coefficient into the sorbent material on the sensors surface. Then the sensor's response can be evaluated as a function of the vapor concentration in the sorbent layer (Equations 25.4 and 25.5).

This approach was taken in the investigation of polymer-coated SAW vapor sensors.[4,11] When this study was begun, it was widely believed that such sensors responded only to the mass of vapor sorbed. In this case, the response was expected to be related to the sorbed vapor according to Equation 25.7:

$$\Delta f_v = \Delta f_s \, C_v \, K/\rho_S \tag{25.7}$$

The response to the vapor, a shift in frequency, is given by Δf_v. The amount of sorbent polymer on the sensor's surface is represented by Δf_s, the frequency shift that occurred when the polymer layer was applied to the bare sensor. The density of the sorbent polymer material is given by ρ_S. If the partition coefficient K is known, then the response Δf_v of a polymer-coated SAW vapor sensor (Δf_s and ρ_S known) exposed to a calibrated vapor stream (C_v known) can be calculated, assuming the response is only due to mass-loading effects.

However, when observed sensor responses were compared with those predicted according to Equation 25.7, it was found that the observed responses were four to six times larger than expected.[4] This result (in combination with other information) showed that these polymer-coated sensors actually responded to modulus decreases in the polymer material that occur when vapor sorbs and swells the material, decreasing polymer chain/polymer chain interactions. A more accurate model was then developed, which in its simplest form is shown in Equation 25.8:

$$\Delta f_v = 4 \, \Delta f_s \, C_v \, K/\rho_S \tag{25.8}$$

The response is due to a combination of mass-loading and swelling-induced modulus changes, with the total response then being four times larger than the response indicated by Equation 25.7.[4] This discovery was possible because the sorption step was understood and quantified.

The same approach could be taken when evaluating the response mechanisms of other sensors that utilize sorbent polymer layers. In this regard, the polymers in Table 25.2 could be used as standards whose sorption properties are known. Many of these polymers are commercially available.[27] Many partition coefficients into these polymers have been measured, and many more can now be predicted using the LSER method.

25.6.8 Estimating Sensor Responses

Once a polymer has been characterized by the LSER method, it is possible to calculate the partition coefficients for many vapors that might be absorbed by that polymer. Since solvation parameters are known for hundreds of vapors (and can be estimated for many more), and 14 diverse polymers have been characterized by the LSER method, it is possible in principle to predict thousands of partition coefficients. Given a quantitative relationship between a sensor's response and the partition coefficient, responses can be estimated without fabricating a sensor and setting up a calibrated vapor stream to test it.

Such estimations can be made for polymer-coated SAW vapor sensors[43] by using Equation 25.8. These estimations provide an easy way to evaluate whether a sensor is likely to have sufficient sensitivity for use in a particular application. Table 25.4 lists such estimations along with permissible exposure limits for the vapors considered. For each vapor, a polymer was selected that provides sensitivity to that vapor, and the partition coefficients for each vapor/polymer pair were calculated using the LSER coefficients in Table 25.2 and solvation parameters for the vapors. Then Equation 25.8 was used to calculate the vapor concentration required to obtain a 10-Hz response, assuming the sensor was coated with a polymer layer to a thickness producing a 250-kHz shift on applying the polymer. The 10-Hz response was selected as the minimum detectable signal assuming a noise level of a few hertz or less.[30]

TABLE 25.4
Estimations[a] for Polymer-Coated SAW Vapor Sensor Sensitivities

Vapor	Polymer	Log K (calc)	Concentration to get 10 Hz response mg/m³ (calc)	ppm (calc)	Exposure limit[b] ppm
Dichloromethane	PECH	2.07	115	33	100
Tetrachloroethene	PIB	2.99	10	1.5	25
Trichloromethane	SXPYR	2.71	20	4	2
Styrene	SXPH	3.62	3	0.7	50
Toluene	SXPH	2.93	14	3.7	100
Benzene	SXPH	2.46	40	13	1
Propanone	SXFA	3.59	4	1.7	750
Propan-2-ol	SXFA	3.92	2	0.8	400
Butanone	SXFA	4.08	1	0.3	200
Formaldehyde	SXFA	2.17	100	81	1
Ethylene oxide	SXFA	2.64	34	19	1

[a] Estimated from partition coefficients predicted by LSER equations for vapor/polymer pairs, and a model for SAW vapor sensor response, assuming the amount of polymer on the sensor is 250 kHz (see text).

[b] Permissible exposure limit based on a time-weighted average, according to regulations of the U.S. Occupational Safety and Health Association.

The results in the table suggest that several of the vapors could easily be detected to concentrations below the exposure limits, but some could not. For example, toluene should be detectable to below 100 ppm, and styrene should easily be detectable below 50 ppm, but it will likely be difficult to detect benzene to concentrations as low as 1 ppm. Among the chlorinated solvent vapors, the calculations indicate that dichloromethane and tetrachloroethene (perchloroethylene) could be detected to concentrations below the permissible limits, but trichloromethane (chloroform) would be more difficult to detect to the concentrations required. Vapors from solvents like propanone (acetone), butanone (methyl ethyl ketone), and isopropanol should be easy to detect well below the permissible levels, but formaldehyde and ethylene oxide will not be detectable with adequate sensitivity. Estimations like these can help to focus sensor development efforts into those applications that are most likely to succeed, and indicate vapors where some other analytical approach should be taken. (Experimental detection limits for some of these vapors using polymer-coated SAW vapor sensors with 15-Hz noise levels have been reported.[26])

25.7 SUMMARY

The science of sorption is relevant to the response mechanisms of a wide range of sensors that use absorbent materials as the chemically selective layer. The responses of polymer-coated acoustic wave vapor sensors, for example, are directly related to the amount of vapor sorbed. An understanding of the interactions that govern sorption, and quantitative models for the sorption process, can help to address many issues in the development of chemical sensors including sensitivity, selectivity, transduction mechanisms, rational material design, and sensor array design. These methods also provide predictive tools that can be used to help estimate the responses of chemical sensors before they are made and tested. This approach is particularly well developed for polymer-coated SAW vapor sensors.

ACKNOWLEDGMENTS

The authors gratefully acknowledge all our students and co-workers who have participated in the development of sorbent polymers for chemical sensors and in the determination of LSER relationships, including Arthur Snow, Gary S. Whiting, Jenik Andonian-Haftvan, Jonathan W. Steed, Ian Hamerton, and Pnina Sasson. We would also like to thank those who generously provided polymer samples for our analysis, including Wilmer Fife and Martel Zeldin for the SXPYR sample, Arthur Snow for PEM and P4V samples, and Jim Griffith for the FPOL sample. J.W.G. also acknowledges the Naval Research Laboratory, where he worked as a research chemist when these studies were begun. The Pacific Northwest National Laboratory is operated for the U.S. Department of Energy by Battelle Memorial Institute under Contract DE-AC06-76RLO 1830.

REFERENCES

1. Grate, J. W., Martin, S. J., and White, R. M., Acoustic wave microsensors. I, *Anal. Chem.*, 65, 940A-948A, 1993.
2. Grate, J. W., Martin, S. J., and White, R. M., Acoustic wave microsensors. II, *Anal. Chem.*, 65, 987A-996A, 1993.
3. Grate, J. W. and Abraham, M. H., Solubility interactions and the selection of sorbent coating materials for chemical sensors and sensor arrays, *Sensors Actuators*, B3, 85-111, 1991.
4. Grate, J. W., Klusty, M., McGill, R. A., Abraham, M. H., Whiting, G., and Andonian-Haftvan, J., The predominant role of swelling-induced modulus changes of the sorbent phase in determining the responses of polymer-coated surface acoustic wave vapor sensors, *Anal. Chem.*, 64, 610-624, 1992.
5. Newman, A. R., Electronic noses, *Anal. Chem.*, 63, 585A-588A, 1991.
6. Gardner, J. W. and Bartlett, P. N., *Sensors and Sensory Systems for an Electronic Nose*, in NATO ASI Series, Kluwer Academic, Dordrecht, 1992.
7. Grate, J. W., Rose-Pehrsson, S. L., Venezky, D. L., Klusty, M., and Wohltjen, H., A smart sensor system for trace organophosphorus and organosulfur vapor detection employing a temperature-controlled array of surface acoustic wave sensors, automated sample preconcentration, and pattern recognition, *Anal. Chem.*, 65, 1868-1881, 1993.
8. Ema, K., Yokoyama, M., Nakamoto, T., and Moriizumi, T., Odour-sensing system using a quartz-resonator sensor array and neural-network pattern recognition, *Sensors Actuators*, 18, 291-296, 1989.
9. Carey, W. P., Beebe, K. R., and Kowalski, B. R., Multicomponent analysis using an array of piezoelectric crystal sensors, *Anal. Chem.*, 59, 1529-1534, 1987.
10. Carey, W. P. and Kowalski, B. R., Chemical piezoelectric sensor and sensor array characterization, *Anal. Chem.*, 58, 3077-3084, 1986.
11. Grate, J. W., Snow, A., Ballantine, D. S., Wohltjen, H., Abraham, M. H., McGill, R. A., and Sasson, P., Determination of partition coefficients from surface acoustic wave vapor sensor responses and correlation with gas-liquid chromatographic partition coefficients, *Anal. Chem.*, 60, 869-875, 1988.
12. Abraham, M. H., Doherty, R. M., Kamlet, M. J., and Taft, R. W., A new look at acids and bases, *Chem. Br.*, 22, 551-554, 1986.
13. Kamlet, M. J., Doherty, R. M., Abboud, J.-L. M., Abraham, M. H., and Taft, R. W., Solubility: a new look, *CHEMTECH*, 16, 566-576, 1986.
14. Abraham, M. H., Scales of hydrogen-bonding. Their construction and application to physicochemical and biochemical processes, *Chem. Soc. Rev.*, 22, 73-83, 1993.

15. Abraham, M. H., Grellier, P. L., Prior, D. V., Duce, P. P., Morris, J. J., and Taylor, P. J., Hydrogen bonding. 7. A scale of solute hydrogen-bond acidity based on log K values for complexation in tetrachloromethane, *J. Chem. Soc., Perkin Trans.,* 2, 699-711, 1989.
16. Abraham, M. H., Grellier, P. L., Prior, D. V., Morris, J. J., and Taylor, P. J., Hydrogen bonding. 10. A scale of solute hydrogen-bond basicity using log K values for complexation in tetrachloromethane, *J. Chem. Soc. Perkin Trans.,* 2, 521-529, 1990.
17. Abraham, M. H., Whiting, G. S., Doherty, R. M., and Shuely, W. J., Hydrogen bonding. XVI. A new solute solvation parameter, pi2H, from gas chromatographic data, *J. Chromatogr.*, 587, 213-228, 1991.
18. Abraham, M. H., Whiting, G. S., Doherty, R. M., and Shuely, W. J., Hydrogen bonding. 13. A new method for the characterisation of GLC stationary phases — the Laffort data set, *J. Chem. Soc. Perkin Trans.,* 2, 1451-1460, 1990.
19. Abraham, M. H., Grellier, P. L., and McGill, R. A., Determination of olive oil-gas and hexadecane-gas partition coefficients, and caculation of the corresponding olive oil-water and hexadecane-water partition coefficients, *J. Chem. Soc. Perkin Trans.,* 2, 797-803, 1987.
20. Abraham, M. H., Grellier, P. L., Hamerton, I., McGill, R. A., Prior, D. V., and Whiting, G. S., Solvation of gaseous non-electrolytes, *Faraday Discuss. Chem. Soc.*, 85 , 107-115, 1988.
21. Abraham, M. H., Whiting, G. S., Doherty, R. M., and Shuely, W. J., Hydrogen bonding. 14. The characterisation of some N-substituted amides as solvents: comparison with gas-liquid chromatography stationary phases, *J. Chem. Soc. Perkin Trans* 2, 1851-1857, 1990.
22. Abraham, M. H., Whiting, G. S., Doherty, R. M., and Shuely, W. J., Hydrogen bonding. XV. A new characterisation of the McReynolds 77-stationary phase set, *J. Chromatogr.*, 518, 329-348, 1990.
23. Abraham, M. H., Hamerton, I., Rose, J. B., and Grate, J. W., Hydrogen bonding. 18. Gas-liquid chromatographic measurements for the design and selection of some hydrogen bond acidic phases suitable for use as coatings on piezoelectric sorption detectors, *J. Chem. Soc. Perkin Trans.,* 2, 1417-1423, 1991.
24. Abraham, M. H., Whiting, G. S., Andonian-Haftvan, J., Steed, J. W., and Grate, J. W., Hydrogen Bonding. XIX. The characterization of two poly(methylphenylsiloxane)s, *J. Chromatogr.*, 588, 361-364, 1991.
25. Conder, J. R. and Young, C. L., *Physicochemical Measurements by Gas Chromatography,* John Wiley & Sons, New York, 1979.
26. Patrash, S. J. and Zellers, E. T., Characterization of polymer surface acoustic wave sensor coatings and semiempirical models of sensor responses to organic vapors, *Anal. Chem.*, 65, 2055-2066, 1993.
27. Abraham, M. H., Andonian-Haftvan, J., Du, C. M., Diart, V., Whiting, G., Grate, J. W., and McGill, R. A., Hydrogen Bonding, Part 29, The characterisation of fourteen sorbent coatings for chemical microsensors using a new solvation equation, *J. Chem. Soc., Perkins Trans.,* 2, 369-378, 1995.
28. Ballantine, D. S., Rose, S. L., Grate, J. W., and Wohltjen, H., Correlation of surface acoustic wave device coating responses with solubility properties and chemical structure using pattern recognition, *Anal. Chem.*, 58, 3058-3066, 1986.
29. Rose-Pehrsson, S. L., Grate, J. W., Ballantine, D. S., and Jurs, P. C., Detection of hazardous vapors including mixtures using pattern recognition analysis of responses from surface acoustic wave devices, *Anal. Chem.*, 60, 2801-2811, 1988.
30. Grate, J. W. and Klusty, M., Surface acoustic wave vapor sensors based on resonator devices, *Anal. Chem.*, 63, 1719-1727, 1991.
31. Abe, H., Yoshimura, T., Kanaya, S., Takahashi, Y., Miyashita, Y., and Sasaki, S., Automated odor-sensing system based on plural semiconductor gas sensors and computerized pattern recognition techniques, *Anal. Chim. Acta*, 194, 1-9, 1987.
32. Abraham, M. H., Whiting, G. S., Doherty, R. M., and Shuely, W. J., Hydrogen bonding. XVII. The characterisation of 24 gas-liquid chromatographic stationary phases studied by Poole and co-workers, including molten salts, and evaluation of solute stationary phase interactions, *J. Chromatogr.*, 587, 229-236, 1991.

33. Snow, A. W., Sprague, L. G., Soulen, R. L., Grate, J. W., and Wohltjen, H., Synthesis and evaluation of hexafluorodimethylcarbinol functionalized polymers as microsensor coatings, *J. Appl. Polym. Sci.*, 43, 1659-1671, 1991.
34. Chang, Y., Noriyan, J., Lloyd, D. R., and Barlow, J. W., Polymer sorbents for phosphorus esters: I. Selection of polymers by analog calorimetry, *Polym. Eng. Sci.*, 27, 693, 1987.
35. Barlow, J. W., Cassidy, P. E., Lloyd, D. R., You, C. J., Chang, Y., Wong, P. C., and Noriyan, J., Polymer sorbents for phosphorus esters. II. Hydrogen bond driven sorption in fluoro-carbinol substituted polystyrene, *Polym. Eng. Sci.*, 27, 703-715, 1987.
36. Grate, J. W., Klusty, M., Barger, W. R., and Snow, A. W., Role of selective sorption in chemiresistor sensors for organophosphorous detection, *Anal. Chem.*, 62, 1927-1924, 1990.
37. Nieuwenhuizen, M. S. and Nederlof, A. J., A SAW gas sensor for carbon dioxide and water. Preliminary experiments, *Sensors Actuators,* B2, 97-101, 1990.
38. Hofle, G., Steglich, W., and Vorbruggen, H., 4-Dialkylaminopyridines as highly active acylation catalysts, *Angew. Chem. Int. Ed. Engl.*, 17, 569-583, 1978.
39. Cumper, S. W. N. and Singleton, A., The electric dipole moments of aniline, aminopyridines, and their N-methyl derivatives in benzene and 1,4-dioxan solutions, *J. Chem. Soc.,* B1096-1099, 1967.
40. Carey, W. P., Beebe, K. R., Sanchez, E., Geladi, P., and Kowalski, B. R., Chemometric analysis of multisensor arrays, *Sensors Actuators*, 9, 223-234, 1986.
41. Muller, R. and Lang, E., Multidimensional analysis for gas analysis, *Sensors Actuators*, 9, 39-48, 1986.
42. Gardner, J. W., Detection of vapours and odours from a multisensor array using pattern recognition. Part 1. Principal component and cluster analysis, *Sensors Actuators,* B4, 109-115, 1991.
43. Grate, J. W., Patrash, S., and Abraham, M. H., Method for estimating polymer-coated acoustic wave vapor sensor sensitivities, *Anal. Chem.,* 67, 2162-2169, 1995.

26 Lipid-Coated Acoustic Devices for Odour Sensing

Isao Karube, Sang-Mok Chang, Satoshi Sasaki, and Kenji Yokoyama

CONTENTS

26.1 INTRODUCTION

Since Sauerbrey[1] developed the empirical equation for the relationship between the frequency shift of the quartz resonator and the mass of substance deposited on its surface, much attention has been paid to piezoelectric crystal detectors as simple, cheap, sensitive, and reliable detectors.[2-5]

$$\Delta f = -2.3 \times 10^6 f^2 \Delta m/A \tag{26.1}$$

where Δf is the change in frequency due to deposited mass (Hz), f is the resonant frequency of the piezoelectric crystal (MHz), m is the mass of the substance deposited on the surface (g), and A is the area coated (cm^2).

Piezoelectric crystal resonators have been applied to both gas and liquid phase analysis. After King's proposal[2] that the coated piezoelectric crystal can be used for vapour detection, extensive research has been performed on gas sensors using a piezoelectric crystal.[6] (See Chapter 9). However, most of the devices reported were intended to detect a specific odorant with a selective coating film, unlike the olfaction system, which has the versatility to detect all kinds of odorants.

The olfactory reception of odorants is not very well understood. Nomura et al.[7,8] emphasized the importance of lipids in olfactory cells for odorant detection. They hypothesized that lipid layers play an important role in the detection of odorants in olfactory cells even if the

0-8493-8905-4/97/$0.00+$.50
© 1997 by CRC Press, Inc.

lipid itself does not have a specificity to odorants. They deduced the pattern recognition mechanism of odour discrimination from these hypotheses. Building on the results of this study, Muramatsu and co-workers reported the application of a lipid-coated AT-cut crystal for the determination of odorants.[9] Their results, normalized to the amount of coating, show that lipid-coated crystals can be used to detect odorants.

A promising way towards mimicking the olfactory system and towards the construction of an artificial odorant sensing system is neural-network pattern recognition in combination with an array of sensors with sensitive but low-selectivity coatings. The importance of pattern recognition for the solutions to a wide range of data analysis problems have been discussed by Kowalski and Bender[10] and research has been done using an array of gas sensors with different sensitivities. Such studies have been performed using quartz crystal[11] surface acoustic wave devices[12] and electrochemical cells.[13] Both conventional multivariate analysis and neural networks have been employed in pattern recognition. Approaches towards the goal of the "electronic nose" are described in Chapters 23 to 27.

The sensitivity of piezoelectric detectors is directly proportional to the square of resonant frequency, and inversely proportional to the active area. Therefore, the surface acoustic wave (SAW) device is considered to be an excellent transducer for sensing chemical vapours, because the oscillation frequency of the SAW device is above a level of several hundred mega hertz, that is two or three orders higher than that of an AT-cut resonator, and the active area of a SAW device is very small. Hence higher sensitivity is expected for SAW devices. Besides the advantage of sensitivity, SAW devices can be mass produced at relatively low cost with precise and reproducible characteristics and be miniaturized through the photolithographic techniques used in the manufacture of microelectronic circuits. In addition, the lithographic fabrication capability easily permits a complex circuit to be present on the crystal surface of the same substrate.[14,15]

The first studies regarding the use of SAW devices as gas sensors were reported in 1979.[16] Their operating principles and properties have been discussed more precisely by Wohltjen and co-workers.[17,18] They derived the empirical equation for the relationship between the shift of resonant frequency of a SAW oscillator and the mass of coating film:

$$\Delta f = K \times f^2 \times \Delta m/A \tag{26.2}$$

where Δf is the change in frequency due to deposited mass (Hz), f is the resonant frequency of the SAW device (MHz), Δm is the mass of the substance deposited on the surface (g), and A is the area coated (cm^2). This equation is the same as that of the quartz resonator.

SAW devices are classified as SAW delay line and SAW resonator. Most of the SAW sensors for physical, chemical, and biological quantities are based on the SAW delay line. However, the SAW resonator offers some advantages over the SAW delay line, particularly at higher oscillator frequencies,[14,15] so that we used the resonator device for the studies described below. If the surface of the SAW device is modified with a thin film capable of adsorbing a particular species from the gaseous environment, surface accumulation of the species results in perturbation of the wave velocity (frequency) and attenuation of the wave.

In this chapter, odorant sensors based on lipid-coated SAW resonators[19-21] are described. Both solvent casting and Langmuir-Blodgett deposition techniques were used. Subsequently, an odorant sensing system using an array of lipid-coated piezoelectric crystals and neural network pattern recognition with back-propagation algorithm[22] is introduced.

26.2 SAW DEVICE SENSORS WITH SOLVENT-CAST FILMS

26.2.1 Preparation and Testing of PE-Coated Devices

The authors investigated the properties of a phosphatidylethanolamine (PE) coated SAW resonator as a sensing transducer using the change in amplitude, delay time, and frequency of the wave as indicators. The performance of the PE-coated SAW resonator as a chemical vapour sensor was examined.

The schematic diagram of the experimental equipment is shown in Figure 26.1a. A 310-MHz SAW resonator was used as a piezoelectric resonator. The SAW resonator was fixed into the wall of the vessel which had two valves for nitrogen gas inlet and outlet. The resonant frequency of the SAW resonator was measured using a network spectrum analyzer. The resonant frequency was measured at intervals of about 30 s.

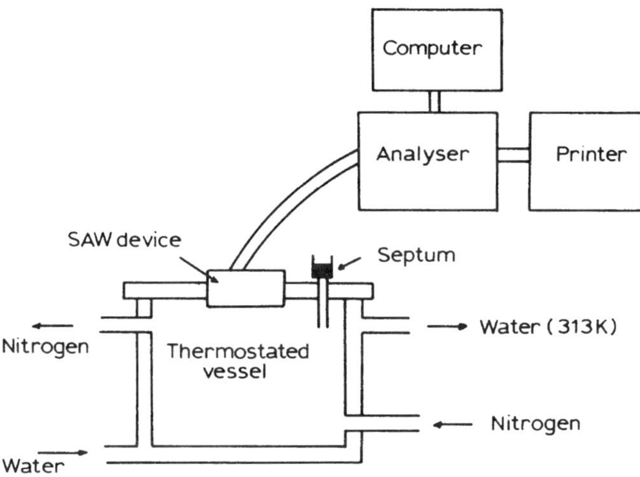

FIGURE 26.1a Experimental setup for study with SAW resonator devices carrying solvent-cast coatings. (From *Biosens. Bioelectron.*, 6, 9, 1991. With permission.)

PE was cast onto the surface of the SAW resonator. Amyl acetate, citral, β-ionone, and menthone were monitored as odorants. The alcohols methanol, ethanol, propanol, and butanol were also used to test the SAW sensors.

The SAW resonator was fabricated on a Y cut (cut angle = 36°) X propagating quartz. The SAW device was a two-port resonator (Figure 26.1b). Aluminium electrode metallization was used. The interdigitated transducer consisted of 55 pairs having half wavelength finger spaces of 5.1 μm, and the grating reflector consisted of 230 grooves having half wavelength finger spacings. The gap between the electrodes was 65 μm wide, because the insertion loss is smallest at this distance. For the main part of the study PE was used as the vapour-sensitive coating. The coating material was dissolved in chloroform (0.2 mg/ml). The film was formed by solvent evaporation, and covered the entire surface.

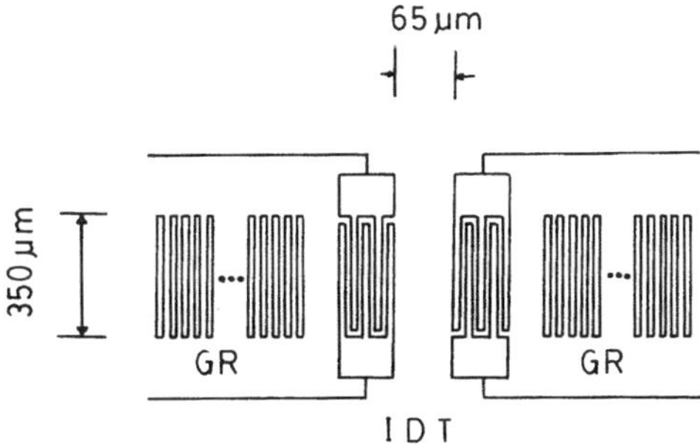

FIGURE 26.1b Two-port SAW resonator. (From *J. Biotech.*, 16, 211, 1990. With permission.)

This film formed by casting from chloroform solution had an average film mass loading of 60 μg/cm² (dry weight). The device was allowed to rest in the clean, dry air for about 3 h prior to testing. After positioning the SAW resonator, nitrogen gas was passed into the vessel and then was stopped when the resonant frequency reached steady state. Subsequently, the valves of the vessel were closed and an odorant was injected by a microsyringe. The odorant was vaporized in the vessel by circulating 40°C water in the vessel jacket. The concentration of the odorant was calculated from the vaporized odorant volume and the vessel volume (vol/vol). The concentrations of amyl acetate, citral, β-ionone, and menthone were controlled by diluting in methanol. A 3-μl sample of methanol mixture was injected. When the resonant frequency response was saturated, nitrogen gas was passed into the vessel again to flush out the vapour. Once the resonant frequency showed a stable value, then the next measurement was performed.

Figure 26.2a shows that the typical frequency changes depended on the amount of coated lipid. The insertion loss and the delay time shift at resonant frequency, and the frequency shift, increased with the amount of coated lipid due to the dissipation of energy in the coating from the vibrating crystal. The delay time measured by the network analyzer is calculated as follows;

$$\text{delay time} = -\Delta\theta/2\pi\ \Delta f \qquad (26.3)$$

where Δθ is the phase shift (deg), and Δf (Hz) is the frequency aperture.

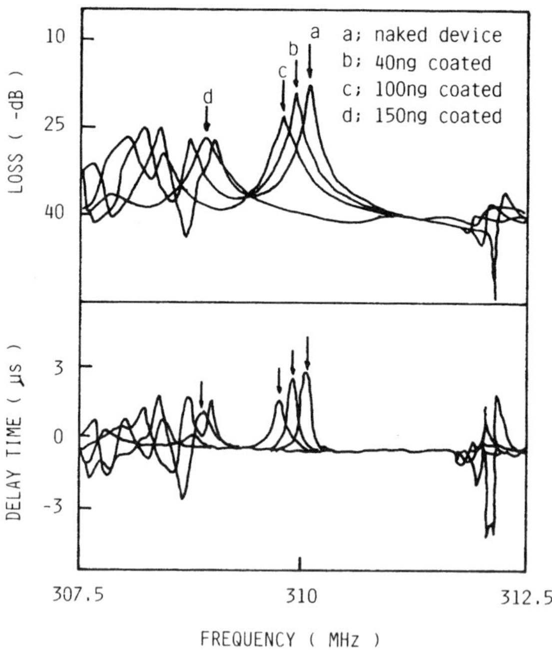

FIGURE 26.2a Typical insertion loss and delay time vs. frequency for two-port SAW resonator with PE-coating (phosphatidylethanolamine). (From *Biosens. Bioelectron.*, 6, 9, 1991. With permission.)

Therefore, the delay time means the phase change at a given frequency in this case. The delay time values at the resonant frequency show a maximum even for PE-coated devices, which means that the phase changes at resonant frequency are maximal and the resonant frequency is unaffected.

The results showed a linear relationship in the range 20 to 100 ng of PE (Figure 26.2b). However, the signal/noise ratio became extremely low above 100 ng of PE, due to a rapid increase of the insertion loss and due to the resultant low Q value (the high degree of slope of the wave). Hence we coated about 100 ng (dry weight) of PE onto the surface of the device.

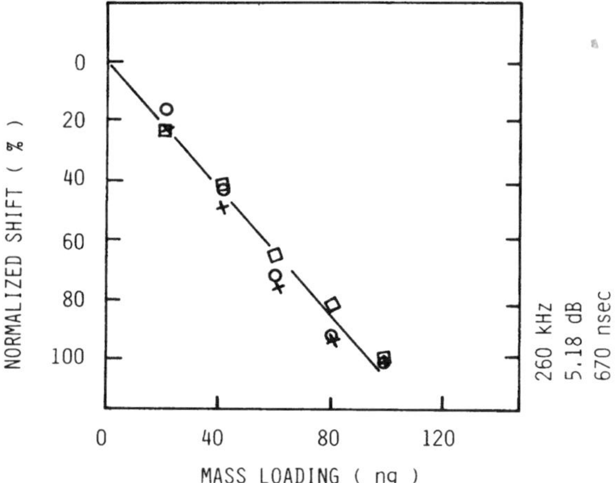

FIGURE 26.2b Normalized shift of insertion loss, delay time, and frequency as a function of PE-coating weight. (From *Biosens. Bioelectron.*, 6, 9, 1991. With permission.)

26.2.2 Response of PE-Coated SAW Devices to Vapours

Figure 26.3 shows a typical response profile obtained from two consecutive on-off exposures to 790 ppm (vol/vol) of butanol. It was shown that the response is reproducible as confirmed by repeated duplication. However, the baseline frequency of the sensor exhibited slow drift which is believed to be related to droplets remaining on the coating.

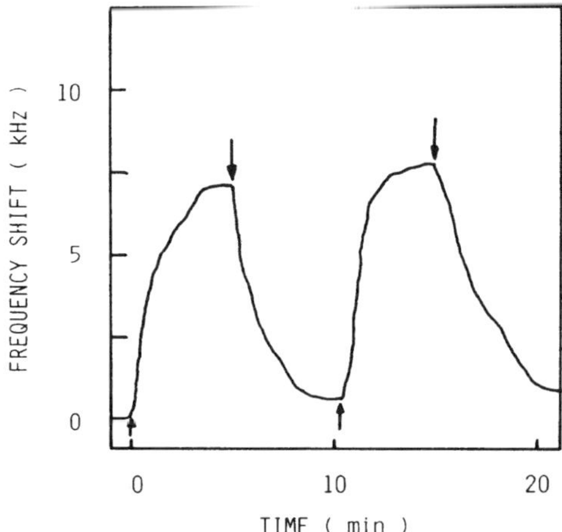

FIGURE 26.3 Typical response of PE-coated SAW resonator to butanol injections. (From *Biosens. Bioelectron.*, 6, 9, 1991. With permission.)

Figure 26.4a shows the correlation between resonant frequency shift and odorant concentration. The results show that the minimum concentration required to give a measurable frequency change and the sensitivity differ between individual odorants. Results for the alcohols are shown in Figure 26.4b. The sensitivity represents the slope obtained from a linear least squares fit of replicate data sets of response. The values for threshold and sensitivity are about 0.1 ppm and 28 kHz/ppm for β-ionone, 0.5 ppm and 14 kHz/ppm for citral, 2 ppm and 1.1 kHz/ppm for menthone, 10 ppm and 0.2 kHz/ppm for amyl acetate, respectively. The frequency shift is about 20 times that obtained with a 9-MHz AT-cut crystal in our laboratory, but the lower detection limit is very similar. These results were thought to be due to the high frequency and the small active surface area. However, there are good correlations between these results and the olfactory threshold values of biological cells observed by several researchers,[7,8,23] who measured the changes in the surface pressure of lipid monolayers or the membrane potential changes of liposomes on addition of various odorants in a liquid phase. The structure of odorants is extremely diverse and it is difficult to find the molecular recognition mechanism of lipid layers in terms of chemical structure. However, it was suggested in their reports that the changes were induced by odorant adsorption onto the hydrophobic region of the membrane, the resultant conformation change causing variations in the surface charge environment. It is considered that these results reflect the equilibrium between the lipid membrane and the gas or liquid phase. From these results, it follows that there is a promising similarity between the mechanism of lipid monolayer surface pressure change, liposome membrane potential change, and the resonant frequency change of the SAW resonator.

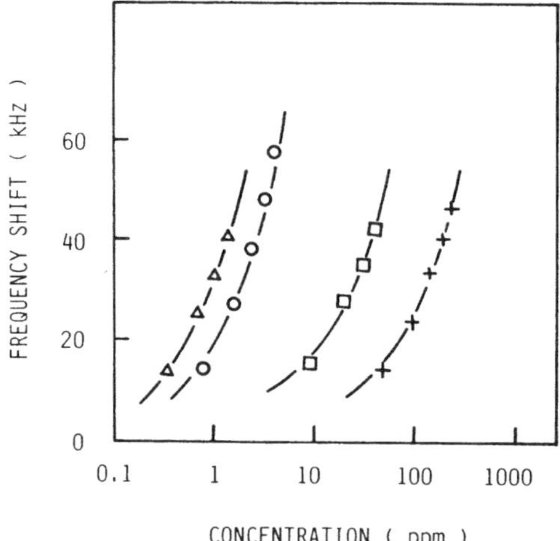

FIGURE 26.4a The correlation between odorant concentration and resonant frequency shifts for a phosphatidylethanolamine-coated SAW resonator. Odorants: (Δ) β-ionone, (○) citral, (□) menthone, (+) amyl acetate. (From *Biosens. Bioelectron.*, 6, 9, 1991. With permission.)

Figure 26.4b shows the correlation between resonant frequency shift and concentration of alcohols for the PE-coated SAW resonator. The results show that the minimum concentration required to give a measurable frequency change and the sensitivity are different among individual odorants. As for the data shown in Figure 26.6, the sensitivity represents the slope obtained from a linear least squares fit of replicate data sets of response. The threshold and sensitivity values are about 0.1% and 14.6 kHz/% for butanol, 0.35% and 5.68 kHz/% for propanol, 1.34% and 1.49 kHz/% for ethanol, 2.42% and 0.83 kHz/% for methanol, respectively. This result also agrees with the results of Kurihara and co-workers.[7,23] As the length of the hydrocarbon chain of the alcohol increased, the minimum concentration required to give a measurable membrane potential change decreased linearly in their study. The dielectric constant considerations allow this behavior to be predicted, at least qualitatively. Lipid compounds such as PE are quite hydrophobic and are unlikely to accommodate much polar solvent in the lipid layers. Present results also lead to the same conclusion.

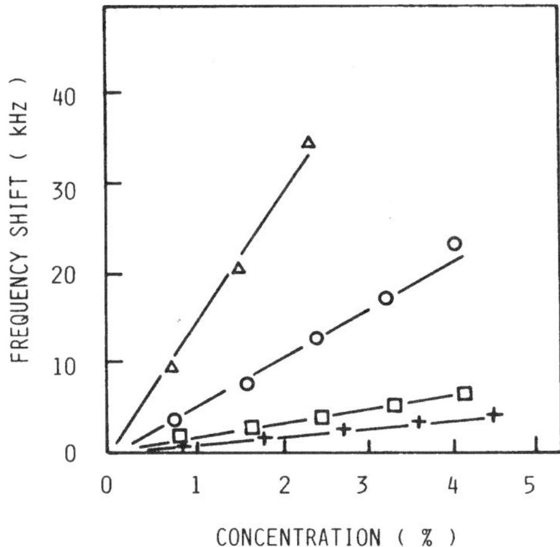

FIGURE 26.4b Correlation between alcohol concentration and resonant frequency shifts for phosphatidylethanolamine-coated SAW resonator; (Δ) butanol, (○) propanol, (□) ethanol, (+) methanol.

26.2.3 SAW Devices Coated With a Range of Lipids

Odorant molecules are mostly lipophilic and therefore have affinity to lipids. Despite the data about different affinities to a mixture of phospholipids,[8] there is no common explanation for specific reception.

Kurihara and co-workers[7,8,23] investigated the role of lipids in olfactory cells for odorant detection. They measured membrane potential changes of liposomes and the response of the olfactory cell on the addition of odorants. The experiments showed a corresponding relationship between the minimum concentration to induce a response from the liposome and that to induce response from the olfactory cell. They hypothesized that the lipid layer acts in the detection of an odorant in the olfactory cell even if the lipid layer does not have a specificity to odorants. They deduced the following pattern recognition mechanism of odour discrimination from these results. Lipid composition of a receptor membrane of an olfactory cell is different from those in the other olfactory cells. Hence, each olfactory cell has an individual response in terms of sensitivity to various odorants. The relative sensitivity of different cells to an odorant is specific. The response profile at the cell level is transformed into a firing pattern among various olfactory axons, and the quality of the odour is recognized in the brain. Recently, we reported on the application of a lipid-coated AT-cut crystal for the determination of odorants.[9] From these results, which were normalized to the amount of coating, it was known that lipid-coated acoustic devices can be used to detect odorants.

In this section, we investigated the properties of a set of SAW resonators as odorant sensor. SAW resonators coated with four types of lipids were examined as chemical vapour sensors. The identification of odorants is discussed by comparing the behavior of the normalized resonant frequency shift pattern depending on the phospholipid coating.

Figure 26.5 shows the correlation between resonant frequency shift and odorant concentration for an asolectin-coated SAW resonator. The concentration was plotted logarithmically to include the four odorants for comparison. The results demonstrate that (as in the case of PE-coatings) the lowest concentration required to give a measurable frequency change differs among individual odorants. The sensitivity represents the slope obtained from a linear least squares fit of a replicate data set of responses. The values are about 7 ppm and 45 Hz/ppm for β-ionone, 9 ppm and 35 Hz/ppm for citral, 25 ppm and 12 Hz/ppm for menthone, and 110 ppm and 2.6 Hz/ppm for amyl acetate, respectively.

The correlation between resonant frequency shift and concentration of alcohols for the asolectin-coated SAW resonator was also investigated. The lowest concentration required to give a measurable frequency change is about 0.2 to 0.5%. This result is in agreement with the data obtained by Nomura and Kurihara.[7]

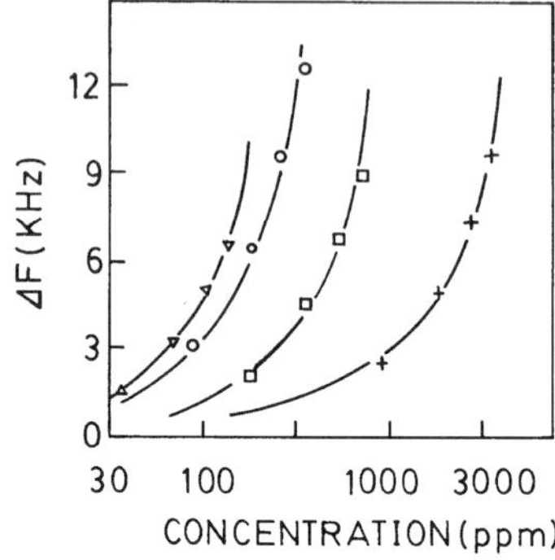

FIGURE 26.5 Correlation between concentration of odorants and resonant frequency shifts for the asolectin-coated SAW resonator; (Δ) β-ionone, (○) citral, (□) menthone, (+) amyl acetate. (From *J. Biotech.,* 16, 211, 1990. With permission.)

Also, other lipids were coated onto the SAW device for use as an odorant sensor. The responses were different for each lipid. Therefore, the frequency shift with the different lipids was represented as a pattern for each odorant (Figure 26.6a). The patterns cannot be compared directly with each other due to the two different vapor concentrations and due to the difference in sensitivity to the vapors. Normalization is necessary for comparison. Therefore, we scaled the response as follows.

$$P(i,j,k) = \Delta f(i,j)/\Delta f(i,k) \tag{26.4}$$

where P is the pattern factor, i is the kind of odorant, j is the kind of lipid, and k is the reference lipid. Cholesterol was used as the reference lipid, because the cholesterol-coated SAW device showed the highest response (on average) The results after normalization procedure are shown in Figure 26.6b. The normalized pattern can be used for the identification of an odorant. The patterns are usually compared by the addition of squares of the difference in the values for each film between two patterns and the sum is used as reference index. In this study, we assumed that the recognition of odorants is related to pattern recognition. Therefore, the normalized pattern has to be used as an index of odorants. The pattern itself is specific and represents a pronounced pattern for each odorant.

From these results, it follows that a lipid-coated SAW resonator responds to different odorants. Using a number of different lipids for coating the surfaces of SAW resonators, odorants can be identified by a computerized pattern recognition algorithm. This approach could open the door to a wide range of sensing systems for the detection of odorants.

26.3 SAW DEVICE ODORANT SENSORS USING LANGMUIR-BLODGETT FILMS

26.3.1 Preparation and Testing

The Langmuir-Blodgett (LB) technique can be used for the preparation of ordered monomolecular films and the production of multilayered systems with the required number of

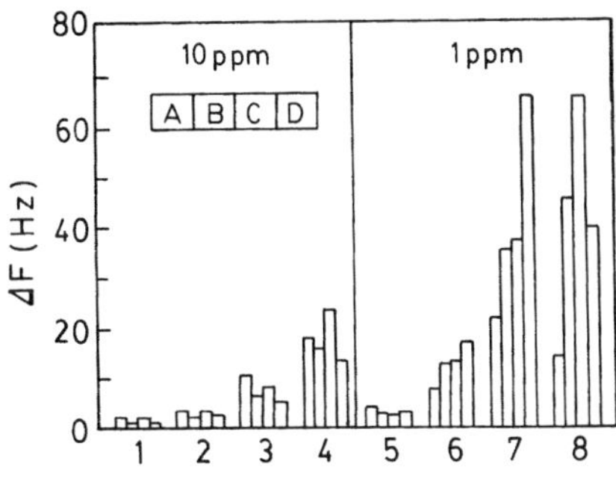

a

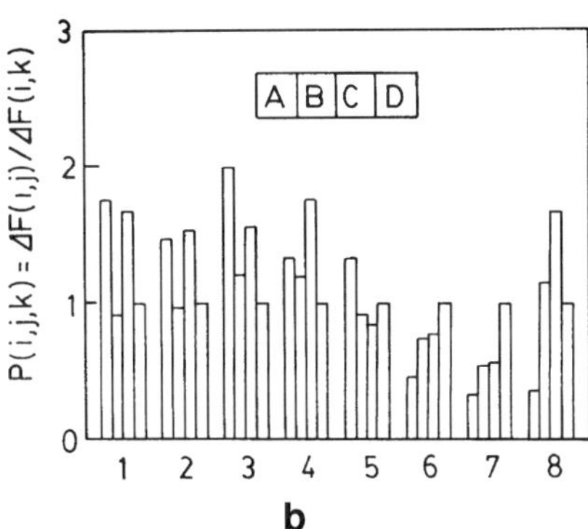

b

FIGURE 26.6a,b Pattern of resonant frequency shifts with the following coating lipids: (A) phosphatidylethanolamine/PE, (B) asolectin/AS, (C) lecithin/LE, (D) cholesterol/CH, for the odorants (1) methanol, (2) ethanol, (3) propanol, (4) butanol, (5) amyl acetate, (6) menthone, (7) citral, (8) β-ionone. (a) As measured. (b) Normalized as per Equation 26.4. (From *J. Biotech.*, 16, 211, 1990. With permission.)

monomolecular layers. The LB technique has been applied to the construction of gas sensors by several groups.[24,25]

In this section, the LB technique was applied to produce uniform reproducible layers of sufficient thinness to keep the insertion losses due to the mass loading low. Phospholipids and a fatty acid have been used for thin coating of SAW devices. The loading efficiency has been controlled by measuring the frequency shift and insertion loss. We investigated the properties of a SAW resonator as an odorant sensor. The identification of odorants is discussed by comparing the behaviour of their normalized resonant frequency shift patterns, which are dependent on the phospholipid used.

The lipids were first dissolved in a chloroform solution (2 mM). The solution was then spread onto a clean water surface. After evaporation of the chloroform, the molecule film was compressed by means of a moveable barrier until it formed a closely packed structure. A SAW device was then passed through the air-water interface, and a monolayer of lipid was deposited at each pass onto the surface of the SAW device.

The deposition of monolayers was performed at a surface pressure of 15 mN/m by the horizontal lifting method. The quality of the phospholipids was checked by measuring their isotherms using an LB trough. The speed of the film lift was kept constant at 6 mm/min.

The scheme of the experimental setup is shown in Figure 26.7. The coated device was placed in clean dry air for 3 h prior to measurement of odorants. The SAW resonator was fixed on top of a small vessel with two valves. Following positioning of the SAW device, the vessel was flushed with nitrogen gas until the resonant frequency reached a steady state. Subsequently, the nitrogen stream was stopped and the odorant was injected by a permeater. It is very important and absolutely essential that the system generates and delivers a precise and accurate concentration of odorant to the detector during the development and testing of any prototype odorant sensor. The principle of odorant generation used in this work is a dynamic system based on the difference of liquid diffusion coefficient with temperature.[26] The temperature and odorant concentration of the gas stream were controlled by the permeater.

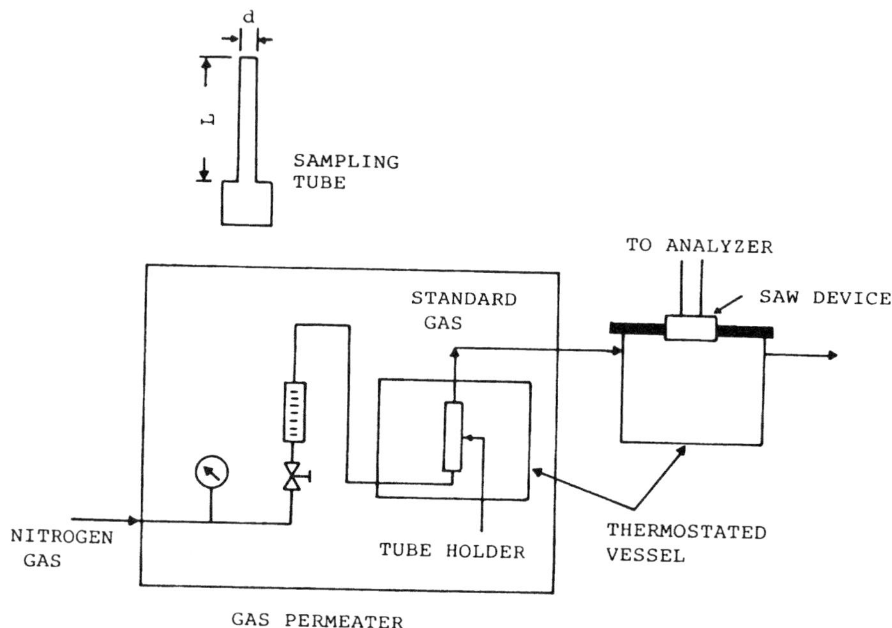

FIGURE 26.7 Flow system for study with SAW resonator devices carrying Langmuir-Blodgett (LB) films. (From *Anal. Chim. Acta.*, 249, 323, 1991. With permission.)

Using the deposition of monolayers by the horizontal lifting method it was possible to cover the SAW device and to make it reproducible for up to 40 monolayers of the X-type structure. The mass loading could be determined with high precision by the frequency change of the SAW device. Figure 26.8a shows that the typical frequency characteristics are dependent on the number of deposited monolayers. The resonance frequency decreases whereas the insertion loss due to the dissipation of energy increases with the number of monolayers deposited.

Figure 26.8b shows the correlation between the number of monolayers and the resonant frequency shift. The results show a linear relationship in the range up to 40 LB layers of phosphatidylcholine (PC). However, the signal/noise ratio became extremely low above 20 layers of phosphatidylcholine, because the insertion loss became so high and due to the resultant low Q value. Based on the stability analysis, the optimum number of layers was found to be between 10 and 20. This was dependent upon the surface pressure and molecular weight of the deposited material; the frequency shift was about 200 kHz.

26.3.2 Response of PC-Coated SAW Devices to Vapours

Figure 26.9 shows typical response profiles obtained from consecutive exposures to 148 ppm of acetoin. The response is quite reproducible and changes linearly with consecutive exposures to acetoin.

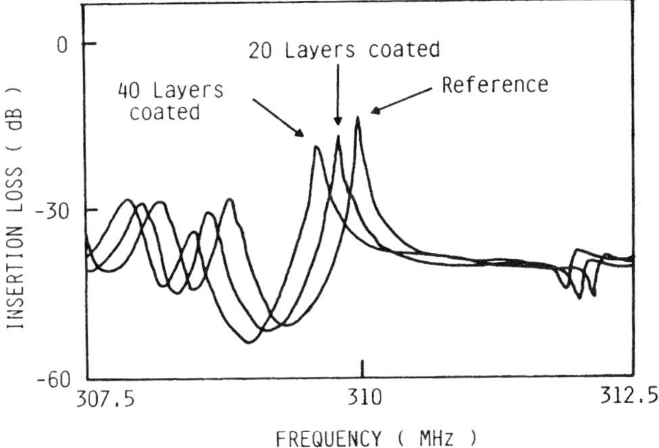

FIGURE 26.8a Typical insertion loss vs. frequency for two-port SAW resonator coated with LB-films of phosphatidylcholine.

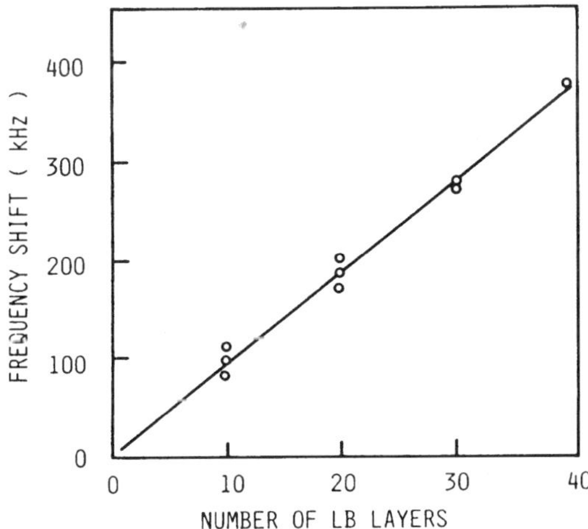

FIGURE 26.8b Correlation between frequency shifts and the number of LB layers for phosphatidylcholine deposition on the surface of the SAW resonator. (From *Sensors Actuators.*, B5, 53, 1991. With permission.)

We measured the frequency shift of the SAW device following the adsorption of odorants onto the coating film. Figure 26.10a shows the correlation between resonant frequency shift and odorant concentration for a phosphatidylcholine (PC)-coated SAW resonator. The results demonstrate that the lowest concentration required to give a measurable frequency change is different for individual odorants just as in the case of the solvent-cast lipid films. The sensitivity represents the slope obtained from a linear least squares fit of replicate data sets. The values for threshold and sensitivity are about 3 ppm and 66 Hz/ppm for menthone, 24 ppm and 6.3 Hz/ppm for amyl acetate, and 35 ppm and 4.0 Hz/ppm for acetoin, respectively. There are good qualitative correlations between these results and olfactory threshold values in biological cells, as observed by Nomura et al.[7,8] and Muramatsu.[9]

Figure 26.10b shows the correlation between resonant frequency shift and concentration for the alcohols using a phosphatidylcholine-coated SAW resonator. The lowest concentration

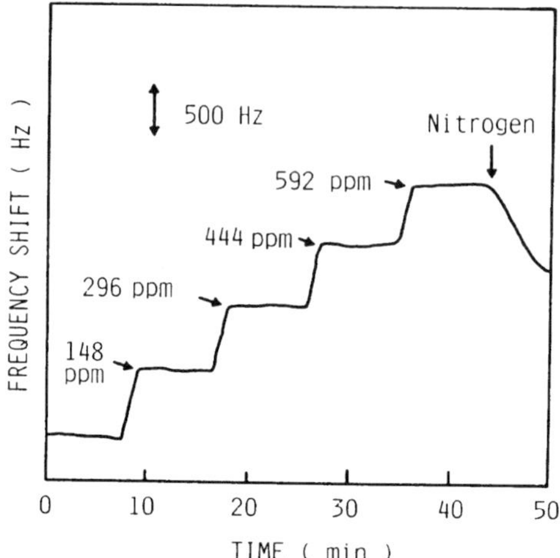

FIGURE 26.9 Typical response of phosphatidylcholine-coated SAW resonator to acetoin. (From *Sensors Actuators.*, B5, 53, 1991. With permission.)

required to give measurable frequency change decreased in the following order: ethanol, propanol, and butanol. This result is in agreement with the data obtained by Nomura et al.[7,8]

26.3.3 SAW Devices With a Range of L-B Lipid Films

Other lipids were also coated onto a SAW device and used to produce odorant sensors. Although the minimum concentrations of odorants required to give a response were almost the same for each film, the amount of odorant adsorbed depended on its concentration. At low concentrations, it is considered that monolayer adsorption occurs regardless of whether specific chemical or physical interactions take place. The frequency shift is affected by the coating film used, but this effect is less than that of the odorants. These results show that there is an affinity difference between odorants for specific phospholipids and to a lesser extent between phospholipids for each odorant.

The frequency shift with the different lipids was represented with an individual pattern for each odorant. The patterns cannot be compared directly with each other because of the different vapor concentrations used. Normalization is necessary for the comparison. Therefore, we normalized the response so that the sum of responses for one odorant is unity.

$$P(i,j) = \Delta F(i,j) \Big/ \sum_j \Delta F(i,j) \tag{26.5}$$

where P is the pattern factor, i is the kind of odorant, j is the kind of lipid.

The results after the normalization procedure are shown in Figure 26.11. The distribution itself is specific and represents a pronounced pattern for each odorant. The normalized pattern can be used for the identification of odorants. Further research on the basis of monolayer properties of phospholipids and fatty acids may reveal an explanation for the different odorant affinities. However, the structure of odorants is extremely diverse and it is difficult to find a molecular recognition mechanism by lipid layers at the chemical structure level.

From these results, it follows that SAW resonator devices carrying lipid films deposited with the L-B technique can monitor different odorants. As in the case of solvent-cast lipids, it is possible to use a range of lipids to coat the surfaces of SAW resonators and odorants can be identified by a computerized pattern recognition algorithm.

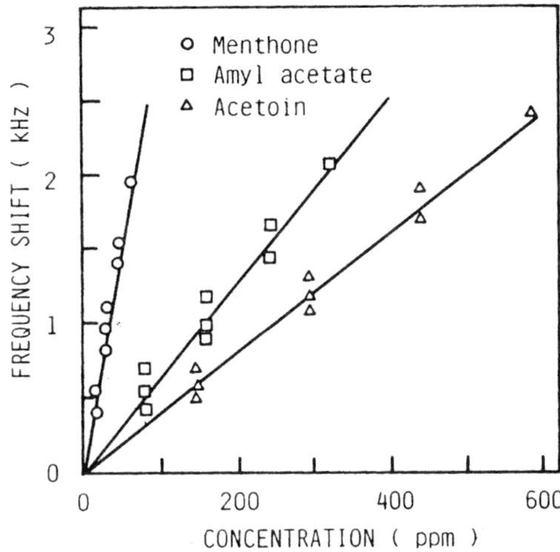

FIGURE 26.10a Correlation between odorant concentration and resonant frequency shifts for phosphatidylcholine-coated SAW resonator.

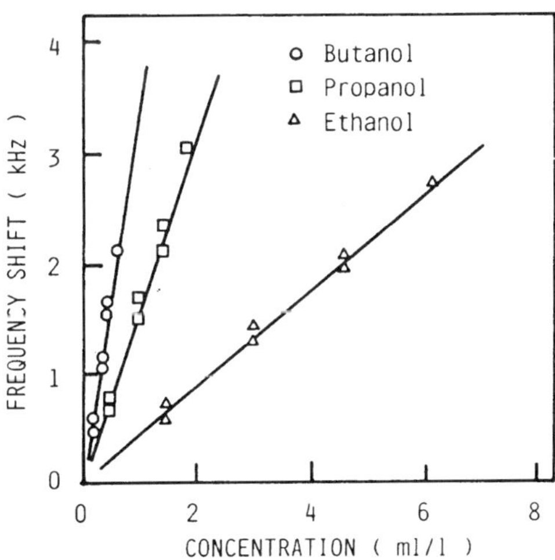

FIGURE 26.10b Correlation between alcohol concentration and resonant frequency shifts. (From *Sensors Actuators.*, B5, 53, 1991. With permission.)

26.4 ODOUR-SENSING SYSTEMS BASED ON AN ARRAY OF PIEZOELECTRIC CRYSTALS AND NEURAL NETWORK PATTERN RECOGNITION

A schematic diagram of the odorant sensing system using an array of piezoelectric crystals is shown in Figure 26.12. The lipid-coated AT-cut quartz crystal resonators were placed in a 10 ml vessel with two valves for nitrogen gas inlet and outlet. The electrodes were prepared by deposition of thickness of 200 Å of chromium and 2000 Å of gold in turn by vacuum vapour deposition on both sides of a quartz crystal. The resonant frequency was

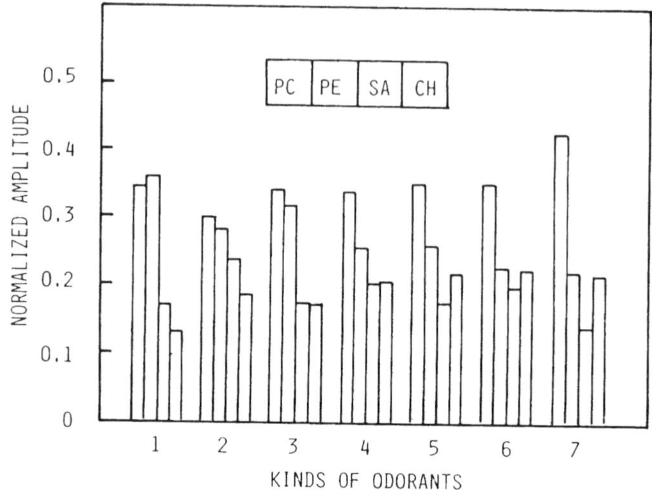

FIGURE 26.11 Normalized patterns (as per Equation 26.5) of resonant frequency shifts for the coatings phosphatidylcholine (PC), phosphatidylethanolamine (PE), stearic acid (SA), cholesterol (CH) in response to the following odorants: (1) methanol, (2) ethanol, (3) propanol, (4) butanol, (5) acetoin, (6) amyl acetate, (7) menthone. (From *Sensors Actuators.*, B5, 53, 1991. With permission.)

measured using a six-channel frequency counter connected in-line to a personal computer. The coating material was diluted with chloroform (5 mg/ml) and subsequently a thin film was coated on and formed by solvent evaporation. The entire surface was covered with the film. The coated film led to a frequency shift of about 230 kHz. Following positioning of the lipid-coated quartz crystal, the vessel was flushed with nitrogen gas until the resonant frequency reached a steady state. Subsequently, the nitrogen stream was stopped and the odorant was injected by a permeater. The temperature and odorant concentration of the gas stream were controlled by the permeater. Nitrogen gas was used as the carrier stream into the detection vessel.

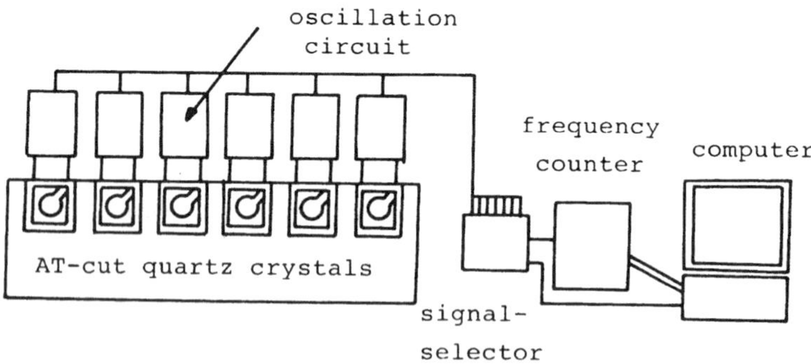

FIGURE 26.12 Odorant detector using an array of piezoelectric quartz crystals. (From *Anal. Chim. Acta.*, 249, 323, 1991. With permission.)

Artificial neural networks are biologically inspired, that is, they are composed of elements that perform in a manner analogous to the most elementary functions of the biological neuron. The schematic diagram of the fundamental model of neuron is shown in Figure 26.13a. Each neuron receives multiple input signals, transforms the signals to electrochemical signals, and transmits the electrochemical signals over the neural pathways only when the summation of input signals exceeds the threshold value. One neuron receives signals from other neurons at a connection point called a synapse. On the receiving side of the synpase, these input signals are conducted to the cell body. There they summed come together, some input signals tending to excite the cell and others tending to inhibit its firing, compared with the threshold value. The synaptic strength and threshold value are thought to be affected and changed by this processing reaction. The nervous system reacts as a result of the neural network system.

In the model neural network system (Figure 26.13b), the weighting factor w is the most important parameter. As the value of w changes, a neural network converts its interconnecting pattern to another pattern. The type of pattern is decided on the basis of a rule of the information theory. In an artificial neuro-computer system, the input signal x is modulated to xw. The value of w is predetermined from the relationship between the output and standard signals, called teaching signals.

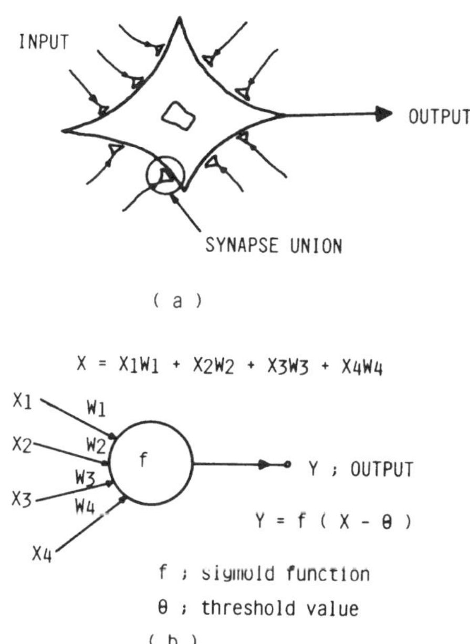

FIGURE 26.13a,b Neural networks: (a) bio-neuron unit; (b) model of neuron unit. (From *Anal. Chim. Acta.*, 249, 323, 1991. With permission.)

On the other hand, in the natural neurons, an input signal is assumed to be converted to a value derived from a more complicated function g(x) rather than a simple representation such as xw. If a converting function (or activation function) such as the natural neuron system is used, one can produce an artificial neural network. In this study, a three-layer neural network was used to recognize the various odorants automatically with the back-propagation algorithm presented clearly and precisely by Rumelhart et al.[27] A sigmoid is used as an activation function in the back-propagation algorithm, because the sigmoid function compresses the sum of input signals so that the output lies between 0 and 1. Coefficients for the back-propagation algorithm can be chosen arbitrarily, but here the values as in the NEC Neuro-07 software were adopted. The structure of this neural network is shown in Figure 26.13c. The number of input layer units was six, which corresponds to the number of sensors, and the number of output layer units was seven, which corresponds to the number of odorants measured. The teaching signals are composed of character symbols and seven-bit data, which correspond to the number of odorants measured. The

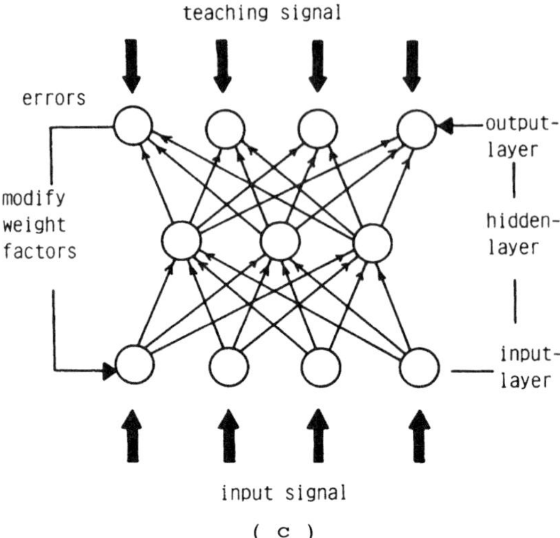

FIGURE 26.13c Hierarchical model of neural network for back-propagation algorithm. (From *Anal. Chim. Acta.*, 249, 323-329. With permission.)

number of intermediate layer (hidden layer) units is decided by the trial and error method in order to accelerate and improve the convergence of the learning process; we used seven units. The initial values for the connecting weight factors w in the neural network are random numbers between –1 and 1.

Responses of an array of lipid-coated AT-cut crystals to odorants were investigated. The correlation between resonant frequency shift and odorant concentration for a PE-coated AT-cut resonator was explored. The results demonstrated that as in the earlier studies the lowest concentration required to give a measurable frequency change differs among individual odorants. The sensitivity represents the slope obtained from a linear least-squares fit of four sets of responses. The values of these parameters are about 1 ppm and 5.3 Hz/ppm for menthone, 7 ppm and 0.6 Hz/ppm for amyl acetate, and 15 ppm and 0.27 Hz/ppm for acetoin, respectively. Again, there are good qualitative correlations between these results and olfactory threshold values in biological cells, as observed by Nomura and Kurihara[7,8] and Muramatsu.[9]

The correlation between resonant frequency shift and concentration of various alcohols for a PE-coated At-cut resonator was also investigated. The lowest concentration required to give measurable frequency change decreased in the order: ethanol, propanol, butanol, in agreement with the results obtained by Nomura and Kurihara,[7,8] who found that the lowest concentration required to give a measurable membrane potential change decreased linearly when the length of the hydrocarbon chain of the alcohol was increased.

The correlations between resonant frequency shift and vapour concentration for other lipid-coated AT-cut quartz crystals were also investigated. Each vapour produced a characteristic response. The frequency shift produced by each vapour for the acoustic devices with the different lipids was represented as a pattern. The patterns cannot be compared directly with each other owing to the different vapor concentrations, and thus the response was normalized so that the sum of each response was unity.

The results after normalization procedure are shown in Figure 26.14. The pattern itself is specific and represents a pronounced pattern for each alcohol or odorant. The normalized pattern can be used for the identification of vapours.

Recognition of vapours was attempted using neural network pattern recognition. The normalized patterns were processed using a three-layer neural network as shown in Figure 26.13c. The procedures and results of the learning process are shown in Figure 26.15a. The normalized patterns are transferred to the input layer as input signals, and the teaching signals

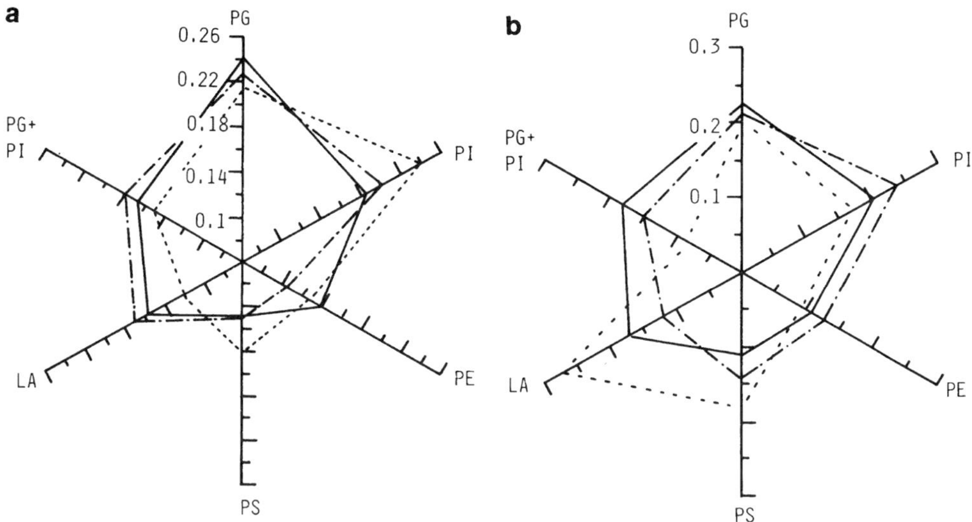

FIGURE 26.14a,b Normalized patterns of resonant frequency in response shifts to (a) alcohols (— methanol, –·–·– ethanol, - - - - n-propanol), (b) odorants (— acetoin, –·–·– amyl acetate, - - - - menthone). Lipid coatings: PG: phosphatidylglycerol, PI: phosphatidylinositol, PE: phosphatidylethanolamine, PS: phosphatidylserine, LA: lipid A. (From *Anal. Chim. Acta.*, 249, 323, 1991. With permission.)

are composed of character symbols and seven-bit data which are "on" (1) at the position of the odorant concerned and "off" (0) at the other positions. The position corresponding to methanol is "on" and other positions are "off" in the teaching signal shown in Figure 26.15a. The shaded areas indicated by the squares for the units are proportional to the activity levels, which are accumulated by the converting function of the last layer. The input signals and teaching signals are processed and connected into the neural network repeatedly, and the neural network is ordered such that the output layer indicates an approximation to the accurate character symbol as a result of training. As shown in Figure 26.15a, the output layer at first indicates a random symbol, but eventually indicates the more accurate symbol according to the learning processes. The indicated result of the relatively accurate symbol means that the neural nework is ordered satisfactorily.

When the input signals for the seven kinds of odorants using responses to a sequence of seven pure compounds were placed in the network, the output layer showed the activity levels indicated by the character symbols as shown in Figure 26.15b. The fact that the relatively large squares are aligned on the diagonal and that relatively accurate symbols are indicated means that this system can be used for the pattern recognition of pure alcohols and odorants.

Using this algorithm, odorants could be recognized at above 70% probability. The remaining uncertainty was primarily caused by the deviation of sensor responses even if pure compounds were used.

From these results, it follows that a multichannel lipid-coated AT-cut quartz crystal array can monitor different pure odorants. Using a number of different lipids for the coating of surfaces of quartz crystals, odorants can be identified by a neural network pattern recognition algorithm, where transformation of a nonrecognizable signal pattern to a recognizable symbol is called pattern recognition. This approach may open up a wide field of developments in the detection of odorants.

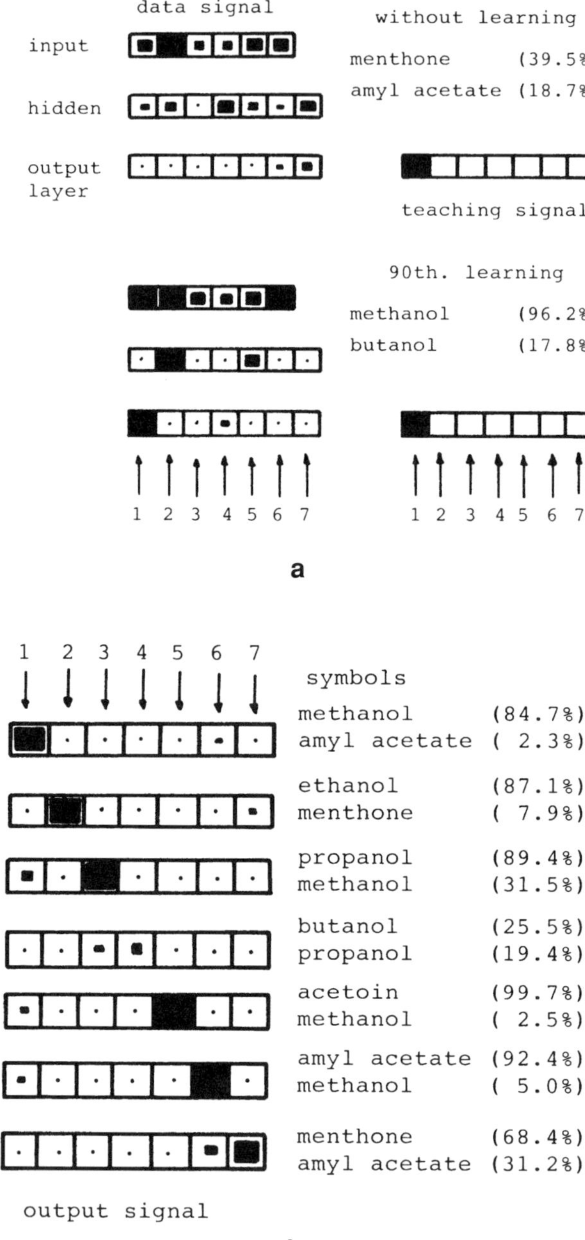

FIGURE 26.15a,b Schematic diagram of neural network learning process towards odorant recognition: 1, methanol; 2, ethanol; 3, n-propanol; 4, n-butanol; 5, acetoin; 6, amyl acetate; 7, menthone. (a) Activity in the network layers without learning and after the 90th learning process. (b) Results of output layer units after 200 learning processes.

REFERENCES

1. Sauerbrey, G., Use of a quartz vibrator for weighing thin films on a microbalance, *Z. Phys.*, 155, 206, 1955.
2. King, W. H., Analytical uses of the piezoelectric crystal, *Anal. Chem.*, 36, 1735, 1964.
3. Guilbault, G., Piezoelectric crystal detectors in analytical chemistry, *Anal. Proc.*, 19, 68, 1982.

4. Muramatsu, H., Kajiwara, K., Tamiya, E., and Karube, I., Piezoelectric immunosensor for the detection of *Candida albicans* microbes, *Anal. Chim. Acta,* 188, 257, 1986.
5. Muramatsu, H., Dicks, J. M., Tamiya, E., and Karube, I., Piezoelectric crystal biosensor modified with protein A for determination of immunoglobulins, *Anal. Chem.,* 159, 2760, 1987.
6. Guilbault, G. and Lung, J. H., Gas phase biosensors, *J. Biotechnol.,* 9, 1, 1988.
7. Nomura, T. and Kurihara, K., Liposomes as a model for olfactory cells. Changes in membrane potential in response to various odorants, *Biochemistry,* 26, 6135, 1987.
8. Nomura, T. and Kurihara, K., Effects of changed lipid composition on responses of liposomes to various odourants. Possible mechanism of odour discrimination, *Biochemistry,* 26, 6141, 1987.
9. Muramatsu, H., Tamiya, E., and Karube, I., Detection of odorants using lipid-coated piezoelectric crystal resonators, *Anal. Chim. Acta,* 225, 399, 1989.
10. Kowalski, B. R. and Bender, C. F., Pattern recognition. A powerful approach to interpreting chemical data, *J. Am. Chem. Soc.,* 9, 5632, 1972.
11. Carey, W. P., Beebe, K. R., Kowalski, B. R., Illman, D. L., and Hirschfeld, T., Selection of adsorbates for chemical sensor arrays by pattern recognition, *Anal. Chem.,* 58, 149, 1986.
12. Ballantine, D. S., Rose, S. L., Grate, J. W., and Wohltjen, H., Correlation surface acoustic wave device coating responses with solubility properties and chemical structure using pattern recognition, *Anal. Chem.,* 58, 3058, 11986.
13. Stetter, J. R., Jurs, P. C., and Rose, S. L., Detection of hazardous gases and vapors. Pattern recognition analysis of data from electrochemical sensor array, *Anal. Chem..* 58, 860, 1986.
14. Ash, E. E., Fundamentals of signal processing devices, in *Acoustic Surface Waves,* Oliner, A. A., Ed., Springer-Verlag, New York, 1978, 115.
15. Morgan, D. P., *Surface-Wave Devices for Signal Processing,* Elsevier, Amsterdam, 1985.
16. Wohltjen, H. and Dessy, R., Surface acoustic wave probe for chemical analysis. I. Introduction and instrument description, *Anal. Chem.,* 51, 1458, 1979.
17. Wohltjen, H., Mechanism of operation and design considerations for surface acoustic wave device vapour sensors, *Sensors Actuators,* 5, 307, 1984.
18. Wohltjen, H., Snow, A. W., Barger, W. R., and Ballantine, D. S., Trace chemical vapor detection using SAW delay line oscillators, *IEEE Trans. Ultrason. Ferroelect. Freq. Control,* UFFC-34, 172, 1987.
19. Chang, S. M., Tamiya, E., and Karube, I., Chemical vapour sensor using a SAW resonator, *Biosens. Bioelectron.,* 6, 9, 1991.
20. Chang, S. M., Ebert, B., Tamiya, E., and Karube, I., Detection of chemical vapour using lipid-coated SAW resonator oscillator, *J. Biotechnol.,* 16, 211, 1990.
21. Chang, S. M., Tamiya, E., Karube, I., Sato, M., and Masuda, Y., Odorant sensor using lipid-coated SAW resonator oscillator, *Sensors Actuators,* B5, 53, 1991.
22. Chang, S. M., Iwasaki, Y., Suzuki, M., Tamiya, E., Karube, I., and Muramatsu, H., Detection of odorants using an array of piezoelectric crystals and neural-network pattern recognition, *Anal. Chim. Acta,* 249, 323, 1991.
23. Koyama, N. and Kurihara, K., Effect of odorants on lipid monolayers from bovine olfactory epithelium, *Nature,* 236, 402, 1972.
24. Roberts, G. G., Holcroft, B., Barraud, A., and Richard, J., The properties of conducting tetracyanoquinodimethane Langmuir-Blodgett films, *Thin Solid Films,* 160, 53, 1988.
25. Jay, W. G., Susan, R. P., and William R. B., Langmuir-Blodgett films of a nickel dithiolene complex on chemical microsensors for the detection of hydrazine, *Langmuir,* 4, 1293, 1988.
26. Lugg, G. A., Diffusion coefficients of some organic and other vapors in air, *Anal. Chem.,* 40, 1072, 1968.
27. Rumelhart, D. E., Hinton, G. E., and Williams, R. J., Learning representations by back propagating errors, *Nature,* 323, 533, 1986.

27 Pattern Analysis Techniques

Julian W. Gardner and Evor L. Hines

CONTENTS

27.1 INTRODUCTION TO PATTERN ANALYSIS

27.1.1 Nature of Sensor Array Data

Computational pattern analysis techniques are being widely used today in fields of research within the physical, chemical, and engineering sciences. There is a large number of pattern analysis techniques currently available, yet it is essential to start by understanding the nature of the data being analysed. Only by a good understanding of the fundamental nature of the data can one select an appropriate analysis technique from this large and growing choice. This chapter is concerned with the analysis of signals, usually analogue, generated by odour sensors being applied in the areas of medicine, food, and the environment. There is a wide variety of sensors employed today, such as thermal (e.g., a thermometer), radiation (e.g., a photodiode), mechanical (e.g., a pressure sensor), magnetic (e.g., a Hall probe), and chemical (e.g., an ISFET; see Chapter 6 in this book).[1] The last class of sensor includes the odour sensors of interest here.

Now let us consider an array of discrete sensors, where each sensor i produces a time-dependent output signal $x_{ij}(t)$ in response to an odour j. The response of a set of n sensors

0-8493-8905-4/97/$0.00+$.50
© 1997 by CRC Press, Inc.

can now be represented by a vector $x_j(t)$ where each component corresponds to the output from an individual sensor:

$$\boldsymbol{x}_j(t) = (x_{1j}(t), x_{2j}(t), \ldots, x_{nj}(t)) \tag{27.1}$$

It is common practice to use the steady-state values of an odour sensor rather than its transient response. In other words, the sensor output is allowed to reach a constant, asymptotic value when the input signal is fixed. The response vector can now be represented by a time-independent parameter $\boldsymbol{r}_j$. This parameter may be defined as simply the absolute change in the sensor signal with measurand j, i.e.,

$$\boldsymbol{r}_j = \left(r_{1j}, r_{2j}, \ldots, r_{nj}\right) \text{ where } r_{ij} = \underset{t \to \infty}{\text{Limit}} \left[x_{ij}(t) - x_{ij}(t=0)\right] \tag{27.2}$$

The choice of the response parameter is fundamental to the subsequent performance of the pattern analysis method. A discussion of this is presented in Section 27.2.1. The response of an array of odour sensors to a set of m odours can now be regarded as a set of m vectors which are best represented as a response matrix $\tilde{\boldsymbol{R}}$.

$$\tilde{\boldsymbol{R}} = \begin{pmatrix} r_{11} & r_{12} & \cdots & r_{1m} \\ r_{21} & r_{22} & \cdots & r_{2m} \\ \vdots & \vdots & \vdots & \vdots \\ r_{n1} & r_{n2} & \cdots & r_{nm} \end{pmatrix} \tag{27.3}$$

Each column represents the response vector associated with a particular measurand, while the rows represent the response of an individual sensor to the different measurands. The complexity of the pattern analysis problem relates to the number of non-zero terms within the response matrix $\tilde{\boldsymbol{R}}$. For example, if one had an array of n independent odour sensors, that is each sensor responded to only one class of measurand j, then all terms off the leading diagonal will be zero:

$$\tilde{\boldsymbol{R}} = \begin{pmatrix} r_{11} & 0 & \cdots & 0 \\ 0 & r_{22} & \cdots & 0 \\ \vdots & \vdots & \vdots & \vdots \\ 0 & 0 & \cdots & r_{nm} \end{pmatrix} \tag{27.4}$$

When a set of sensors is independent, then the response matrix is a convenient way of handling the data and there is no need to carry out sophisticated pattern analysis. The exception to this is when an array of identical sensors is used to generate a 2-d spatial map. For instance, a solid-state camera produces an optical image which can then be analysed for spatial information such as the shapes of objects. In contrast, odour sensors do not behave as completely independent sensors; instead, an individual sensor will respond to a variety of odours but with varying sensitivity. So the off-diagonal terms of the response matrix are non-zero, but smaller than the diagonal terms. It is under these conditions that a pattern analysis technique is usually employed to process the signals generated by an array of sensors and thereby extract information.

27.1.2 Classification of Analysis Techniques

The signals generated by an array of odour sensors may be processed using a variety of techniques. Figure 27.1 illustrates the basic data-processing structure of an electronic nose. When a set of odours (j:1-m) is introduced to an array of n odour sensors, the sensor output $\tilde{x}_{nm}$ is preprocessed or conditioned so that the response matrix $\tilde{\boldsymbol{R}}_{nm}$ can be fed into a pattern recognition (PARC) engine. In some situations the response vectors are linearly dependent upon the concentration of the odour signal, for instance when a conducting polymer sensor responds to sub-ppm levels of methanol. However, in other situations it may be necessary to linearise the concentration-dependence via a mathematical function, for instance when using a metal oxide semiconducting sensor to measure supra-ppm levels of ethanol. There are a variety of PARC methods available, but the linear ones are easiest to implement. However, the application of a linear PARC method to a nonlinear response matrix may lead to a significant reduction in accuracy.

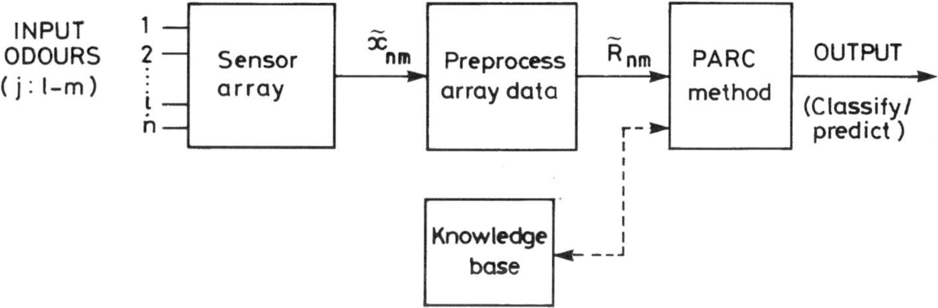

FIGURE 27.1 Basic structure of a data processing system for an electronic nose.

The nature of the PARC engine is usually classified by the terms "parametric or nonparametric" and "supervised or unsupervised". A parametric technique is based upon the assumption that the sensor data can be described by a probability density function (PDF) which *a posteriori* defines its spread of values. The most likely assumption made is that the sensor data are normally distributed with a known mean and variance. This assumption permits the application of several techniques, such as linear discriminant analysis (see Section 27.3.2). With this type of technique, it is necessary to create a knowledge base which contains the appropriate PDFs. This requires a supervised PARC method in which a set of known odours are systematically introduced to the electronic nose, which then classifies them according to known descriptors (e.g., odour type A or B, or woody, grassy, etc.). A supervised PARC scheme can be regarded as either a training or classification programme. In some cases, a PARC scheme is applied which predicts or identifies unknown odours from a knowledge base. This is referred to as an unsupervised or testing scheme. The idea of testing using unclassified response vectors is well established and often referred to as cross-validation. PARC methods that do not assume a PDF are known as nonparametric techniques, and some of these are also unsupervised such as cluster analysis (CA, Section 27.4.2). These techniques attempt to discriminate between different response vectors and subsequently group them into distinct clusters. Such methods are in a sense a type of preprocessor because they extract crucial features and often need to be used with a supervised classification method to predict group membership.

There is enormous interest at the moment in the application of artificial neural networks (ANNs) to odour classification (Section 27.5). This is due to the belief that ANNs can handle nonlinear, nonparametric data and be applied in a supervised mode, unsupervised mode, or a combination of them both. Clearly, they are attractive here because they are closer to mimicking the human olfactory system than a linear (unadaptive) classical multivariate technique. In addition, it is possible to train the ANNs using fuzzy rather than crisp data generated from an organoleptic panel.

Table 27.1 lists some of the different pattern analysis methods that have been applied to electronic noses. The table classifies the methods according to their basic properties and type of sensors employed. The first six methods in the table are discussed in detail below in the context of odour sensing. The seventh method, fuzzy logic, is treated in Chapter 20 of this book. A recent review article discussed the history of electronic noses,[2] while readers interested in the application of PARC methods in the wider field of gas sensing are referred to Reference 3.

TABLE 27.1
Some Common Pattern Analysis Techniques Used in Electronic Noses

Method	Parametric	Supervised	Linear	Sensors
Partial least squares (PLS)	Yes	Yes	Yes[a]	MO, CP, P
Principal component regression (PCR)	Yes	Yes	Yes	MO, CP
Discriminant function analysis (DFA)	Yes	Yes	Yes[a]	MO, CP
Principal component analysis (PCA)	No	Yes	Yes	MO, CP, P
Cluster analysis (CA)	No	No	Yes[a]	MO, CP, P
Artificial neural networks (ANNs)	No	Yes[b]	No	MO, CP, P
Fuzzy logic (FL)	No	No	No	MO

Note: MO: metal oxide; CP: conducting polymers; P: BAW or SAW sensor.

[a] Nonlinear versions of these techniques have been developed but are based upon simple mathematical functions (e.g., non-Euclidean metrics in cluster analysis).

[b] The commonly used back-propagation technique has a supervised training stage; however, other paradigms are unsupervised (e.g., Kohonen).

27.2 DATA PREPARATION AND DISPLAY

27.2.1 Data Preprocessing

It is important to examine carefully the data generated by an array of odour sensors so that the most informed choice of sensor, preprocessing, and PARC method is made. By plotting out the responses r_{ij} of each sensor i to odour j, it is possible to identify quickly those sensors which clearly generate small and noisy signals. A more sophisticated method is to examine the regression and correlation matrices of the sensor response matrix, and to eliminate those sensors which have small regression terms or exhibit a high degree of linearity with other sensors (although caution is needed when applying parametric analysis of variance techniques to nonlinear nonparametric odour data!). In addition, it is possible to identify spurious responses that are either much larger or smaller than the expected response. These outliers should be examined and understood before applying sophisticated PARC techniques.

In the human olfactory system the sensitivity to odour intensity is poor and generally follows a logarithmic relationship. However, the loss of sensitivity is compensated for by an excellent power to discriminate similar complex odours. Thus preprocessing of the response vectors should be designed to help analyse data from a specific problem, such as to linearise the output from the sensors, or perhaps compensate for concentration-fluctuations in the response vectors by a normalisation procedure. For example, when analysing data from metal oxide odour sensors, the fractional change in conductance performs well as a sensor parameter with linear and nonlinear PARCs. Moreover, when trying to discriminate between very similar complex odours it may be useful to normalise the length of the response vector and thus eliminate the variation in the concentration vector length. Figure 27.2 illustrates the effect of normalising the response vector according to the formula below,

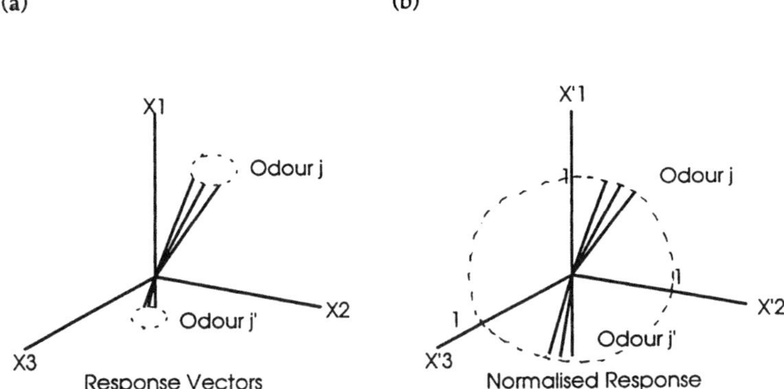

FIGURE 27.2 Effect of array normalisation as a preprocessing method to enhance the discrimination of similar complex odours.

$$r'_{ij} = \frac{r_{ij}}{\sqrt{\sum_{i=1}^{i=n} r_{ij}^2}} \tag{27.5}$$

The effect of this is to place the end of all response vectors onto the surface of an (n-1)-dimensional hypersphere and reduce the effect of concentration fluctuations. This has been shown to improve the classification performance in respect of response vectors from similar alcohols and beers in a 12-element tin oxide-based electronic nose,[4] but again, caution is needed as it can enhance the noise in the case of small response vectors.

27.2.2 Data Display

The graphical display of the response vectors can help the analyst to preprocess the odour data and assess its validity. To this end the so-called polar, radar, or spider plot displays multivariate data in a rapid and simple manner. This consists of plotting the response of each sensor as the radial parameter with the angle indicating the position of the sensor in the array. For example, Figure 27.3 shows a polar plot of the fractional change in conductance of an array of 12 polymeric sensors in an electronic nose.[5] Our own brain rapidly carries out its own spatial pattern recognition on the polar plots and so assesses their similarity. In this case it is clear that Brazilian and Colombian roasted coffee beans have quite different response vectors that could easily be classified by an artificial neural network analysis. However, it is more common to analyse very similar response vectors, in which case it is necessary to extract features (e.g., principal component scores) which can be used to discriminate between different odours.

27.3 PARAMETRIC ANALYSIS TECHNIQUES

27.3.1 Linear Calibration Methods

The problem of multivariate calibration is well known and a subject discussed in standard textbooks.[6] In the chemical sciences, a common problem of interest is to calibrate the response

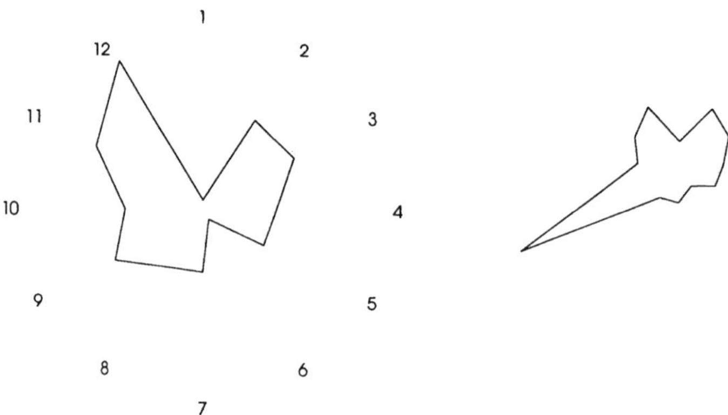

FIGURE 27.3 Polar resistance plots of response vector for Brazilian and Colombian roasted coffee beans using a 12-element polymer electronic nose.

of an analytical instrument such as a mass spectrometer. This is a similar problem to that of processing the data from a chemical sensor array to obtain the concentrations within a multicomponent mixture. For example, a gaseous mixture of CO_2, H_2, and CH_4 is often of interest as a fire hazard in coal mines. Thus, it is desirable to determine the individual gas concentrations from a multivariate data set. Two common methods are partial least squares (PLS) and principal component regression (PCR) which assume that a linear inverse model can be applied to the data. In this model the concentration vector $\boldsymbol{c}$ is related to the response matrix by

$$\boldsymbol{c} = \tilde{\boldsymbol{R}}\boldsymbol{M} + \mathbf{e} \tag{27.6}$$

where $\boldsymbol{M}$ is a regression vector containing all the model parameters, and $\boldsymbol{e}$ is an error vector containing the concentration residuals. The regression vectors are estimated in PLS and PCR by finding a pseudo-inverse response matrix in terms of orthonormal and diagonal matrices.[7] The main difference between PLS and PCR methods is that PLS incorporates information about the concentration vector whereas the principal component analysis (PCA) part of the PCR does not. This is important when analysing data to classify odours rather than predict chemical concentrations. To start with, odour strengths or intensities are subjective and so cannot be quantified in the same way that a gas concentration can. It is believed that the concentration-vector only weakly influences our perception of odours (log-dependency) due to complex neural preprocessing. Consequently, most research has focused on the use of other types of classification methods for electronic nose data, such as discriminant analysis and cluster analysis.

27.3.2 Linear Discriminant Analysis

Discriminant function analysis (DFA) is a parametric pattern analysis method that has been used to analyse electronic nose data. DFA assumes that the data are multinormal-distributed (unlike PCA or CA) and then determines the discriminant functions Z_j. Each discriminant function is calculated for which the F-ratio on the analysis of the variance is maximised subject to Z_p being uncorrelated with Z_p .. Z_{p-1} within groups. The problem is similar to the eigenvalue problem. The discriminant functions are related to the sensor responses by the following (linear) equation:

$$Z_p = a_{1p}\boldsymbol{r}_{1j} + a_{2p}\boldsymbol{r}_{2j} + \ldots + a_{np}\boldsymbol{r}_{nj} \tag{27.7}$$

Once the regression coefficients $a_{ip}/\boldsymbol{r}_{ip}$ have been computed on the known data (supervised learning), then they can be used to form the classification functions which predict the group membership of unknown response vectors. The latter process is referred to as cross-validation. Figure 27.4 shows the results of the application of DFA to the response (fractional change in conductance) vectors obtained when an array of 12 tin oxide sensors sample the headspace of 3 different commercial coffees.[8] Plots of the first two discriminant functions show reasonable separation of the three groups. The observed classification rate was 90% on the entire data set, falling to 81% when half the data set is used to cross-validate. Array normalisation gave some improvement, with the classification rate increasing from 90 to 96% on this data set.

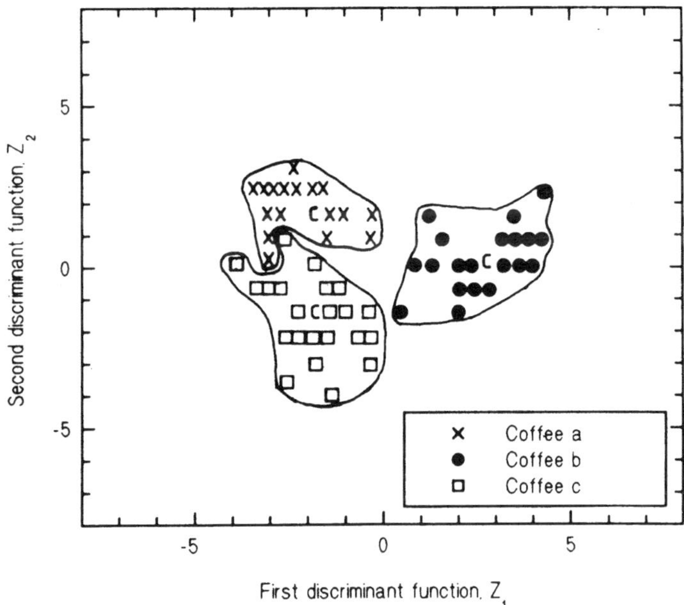

FIGURE 27.4 Results of linear DFA on the analysis of three commercial roasted coffees using a 12-element tin oxide electronic nose (c denotes the centroid of a group of points). (From Gardner, J. W. et al., *Sensors Actuators,* B6, 71, 1992. With permission.)

27.3.3 Nonlinear Parametric Techniques

The use of a linear pattern analysis method on nonlinear sensors is acceptable when the concentration vector is fairly constant. In other words, when analysing complex odours of a very similar nature (e.g., a spiked and control sample) the lengths of the response vectors are similar so that the relevant part of nonlinear response space may be approximated by a linear region. When covering a wider region of the response space (or solving the multicomponent gas mixture problem), then most sensors have a nonlinear concentration response and so a nonlinear technique is required. Nonlinear parametric techniques tend to assume either a simple analytical concentration relationship (such as quadratic) or approximate the response space by a series of linear functions. There are several nonlinear parametric techniques that have been applied to related problems in analytical chemistry.[9] For example, multivariate adaptive regression splines (MARS) methods have been used to analyse simple gas mixtures with some success. However, there are several problems associated with applying these techniques to electronic nose data. Firstly, they not only assume a constant PDF (e.g., normal), but assume a response space which varies smoothly and monotonically in a simple analytical fashion. When more complicated functions are used to analyse data the mathematical complexity of the problem is greatly increased, as is the effort required to determine the modeling vectors (i.e., knowledge base). In some situations it may be possible to linearise the response vectors by preprocessing; however, this generally only works when there is a mixture of a small number of independent odorant molecules. In practice, there are hundreds, if not thousands, of molecules present in a mixture which interact to give a highly nonlinear response space which cannot be described by a straightforward PDF. More interest has thus been shown in the application of unsupervised methods, such as PCA and CA, which do not make underlying assumptions about the distribution. CA has the added advantage that nonlinear (non-Euclidean) metrics can be used in a straightforward manner to map out nonlinear response space.

27.4 CLASSICAL NONPARAMETRIC TECHNIQUES

27.4.1 Principal Component Analysis

PCA is a powerful (linear) supervised PARC method that has been used by various researchers to discriminate the response of an electronic nose to simple and complex odours (e.g., alcohols, beers, coffees). The method basically consists of expressing the response vectors $\boldsymbol{r}_j$ in terms of linear combinations of orthogonal vectors, and is sometimes referred to as vector decomposition. Each orthogonal (principal) vector accounts for a certain amount of variance in the data with a decreasing degree of importance. The scalar product of the orthogonal vectors with the response vector gives the value of the principal components X_p.

$$X_p = \alpha_{1p} r_{1j} + \alpha_{2p} r_{2j} + \ldots + \alpha_{np} r_{nj} \tag{27.8}$$

The variance of each principal component, X_p, is maximised under the constraint that the sum of the coefficients of the orthogonal vectors (often called eigenvectors) is set to unity, and the eigenvectors are uncorrelated. There is often a high degree of sensor collinearity within data obtained from electronic noses. This means that the majority of the information held in response space can often be displayed using a small number of principal vectors, thus describing perhaps a 12-dimensional problem by a 2- or 3-dimensional plot. Figure 27.5 illustrates how well this technique works when analysing the response from an array of tin oxide sensors.[10] As tin oxide sensors respond in a similar manner, over 80% of the variance is described by only two principal components, X_1, and X_2. It can be seen in Figure 27.5 that three distinct groups are apparent and are associated with lagers (group A), beers (group B), and spirits (group C). The discrimination of beverages within each group is harder, but some success has been reported for the analysis of Japanese beers and whiskies. Although PCA is useful as a tool with which to display the performance of an electronic nose, CA is perhaps more important because it is an unsupervised technique for enhancing the differences between the response vectors.

27.4.2 Cluster Analysis

CA is an unsupervised, nonparametric technique that is widely used to discriminate between response vectors in n-dimensional space, and identify clusters or groups to which unknown vectors are likely to belong. First a distance metric $d_{jj'}$ is calculated between data points j and j′ according to:

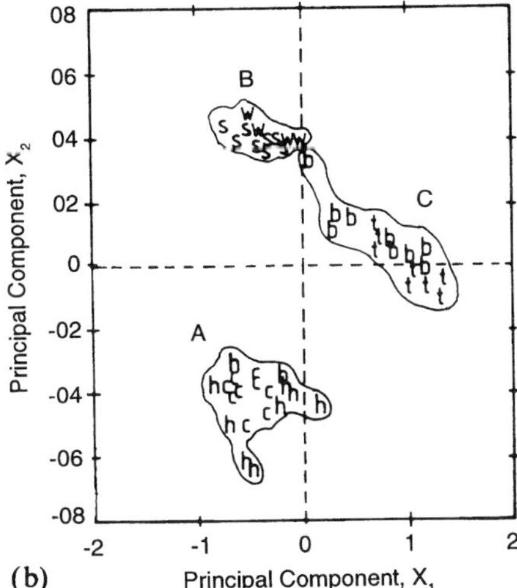

FIGURE 27.5 Results of a PCA analysis of the response (normalised fractional conductance change) of a 12-element tin oxide electronic nose to two beers (labeled w and s), two lagers (labeled h and c), and two spirits (labeled t and b). (From Gardner, J. W. et al., *Sensors Actuators,* B4, 109, 1991. With permission.)

$$d_{jj'} = \left(\sum_{k=1}^{N} \left(r_j - r_{j'} \right)^N \right)^{1/N} \tag{27.9}$$

The exponent N is normally set to 2 which is the Euclidean (linear) metric, and there seems to be little to be gained from using a nonlinear metric when analysing electronic nose data. The proximity of all points relative to each other is then found by computing a so-called similarity value $S_{jj'}$, for example,

$$S_{jj'} = 1 - \frac{d_{jj'}}{\max\left\{d_{jj'}\right\}} \tag{27.10}$$

In this case the distance metric is divided through by the maximum separation between all the data points (also called the complete linkage method), so the similarity value is zero for the furthest neighbours and close to unity for the nearest neighbours. There are a variety of linkage methods possible, and chemometric packages often offer several. However, the choice of metric and linkage usually has a marginal effect on the results. Figure 27.6 shows the display of the results of a CA (Euclidean metric, complete linkage) on the response of a tin oxide electronic nose to a series of alcohols. The dendrogram (branching diagram in the style of a family tree) connects up response vectors with the nearest similarity value and thus illustrates how the odours are interrelated.

CA has also been used to analyse the response of a polymer electronic nose to coffee aromas, with some degree of success.[11] It is an easy method to use and rapidly provides the user with pertinent information. However, the nature of electronic nose data is such that it is often desirable to use a more powerful pattern analysis method. Typically, a method is required which can not only cope with nonlinear, nonparametric data, but which can also generate a metric which can adapt locally to regions of closely packed response vectors and so give superior predictive performance. This has led to the rapid and widespread application of artificial neural networks to the analysis of patterns generated by electronic noses.

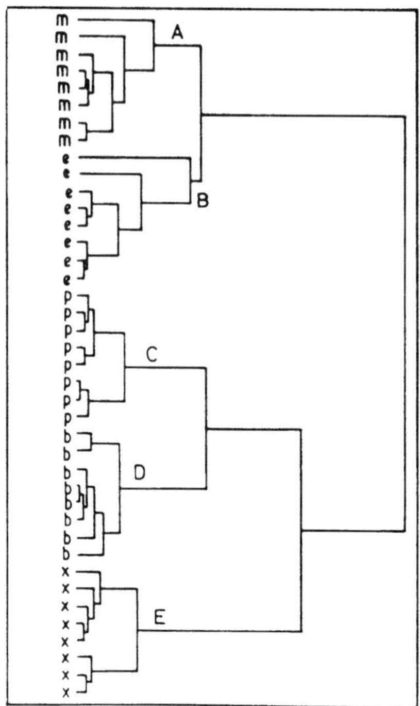

FIGURE 27.6 Dendrogram showing the results of a CA on the response of a 12-element tin oxide electronic nose to samples of methanol (m), ethanol (e), propanol (p), butanol (b), and methyl-butanol (x). (Euclidean metric, complete linkage.) (From Gardner, J. W. et al., *Sensors Actuators,* B4, 109, 1991. With permission.)

27.5 ARTIFICIAL NEURAL NETWORKS

27.5.1 Introduction to Multilayer Perceptron

Artificial neural networks (ANNs) consist of parallel interconnected, and usually adaptive, processing elements. The hierarchical organisation or architecture of these elements is based upon a physical model of the biological nervous systems.[12] The processing elements represent the biological or olfactory neurones, and their interconnections, the synaptic links. Consideration of the olfactory process[13] prompted our adoption of a three-layer network architecture, and other workers have adopted the same topology. It has also been suggested by Lippman (that a three-layer network has sufficient computational degrees of freedom to solve any problem.[14] In a three-layer network, the processing elements are organised into three distinct groups or layers; namely, input, hidden layer, and output. The three-layer network which was used to model our 12-element artificial nose is shown in Figure 27.7. The input layer in this case consists of 12 processing elements, corresponding to the odour sensors (olfactory receptors) in an electronic nose, set to the value of the array normalised response r_{ij}'. The hidden layer, so called because it is not readily accessible, possesses a number of processing elements (glomeruli nodes) which are to be determined experimentally. The output layer has a number of output elements (mitral cells), N, that are determined by the number of odours or vapours analysed. In this case there are five classes of odour so we have five output neurones. The interconnectivity and learning rules of the processing elements determine the performance of a particular architecture.

ANNs have a number of possible advantages over conventional methods (e.g., PCA) in terms of their adaptability (learning, self-organisation, generalisation, and training); noise

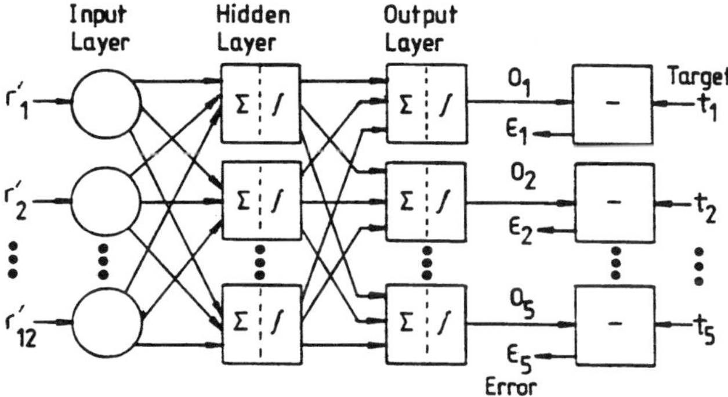

FIGURE 27.7 Structure of a fully connected three-layer back-propagation network used to process data from a 12-element tin oxide electronic nose for five odour classes. (From Gardner, J. W. et al., *Meas. Sci. Technol.*, 1, 446, 1990.)

tolerance; fault tolerance; distributed associated memory; inherent parallelism generating a high speed of operation subsequent to training; and, importantly, they are amenable to VLSI implementation.[15] Disadvantages include the fact that the training time can be long and may increase rapidly with the size of the network, and it is difficult to interpret the network output.[16] Although there are many ANN paradigms under investigation,[17] the Multi-Layer Perceptron (MLP) is perhaps the most significant because of its widespread use as a predictive classifier. The application of ANNs to classification problems requires far less restrictive assumptions than conventional methods about the nature of the input vectors.

The network shown in Figure 27.7 was designed to analyse a set of five vapours: methanol, ethanol, butanol, propanol, and 2-methyl-1-butanol. The response of each sensor i to measurand j was array normalised using Equation 27.5. The normalisation procedure has the desired property of scaling the response values between 0 and 1.

27.5.2 Back-Propagation Algorithm

Various algorithms can be used to train this three-layer network, but the ubiquitous back-propagation (BP) technique is perhaps the most important. This technique relies on two stages, the first being the learning phase during which the network learns how to recognise each of the known odour classes presented in the training data. The second phase is the so-called recall phase (i.e., prediction or validation) during which the trained network is used to classify unknown odours from the same classes as those from which the training set was derived. In the case of the three-layer network considered here, the input to the ith unit, from the jth odour, in the lth layer may be written as r_{ijl}. Then the odour signals, r_{ij0}, are presented to the input layer (l=0) to be learnt. In a feed-forward learning process, the signals r_{ijl} are calculated from a sigmoid activation function F and the difference between the sum of the outputs $r_{jk(l-1)}$ from units k in the layer below l–1, multiplied by a weighting w_{ikl} and a threshold weight w_{i0l},

$$r_{ijl} = F\sum_{k}\left[w_{ikl}r_{jk(l-1)} - w_{i0l}\right] \tag{27.11}$$

The calculation is carried out for each layer feeding the values through to the output layer. In the back-propagation process these weights w_{ikl}, and thresholds w_{i0l} are interactively changed to minimise the difference between the ideal output t_{ij} and the actual output r_{ijl} for each odour. In the output layer, the differences δ_{ik} is evaluated using,

$$\delta_{ik} = (t_{ij} - r_{ijl})(1 - r_{ijl}) \tag{27.12}$$

Then the synapse weightings in the layer below are changed by $\eta\delta_{ik}r_{ij(l-1)}$. The parameter η determines the learning rate of the process and was set to a value of 0.6 here. The threshold of each unit, w_{i0l}, is changed by $-\eta\delta_{ik}$ on each iteration.

TABLE 27.2
Ideal Target Output t_{ij} of a Neural Network for Alcohol Classification

	Output class p				
Sample p	t_{1j}	t_{2j}	t_{3j}	t_{4j}	t_{5j}
Methanol	1	0	0	0	0
Ethanol	0	1	0	0	0
Propanol	0	0	1	0	0
Butanol	0	0	0	1	0
Methyl-propanol	0	0	0	0	1

Table 27.2 shows the ideal, or target, values of the processing elements, t_{ij}, in the output layer when classifying the set of five alcohols. An important objective is to decide whether the BP algorithm can successfully recognise each odour, and to determine the extent to which the output values converge to the ideal values and the ability of the network to generalise, i.e., recognise similar input patterns to the ones on which it was trained. This was established by using the v-fold validation technique. Here v is set to one and the technique is thus equivalent to the leaving out one procedure,[18] as follows:

1. Compile a training data set.
2. Train the network (see Figure 27.7) until satisfactory convergence is achieved. It is customary to use an output element value of 0.9 to show good convergence; however, we adopted a slightly lower level, 0.8, because our experience[19] has shown that this is acceptable for a good compromise between network convergence and the ability of the network to generalise.
3. After convergence, the network's ability to generalise is tested by an unknown input vector.

The procedure in steps 1 to 3 can be repeated by using another vector for testing. In this case the outputs generated during testing were typically of the order of 0.8 or above compared with an ideal value of 1.0, and of the order of 0.2 or below compared with an ideal value of 0 (see Figure 27.8).[20] These results show that the network discriminates well between these odours (i.e., alcohols). The level of classification represents an advance on the work of Huang and Lippman who suggest that it is satisfactory to select the largest output which is greater than 0.5 as the correct one.[21] Although a BP neural network can readily learn electronic nose data, there are several aspects that need further consideration. For example, how can the optimal number of hidden layers, hidden units, and output units be found quickly and easily? Our experiments to-date have shown that variations in the number of hidden units, above or below a certain level, do not have a significant effect on the network performance, except for the effect on training time requirements. However, the automatic design of efficient networks is highly desirable.

27.5.3 Genetic Algorithm

MLPs are usually trained (e.g., BP) after both the neural network architecture and the initial values of various network parameters have been defined. Since the success of the training

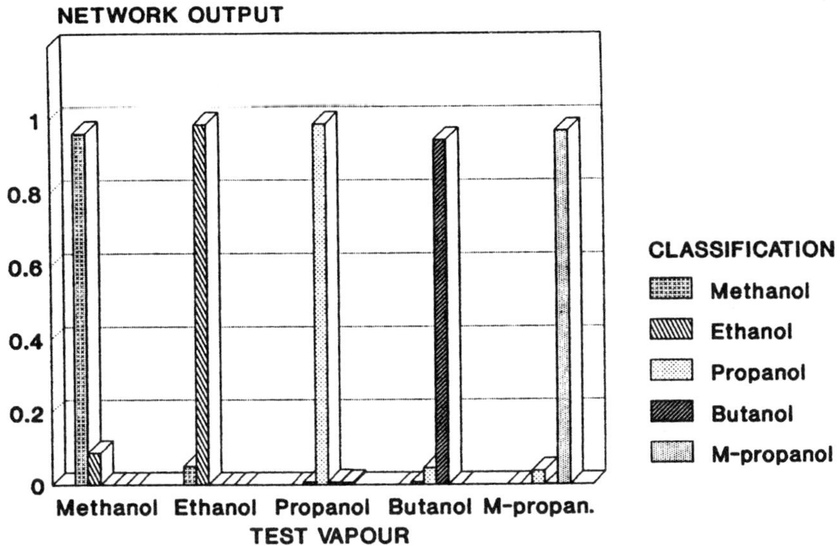

FIGURE 27.8 Results of the classification of five alcoholic odours using the network in Figure 27.7. (From Gardner, J. W. et al., *Meas. Sci. Technol.*, 1, 446, 1990. With permission.)

process in terms of a fast rate of convergence and good generalisation can be affected by the choice of the architecture and initial network parameters, much time may be spent in searching for the optimal ANN. An alternative method is to use a genetic algorithm (GA) to determine automatically a suitable network architecture and a set of parameters from a restricted region of design space.

Learning using the BP algorithm involves two phases. During the first phase, each input response vector is fed into the network in turn, producing corresponding output vectors which are compared with target outputs to give the error at each of the output nodes. In the second phase, the error signal is passed backwards through all units and weight changes are made accordingly, whence

$$E = 0.5 \sum_{p} \sum_{i} \left(t_{pi} - y_{pi} \right)^2 \tag{27.13}$$

$$\Delta w(n+1) = -\eta \nabla E(n) + \alpha w(n) \tag{27.14}$$

where $w(k)$ is the weight vector at the kth iteration, $\nabla E(n)$ is the gradient of the error, E, evaluated at $w(n)$, η and α are constants referred to as the learning rate and the momentum coefficient, respectively, $\boldsymbol{t}_p$ and $\boldsymbol{y}_p$ are the target and the calculated network output corresponding to the pth input vector, respectively. Network training may be stopped when either the number of training cycles reaches the maximum specified or the total sum of squared error (TSSE), E, is below a specified value. The BP is a gradient descent optimisation technique which tries to minimise the TSSE, E, defined by Equation 27.13. The step length or learning rate, and the momentum coefficient are predetermined constant parameters of the algorithm and the choice of their value will affect the rate of convergence as well as the pattern recognition error.

In order to increase the rate of convergence, a number of improvements have been suggested. The adaptive back-propagation algorithm[22] (ABP) which modifies the values of the learning rate and the momentum coefficient has been shown to give the best performance on a number of data sets.[23] The training performance, in terms of the rate of convergence and the network error value, is generally affected by the choice of the initial values of the learning rate, momentum coefficient and weights, and the network architecture. Unfortunately, all these have to be predetermined before applying ABP.

Genetic algorithms are heuristic search algorithms based on the mechanics of natural selection.[24] They use nature's basic philosophy of survival — the fittest survive and the worst die off. GAs work on the coding of the parameters rather than the parameters themselves. The structure of the system we are concerned with is mapped into a string of symbols (called chromosomes) — usually binary strings consisting of 0s and 1s. Each range of parameter values may be mapped onto a binary string, which when concatenated form a chromosome. GAs are then applied to search populations of chromosomes.

Several genetic operators can be identified; the ones which are most commonly used in simple GAs being parent selection (an artificial version of natural selection), crossover (recombination of parents' genetic material to make children), and mutation (reintroduction of genetic diversity by random modification of chromosomes). Simple GAs that only use these three operators have been found to be satisfactory in the work described here; however, several other more sophisticated operators may also be employed.

Members of the population are assigned fitness values according to the evaluation of the fitness function to measure how well-suited the parameter values encoded in the chromosome are for the application. The higher the fitness value of a chromosome the greater the chance it has to breed.

The parameters which need to be searched by GA in our network training are the range of initial weights (R), initial values of learning rate and momentum coefficient, and the network architecture. The initial weights are generated using a uniform random number generator in the range $[-R, R]$. The network architecture is described by the number of hidden layers (h), the number of nodes in each layer (n_i: i=0, 1, ..., h) and by the connectivity of nodes, that is, which node is connected to which. Since we are using the back-propagation algorithm to train the neural networks, the neural networks are restricted to a feed-forward MLP. The MLP may be randomly or fully connected. In a fully connected MLP every node in a layer is connected only to all the nodes in the next higher layer.

Since the range, learning rate, and momentum terms are all real numbers, the mapping of these values to bit strings can easily be achieved using a linear transformation of the real numbers to binary values using Equation 27.15:

$$b = Integer\left[\left(2^n - 1\right)\frac{x - x_0}{x_m - x_0}\right] \tag{27.15}$$

where x_0 and x_m are the minimum and the maximum values of the parameter, n is the length of the binary string, b is the binary representation of the parameter value x. The parameter transformed using Equation 27.15 is discretised to only 2^n possible values in the interval $[x_0, x_m]$. The integer values, h and n_i, are represented by their equivalent binary values. Gray-coding is often claimed to be better than binary coding for GAs.[25] Thus, the binary representations are gray-coded in the approach described here.

It is the representation of the connectivity that requires most attention since it does not actually have a numerical value. There are only two possible values for a connection from one node to another node: the connection exists or it does not exist. Thus, a single connection can be represented by a binary digit. One way of representing the connectivity is to construct a positional binary string for every possible connection in the network. For example, assume we have a network with 3 inputs, 2 outputs and a maximum of 1 hidden layer having a maximum of 5 nodes. Then each of the input nodes can be connected to any hidden or output nodes and thus the maximum number of connections from any one of the input nodes is $5 + 2 = 7$. Similarly, the maximum number of connections from any one of the hidden nodes is 2. The maximum number of connections in the network is $(3 \times 7) + (5 \times 2) = 31$. We now construct a binary string of length 31, representing each possible connection in the network by a single bit. Figure 27.9 shows a 3-5-2 randomly connected neural network, and its binary representation is shown in Figure 27.10. The connections from the first node in the input layer to any of the nodes in the hidden or output layers are represented by the first 7 bits (the first 5 bits for the connections to each of the 5 hidden nodes, the next 2 bits for the connections to each of the 2 output nodes), from the second input node by the next 7 bits and so on. The position of a bit in the string will determine the connection of which two nodes is represented by the bit. A bit value of 1 means that the connection exists and a bit value of 0 means the connection does not exist. Once the string is initialised, a network can be constructed by examining each bit in the string. One potential problem with this method of representation of connectivity, however, is that the network constructed by interpreting the string may not be meaningful (for instance, networks with no forward path between the input and output nodes). Therefore, a consistent method of constructing a meaningful network from the representation must be used.

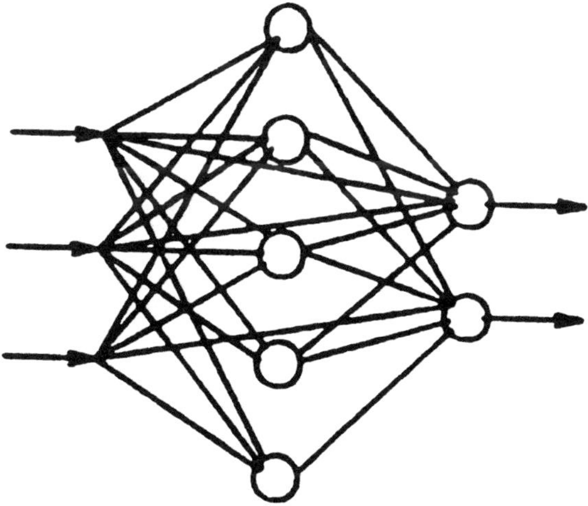

FIGURE 27.9 A 3-5-2 randomly connected feed-forward network.

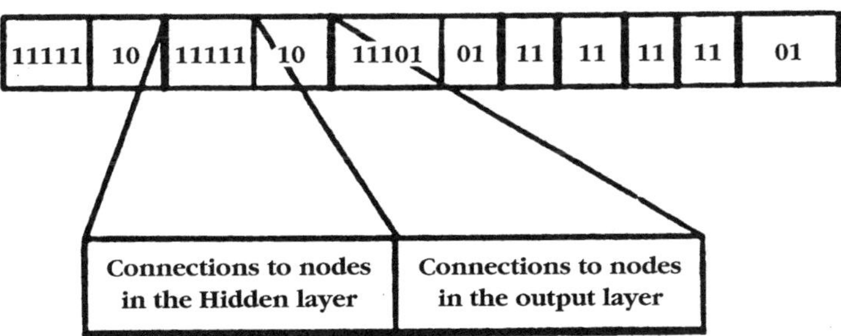

FIGURE 27.10 Binary representation of the network in Figure 27.9.

A chromosome is constructed by concatenating the representations of all the parameters, giving a long string. A chromosome can thus be interpreted to give the initial parameter values and architecture of the network which can be trained by ABP or BP.

The performance of the ith chromosome, or of the network represented by it, is evaluated using the fitness function:

$$F(c_i) = au(c_i) + b \tag{27.16}$$

where F is the fitness function, u is the objective function which we want to optimise, a and b are transformation parameters dynamically adjusted to avoid premature convergence. The performance of a network can be evaluated with respect to its different attributes. Different performance measures for a network can be evaluated depending on the relative interest in the attributes. The objective function can be defined as a weighted sum of the various performance measures. The weights can then be adjusted to reflect the interest in any of the performance measures. Here the objective function, u, for chromosome c_i is defined by

$$u(c_i) = \frac{K}{\sum_j w_j v_j(c_i)} \tag{27.17}$$

where v_j is a performance measure with respect to the jth network attribute, w_j is a non-negative significance measure attached to the performance of the jth attribute, and K is a constant.

In the sensor data classification problem, the performance measures used in the objective function are based on the network prediction error, the speed of convergence, the size of the network, and the level of generalisation achieved. Except for the prediction error, all the other measures are expressed as unitless ratios. The performance of the network with respect to the speed of convergence is expressed as a ratio of the number of epochs for which the network was trained before training terminates to the maximum number of epochs specified. In terms of size, the number of nodes and the number of weights expressed as fractions of their respective maximum specified values were used. The ratio of the number of misclassified patterns to the total number of input patterns, using both the training and the testing data sets, is used to express generalisation performance. For good generalisation, this ratio has to be smaller. Since the objective function (Equation 27.17) is inversely related to the performance measures, larger performance values will result in smaller values of the objective function. The weights, w_j, (in Equation 27.17) are actually cost factors attached to each of the performance measures. Thus, the larger the weight value attached to an attribute's performance measure, the more the emphasis is placed on the attribute being smaller.

This procedure has been used to analyse the alcohol data set. Table 27.3 shows the required specifications for the problem in this simulation. Although the results are not conclusive yet, it was observed that normalising the input improves performance of the network. The normalisation ranges specified in Table 27.3 were chosen from repeated training of the network problem.

The alcohol classification problem was studied previously.[26] After repeated experiments (using both the BP and ABP methods of network training), a 12-7-5 fully connected feed-forward network with initial weight range [–1,+1], learning rate 1.0, and momentum coefficient of 0.7 was found to give good results. In our simulation, we restricted the network to a maximum of 2 hidden layers each having a maximum of 20 units.

The full results obtained are summarised in Table 27.4. The table shows the ten best networks that the GA selected for the problem — 100% correct classifications during training as well as testing were achieved for the alcohol problem with a network error of less than 1%.

The shift in the fitness curve (Figure 27.11) and the increasing trend in average population fitness (Figure 27.12) show that networks with good performance are generated as the number of generations increases. When the algorithm converges, the fitness curve will be flattened and the change in the average population fitness will be small.

TABLE 27.3
Specifications Used in the Genetic Algorithm Simulations for Alcohols

Parameter	Value
Maximum number of hidden layers	2
Maximum number of units in each hidden layer	20
Input normalisation range	−1, +1
Maximum number of training cycles	500
Minimum error (TSSE) to terminate training	0.01
Number of generations	15
Population size	100
Cross-over probability	0.9
Mutation probability	0.01
Number of training data sets	35
Number of test data sets	5

TABLE 27.4
The Ten Best Network Parameters Selected by a Genetic Algorithm for Classifying Alcohols

Rank	Network	Links	Epoch	η	α	r	Error (%)	Fitness
1	12-3-5	62	65	0.507	0.826	0.763	0.99	14.59
2	12-11-5	129	61	0.310	0.956	0.835	0.91	12.97
3	12-1-11-5	137	61	0.310	0.949	0.084	0.90	12.59
4	12-10-5	114	68	0.295	0.809	0.946	0.95	12.51
5	12-12-5	135	73	0.348	0.980	0.145	0.82	12.18
6	12-14-5	158	63	0.172	0.866	0.794	0.99	12.13
7	12-12-5	134	78	0.652	0.970	0.145	0.94	11.72
8	12-7-8-5	177	69	0.471	0.892	0.061	0.89	11.67
9	12-11-5	123	88	0.530	0.742	0.036	0.81	11.33
10	12-6-15-5	273	59	0.961	0.802	0.038	0.88	10.85

GAs can be applied to find an appropriate architecture and a set of suitable network parameters all in parallel. The results demonstrate that no simplifying assumptions, such as linearity, etc., on the function to be optimised are required, except for a search space of possible values with some measure of performance which may be highly complicated and nonlinear. The domain-independent nature of GAs has also been demonstrated. Two problems, namely, a search for suitable network parameters having numerical values (such as the learning rate), and a search for the suitable network architecture representing nonnumerical values (such as the existence of a connection link between two nodes), have been shown to be combined together as one problem. Since input normalisation has been observed to affect the rate of convergence, the input transformation range may be added to the GA parameters set, simplifying the preprocessing work for finding a suitable normalisation range.[27]

27.7 CONCLUDING REMARKS

A considerable number of pattern analysis techniques have been used to analyse response vectors produced by metal oxide, polymer, and SAW electronic noses. Of all these techniques,

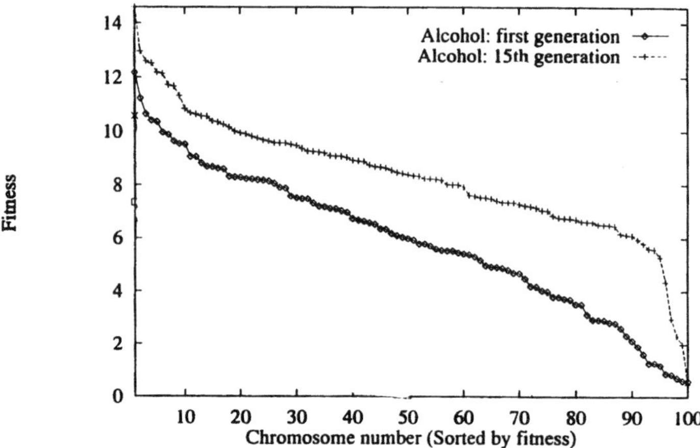

FIGURE 27.11 Fitness of chromosomes in the classification of alcoholic odours.

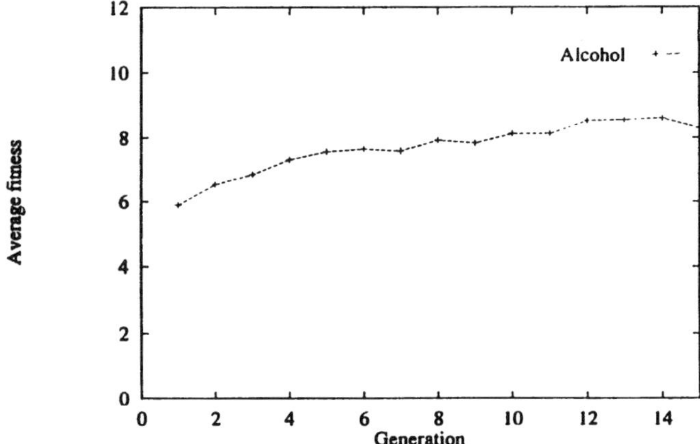

FIGURE 27.12 Average population fitness in the classification of alcoholic odours.

the back-propagation neural network has arguably been the most successful. The technique has been shown to perform well in a variety of applications. Yet, all these techniques are quite crude when compared with the neural processing that takes place in the human olfactory system. First, there is a very large number of olfactory receptors (about 100,000,000) which provide a high level of redundancy. In fact, these cells only live for about 20 days on average and so any effect of poisoning or drift is relatively short-lived. Secondly, there is a massively parallel secondary processing structure which has many layers (perhaps as many as five). This olfactory processor has neural weights which are modified by the presence of certain chemicals even after the electrical connections have grown into place. In addition, new connections can be formed as the nose is trained against a particular problem. Finally, one striking difference exists; the human nose is a *differential* signal processor, that is, the nose can only detect an increase (or decrease) in the intensity of a smell. Moreover, the smell can only be detected for a matter of seconds, after which it can no longer be smelt. Thus, a closer analogue to the human olfactory system requires the use of an adaptive AC filter which removes the DC component from the odour sensors, yet generates an output which is independent of the ambient odour level. This type of device, combined with a fuzzy classification function, will bring us much closer to an instrument that not only behaves like the human nose, but would also find much wider application in areas such as the monitoring of environmental pollution.

ABBREVIATIONS

ABP	Adaptive back-propagation
ANN	Artificial neural network
BAW	Bulk acoustic wave
BP	Back-propagation
CA	Cluster analysis
CP	Conducting polymer
DFA	Discriminant function analysis
FL	Fuzzy logic
GA	Genetic algorithm
ISFET	Ion-selective field effect transistor
MARS	Multivariate adaptive regression splines
MLP	Multilayer perceptron
MO	Metal oxide
P	Piezoelectric
PARC	Pattern recognition
PCA	Principal component analysis
PCR	Principal component regression
PDF	Probability density function
PLS	Partial least squares
SAW	Surface acoustic wave
TSSE	Total sum of squared error
VLSI	Very large scale integration

REFERENCES

1. Gardner, J. W., *Microsensors: Principles and Applications,* John Wiley & Sons Ltd., Chicester, 1994, chap. 1.
2. Gardner, J. W. and Bartlett, P. N., A brief history of electronic noses, *Sensors Actuators,* B18, 221, 1994.
3. Gardner, J. W. and Bartlett, P. N., Pattern recognition in gas sensing, in *Techniques & Mechanisms in Gas Sensing,* Moseley, P. T., Norris, J., and Williams, D., Eds., Adam-Hilger, Bristol, 1981, chap. 14.
4. Gardner, J. W., Detection of vapours and odours from a multisensor array using pattern recognition. 1. Principal component and cluster analyses, *Sensors Actuators,* B4, 109, 1991.
5. Gardner, J. W., Intelligent ChemSADs for artificial odour-sensing of coffee and lager beers, 11th Int. Symp. Olfaction & Taste, Sapporo, Japan, July 12-16, 1993.
6. Martens, H. and Naes, T., *Multivariate Calibration,* John Wiley & Sons, New York, 1989.
7. Manly, B. F. T., *Multivariate Statistical Methods,* Chapman & Hall, London, 1986.
8. Gardner, J. W., Shurmer, H. V., and Tan, T. T., Application of an electronic nose to the discrimination of coffees, *Sensors Actuators,* B6, 71, 1992.
9. Sekulic, S., Seaholtz, M., Wang, Z., and Kowalski, B. R., Nonlinear multivariate calibration methods in analytical chemistry, *Anal. Chem.,* 65, 835, 1993.
10. Gardner, J. W. and Bartlett, P. N., Pattern recognition in odour sensing, in *Sensors & Sensory Systems for an Electronic Nose,* Gardner, J. W. and Bartlett, P. N., Eds., NATO ASI Series, Kluwer Academic, Dordrecht, chap. 11.
11. Bartlett, P. N., Blair, N., and Gardner, J. W., Electronic noses, principles, applications and outlook, Assoc. Sci. Int. Café, 15e Colloque, Montpellier, 616, 1993.
12. Kohonen, T., *Neural Networks,* 1, 3, 1988.

13. Gardner, J. W. and Hines, E. L., *IEE Colloquium,* Digest no 1988/130, 6, Dec. 7, 1988.
14. Lippman, R. P., *IEEE ASSP,* 4(2), 4, 1987.
15. Rumelhart, D. E. and McClelland, J. L., *Parallel Distributed Processing,* MIT Press, Cambridge, MA, 1986, 318.
16. Debenham, R. M. and Garth, S. C. J., *IEE Colloquium,* Digest no 1989/83, 18, May 6/1, 1989.
17. Hecht-Nielsen, R., *IEEE Spectrum,* 36, 1988.
18. Duda, R. O. and Hart, P. E., *Pattern Classification and Scene Analysis,* John Wiley & Sons, New York, 1973.
19. Hines, E. L. and Hutchinson, R., Proc. IEE Image Processing Conf., University of Warwick, July 18-20, 39, 1989.
19a. Anthony, D. M., Hines, E. L., Taylor, D., and Barham, J., IEE Image Processing Conf., University of Warwick, U.K., July 18-20, 338-342, 1989.
20. Gardner, J. W., Hines, E. L., and Wilkinson, M., The application of artificial neural networks in an electronic nose, *Meas. Sci. Technol.,* 1, 446, 1990.
21. Huang, W. Y. and Lippman, R. P., Int. Conf. on Neural Networks, San Diego, June, 1987, 485, 1987.
22. Chan, L. W. and Fallside, F., An adaptive training algorithm for back propagation networks, *Comput. Speech Lang.,* 2, 205, 1987.
23. Hines, E. L., Gardner, J. W., Fung, W., and Fekadu, A. A., Improved rate of convergence in a MLP based electronic nose, 2nd Irish Neural Network Conf., Queen's University, Belfast, June, 1992.
24. Goldberg, D. E., *Genetic Algorithms in Search, Optimization and Machine Learning,* Addison-Wesley, Reading, MA, 1989.
25. Davis, L., *Handbook of Genetic Algorithms,* Van Nostrand Reinhold, New York, 1991.
26. Gardner, J. W., Hines, E. L., and Tang, H., Detection of vapours and odours from a multisensor array using pattern recognition technique. 2. Artificial neural networks, *Sensors Actuators,* B9, 9, 1992.
27. Fekadu, A. A., Hines, E. L., and Gardner, J. W., Genetic algorithm design of neural network based electronic nose, in *Artificial Neural Nets and Genetic Algorithms,* Albrecht, R. F., Reeves, C. R., and Steele, N. C., Eds., Springer-Verlag, New York, 1993, 691-698.

INDEX

Index

B

C

D

E

F

G

J

K

L

N

O

Q

R

U

V

W